Textbook of
Travel Medicine
and
Health

Second Edition

Textbook of
Travel Medicine
and
Health

Second Edition

Herbert L. DuPont, M.D.
Chief, Internal Medicine Service
St. Luke's Episcopal Hospital
Houston, Texas

Robert Steffen, M.D.
Professor of Travel Medicine
Institut für Sozial-und Präventivmedizin der Universität
Zurich, Switzerland

2001

B.C. DECKER INC.
Hamilton • London

B.C. Decker Inc.
20 Hughson Street South
P.O. Box 620, L.C.D.1
Hamilton, Ontario L8N 3K7
Tel: 905-522-7017; 1-800-568-7281
Fax: 905-522-7839
e-mail: info@bcdecker.com
Website: www.bcdecker.com

00 01 02 03 /UTP/ 9 8 7 6 5 4 3 2 1

ISBN   1-55009-037-9

Printed in Canada

Sales and Distribution

United States
B.C. Decker Inc.
P.O. Box 785
Lewiston, NY 14092-0785
Tel: 905-522-7017 / 1-800-568-7281
Fax: 905-522-7839
E-mail: info@bcdecker.com
Website: www.bcdecker.com

Canada
B.C. Decker Inc.
20 Hughson Street South
P.O. Box 620, L.C.D. 1
Hamilton, Ontario L8N 3K7
Tel: 905-522-7017 / 1-800-568-7281
Fax: 905-522-7839
E-mail: info@bcdecker.com
Website: www.bcdecker.com

Japan
Igaku-Shoin Ltd.
Foreign Publications Department
3-24-17 Hongo
Bunkyo-ku, Tokyo, Japan 113-8719
Tel: 3 3817 5680
Fax: 3 3815 6776
E-mail: fd@igaku.shoin.co.jp

UK, Europe, Scandinavia, Middle East
Harcourt Publishers Limited
Customer Service Department
Foots Cray High Street
Sidcup, Kent
DA14 5HP, UK
Tel: 44 (0) 208 308 5760
Fax: 44 (0) 181 308 5702
E-mail: cservice@harcourt_brace.com

Singapore, Malaysia, Thailand, Philippines, Indonesia, Vietnam, Pacific Rim
Harcourt Asia Pte Limited
583 Orchard Road
#09/01, Forum
Singapore 238884
Tel: 65-737-3593
Fax: 65-753-2145

Foreign Rights
John Scott & Company
International Publishers' Agency
P.O. Box 878
Kimberton, PA 19442
Tel: 610-827-1640
Fax: 610-827-1671

CONTRIBUTORS

REMON R. ABU-ELYAZEED, M.D., PH.D.
Head, Epidemiology Division, United States Naval
Medical Research Unit No. 3, Cairo, Egypt
*12.1. Risk to Travelers by Region and Environmental
Factors: Northern Africa*

ABU SALEH M. ABDULLAH, M.B.B.S., M.P.H.,
PH.D.
Department of Community Medicine, The University of
Hong Kong, China
*12.9. Risk to Travelers by Region and Environmental
Factors: East Asia*

JAVIER A. ADACHI, M.D.
Center for Infectious Disease, University of Texas –
Houston Medical School; Universidad Peruana
Cayetano Heredia, Lima, Peru
*12.7. Risk to Travelers by Region and Environmental
Factors: Tropical South America*

VERNON E. ANSDELL, M.D., F.R.C.P.,
D.T.M.&H.
Associate Professor, University of Hawaii School of
Public Health; Tropical and Travel Medicine, Kaiser
Permanente, Hawaii; Honolulu, Hawaii
14.2. Seafood Infection and Intoxication

DEANNA ASHLEY, M.B., B.S., D.P.H.,
D.M.(PAED)
Associate Director, Department of Community
Health and Psychiatry, University of the West Indies,
Mona; Director of Health Promotion and Protection,
Ministry of Health, Jamaica
*12.6. Risk to Travelers by Region and Environmental
Factors: Caribbean Middle America*

PAUL S. AUERBACH, M.D., M.S., F.A.C.E.P.
Clinical Professor of Surgery, Division of
Emergency Medicine, Department of Surgery,
Stanford University Medical Center, Stanford,
California
14. Marine Hazards

ELIZABETH D. BARNETT, M.D.
Assistant Professor of Pediatrics, Maxwell Finland
Laboratory for Infectious Diseases, Boston Medical
Center, Boston, Massachusetts
*22.2. Principles and Practices of
Immunoprophylaxis*

RON H. BEHRENS, M.D., F.R.C.P.
Senior Lecturer, London School of Hygiene and
Tropical Medicine; Consultant in Tropical and
Travel Medicine, Travel Clinic, Hospital for
Tropical Diseases; London, United Kingdom
36. Traveling with Children

PHILIPPE BEUTELS, M.SC.
Research Fellow; Health Economist – Commercial
Engineer, Center for the Evaluation of Vaccination;
Epidemiology and Community Medicine, University
of Antwerp; WHO Collaborating Center for the
Prevention and Control of Viral Hepatitis; Antwerp,
Belgium
5. Economic Evaluation in Travel Medicine

MAURO BODIO, DR.PHIL.,DIPL.BIOL.
Swiss Tropical Institute; Basel, Switzerland
30. Envenoming and Poisoning Caused by Animals

ALAIN R. BOUCKENOOGHE, M.D., M.P.H.,
D.T.M.
Assistant Professor in Medicine, Baylor College of
Medicine; Houston Veteran Affairs Medical Center,
Houston, Texas
*12.2. Risk to Travelers by Region and Environmental
Factors: Sub-Saharan Africa*

DAVID J. BRADLEY, M.D., F.R.C.P., F.R.C.PATH.,
F.F.P.H.M.
Professor of Tropical Hygiene, London School
of Hygiene and Tropical Medicine; Director,
Malaria Reference Laboratory of PHLS; London,
England
Foreword

JUAN PABLO CAERIO, M.D.
Catholic University of Cordoba; Division of
Infectious Diseases, Hospital Privado de Cordoba;
Cordoba, Argentina
*12.8. Risk to Travelers by Region and Environmental
Factors: Temperate South America*

GIAMPIERO CAROSI, M.D., PH.D.
Director, Clinic of Infectious and Tropical Diseases,
University of Brescia, Brescia, Italy
26. Bacterial Infections

RODNEY Y. CARTWRIGHT, M.B., F.R.C.PATH.
Consultant Medical Microbiologist; Medical
Advisor United Kingdom Federation of Tour
Operators; Guildford, England
17. Hotel Swimming Pool Hygiene and Safety

ERIC CAUMES, M.D.
Infectious and Tropical Diseases Service, Hôpital
Pitié Solpetriere
*42.5. Dermatologic Problems Abroad and on
Returning*

MARTIN S. CETRON, M.D.
Division of Global Migration and Quarantine, CDC;
Emory University School of Medicine and Rollins
School of Public Health; Atlanta, Georgia
*43. Investigation and Management of Infectious
Diseases on International Conveyances (Airplanes
and Cruise Ships)*

SANTANU CHATTERJEE, M.B.B.S., D.T.M.H.
Consultant Physician, Travel and Tropical Medicine;
Physician, Wellesley Medicentre, Calcutta; Calcutta,
India
*12.11. Risk to Travelers by Region and
Environmental Factors: Middle South Asia*
*42.3. Medical Emergencies for International Visitors
to Developing Countries*

ROBERT T. CHEN, M.D., M.A.
Chief, Vaccine Safety and Development Activity,
Centers for Disease Control and Prevention,
Atlanta, Georgia
*22.2. Principles and Practices of
Immunoprophylaxis*

CHRISTOPHER P. CONLON, M.A., M.D., F.R.C.P.
Honorary Senior Lecturer, University of Oxford;
Nuffield Department of Medicine, John Radcliffe
Hospital; Consultant Physician, Oxford Radcliffe
Hospitals NHS Trust; Oxford, United Kingdom
39. The Immunocompromised Traveler

BRADLEY A. CONNOR, M.D.
Clinical Assistant Professor of Medicine, Weill
Medical College of Cornell University; Assistant

Attending Physician, The New York - Presbyterian
Hospital; New York, New York
20.4. Persistent Travelers' Diarrhea

JONATHAN H. COSSAR, M.D., CH.B.
Honorary Clinical Senior Lecturer, University of
Glasgow; Research Associate, Scottish Centre for
Infection and Environmental Health (SCIEH);
General Practitioner; Glasgow, Scotland
2. Health Risks Abroad: General Considerations
2.1. Morbidity and Mortality
2.2. Surveillance of Travel-Related Disease
*12.13. Risk to Travelers by Region and
Environmental Factors: Northern Europe*

JOHN COTTRELL-DORMER, M.B.B.S.
Medical Director, The Travel Doctor TMVC,
Sydney, Australia
32. Very Short-Term Travel

ED W. CUPP, PH.D.
Professor of Medical/Veterinary Entomology,
Department of Entomology and Plant Pathology,
Auburn University, Alabama
21.2. Malaria: Protection Against Mosquitoes

ALEXANDER GRAHAM DAWSON, M.D.
Wellington, New Zealand
31. Medical Aspects of Air Travel

FLOYD W. DENNY, JR., M.D.
Professor of Pediatrics, University of North Carolina
School of Medicine; University of North Carolina
Hospitals; Chapel Hill, North Carolina
23. Respiratory Tract Infections

BRADFORD L. DESSERY, B.A., R.N.
University of California – San Diego Medical
Center; International Traveler's Clinic, San Diego,
California
38. The Aged, Infirm, or Handicapped Traveler

DANIEL ANDRES DICESARE, M.D.
16. Diseases and Disorders Caused by the Sun

HERBERT L. DUPONT, M.D.
Clinical Professor, Baylor College of Medicine,
University of Texas; Chief, Internal Medicine, St.
Luke's Episcopal Hospital; Medical Director, St.
Luke's Travel Medicine; Houston, Texas
Preface
1. Travel Medicine as a Unique Medical Specialty
44. Travel Medicine 2010

ROBERT L. DUPONT, M.D.
Clinical Professor of Psychiatry, Georgetown
University School of Medicine; Rockville, Maryland
28. Psychiatric Illness and Stress

ROBERT EDELMAN, M.D.
Professor, Department of Medicine and Pediatrics
and Center for Vaccine Development, University of
Maryland School of Medicine; Director, Travelers'
Health Clinic, University of Maryland Medical
Center; Baltimore, Maryland

*22.4. Future Nonenteric Nonmalarial Vaccines for
Travelers*

CHARLES D. ERICSSON, M.D.
Professor of Medicine, Head, Clinical Infectious
Diseases, University of Texas Medical School at
Houston; Medical Director, Travel Medicine Clinic
at Herman Hospital, Houston, Texas

*20.2. Prevention of Travelers' Diarrhea: Risk
Avoidance and Chemoprophylaxis*

JOHN A. FREAN, M.B., B.CH., M. MED.,
D.T.M.& H., M.SC.
Senior Lecturer, Department of Clinical
Microbiology and Infectious Diseases, University
of the Witwatersrand; Senior Pathologist, South
African Institute for Medical Research,
Johannesburg, South Africa

*12.3. Risk to Travelers by Region and Environmental
Factors: Southern Africa*
*42.4. Diagnostic and Management Approaches in
Returning Travelers*

DAVID O. FREEDMAN, M.D.
University of Alabama at Birmingham; Director,
UAB Travelers Health Clinics; Birmingham,
Alabama

8. Information Sources in Travel Medicine

HASSAN GHAZNAWI, M.B., B.S., M.P.H., DR.P.H.
Professor of Community Medicine, College of
Dentistry, King Abdul Aziiz University, Jeddah,
Saudi Arabia

35. The Migrant as a Traveler

KEE-TAI GOH, M.B.B.S., M.SC., M.D., F.A.M.S.
Quarantine and Epidemiology Department/Institute
of Environmental Epidemiology, Ministry of the
Environment; Fellow, Academy of Medicine;
Associate Professor, Faculty of Medicine, National
University of Singapore; Singapore

*12.10. Risk to Travelers by Region and
Environmental Factors: Eastern South Asia*

SHERWOOD L. GORBACH, M.D.
Professor of Community Health and Medicine, Tufts
University; Community Health/Nutrition Infection
Unit, Boston, Massachusetts

*20.1. Travelers' Diarrhea: Epidemiology and
Clinical Aspects*

ROBERT D. GRENFELL, M.B.B.S., M.P.H.,
F.A.F.P.H.M.
Public Health Physician, Grenfell Health
Consulting, Horsham; Victoria, Australia

*29. Travel-Related Injuries (Motor Vehicle Crashes,
Falls, Drownings): Epidemiology and Prevention*

PETER H. HACKETT, M.D.
Emergency Medicine, St. Mary's Medical Center,
Grand Junction, Colorado; Affiliate Professor,
Department of Medicine, University of Washington
School of Medicine, Seattle

13. Medical Problems of High Altitude

HENRYK HANDSZUH, M.SC.
Chief, Quality of Tourism Development, World
Tourism Organization, Madrid, Spain

7. Tourism Patterns and Trends

STEPHEN W. HARGARTEN, M.D., M.P.H.
Professor and Chairman, Department of Emergency
Medicine, Medical College of Wisconsin,
Milwaukee, Wisconsin

*29. Travel-Related Injuries (Motor Vehicle Crashes,
Falls, Drownings): Epidemiology, and Prevention*

CHRISTOPH F.R. HATZ, M.D., D.T.M.& H.
University of Basel, Head, Department of Medicine,
Swiss Tropical Institute, Basel, Switzerland

25.2. Other Important Viral Infections

ADELAIDE A. HEBERT, M.D.
Professor and Vice Chairman, Department of
Dermatology, University of Texas – Houston
Medical School

16. Diseases and Disorders Caused by the Sun

ANTHONY JOHNSON HEDLEY, M.D., F.R.C.P.
Department of Community Medicine, University of
Hong Kong, China

*12.9. Risk to Travelers by Region and Environmental
Factors: East Asia*

JON HELTBERG, M.D.
Chief Psychiatrist, S.O.S. International,
Copenhagen, Denmark

28. Psychiatric Illness and Stress

DAVID R. HILL, M.D., D.T.M.&H.
Professor of Medicine, University of Connecticut
School of Medicine; Director, International
Traveler's Medical Service, University of
Connecticut Health Center, Farmington, Connecticut

*10.2. Travel Medicine and the Travel Medicine
Clinic: Travel Clinics in the United States and
Canada*

SUBHASH K. HIRA, M.D., M.P.H.
Professor of Infectious Diseases, University of
Texas, Houston, Texas; Director, Aids Research and
Control Centre, Mumbai, India; Professor-Director,
Department of Infectious Diseases, MGM Medical
College, New Mumbai, India
24. Sexually Transmitted Infections

JAMES M. HUGHES, M.D.
Clinical Associate Professor of Medicine, Division
of Infectious Diseases, Department of Medicine,
Emory University School of Medicine; Adjunct
Professor, Department of Epidemiology, Rollins
School of Public Health, Emory University; Staff
Physician, Division of Infectious Diseases,
Department of Medicine, Emory University School
of Medicine, Atlanta Veterans Administration
Hospital; Director, National Center for Infectious
Diseases, Centers for Disease Control and
Prevention; Atlanta, Georgia
Introduction

MARGARETHA ISAÄCSON, M.B., B.CH.,
D.SC.(MED), D.P.H., D.T.M.& H.,
F.A.C.T.M.(HON.)
Emeritus Professor of Tropical Diseases, The South
African Institute for Medical Research; University
of the Witwatersrand, Johannesburg, South Africa
*42.4. Diagnostic and Management Approaches in
Returning Travelers*

NANCY PIPER JENKS, M.SC., C.S., F.N.P.
Research Fellow, Center for the Evaluation of
Vaccination; WHO Collaborating Center for the
Prevention and Control of Viral Hepatitis;
Epidemiology and Community Medicine,
University of Antwerp, Antwerp, Belgium
5. Economic Evaluation in Travel Medicine

THOMAS JUNGHANSS, M.D., M.SC., P.H.D.C.
Consultant Physician, Tropical Medicine Unit,
Department of Tropical Hygiene and Public Health,
University Hospital, Heidelberg, Germany
30. Envenoming and Poisoning Caused by Animals

S. PATRICK KACHUR, M.D., M.P.H.
Malaria Epidemiology Branch (proposed), Division
of Parasitic Diseases, Centers for Disease Control
and Prevention, Atlanta, Georgia
21.1. Malaria Epidemiology

INGEGERD KALLINGS, M.D.
Chief, WHO Collaborating Center for Legionella
Infections, Department of Bacteriology, Swedish
Institute for Infectious Disease Control, Stockholm,
Sweden
23. Respiratory Tract Infections

JAY S. KEYSTONE, M.D., M.SC. (CTM),
F.R.C.P.C.
Professor of Medicine, University of Toronto; Staff
Physician, Centre for Travel and Tropical Medicine,
Toronto General Hospital, Toronto, Ontario, Canada
2. Health Risks Abroad: General Considerations
2.1. Morbidity and Mortality
2.2. Surveillance of Travel-Related Disease
9. Compliance with Travel Health Recommendations

JUDITH R. KLEIN, M.D.
14. Marine Hazards

HERWIG KOLLARITSCH, M.D.
Head, Department of Specific Prophylaxis and
Tropical Medicine, University of Vienna, Vienna,
Austria
20.3. Treatment of Traveler's Diarrhea
22.1. The Commercially Available Vaccines

PHYLLIS E. KOZARSKY, M.D.
Associate Professor of Medicine (Infectious
Diseases), Emory University School of Medicine;
The Emory Clinic; Atlanta, Georgia
37. Pregnancy, Nursing, Contraception, and Travel

JACK P. LANDOLT, PH.D.
Defence and Civil Institute of Environmental
Medicine, Toronto, Ontario, Canada
31.1. Motion Sickness

CLAUDINE LEUTHOLD, PHARM.D.
Project Manager and Medical Database Department
manager, Astral, Geneva
8. Information Sources in Travel Medicine

MYRON M. LEVINE, M.D., D.T.P.H.
Professor and Director, Center for Vaccine
Development, Division for Geographic Medicine,
Department of Medicine Division of Infectious
Diseases and Tropical Medicine, Department of
Pediatrics, University of Maryland; Attending
Physician, University of Maryland Medical Center,
Baltimore, Maryland
22.3. Enteric Vaccines: Present and Future

HANS O. LOBEL, M.D., M.P.H.
Medical Epidemiologist, Malaria Section,
Epidemiology Branch, Division of Parasitic
Diseases, National Center for Infectious Diseases,
Centers for Disease Control and Prevention, Atlanta,
Georgia
21.1. Malaria Epidemiology

THOMAS LÖSCHER, M.D.
Professor, Faculty of Medicine, University of
Munich; Head, Department of Infectious Diseases
and Tropical Medicine, Central University Hospital;
Munich, Germany
27. Parasitic Tropical Infections

LOUIS LOUTAN, M.D., M.P.H.
Priva Docent, Faculty of Medicine, Geneva
University Medical School; Head, Senior
Consultant, Travel and Migration Medicine Unit,
Department of Community Medicine, Geneva
University Hospital; Geneva, Switzerland
35. The Migrant as a Traveler

LESLIE C. LUCCHINA, M.D.
Instructor in Dermatology, Harvard Medical School,
Boston, Massachusetts
*42.5. Dermatologic Problems Abroad and on
Returning*

SUSAN A. MALONEY, M.D., M.H.S.
Division of Global Migration and Quarantine;
Centers for Disease Control and Prevention; Atlanta,
Georgia
*43. Investigation and Management of Infectious
Diseases on International Conveyances (Airplanes
and Cruise Ships)*

LEONARD C. MARCUS, V.M.D., M.D.
Adjunct Associate Professor of Medicine, University
of Massachusetts; Clinical Associate Professor,
Department of Environmental and Population
Health, Tufts University School of Veterinary
Medicine; Travelers' Health and Immunization
Services, Newton, Massachusetts
*11. Environmental Degradation: Medical Impact on
Tourism and Tropical Medicine*

PER-ANDERS MÅRDH, PROF., M.D., PH.D.
Lund University, Lund, Sweden; Department of
Bostetrics and Gynecology, Healthy Travel and
Tourism Centre, Simrishamn, Sweden
24. Sexually Transmitted Infections

ALBERTO MATTEELLI, M.D.
Adjoint Director, Division of Infectious Diseases,
Teaching Hospital of Brescia, Brescia, Italy
26. Bacterial Infections

LEENA MATTILA, M.D.
National Public Health Institute, Laboratory of
Enteric Pathogens, Finland
*20.2. Prevention of Travelers' Diarrhea: Risk
Avoidance and Chemoprophylaxis*

JACK MELLING
41. Biologic and Chemical Terrorism

**DAVID R. MURDOCH, M.B., CH.B., D.T.M.&H.,
F.R.A.C.P., F.R.C.P.A.**
Clinical Microbiologist, Microbiology Unit,
Canterbury Health Laboratories, Christchurch,
New Zealand
13. Medical Problems of High Altitude

GERALD S. MURPHY, M.D.
Head, Viral and Rickettsial Disease Department,
Naval Medical Research Center; Silver Spring,
Maryland
20.3. Treatment of Travelers' Diarrhea

PAT MURPHY, M.ED.
Clinical Ethicist, Health Care Ethics Service, St.
Boniface General Hospital; Winnipeg, Manitoba
4. Philosophical and Ethical Considerations

JAMES J. MWENEUANYA, M.B., B.S.
Department of Pediatrics, College of Medicine,
University of Malawi; Lecturer, Wellcome Trust
Malaria Laboratories, Blawtyre, Malawi;
Department of Pediatrics, Queen Elizabeth Central
Hospital, Blawtyre, Malawi, Africa
21.4. Malaria Treatment

KARL NEUMANN, M.D.
Associate Clinical Professor of Pediatrics, Cornell
Medical School; Associate Clinical Attending
Pediatrician, The New York Hospital, Forest Hills,
New York
36.Traveling with Children

BO NIKLASSON, M.D., PH.D.
Professor, Swedish Institute for Infectious Disease
Control, Stockholm, Sweden
25.1. Arboviruses and Zoonotic Viruses

PABLO C. OKHUYSEN, M.D.
Associate Professor of Medicine, Division of
Infectious Disease, University of Texas – Houston
Medical School; Memorial Hermann Hospital;
Lyndon B. Johnson General Hospital; Houston, Texas
*12.5. Risk to Travelers by Region and Environmental
Factors: Mainland Middle America*

WILHELMUS J. OOSTERVELD, M.D., PH.D.
Professor in Otorhinolaryngology, University of
Amsterdam; Vestibular Department, ENT Clinic,
Academic Medical Center, Amsterdam, The
Netherlands
31.1. Motion Sickness

STEPHEN M. OSTROFF, M.D.
Associate Director for Epidemiologic Science,
National Center for Infectious Disease, Centers for
Disease Control and Prevention; Atlanta, Georgia
19. Emerging Infectious Diseases and Travel

WALTER PASINI, M.D.
Professor in Occupational Health, University of
Pavia, Italy; Director, WHO Collaborating Center
for Tourist Health and Travel Medicine, Rimini, Italy
*12.14. Risk to Travelers by Region and
Environmental Factors: Southern Europe*
40. Travel for Health

HEIKKI PELTOLA, M.D., D.T.M.
Professor of Infectious Diseases, University of
Helsinki; Head of Pediatric Infectious Diseases,
Hospital for Children and Adolescents; Helsinki
University Central Hospital; Helsinki, Finland
*20.1. Travelers' Diarrhea: Epidemiology and
Clinical Aspects*

KEITH J. PETRIE, PH.D.
Associate Professor, Department of Health
Psychology, Faculty of Medicine and Health
Sciences, The University of Auckland; Auckland,
New Zealand
31.2. Jet Lag

BRUNO P. PETRUCCELLI, M.D.
Major, Medical Corps, United States Army,
Washington, District of Columbia
20.3. Treatment of Travelers' Diarrhea

PENELOPE A. PHILLIPS-HOWARD, PH.D.
Centers for Disease Control and Prevention, Kenyan
Medical Research Centre, Kisumu, Kenya, Africa
*21.5. Malaria: Emergency Self-Treatment by
Travelers*

PIERRE J. PLOURDE, M.D., F.R.C.P.C.
Assistant Professor, Internal Medicine and Medical
Microbiology, University of Manitoba; Director,
Infection Control, St. Boniface General Hospital;
Winnipeg, Manitoba
4. Philosophical and Ethical Considerations

DANIEL REID, O.B.E., M.D., F.R.C.P., F.F.P.H.M.,
D.P.H.
Honorary Professor, University of Glasgow,
Glasgow, Scotland; Visiting Professor, University of
Strathclyde, Strathclyde, Scotland; Honorary Senior
Lecturer, University of Edinburgh, Edinburgh,
Scotland; Honorary Senior Lecturer, Department of
Infectious and Tropical Diseases, Ruchill Hospital,
Glasgow, Scotland
2. Health Risks Abroad: General Considerations
2.1. Morbidity and Mortality
2.2. Surveillance of Travel–Related Disease

EDWARD R. RENSIMER, M.D., F.A.C.P.
Assistant Clinical Professor of Medicine, University
of Texas School of Medicine, Houston; Director,
International Medicine Center, Houston, Texas
*42.2. Medical Care for International Visitors to the
United States and Canada*

MICHEL REY, M.D.
President, Society of Travel Medicine, Paris, France;
Professor Emeritus, Centre Hospitalier Regional
Universitaire de Clermont-Ferrand, France
*22.2. Principles and Practices of
Immunoprophylaxis*

MARC R. ROBIN, A.N.P., R.N.
Sharp Reese Stealy, International Traveler's Clinic,
San Diego, California
38. The Aged, Infirm, or Handicapped Traveler

PATRICK RODRIGUEZ-REDINGTON, M.D.
Head, Passenger Medical Services, Service Medical
Air France, Paris, France
*10.1. Travel Medicine and the Travel Medicine
Clinic: Travel Clinics in Europe*

PHILIP ROGENMOSER, M.D, F.M.H.
Tropical Medicine, F.M.H.; Swiss Air Ambulance,
Rega, Zurich-Airport, Switzerland
*42.1. Medical Emergencies Abroad: Indications for
and Logistics of Aeromedical Evacuation*

TILMAN A. RUFF, B.S. (HONS), M.B., F.R.A.C.P.
Honorary Associate Physician, Victorian Infectious
Diseases Service, Royal Melbourne Hospital;
Director, Clinical Medical Affairs, SmithKline-
Beecham Biological, Australia/New Zealand/
Oceania; Medical Advisor, International
Department, Australian Red Cross
*12.15. Risk to Travelers by Region and
Environmental Factors: Pacific Islands, New
Zealand and Antartica*
*12.16. Risk to Travelers by Region and
Environmental Factors: Australia*

ERICH W. RUSSI, M.D.
Professor of Medicine, University of Zurich;
University Hospital of Zurich; Zurich, Switzerland
14.1. Diving-Related Health Problems

TARÁZ SAMANDARÍ, M.D., PH.D.
Assistant Professor of Medicine, University of
Maryland at Baltimore, Department of Geographic
Medicine; Baltimore, Maryland
*22.4. Future Nonenteric Nonmalarial Vaccines for
Travelers*

PETER V. SAVAGE, B.S., J.D.
Vice-President, Passport Health Inc., Baltimore,
Maryland
18. Threats of Security During International Travel
*42.1. Medical Emergencies Abroad: Indications for
and Logistics of Aeromedical Evacuation*

ARTHUR L. SCHIFF, ESQ., B.A., L.L.B.
3. Travel Industry and Medical Professionals
3.1. Responsibilities and Ideal Interaction
3.2. Legal Aspects of Travel Health

PATRICIA SCHLAGENHAUF, PH.D.
Research Scientist, Institute for Social and
Preventive Medicine, University of Zurich; Zurich,
Switzerland
*21.5. Malaria: Emergency Self-Treatment by
Travelers*

G. DENNIS SHANKS, M.D., M.P.H.
Director, United States Army Component, Armed
Forces Research Institute of Medical Sciences;
Bangkok, Thailand
21.3. Malaria Prevention

DAVID R. SHLIM, M.D.
Jackson Hole Travel and Tropical Medicine; Editor-
in-Chief, Medicine Planet, Inc.; Kelly, Wyoming
33. Expatriates and Long-Term Travelers

ROBERT STEFFEN, M.D.
Professor and Head, Division of Epidemiology and
Prevention of Communicable Diseases, Institute for
Social and Preventive Medicine, Professor of Travel
Medicine, Head, Travel Clinic, University of Zurich;
Zurich, Switzerland
Preface
1. Travel Medicine as a Unique Medical Specialty
44. Travel Medicine 2010

ANDREA SUHNER, PH.D.
Research Associate, Laboratory of Human
Chronobiology, Cornell Medical School; White
Plains, New York
31.2. Jet Lag

ADEL SULAIMAN, M.D.
Clinical Instructor in Medicine, State University of
New York/Buffalo; Williamsville, New York
*12.12. Risk to Travelers by Region and
Environmental Factors: Western South Asia*

ANN-MARI SVENNERHOLM, M.D., PH.D.
Professor, Department of Medical Microbiology
and Immunology, Göteborg University, Göteborg,
Sweden
22.3. Enteric Vaccines: Present and Future

MARCEL TANNER, PH.D., M.P.H.
Professor and Director, Swiss Tropical Institute,
Basel, Switzerland
*21.6. Malaria Vaccines – Current Status and
Development*

DAVID N. TAYLOR, M.D.
Walter Reed Army Institute of Research, Division of
Communicable Diseases and Immunology; Silver
Spring, Maryland
20.3. Treatment of Travelers' Diarrhea

DOMINIQUE TESSIER, M.D.
Medical Director of Travel Medisus, Montréal,
Québec, Canada
6. Pretravel Planning

CHULE THISYAKORN, M.D.
Professor of Pediatrics, Chulalongkorn University
Hospital, Bangkok, Thailand
25.2. Other Important Viral Infections

USA THISYAKORN, M.D., M.P.H.
Chief Executive Officer, VEI, Inc.; Great Falls,
Virginia
25.2. Other Important Viral Infections

THEODORE F. TSAI, M.D., M.P.H.
Clinical Research, Wyeth Lederle Vaccines; Pearl
River, New York
25.1. Arboviruses and Zoonotic Viruses

THOMAS H. VALK, M.D., M.P.H.
Chief Executive Officer, VEI Incorporated, McLean,
Virginia
28. Psychiatric Illness and Stress
33. Expatriates and Long-Term Travelers

PIERRE VAN DAMME, M.D., P.R.D.
Professor, Epidemiology and Community
Medicine, University of Antwerp; Director, WHO
Collaborating Center for the Prevention and Control
of Viral Hepatitis; Antwerp, Belgium
5. Economic Evaluation in Travel Medicine

ALFONS VAN GOMPEL, M.D.
Associate Professor, Tropical Medicine; Chief
Physician of the Travel Clinic, Institute of Tropical
Medicine; Antwerp, Belgium
37. Pregnancy, Nursing, Contraception, and Travel

ERIC L. WEISS, M.D., D.T.M.& H.
Associate Chief, Division of Emergency Medicine;
Director, Stanford Travel Medicine Service,
Stanford University; Stanford, California
15. Medical Risks of Temperature Extremes
43.1. Epidemiologic Alert at International Airports

CHRISTOPHER J.M. WHITTY, M.A., M.SC.,
M.R.C.P., D.T.M.&H.
Lecturer, Department of Medicine, University of
Malawi; Consultant in Medicine, Queen Elizabeth
Central Hospital, Blawtyre, Malawi, Africa;
Lecturer, London School of Hygiene and Tropical
Medicine; Senior Registrar, Hospital for Tropical
Diseases, London, United Kingdom
21.4. Malaria Treatment

GERHARD WIEDERMANN, M.D.
Professor Emeritus (retired), Department for
Specific Prophylaxis and Tropical Medicine,
University of Vienna; Vienna, Austria
22.1. The Commercially Available Vaccines

HENRY WILDE, M.D., F.A.C.P.
Professor of Medicine, Chulalongkorn University;
Queen Saovabha Memorial Instiute; Bangkok,
Thailand

25.2. Other Important Viral Infections
26. Bacterial Infections

JOAN L. WILLIAMS, R.N., M.S.
Clinical Coordinator, St. Luke's Travel Medicine,
St. Luke's Episcopal Hospital, Houston, Texas

12.4. Risk to Travelers by Region and Environmental
Factors: North America

MARY ELIZABETH WILSON, M.D., F.A.C.P.
Associate Professor of Medicine, Harvard Medical
School; Associate Professor of Population and
International Health, Harvard School of Public
Health; Chief of Infectious Diseases, Mount Auburn
Hospital, Cambridge, Massachusetts

27. Parasitic Tropical Infections

ROSMARIE WYSS, M.D., F.M.H.
Occupational Health Specialist in Travel Medicine
and Aviation Medicine, Swissair, Zurich,
Switzerland

32. Very Short-Term Travel

STEPHEN C. ZELL, M.D.
Professor of Medicine, University of Nevada School
of Medicine; Washoe Medical Center, Reno, Nevada

34. Expedition Participants

INTRODUCTION

As a result of improvements in sanitation and overall living conditions during the early part of the 20th century and the subsequent introduction of many vaccines and antibiotics, considerable complacency has developed regarding infectious diseases, which many regarded as either preventable by immunization or treatable by antibiotics. However, infectious diseases remain the leading cause of death worldwide. In the United States, infectious diseases are the third leading cause of death. The World Health Organization estimates that approximately 17 million (33%) of the 52 million deaths that occurred worldwide in 1997 were caused by microbial agents. In addition, the last 25 years have produced a series of reminders regarding the challenges that infectious diseases will continue to pose domestically and globally.

Experiences with these and other emerging and re-emerging diseases should have alerted clinicians, microbiologists, researchers, public health officials, policy makers, and the public to the critical importance of ensuring the capacity to detect, respond to, and control these infections. The Institute of Medicine (IOM) published a report entitled "Emerging Infections: Microbial Threats to Health in the United States" in the fall of 1992. This report, developed under the leadership of Drs. Joshua Lederberg and Robert Shope, emphasized the global context of emerging infectious diseases, highlighted this complacency regarding emerging infections, and identified six important factors in disease emergence and re-emergence. One of these factors was the dramatic increase in the frequency and speed of global travel and commerce. The others included changes in human demographics and behaviors, advances in technology and industry, economic development and changes in land use, microbial adaptation and change, and deterioration in the public health system at the local, state, national, and global levels. The IOM committee made 15 recommendations that stressed the need to improve surveillance and response capacity and identified research issues and training priorities.

A number of recent domestic challenges occurred in an international context, providing a reminder that we do indeed live in a "global village." For example, several food-borne outbreaks have been international in scope (e.g., *Cyclospora* gastroenteritis in the United States and Canada associated with raspberries imported from Guatemala), and drug resistance is well recognized as a global problem (e.g., the continued emergence and intercountry spread of penicillin resistance in *Streptococcus pneumoniae* and the recent identification of *Staphylococcus aureus* infections caused by strains with partial resistance to vancomycin in Japan, France, and the United States).

Internationally, a number of outbreaks have provided similar reminders. Examples include plague in India and Hendra virus infection in Australia in 1994, Ebola hemorrhagic fever in Zaire and leptospirosis in Nicaragua in 1995, a new variant of Creutzfeldt-Jakob disease in the United Kingdom, a large outbreak of *Escherichia coli* O157:H7 hemorrhagic colitis in Japan in 1996, avian influenza in Hong Kong in 1997, and amebiasis in Georgia in 1998. Each of these outbreaks illustrates the need for clinicians to be aware of emerging diseases in other countries, the critical importance of adequate surveillance and response capacity, the critical role of the diagnostic laboratory, and the global implications of local problems.

The ability to address these emerging and re-emerging microbial threats requires adequate surveillance and response capacity, ongoing research programs, effective prevention and control programs, and strengthening of the public health system locally, at the state and national levels, and internationally. The challenges that these diseases will continue to pose demand a multidisciplinary approach and a supply of trained health professionals.

Clinicians involved in travel medicine are uniquely positioned both to recognize emerging infectious diseases acquired by travelers and to take action to prevent infectious diseases in travelers. These professionals are in a unique position to help bridge the gap between clinical medicine and public health. They need skills in both risk assessment and risk management. They need communication skills to advise the broad array of individuals who travel abroad for business, pleasure, education, and visits with family and friends. They must be skilled in the differential diagnoses of a broad array of syndromes. Finally, they must be alert to the possibility that one of their patients may be part of an epidemic abroad that may require public health action. This book, the scope of which has been expanded far beyond that of the first edition, should serve as a valuable source of information for them and their colleagues in related disciplines as they strive to prevent, diagnose, and treat the myriad of potential infectious and noninfectious diseases and conditions that travelers may experience as we enter the next millennium.

James M. Hughes, M.D.

FOREWORD

We human beings have chosen to call ourselves *Homo sapiens* in our immodest way, although a historian has made a case for *Homo ludens* from what he sees as our essentially playful nature. However, on the evidence, the right name is surely only *Homo vagans*, in recent decades at least, as human beings are remarkable for the scale and frequency of their wanderings. Moreover, these contrast with those of most other species by their irregularity and diversity. Total tourist journeys per year are estimated at over 5 billion, equal to the world's population, and on top of these are all of the movements in search of work and the unhappy and unwilling migrations of refugee populations.

These words from the first edition remain true, but in the mere 3 years since they were written, the subject of travel medicine—the response of physicians and other health professionals to the health hazards of travel—has evolved and matured to a striking degree.

Travel medicine began with a limited vision, with a focus on tourists and their individual needs in traveling to more or less distant places. It was preventive medicine, but with an individual focus, and as such it had some ambivalence, because prevention is as much an action of society as of the individual. The focus has widened: most of the hazards of the traveler are environmental (other than jet lag), and due attention needs to be paid to the environment both of travel and at the destination. Indeed, travel can be viewed as a process of environmental change but where the traveler changes environments, rather than the environment of a static person changing over time. A widespread problem today is when those who lived many years in a place migrate to another and settle there. In due course, they or their children visit their former home, but the health risks may have changed, without their knowledge, in the intervening years. The two aspects of environmental change are here combined.

The initial focus of travel medicine was on short-term travel. But those who move elsewhere for several years both encounter different levels of hazard and, at least as important, perceive them differently. These aspects have to be added to those faced by health workers, to whom it is already clear that a great deal of expert knowledge is needed: the hazards from sitting on a beach on the Cote d'Azur differ greatly from those encountered while exploring forests in Guatemala, and the range of destinations and risks is far beyond the personal experience of individual practitioners. The needs of forced migrants, whether refugees driven from their homes by violence or those who go to new countries to earn the means of survival, are still more demanding. Even so, travel medicine practitioners will increasingly be used as those best able to cope with their needs, and the experience will serve to broaden what could otherwise become a rather restricted field.

The public/private ambivalence adds to the complexity of travel medicine: people expect centrally defined vaccine and other schedules at the public health level, but individual travel advice has more the character of clinical practice, where each patient has and expects a personal set of recommendations to fit a particular journey and person, yet may complain about the resulting diversity of advice seen in fellow travelers. Travel medicine is peculiarly vulnerable to economic pressures, as the extent to which so many people take prophylactic vaccines and medicines can affect the fortunes of both manufacturers and travelers. Moreover, simple advice may take a lot of time. At first sight, travel medicine deals largely with people in an optional aspect of their lives and may mistakenly be viewed as an optional extra, like some forms of plastic surgery. However, the outcome of neglecting health precautions for travel may be death or prolonged disability. Most deaths from imported disease in travelers are avoidable.

The subject is, by its very nature, international in scope. It is clear that, for the optimal health of travelers, attention needs to be paid to the destination environment and means of transport, as well as to the travelers themselves. This second edition begins to widen the scope of travel medicine while still focusing on tourists, in order to address their needs in a very full and comprehensive way. But as travel medicine matures, its approach and scientific basis must consider the whole range of human migration in relation to health. This is reflected in the scope and content of this invaluable book.

David J. Bradley, M.D.

PREFACE

There are two principal reasons for the existence of this text: to provide medical and travel authorities with guidelines and recommendations to help prevent disease and ensure optimal medical care of the traveling public and to help define the boundaries of this new and expanding field of travel medicine. It is our hope that compiling the best available information into a single source will assist those in charge to protect the traveler's health interests.

Currently, the temptation exists to define travel medicine broadly, making the discipline appear nebulous and diffuse. Our purpose here is to describe boundaries for travel medicine. We provide principles of health promotion among the traveling public. There are several areas that are of special concern in travel medicine—the environment and modes of travel, health promotion and disease prevention, travel for disadvantaged persons, malaria and other tropical and febrile illnesses, HIV/AIDS, sexually transmitted disease, diarrhea, hepatitis, psychoneurologic disorders, and accidents—all of which are discussed in the book. Perhaps this text will encourage the standardization and dissemination of the best and latest information for medical personnel, as well as for the lay traveler. We encourage the reader to solicit other sources as well, which deal with tropical, migration, and military medicine, all of which overlap travel medicine to some extent.

An essential aspect of the book is the international orientation of the chapters. Where possible, authorities from both sides of the Atlantic were teamed to coauthor chapters, to address the differences that exist in important areas of the discipline. In some instances, little information was available in the medical literature to help guide the authors.

The second edition of the *Textbook of Travel Medicine and Health* has been expanded by the inclusion of 13 new chapters. We now include a "Disease Risks by Region" section detailing important health risks occurring in 15 regions of the world. Also new to this edition are "Environmental Degradation: Medical Impact on Tourism and Tropical Medicine," "Diseases and Disorders Caused by the Sun," "Seafood Infections and Intoxication," "Hotel Swimming Pool Hygiene and Safety," "Threats of Security During International Travel," "Emerging Infections Diseases and Travelers," "Protection Against Mosquitoes," "The Migrant as a Traveler," "The Immunocompromised Traveler," "Biological and Chemical Terrorism," "Dermatologic Problems Abroad and On Returning," and "Epidemiologic Alert at International Airports."

Travel medicine is a dynamic field, and this information will need updating from other sources, as new information becomes available. We look forward to presenting you with this new information through the publication of subsequent editions of the *Textbook*.

We wish to thank the many authors who have dedicated their time and effort to writing these chapters. Without their scientific and clinical expertise, neither the discipline of travel medicine nor this book would exist.

Herbert L. DuPont, M.D.
Robert Steffen, M.D.

ACKNOWLEDGMENT

Ms Kathryn Eslinger-Lutz, Ms Christa D. Lynch, and Ms Barbara S. Kelly are gratefully acknowledged for their numerous contributions to the development of this text.

DEDICATION

"To all travel health professionals: may they be successful and achieve satisfaction in their work, and may they enjoy their own travels."

CONTENTS

Chapter 1

TRAVEL MEDICINE AS A UNIQUE MEDICAL SPECIALTY

HERBERT L. DUPONT AND ROBERT STEFFEN

INTRODUCTION

The public is leaving home to enter new territories with increasing frequency. These individuals are put at increased risk for illness or injury because of the occurrence of diseases endemic to the regions being visited or because of the greater likelihood of accidents while on the move, especially when in areas where the regard for public safety is lacking.

A number of factors serve as stimuli for the development of travel medicine as a new medical discipline. The first factor relates to the economic considerations of travel. Travel-related activities generate huge sums of money for the travel industry and for the host regions. It is in the interest not only of the traveler but also of the travel industry and of the host country to reduce illness where the objective is the encouragement of additional travel. A second factor relates to available research studies that have helped to characterize risks of acquisition of illness. These studies serve as the basis for current control and prevention programs. The third factor relates to these disease reduction or elimination approaches employing preventive strategies administered before or during travel. The fourth factor important to the development of travel medicine is that many health risks are sufficiently predictable that it is possible to arm the traveler with medications to employ in case one of the more common illnesses develops during travel. The fifth factor relates to the need to have an educated medical capability at home to appropriately deal with health problems among individuals when they return home from areas of the world with uniquely endemic medical conditions.

WHAT CONSTITUTES THE SPECIALTY?

Nearly all medical groups and many nonmedical groups and individuals have an interest in the travelers' health and welfare, serving to make the subject of travel medicine interdisciplinary and hard to define. In its broad application, travel medicine extends beyond the immediate health of the traveling public. The environment into which individuals move, whether it be transient (mode of transportation) or more permanent (travel destination), is an important consideration. The health of the local setting or host region is also influenced by travel patterns where natural resources may be depleted, and the health of the local population may be given a lower priority than the pleasure and well-being of the foreign guest.

Although it is tempting to be expansive in thinking of the area of travel medicine, the interrelating subjects and issues are too numerous to include in the general discipline. Without restriction, the impact of our work in the area will be limited. Travel medicine is best restricted to the topics that directly influence the health and medical welfare of travelers whether they are visiting regional areas or international settings. Travel medicine is also concerned with the host region into which there is a temporary translocation of persons. The concerns include both the physical and psychological well-being of the traveler and host country population. Health promotion and disease prevention are the cornerstone of the specialty. These become daunting tasks when one considers the myriad of risks to which the traveler is exposed and the increasing movement of disadvantaged persons such as infants, the elderly or infirm, the pregnant, or the chemically dependent.

Although travelers are the major focus, the lessons learned are applicable to other populations, including foreign diplomats, expatriates and refugees, and military populations.

SPECIAL AREAS OF CONCERN

Areas of concern are identification of diseases and disorders of risk in various regions of the world, prevention of disease through education and behavior change and immunoprophylaxis, chemoprophylaxis, and self-treatment of certain diseases. Virtually all travelers to endemic areas have to be concerned with special health risks, including malaria and other tropical and febrile infections, HIV/AIDS and other sexually transmitted diseases, diarrhea, hepatitis, respiratory diseases, psychoneurologic disorders, and accidents. If appropriate, travelers need to be educated about the effects of high altitude, temperature extremes, and excessive sunlight, as well as about marine hazards and jet lag. Medical personnel at home need to be trained in the areas of travel medicine and clinical tropical medicine to be able to deal with illness in the returning traveler, considering the bacterial, rickettsial, parasitic, and viral threats to international travel. Issues that are more recently becoming important include threats of security during travel including kidnapping, random acts of violence, and biologic and chemical terrorism.

SOURCES OF INFORMATION

There are numerous sources of information. The World Health Organization (WHO) and the U.S. Centers for Disease Control and Prevention (CDC) prepare regularly updated publications dealing with travel medicine issues and recommendations. Travel medicine clinics exist in most of the industrialized world and in many urban centers in the developing world. Computer programs are available that are regularly updated with WHO and CDC information to be as current as practical. Textbooks, including this one, are useful sources of valuable information, although they need to be updated on a regular basis to be complete. Newspapers and magazines may offer useful articles dealing with health threats for travelers.

REASONS FOR PREPARING THE *TEXTBOOK OF TRAVEL MEDICINE AND HEALTH*

Travel medicine issues are not new to the medical profession or to the lay public. The needed medical information in the area of travel medicine is not readily available in one source to practitioners. Also, travel medicine as a medical discipline remains arbitrarily defined with differences from place to place and from country to country. Travel medicine is only slowly becoming known by the medical community. Hence, information given to the traveling public is often inadequate or erroneous. The *Textbook of Travel Medicine and Health* is being developed to provide a single source of information in the area for physicians and paramedical personnel interested in the medical problems of travelers. Also, the text has been developed to help better define the medical specialty and to set some limits for the discipline. Whenever feasible in the preparation of the chapters, we have coupled experts from two continents to cover the topics compre-

hensively, which is intended to provide a range of appropriate recommendations.

The text begins with a detailed look at the issues of travel and tourism patterns, the travel industry and medical professionals, a description of health risks abroad, sources of travel medicine information including publications and the growing number of clinics dedicated to the area, and pretravel planning. Disease risk by region is offered by coupling an expert in the region with region-specific material developed by WHO. The environment is considered in detail with discussion of climatologic factors, marine hazards, and extremes of temperature and altitude. A chapter dealing with threats of security during international travel is designed to offer travel medicine specialists and tourists up-to-date advice in reducing and dealing with security risks. Special medical conditions that occur with frequency during international travel are discussed, including travelers' diarrhea, malaria, vaccine-preventable diseases, respiratory tract infections, sexually transmitted diseases, and viral, bacterial, and parasitic infections, as well as psychiatric illness and stress. For the travel medicine practitioner, considerations important to ensuring the health of special travelers such as airline crews and short-term business persons, expatriates and expedition participants, infants and young children, pregnant and nursing women, the aged, and handicapped and infirm travelers are addressed. The growing problem of biologic and chemical terrorism is discussed, and outbreak investigations and epidemiologic alerts at airports are topics presented. Suggested approaches to dealing with a person acquiring illness while outside his/her own region or presenting for medical evaluation upon returning home are provided. Finally, the text ends with a discussion of the probable future of this most exciting area of medicine.

As with all medical areas, the knowledge base for travel medicine is in a state of continual evolution. Although this text and other references will provide an important perspective on the subject and most of the information will remain useful for an important period of time, for some of the evolving areas it will be necessary to consult more up-to-date sources for changing recommendations on disease risks and prevention strategies.

Chapter 2

HEALTH RISKS ABROAD: GENERAL CONSIDERATIONS

DANIEL REID, JAY S. KEYSTONE, AND JONATHAN H. COSSAR

2.1 MORBIDITY AND MORTALITY

The history of epidemics is the history of wars and wanderings.[1] It has, of course, been recognized since biblical times that when humans move from one environment and climate to another, this often results in consequences to their health ranging from trivial illness to death.

One of the earliest references to travel-related disease is that describing the epidemics that afflicted the Philistines around 1190 BC when they battled with the Israelites for the Ark of the Covenant. As the Philistines moved from place to place after capturing the Ark, further outbreaks of illness (which might have been due to bacillary dysentery[2]) occurred at these locations. The Athenian plague, which started in 430 BC, has been described in some detail by Thucydides. It caused tremendous mortality among the civilian and military population of Athens and was probably spread via the trade routes as the inhabitants of the Port of Piraeus were the first to be affected—the disease having spread from Ethiopia, Egypt, and throughout the greater part of the Persian Empire.[3] The cause of this dramatic outbreak is unclear, and various suggestions—bubonic plague, smallpox, influenza, or measles—have been made. Whatever the cause, this episode is seen as being a contributory factor in the weakening of Athen's power.

It was the 14th-century pandemic of plague that resulted in ships, crews, travelers, and cargoes being detained for 40 days—hence "quarantine" from the Italian, *quaranta giorni*, meaning "40 days."[4] These precautions, which were organized as early as 1348 in Venice, 1377 in Ragusa, and 1383 in Marseilles, are an indication of the apprehension experienced by countries of the distinct possibility of disease being introduced from the trade routes. This fear was well founded as witnessed by the Black Death, which resulted in the death of at least one-quarter of the population of Europe.[5] The Black Death, which was the hemorrhagic form of plague, started in Asia and crossed to Europe through Turkey and the Mediterranean ports in 1347, and during the next 3 years spread throughout the European continent. It reached Britain the following year, and it is estimated that between one-quarter and one half of the population succumbed.

Examples of other travel-related infections occurring in former times are not hard to find. The Americas saw the introduction of smallpox, syphilis, and measles soon after the arrival of Columbus, and the Spanish conquest of Mexico owes much of its success to an epidemic of smallpox that destroyed almost half of the Aztec population.[5] Diarrheal diseases, including cholera, have always been an affliction of travelers, as the terms "Delhi belly," "Montezuma's revenge," "Rangoon runs," and "Hong Kong dog" testify. It is little wonder that the 18th-century English diarist Fanny Burney poignantly wrote in 1792 that "traveling is the ruin of all happiness."[6]

MORBIDITY

Illness among travelers depends on a variety of factors such as the age and lifestyle of the traveler, country visited, and climatic factors. Also, the span of illness is considerable, ranging from the usually non–life-threatening conditions such as vomiting and diarrhea to the potentially dangerous diseases such as legionellosis, rabies, and malaria.

On the basis of the many studies that have now been carried out, it is possible to obtain a consensus about the degree of risk experienced by different groups. Among the highest attack rates reported are those by Steffen and colleagues,[7,8] who observed that up to 75% of short-term Swiss travelers to the tropics or subtropics report some health impairment. Few of these self-reported health problems were severe; only 5% required medical attention. Less than 2% were unable to work for a mean duration of 15 days, and less than 1% required hospital admission. Nevertheless, 5 in 10,000 travelers needed to be evacuated by air (Figure 2.1–1).[9]

A series of studies of 14,227 Scottish holidaymakers showed that the overall attack rate was 38%: 27% suffered from alimentary symptoms, 5% suffered from respiratory illness, and 6% had both.[10–14] In a Finnish investigation of 2,665 travelers, 18% reported illness.[15]

When age was considered in the Scottish studies, the highest attack rates of illness were recorded by those aged under 40 years, with 41% of the 10 to 19 years age groups, 48% of the 20 to 29 years age groups, and 38% of the 30 to 39 years age groups reporting illness (Table 2.1–1).

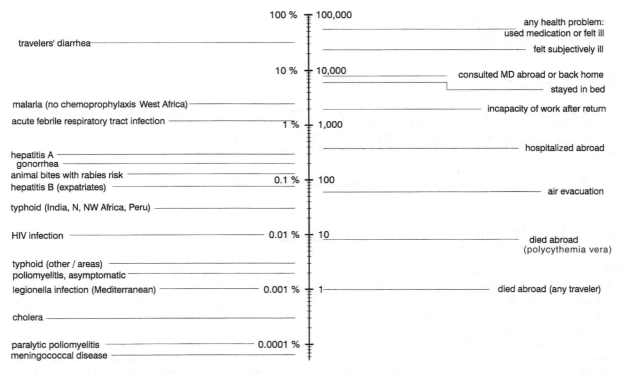

Figure 2.1–1.   Incidence rate per month of health problems during a stay in developing countries.[8]

Thereafter, attack rates showed a progressive diminution with increasing age. In short-term Swiss travelers to developing countries, the highest attack rate (20%) was also in the 20 to 29 years age group.[8]

When the country of destination was considered, there was a general indication that the further south one traveled and, to some extent, the further east in Europe and beyond, the higher the rate of illness (Table 2.1–2). This generally remained true both in the summer and in winter. Examples in support of this trend were the 77% attack rate reported by tourists to Northern Africa in the summer and the 57% rate for those traveling to Eastern Europe. In Swiss travelers, the highest attack rate of ill-ness (21%) was noted in those returning from East Africa, Sri Lanka, and the Far East, and almost three times that of travelers returning from the Greek Islands.[8] Reports of illness are less frequent during the winter months.[16] The incidence of illness recorded in various studies is summarized in Table 2.1–3.

TRAVELERS' DIARRHEA

Undoubtedly, the most common health problem encountered by travelers to foreign countries, especially in developing regions, is diarrhea.[17] This problem is dealt with in Chapter 20 (Travelers' Diarrhea).

Table 2.1–1.   AGE OF TRAVELERS AND REPORTS OF ILLNESS OF SCOTTISH PACKAGE HOLIDAY TRAVELERS

AGE GROUP (YR)	TOTAL	UNWELL (%)
0–9	550	33
10–19	1,974	41
20–29	3,033	48
30–39	2,028	38
40–49	2,297	32
50–59	2,381	28
≥60	1,239	20
Not known	725	32
Total	14,227	37

Table 2.1–2.   AREA VISITED, SEASON, AND REPORTS OF ILLNESS AMONG SCOTTISH PACKAGE HOLIDAY TRAVELERS*

AREA VISITED	SUMMER ATTACK RATE	WINTER ATTACK RATE
Europe (north)	19	20
Europe (east)	57	12
Mediterranean (southern Europe)	34	19
Mediterranean (North Africa)	77	32
Average attack rates	37	20

*All values are percentages.

Table 2.1–3.   INCIDENCE OF VARIOUS HEALTH IMPAIRMENTS IN TRAVELERS

	AUTHOR				
CHARACTERISTIC	GANGAROSA[57] (1969/1970)	STEFFEN[7] (1976/1977)		REID[11] (1977)	PELTOLA[15] (1979/1980)
Population					
Origin	U.S.	Switzerland		Scotland	Finland
Destination	Europe	Tropics	U.S. Canada	Spain North Africa	Spain North Africa
Duration of stay	N/A	Usually 2–3 wk		Usually 2–3 wk	1–2 wk
Number	9,492	10,555	1,379	2,211	2,665
Any health complaint (%)	20	75	6	43	48
Diarrhea	11 (4–12)	34 (20–53)	6	34	18 (5–37)
Constipation	N/A	14	20	N/A	N/A
Respiratory infection	10	13	8	6	10
Insomnia	N/A	11	7	N/A	N/A
Headache	N/A	8	8	N/A	6
Sunburn/dermatosis	N/A	6	3	4	10

N/A = not available.

MALARIA

Malaria is a particularly serious problem for those traveling to areas where this disease is prevalent. This problem is dealt with in Chapter 21 (Malaria).

VACCINE-PREVENTABLE DISEASES

For many immunizable diseases, risk estimates for travel are not known. The most frequent immunizable disease in travelers, hepatitis A, has a reported monthly incidence rate of 3 cases per 1,000 Swiss travelers.[18] This rate increased to 20 per 1,000 for those who abandon the usual tourist routes and eat or drink under poor hygienic conditions.[19] Another study of Swedish travelers reported a rate of 6 to 109 per 1,000 travelers for a mean stay abroad of 2 weeks.[20] Among 3,322 Swiss aircrew members who spent an average of 45 nights in developing countries, the incidence was 12.2/1,000, a more than 10 times greater incidence than for those who did not fly to high-risk countries.[21]

Although the risk of hepatitis B appears to be low for short-stay tourists, long-term overseas workers are at considerable risk for infection. For U.S. missionaries serving in Africa, the attack rates of hepatitis were highest during the first 2 years of service, when 28% and 11% were infected with hepatitis A and B, respectively.[22] Over the next decade, the median annual attack rates were 5.4% for hepatitis A and 1.2% for hepatitis B. Steffen[23] noted that professional workers in developing countries had a monthly incidence of symptomatic or asymptomatic hepatitis B of 80 to 420 per 100,000, with symptomatic disease occurring in 20 to 60 per 100,000.

Several surveys have documented the attack rate of typhoid fever in travelers to be approximately 1:30,000.[24,25]

In India, Senegal, and North Africa, a 10-fold greater risk was found, especially for those traveling off the usual tourist routes.[26] A review of typhoid fever cases in the United States between 1985 and 1994 showed that 72% reported international travel within 30 days before onset of illness. In 1994, 37% of cases arose from trips to the Indian subcontinent and 23% to Mexico. The incidence of typhoid fever in U.S. citizens traveling to the Indian subcontinent was at least 18 times higher than for any other geographic region. Recent cases were more likely to be resistant to ampicillin, chloramphenicol, and trimethoprim-sulfamethoxazole.[27]

Cholera is a rare infection in travelers with attack rates estimated to be 1 in 500,000 travelers.[28] In Japan, where regular microbiologic screening for cholera is carried out among returned travelers with diarrhea, the overall incidence of cholera was 5 per 100,000 and 13 per 100,000 in Japanese travelers returning from Bali.[28] In the United States, a 10-fold increase in cholera cases noted by the Centers for Disease Control was due to the proximity of the Latin American outbreak; among U.S. residents it occurred most often in those returning to visit their country of origin.[29] Although the disease no longer poses a threat to countries with a minimum standard of healthy living, it remains a challenge to those where access to safe drinking water and adequate sanitation cannot be ensured.[30] It remains a global threat, and epidemics with substantial numbers of cases and mortality have occurred in recent years (e.g., in the Horn of Africa there has been a dramatic cholera epidemic with case-fatality rates as high as 20%).[31]

Travel overseas may put the unprotected person at substantial risk for measles. Although impressive progress has been made toward achieving global morbidity and mortality reduction targets, measles still remains endemic in many countries despite the widespread availability of a safe and effective vaccine since 1963. In 1997, 702,298 cases were notified, with Africa reporting a rate of 47.5 per 100,000 population.[32]

There have been further achievements with polio eradication, and a 90% decrease in the number of cases has been notified during the last decade. In 1988, poliovirus circulated widely in all continents except Australia, but by 1998 the Americas were polio-free and transmission had been interrupted. Despite this progress, however, wild poliovirus was still present in many countries in 1998, and 5,108 cases were reported to the World Health Organization.[33]

The risk of acquiring Japanese encephalitis among travelers is uncertain. The chance that a traveler to Asia will develop the disease is probably small; only 5 cases among Americans traveling or working in Asia are known to have occurred since 1981.[31] On the other hand, it has been calculated that the risk of a nonimmunized person becoming infected in a rural area where Japanese encephalitis is endemic is 1 in 5,000 per month of exposure.[34]

Cruise ships appear to be ideal "floating reservoirs" for the transmission of air-borne pathogens. The largest outbreak of travel-related influenza occurred in the summer of 1998 in Alaska and the Northwest Territories of Canada among cruise ship passengers and staff.[35] Recently in the Caribbean, an outbreak of rubella occurred among cruise ship crew,[36] and in a separate incident, legionella caused serious illness among ship passengers exposed to a contaminated whirlpool spa.[37]

Rabies has been reported in travelers, but sufficient data are unavailable to determine rates of exposure. Animal bites among travelers have been estimated to occur in the range of 0.2% to 0.4% per month of travel.[38] A recent survey of 1,882 foreign travelers in Thailand showed that a dog lick or bite was experienced by 8.9% and 1.3% of travelers, respectively, during an average stay of 17 days in the country.[39] Considering that up to 6.8% of street dogs in Thailand carry the rabies virus, the results of this study showed that the risk for rabies among travelers may be considerable.[40]

SEXUALLY TRANSMITTED DISEASES

Casual sexual contacts abroad play an important role in the transmission of sexually transmitted diseases (STDs) and HIV infection.[41,42] Because of the global epidemic of HIV and STDs, available data on the sexual behavior of travelers are disturbing. In one study, 5% of short-term travelers had had casual sex contacts, of whom half were unprotected by condoms.[43] When 354 British travelers were surveyed, 4.8% admitted to having had casual sex while abroad, compared with 6.4% of 484 Swiss travelers.[44] A recent cross-sectional survey of U.K. travelers attending a tropical disease clinic showed that 18.6% had had new sexual partners during their most recent trip abroad.[42] Almost two-thirds of those who were sexually active did not use condoms on every occasion, and 5.7% contracted STDs. Although it is commonly believed that women do not usually engage in casual sex during travel,

a recent study of 996 Swedish women attending a family planning clinic showed that 28% of women had experienced casual sex during travel; they were most often single, had broken relationships, were smokers, and used alcohol and cannabis at a higher frequency.[45]

Long-term overseas workers appear to put themselves at greater risk than do short-term travelers. Among HIV-negative Belgian men working in Central Africa, 51% and 31% reported casual sex with local women or prostitutes, respectively.[46] A study of almost 2,000 Dutch expatriates working in sub-Saharan Africa showed that 31% of males and 13% of females had casual sexual contacts with African partners, and consistent condom use was reported by less than 25% of study participants.[47] The prevalence of HIV among overseas workers was noted to be 8.6% among Danish volunteers and ranged from 0.4% to 1.1% in Dutch and Belgian expatriates, respectively. These rates are 100- to 500-fold greater than those noted in comparable populations in these countries.[47] These high rates of HIV were not found among U.S. Peace Corps volunteers working in West Africa between 1988 and 1993. In spite of the previously reported high rates of sexual intercourse with host country nationals and the low consistent use of condoms among Peace Corps volunteers, only 3 of 2,491 subjects were infected with HIV-1 and none with HIV-2.[48]

SCHISTOSOMIASIS

Travelers to Africa appear to be at increased risk of schistosomiasis as judged by the numerous outbreaks of infection reported recently.[49-52] In Malawi, among 305 U.S. citizens and 650 non-U.S. foreign nationals, 33% had serologic evidence of current or past schistosomiasis.[51] Between 1991 and 1994, 238 cases of schistosome infection were documented among travelers returning from sub-Saharan Africa who attended The Hospital for Tropical Diseases in the U.K.[52]

MORTALITY

Travel-related deaths can occur on the way to the destination, within the country being visited, or soon after return.

In colonial times, mortality was very high among overseas travelers of whom the majority worked for prolonged periods as missionaries, military personnel, and colonial administrators; short-stay overseas vacations were the exception.

Travel was much more hazardous, with significant mortality taking place en route to the destination on the long sea voyages undertaken on sailing ships or the slow overland journeys through inhospitable environments. In these times, the traveler was much more susceptible to infection because of the lack of appropriate immunizations and other means of protection; death in these early travelers was often due to infection. For example, of 1,427 Presbyterian missionaries who traveled abroad between 1873 and 1929, 11% died in service, mostly from infection.[53]

Although a large number of travelers become infected abroad nowadays, it is paradoxical that there are so few

Table 2.1–4. DEATHS RELATED TO INTERNATIONAL TRAVEL*

CAUSE OF DEATH	HARGARTEN[59] (n = 2,463) (1991)	SNIEZEK[60] (n = 17,988) (1991)	PROCIV[54] (n = 421) (1995)	PAIXAO[55] (n = 952) (1991)
Cardiovascular	49.0	45.0	35.0	68.9
Injury	22.0	23.0	26.0	20.7
Infectious disease	1.0	—	2.4	3.6
Cancer	5.9	—	—	—
Suicide/homicide	2.9	17.0	8.2	—
Medical	13.7	—	—	—
Other/unknown	5.5	—	17.0	7.0

*All values are percentages.

infection-related deaths; infection has been eclipsed by other causes (Table 2.1–4).

In a study of 421 deaths among Australian travelers, only 10 (2.4%) were attributed to infection,[54] and in a Scottish study involving 952 persons who died abroad, infection occurred in 34 (3.6%).[55] Men die more frequently than women do while abroad—almost 4:1 and 3:1 in the Australian and Scottish studies, respectively.

By far the most common cause of death was cardiovascular disease, usually myocardial infarction (35% in the Australian study and 68.9% in the Scottish). Among American travelers, cardiovascular problems among male travelers aged over 60 years accounted for 50% of reported deaths.[56]

Trauma has emerged as an important cause of death in travelers, and various studies have pointed to the fact that motor vehicle accidents and other injuries cause sig-

Table 2.1–5. INJURY DEATHS RELATED TO INTERNATIONAL TRAVEL

CAUSE OF DEATH	HARGARTEN[59] (n = 601) (1991)	SNIEZEK[60] (n = 17,988) (1991)	PROCIV[54] (n = 100) (1995)
Motor vehicle	26.8	37.0	28.3
Drowning	16.1	15.0	—
Air crash	7.2	7.0	—
Homicide	8.6	11.0	8.2
Suicide	3.4	6.0	
Poisoning	6.5	—	—
Burns	3.6	2.0	—
Electrocution	0.5	—	—
Water transport	—	4.0	—
Others	27.4	—	43.0

nificant mortality (Table 2.1–5).[54–62] In American travelers, motor vehicle accidents accounted for 25% of all deaths, with other injuries and accidents such as drowning and falls from a height causing 10%.[56] Among Australian travelers, accidents (mainly traffic accidents) accounted for 18% of deaths, and in Scottish travelers 21%. When those with cardiovascular disease are compared with those who had injuries or accidents, there is a marked preponderance of older persons in the former and younger persons in the latter.

It is likely that the recent increase in the number of elderly people taking foreign holidays (often for prolonged periods of time—indeed, some tour operators cater specifically for this age group) has made a major contribution to the preponderance of cardiovascular deaths. Although it is possible that those who succumb to cardiovascular illness would have died anyway had they stayed at home, perhaps more consideration should be given to the question of whether those with preexisting cardiovascular problems are wise to seek very warm climates, which may present an added workload to an already stressed heart.

It is not surprising that most injuries and accidents occur in younger age groups who are often involved in more active pursuits. Traumatic deaths such as road traffic accidents do seem to be a major hazard for younger travelers, and more attention should be drawn to ways in which they can avoid hazardous situations. However, in a recent study of motorbike accidents in Bermuda, older travelers were at particular risk of injury, especially those in the 50 to 59 years age group.[58]

Also in the case of older persons, there is a need for judicious consideration of their holiday destination, especially if they have cardiovascular problems. Since, in practice, no preventive measures guarantee safety, adequate health insurance should be obtained before venturing abroad.

2.2 SURVEILLANCE OF TRAVEL-RELATED DISEASE

The surveillance of travel-related disease is no different from the surveillance of any other group of diseases. It has the same key elements: (1) the collection of pertinent data, (2) the orderly consolidation and evaluation of these data, and (3) the prompt dissemination of the information especially to those who can take appropriate action.

COLLECTION OF PERTINENT DATA

This step involves the prompt dispatch of data giving details about travelers who have become ill. Much useful material is sent by microbiologic and other laboratories that report as part of national surveillance programs. This is often the main source of important travel-related diseases such as malaria, dengue fever, dysentery, typhoid, and other enteric diseases. Reference laboratories are especially important in sending detailed information about particular organisms that have been isolated from infected patients.

In many countries, there is a legal requirement for medical practitioners to notify public health authorities about certain infections including the location in which they were acquired. Therefore, these notifiable diseases are pertinent to the surveillance of travel-related diseases. Through the recording of notifiable diseases over many years, trends can be observed.

Information on noninfectious travel-related diseases can also be obtained from a variety of sources. Admission to accident and emergency departments can give a useful indication about traumatic problems affecting travelers (e.g., road traffic accidents). Hospital admissions will give data on the especially serious conditions that involve more complex investigation and treatment.

Data may also be available about travelers who require repatriation because of the severity of their illnesses or injuries, while the extent of travel-related mortality can be determined by an examination of death certificates issued in connection with those who have succumbed abroad.[55] Because illness incurred by travel may result in claims to insurance companies, information from this source may give another valuable insight into the extent of travel-related problems.

Information about special groups of travelers (e.g., package tourists, volunteers, and expatriates) may be sought by conducting prospective surveys designed to obtain specific information about morbidity and mortality associated with travel. Various studies in different countries have been undertaken in recent years to assess the rates of illness in overseas travellers. Examples of these studies are given in Table 2.1–3.

ORDERLY CONSOLIDATION AND EVALUATION OF THESE DATA

The reporting of illness or death in travelers usually involves the recording of entities such as the date of onset, diagnosis (with or without laboratory back-up), location in which illness occurred, and outcome.

Appropriate interpretation and analysis of this information is needed to establish such features as the time, place, and persons involved, as well as the manifestations of the disease. When combined with information about the population from which the sample was drawn, then using this as a denominator, morbidity and mortality rates can be calculated. Properly interpreted surveillance data can give important insights into the cause, risk factors, transmission, seasonal patterns, and control of travel-related disease. Proper analysis is important to avoid the pitfall of associating a disease with events that are not involved with this actual causation.

PROMPT DISSEMINATION OF THE INFORMATION ESPECIALLY TO THOSE WHO CAN TAKE APPROPRIATE ACTION

Data on travel-related disease should not be collected just for their own sake; one of the responsibilities of a travel surveillance unit is to ensure that it does not become a dustbin for heaps of unused information. Unless appropriate and timely feedback of the information is given to its providers and to those who need the information so that effective action can be taken, its quantity and quality will rapidly dwindle.

The outlets for surveillance information on disease risks for travelers are many. Published material appears at frequent and regular intervals in periodicals ranging from the World Health Organization's *Weekly Epidemiological Record* to various national publications. These provide valuable guidance about the current infections prevalent in different countries and should be available to those giving health advice to travelers. Also, information from sending countries about illnesses experienced by travelers who have recently returned from abroad can usefully augment reports received from destination countries. It is important to ensure that data derived from a source outside the country to which the infected traveler has returned are reported back to that country so that appropriate measures can be taken to deal with the problem.

With the upsurge of interest in and availability of rapid information transfer by electronic means, the dissemination of reports about travel-related disease has been greatly facilitated. Disease outbreaks can be notified and updated and the information shared across the world in a matter of minutes via the Internet. Both the input and the output of surveillance data can thus be much more rapid, giving a better chance for effective action to take place.

REFERENCES

1. Christie AB. Infectious diseases: epidemiology and clinical practice. Edinburgh, London, and New York: Churchill Livingstone, 1974.
2. Shrewsbury JFD. The plague of the Philistines and other medico-historical essays. London: Gollancz, 1964.
3. Cossar JH. Influence of travel and disease: an historical perspective. J Travel Med 1994;1:36–39.
4. Dorolle P. Old plagues in the jet age. International aspects of present and future control of communicable disease. BMJJ 1968;4:789–792.
5. Paul H. The control of disease. Edinburgh and London: Churchill Livingstone, 1964.
6. Burney F. Cecilia, Book 4.
7. Steffen R, van der Linde F, Meyer HE. Erkrankungsrisiken bei 10,500 Tropen- und 1300 Nordamerika-Touristen. Schweiz Med Wochenschr 1978;108:1485–1495.
8. Steffen R, Rickenbach M, Willhelm U, et al. Health problems after travel to developing countries. J Infect Dis 1987;156: 84–91.
9. Wenker O. Repatrierungs fluge der REGA 1983. Thesis, University of Zurich.
10. Reid D, Grist NR, Najera RJ. Illness associated with package tours: a combined Spanish-Scottish study. Bull WHO 1978;56: 117–122.
11. Reid D, Dewar RD, Fallon RJ, et al. Infection and travel: the experience of package tourists and other travelers. J Infect 1980;2:356–370.
12. Cossar JH, Reid D, Fallon RJ, et al. A cumulative review of studies on travelers, their experience of illness and the implications of these findings. J Infect 1990;21:27–42.
13. Dewar RD, Cossar HH, Reid D, Grist NR. Illness amongst travelers to Scotland: a pilot study. Health Bull (Edinb) 1983; 41:155–162.
14. Cossar JH, Reid D, Grist NR, et al. Illness associated with travel. Travel Med Int 1985;3:13–18.
15. Peltola H, Kyronseppa H, Holsa P. Trips to the South—a health hazard. Scand J Infect Dis 1983;15:375–381.
16. Cossar JH, Dewar RD, Reid D, Grist NR. Travel and health: illness associated with winter package holidays. J R Coll Gen Prac 1988;33:642–645.
17. DuPont HL, Khan FM. Travellers' diarrhea: epidemiology, microbiology prevention and therapy. J Travel Med 1994;1: 84–93.
18. Steffen R, Lobel HO. Epidemiologic basis for the practice of travel medicine. J Wilderness Med 1995;5:56–66.
19. Steffen R, Kane MA, Shapiro CN, et al. Epidemiology and prevention of hepatitis A in travelers. JAMA 1994;272:885–889.
20. Christenson B. Epidemiological aspects of acute viral hepatitis A in Swedish travelers to endemic areas. Scand J Infect Dis 1985;17:5–10.
21. Gutersohn T, Steffen R, Van Damme P, et al. Hepatitis A infection among air crews: risk of infection and cost-benefit analysis of hepatitis A vaccination. Aviat Space Environ Med 1996;67:153-156.
22. Lange WR, Frame JD. High incidence of viral hepatitis among American missionaries in Africa. Am J Trop Med Hyg 1990; 43:527–533.
23. Steffen R. Risks of hepatitis B for travellers. Vaccine 1990; 8:31–32.
24. Steffen R. Typhoid vaccine for whom? Lancet 1982;1:615–616.
25. Taylor DN, Pollard RA, Blake PA. Typhoid in the United States and the risk to international travelers. J Infect Dis 1983; 148:615–616.
26. Steffen R. Travel medicine—prevention based on epidemiological data. Trans R Soc Trop Med Hyg 1991;85:156–162.
27. Mermin JH, Townes JM, Gerber M, et al. Typhoid fever in the United States, 1985–1994. Arch Intern Med 1998;158: 633–638.
28. Wittlinger F, Steffen R, Watanabe H, Handszuh H. Risk of cholera among Western and Japanese travelers. J Travel Med 1995;2:154–158.
29. Mahon BE, Mintz ED, Green KD, et al. Reported cholera in the United States 1990–94. JAMA 1996;276:307–312.
30. World Health Organization. The 50th anniversary of W.H.O. Wkly Epidemiol Rec 1998;73:145–147.
31. World Health Organization. Cholera in 1997. Wkly Epidemiol Rec 1998;73:201–208.
32. World Health Organization. Measles: progress towards global control and regional elimination, 1990–1998. Wkly Epidemiol Rec 1998;73:389–394.
33. World Health Organization. Performance of acute flaccid paralysis (AFP) surveillance and incidence of poliomyelitis, 1998–1999. Wkly Epidemiol Rec 1999;74:81–84.
34. Centers for Disease Control. Inactivated Japanese encephalitis virus vaccine. Recommendations of the advisory committee on immunization practices (ACIP). MMWR Morb Mortal Wkly Rep 1993;42:1–15.
35. Centers for Disease Control. Update: outbreak of influenza A infection—Alaska and the Yukon Territory, July–Aug, 1998. MMWR Morb Mortal Wkly Rep 1998;47:685–688.
36. Center for Disease Control. Rubella among crew members of commercial cruise ships—Florida, 1997. MMWR Morb Mortal Wkly Rep 1998;46:1247–1250.
37. Jernigan DB, Hofmann J, Cetron M, et al. Outbreak of legionnaires' disease among cruise ship passengers exposed to a contaminated whirlpool spa. Lancet 1996;347:494–499.
38. Bernard KW, Fishbein DB. Pre-exposure rabies prophylaxis for travellers; are the benefits worth the cost? Vaccine 1991;9: 833–836.
39. Phanuphak P, Ubolyam S, Sirivichayakul S. Should travellers in rabies endemic areas receive pre-exposure rabies immunisation? Ann Med Interne (Paris) 1994;145:409–411.
40. Sperizh RO, Morris JH, Lawhashwasdik. Rabies study SEATO. Medical Residence Laboratory, Annual Report, 1996.
41. De Schrijver A, Meheus A. International travel and sexually transmitted diseases. World Health Statistics 1989;42:90–99.
42. Hawkes S, Hart GJ, Johnson AM, et al. Risk behaviour and HIV prevalence in international travellers. AIDS 1994;8:247–252.
43. Stricker M, Steffen RH, Gutzwiler F, et al. Fluchtige Sexuelle Kontakte von Schweizer Touristen in den Tropen. Munch Med Wochenschr 1990;132:175–177.
44. Laga M. Risk of infection and other sexually transmitted diseases for travellers. In: Lobel HO, Steffen R, Kozarsky PE, eds. Travel medicine 2. Proceedings of the Second Conference on International Travel Medicine. Atlanta: International Society of Travel Medicine, 1992:201–203.
45. Arvidson M, Kallings I, Nilsson S, et al. Risky behavior in women with history of casual travel sex. Sex Transm Dis 1997; 24:418–421.

46. Bonneux L, van der Stuyft P, Taelman H, et al. Risk factors for HIV infections among European expatriates in Africa. BMJ 1988;297:581–584.

47. Houweling H, Coutinho RA. HIV infections, needlesticks and sexual behaviour among Dutch expatriates in sub-Saharan Africa. In: Lobel HO, Steffen R, Kozardsky PE, eds. Travel medicine 2. Proceedings of the Second Conference on International Travel Medicine. Atlanta: International Society of Travel Medicine, 1991:204–206.

48. Eng TR, O'Brien R, Bernard KW, et al. HIV-1 & HIV-2 infections among U.S. Peace Corps volunteers returning from West Africa. J Travel Med 1995;2:174–177.

49. Visser LG, Polderman AM, Stuiver PC. Outbreak of schistosomiasis among travelers returning from Mali. West Afr Clin Infect Dis 1995;20:280–285.

50. Jelinek T, Nothdurft HD, Loscher T. Schistosomiasis in travelers and expatriates. J Travel Med 1996;3:160–164.

51. Cetron MS, Chitsulo L, Sullivan JJ, et al. Schistosomiasis in Lake Malawi. Lancet 1996;348:1274–1278.

52. Day JH, Grant AD, Doherty JF, et al. Schistosomiasis in travellers returning from sub-Saharan Africa. BMJ 1996;313:268–269.

53. Cossar JH. Studies on illness associated with travel. Thesis, University of Glasgow, 1987.

54. Prociv P. Deaths of Australian travellers overseas. Med J Aust 1995;163:27–30.

55. Paixao MLT, Dewar RD, Cossar JH, et al. What do Scots die of when abroad? Scott Med J 1991;36:114–116.

56. Jong EC, McMullen R. The travel and tropical medicine manual. Philadelphia: WB Saunders, 1995.

57. Gangarosa EJ, Kendrick MA, Loewenstein MS, et al. Global travel and travellers' health. Aviat Space Environ Med 1980;51:265–270.

58. Carey MJ, Aitken ME. Motorbike injures in Bermuda: a risk for tourists. Ann Emerg Med 1996;28:424–429.

59. Hargarten SW, Baker TD, Guptill K. Overseas fatalities of United States citizen travellers: an analysis of deaths related to international travellers. Ann Emerg Med 1991;20:622–626.

60. Sniezek JE, Smith SM. Injury mortality among non-US residents in the United States 1979–1984. Int J Epidemiol 1991;19:225–229.

61. Guptill KS, Hargarten SW, Baker TD. American travel deaths in Mexico: causes and prevention strategies. West J Med 1991;154:169–171.

62. Odero W, Garner P, Zwi A. Road traffic injuries in developing countries: a comprehensive review of epidemiologic studies. Trop Med Int Health 1997;2:445–460.

Chapter 3

TRAVEL INDUSTRY AND MEDICAL PROFESSIONALS

ARTHUR L. SCHIFF

INTRODUCTION

This chapter will describe the commercial travel industry as it exists in the late 1990s and suggest ideal health advice interactions between the traveler, various elements of the travel industry, and the medical profession, including "family" physicians and operators of travel medicine clinics. The chapter will also comment on the role assumed by international organizations and by national governments in providing health advice to travelers, and will summarize the legal responsibilities borne by travel industry and medical professionals as required in various parts of the world.

3.1 RESPONSIBILITIES AND IDEAL INTERACTION

TRAVELER/TRAVEL INDUSTRY

DESCRIPTION

The commercial travel industry has developed enormously throughout the world in the 40 plus years since the advent of the modern passenger jet aircraft. Business and vacation travelers now number many millions annually, spending $4 trillion per year and creating jobs for one in nine workers throughout the world.

A global industry of this size obviously has had to develop methods of putting travelers together with companies providing travel services in cities and countries throughout the world. Indeed, a highly integrated, interconnected travel industry has developed.

The industry consists of three basic levels or components: suppliers of travel services, tour operators, and retail travel agents. Suppliers include air carriers, cruise lines and other providers of transportation, hotel/motel companies, vacation resorts, car rental companies, restaurants, and other entities actually responsible for delivering transportation and accommodations to the traveling public.

Tour operators, sometimes known as wholesalers, group operators, or charter operators, often purchase (or are allocated) blocks of travel services from travel suppliers and package them together as "package tours." The tours, as well as the services offered directly by suppliers, are marketed and sold through retail travel agents.

Retail travel agents are generally independent companies promoting and selling the tours and services offered by suppliers, tour operators, wholesalers, and thousands of others providing travel services to the traveling public. Retail agents earn their compensation either through commissions paid by suppliers and tour operators or, increasingly, by service charges paid by consumers who purchase travel services through the retail agents.

Since suppliers, tour operators, and retail travel agents all communicate with the traveling public, each can be an important source of health advice and precaution.

PRETRAVEL HEALTH ADVICE BY TRAVEL PROFESSIONALS*

Almost all health problems related to travel are preventable. To a large extent, however, travelers are often unaware of the health risks and/or lack an understanding

---

*Material in this section and in the section below dealing with the interaction between the family physician, the travel medicine specialist, and the travel clinic relies heavily on a report prepared in April 1993 by the Subcommittee on Minimum Standards for Health Advice of the Travel Industry and Public Education Committee (TIPEC) of the International Society of Travel Medicine and on consensus statements on standards for travel health advice adopted in Europe (1994) and North America (1996) by travel health practitioners and government experts brought together by the International Society of Travel Medicine.

of the measures necessary to avoid them. Travel professionals with whom travelers interact in the travel planning stage thus have a significant opportunity to provide information and advice necessary to achieve prevention.

Retail Travel Agents Since their income is usually dependent on the successful sale of travel, agents have a commercial interest in "completing the deal" and are often perceived as being reluctant to pass on discouraging health information. Agents respond that they rely on repeat business, which demands that they show concern for the client's overall interests, and they point out further that they are not medically qualified and therefore cannot be expected to give specific medical advice.

Nevertheless, at a minimum, retailers should reasonably be expected to provide the following:

1. *Vaccination certificates*. Agents should provide their clients with information about vaccinations that are a legal condition of entering a country. They should be absolutely clear that these requirements exist not for the protection of their clients but as a protective measure for the population of the receiving countries.

2. *Vaccination recommendations*. Agents should, where possible, state that additional vaccinations may be strongly advised for a particular destination and identify to the traveler a written or telephone source of further advice that would apply to the specifics of their trip.

   Examples may be given of the diseases for which vaccinations may be recommended, but decisions such as whether a particular vaccine is or is not contraindicated are medical matters best left to medical professionals. Where a country's health department has made recommendations, these should be followed.

3. *Malaria prevention*. Any travel agent booking a ticket to a malarial country or region as a transit or final destination should inform the traveler that risk exists and that tablets and precautions to reduce insect bites may be necessary. Information about a source that can offer further advice should be provided. Where there is a national channel for malaria information (e.g., the Centers for Disease Control [CDC] hotline in the U.S. or the Malaria Reference Laboratory in the U.K.), this information should be provided. Travel agents should not be expected to provide details regarding geographic areas of drug resistance but should be expected to mention that tablets, on their own, may be an insufficient form of prevention.

4. *Additional health advice*. Retail agents cannot reasonably be expected to offer specific medical advice. However, they should not minimize health risks and should be expected to state that "additional health precautions may be advisable," particularly regarding adjustment to local climate conditions and the prevention of AIDS. Agents should be able to identify one or more sources of information: government health department leaflets, books, telephone hotlines, travel clinics, or general practitioners. Retail agents

should be clear that it is the quality of pretravel advice, rather than any vaccinations or tablets that a traveler takes, that will have the greatest effect on the outcome of the trip as far as health is concerned.

Tour Operators Tour operators should identify in their brochures possible health risks by destination and should encourage travelers to obtain specific prevention advice at an early stage. Tour operators should ensure that retail agents who sell their travel arrangements adhere to the recommendations above and that they make travelers aware of any specific health risks that apply to the particular destinations and types of trips being sold.

Where inclusive tours are offered with meals and where accommodation and travel are sold as a package, tour operators should establish a framework for monitoring illness, accident, and injury suffered by those to whom they provide services and make this information available to government agencies and medical professionals with a legitimate interest. Tour operators should act on the results of the information they obtain and make the results available to future clients and to suppliers whose services they use so that appropriate additional precautions can be taken (e.g., to hotels with a high experience of diarrhea). Moreover, they should also take steps to improve or correct tourist facilities for which they are responsible or are able to influence, such as food hygiene standards in hotels that they commonly use. Finally, tour operators should identify for clients the general quality of the medical environment at their destinations and make known the possibility of contracting for medical repatriation through travel insurance.

Airlines, Other Common Carriers, and Carrier Staff Airlines, like other sellers of travel, should provide information about vaccinations that are a legal condition of entry to the destination country. Moreover, airlines should also provide health education information for consultation in-flight, either by leaflet or as an in-flight video. Airline staff should notify travelers when their itinerary includes a malarial area. This should be done both at time of booking and either at check-in or as an in-flight announcement prior to landing. The possible need for tablets and/or antimosquito measures should be mentioned.

PHYSICIANS/TRAVEL CLINICS

DESCRIPTION

Even as the travel industry has experienced significant growth during the latter part of the 20th century, the number of and interest in travel clinics in North America, Europe, Asia, and elsewhere have grown even more dramatically.

IDEAL INTERACTION BETWEEN "FAMILY PHYSICIAN," TRAVEL MEDICINE SPECIALIST, AND TRAVEL CLINIC

General practitioners—family doctors—are in a unique position to be aware of any adverse factors in a traveler's medical history that might make special precautions necessary, and they should take appropriate action even if it means discouraging a particular trip. Most importantly, family physicians should be aware that healthy travel is not simply a matter of providing vaccinations and tablets but also that traveler education is generally the most important element of protection. They should devote part of their consultation to education or at least to identifying for the traveler sources of travel health information such as leaflets, books, telephone and/or computer information services, and other educational materials. If family physicians are not prepared to provide such educational referrals, they should refer the patient to a travel clinic or elsewhere.

For their part, travel medicine specialists and travel clinicians should not hesitate to communicate with the traveler's own general practitioner regarding a specific course of treatment that seems indicated by a particular destination.

TRAVELERS/GOVERNMENTS

DESCRIPTION/IDEAL ROLE

Governments in countries all over the world, to a greater or lesser degree, currently assume a number of basic responsibilities for promoting safe health conditions for their own citizens and for travelers. They build roads that are safe to drive on, build or supervise the establishment of sanitation and sewerage systems, ensure the cleanliness of drinking water, protect against beach pollution, operate or supervise a public or private hospital system, and take responsibility for disease surveillance and control and for notification of international organizations and other nations.

Governments of countries from which travelers leave have the further obligation to disseminate accurate and timely travel health precautions and health information. Clearly, developed countries do a more comprehensive job in this area.

International organizations including the World Health Organization, the CDC, and others also play a role in protecting the traveler. They monitor health conditions around the world, evaluate and verify what is reported, disseminate needed information, and provide travel health advice and warnings in written, telephonic, and computerized formats.

3.2 LEGAL ASPECTS OF TRAVEL HEALTH

LEGAL REQUIREMENTS FOR PROVIDING PRETRAVEL HEALTH INFORMATION TO TRAVELERS

As might be anticipated, the governments of the world have expressed varying degrees of concern regarding the provision of pretravel health information to citizens about to travel.

EUROPEAN COMMUNITY CODE REQUIREMENTS

By far the most specific travel health requirements are those of the nations of the European Community (E.C.). On June 13, 1990, the European Community Council adopted a directive on package travel, package holidays, and package tours (90/314/EEC). The directive, which required that E.C. countries adopt their own laws implementing the directive's policies by December 31, 1992, established the following:

2. "When a [tour] brochure is made available to the consumer, it shall indicate...adequate information concerning:

(e) general information on passport and visa requirements for nationals of the Member State... and health formalities required for the journey and the stay" (Art. 3).

1(a) "The organizer and/or the retailer shall provide the consumer...with information of the health formalities required for the journey and the stay" (Art. 4).

For the first time, E.C. governments would now require that travelers, at least those purchasing package tours, be informed of health measures required for their travel.

The E.C. countries have, by now, adopted implementing national laws. In Ireland, for example, the Package Holidays and Travel Trade Act (effective October 1, 1995) implemented the 1990 EU Package Holiday Directive. Section 10 provides that any consumer tour brochure must contain:

"(vi) health formalities for both the journey and the stay...."

Failure by a tour organizer or travel agent to include the required information in the brochure can make the organizer or retail agent guilty of an "offense."[1]

Similarly, in the United Kingdom, the Package Travel Regulations of 1992 require that any tour brochure must contain "information about health formalities required for the journey and the stay" (Regulation 7[2][b]). In France, the law of July 13, 1992, and the decree of June 15, 1994, revised the responsibilities of travel agents to include "...[informing] the consumer, in writing and before signing the contract, of the administrative and medical formalities necessary to cross borders..."

French enforcement decrees will be necessary before it is entirely clear what level of disclosure is required of French travel agents, but some French companies are already assuming that "medical formalities for crossing borders" will include the following:

1. health measures necessary for incident-free travel and stay (e.g., obligatory and advisable vaccinations) and information about areas with a risk for malaria,
2. health information of a general nature that is useful for incident-free travel and stays, and
3. address and telephone number of appropriate medical information center.

E.C. regulations regarding pretravel health advice are far ahead of those promulgated elsewhere in the world. Nevertheless, it remains unclear how aggressively they will be interpreted and enforced in the years ahead. Of course, it must be remembered that they apply only to E.C. consumers purchasing package tours.

U.S. STATUTORY AND COMMON LAW REQUIREMENTS

In the United States, and in many other parts of the world, legal requirements are a mixture of laws enacted by legislative bodies at various levels (federal, state, county, city, etc.), regulations adopted by administrative bodies to implement and clarify laws, judicial decisions by state and federal courts determining a law's constitutionality, and interpreting the laws as they apply to specific fact situations.

To date, neither the U.S. Congress nor the legislature of any U.S. state has enacted a law requiring the provision of any specific travel health advice to U.S. travelers. Nevertheless, expanding concepts of "negligence" jurisprudence may already provide for monetary liability for a seller of travel that fails to provide the pretravel health guidance expected of the "reasonably prudent" tour operator or retail agent.

Under what circumstances would the failure to provide travel health guidance result in legal liability for a U.S. travel seller? Each specific set of circumstances will require the standard of care for those circumstances that one would expect of the average, careful seller of travel. For example, liability might be found where the CDC was advising the travel trade of an outbreak of malaria in a country in South America and a retail agent sold a vacation package to that country without at least advising of

the outbreak and the need to get further information about necessary precautions.

It will be recognized, therefore, that to the extent that health information becomes increasingly available to the travel trade through computer reservation systems, the Internet, and otherwise in countries that apply "common law" principles (e.g., negligence concepts) to determine liability, travel sellers will need to become increasingly systematic in providing pretravel health advice to their customers.

LEGAL REQUIREMENTS ELSEWHERE

With some exceptions, the nations of the world have chosen to be governed by concepts of civil law, common law, or some combination thereof.

In those countries in which the legal regime stems from the Anglo-American system, developing concepts of negligence will govern liability, with judges in each nation putting their own national "spin" on the standards of health advice required of travel sellers.

In civil law countries, taking their legal standard from Europe, national legislatures can increasingly be expected to establish minimum statutory requirements like those set forth in the E.C.'s Directive on Package Travel for pretravel health advice.

PENALTIES FOR VIOLATION

In some E.C. nations, regulations make a knowing failure to include accurate health advice in brochures a potential criminal offense, although it remains to be seen how aggressively these rules will be enforced. Nevertheless, failure to advise can subject the travel industry violator in Europe or North America to heavy civil financial damages should liability be found and severe injury or death result. Money damages in each case will depend on the facts and circumstances involved, the severity of injury and/or loss of property, and the emotional reaction of judge or jury.

CONFLICTING INCENTIVES FOR TRAVEL PROFESSIONALS IN PROVIDING PRETRAVEL HEALTH ADVICE

It is often suggested that sellers of travel believe that providing health warnings to prospective travelers will serve to discourage the purchase of discretionary vacation travel. Although no determinative studies have been made, human experience suggests that people warned of the possibility of disease at a vacation destination are likely to decide not to travel there. Human experience likewise suggests, however, that vacation planners, warned of health risks at one destination, will, rather than cancel vacation plans altogether, simply choose another destination. That is the experience reported by most professional retail agents. Although suppliers of travel services (hotels, car rental companies, etc.) in an infected city or country and tour operators who have organized tours to such regions might well have a financial incentive to remain silent in the face of negative health information at their travel destination, retail agents who offer vacation products all over the world can simply suggest a noninfected alternative.

POTENTIAL LEGAL LIABILITY FOR FAILING TO PROVIDE REQUIRED HEALTH ADVICE

Just as economic pressure to sell a particular travel service may create some incentive for some sellers of travel to remain silent regarding health precautions, it may be presumed that increasingly clear legal standards requiring pretravel health advice and carrying the potential for monetary damages will serve as an effective counter-incentive. Such balancing of risks and rewards by sellers in the marketplace is certainly to be expected, at least in the capitalist world, and the creation of incentives by governments to encourage desirable conduct by business people (e.g., pretravel health precautions) is to be encouraged.

POTENTIAL LIABILITY FOR PROVIDING INCORRECT ADVICE

Sellers of travel are not medical professionals and are not expected to advise travelers with regard to specific treatments required in specific medical circumstances. Indeed, travel professionals expose themselves to potentially severe liability by providing medical advice that proves to be wrong.

Thus, the challenge for the travel professional is to recognize the circumstances in which pretravel health advice and precautions are required and to provide guidance that will raise the appropriate medical questions for the traveler and his general practitioner or travel medicine specialist, while not going beyond his/her area of expertise and into the realm of making specific medical recommendations. For most travel professionals, with neither the medical training nor the time to become knowledgeable regarding medical advice, adopting practices that avoid the risks of liability on either side will be challenging but, ultimately, not difficult.

PRETRAVEL HEALTH ADVICE AS A "VALUE ADDED" IN TRAVEL MARKETING

Although the growth of the worldwide travel industry shows every indication of making tourism the largest industry in the world by the year 2000, it has become clear that government deregulation in the U.S., Europe, and elsewhere and the resulting growth in competition in the marketplace have forced travel companies at every level to re-engineer and to reduce costs in order to regain and retain profitability. Indeed, after years of serious losses in the hundreds of millions of dollars, since February 1995 the major U.S. carriers have imposed cuts and caps on the commissions they pay to retail agents on individual air tickets, with the effect that commission income for North American agents and others has dropped perhaps as much as 40%.

Some retailers immediately began charging fees to their clients for providing specialized (and, in some cases, not so specialized) services, and all began looking for new ways to separate themselves from their competition.

In such an environment, it becomes clear that knowledgeable retailers and tour operators, recognizing their increasing legal obligation to provide at least the minimum pretravel health precautions, can turn the obligation into a value added for their clients by marketing their companies as proficient in the basics of travel health. Such proficiency would begin with knowledge of necessary immunizations but would also include general advice on disease prevention (particularly malaria), sensitivity to the travel needs of clients with respiratory and coronary conditions, and advice to clients on ways of protecting themselves from sexually transmitted diseases and on changing health risks around the world. Most importantly, travel health expertise would assume the ability to refer travelers to travel health clinics and other appropriate health authorities.

In a world increasingly health conscious, it can be assumed that many travelers will be prepared to reward travel industry professionals who, in addition to choosing just the right hotel on just the right island, can help them steer clear of travel health risks.

REFERENCE

1. Yaqub B. European travel law. New York: John Wiley & Sons, 1997.

Chapter 4

PHILOSOPHICAL AND ETHICAL CONSIDERATIONS

PIERRE J. PLOURDE AND PAT MURPHY

INTRODUCTION

Tourism is undoubtedly one of the fastest-growing industries at the end of the 20th century. It is often used as a reliable indicator of economic growth in both developed and developing countries. With other aspects of world economies struggling, tourism is seen by many nations as a quick and easy solution to combating economic difficulties. Increasingly, countries are choosing to develop and promote their natural resources to attract more tourists in what has become a very competitive market. This has posed new philosophical and ethical challenges to the travel and tourism industry, the traveler, prospective destination host cultures, and travel health professionals. Meeting in Manila on May 22, 1997, under the auspices of the World Tourism Organization, a United Nations agency, world tourism leaders made a commitment to work toward the formulation and adoption of a "Global Code of Ethics for Tourism" by the year 2000. It will focus on both the responsibility of host nations and communities and the traveling individual, recognizing the need to address global ethics in respect of the continuous and new challenges faced by global tourism development. This chapter seeks to raise philosophical and ethical issues with respect to travel, tourism, and travel medicine from the perspective of the travel industry, the traveler, the host culture, and the health care professional.

TRAVEL INDUSTRY

Ethical tensions are inherent to the nature of any industry that balances the "good of the market" versus the "good of the people." According to the World Travel and Tourism Council, travel and tourism has overtaken the auto, steel, electronics, and agricultural industries and is now regarded as one of the largest global industries.[1] With more than 100 million people in the tourism industry serving an annual tourist population of around half a billion, this enterprise generates an estimated annual economic force of U.S.$2–3.5 trillion.[2,3] The ethical tension arises from the fact that the tourism industry has and continues to function without a code of ethics, although many of the problems faced by the tourism industry are ethical in nature,[4] including destruction of the environment, pollution, depletion of natural resources, economic imperialism, and sexual exploitation. The lack of ethical standards is understandable when the immensity and diversity of the industry are taken into consideration. Tourism has been defined as "the industry of the holiday companies, travel agents, transport firms, building companies, caravan manufacturers, cable railway operators, ski manufacturers, souvenir sellers, the car industry, banks, insurance companies...an industry with its own laws, its own legitimacy."[5] Each sector of the tourism industry is competing for a greater share of the market, using whatever marketing methods work to reach target economic goals, where market precepts, not ethics, predominate.

Responding to these ethical tensions, there has been a recent recognition of the need to consider the concept of sustainable tourism if the economic gains of the tourism industry are to continue being realized. Sustainable tourism is defined as the development of global tourism capacity and the quality of its products without adversely affecting the environment that maintains and nurtures the industry.[6] Within this framework has emerged a branch of tourism known as ecotourism, now comprising up to 10% of the tourism industry.[7] Ecotourism is defined as "responsible travel to natural areas which conserves the environment and improves the welfare of local people."[8] According to the Canadian Environmental Advisory Council, ecotourism should promote positive environmental ethics, be biocentric rather than homocentric in philosophy, and should benefit the wildlife and the environment socially, economically, scientifically, managerially, and politically.[9] The ethic of ecotourism has generated considerable interest in the travel industry, partly because of increasing consumer interest and economic impact but also due to increasing concern with the conservation and sustainable development of tourism's most valuable resource, the natural environment, which primarily attracts tourists. However, the popularity of ecotourism has also given rise to a plethora of "ecotourism" companies that do not meet the standards of minimal environmental impact, maximal benefits for tourist areas, and conservation ethics.[10] Currently, although proposals have been made to monitor the level of sustainable development and conservation practiced by the tourism industry,[11–13] there still exists no regulatory body or mechanism with which to evaluate the impacts of tourism.

TRAVELER

Until recently, the subject of ethics was rarely found in tourism literature. Largely as a result of a growing concern over alleged irresponsible practices by tourists, the tourist industry, and governments, myriads of codes of ethics have been developed primarily aimed at tourists and secondarily to the tourist industry.[14] These codes generally address ethical principles focusing on a sense of responsibility rather than precise conduct, an exhortation and moral suasion rather than an enforceable set of rules (Table 4–1). According to Dean, "codes are meant to translate the more formal philosophical theories of ethics into a set of guidelines that can be applied to the day to day decision making."[15] Part of the tourist's responsibility when entering a foreign culture is to learn from and have respect for the host culture and customs. Travelers are usually primarily concerned with the risks that travel will expose them to, such as theft, assault, accidental trauma, and infection. Rarely does the idea that the traveler poses a potential risk or danger to the host population and their environment receive much consideration. Discussion of such hazards including the spread of infection from tourists to local indigent populations, introduction of pollution by tourists, increased use of valuable resources by tourists including water and electricity, increased costs of living and inflation of land values resulting from tourists' demands, conflicts created by the display of leisure and prosperity amid the pervasive poverty of many receiving host cultures, sexual exploitation by tourists of local populations, and lack of economic opportunities by local populations who generally do not enjoy ownership in the tourism industry are rarely part of pretravel discussions. Tourists are mostly interested in getting a break from the stresses of (usually Western) society and are not interested in discussing or being reminded of such challenging ethical issues. Nevertheless, a growing resentment toward tourists in some receiving host cultures[16] and the magnitude of tourism-related disease transmission demonstrated by infectious agents with prolonged infectious periods such as HIV[17] necessitate that ethical behaviors of the traveler be appropriately addressed. The problem rests in how and by whom this issue should be addressed. Strict rules or codes of conduct for travelers will not be easily imposed or enforceable and therefore may not ultimately be useful. However, those disseminating pretravel advice, including travel medicine specialists, travel agents, and tourism companies, will need to consider what constitutes adequate education and information concerning travel ethics, that travelers may be equipped not only with appropriate disease prevention messages but also with an ethic that will ensure preservation of the host culture and its environment, ultimate survival of the tourism industry, and a safer and more rewarding experience for all travelers.

Table 4–1. **CODE OF ETHICS FOR TOURISTS**[*]

1. Travel in a spirit of humility and with a genuine desire to learn more about the people of your host country. Be sensitively aware of the feelings of other people, thus preventing what might be offensive behavior on your part. This applies very much to photography.

2. Cultivate the habit of listening and observing, rather than merely hearing and seeing.

3. Realize that often the people in the country you visit have time concepts and thought patterns different from your own. This does not make them inferior, only different.

4. Instead of looking for the "beach paradise," discover the enrichment of seeing a different way of life, through other eyes.

5. Acquaint yourself with local customs. What is courteous in one country may be quite the reverse in another—people will be happy to help you.

6. Instead of the Western practice of "knowing all the answers," cultivate the habit of asking questions.

7. Remember that you are only one of thousands of tourists visiting this country and do not expect special privileges.

8. If you really want your experience to be a "home away from home," it is foolish to waste money on traveling.

9. When you are shopping, remember that the "bargain" you obtained was possible only because of the low wages paid to the maker.

10. Do not make promises to people in your host country unless you can carry them through.

11. Spend time reflecting on your daily experience in an attempt to deepen your understanding. It has been said that "what enriches you may rob and violate others."

[*]Issued by the Ecumenical Coalition on Third World Tourism, Bangkok, Thailand.

HOST CULTURE

The roots of global opposition to tourism can be traced back to a conference, convened once again in Manila (1980), by religious leaders from developing countries who were concerned about the negative impact of tourism on their hosting cultures. Out of this gathering came the bold statement, known as the "Manila statement," asserting that "tourism does more harm than good to people and to societies of the Third World." Subsequently, the Ecumenical Coalition on Third World Tourism was instituted and has since become a foremost international organization advocating for responsible tourism (see Table 4–1).

The benefits of tourism to host cultures are often listed as primarily economic including generation of foreign exchange, employment creation, an added source of income for host government through taxation of tourists, and improvement of local economic structures. Other indirect benefits also include improved roads, availability of electricity, access to hospitals, improved water and sewage systems, and better health. Are these benefits, in fact, realized, and what tourism-related risks are host cultures subject to? Although few systematic studies can be found in the literature to answer these questions, it is important to briefly consider these two issues.

First, are the proposed benefits of tourism realized by host cultures? Although there are numerous potential economic benefits of tourism for host cultures, current evidence suggests that these benefits are not realized. The majority of revenues generated by tourism in the developing world are repatriated by transnational corporations in developed countries. This "tourism industry leakage," as it is referred to, largely results from Western ownership of many hotels, resorts, restaurants, travel agencies, airlines, and car rental agencies used by tourists in developing countries.[18] In addition, many of the commodities used by the tourism industry sector in developing countries, including building supplies, construction equipment, food, and beverages, are also imported. Despite these leakages, tourism may still benefit local cultures through employment generation. However, this potential benefit has also been questioned.[18] Since tourists visiting developing countries have stronger currencies, and subsequently greater purchasing power, local inflation soars and local currencies are devalued. Consequently, local populations employed by the tourism sector may, in reality, receive grossly inadequate salaries for the more menial jobs that they are often assigned.[19] More financially lucrative managerial, financial administrative, and public relations opportunities are reserved for foreigners.[20] Finally, the added foreign exchange generated through taxation of tourists by developing country governments is largely used to service huge debts owed to developing country financial institutions. Therefore, the economic benefits of tourism to local host cultures may be overstated.

Second, are the indirect benefits of tourism realized by host indigenous peoples? Improved transportation, electricity, water, and sewage systems are often mentioned as an indirect benefit of the tourism industry. However, tourists consume disproportionately more water, food, and electricity than local populations, resulting in reduced availability of these resources to local populations.[19] Evidence also suggests that the health of local populations may be worsened by the influx of tourists.[20,21] As mentioned, tourism may have contributed to the introduction and spread of HIV in at least one instance.[17] It is unlikely that tourist revenues are used to improve the health status of local populations.

In addition to unrealized potential benefits, what other tourism-related risks are host cultures subject to? The environmental costs of tourism such as disruption and destruction of ecosystems, pollution, land erosion, depletion of natural resources (food, water, land, fossil fuels), and waste created by disposables have been well documented.[20,22] The social costs of tourism are not so clearly linked to the tourism industry. The loss of cultural traditions and local languages and the increase in problems such as burglary, robbery, prostitution, gambling, and violent crimes have all been attributed to tourism.[23–25] Increases of drug and alcohol abuse with subsequent increases in sexually transmitted diseases are clearly linked to tourism in the developing world.[26] Local peoples are also ultimately denied access to those natural resources that have attracted the tourist in the first place.[27] For tourism to be sustainable in the long term, the benefits to local host cultures will need to outweigh these significant risks.

TRAVEL HEALTH PROFESSIONALS

Ethical tensions aside, an inevitable consequence of a thriving global tourist sector is an increasing recognition of travel medicine as a unique branch of medicine requiring that its practitioners attain a wide breadth of knowledge exceeding the content of most undergraduate medical education curricula. Traditional undergraduate medical education focuses on local disease epidemiology, teaching future physicians content relevant to the practice of medicine within national borders. Specialists in travel medicine must also develop and maintain a global awareness of emerging infectious diseases and antibiotic-resistance patterns, up-to-date knowledge of disease outbreaks, and knowledge of global climatic, ecologic, and even political changes. As travel medicine is not recognized as a separate specialty by colleges of physicians or boards of medicine, standards for its practice do not currently exist. The issue of certification is further complicated by the fact that travel medicine professionals constitute a wide variety of practitioners including physicians, nurses, pharmacists, hygienists, social psychologists, and public health and other allied health personnel primarily responsible for the dissemination of pretravel health advice. An ideal continuum of care model should also provide access to post-travel consultation should it be necessary for the returned traveler. Post-travel assessment is necessarily more specialized as it usually requires input from physicians, with access to specialized travel clinics often restricted to urban academic health institutions. Post-travel care is the subject of textbooks of tropical medicine and is governed by traditional health care provider-patient interactions. However, the interaction between provider and client in a pretravel assessment scenario is somewhat different and may be governed by different precepts.

The relationship between health care professional and traveler challenges both traditional and current understandings of the "therapeutic relationship." This is significant in that how one understands this relationship will largely determine what one takes to be the professional's obligations, the perceptions of the client's role, and the goals of the professional-client interaction.[28] For example, within what is commonly referred to as the *paternalistic* model, the clinician assumes the role of the patient's guardian, identifying what is best for the individual. The patient's role is limited to simply accepting or rejecting the clinician's determination. Within an *informative* model of the therapeutic relationship, the clinician's role is that of the "technical expert." Absent any reference to what the clinician understands to be in the patient's best interest, the patient's values alone direct what will transpire. Similarly, within the *interpretive* model, the clinician's role is to provide the patient with information and the risks/benefits of possible interventions. Further to this, however, the clinician acts as a counselor to the patient, attempting to help the patient identify what he/she sees as most important in any given situation. Finally, within the *deliberative* model, the clinician acts as a teacher, informing the patient about possible courses of action, and goes the next step of recommending why one course of action might be preferable to others that are equally possible.

When the traveler presents to a health care professional for pretravel advice, the traveler does not consider himself/herself a patient per se but a healthy client seeking information. Hence, the informative, interpretive, or deliberative model may be more appropriate to this interaction. The information shared, recommendations given, and decisions taken within the context of that relationship end in a person. Regardless of whether the traveler's status changes to that of "patient" during or post-travel, the fact that a relationship has been established between health care professional and traveler has ethical significance in itself. Although different from what we might typically understand as "therapeutic," the health care professional-traveler relationship is a relationship of trust and subject to the same obligations and duties.

What pretravel advice should fall within the responsibility of the health care professional? Are pretravel clinics obliged to educate the traveler with respect to ethical patterns of behavior and cross-cultural interactions, as well as disease-preventing behaviors? Should pretravel advice be a prerequisite for travel to certain destinations? In reality, pretravel health advice is sought by less than half of travelers journeying from a developed to a developing country.[29] When it is obtained, travelers primarily seek advice from previous travelers, travel agents, tour groups, or embassies/consulates of host countries, often receiving inaccurate information.[30–33] Unfortunately, travelers receiving pretravel advice from private physicians also often do not receive appropriate information.[34,35] In North America, the most accurate pretravel health information is received from public health nurses specifically trained in and hired for their expertise in preventive medicine education.[34] However, even within these specialized settings, inaccurate pretravel advice on immunizations and antimalarials has been observed in more than one-quarter of travel clinics.[34] It is, therefore, apparent that, regardless of the source, it is difficult for travelers to obtain accurate and up-to-date pretravel information. With respect to disease prevention messages, there is clearly a need to improve the education of health care professionals. This may be accomplished by including travel medicine in health sciences curricula, improving and increasing continuing medical education programs for travel health advisors, and better standardization of recommendations. With respect to ethical travel messages, more attention will need to be given to appropriate sources and content of ethical recommendations.

CONCLUSION

Tourism will continue to be a global growth industry. Comprehensive pretravel assessment goes far beyond personal health risks to the individual traveler. Should the ethical aspects of travel and tourism fall within the scope of the travel medicine specialist? What should be the role of the tourism industry, coming under increasing scrutiny by societies? Tourism that markets and sells to the tourist as the primary target population of interest, ignoring envi-

ronmental and sociocultural risks to host cultures, may reach short-term profit goals but will ultimately not be sustainable. Global codes of ethics for tourists and the tourist industry will only be effective to the extent that travel health professionals increase their awareness of current ethical issues concerning tourism and subsequently educate the tourist industry and the potential traveler.

REFERENCES

1. World Travel and Tourism Council. The WTTC report: travel and tourism in the world economy. Brussels, 1992.
2. Whitney DL. Ethics in the hospitality industry: an overview. In: Hall SSJ, ed. Ethics in hospitality management: a book of readings. East Lansing, MI: Educational Institute of the American Hotel & Motel Association, 1992.
3. Exploring tourism [editorial]. The Nation 1997;265:3.
4. Payne D, Dimanche F. Towards a code of conduct for the tourism industry: an ethics model. J Business Ethics 1996;15:997–1007.
5. Krippendorf J. Towards new tourism policies. In: Medlick S, ed. Managing tourism. Oxford: Butterworth-Heinemann, 1991:309.
6. Hawkes S, Williams P. The greening of tourism—from principles to practice, GLOBE'92 Tourism Stream: case book of best practice in sustainable tourism. Sustainable Tourism, Industry, Science and Technology, Canada and the Centre of Tourism Policy and Research, Simon Fraser University, British Columbia, 1993.
7. Frank P, Bowerman J. Can ecotourism save the planet? Conde Nast 1994;Dec:134–137.
8. Western D. Defining ecotourism. In: Lindberg K, Hawkins DE, eds. Ecotourism: a guide for planners and managers. North Bennington, VT: The Ecotourism Society, 1993:7–11.
9. Canadian Environmental Advisory Council. A protected areas vision for Canada. Cat. No. EN 92-14/1991E. Ottawa: Minister of Supply and Services Canada, 1991.
10. Arlen C. Ecotour, hold the eco: polluting rivers and bagging wildlife may be on the agenda. U.S. News & World Report 1995;May 29:61–63.
11. Hiller H. Environmental bodies edge closer to green ratings for travel. The Ecotourism Society Newsletter 1991;(Summer):1.
12. Holland R. Rating and recommending ecotourism enterprises [abstract]. Presented at First World Congress on Tourism and the Environment (Belize City), Belize, April 1992.
13. Shores JN. The challenge of ecotourism: a call for higher standards [abstract]. Presented at Fourth World Congress on National Parks and Protected Areas (Caracas), Venezuela, February 1992.
14. Malloy DC, Fennell DA. Codes of ethics and tourism: an exploratory content analysis. Tourism Management 1998;19:453–461.
15. Dean PJ. Making codes of ethics "real." J Business Ethics 1991;10:99–110.
16. Chandrapurkar J. Tourists' haven, locals' hellhole. Herald (Calangute, Goa) 1997;(July 18).
17. Figueroa JP, Brathwaite A, Ward E, et al. The HIV/AIDS epidemic in Jamaica. AIDS 1995;9:761–768.
18. Hundt A. Impact of tourism development on the economy and health of Third World nations. J Travel Med 1996;3:107–112.
19. Ascher F. Tourism: transnational corporations and cultural identities. Paris: UNESCO, 1985.
20. Stonich S, Sorensen JH, Hundt A. Ethnicity, class, and gender in tourism development: the case of the Bay Islands, Honduras. J Sustainable Tourism 1995;3:1–28.

21. Bezruchka S. Tourism and the health of local populations [editorial]. Wilderness and Environmental Medicine 1997;8:73–74.

22. Green H, Hunter C. The environmental impact assessment of tourism development. In: Johnson P, Thomas B, eds. Perspectives on tourism policy. London: Mansell, 1992:29–48.

23. Mathieson A, Wall G. Tourism: economic, physical and social impacts. New York: Longman, 1982.

24. Harrison D, ed. Tourism and the less developed countries. New York: Halstead Press, 1992.

25. Hitchcock M, King VT, Parnwell MJG, eds. Tourism in South-East Asia. New York: Routledge, 1993.

26. Hobson JSP, Dietrich UC. Tourism, health and quality of life: challenging the responsibility of using the traditional tenets of sun, sea, sand, and sex in tourism marketing. Journal of Travel and Tourism Marketing 1994;3(4):21–38.

27. McKee DL, Tisdell C. Developmental issues in small island economies. New York: Praeger, 1990.

28. Emanuel EJ, Emanuel LL. Four models of the physician-patient relationship. JAMA 1992;267:2221–2226.

29. Lobel HO, Campbell CC, Pappaioanou M, Huong AY. Use of prophylaxis for malaria by American travelers to Africa and Haiti. JAMA 1987;257:2626–2627.

30. Centers for Disease Control. Imported malaria among travelers—United States. MMWR Morb Mortal Wkly Rep1984;33: 388–390.

31. Demeter SJ. An evaluation of sources of information on health and travel. Can J Public Health 1989;80:20–22.

32. Nettleman MD, Wenzel AH. Health advice for travelers from embassies and consulates [letter]. N Engl J Med 1990;322:136.

33. Sawyer LJ, Keystone JS. Travel advice from embassies and consulates of developing countries. Can Med Assoc J 1987; 136:693.

34. Keystone JS, Dismukes R, Sawyer L, Kozarsky PE. Inadequacies in health recommendations provided for international travelers by North American travel health advisors. J Travel Med 1994;1:72–78.

35. Townend M. Sources and appropriateness of medical advice for trekkers. J Travel Med 1998;5:73–79.

Chapter 5

ECONOMIC EVALUATION IN TRAVEL MEDICINE

PHILIPPE BEUTELS, PIERRE VAN DAMME, AND NANCY PIPER JENKS

The practice of travel medicine would benefit from the formulation of guidelines indicating how to make the optimal choice among different options. The need for such a rational decision process has become more urgent as the potential economic costs of misallocating resources becomes more significant. On the one hand, the growing popularity and accessibility of high-endemic travel destinations has greatly increased the population of those vulnerable to travel-related illness. On the other hand, the expansion of the availability of various preventive measures for traveler's diseases has greatly increased the number of possible preventive options. Against this background, economic evaluations are an essential instrument in decision making and in providing guidelines for the optimal use of scarce resources in travel medicine.

PRINCIPLES OF ECONOMIC EVALUATION

Economic evaluation can be empirical or model based in approach. In the empirical approach, as in clinical research, a (randomized) comparative experiment is set up in which the differences in costs and effects are statistically tested in a real-life situation.[1] In a model-based approach, computer simulations are used to represent reality with respect to an intervention. Input data for such models are of an epidemiologic, medical, demographic, and economic nature. For economic evaluations in travel medicine, complicated by many uncertain parameters and future projections, the model-based approach is most commonly applied.

A basic principle of economics is that in an environment of scarce resources, optimal choices have to be made in the allocation of resources. This principle also applies to the provision of health care. Even if health for all would be technically feasible from a purely medical point of view, it is economically impossible to cure or prevent all illnesses and infections. An economic evaluation combines medical effectiveness of an intervention and the costs of that intervention with the goal of identifying the most cost-effective choice between different alternatives.[1] As such, it can be an important factor in the decision-making process for the public health sector (e.g., establishing reimbursement levels, introducing new treatments or prevention strategies) and for the private sector (e.g., formu-

lating policies in hospitals, managed care practices, or price setting in the pharmaceutical industry). While categorizing costs, a distinction is made between direct and indirect costs (Table 5–1).

The listings in italics in Table 5–1 are often not taken into account because they are difficult to estimate and/or because they can be relatively small in comparison to the other costs. It should be noted that costs in an economic sense are opportunity costs: they represent a sacrifice of the next best alternative application. This entails that economic costs are not limited to financial expenses but can also include goods and services that are not expressed in monetary terms. Market prices are often used as a proxy when opportunity costs are not known. If particular goods and services are not traded on a market (e.g., work of volunteers), ("shadow") prices of a similar activity can be used instead (e.g., wage of unskilled labor). In practice, direct costs of medical treatment are usually estimated on the basis of invoices and patient files. If the means with which an intervention is taking place are stipulated accurately, intervention costs can be estimated quite easily as well. Typical costs in travel medicine, such as mosquito netting, water purification tablets, prophylactic medication, and standby treatment medications, can be categorized under intervention costs. If post-travel costs arise as

Table 5–1. COST CATEGORIES IN AN ECONOMIC EVALUATION OF A MEDICAL INTERVENTION

Direct costs

   Treatment costs directly related to medical consumption (consultations, medication, diagnostic tests, surgery, etc.)

   Intervention costs directly related to the implementation of an intervention (e.g., information campaign, new medication or therapy), also for treatment of adverse events

   Personal direct costs (transport, home treatment, special education, etc.)

Indirect costs

   Costs of lost productivity (outside the health care sector)

   Costs in life-years gained (treatment for disorders acquired during prolonged lifetime)

   Personal indirect costs (opportunity costs of travel and waiting, costs of pain and suffering)

Adapted from Lapré and Rutten.[2]

part of standard therapeutic measures for some travel-associated disorders (e.g., long-term travelers screened on return for schistosomiasis, HIV, parasites in stool, etc.), then these costs should be included in the intervention costs. Treatment costs for disease acquired abroad or at home as well as medical evacuation costs, if applicable, are part of direct medical treatment costs.

The assessment of indirect costs of productivity losses, however, remains difficult. These costs arise whenever an individual interrupts his normal activities in society because of illness or premature mortality. During his illness or for the rest of his natural lifetime, this individual's contribution to society is temporarily lost, leading to a decrease in productivity in society as a whole. There are several theoretical methods to assess the costs of lost productivity, but they are often impracticable.[1,2] The easiest method departs from gross wages: one's earnings are then considered to be a good estimate of one's contribution to society. An objection to this method is that it discriminates on the basis of income because an intervention could turn out to be more advantageous for target groups of individuals with a higher income. However, this method could be useful to calculate the average loss in productivity in large heterogeneous target groups. In travel medicine, indirect costs could also be quantified based on the value travelers attribute to each day that they remain disease free when traveling.

The first step in an economic evaluation is determining the perspective of the analysis. If the analysis is performed from the health care payer's point of view, only direct costs need to be taken into account. However, from society's viewpoint, indirect costs are also relevant. Other viewpoints are those of the patient, hospitals, travel clinics, managed care practices, insurance companies, other private companies, etc. For each of these alternative viewpoints, other costs and effects may be relevant. This implies that it is theoretically possible that an intervention is cost effective for one party involved, whereas it is not for another. For each strategy, the relevant costs and benefits are determined and information on them is collected. Finally, costs and benefits are calculated for each strategy, relative (incremental) to another strategy.

A complete economic evaluation should not only include inputs (or costs) and outputs (or consequences), but also should compare different alternatives for an intervention. Table 5–2 presents a helpful way of determining this. If the answer to either of the two questions is negative, the evaluation becomes either descriptive (e.g., only measuring costs or disease incidence in a completely immunized group without relating it to an unimmunized group) or one sided (e.g., making either only a cost analysis or an effectiveness analysis). Only if both requirements are met can there be mention of a complete economic evaluation.[1]

Depending on how health gains are measured, a distinction can be made between different methods of evaluation. A cost-minimization analysis compares the costs of equally effective alternatives without quantifying the health gains. It differs from a cost analysis in that the effectiveness is known to be equal. In a cost-effectiveness analysis, health gains are measured in one-dimensional natural units (e.g., infections prevented, deaths averted, life-years saved). By weighing the life-years saved for quality, in a cost-utility analysis, health gains can be measured in quality adjusted life-years, healthy year equivalents, or disability adjusted life-years. In a cost-benefit analysis, health gains are converted into monetary units.[1] The most widely used methods for economic evaluation in travel medicine are cost-effectiveness and cost-benefit analysis. However, one should be aware that some so-called cost-benefit analyses are, in fact, cost-comparison analyses in which health gains are not monetarized.[3] The effects in which health gains are expressed should represent the final results or clinical endpoints of an intervention as adequately as possible to enable comparison between different interventions.[4] If, hypothetically, the cost effectiveness of typhoid fever vaccination were $10,000 per case prevented, whereas rabies prophylaxis is evaluated at $30,000 per case prevented, instinctively, if a choice needs to be made, typhoid fever vaccination is opted for because it is more cost effective (i.e., less costly to prevent one case). However, can a case of rabies be compared with a case of typhoid fever? Therefore, to make that judgment, it would be preferable to express the avoided effects, for instance, in life-years saved instead of infections prevented. Nevertheless, while comparing different alternatives for the same intervention (e.g., antibiotics and a vaccine against traveler's diarrhea), using costs per case avoided is perfectly acceptable.

In order to express time preference and to account for uncertainty with regard to the future, future costs and benefits are usually discounted (or scaled down) to their

Table 5–2. OVERVIEW OF EVALUATION METHODS WITHIN THE HEALTH CARE SECTOR

	ARE COSTS (INPUTS) AS WELL AS CONSEQUENCES (OUTPUTS) INVESTIGATED?		
	ONLY OUTPUTS	ONLY INPUTS	INPUTS AND OUTPUTS
No comparison of different alternatives	Description of outcomes	Description of costs	Description of costs and outcomes
Comparison of different alternatives	Efficacy or effectiveness analysis	Cost analysis	Full economic evaluation Cost-minimization analysis Cost-effectiveness analysis Cost-utility analysis Cost-benefit analysis

Adapted from Drummond et al.[1]

present value. In other words, costs and benefits are considered less important the further they arise in the future. Discounting can be regarded as a technical correction, which puts costs and benefits occurring at different points in time on the same basis of comparison. As such, it is nothing but an inverse interest calculation. The higher the discount rate, the more importance is given to events in the present as opposed to future events. Discount rates in economic evaluations of health care vary from 0% to 10%. Traditionally, the 5% discount rate is the most widely used. Lately, it has been suggested to lower the discount rate in some countries in the base case calculations to 3%.[5] The introduction of the concept of discounting is important: it is said to disadvantage prevention versus curation.[6] Furthermore, within the field of infectious diseases, prevention of infections with serious complications long after the moment of vaccination is disadvantaged in comparison to infections with immediate repercussions (e.g., hepatitis B versus influenza).

Given the uncertainty with respect to some crucial input parameters, it is important to check the robustness of the findings by varying these input values within reasonable bounds in a sensitivity analysis. Parameters for which results prove to be sensitive should be estimated as accurately as possible, and ways of improving estimation of these parameters should be investigated. Threshold analysis also provides policy makers with valuable information by calculation of the respective threshold values; these are points at which the decision maker becomes indifferent to various alternatives, viewing them as equally efficient.

The main difficulty in economic evaluations is not about methodology but about data availability. To perform a good analysis, data on (age-specific) prevalence and incidence, coverage over multiple interventions and/or doses, protection and/or effectiveness rates, adverse events, treatment profiles, disease progression, and all associated costs are needed. Unfortunately, very few of these data are readily available. It is in the interest of all organizations in the health care sector (including travel clinics) to monitor and manage the enormous potential of data, which are now not being registered or neglected until they have become obsolete.[7] This is why there are to date relatively few economic evaluations in the field of travel medicine. In the next paragraphs, in which some travel-associated diseases are discussed, it will become clear why data gathering is such an important aspect in the process of economic evaluation.

HEPATITIS A

In this section, we will try to demonstrate the usefulness of economic evaluation in travel medicine by elaborating the example of hepatitis A vaccination.

A very common travel-related disease, hepatitis A is prevalent wherever standards of hygiene and sanitation are poor. Several economic evaluations on hepatitis A in travelers have been performed. Quite a few of these are vague because of many parameters that are neglected (e.g., incidence in the home country, disease evolution parameters) or because the underlying methodology is not clearly explained. The following is an example of what we consider a solid and complete economic evaluation on the subject by Tormans et al.,[8] resulting in a number of practical and useful recommendations. A problem to start with is how to define an average traveler from a low-endemic region to a high-endemic region: in the study presented here, the average traveler profile is based on a survey in four different travel clinics in Belgium. On average, this traveler is 35 years old and is expected to travel three times in the next 10 years to a high-endemicity area for periods of 25 days. In terms of prevention, there were different options: (1) doing nothing, (2) passive immunization of all travelers with immunoglobulins, (3) active immunization of all travelers, and (4) screening for HAV antibodies and active immunization of susceptible travelers only.

Table 5–3 gives the input data that were necessary to perform this economic evaluation. As mentioned above, gathering and estimating these data accurately was the most time-consuming aspect of the evaluation.

In this particular study, two hepatitis A vaccines were considered for active immunization of adult travelers: the Havrix 720® (two-dose schedule) and the Havrix 1440® (three-dose schedule) vaccine. All strategies were analyzed relative (incremental) to doing nothing. The baseline results showed that the cost-effectiveness ratio of any of the immunization strategies is relatively high when compared to the cost effectiveness of interventions for other vaccine-preventable diseases. With a cost-effectiveness ratio of $23,333 per discounted life-year saved, HAV vaccination of travelers is less attractive to the Belgian health care payer than, for instance, universal hepatitis B vaccination ($710 per discounted life-year saved).[9,10]

The main conclusion of this study is therefore that hepatitis A immunization (active or passive) for the defined "average traveler" is not a cost-effective intervention (even with inclusion of indirect costs, expressing society's viewpoint) and is not first in line when it comes to reimbursement by the authorities. Table 5–4 shows that vaccination with Havrix 1440 is—compared with the other alternatives—the most cost-effective preventive strategy against HAV. Passive immunization was the least appropriate option according to these baseline results. However, by multiple parameter variations, threshold analyses gave clear indications of the optimal prevention strategy for different travel profiles. In Figure 5–1, the incremental cost-effectiveness ratios for active (with Havrix 720) and passive immunization are presented for travelers from low-endemic (e.g., North America, Western Europe) to high-endemic regions. The travel frequency on the horizontal axis is varied from once to 10 times in the next 10 years. For those who do not undertake more than two trips of 25 days during a 10-year period, passive immunization is the most cost-effective strategy. For travelers who are expected to journey more than twice in 10 years, active immunization before the first trip is the most cost-effective option.

Adding similar calculations for travelers leaving from moderate-endemic regions, Table 5–5 presents practical general recommendations for the choice between active and passive immunization in relation to travel fre-

Table 5–3. OVERVIEW OF BASELINE INPUT DATA

GENERAL DATA

Number of individuals in target group	100,000
Time horizon	10 years
Mean age of target group	35 years
Travel frequency	3 times in 10 years
Duration of stay abroad per trip	25 days

EPIDEMIOLOGIC DATA

Very low-endemic region	
HAV prevalence	20%
HAV annual incidence	0.003%
Low-endemic region	
HAV prevalence	25%
HAV annual incidence	0.01%
Moderate endemic region	
HAV prevalence	45%
HAV annual incidence	0.05%
Developing countries (high-endemic region)	
HAV annual incidence	3.6%

CLINICAL DATA

Symptomatic hepatitis	90%
Mild hepatitis	50%
Moderate hepatitis	30%
Severe hepatitis	19.9%
Fulminant hepatitis	0.1%
Relapse after mild hepatitis	9%
Relapse after moderate hepatitis	7%
Relapse after severe hepatitis	2%

IMMUNIZATION DATA

Vaccine Havrix 720 El.U	2 doses, 1 booster
Compliance (1st, 2nd, 3rd dose)	100%, 60%, 50%
Duration of protection	1, 2, 10 years
Protection rate	90%, 98%, 99%
Vaccine Havrix 1440 El.U	1 dose, 1 booster
Compliance (1st, 2nd dose)	100%, 60%
Duration of protection	1, 10 years
Protection rate	95%, 99%
Immunoglobulins (passive immunization)	
Compliance (first dose, next doses)	100%, 50%
Duration of protection	90 days
Protection rate	85%

SCREENING DATA

Sensitivity of screening test	99%
Specificity of screening test	99%

ECONOMIC DATA (US$)

Unit costs for treating	
Mild hepatitis	342
Moderate hepatitis	434
Severe hepatitis	2,216
Fulminant hepatitis	22,152
Relapsing hepatitis	434
Unit costs for	
Vaccination	40
Screening	30
Passive immunization	24
Discount rate	5%

Adapted from Tormans et al.[8] and Van Doorslaer et al.[31]

Table 5–4. INCREMENTAL DIRECT MEDICAL COSTS AND EFFECTS COMPARED TO DOING NOTHING (1993 US$)

STRATEGY	COSTS INCURRED	NUMBER OF INFECTIONS PREVENTED	COSTS PER INFECTION PREVENTED
Havrix 1440	8,402,170	556	15,106
Screening + Havrix 1440	9,162,158	551	16,638
Havrix 720	9,660,144	475	20,330
Screening + Havrix 720	10,113,560	470	21,500
Immunoglobulins	6,644,974	304	21,840

Target group = 100,000 travelers leaving from a low-endemic country to a high-endemic region.
Travel behavior = three times 25 days during the next 10 years.
Adapted from Van Doorslaer et al.[31]

quency, duration of stay abroad, and region of origin. If duration of stay abroad is less than the threshold value of 180 days, passive immunization remains the most cost-effective strategy for a single journey. For individuals with an expected travel frequency of twice in a 10-year period, recommendations depend on the region of origin. When the duration of stay abroad is less than 90 days, passive immunization is the most cost-effective alternative for travelers from a low- or very low-endemic region, whereas this is never the case for travelers from a moderately endemic region.

If active immunization is chosen over administering immunoglobulins, the question remains as to whether a screening test should be carried out prior to active immunization in order not to waste the costs of vaccination on protected travelers, who already acquired natural immunity.

Basically, three parameters that have an important influence on this decision were singled out: (1) the expected prevalence of HAV immunity in the target group (mostly dependent on patient's age and degree of endemicity), (2) the cost of the screening test, and (3) the cost of the vaccine. Although other means of testing for

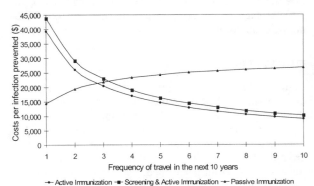

Figure 5–1. Cost effectiveness in relation to travel frequency. Adapted from Tormans et al.[8]

Table 5–5. HAV IMMUNIZATION RECOMMENDATIONS IN RELATION TO TRAVEL FREQUENCY AND REGION OF ORIGIN

| | EXPECTED TRAVEL FREQUENCY IN 10 YEARS | | |
REGION OF ORIGIN	ONCE	TWICE	THREE TIMES OR MORE
Very low-endemic or low-endemic region	Ig: < 180 days Vaccine: ≥ 180 days	Ig: < 90 days Vaccine: ≥ 90 days	Vaccination
Moderate endemic region	Ig: < 180 days Vaccine: ≥ 180 days	Vaccination	Vaccination

Adapted from Tormans et al.[8]
Ig = immunoglobulins.

HAV antibodies, such as questionnaires and saliva tests, have been reported to be useful in that these avoid the need for a needle puncture, blood tests are preferred because of their superior accuracy. Since the sensitivity and specificity of blood tests are close to 100%, these parameters were kept constant in view of the decision of whether to screen first. It becomes immediately apparent in Figure 5–2 how these parameters relate to each other. Each line connects break-even points of combined threshold values for HAV prevalence (vertical axis) and the screening test price (horizontal axis), for which the costs per infection prevented are equal for vaccination with and without prior screening. Each line divides the diagram into two areas: for all combinations below each line, vaccination without prior screening is the most cost-effective strategy; above each line, prior screening is optimal. The lower the costs of vaccination, the steeper the slope of the break-even line and the smaller the area becomes in which the optimal decision includes prior screening.

An example can easily clarify the usefulness of the data presented in Figure 5–2. For German travelers, the HAV prevalence rates by age group are as follows: <20 years: 5%; 21 to 30 years: 5%; 31 to 40 years: 13%; 41 to 50 years: 28%; 51 to 60 years: 50%.[11] With a cost for screening of $30 and vaccination costs per dose of $40, immediate vaccination is the most cost-effective option for HAV prevalence rates below 35%. Therefore, it could be recommended that German travelers older than 50 years be systematically screened before vaccination. Sim-

ilarly, recommendations for different countries or regions could be tailored to the local age-related immunity data.

It needs to be said that this example is given here in the first place to indicate how the theory in the previous section can be applied to the practice of travel medicine. The actual use of part of the results of this study may be of limited relevance as some of the considered alternatives are no longer an option in a number of countries.

In another cost-effectiveness analysis of hepatitis A prevention in French tourists, vaccination was associated with much higher costs per symptomatic case avoided (between F 168,000 and F 280,000) than in previous studies.[12] This is mainly a consequence of the authors' very low estimate of the annual incidence of symptomatic hepatitis A (0.0145% while in France and 25 times higher while abroad). At the average age of French travelers of 42 years, 77% of them have already acquired natural immunity, so that pretravel screening is generally more cost effective than immediate vaccination.[12] A more restricted study looked specifically at the choice between active and passive immunization of frequent travelers, assuming that the decision to immunize had already been taken. Active was found to be preferable to passive hepatitis A immunization when the anticipated travel frequency to a high-risk area exceeds five trips during the next 10 years.[13]

OTHER TRAVEL-RELATED DISEASES

Malaria is a common and serious tropical disease. Each year, while visiting endemic countries, more than 10,000 travelers fall ill after returning to their home country. About 1% of these travelers who contracted *Plasmodium falciparum* infection die.[14,15] Early diagnosis and adequate (standby) treatment could prevent most of these deaths. Behrens and Roberts[16] calculated benefit-cost ratios (BCRs) for malaria prophylaxis of 5.3 for chloroquine and proguanil and 1.7 for mefloquine, indicating that malaria prophylaxis in travelers is a cost-saving intervention. This is due to the substantial morbidity (and mortality) associated with malaria, giving rise to high treatment costs, which, in combination with a relatively high incidence rate and easily provided (cheap) chemoprophylaxis, results in savings. In another study by Schlagenhauf et al., the use of standby treatment for malaria was examined.[14] The authors calculated a cost-effectiveness ratio that compared very favorably with other inter-

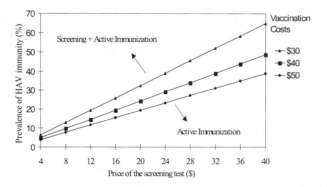

Figure 5–2. Active immunization with or withour prior screening in relation to three parameters.
Adapted from Tormans et al.[8]

ventions. Based on their data, a BCR of 0.56 can be calculated, which means that 56% of the investment can be recovered by savings in treatment costs for avoided malaria cases (Schlagenhauf, personal communication, 1995). More recently, a number of cost-effectiveness evaluations of antimalaria bednet programs on a nationwide scale have been published. Although such programs are obviously not aimed specifically at travelers, these evaluations could provide useful information for future travel-related analyses on the subject.[17–19]

Low incidence of typhoid and the rather high costs of oral and intramuscular vaccines explain the unfavorable results of economic evaluation of typhoid prevention in travelers. Behrens and Roberts[16] found for typhoid fever BCRs of less than 1 for both the oral Ty 21a vaccine (BCR: 0.045) and the intramuscular Typhoid Vi vaccine (BCR: 0.055). It is, of course, not necessary for an intervention to be cost saving (i.e., having BCRs > 1) to justify its initiation, but a relatively poor ratio of benefits to costs may be an indication of the low priority of this prevention from an economic point of view. The unfavorable outcomes for typhoid prevention have already been indicated in 1982 by Steffen,[20] who estimated the cost effectiveness of typhoid vaccinations at $100,000 US to $300,000 US per illness case prevented in Swiss or American travelers going to endemic areas.[20]

MacPherson and Tonkin[21] and Morger et al.,[22] in two separate publications, analyzed that 5 million to 29 million US$ would be the cost of preventing a single case of cholera in North Americans traveling to endemic regions. Here, too, the small overall risk of one case of cholera per 500,000 journeys to endemic regions provides the main explanation for this unattractive ratio.

In a well-wrought analysis, LeGuerrier et al.[23] found that pre-exposure rabies prophylaxis in North American travelers headed for endemic areas would cost 417 million CAD$ to 5 billion CAD$ per life-year gained. In children, the costs per case prevented per year of stay would total 275,000 CAD$. Their analysis confirmed earlier findings that postexposure rabies prophylaxis (POST-EP) is more cost effective than pre-exposure rabies prophylaxis (PRE-EP), and that the main analytic problem is the lack of data about actual rabies exposure risks.[23–25] Even while using unconservative estimates regarding pre- and post costs, they showed that PRE-EP would not become more cost effective to travelers than POST-EP unless at least 37.5% of them were exposed to rabies, which is still a much higher risk than the highest available estimates.

Furthermore, an analysis by Wilson and Fineberg[26] showed that it would cost 9 million US$ to avert one case of rabies and 4 million US$ to avert one case of Japanese encephalitis.

Financial data have also been used to show that prophylaxis of travelers' diarrhea is indicated for selected high-risk groups only; otherwise, limited self-treatment was found to be preferable.[27,28]

We have to date no knowledge of other published economic evaluations for travelers about diphtheria, yellow fever, tetanus, or polio.

CONCLUSION

The most important aspect of travelers' pretrip preparation may actually be educational and not prescriptive. In other words, it may consist of informing travelers about necessary precautions rather than vaccination. After all, most travel-related infections are not vaccine preventable.[29] The problem in terms of evaluation here is that it is much more difficult to measure the impact of providing educational material to a traveler than to measure the immune response to a vaccination. Collecting the information that would make such a measurement possible requires a different approach to data collection. Until such data are available, it will remain extremely difficult to make a proper evaluation of the real impact and relative importance of educating the traveler. Clearly, prevention by vaccination and prophylactic medication is—despite imperfections—the most confident way of preventing life-threatening travel incidents, but it may not necessarily be the most cost-effective way. Present evaluations indicate that the economically most attractive prevention for travelers is malaria prophylaxis, whereas hepatitis A prevention can be cost effective for travelers with a certain profile. There is no evidence that other preventive measures may be cost effective for the health care payer or for society. However, travelers may place a higher value on the peace of mind of knowing that they will not contract a serious illness, so that, on the personal level, the costs of vaccination should be balanced against the personal costs of a ruined trip for the individual embarking on international travel. In this respect, it seems that the current trend of cheaper exotic holidays may be instrumental in increasing numbers of less well-off travelers who leave unprepared, as they are not willing to pay a relatively large part of their package deal on prophylaxis and are more easily prepared to take a certain voluntary risk.[30] It seems that public and private insurers should keep an eye on the impact of this on the general health care costs and intervene by readjusting copayment for travel prophylaxis if appropriate.

The main conclusions of this chapter are twofold. In the first place, it is clear that the methodology exists to perform an economic evaluation of different travel-related interventions. Second, however, it will not be possible to apply this methodology in practice until data are available that allow one to differentiate the impact in terms of costs and effects of various interventions. In this context, we feel that it is in the interest of travel clinics to start or continue monitoring their data so that solid economic evaluations become possible in the future. In order to accomplish this, standardization of data inventory is urgently needed.

REFERENCES

1. Drummond M, O'Brien B, Stoddart G, et al. Methods for the economic evaluation of health care programmes. 2nd Ed. Oxford: Oxford University Press, 1997.
2. Lapré R, Rutten F, eds. Economics of health care [in Dutch]. Utrecht: Lemma, 1993.

3. Zarnke KB, Levine MAH, O'Brien B. Cost-benefit analyses in the health care literature: don't judge a study by its label. J Clin Epidemiol 1997;50:813–822.

4. Drummond M. Output measurement for resource allocation decisions in health care. In: McGuire A, Fenn P, Mayhew K, eds. Providing health care. The economics of alternative systems of finance and delivery. Oxford: Oxford University Press, 1991:99–119.

5. Weinstein MC, Siegel JE, Gold MR, et al. for the panel on Cost-Effectiveness in Health and Medicine. Recommendations of the panel on Cost-Effectiveness in Health and Medicine. JAMA 1996;276:1253–1258.

6. Phillips KA, Holtgrave DR. Using cost-effectiveness/cost-benefit analysis to allocate health resources: a level playing field for prevention? Am J Prev Med 1997;13(1):18–25.

7. Jenks N, Van Damme P, Beutels P. Data management systems: are travel medicine clinics tracking and using their data [abstract]? Fifth International Conference on Travel Medicine, Geneva, March 24–27, 1997.

8. Tormans G, Van Damme P, Van Doorslaer E. Recommendations for prevention of hepatitis A based on a cost-effectiveness analysis. J Travel Med 1994;1:127–135.

9. Beutels P, Tormans G, Van Damme P, et al. Universal hepatitis B vaccination in Flanders: cost-effective [in Dutch]? Tijdschr Soc Gezondheidsz 1996;74:270–279.

10. Beutels P. Economic evaluations applied to hepatitis B vaccination: general observations. Vaccine 1998;6(Suppl):S84–S92.

11. Bienzle U, Bock HL, Meister W, et al. Anti-HAV seroprevalence in German travellers and hepatitis A vaccination in immune subjects. Lancet 1993;341:1028.

12. Severo C, Fagnani F, Lafuma A. Cost-effectiveness of hepatitis A prevention in France. PharmacoEconomics 1995;8(1):46–61.

13. Fenn P, McGuire A, Gray A. An economic evaluation of vaccination against hepatitis A for frequent travellers. J Infect 1998;36:17–22.

14. Schlagenhauf P, Steffen R, Tschopp A, et al. Behavioural aspects of travelers in their use of malaria presumptive treatment. Bull World Health Organ 1995;73:215–221.

15. World Health Organization. International travel and health: vaccination requirements and health advice. Geneva: WHO, 1995.

16. Behrens R, Roberts J. Is travel prophylaxis worthwhile? Economic appraisal of prophylactic measures against malaria, hepatitis A, and typhoid in travellers. BMJ 1994;309:918–922.

17. Aikins MK, Fox-Rushby J, D'Alessandro U, et al. The Gambian national impregnated bednet programme: costs, consequences and net cost-effectiveness. Soc Sci Med 1998;46:181–191.

18. Graves PM. Comparison of the cost-effectiveness of vaccines and insecticide impregnation of mosquito nets for the prevention of malaria. Ann Trop Med Parasitol 1998;92:339–410.

19. Kirigia JM, Snow RW, Fox-Rushby J, et al. The cost of treating paediatric malaria admission and the potential impact of insecticide-treated mosquito nets on hospital expenditure. Trop Med Int Health 1998;3:145–150.

20. Steffen R. Typhoid vaccine, for whom [letter]? Lancet 1982;1:615.

21. MacPherson DW, Tonkin M. Cholera vaccination: a decision analysis. Can Med Assoc J 1992;146:1947–1952.

22. Morger H, Steffen R, Schar M. Epidemiology of cholera in travellers, and conclusions for vaccination recommendations. BMJ 1983;286:184.

23. LeGuerrier P, Pilon PA, Deshaies D, et al. Pre-exposure rabies prophylaxis for the international traveller: a decision analysis. Vaccine 1996;14:167–176.

24. Bernard-KW; Fishbein-DB. Pre-exposure rabies prophylaxis for travellers: are the benefits worth the cost? Vaccine 1991;9:833–836.

25. Mann JM. Routine pre-exposure rabies prophylaxis: a reassessment. Am J Public Health 1984;74:720–722.

26. Wilson ME, Fineberg HV. Analysis of benefits and costs for three multidose vaccines in travelers: hepatitis A, rabies and Japanese encephalitis. In: Proceedings of the Third Conference on International Travel Medicine, Paris, 1993:159.

27. Thomson MA, Booth IW. Treatment of traveler's diarrhea—economic aspects. PharmacoEconomics 1996;9:382–391.

28. Reves RR, Johnson PC, Ericsson CD, et al. Cost-effectiveness comparison of the use of antimicrobial agents for treatment of prophylaxis of traveler's diarrhea. Arch Intern Med 1988;148:2421–2427.

29. Wilson M. Critical evaluation of vaccines for travelers. J Travel Med 1995;2:239–243.

30. Fair R, Nathwani D. Travel medicine—at what cost and who pays? Scott Med J 1996;41:141–142.

31. Van Doorslaer E, Tormans G, Van Damme P. Cost-effectiveness analysis of vaccination against hepatitis A in travelers. J Med Virol 1994;44:463–469.

Chapter 6

PRETRAVEL PLANNING

DOMINIQUE TESSIER

As travel evolved over the last century, the needs of travelers changed. Nowadays, travelers are a heterogeneous group composed of vacationers, business people, migrants, workers, students and teachers, young retired persons, and volunteers. Their needs for medical services increased and became more specific. To help protect the health of those traveling abroad, pretravel advice by expert health care professionals is needed. Unfortunately, many are ill equipped to provide accurate recommendations and prescriptions. This chapter will try to assist health care practitioners in the delivery of quality pretravel counseling.

The health care professional giving pretravel advice should be aware that the knowledge needed is far beyond tropical medicine or infectious diseases alone. It should include acclimatization advice, counseling on blood and body fluid exposure protection, environment risks, prevention of trauma (particularly related to sports and road accidents), special care needed by pregnant women, sexual protection, marine and land envenomation, insect-borne disease prevention and treatment, and vaccine-preventable diseases. Currently available guidelines should be known and used and resources to keep up with new developments available and effective. Even if no certification is yet required for the practice of travel medicine, good standards of practice are the usual rule in most countries.

PRETRAVEL COUNSELING

The pretravel consultation can be divided into questions you need to ask and areas you need to cover. A minimum of information is required to determine vaccination requirements (see Chapter 22 on Vaccine-Preventable Diseases) and prescribe malaria chemosuppression (see Chapter 21 Malaria) or antibiotics for the prevention and treatment of travelers' diarrhea (see Chapter 20 Travelers' Diarrhea). These are certainly the most common concerns, but it would be simplistic to reduce travel medicine to these only as experts in travel medicine should offer a lot more to travelers.

INFORMATION TO OBTAIN FROM TRAVELERS

All consultation should begin with the gathering of basic information concerning travel (Table 6–1). To correctly advise travelers, it is important to ask about all countries to be visited, with questions regarding stay, particularly at night, in rural or urban areas. It is also important to know the exact period and duration of the travel, with special attention given to season, which may influence the risk of acquisition of malaria and other vector-borne diseases and the risk of transmission of other infectious diseases. Travelers at five-star hotels and campers are not exposed to the same risks. Many tourists book accommodation in beautiful hotels near the beach for most of their travel but would like to include a stay in rural accommodation

Table 6–1. WHAT TO ASK?

INFORMATION TO OBTAIN FROM TRAVELERS

Where (specific destination, altitude, malaria endemic areas)

Why (business, pleasure, veterinarian, adoption)

When (season, time before departure)

How long (duration)

What (type of travel, hotels, camping, special activities planned, trekking, diving)

Who: health status, medication, allergies, immune status, family, pregnancy (actual or planned), previous immunizations, special needs, previous experience with travel (malaria prophylaxis, altitude)

PURPOSE OF TRAVEL

Leisure, business, family obligations, military, airline crew, expedition, cooperation, expatriation, international adoption

HEALTH STATUS OF THE TRAVELER

Medical evaluation should include:

Medical examinations (general, dental, eyes, Pap smear, mammograms, and EKG)

Immunizations (mandatory, recommended, specials, how to receive it abroad)

Vector precautions

Cardiopulmonary problems

Allergies (Medic-Alert, epinephrine (adrenaline) auto-injectors or kit, picture of allergens)

Anti-HIV and other tests requested? (country, employer)

Psychological evaluation

Likelihood of pregnancy and complications and risks

Age-related particularities

Handicaps

in a hut or go hiking and camping. Travelers returning to their native country to visit family will often venture to more remote areas and take fewer precautions concerning food hygiene.

The purpose of the trip is an essential piece of information. Veterinarians may be more exposed to rabies, farmers to Japanese encephalitis, children of people providing aid to developing countries attending a local school to tuberculosis, cave explorers to rabies, and the so-called sexual tourist to HIV, hepatitis, and other sexually transmitted diseases (STDs). In addition, a business person on an important trip may be severely affected by moderate diarrhea or a speaker may feel unable to give his presentation because of dizziness or medication-induced anxiety. Frequent short-term travelers such as airline crew, immigration officers who accompany deportees, and some business persons will require less stringent recommendations. Even if these frequent travelers choose to be on antimalarials continuously, most, and some long-term travelers, will eventually stop taking them. If the traveler is not questioned about that possibility, an opportunity to discuss acceptable alternatives will be missed. The best alternative is usually better than nothing. Don't be too strict.

Persons providing aid to developing countries and new citizens returning to their homelands need more counseling regarding malaria protection. They should be informed about the controversies regarding malaria chemoprophylaxis. Accurate information, including a realistic view concerning side effects and alternatives, will help the traveler to make up his/her own mind when faced with an assertive fellow provider of aid to a developing country or national urging him to stop that poison. This is particularly true for malaria chemoprophylaxis.

HEALTH STATUS OF THE TRAVELER

Travelers themselves need to be evaluated. The travel health advisor should inquire about the traveler's present health status, history of significant medical problems, previous immunizations, use of antimalarials in the past, experience at altitude, current or occasional medications, allergies, immune status, and likelihood of pregnancy.

The health care professional must keep in mind that the purpose of the consultation is not meant to discourage clients from traveling but rather to provide them with the best counseling possible according to their health status and the type of travel planned. As an example, a severely immunosuppressed person unable to take live vaccines may still decide to venture into yellow fever endemic areas even without the appropriate immunization. This could be a dream come true that cannot be postponed. The traveler would need to know the ways to prevent mosquito bites, where to get products that may not still be available in his country (such as permethrin), and how, when, and where to use them. What to do and where to consult in case of emergency should also be covered.

Psychological evaluation is too often skipped or done rapidly. A careful evaluation is advised for all mid- or long-term residents. Those traveling alone are at the greatest risk.

For long-term travelers such as overseas workers, counseling regarding readaptation when the traveler returns is also helpful (see Chapter 33 Expatriates and Long-Term Travelers).

Pregnancy deserves more than passing attention (see Chapter 37 Pregnancy, Nursing, Contraception, and Travel). The possibility of an actual or future pregnancy should be assessed before choosing immunizations: a plan for a future pregnancy may motivate one to immunize earlier or give boosters with live vaccines. Pregnancy also influences the choice of medication for prevention and treatment of numerous conditions (i.e., malaria or diarrhea).

HEALTH EVALUATION

All individuals traveling frequently or planning a long stay abroad should have a pretravel health evaluation. Depending on age and general health, it could include a physical, dental, and ophthalmic examination, Pap smear, mammogram, tuberculin test, and an electrocardiogram. This, of course, takes some time. Even if the departure is imminent, some tests can be done and are usually worth doing. Ideally, a copy of significant laboratory results should be carried by the traveler or forwarded when available. Many travelers with a history of possible hepatitis postpone serologic testing because they always leave at the last minute. Even if not useful for the current trip, results would be useful for future planning.

Some medical examinations and tests are required for entry into certain countries, by schools and by employers. Increasingly, HIV testing is required by more and more countries especially for students, overseas workers, or even in some cases for all foreigners. If that type of service cannot be provided by a center, a list of references should be available and offered to the traveler.

Cardiopulmonary conditions that are not stable can result in major problems during travel, especially during overseas flights. If a person cannot walk up a single flight of stairs without dyspnea, oxygen should be recommended during air travel. Arrangements with the airline can easily be made by the physician, preferably 1 week in advance. A nasal canula, when available, is often more comfortable than a mask. Since high-altitude destinations can also lead to severe problems, this issue should be discussed (see Chapter 13 Medical Problems of High Altitude). Defibrillators are appearing on airlines but are still far from frequent.

Allergies and anaphylaxis are potentially severe problems for a traveler. Allergy to eggs and antibiotics should be investigated before immunizations. Food allergy in a country where the traveler can hardly make himself understood is a life-threatening condition. Carrying pictures of the ingredients to be avoided could help but will not guarantee the safety of meals. In such circumstances, it is advisable to carry adrenaline. When traveling, all asthmatics should carry inhalers even if their latest crisis occurred several months or years ago. Although many airline companies are now banning peanuts on board, no guarantee can be given as other passengers may have some with them. Severely allergic children should be warned and supervised carefully. Cooperation of nearby passengers can usually be obtained easily.

Many travelers are not even familiar with the special services offered by airlines or hotels such as special meals, accompanying person rebates, and rooms accommodating wheelchairs. It is the role of health care workers to inform them about such services. Every person with a specific medical condition should be encouraged to wear a Medic Alert bracelet.*

Being elderly is not a contraindication for travel. However, age will be associated with other health factors. The traveler's health status, more than age, should be the primary consideration during the pretravel evaluation.

More detailed information may be found in the following chapters of this book that deal with travelers and the environment, infectious health risks abroad and preventive measures, noninfectious health risks and preventive measures, and special risk groups.

HEALTH DURING TRAVEL

Maintaining the good health of travelers while abroad is the major purpose of travel medicine (Table 6–2). It is important to individualize counseling regarding water and food intake, illness abroad, the common cold, malaria,

*A bracelet is engraved with the wearer's allergies or other medical conditions to alert medical practitioners in situations of emergency.

birth control, STD, HIV prevention, Medic Alert, and the need to carry epinephrine (adrenaline) and first-aid kits.

ADOPTION

International adoption is easier and a lot more frequent nowadays. Future parents are often very anxious and may know only at the last minute the age and sex of the child. The child's weight or any other basic information is seldom available. Many parents wish that they could travel with an entire pharmacy to cover all possible diseases. Reassurance is essential as most problems encountered during the trip (i.e., scabies and dermatitis) are not urgent or life threatening. It is usually acceptable to prescribe an antibiotic for acute diarrhea in certain countries where health care is inadequate or medications may be difficult to find or administered parentally, increasing the risk of hepatitis B and C, HIV, and other blood-borne diseases. The prescription must indicate the dosage for different weight ranges.

BEHAVIOR

The pretravel visit would not be thorough without basic information on prevention and risk behavior. Physical precautions against vectors, sun exposure, accidents involving motor vehicles, bites, altitude, water (i.e., diving, parasites, tides, sand, and drowning), alcohol consumption and drugs, and personal violence and sexual risk factors

Table 6–2.   QUICK REMINDERS—PRACTICAL TIPS

Food	The consumption of uncooked or not freshly prepared foods such as salads, raw vegetables, or open fruit should be avoided completely following the popular advice: "Cook it, boil it, peel it, or forget it!" Cooked food should be well done and eaten immediately. Attention should be paid that prepared foods are not contaminated by dirty surfaces, water, or insects.
Water	If there is no safe drinking water, only industrially bottled water and beverages or those prepared with boiled water like coffee or tea should be consumed. Alternatively, sufficient chlorination or treatment with disinfectants can be used. Ice cubes are especially risky as the purity of the water is never guaranteed. Fresh milk must be boiled before drinking.
Dehydration	In hot climates, it is important to maintain a sufficient fluid balance. Thirst, especially in elderly persons, is often not a good indicator for sufficient fluid uptake. As a rule, the urine color should be light. Alcohol consumption during daytime should be avoided completely.
Sun	Too much insolation might especially affect small children. Therefore, sufficient measures for sun protection (hat, cap, sunglasses, sun creams) should be mandatory.
Mosquitoes	Protection against mosquito bites is especially important in malarious areas. However, many other diseases are transmitted by bloodsucking insects. Therefore, the use of insect repellents and other precautions against vectors should be emphasized. In dengue-endemic areas, a sunscreen that incorporates a mosquito repellent can be used.
Walking	Walking barefoot or other direct skin contact with sandy or soily floors can lead to infection with sand fleas. Soils contaminated with animal or human excrement bear the risk of transmitting worm larva such as hookworms or strongyloides. Children in particular should wear shoes or sandals and not play on such risky grounds.
Sexual activities	Considering the high risk of acquiring HIV infection or other sexually transmitted diseases in many favorite holiday destinations, casual sexual contacts should be avoided completely or at least protected by safer sex practices (i.e., careful use of condoms). Birth control should be covered.
Envenomation	In areas with venomous animals (snakes, scorpions, spiders, or other biting animals), one should avoid touching or walking on what cannot be seen. At night, a light is very useful. Robust shoe wear and long sleeves and trousers are recommended.
Injuries	Motor vehicle accidents, violence and aggressions, drowning, sports-related injuries, animal bites, and other accidents are unwanted but frequent parts of a trip. The purchase on health insurance should be considered and common sense used as the first prevention tip. Too often, alcohol and/or drug consumption are related.
Altitude	Air travel, high-altitude destination, trekking, and mountain climbing may need special counseling. All travelers should be encouraged to drink a lot, avoiding caffeine and alcohol.

should be dealt with in a realistic way. One should never guess which traveler is at risk and therefore requires that type of information. Polite but direct questioning should be used to obtain the required answers. The attention of the traveler is more likely to be secured if the situations discussed are those involving unplanned, unprotected sex. For example, the sentence "In a bar, after an exhausting day and a few drinks,..." may elicit the desired response: "Well, that's exactly how it once happened!"

If possible, see the traveler more than once before his/her trip. For both the traveler open to additional counseling and for the wise, frequent traveler who has no time to listen to details, the following travel advice is recommended: travel lightly, use luggage with wheels, and eat lightly during the flight. On business travel, limit alcohol and caffeine intake but drink copious amounts of other liquids, limit sun exposure, respect your limits and listen to your body, accept help (i.e., wheelchair and preboarding), and wear sensible shoes.

TRAVEL KIT

For the traveler who plans to visit a remote area or to travel for an extended period of time, it is usually a good idea to carry a first-aid kit. Families should also have one. The content will be influenced by the length and conditions of stay, country visited, number of travelers in the group, potential risks to health, and health and experience of the traveler. In most cases, a minimal kit, as described in Table 6–3, will be sufficient. Many prepared kits are available in specialized stores and pharmacies. They are usually expensive and very often not adapted to the specific needs of travelers. For example, kits may contain plasma and intravenous products but will rarely include basic yet essential items such as a thermometer. Health care professionals counseling travelers should weigh not only the potential risks to health but also the ability of the travelers to use what they bring along.

For all travelers carrying needles and syringes, a letter on official stationery, signed by the attending physician, should be provided. An example in French, English, Spanish, and Portuguese is shown in Figure 6–1.

When traveling with children, childproof safety containers are essential. Pill cutters are helpful. When carrying medications from one country to another, it is preferable to use the original bottle labeled at the pharmacy. Never mix medications together in unidentified containers. This could raise the suspicions of some customs officers. It is also preferable to keep medications in a carry-on bag and not to send them with the checked luggage. Medication could be lost or exposed to freezing, depressurization, or sun radiation. These conditions could alter the efficacy or safety of the products. Inhalers and liquids are particularly vulnerable.

INSURANCE

Most travelers should obtain health insurance for travel before leaving home. The role of the health care profes-

Table 6–3.   TRAVEL KIT

MINIMAL FIRST-AID KIT

Thermometer
Personal medication
Acetaminophen
Sunblock (skin and lips, SPF 15 or more)
Self-treatment for diarrhea
Iodine drops (white, for water treatment and wounds)
Condoms
Bandages
Scissors
Safety pins

USUALLY NEEDED FOR MOST TRAVELERS

Malaria prophylaxis (medications, nets, and repellents)
Birth control
Pain killers/anti-inflammatory
Moleskin (for walkers and trekkers)
Gauze (plain, elastic)
Nonadhering dressing
Adhesive tape
Gloves
Disinfectant gauze
Antibiotics
Antihistamine
Ear drops
Rehydration powder

EXTRAS FOR SPECIAL TRAVELERS

Syringes and needles
Matches, flashlight, and knife
Altitude medication
Laxative
Antacid
Decongestant
First-aid manual
Extra pair of glasses
Tropical and/or per os steroid, antibiotics and antifungals
Narcotics for analgesia
Ear and eye antibiotic drops
Motion sickness medication
Epinephrine (adrenaline) auto-injector or kit

sional should be limited to the recommendation of a particular health coverage and not to discuss the different types of insurance available. However, if questions should arise, it is advisable to know the options offered on the market.

The cost of health care services during travel can be covered by the usual insurance provider at home (private or public) or, in most cases, purchased for the sole purpose of the travel. In every case, coverage should be thoroughly assessed before departure. One should stress the importance of reading all of the fine details in an insurance policy. A signed contract is highly preferable over a glossy pamphlet. If traveling in developing countries with poor or nonexisting health services, emergency evacuation should usually be included in the contract. A somewhat minor problem can degenerate into a frightening, major emergency when none of the health care professionals can understand the traveler. To avoid the problem, the International Association for Medical Assistance to Travelers (IAMAT) booklet is a good resource.

CERTIFICAT MÉDICAL - MEDICAL CERTIFICATE - CERTIFICADO MÉDICO

En faveur de: _____

(In favor of: - *A favor de: - Em favor de:*) _____

DATE: 20

(Date: - *Fecha: - Data:*) _____

OBJET: Médicaments, trousse médicale, seringues et aiguilles

Object : medication, medical kit, syringes and needles

Objeto : medicamentos, botiquin, médico, jeringas y aguyas

Objeto : medicamentos, kit de primeiros socorros, seringas e agulhas

Nous, médecins dûment autorisés, attestons que la personne ci-dessus mentionnée, transporte avec elle des médicaments, une trousse médicale, des seringues et des aiguilles stériles pour son usage personnel au cours du voyage. Tous ces objets ne sont pas destinés à la vente et ont fait l'objet d'une ordonnance médicale personnelle.

We, fully accreditated doctors, attest that the person mentioned above is carrying with her/him medication, medical kit, sterilized syringes and needles for personal use during their trip. All those objects are not for retail sale and were prescribed for personal medical use.

Nosotros, médicos debidamente autorizados, certificamos que la persona arriba mencionada transporta medicamentos, un botiquin médico, jeringas y agujas estériles para su uso personal durante el viaje. Todos esos objetos no son destinados a la venta y son parte de una prescripcion médica personal.

Nos, médicos devidamente autorizados, certificamos que a pessoa acima mencionada transporta medicamentos, kit de primeiros socorros, seringas e agulhas estéreis para seu uso pessoal durante a viagem. Todos esses objetos não são destinados à venda e são parte de sua prescrição médica.

Le directeur médical

Dr Fernand Turgeon

par D^r / D^{re}

_____

Figure 6–1.   Official travel letter.

Preexisting medical conditions are not precluded from insurance coverage. A higher premium can be offered or the preexisting condition would not be covered but accidents and other problems would be. HIV-infected patients and persons with cardiopulmonary problems or cancer can and should obtain insurance before travel.

A pregnant woman should ascertain whether her insurance policy will acknowledge the fact that she was pregnant before the departure and still provide coverage. The document should also indicate coverage for a newborn, even if premature. Expensive surprises await parents who forget to do so.

Obviously, there is no need to insist on insurance coverage when health care is unavailable. If health care cannot be purchased abroad, the only insurance required may be coverage to ensure a fast return home.

BIBLIOGRAPHY

Access Travel. A guide to the accessibility of airport terminals. Available from Airport Operators International, 1700 K Street NW, Washington, DC 20006 (for disabled travelers).

Auerback PS. Medicine for the outdoors: a guide to emergency medical procedures and first aid. Boston: Little, Brown, 1991.

Barry M, Bia F. Pregnancy and travel. JAMA 1989;261:728–731.

Berger SA. Emporiatrics versus geographic medicine; interface or spectrum? J Travel Med 1995:2:153.

Bewes PC. Trauma and accidents: practical aspects of the prevention and management of trauma associated with travel. Ber-Med-Bull 1993;49:454–64.

Bruneau A. Partir en sant ... revenir enchante: guide medical du voyageur. Montreal: Hurtubise, 1994.

Comite consultatif quebecois sur la sante des voyageurs (CCQSV). Guide d'intervention sante-voyage: situation epidemiologique et recommandations. Quebec City: Ministere de la Sante et des Services Sociaux, 2000.

Cossar JH, Reid D. Health hazards of international travel. World Health Stat Q 1989;42:61–69.

DuPont HL, Ericsson CD. Prevention and treatment of traveller's diarrhea. N Engl J Med 1993;328:1821–1827.

Gill-GV, Redmond S. Insulin treatment, time-zones and air travel: a survey of current advice from British Diabetic Clinics. Diabetes Med 1993;10:764–767.

Goodwin K, Brennan D. Advice for business travel: the wider picture. Occup Health (Lond) 1994;46:200–203.

Health advice for living overseas. Ottawa: CUSO, Health Support Service, 1994.

Health hints for the tropics. 11th Ed. American Society of Tropical Medicine, 1993.

Keystone JS, ed. Don't drink the water! Ottawa: Canadian Public Health Association and The Canadian Society for International Health, 1994.

Lechky O. Resources avilable to help family physicians provide advice to travellers. Can Med Assoc 1995;153:996–998.

Ostrowski M, Tessier D, Keystone JS. Information for the patient: travelling with HIV. Can Med Assoc J 1995;6:291–295.

Societe de medecine des voyages. Medecine des voyages: guide d'information et de conseils pratiques. Ed du Format Utile, France 1995.

Steffen R, Van der Linde F. Intercontinential travel and its effect on pre-existing illnesses. Aviat Space Environ Med 1981; Jan:57–58.

World Health Organization. Vaccination certificate requirements and health advice for international travel. Geneva: WHO, 1999.

Committee to Advise on Travel and Tropical Medicine (CATMAT). Travel medicine recommendation: dengue fever and international travel. Canada Communicable Disease Report. Vol. 22-4, February 1996.

Canadian recommendations for the prevention and treatment of malaria among international travellers 1997. Canada Communicable Disease Report, Suppl 23S5, October 1997.

An Advisory Committee Statement (ACS) Committee to Advise on Tropical Medicine and Travel (CATMAT). Statement on Japanese encephalitis vaccine. Canada Communicable Disease Report, Vol. 24 (ACS-3), August 15, 1998.

Human rabies prevention — United States. 1999 recommendations of the Advisory Committee on Immunization Practices (ACIP). Morb Mortal Wkly Rep January 8, 1998, Vol. 48, no. RR-01.

Management of possible sexual, injecting-drug-use, or other nonoccupational exposure to HIV, including considerations related to antiretroviral therapy. Public Health Service statement. MMWR Morb Mortal Wkly Rep September 25, 1998, Vol. 47, no. RR-17.

HIV prevention through early detection and treatment of other sexually transmitted diseases. United States recommendations of the Advisory Committee for HIV and STD Prevention. MMWR Morb Mortal Wkly Rep July 31, 1998, Vol. 47, no. RR-12.

Measles, mumps and rubella: vaccine use and strategies for elimination of measles, rubella and congential rubella syndrome and control of mumps: recommendations of the Advisory Committee on Immunization Practices (ACIP). MMWR Morb Mortal Wkly Rep May 22, 1998, Vol. 47, no. RR-08.

Prevention and control of influenza: recommendations of the Advisory Committee on Immunization Practices (ACIP). MMWR Morb Mortal Wkly Rep May 1, 1998, Vol. 47, no. RR-06.

Dubowitz G. Effect of temzepam on oxygen saturation and sleep quality at high altitude: randomized placebo controlled crossover trial. BMJ 1998;316:587–589.

Prevention of varicella. Recommendations of the Advisory Committee on Immunization Practices (ACIP). MMWR Morb Mortal Wkly Rep July 12, 1996, Vol. 45, no. RR-11.

Chapter 7

TOURISM PATTERNS AND TRENDS

HENRYK HANDSZUH

The World Tourism Organization (WTO) predicts that 21st-century tourism will be the antidote to "high-tech" living. The year 2020 will see the penetration of technology into all aspects of life. It will become possible to live one's days without exposure to other people. But this bleak prognosis has a silver lining for the tourism sector. People in the high-tech future will crave the human touch, and tourism will be the principal means to achieve this.

Tourism companies that manage to provide "high-touch" products will prosper. Upscale, luxury services that pamper and spoil their customers have a bright future in the upcoming century. At the same time, there are good prospects for low-budget destinations and packages. Self-catering holiday facilities, for example, offer plenty of opportunities for socializing among families and friends.

$5 BILLION A DAY INDUSTRY

WTO predicts that 1.5 billion tourists will be visiting foreign countries annually by the year 2020, spending more than 2 trillion U.S. dollars—or 5 billion U.S. dollars every day. These forecasts represent nearly three times more international tourists than the 625 million recorded in 1998 and nearly five times more tourism spending, which last year topped 444 billion U.S. dollars.

Tourist arrivals are expected to grow by an average 4.3% a year over the next two decades, whereas receipts from international tourism will climb by 6.7% a year.

To factor in domestic tourism, WTO multiplies arrivals by 10 and quadruples receipts, which brings us to the grand totals of 16 billion tourists spending 8 trillion U.S. dollars in 2020.

Tourism in the 21st century will not only be the world's biggest industry, it will also be the largest by far that the world has ever seen. Along with its phenomenal growth and size, the tourism industry will also have to take on more responsibility for its extensive impacts—not only its economic impact but also its impact on the environment, societies, and cultural sites, all of which will be increasingly scrutinized by governments, consumer groups, and the traveling public.

GROWTH OF LONG-HAUL TRAVEL

WTO forecasts that tourists of the 21st century will be traveling further afield on their holidays, often to China and even to outer space. The percentage of long-haul travel is predicted to increase from 18% in 1995 to 24% by 2020.

China will be the world's number one destination by the year 2020 and will also become the fourth most important generating market. Currently, it does not even figure among the world's top 20 generating countries. Other destinations predicted to make great strides in the tourism industry are Russia, Hong Kong, Thailand, Singapore, Indonesia, and South Africa.

Short pleasure voyages to outer space will become a reality by 2004 or 2005. It is expected that space trips will last up to 4 days and cost on average 100,000 U.S. dollars. NASA, the U.S. space agency, has recently surveyed the travel industry for interest in space tourism, and some U.S. companies are already taking reservations and deposits from private citizens hoping to become the first tourists in outer space.

But although some travelers may be suiting up for space voyages, the vast majority of the world's population will never leave their own countries, not even by the year 2020: only 7% of the world's population will be traveling internationally by that year, up from 3.5% in 1996—still just the tip of the iceberg.

TRENDS

EUROPE

Europe will remain by far the leading inbound tourism region as well as the main generator of international trips. International arrivals in Europe will reach 717 million by 2020—more than twice as many as last year.

Overall, tourism to Europe is predicted to grow more slowly than the world average, at a rate of 3.1% annually, although some countries will fare better than others. Central and Eastern European countries will become the new motor for Europe, feeding and being fed by other European and long-haul generating markets. Tourism to Central and Eastern Europe will grow by 4.8% a year and will surpass 200 million arrivals by 2016—a doubling in just 15 years.

The Eastern Mediterranean countries of Cyprus, Turkey, and Israel are also expected to show good growth of 4.6% a year. Tourism to the United Kingdom is forecast to grow by 4% annually, just under the world average. Reflecting world patterns and increasing air travel, Europeans will be taking trips more frequently and further from home. Total outbound travel from European countries is predicted to reach 771 million trips a year by 2010, again more than twice as many as last year.

Table 7–1. WORLD'S TOP DESTINATIONS—2020

COUNTRY	TOURIST ARRIVALS (MILLIONS)	% GROWTH RATE PER YEAR 1995–2020
1 China	137.1	8.0
2 United States	102.4	3.5
3 France	93.3	1.8
4 Spain	71.0	2.4
5 Hong Kong SAR	59.3	7.3
6 Italy	52.9	2.2
7 United Kingdom	52.8	3.0
8 Mexico	48.9	3.6
9 Russian Federation	47.1	6.7
10 Czech Republic	44.0	4.0

Source: World Tourism Organization.

Table 7–2. WORLD'S TOP GENERATING MARKETS—2020

COUNTRY	TOURIST ARRIVALS GENERATED WORLDWIDE (MILLIONS)	MARKET SHARE %
1 Germany	163.5	10.2
2 Japan	141.5	8.8
3 United States	123.3	7.7
4 China	100.0	6.2
5 United Kingdom	96.1	6.0
6 France	37.6	2.3
7 Netherlands	35.4	2.2
8 Canada	31.3	2.0
9 Russian Federation	30.5	1.9
10 Italy	29.7	1.9

Source: World Tourism Organization.

Long-haul travel to countries outside of Europe will grow by 6.1% a year in the upcoming decades to reach 15% of all trips taken by Europeans or 115,600,000 departures. Long-haul travel currently accounts for 12% of European outbound travel or about 42 million trips a year.

AFRICA

By 2020, the volume of international tourist arrivals in Africa will reach 75 million, almost four times the 20 million recorded in 1995. Southern Africa (at 7.3% per annum growth 1995–2020) will continue to be the leader, followed by Eastern Africa (5.3% per annum). By 2002, Southern Africa is expected to reach 10 million arrivals, five times the level of 1990.

Although any form of international travel will remain outside the financial ability of the great majority of Africans, there will be substantial growth in intraregional travel, which will grow from 58% to 64% between 1995 and 2020. Africa's share of global tourist arrivals will rise from 3.6% in 1995 to 4.7% by 2020.

Arrivals from the Americas (5.4% per annum) will grow faster than those from Europe (4.5%), but European arrivals will account for considerably more trips to the region (19 million in 2020). Growth in arrivals from Central/Eastern Europe and East Mediterranean Europe will be the strongest.

EAST ASIA AND THE PACIFIC

Even allowing for a slowdown during 1995–2000 because of the region's economic difficulties, WTO forecasts an overall average rate growth in international arrivals in the region amounting to 7.0% annually between 1995 and 2020. Thus, the volume of arrivals is forecast to reach 438 million, 5.5 times more than in 1995. East Asia and the Pacific will overtake the Americas as the second largest inbound region (after Europe) by 2005.

Already in 1995, almost four of five arrivals in the region were intraregional. This share will increase even further to 83% in 2020, whereas the long-haul share will decline from the present 21% to 17%.

SOUTH ASIA

By 2020, the number of international tourist arrivals in the region will reach 19 million, almost 4.5 times the level of 1995. The 10 million mark will be achieved in 2009.

Over the period to 2020, inbound arrivals will continue to be the strongest from long-haul markets (growth of 6.6% per annum), whereas intraregional arrivals will expand at just 4% per annum. Arrivals from the Americas and Europe will grow at 6.9% and 6.7% per annum, respectively.

AMERICAS

WTO forecasts a continued modest rate of growth in international tourist arrivals in the Americas with an average annual increase between 1995 and 2020 of 3.8%. By 2001, the Americas region will receive more arrivals than it generates, a gap that will progressively widen to 2020. By 2020, the volume of arrivals will total 284 million, 2.5 times the level of 1995.

The future for the Americas subregions shows less variance than in the recent past. The highest rate of growth will be achieved by South America (4.9% per annum), whereas the lowest will be in North America (3.6% per annum). The Caribbean will double its tourist arrivals between 1995 and 2011. The share of long haul will rise from 23% to 38% between 1995 and 2020.

MIDDLE EAST

WTO forecasts a continued, significantly above global average rate of growth in international tourist arrivals in the countries of the Middle East, with an average rise between 1995 and 2020 of 6.7% per annum, to reach almost 69 million arrivals in 2020, five times the level recorded in 1995.

MEGATRENDS

Although the growth of tourism, including trips for leisure (holiday), business, learning, and other purposes, will be unstoppable in the 21st century due to a combination of technological, demographic, economic, cultural, and other factors, increased benefits cannot be taken for granted. No destination or tourism operator can afford to sit back and wait for more tourists to arrive. Competition among destinations will also become increasingly fierce. It will be based on the criteria of quality and sustainability in a broad sense addressing the interests of travelers, tourism staff, and local communities.

The WTO Tourism 2020 Vision outlines a series of megatrends that will shape the tourism sector in the foreseeable future:

Technology

- information technology development,
- advances in transport technology, and
- smart cards.

Economic Factors

- continued moderate-to-good rates of global economic growth;
- volatile economic performance in large areas (e.g., recently in Asia, Russia), thus causing quick mass-scale shifts in demand for leisure and business travel;
- emerging importance of new economies, in particular in Central Europe, parts of Asia and Africa, and Latin America;
- widening gap between rich-poor countries;
- harmonization of currencies (U.S.-dollar and Euro-based economies); and
- creation and enlargement of economic groupings (e.g., the European Union).

Demographic Factors

- further erosion of the traditional Western household: more single-member households, late marriages, more single-parent families, more single-child families, population aging; and
- emigration pressure from South to North.

Demography will favor tourism due to increased disposable time to travel and a desire to compensate "single" life at home with meeting other people opportunities when traveling. Important parts of employment and immigration will tend to look for and find jobs in the tourism sector.

Political Factors

- removal of administrative barriers to international travel,
- polarization of political power and influences, and
- political integration.

The latter will boost affinity exchanges and trips in many areas: school, training, science, business, culture, and local communities.

Globalization <=> Localization

- growing power of global corporations and international market forces,
- reduced control by national governments,
- conflict between modernity and identity, and
- demands to preserve ethnicity, religion and social structures confronted with pressure by media, and market approaches to use values as commodities.

The problems emphasized above are commonly attributed to developing countries confronted with the Western type of tourism, but the countries of the North do not escape such problems either.

Socioenvironmental Awareness

- increased public sensitivity and
- media focus on disasters and infringements in the environmental area.

As tourism, especially under its leisure coverage, is regarded as a commodity, it may become an object of trade negotiations. It is possible that, in the future, the volumes of tourism will have to be delimited by taking into consideration the established carrying capacity (of areas, resources, facilities, etc.).

Living and Working Environments

- growing urban congestion.

The more people concentrate in urban areas, the more they experience the need to travel to the countryside, rural areas, and small traditional towns to experience parallel and past "authenticity." This creates the demand for more transport facilities between the city and the hinterland.

Change from "Service" to "Experience" Economy

- focus switching to delivering unique leisure experiences that personally engage the consumer.

This is a long-term perspective that will engage only a limited percentage of consumers.

Tourist Safety and Security   Many actual and potential tourism destinations are concerned or associated with safety and security problems derived from social unrest, delinquency, terrorism, natural disasters, and health hazards.

Quality   Tourist safety and security is a basic condition for quality. Quality is an overriding concept that best reflects all of the other concerns and determinants shaping tourism demand. The objective is the quality of tourism experience interacting with all ingredients of the tourism product and involving all of its factors.

The present article is an adapted summary of WTO's "Tourism 2020 Vision: A New Forecast from the World Tourism Organization" (revised and updated).

Chapter 8

INFORMATION SOURCES IN TRAVEL MEDICINE

DAVID O. FREEDMAN AND CLAUDINE LEUTHOLD

INTRODUCTION AND OVERVIEW

Travel medicine providers need to be familiar with constantly changing disease risk patterns in over 220 different countries. Travel medicine practices are expanding and multiplying. The knowledge on which interventions are based is evolving rapidly as more data on increasing numbers of travelers are disseminated through publication in the literature. Travelers are finding ever more exotic and previously unvisited locales to go to. In addition, these travelers are bringing ever more sophisticated amounts of information into the pretravel medical encounter.

At the present time, keeping current primarily means using the wide array of resources available on the Internet or through frequently updated software packages or other electronic media. These resources have yet to replace books, print journals, newsletters, and institutional bulletins. However, the delays inherent in producing print media mean that these are now primarily reference sources for detailed reading on a particular topic. Not only are essentially all of the most important authoritative national and international surveillance bulletins, outbreak information, and official recommendations available on the World Wide Web, but they are often available electronically prior to appearance in print. Patients almost everywhere have open access to these medical information resources on the Internet. Travel medicine providers who are not current with what is posted on the popular and authoritative Internet sites will be at a disadvantage when interacting with their patients.

This chapter will provide lists and background information on key travel medicine-oriented information resources targeted to travel medicine professionals. Selected consumer-targeted resources will be outlined briefly. Electronic media will be emphasized over print media so that when available in both formats, information will be provided on how to locate the electronic version of that resource. In essentially all cases, this will then allow the user to also locate the print version of that resource should it be necessary. By their nature, electronic resources change both location (Web sites) and content (Web sites and software packages) more frequently than can be compensated for in a printed resource

text such as this. The electronic resources discussed below were current at press time but inevitably some information will be outdated by the time this chapter is in the hands of the reader.

REFERENCE TEXTS

The first section of Table 8–1 lists selected core reference texts with primary emphasis on comprehensive approaches to travel medicine and to keeping travelers alive and healthy. The key resource texts listed in the next section are not specifically aimed at travel medicine providers but are helpful in providing detailed background information on infectious diseases, epidemiology, and pharmacology that may be helpful in dealing with select or unusual patients. Some special groups of patients may be more frequent in certain health care settings, and the listed publications may be worthwhile for providers who see many of a particular type of traveler. Many World Health Organization (WHO) and Pan American Health Organization (PAHO) publications are appropriate to travel medicine. Several select publications are listed and information on how to access the listings of the complete set of publications is provided. Both the Centers for Disease Control (CDC) and WHO Yellow Books are available over the Internet (Table 8–2), but due to the frequent use both of these publications see in many settings, most providers still prefer to keep a hard-copy bound version on hand. Many very high-quality travel medicine reference booklets are produced by national or regional societies or governmental entities. As these are not easily publicized or available across national boundaries, they will not be considered here. Several popular English-language books targeted at consumers are listed and several others are listed under their Internet location (see Table 8–2). Health care providers need to be aware of what their patients are reading in order to be able to understand concerns and correct any misunderstandings that sometimes can arise from a lay literature that is of varying quality.

JOURNALS

Table 8–3 lists selected English-language journals that consistently and frequently feature articles on travel medicine. Many of these journals give free Internet access

---

Statement of potential conflicts of interest: D. Freedman is a paid consultant to Shoreland, Inc., Milwaukee, U.S.A. C. Leuthold is employed full-time as a project manager for Astral, Inc., Geneva, Switzerland.

Table 8–1.   BOOKS

GENERAL TRAVEL MEDICINE

Cook GC. Travel associated disease. London: Royal College of Physicians of London, 1995.

Freedman DO. Travel medicine. Infectious Disease Clinics of North America. Philadelphia: WB Saunders, 1998. http://www.wbsaunders.com/

Jong EC. Travel medicine. Medical Clinics of North America. Philadelphia: WB Saunders 1999. http://www.wbsaunders.com/

Jong EC, McMullen R. The travel and tropical medicine manual. 3rd Ed. Philadelphia: WB Saunders, 2000. http://www.wbsaunders.com/

Thompson RF. Travel and routine immunizations. Milwaukee, WI: Shoreland, 2000. http://www.shoreland.com

U.S. Department of Health and Human Services, Centers for Disease Control and Prevention. The "CDC Yellow Book." Health information for international travel. 1995–2000 Ed. Order from the U.S. Government Printing Office. Catalogue number 017-023 00202-3. Superintendent of Documents, PO Box 371954, Pittsburgh, PA 15250 7954. Fax: 202-512-2250. Tel: 202-512-1800. http://www.access.gpo.gov. New edition in 2001.

KEY RESOURCE TEXTS

Chin J. Control of communicable diseases manual. 17th Ed. Washington, DC: American Public Health Association, 2000. http://www.apha.org

Gilles HM, Warrell DA. Bruce-Chwatt's essential malariology. 3rd Ed. New York: Oxford University Press, 1993.

Parfitt K, ed. Martindale the complete drug reference. 32nd Ed. London: PhP Pharmaceutical Press, 1999.

2000 Red Book. Report of the Committee on Infectious Diseases. Elk Grove, IL: American Academy of Pediatrics, 2000. http://www.aap.org/pubserv

Wilson ME. A world guide to infections. New York: Oxford University Press, 1991.

SPECIAL GROUPS OF TRAVELERS

Auerbach PS. Wilderness medicine. Management of wilderness and environmental emergencies. 3rd Ed. St. Louis: Mosby, 1995. http://www.mosby.com

Backer HD. Wilderness first aid: emergency care for remote locations. Sudbury, MA: Jones and Bartlett, 1998. http://www.jbpub.com

Herzstein JA. International occupational and environmental medicine. St. Louis: Mosby, 1998. http://www.mosby.com

Hultgren H. High altitude medicine. Stanford, CA: Hultgren Publications, 1997. http://www.highaltitudemedicine.com

Refugee health. Medecins Sans Frontieres. London: Macmillan Education, 1997. http://www.msf.org

WHO PUBLICATIONS

Contact: WHO, Distribution and Sales, CH-1211 Geneva 27, Switzerland. Tel: 41 22 791 24 76. Fax: 41 22 791 48 57. E-mail: publications@who.ch. List of country sales agents: http://www.who.int/dsa/cat97/zsale.htm

International medical guide for ships. Including the ship's medicine chest. 2nd Ed. 1988. Order no. 1152078.

WHO technical report series. Many disease specific reports. See listing: http://www.who.int/dsa/cat97/ztrs.htm

WHO Yellow Book. International travel and health: vaccination requirements and health advice. Situation as of 1 January 2000. Order no. 1180000. Annual update.

PAN AMERICAN HEALTH ORGANIZATION PUBLICATIONS

List of sales agents at http://www.paho.org e-mail sales@paho.org

Health in the Americas. Washington, DC: Pan American Health Organization, 1998. Scientific publication no. 569. www.paho.org

CONSUMER-ORIENTED BOOKS

Dawood R. Traveler's health. Oxford: Oxford Paperbacks, 1992.

Rose SR. 2000 International travel health guide. Northampton, MA: Travel Medicine, 2000. http://www.travmed.com

Savage P. The safe travel book. A guide for the international traveller. New York: Macmillan, 1993. http://www.macmillan.com

to their tables of contents and sometimes abstracts (see Table 8–2).

TRAVEL CLINIC SOFTWARE

In the past decade, electronic information systems for travel health counseling have become widely used and increasingly sophisticated. These systems allow the user to query large electronic databases containing information on disease risk, epidemiology, and vaccine recommendations across the more than 200 countries in the world. Since the majority of providers who counsel patients do this as only one component of a larger practice, these systems allow a rapid, convenient means of accessing a large body of changing information.

Table 8–2.   TRAVEL MEDICINE WEB SITES

AUTHORITATIVE TRAVEL MEDICINE RECOMMENDATIONS

CDC Home Travel Information	http://www.cdc.gov/travel/index.htm
CDC Yellow Book 1999–2000	http://www.cdc.gov/travel/yellowbk99.pdf
WHO Yellow Book 2000	http://www.who.int/ith/
Health Canada Travel Medicine	http://www.hc-sc.gc.ca/hpb/lcdc/osh/tmp_e.html
Swiss Travel Medicine Recommendations (German, French)	http://www.admin.ch/bag/infekt/prev/reisemed/
Robert Koch Institute Guidelines (German)	http://www.rki.de/GESUND/STIKO/STIKO.HTM
German Tropical Medicine Society (German)	http://www.dtg.mwn.de/index.htm
Italian Recommendations (Italian)	http://www.sanita.interbusiness.it/malinf/
Belgium-Prince Leopold Institute Recommendations (French)	http://www.itg.be/travel/LIJSTF.htm
U.K. 1997 Malaria Guidelines	http://www.phls.co.uk/advice/cdrr1097.pdf
Aircraft Disinsection Policies	http://ostpxweb.dot.gov/policy/safety/disin.htm

TRAVEL WARNINGS AND CONSULAR INFORMATION

U.S. State Department Advisories	http://travel.state.gov/travel_warnings.html
U.K. Consular Information	http://www.fco.gov.uk/travel/
Canada Advisory Reports	http://www.dfait-maeci.gc.ca/travelreport/menu_e.htm
Australia Consular Sheets	http://www.dfat.gov.au/consular/advice/advices_mnu.html
Germany Consular Information (German)	http://www.auswaertiges-amt.de/5_laende/index.htm
Swiss Travel Warnings (German, French)	http://www.dfae.admin.ch/site/f/schweiz/hinweise/reisehinweise.html
France Travel Warnings (French)	http://www.france.diplomatie.fr/voyageurs/etrangers/avis/conseils/default.asp

SURVEILLANCE AND EPIDEMIOLOGIC BULLETINS

MMWR Weekly and Summaries	http://www2.cdc.gov/mmwr/
WHO Weekly Epidemiological Record	http://www.who.int/wer/
EuroSurveillance Weekly	http://www.eurosurv.org/update/
EuroSurveillance Monthly	http://www.ceses.org/eurosurv/
U.K. CDR Weekly	http://www.phls.co.uk/publications/cdrw.htm
Canada Communicable Disease Report	http://www.hc-sc.gc.ca/hpb/lcdc/publicat/ccdr/index.html
Australia Communicable Diseases	http://www.health.gov.au/pubhlth/cdi/cdihtml.htm
U.S. Military Surveillance	http://www.geis.ha.osd.mil/
SCIEH Weekly Report (Scotland)	http://www.show.scot.nhs.uk/scieh/report.htm
France SentiWeb (French)	http://www.b3e.jussieu.fr/sentiweb/en/
French Weekly Surveillance Bulletin (French)	http://www.rnsp-sante.fr/beh/index.html
Swiss Infectious Disease Statistics (German, French)	http://www.admin.ch/bag/infreporting/
Robert Koch Institute Bulletin (German)	http://www.rki.de/INFEKT/EPIBULL/EPIBULL.HTM
Italy Bulletin (Italian)	http://www.sanita.interbusiness.it/malinf/BollEpid/indice.htm
Netherlands Surveillance Bulletin (Dutch)	http://www.isis.rivm.nl/inf_bul/home_bul.html
Finland Bulletin (Finnish)	http://www.ktl.fi/ttr/
Spain Bulletin (Spanish)	http://cne.isciii.es/bes/bes.htm
Sweden Bulletin/Statens (Swedish)	http://www.ssi.dk/en/index.html
South Ireland Bulletin	http://www.ucc.ie/ucc/faculties/medical/infoscan/
Portuguese Bulletin (Portuguese)	http://www.dgsaude.pt/
Hong Kong Bulletin	http://www.info.gov.hk/dh/diseases/content.htm
Japan Bulletin	http://idsc.nih.go.jp/iasr/index.html
Norway Bulletin (Norwegian)	http://www.folkehelsa.no/
FluNet—WHO	http://oms2.b3e.jussieu.fr/flunet/

EMERGING DISEASES AND OUTBREAKS

WHO EMC Home	http://www.who.int/emc/index.html
EMC Outbreak	http://www.who.int/emc/outbreak_news/index.html
ProMed	http://www.promedmail.org

continued

Table 8–2.   Continued

INTERNATIONAL AGENCIES

WHO Main Page	http://www.who.int/
WHO Infectious Disease Health Topics	http://www.who.int/health-topics/idindex.htm
WHO Fact Sheets	http://www.who.int/inf-fs/en/index.html
CDC Health Topics A to Z	http://www.cdc.gov/health/diseases.htm
Pan American Health Organization (PAHO)	http://www.paho.org/
International Civil Aviation Organization (ICAO)	http://www.icao.int/
International Air Transport Association (IATA)	http://www.iata.org/
U.S. FAA Aviation Certification Program	http://www.faa.gov/avr/iasa/index.htm

CONSUMER TRAVEL HEALTH

Travel Health On-line	http://www.tripprep.com
Fit For Travel (Munich; in German)	http://www.fit-for-travel.de/
Fit For Travel (Munich; in English)	http://www.fit-for-travel.de/en/index.html
Fitfortravel (SCIEH Scotland) (unrelated to original Fit For Travel Website)	http://www.fitfortravel.scot.nhs.uk/
SafeTravel Switzerland	http://www.safetravel.ch/
High Altitude	http://www.high-altitude-medicine.com
Lonely Planet Health	http://www.lonelyplanet.com/health/health.htm
Highway To Health	http://www.highwaytohealth.com/
MASTA	http://www.masta.org/home.html
MASTA Australia	http://www.masta.edu.au/maps.html
TMVC Australia	http://www.tmvc.com.au/info.html
Medicine Planet	http://www.medicineplanet.com

DISABILITY RESOURCES

American Diabetes Association	http://www.diabetes.org/
SATH	http://www.sath.org/
Acess-able Page	http://www.access-able.com/
Mobility International	http://www.miusa.org
Disabilities Newsletter	http://www.sasquatch.com/ableinfo/

OVERSEAS ASSISTANCE

AEA	http://www.aeaintl.com/
International SOS	http://www.intsos.com/index.htm
IAMAT	http://www.sentex.net/~iamat/
State Department Medevac Resources List	http://travel.state.gov/medical.html

MAPS AND COUNTRY INFORMATION

CIA World Factbook	http://www.odci.gov/cia/publications/factbook/index.html
State Department Background Notes	http://www.state.gov/www/background_notes/index.html
Links to Map Libraries	http://www-map.lib.umn.edu/map_libraries.html
Map-Related Web Sites	http://www.lib.utexas.edu/Libs/PCL/Map_collection/map_sites/map_sites.html
UN Maps	http://www.un.org/Depts/Cartographic/english/htmain.htm
PCL Map Collection	http://www.lib.utexas.edu/Libs/PCL/Map_collection/Map_collection.html

SECURITY

U.S. State Department OSAC	http://www.ds-osac.org/
Kroll Associates	http://www.krollworldwide.com/home.cfm
Control Risks Group	http://www.crg.com/

continued

Table 8–2.   Continued

PROFESSIONAL SOCIETIES

International Society of Travel Medicine (ISTM)	http://www.istm.org
ISTM Directory of Travel Clinics	http://www.istm.org/disclinics.html
American Society of Tropical Medicine and Hygiene (ASTMH)	http://www.astmh.org/
ASTMH Directory of Travel Clinics	http://www.astmh.org/clinics/clinindex.html
Royal Society of Tropical Medicine and Hygiene (RSTMH)	http://www.rstmh.org/
Canadian Society of International Health	http://www.csih.org/
Divers Alert Network	http://www.diversalertnetwork.org/home.htm
Wilderness Medical Society	http://www.wms.org/
Malaria Foundation	http://www.malaria.org/
Undersea and Hyperbaric Medicine Society	http://www.uhms.org/

JOURNALS WITH TRAVEL MEDICINE CONTENT

Journal of Travel Medicine	http://www.istm.org/jtm.html
Emerging Infectious Diseases Journal	http://www.cdc.gov/ncidod/eid/index.htm
American Journal of Tropical Medicine and Hygiene	http://www.ajtmh.org/
Transactions RSTMH	http://www.rstmh.org/pgs/tmframe1.htm
Tropical Medicine and International Health	http://www.blacksci.co.uk/~cgilib/jnlpage.bin?Journal=TMIH&File=TMIH&Page=aims
Medical Letter	http://www.medicalletter.com/
The Lancet	http://www.thelancet.com/
British Medical Journal	http://www.bmj.com/bmj/

ACADEMIC TRAINING IN TRAVEL MEDICINE

Medicus Mundi Switzerland	http://www.medicusmundi.ch/
HealthTraining.org Directory	http://www.healthtraining.org
London School of Hygiene and Tropical Medicine	http://www.lshtm.ac.uk/
Gorgas Memorial Institute	http://www.gorgas.org
Liverpool School of Tropical Medicine	http://www.liv.ac.uk/lstm/lstm.html
Swiss Tropical Institute	http://www.sti.unibas.ch/kurse.htm
Tulane Tropical Medicine	http://www.tropmed.tulane.edu/tropmed.htm
James Cook University	http://www.jcu.edu.au/school/phtm/PHTM/putravel.htm
Mahidol Tropical Medicine	http://www.mahidol.ac.th/mahidol/tm/h-tromed.htm
University of Glasgow	http://www.dph.gla.ac.uk/Teaching.htm

Table 8–3.   JOURNALS FREQUENTLY PUBLISHING PAPERS ON TRAVEL MEDICINE

Journal of Travel Medicine	*Clinical Infectious Diseases*
American Journal of Tropical Medicine and Hygiene	*Wilderness and Environmental Medicine*
Tropical Medicine and International Health	*Aviation, Space, and Environmental Medicine*
Transactions of the Royal Society of Tropical Medicine and Hygiene	*Journal of Occupational and Environmental Medicine*
Lancet	*Annals of Tropical Medicine and Parasitology*
British Medical Journal	*Journal of Tropical Medicine and Hygiene*
Journal of the American Medical Association	*Bulletin of the World Health Organization*
Emerging Infectious Diseases Journal	*Pan American Journal of Public Health*
Journal of Infectious Diseases	

Most high-quality systems now have at least two major components: (1) displays of information including country-by-country information on health risks within a given country, country-by-country vaccine recommendations, and disease-by-disease fact sheets for major dis- eases; and (2) an itinerary maker feature that, after input of a complete patient itinerary, prints out summary rec- ommendations for the entire itinerary in the order of travel. These printouts generally include a vaccination plan, malaria recommendations, destination risks, and in-country resources and are individualized with the name of the patient and the clinic. In addition, detailed country-by-country disease maps, especially for malaria or yellow fever, are important features to consider in evaluating a system. Printouts of these can be important in educating patients who may have indefinite or changeable itineraries. Many software packages also now include global distribution maps for a number of important tropical diseases. As described individually in Table 8–4, a number of other important and useful features are included in many of the available packages.

The available electronic databases are mainly PC based and are accessed in a number of differing ways as listed for individual packages in Table 8–4. These include directly from a PC hard disk, from CD-ROM, from a local area network, via on-line dial-up modem connection, via Intranet, or increasingly via Internet Web-based browser access. Several vendors offer multiple different access options for the same database software. Ease of use of each of the different formats is largely a function of local circumstances: (1) the availability of high-speed modem lines, (2) the availability of high-quality and high-speed

Table 8–4. TRAVEL CLINIC SOFTWARE

CATIS

Country/Language:	Canada/English
Reference/Distribution:	Computerized-Assisted Travel Information System (CATIS). Dr. David Lawee. Travel Information & Supplies. PO Box 41003, 2795 Bathurst St. Toronto, Ontario, Canada M6B 4J6. Tel/fax: 416-785-6219.
Content:	Country-by-country vaccine recommendations, plus disease risk information both textual or illustrated with colored maps. Brief disease and vaccine fact sheets. Comparison maps for CDC, WHO, CATMAT; malaria recommendations. Itinerary maker feature requires responses to a multiscreen detailed questionnaire even if patient and itinerary are uncomplicated. Requires patient to have detailed knowledge of in-country itinerary. Printout generated accounting for traveler health status. Printed prescription for malaria prophylaxis with calculation of dosage, number of tablets required, and schedule of administration. No country background or emergency contact information.
Target audience:	Specialized travel clinic and health professionals
Type/Material:	PC only, DOS or Windows 95 NT, install from CD-ROM onto hard disk
Update/Price:	Periodic updates at unspecified intervals/Canadian $525.00 (DOS) or $750 (Windows 95 NT) + taxes C$125/175 annual for updates

GIDEON

Country/Language:	Israel, USA/English
Reference/Distribution:	Global Infectious Disease & Epidemiology Network (GIDEON). Dr. Steven Berger. E-mail: mberger@post.tau.ac.il. http://www.Cyinfo.com
	Israel: C.Y. Informatics, 34 Keren Hayesod St, Ramat Hasharon, Israel, 47248, Tel: 972-3-549-1120, Fax: 972-3-549-2956.
	USA: Gideon USA, 15 Oak Street, Beverly Farms, MA 01915. Tel: 1-800-316-8585, 978-927-3808, Fax: 978-927-1308
Content:	Most detailed database available containing epidemiologic and diagnostic information on over 300 common and exotic infectious diseases as they occur in over 200 countries. Algorithm links key clinical features and epidemiologic profiles in individual patients to give ranked differential diagnoses based on likelihoods. Useful for answering important epidemiologic questions but not targeted for use in routine pretravel consultation.
Target audience:	Health professionals, clinical laboratories
Type/Material:	PC, Windows
Update/Price:	Quarterly/$395 (single user), $895.00 and up (site license)

MASTA

Country/Language:	United Kingdom/English
Reference/Distribution:	The Medical Advisory Service for Travellers (MASTA), London School of Hygiene and Tropical Diseases, Keppel Street, London WC1E 7HT. Tel: 0171-631-4408. Public access 09068 224100.
Content:	Itinerary maker interface generates an immunization, malaria prophylaxis schedule taking into account past immunizations. General disease brief for the itinerary. Risk evaluation for 84 conditions in any of the 230 countries under different living conditions. Recent epidemiologic news. Seasonal disease inquiry, disease-by-disease fact sheets.
Target audience:	Health professionals, individual travelers
Type/Material:	On-line access via PC or terminal with a modem. Travelers access via automated telephone voice mail questionnaire. Printed summary recommendations then mailed. Only in U.K.
Update/Price:	Dial-up service: annual/£895.00. Printout by mail to public—no charge.
Comment:	Available with some modification in Germany (in German) via dial-up modem from Centrum für Reisemedizin (CRM), Oberrather Strasse 10, D-40472 Düsseldorf. Tel: 49-211-90-42-960, Fax: 49-211-90-42-969. DM 230 then DM 360/year. Also in South Africa and Australia.

continued

Table 8–4. Continued

MEDITRAVEL and EDISAN

Country/Language:	France/French
Reference/Distribution:	Pr A. Bourgeade, Dr H. Chaudet, CD-Conseil, rue Le Sueur 18, F-75116 Paris. Tel: 33-1-40-67-78-72, Fax: 33-1-40-67-78-79, E-mail: conseil@calva.net
Content:	Country-by-country information on recommended vaccines and disease risks. 1500 country-disease risk maps for multiple diseases. Disease risk map for malaria only. Disease-by-disease fact sheets. Drug and vaccine information sheets. Background information, geopolitical map, and emergency contact information (French and Swiss embassies) in the destination country. Destination medical resources including medical facilities, practitioners, and pharmacies. No itinerary maker feature or integrated printout for multicountry itinerary. Does not account for underlying health problems.
Target audience:	Health professionals, travel clinics, private companies
Type/Material:	Meditravel: CD-ROM, Macintosh, Windows and hard disk. EDISAN: CD-ROM only, Mac 7.5.5 or greater, Windows 95/98 or NT 4.0 or greater.
Update/Price:	Meditravel: Biannual on CD-ROM/$170/year. EDISAN: Every 6 weeks/$2,000 + $850/year. Accompanied by printed "Guide Edisan" medical reference guide.
Comment:	Meditravel is an abbreviated version of the EDISAN database with less detail on medical facilities and emergency logistics. Quarterly newsletter with both products.

TRAVAX

Country/Language:	USA/English
Reference/Distribution:	Shoreland, Inc., P.O. Box 13795, Milwaukee, WI 53213-0795, USA. Tel: 414-290-1900 (800-433-5256 in USA and Canada), Fax: 414-290-1907, E-mail: sales@shoreland.com, Internet: www.shoreland.com. Since 1986.
Content:	Basic travel health recommendations. Country-by-country information for disease risks, vaccine recommendations, current disease outbreaks. Disease-by-disease fact sheets. Very detailed malaria, yellow fever, and cholera risk maps by country. Health-related entry requirements. Detailed country profiles including geography and climate. Crime, security, and other associated information. Contact information for U.S., Australian, and Canadian embassies and consulates. List of Internet URLs for U.S. State Department resources. Itinerary maker feature considers order of travel and presents summary recommendations for entire itinerary. Printout for each country can be customized to allow physician-added comments and allows deletion of sections not of use to an individual patient.
Target audience:	Health professionals, corporate medical departments
Type/Material:	PC software on diskettes (installs to local or network hard disk drive) for Windows 3.1, 95, 98, NT
Update/Price:	Weekly/$895 or monthly/$595.00 for single user. Other license fees vary by number of sites/users. Weekly service packaged with monthly literature reviews, clinic operations manual, and printed reference materials. E-mail updates available. Internet/direct subscription available via Web browser beginning in 2000.
Comment:	The original and most widely used in U.S./Canada PC-based travel medicine software. Travax EnCompass, an expanded (detailed overseas medical facility data) wholly Internet-based version, is available to corporations with licenses beginning at $6,000/yr.

TRAVAX (independent from Shoreland product)

Country/Language:	United Kingdom (Scotland)/English
Reference/Distribution:	Provided within the National Health Service, available from the Scottish Center for Infection and Environmental Health, Ruchill Hospital, Glasgow G3 7LN. travax@scieh.tcom.co.uk. www.nxl.co.uk/scieh
Content:	Basic travel health recommendations. Country-by-country information for disease risks, vaccine recommendations, current disease outbreaks. Disease-by-disease fact sheets. No maps or itinerary maker feature. Vaccine and medication details and dosing. Not dogmatic; presents data and encourages users to advise based on personal experience and skills.
Target audience:	All health professionals
Type:	Password-protected Internet access via Web browser.
Update/Price:	Continuous/free via National Health Service for qualified practitioners
Comment:	Limited part of the database available to the public for free via the Internet (see Table 8–2)

TRAVEL CARE

Country/Language:	USA/English
Reference/Distribution:	International SOS Assistance, Inc. Dr. Robert L. Weston, 8 Neshaminy Interplex, Suite 207, Trevose, PA 19053, USA. Tel: 215-633-6606, Fax: 215-244-2213. http://www.travelcare.com (free demonstration available at this site). Corporate@intsos.com
Content:	State Department advisories, basic travel health recommendations, country-by-country disease information. Disease-by-disease fact sheets. Disease-by-disease color maps of global distribution for over 10 tropical diseases. Color country-by-country malaria maps. Vaccine-by-vaccine data sheets. Itinerary maker feature considers order of travel and presents summary recommendations for entire itinerary. High-quality printout can incorporate underlying health conditions if necessary.

continued

Table 8–4.   Continued

Target audience:	Corporate medical departments, academic and government institutions, health care enterprises
Type/Material:	Password-protected Internet access via Web browser. Integrated into package of international medical assistance products
Update/Price:	Daily database update
Comment:	Highly attractive and friendly graphical user interface

TROPIMED (GERMANY AND SWITZERLAND)
ADVICE FOR TRAVELERS on CD-ROM (U.S. Adaptation)

Country/Language:	3 versions: (1) Germany, (2) Switzerland, (3) USA: German, French/German, English
Reference/Distribution:	(1) Institut für Tropenmedizin, Berlin, Pr. Bienzle, Dr. Schönfeld/ASTRAL, Rue Pedro-Meylan 7, CP 142, CH-1211 Geneva 17. Tel: 41-22-718-96-40, Fax: 41-22-718-96-41, E-mail: info@astral.ch. Since 1992.
	(2) Institute for Social and Preventive Medicine, University of Zurich, Professor R. Steffen/ASTRAL, Rue Pedro-Meylan 7, CP 142, CH-1211 Geneva 17. Tel: 41-22-718-96-40, Fax: ++41-22-718-96-41, E-mail: info@astral.ch. Since 1992.
	(3) Professor Murray Wittner, Albert Einstein College of Medicine and the Editors of The Medical Letter, Inc., 1000 Main Street, New Rochelle, New York, 10801-7537. Tel: 800-211-2769, Fax: 914-632-1733, www.medicalletter.com.
Content:	Basic travel health recommendations. Country-by-country information for disease risks, vaccine recommendations. Disease-by-disease fact sheets with risk by country. Country-by-country colored maps for malaria and other selected diseases. Country profiles including geography and climate. Itinerary maker feature considers order of travel and presents summary recommendations for entire itinerary. Allows tailoring to previous vaccine history, health status, and specific vaccine type and name. Printout indicates the vaccines for which the time left before departure is not sufficient. Depending on program version, embassy addresses of the departure country (Germany, Switzerland, USA) with Internet links to these resources. Addresses of vaccination centers for yellow fever (Germany, Switzerland).
Target audience:	Health professionals
Type/Material:	Software on diskettes or CD-ROM/Windows 3.11, 95, 98 NT
Update/Price:	Biannual / (1) DM 270. 00, (2) SF 230. 00, (3) US $160, Faxnews: (1) DM 50. 00, (2) SF 30.00 (3) U.S. Available to the public at www.medicalletter.com.
Comment:	Each version tailored to national guidelines in that country by a national expert. Data updated by monthly epidemiologic news bulletin with recommendations faxed to subscribers. Most used software in Switzerland.

Internet access, (3) the user's capacity to install and regularly update software onto a PC hard disk, and (4) the relative cost of each of these under local conditions.

The database packages listed in Table 8–4 represent the more widely used and available high-quality systems. The quality and timeliness of the information contained in a software package should be the premier consideration. The listed databases all contain high-quality information and the recommendations generated consistently represent those of authoritative national or international bodies. In case of discrepancy between WHO, CDC, and national bodies, many of the software packages highlight these differences and allow for selection of one or the other in generating a final report.

TRAVEL MEDICINE WEB SITES

Those not already familiar with technical aspects of accessing the Internet or the World Wide Web should refer to one of many excellent instructional review articles available to the medical professional.[1–6]

Only selected Web sites that have data of generally high quality and are of broader international interest to travel medicine providers are referenced in Table 8–2. Checking more than one authoritative site on a specific issue is always recommended. First, authoritative recommendations still contain some element of opinion. Thus, even major sources like the CDC and the WHO can disagree on some issues. Second, because of changing disease patterns, what was accurate yesterday may not be accurate today, and some sites are updated more frequently than others. Fortunately, most sites now put an indicator at the bottom of each page stating when the last update was. Always be suspicious of information on a Web page that carries no date. For resources that are not referenced directly in Table 8–2, remember that availability on the World Wide Web does not in itself confer any credibility on information that is presented. Just about anybody can put up an Internet site, and many individuals with much to say but with few credentials do so.

The URLs listed in Table 8–2 are grouped by general category. The sites maintained by the CDC and the WHO contain the most comprehensive primary information. Many important subsidiary Web pages on these sites are not specifically listed in the table but are easily accessible from the CDC and WHO pages that are listed. The sites maintained by the major professional societies, especially that of the International Society of Travel Medicine, also generally contain numerous hyperlinks to other sites. Use of these already existing hyperlinks will save the user time in avoiding having to key in the URLs himself or herself. The consumer-oriented sites are widely accessed by patients as a primary source of travel health information so it is important for practioners to be familiar with what their patients are reading.

ELECTRONIC DISCUSSION FORUMS AND LISTSERVS

Listservs are electronic distribution lists that function using e-mail. Anyone who has joined a particular listserv group can e-mail a posting to a central server. The posting is then disseminated to all members who have subscribed to the same list. If the list is unmoderated, then this dissemination is automatic. If the list is moderated, then the moderator or editor must manually approve each posting prior to its dissemination. The moderator serves the purpose of eliminating irrelevant or repetitive postings and allowing for more focused discussions.

Four electronic discussion groups are recommended for travel medicine providers (Table 8–5). To join one of these listservs, an e-mail message must be sent to the server as specified in Table 8–5. Once a person is accepted as a list member, the computer will generate, by e-mail, a list of instructions on how to participate in the discussion for that group. TravelMed is an unmoderated discussion of issues related to the practice of travel medicine (see http://www.istm.org/listserv.html for further information). ProMed-mail is a moderated discussion of emerging infections with the ability to post only a proportion of submissions received. It presently has over 20,000 subscribers.

Some listservs are set up to provide information only and not to allow interactive discussion. For example, with MMWR-TOC, subscribers receive by e-mail each Friday morning the table of contents of that week's CDC *Morbidity and Mortality Weekly Report*. Subscribers can then decide whether to download the whole issue from the CDC server. Similar arrangements are in place for the *Emerging Infectious Diseases Journal*, Eurosurveillance, and the WHO *Weekly Epidemiological Record*. The travel advisories listserv automatically e-mails U.S. State Department Consular Information sheets each time one is updated or changed or when a travel advisory or warning is issued.

Table 8–5.   **LISTSERVS RELEVENT TO TRAVEL MEDICINE PRACTICE**

Discussion groups

Type in the body of the message:	*Send to this address:*
Subscribe TRAVELMED your name*	listserv@yorku.ca
Subscribe TROPMED your name†	listserv@yorku.ca
Subscribe PROMED your name	majordomo@promedmail.org
Subscribe MALARIA your name	listserv@wehi.edu.au

Automated Information Services

Type in the body of the message:	*Send to this address:*
Subscribe MMWR-TOC	listserv@listserv.cdc.gov
Subscribe EID-TOC	listserv@cdc.gov
Subscribe WER-REH	majordomo@who.ch
Subscribe DOSTRAVEL your name	listserv@listserv.uic.edu
Eurosurveillance Weekly	Point Web browser to www.eurosurv.org

*List restricted to members of the International Society of Travel Medicine.
†List restricted to members of the American Society of Tropical Medicine and Hygiene.

REFERENCES

1. Peters R, Sikorski R. Digital dialogue. Sharing information and interests on the Internet. JAMA 1997;277:1258–1260.
2. Pallen M. The World Wide Web. BMJ 1995;311:1552–1556.
3. Peters R, Sikorski R. Navigating to knowledge. Tools for finding information on the Internet. JAMA 1997;277:505–506.
4. Sikorski R, Peters R. Internet anatomy 101. Accessing information on the World Wide Web. JAMA 1997;277:171–172.
5. Sikorski R, Peters R. Medical literature made easy. Querying databases on the Internet. JAMA 1997;277:959–960.
6. Sonnenberg F. Health information on the Internet. Opportunities and pitfalls [editorial; comment]. Comment on: Arch Intern Med 1997;157:209–212. Arch Intern Med 1997;157:151–152.

COMPLIANCE WITH TRAVEL HEALTH RECOMMENDATIONS

JAY S. KEYSTONE

In the Judeo-Christian tradition, the first recorded incident of noncompliance, albeit in a nontraveler, occurred in the Garden of Eden when Eve ate the fruit of the tree of knowledge.[1] In this chapter, compliance is defined as the extent to which a person's behavior (in terms of following medication, dietary, or lifestyle recommendations) coincides with medical or health advice. Since the word *compliance* today is deemed by some to be politically incorrect because it conjures up images of serfdom, the reader is free to substitute for it the term *adherence*.

A review of compliance with health recommendations by travelers should cover such areas as immunizations, malaria chemoprophylaxis and self-treatment, dietary recommendations to prevent travelers' diarrhea, safer sex practices for the avoidance of sexually transmitted disease, use of seat belts in motor vehicles, and a dozen or more do's and don'ts that have been promulgated by health care providers to terrified travelers over the decades. Unfortunately, many of these rules of travel health have not been systematically studied from a compliance perspective. The aim in this chapter is to give the reader an overview of current levels of compliance with a few selected recommendations, highlight the reasons and factors for noncompliance, and provide a well-established framework for scientists and clinicians to draw on as they search for solutions to the problem of noncompliance in the field of travel medicine.

PREVENTION/SELF-TREATMENT OF MALARIA

GENERAL

Only recently has the issue of compliance with recommendations to prevent malaria been addressed in the literature. However, it is important to note that most studies have been retrospective ones in which compliance was determined after exposure, without the investigator knowing for certain what information was provided to travelers before departure to malarious areas. Even when travelers have been provided with pretravel information, recent studies of health care provider knowledge in this area suggest the possibility that travelers might be receiving incorrect or insufficient information on the subject.[2–4] In 1984, a telephone survey of health care providers in Canada showed that malaria advice was correctly given

by only 25% of respondents.[2] Hatz et al. showed recently that among 150 general practitioners in Switzerland and Germany, only 11% of Swiss and 1% of German general practitioners reported correct recommendations for malaria protection and immunizations according to their national standard.[4] With respect to malaria prevention other than with drugs, only 27% of Swiss and 19% of German practitioners recommended three personal protection measures against mosquito bites. Another recent study of primary care physicians in the United States showed that only 12% of those who give pretravel advice were able to provide correct malaria recommendations.[3] Finally, even among travel experts, there is considerable variability in the quality of pretravel advice provided. In 1993, a survey of travel experts across North America showed that malaria recommendations were correctly provided by only 60% to 80% of respondents.[5]

COMPLIANCE WITH MALARIA CHEMOSUPPRESSION

In spite of the limitations of present studies, it is clear that compliance with measures to prevent malaria is a fundamental problem that needs to be addressed by travel health care researchers. The largest study of this subject was reported by Steffen et al.[6] They noted that although 99% of 44,472 travelers were informed about the risk of malaria, 90.3% by a medical source, only 55.4% were fully compliant with chemoprophylaxis. Although the majority of travelers (94.1%) took their antimalarials regularly while abroad, slightly more than half of them did not continue their drugs for a full 4 weeks on their return. Similar results were detected in a U.K. study that showed that 50% of travelers stopped their antimalarials before they were supposed to.[7]

Among 4,042 U.S. travelers to Africa and Haiti, 67.4% used chemoprophylaxis during their trip, but only 42.4% used recommended prophylaxis without interruption.[8] This ranged from 50% of travelers to West Africa to 27.4% of travelers returning from Haiti.

An assessment of compliance among a cohort of 547 Dutch travelers showed that only 60% reported uninterrupted chemoprophylaxis use during and after travel.[9] Noncompliance was associated with youth (<30 years), previous travel experience, travel outside of Africa and nonorganized travel. To assess the veracity of self-reported compliance in patients with malaria, Behrens and his colleagues compared reported prophylaxis compliance with plasma drug levels.[10] Not surprisingly, they found significant discrepancies between reported compliance and expected drug levels. Whether these discrepancies were due to "misreporting" or poor recall of antimalarial dosing is a matter of speculation.

COMPLIANCE WITH ANTIMOSQUITO MEASURES

In general, travelers are almost as compliant with measures to prevent insect bites as they are with malaria chemoprophylaxis. In Steffen et al.'s large survey, 55.6% of European travelers to Africa used one or more measures to prevent mosquito bites.[6] Lobel and his colleagues, in a similar but smaller study of European and North American travelers departing Kenya, found that 75% of 5,489 travelers used at least two antimosquito measures.[11] The results of the latter study contrast with the findings in a 1986 survey of 1,796 U.S. travelers returning from Africa that showed that only 56.5% of travelers used antimosquito measures.[12] Thirty-six percent applied insect repellents, 32% sprayed insecticides, and 25% used a mosquito net or wore long-sleeved shirts and trousers in the evening.

STANDBY THERAPY

Self-treatment of malaria, using standby therapy, came into vogue in 1985 when pyrimethamine-sulfadoxine (Fansidar) was no longer recommended for weekly prophylaxis due to the high incidence of severe cutaneous adverse reactions.[13] Since then, the indications have expanded from its original intended use for travelers who were ill with suspected malaria but out of reach of medical attention to those going without prophylaxis to low-risk malaria areas, to overnighters and short-term travelers, and to those with brief repeated exposures, such as airline crews.[14,15]

Several studies have analyzed compliance issues concerning self-treatment of malaria. In Lobel's study of travelers returning from Kenya, 31% of 5,489 travelers carried drugs to treat malaria and 3% treated themselves.[11] Long-stay travelers (8%) were more likely to use presumptive therapy than were short-stay travelers (0.6%). Weinke and his colleagues recently concluded that standby therapy was used too often when they found that 5% of 880 travelers to Africa used it, 54% before seeing a physician and 39% instead of visiting one.[16] The most comprehensive study of self-treatment was carried out recently by Schlagenhauf et al.[17] In a prospective study of 1,187 Swiss travelers, 123 developed an illness that was compatible with malaria. Two-thirds of those who were ill failed to seek medical attention despite their symptoms and comprehensive pretravel advice. Standby treatment was self-administered by six travelers (4.6%), only one of whom had confirmed malaria. The authors concluded that inappropriate behavior and poor malaria awareness among travelers limited this approach.

FACTORS ASSOCIATED WITH NONCOMPLIANCE

Most malaria chemoprophylaxis studies have looked at factors that might predict noncompliance. As expected, use of prophylaxis has been associated with advice received before travel.[8] However, in one study, the use of chemoprophylaxis was not influenced by the source providing the advice; those informed by health care professionals were just as likely to use chemoprophylaxis as those informed of malaria risk by nonmedical ones. These results contrast with a British study that found that shopping around for information was associated with lower compliance.[7]

Several studies have shown that age, duration of travel, and reasons for travel were associated significantly with compliance.[6–16,18] Compliance increased with age and was inversely proportional to the length of the trip. Tourists traveling on organized tours were significantly more compliant than were business men or individual travelers.[19] Those who visited friends and relatives were especially noncompliant.[9] Experienced travelers who have made several trips abroad were less likely to be compliant than first-time travelers.[4] Finally, as expected, adverse reactions to medications have been associated with noncompliance.[6,7,20,21] When asked directly as to the reasons for their noncompliance, travelers frequently said that they forgot, considered the medications to be unnecessary, were advised to stop by locals or other travelers, were concerned about the potential medication side effects, or were confused because fellow travelers were taking different antimalarials from their own.[7,20]

TRAVELERS' DIARRHEA

For hundreds of years, health care providers have been warning travelers to the developing world to avoid certain food and beverages. However, most studies investigating the benefits of such dietary self-restrictions have demonstrated little or no benefit.[22–24] In a worldwide survey of 16,568 tourists, Steffen and his colleagues showed that "travelers' diarrhea seemed to be more frequent the more one tried to elude it."[25] The authors postulated that this was probably due to recall bias. Although several studies have addressed the efficacy of dietary precautions, few have looked at compliance using cohort studies. In a classic paper, Kozicki and his colleagues evaluated the dietary habits of charter tourists returning from abroad.[26] In the first 3 days of travel, only 2% of 688 travelers adhered strictly to the rules and committed no dietary mistakes. During the study, the median number of mistakes committed was 5, with 13 being the largest number of errors. Seventy percent consumed salads, uncooked vegetables, or fruit that could not be peeled and 53% accepted drinks containing ice cubes. Usually, travelers committed the same food faux pas every day. As expected, the incidence of diarrhea correlated well with the number of dietary mistakes. In a recent similar study of Finnish tourists who vacationed in Morocco, only 5% of 933 subjects adhered to generally accepted dietary recommendations. About 45% made five or more dietary errors during a 1- or 2-week holiday; no association between travelers' diarrhea and the number of dietary errors was observed.[27]

It is clear that food and water precautions are by no means a guarantee of good health during travel and are often impractical.[28] Farthing summed up the situation well when he wrote: "Even if one adhered scrupulously to all of these [food] guidelines, as in practice few people do, one might avoid many episodes of travelers' diarrhea, but major and sometimes unacceptable restraints would be placed on one's eating and drinking behavior and on recreational activities. It is for these reasons that alternative measures for prophylaxis have been sought."[29]

CASUAL SEXUAL CONTACT

Although few prospective studies have evaluated compliance of travelers with respect to abstinence of casual sex during travel or use of safer sex practices, a recent excellent review contains an astonishing number of articles related to sexual behavior among international travelers.[30] The most obvious group to study, albeit not representative of the general public, is military personnel who have received pretravel advice concerning sexual behavior. A study of 1,744 returning U.S. Navy and Marine Corps personnel showed that during a 6-month cruise, 49% had had sexual contact, of whom 92% used condoms, but 27% used them inconsistently.[31] Inconsistent condom use was associated with being Hispanic. A prospective study of high-risk Swiss tourists to the tropics showed that 59.8% had casual sex abroad compared with 3.6% of a comparison group that was not selected to be at high risk for casual sexual contact.[32] Twenty-six percent of the high-risk group did not use condoms or used them inconsistently. Explanations of their behavior included indifference at the decisive moment, belief in the health of their partners, or inconvenience. One of the few prospective studies that examined intended sexual behavior abroad was conducted in Australia among persons seeking pretravel health advice at private clinics in five Australian cities. Only 34% of 213 unaccompanied travelers planning a trip to Thailand indicated a definite intention not to have sex while abroad.[33] Regarding choice of potential partners, 24.5% more men than women said they would have sex with a Thai national, 13.7% of men said they would have sex with a bar girl, and 21.7% more women than men said they would choose a fellow Australian traveler. Eighty-two percent of the sample reported that they would use condoms 100% of the time. A rather disturbing prospective intervention study in Switzerland that assessed the effect of advice on AIDS prevention in travelers found that in spite of innovative preventive medicine techniques, 6% of 2,000 travelers had sex abroad, 38% of whom had unprotected sex.[34]

Although most studies show that younger travelers are most likely to engage in casual sex, a study of 1,378 Hong Kong travelers revealed that older travelers, especially married men, were least fearful of HIV infection and were least likely to use condoms consistently.[35] When condom use was assessed in U.K. travelers recently, a surprising high percentage (75%) used condoms consistently with all casual sexual contacts.[36] For men, patterns of condom use abroad with casual contacts reflected patterns of use at home, whereas for women, perhaps not unexpectedly, patterns of condom use varied according to their partners' background.

The few data on sexual behavior of long-term overseas workers are especially worrisome in view of the current HIV epidemic in many parts of the world. In a study of 1,968 Dutch expatriates working in sub-Saharan Africa, 31% of males and 13% of females had sexual contacts with locals during which fewer than 25% used condoms consistently.[37] In another study of Belgian workers in Central Africa, 51% and 31% reported extramarital sex with local women or prostitutes respectively.[38]

HOW DO WE IMPROVE COMPLIANCE?

Compliance with therapy implies a positive behavior in which the patient is sufficiently motivated to adhere to a recommended therapy or preventive measure because of perceived self-benefit and a positive outcome. Depending on the study design, the group being studied, and the measurement method, reported rates of noncompliance with drug therapy average 40% (range 13% to 93%).[39] These rates are comparable with the compliance of travelers with pretravel health recommendations.

A theoretical framework for explaining the likelihood of an individual's undertaking a preventive health action is the Health Belief Model (HBM) (Fig. 9–1).[40] The theory argues that an individual's decision to undertake a health action is dependent on that individual's perception of (a) level of personal *susceptibility* to that particular illness; (b) the degree of *severity* of its consequences; (c) the health actions and potential *benefits*; and (d) the other *barriers* or costs related to initiating the advocated behavior. The HBM also stipulates that a *cue to action* or stimulus must occur to trigger the appropriate behavior by making the individuals aware of their feelings about the health threat.

Several studies have shown that travelers have inaccurate perceptions of various health risks associated with travel. For example, 45% of 100 U.S. elderly travelers chose air travel as their greatest risk factor,[41] 70% of French travelers were concerned about snake or scorpion bites,[42] and 56% of Canadian travelers perceived their risk of illness to be less than 20% in a 1- to 4-week trip to Africa, Asia, or South America.[43]

For many years, health care providers have paternalistically laid down rules and guidelines for behavior during travel that have been shown to be neither beneficial nor practical. Who among us wants to avoid buffet fruit salads at a first-class hotel in the Caribbean on our once in a year vacation, to wear long-sleeved shirts and trousers in 40°C heat of the tropics, or to spend hundreds of dollars for immunizations for potentially low-risk situations. It is time for travel medicine advisors to put ourselves in

INDIVIDUAL PERCEPTIONS   **MODIFYING FACTORS**   **LIKELIHOOD OF ACTION**

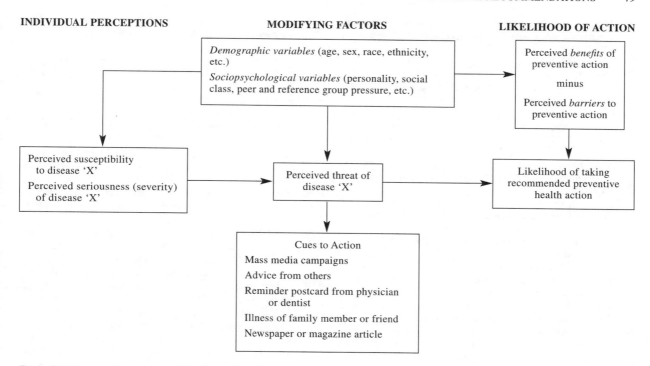

Figure 9–1. Original formulation of the Health Belief Model.

the sandals or flippers of our clients and develop rational, practical, and cost-effective recommendations for prevention of illness during travel. Also, we must do a much better job of cueing travelers about their risks of illness and accidents to increase their likelihood of taking recommended preventive health actions. But, most of all, there is a need for large, multicenter, controlled studies to investigate ways to improve travelers' compliance with health recommendations. It is not only our job, it is our responsibility!

REFERENCES

1. Genesis 2:25–3:24.
2. Keystone JS, Lawee D, McIntyre L, et al. Counseling travelers about malaria. Can Med Assoc J 1984;131:715–716.
3. Lobel HO, Kozarsky PE, Barber M, et al. Pre-travel health advice to international travelers by primary care physicians [abstract 63]. Fourth International Conference on Travel Medicine, Acapulco, April 23–27, 1995.
4. Hatz C, Krause E, Grundmann H. Travel advice—a study among Swiss and German general practitioners. Trop Med Int Health 1997;2:6–12.
5. Keystone JS, Dismukes R, Sawyer L, Kozarsky P. Inadequacies in health recommendations provided for international travelers by North American travel health advisors. J Travel Med 1994;1:72–78.
6. Steffen R, Heusser R, Mächler. Malaria chemoprophylaxis among European tourists in tropical Africa; use, adverse effects and efficacy. Bull World Health Organ 1990;68:313–322.
7. Phillips-Howard PA, Blaze M, Hurn M, Bradley DJ. Malaria prophylaxis: survey of the response of British travelers to prophylactic advice. BMJ 1986;293:932–934.
8. Lobel HO, Campbell CC, Papaioanou M, Huong AY. Use of prophylaxis for malaria by American travelers to Africa and Haiti. JAMA 1987;257:2626–2627.
9. Cobelens FGJ, Leentvaar-Kuijpers A. Compliance with malaria chemoprophylaxis and preventative measures against mosquito bites among Dutch travellers. Trop Med Int Health 1997; 2:705–713.
10. Behrens RH, Taylor RB, Pryce DI, et al. Chemoprophylaxis compliance in travelers with malaria. J Travel Med 1998;5: 92–94.
11. Lobel HO, Phillips-Howard PA, Brandling-Bennett AD, et al. Malaria incidence and prevention among European and North American travelers to Kenya. Bull World Health Organ 1990; 68:209–215.
12. Lobel HO. Malaria and use of prevention measures among United States Travelers. In: Steffen R, Lobel HO, Haworth J, Bradley DJ, eds. Travel medicine. Berlin: Springer-Verlag, 1989:81–89.
13. Centers for Disease Control—revised recommendations of preventing malaria in travelers to areas with chloroquine-resistant *Plasmodium falciparum,* MMWR Morb Mortal Wkly Rep 1985;34:185–195.
14. Schlagenhauf P, Steffen R. Stand-by treatment of malaria in travelers: a review. J Trop Med Hyg 1994;97:151–160.
15. Steffen R, Holdener F, Wyss R, et al. Malaria prophylaxis and self-therapy in airline crews. Aviat Space Environ Med 1990; 111;942–945.
16. Nothdurft HD, Jelinek T, Pechel S, et al. Stand-by treatment of suspected malaria in travellers. Trop Med Parasitol 1995;46:161–163.
17. Schlagenhauf P, Steffen R, Tschopp A, et al. Behavioral aspects of travelers in their use of malaria presumptive treatment. Bull World Health Organ 1995;73:215–221.
18. Phillips-Howard PA, Radalowicz A, Mitchell J, et al. Risk of malaria in British residents returning from malarious areas. BMJ 1990;300:499–503.

19. Held TK, Weinke T, Mansmann U, et al. Malaria prophylaxis: identifying risk groups for non-compliance. Q J Med 1994; 87:17–22.

20. Chatterjee S. Prophylaxis against malaria. BMJ 1995;310:401.

21. Hoebe C, de Munter J, Thijs C. Adverse effects and compliance with mefloquine or proguanil antimalarial chemoprophylaxis. Eur J Clin Pharmacol 1997;52:269–275.

22. Lowenstein MS, Balows A, Gangarosa EJ. Tourists at an international congress in Mexico. Lancet 1973;1:529–531.

23. Chang TW. Travelers' diarrhea. Ann Intern Med 1978;89: 428–429.

24. Ryder RW, Oquist CA, Greenberg H, et al. Travelers' diarrhea, in Panamanian tourists in Mexico. J Infect Dis 1981;144: 442–448.

25. Steffen R, Van der Linde F, Gyr K, Schar M. Epidemiology of diarrhea in travelers. JAMA 1983;249:1176–1180.

26. Kozicki M, Steffen R, Schar M. Boil it, cook it, peel it or forget it: does this rule prevent travelers' diarrhea? Int J Epidemiol 1985;14:169–172.

27. Mattila L, Siitonen A, Kyrönseppä H, et al. Risk behavior for travelers' diarrhea among Finnish travelers. J Travel Med 1995; 2:77–84.

28. Blaser MJ. Environmental interventions for the prevention of travelers' diarrhea. Rev Infect Dis 1986;8(Suppl 2): S142–S150.

29. Farthing MJG. Prevention and Rx of travelers' diarrhea. Aliment. Pharmacol Ther 1991;5:15–30.

30. Mulhall BP. Sex and travel: studies of sexual behavior, disease and health promotion in international travelers—a global review. STD AIDS 1996;7:455–465.

31. Malone JD, Hyams KC, Hawkins RE, et al. Risk factors for sexually-transmitted diseases among deployed U.S. military personnel. Sex Transm Dis 1993;20:294–298.

32. Stricker M, Steffen R, Hornung, R et al. Fluchtige sexuelle Kontakte von Schweizer Touristen in den Tropen. Munch Med Wochenschr 1990;132:175–177.

33. Mulhall BP, Hu M, Thompson M, et al. Planned sexual behavior of young Australian visitors to Thailand. Med J Aust 1993;158:530–535.

34. Gagneux OP, Blöchliger CU, Tanner M, Hatz CF. Malaria and casual sex: what travelers know. J Travel Med 1996;3:14–21.

35. Abdullah ASM, Hedley AJ, Fielding R. Sexual behaviour in travellers. Lancet 1999;353:595.

36. Bloor M, Thomas M, Hood K, et al. Differences in sexual risk behaviour between young men and women travelling abroad from the U.K. Lancet 1998;353:1664–1668.

37. Houweling H, Corotinho RA. Risk of HIV infection among Dutch expatriates in sub-Saharan Africa. Int J STD AIDS 1991;2:252–257.

38. Bonneux L, van der Stuyft P, Tallman H, et al. Risk factors for HIV infections among European expatriates in Africa. BMJ 1988;297:581–584.

39. Bond WS, Hussar DA. Detection methods and strategies for improving medication compliance. Am J Hosp Pharmacol 1991;48:1978–1988.

40. Becker MH, Marman LA, Kirscht JP, et al. Patient perceptions and compliance: recent studies of the Health Belief Model. In: Haynes RB, Taylor DW, Sackett DL, eds. Compliance in health care. Baltimore: Johns Hopkins University Press, 1979:79.

41. Olson Pe, Myers MT, Rumans L, et al. Misperception of travel risks by older travelers [abstract 58]. In: Proceedings of the Third International Conference on Travel Medicine. Paris, France, April 25–29, 1993.

42. Picot N, Receveur MC, Goujon C, et al. Real information needs of the traveller before his departure. Results of a survey by questionnaire. Bull Soc Pathol Exot 1993;86:418–420.

43. McPherson DW, Stephenson BJ. Perception of risk in Canadian travelers [abstract 48]. In: Proceedings of the Third International Conference on Travel Medicine. Paris, France, April 25–29, 1993.

Chapter 10

TRAVEL MEDICINE AND THE TRAVEL MEDICINE CLINIC

10.1 TRAVEL CLINICS IN EUROPE

PATRICK RODRIGUEZ-REDINGTON

Although the term travel clinic is new in Europe, institutions have been advising travelers mainly on malaria and on the compulsory vaccines against smallpox, cholera, and yellow fever for decades. For the latter vaccine, World Health Organization approval in Europe was granted to civilian or military centers for infectious diseases, tropical medicine, or preventive medicine. Air France and British Airways were the first to create travel clinics with the main objective of sparing their passengers long waiting hours in hospital centers. The Air France Center in Paris, created in 1965, is now one of the largest travel clinics worldwide administering more than 100,000 vaccine doses in 1998.

According to a study of 650 travel clinics in Europe, 60% are small and use less than 1,000 doses of yellow fever vaccine per year. Just 8% of the travel health centers perform 57% of all vaccinations for travelers. In France, Germany, and Norway, the majority of travel clinics are in state institutions, whereas most of those in the United Kingdom and the Netherlands are privately owned. In Belgium and Switzerland, the large centers are state owned and the small ones are private.

The activities of the travel clinics vary broadly between countries. Health advice is given to more than 85% of travelers consulting institutions in Switzerland, Norway, Luxembourg, Spain, and Finland. In France, Sweden, and Germany, this rate is 55% to 85%, whereas in the Netherlands, Belgium, and particularly in the United Kingdom and Denmark, this rate is below 55%. About two-thirds of the recommendations are given by a physician and 25% by a nurse, whereas 10% are given by a person trained in travel medicine without prior medical training. Few pharmacies but numerous travelers, family practitioners, and employers request advice by telephone. The proportion of family practitioners seeking advice from travel clinics varies between 10% and 30% in European countries. Larger centers often use taped messages, offering telephone numbers for different destinations. Many travel clinics distribute written advice, particularly in Switzerland, where it has been demonstrated that travelers recall only a small proportion of what they have been told during a travel health advice session.[1]

In Belgium (60% of the centers) and to a lesser extent elsewhere, travel information is also mailed.

Returning travelers are advised and/or examined by 18% of travel clinics in Sweden, but in most European countries, such a service is offered by only 5% of the centers.

The main information sources for European travel clinics stem from the World Health Organization.[2,3] American sources (such as the Centers for Disease Control[4]) and the *Travel Information Manual*[5] are also important sources. In many countries, recommendations are agreed on by expert groups and are therefore distributed nationally.

Of the various on-line or off-line computerized systems being used, the data bank at EDISAN (France) is probably the largest. In various countries, travel clinics are united in networks.

REFERENCES

1. Hanny Georg. Prophylaktische Massnahmen bei Tropenreisen. Dissertation Universität Zürich, 1979.
2. World Health Organization. International travel and health—vaccination requirements and health advice. Geneva: WHO, 1995.
3. World Health Organization. Weekly Epidemiological Record. Weekly publication.
4. Centers for Disease Control. MMWR. Weekly publication.
5. IATA. Travel information manual. Monthly publication.

10.2 TRAVEL CLINICS IN THE UNITED STATES AND CANADA

DAVID R. HILL

The practice of travel medicine varies widely throughout the world; providers of advice range from generalists to tropical disease specialists, and the settings from private offices to medical schools.[1] This diversity makes it difficult to define travel medicine as any one clinic, procedure, or protocol. However, the general setting can be described and an effort made to develop a standard of care for the appropriate practice of travel medicine. In a position paper, Health Canada has set forth their standards for travel medicine.[2] This section will focus on travel clinics within the United States and Canada.

Why choose a travel medicine specialist for the receipt of pretravel advice and preventive measures? This textbook establishes the position that the field of travel medicine encompasses a broad range of clinical medicine not familiar to many primary care health professionals. It is also a field that is constantly changing as new disease patterns are described and new preventive measures become available. In addition, many vaccines may be specialized in both their storage and administration and therefore not readily accessed in a generalist's office. Travel medicine specialists should be able to provide up-to-date information on health conditions throughout the world and give appropriate advice and administer vaccines based on an individual traveler's itinerary and underlying health. The provision of clear, concise advice to many travelers on a consistent basis will likely improve the quality of compliance with preventive measures and translate into improved health for the traveler.

TRAVEL CLINIC SURVEY

Can the current practice of travel medicine be defined? Although there have been studies describing the epidemiology of the travel population, there is very little published information about the actual functioning of travel clinics.[3-5] The most complete survey of travel medicine practices was published in 1996.[1] Members of the International Society of Travel Medicine (ISTM) were contacted in 1994 and asked to complete a survey of their travel medicine services. Worldwide, 341 clinics responded.

Eighty-nine percent of the clinics were located in North America or Western Europe. Most travel medicine was performed in a private office setting (41%), 20% was within a school of medicine, 10% was hospital affiliated, 10% was associated with corporate or student health practices, and 8% was associated with public health departments. Table 10.2–1 presents the affiliations for clinics in the United States. The majority of clinics in Canada are associated with a public health unit.

The greatest variation between clinics occurred in the number of travelers seen each year: 14% of clinics saw ≤ 100 patients per year and 13% more than 5,000. The median number for all clinics was 750 and for U.S. clinics 450. Thus, much of travel medicine was being performed in a private office setting, probably in the context of another practice since a volume of only a few hundred travelers per year would not be sufficient to independently sustain a practice. It might also not be sufficient to sustain an adequate knowledge and experience base for the health professionals working in such settings.[6]

PROVIDER TRAINING

Travel medicine services were almost always directed by physicians (94% of the time), but when clinics were asked who was giving the advice, nurses were providers of advice nearly 60% of the time.[1] In a recent survey from the U.K., over 90% of nurses in the offices of general practitioners were proving advice.[7] The level of training in tropical and travel medicine also varied between countries. Over 60% of all physicians had trained in infectious diseases and/or tropical medicine, but physicians in Canada were more likely to be generalists; in the United States, internists or infectious diseases specialists; and in Europe and the U.K., tropical medicine specialists (Table 10.2–2).

Provider training raises the issue of quality of care in the field. At present, there is no regulation of travel medicine services. Anyone can practice in the field. However, it is clear that the qualifications, level of training, and experience vary widely among providers. The efforts of the American Society of Tropical Medicine and Hygiene (ASTMH) to develop formal training and certification of knowledge in travel and tropical medicine for North America are likely to favorably impact the level and quality of practice. The ISTM is also evaluating training and potential certification. In addition, providers should have experience in the discipline and attend continuing education venues since these are important factors for knowledge in travel medicine.[8]

Table 10.2–1. **AFFILIATION OF UNITED STATES TRAVEL CLINICS (%)***

Private	45
School of medicine	18
Corporate/student health	11
Health maintenance organization	9
Hospital	7
Public health	5
Military	3
Other	2

*Information was obtained on 194 clinics in 1994.[1]

Table 10.2–2.   TRAINING OF TRAVEL MEDICINE PHYSICIAN PROVIDERS*

	U.S. (%)	CANADA (%)
General medicine/family medicine	13%	54%
Internal medicine	25	6
Infectious diseases	39	9
Tropical medicine	7	14
Infectious diseases and tropical medicine	13	14
Other	3	3

*Information was obtained from 320 providers in the United States and 35 providers in Canada.[1]

ACCESSING A TRAVEL CLINIC

Accessing a travel medicine service may be difficult for the average traveler. Initially, they may neither know that they need a specialized service nor be able to discern the quality of the advice they receive. Thus, they may travel without advice or with incorrect advice.[9] Numerous studies have shown that the quality of advice is often inadequate, even among so-called specialists.[4,10–12] Therefore, it is important that as many sources as possible direct travelers to appropriate pretravel care.

One of the most likely reasons for travelers to seek pretravel care is the perception that they need to get "shots." They may be referred to a clinic by a travel agency if there is a history within the community of cooperation between the travel industry and travel medicine. Because a travel agency is frequently the first point of contact for a traveler, these agencies should at least alert the traveler to the potential need for pretravel medical care. The ISTM has developed a position statement in conjunction with the travel industry in North America on a minimum level of health advice that should be provided by travel agencies: travel professionals should advise the traveler of required immunizations and to seek advice from health providers on other destination-specific vaccinations.[13] They should also advise them to seek information about appropriate malaria prevention if traveling to a malaria endemic area.

Travelers may call a health department to inquire where they can receive yellow fever vaccine, the only vaccine required for travel to some countries. In the United States and Canada, yellow fever vaccination may be administered only in approved yellow fever vaccination centers; these are usually travel clinics or health department units. Primary care physicians may refer patients because they do not have the necessary travel vaccines or are not familiar with current malaria prevention recommendations.

Occasionally, travelers will visit Internet sites and identify clinics based on these lists. Three of the most important Internet referral sites are the home pages of the ISTM and the ASTMH and the travel medicine page of the Laboratory Centre for Disease Control (LCDC) in Canada (Appendix). The Canadian Society for International Health also provides a listing of travel clinics. The

ISTM lists clinics only if the clinic personnel are members of the ISTM. As of mid-1999, there were 301 clinics listed in the United States and 39 in Canada. The ASTMH lists providers of tropical and/or travel medicine care who are members of the ASTMH. There were 167 providers listed from the United States and 9 from Canada. The LCDC Web site lists 319 clinics; 55% of these administer yellow fever vaccine. In the United States, however, there are far more providers of travel medicine than those listed on these sites. As an example, in the Hartford, Connecticut area, there is only one clinic listed on either of the ISTM or ASTMH Web sites; however, each regional hospital runs a clinic, many walk-in medical centers provide travel medicine care, and many private offices also provide care, adding up to over 10 places where one can receive pretravel care. The issues raised earlier about quality of care, however, are emphasized again when there are so many providers.

TRAVEL CLINIC SERVICES

Once a travel clinic is identified, what should be the basic level of service? Preventive advice and provision of immunizations should be universal. Vaccination against hepatitis A and B, diphtheria-tetanus, meningococcal meningitis, typhoid fever, measles, mumps, and rubella, yellow fever, rabies, and polio was available in over 80% of clinics worldwide and in 88% and more in clinics in the U.S. and Canada.[1] Advice for the prevention of malaria, insect avoidance, and travelers' diarrhea prevention and therapy was provided in at least 97% of services. A listing of vaccines and topics of prevention that should be available is in Tables 10.2–3 and 10.2–4. A complete com-

Table 10.2–3.   VACCINES*

Recommendations for Travel Clinics

Hepatitis B

Diphtheria/tetanus

Hepatitis A
    Immune globulin
    Parenteral-inactivated

Neiserria meningitidis

Salmonella typhi
    Oral-attenuated
    Whole-cell inactivated
    Vi antigen

Measles-Mumps-Rubella

Yellow fever

Rabies

Polio
    Parenteral-inactivated

Streptococcus pneumoniae

Vibrio cholerae

Hemophilus influenzae

Japanese B encephalitis

*Bacille Calmette-Guérin and tick-borne encephalitis vaccines are not usually available in North America.

Table 10.2–4. TOPICS OF ADVICE

Recommendations for Travel Clinics

Malaria prevention

Insect avoidance

Travelers' diarrhea—prevention and self-treatment

Sexually transmitted diseases, including HIV testing

Water-borne disease, e.g., schistosomiasis

Blood safety

Environmental illness—heat, cold, altitude

Jet lag and motion sickness

Personal safety

Animal bites and rabies avoidance

Travel medical kits

Medical care overseas and travel health insurance

Travel for those with special health needs

Cultural adaptation for expatriate travelers

Table 10.2–5. OPTIONAL TRAVEL CLINIC SERVICES

Telephone advice to physicians and the public

Pretravel physicals

Post-travel care medical care

Clinical laboratory services

Sale of travel medicines items

Pharmacy services

plement of vaccines and information on the prevention of all travel-related illness will help to distinguish the services that are offered by a travel medicine clinic compared with those offered in a generalist's office and, therefore, potentially increase the value of the service.

Other areas of service into which clinics have expanded include telephone advice (given to physicians by 89% of clinics and to the public by 66%),[1] the provision of pretravel physicals and care for ill returned travelers, the sale of travel-related items such as repellents and netting, and a clinic pharmacy (Table 10.2–5). Selling items within the clinic setting was less frequently done in the United States (31%) than in either Canada (42%) or other areas of the world (47%), and directly selling medications was only done 25% of the time in U.S. clinics compared with 43% in other areas of the world.[1]

INFORMATION SOURCES

Up-to-date and accurate information is the key to travel medicine. Without this, recommendations often become based on opinion rather than on information that has been reviewed by experts or is evidence based. Within the United States and Canada, there are several authorities to which every travel medicine service should refer. These resources may be periodicals, commercial computerized information systems, textbooks, and Internet information sites and listserv discussion groups. Some of the Internet sites for the U.S. and Canada are listed in the Appendix and many others in Chapter 8 Information Sources in Travel Medicine and referenced in Blair.[4]

In the U.S., the Centers for Disease Control and Prevention (CDC) establishes most policy about travel medicine. This is disseminated via the publication *Health Information for International Travel*, known as the "Yellow Book."[14] This book can be accessed via the CDC's Internet Web site. Periodic updates are found in the biweekly "blue sheet," which indicates areas within countries of the world that are reporting cholera and yellow fever.[15] The blue sheet, health advisories and updates,

general travel information, and links to other sites such as the World Health Organization (WHO) and the U.S. State Department's travel safety advisories are also on this site. The weekly publication of the CDC, *Morbidity and Mortality Weekly Report* (*MMWR*), has updates and epidemiologic information on many topics of importance to travel medicine practitioners. Critical analysis of vaccines and recommendations for their use are published as supplements to *MMWR* by the Advisory Committee on Immunization Practices.

In Canada, there are similar resources for travel health information (see Appendix). Extensive recommendations for both the traveler and the travel specialist are provided by the Travel Medicine Program of the Laboratory Centre for Disease Control. This can be accessed via the Internet. Health hazard advisories, news, and general travel health advice are also posted on this site. Official, evidence-based clinical practice guidelines are prepared by the Committee to Advise on Tropical Medicine and Travel (CATMAT) and can be found on their Web site. The *Canada Communicable Disease Report* is published biweekly; this reports on outbreaks throughout Canada and the world.

Clinics can access other resources including those published and posted by the WHO. Commercial computerized information sources have also been developed that provide country-specific information on travel health, safety, vaccine requirements, and malaria recommendations. These are referenced in Chapter 8 Information Sources in Travel Medicine.

THE TRAVEL CLINIC VISIT

The recommended services have been outlined and the traveler has accessed the service. What should be the standard for the travel clinic visit? Other chapters in this text describe in detail the actual advice provided and vaccines administered, but Table 10.2–6 details the general content of the visit. Each clinic should develop a standardized form that becomes part of the patient's permanent medical record. This form will ensure that the necessary information is obtained from the traveler, that appropriate areas of advice are covered, and that the immunizations that are given are properly recorded.

There are two areas of information that should be obtained before any decisions are made on vaccination and advice: the patient's travel plans and health history (see Table 10.2–6). The goal is to develop a risk profile

Table 10.2–6. THE TRAVEL CLINIC VISIT

Assessing the risk of travel
  Patient demographics
  Travel plans
    Itinerary
    Duration
    Activities
Assessing the health of the traveler
  Medical history
    Medical conditions
    Medications, and food, insect, or drug allergies
  Vaccination history
Providing advice
Providing vaccines
Documentation

for the traveler: in what activities will he/she be engaging, for how long, and in what types of setting? Is there anything in the patient's health history that will prevent, interfere with, or alter his/her plans? As many as 25% of travelers have an underlying medical condition, and almost 15% are aged 65 years and older and 5% younger than 12 years.[3] Fortunately for most, the planned trip can be undertaken safely as long as the appropriate preventive measures are reviewed and practiced. It should be clear that a 3-day business trip to Nairobi, Kenya, presents a very different health risk compared with a 2-month research stay on the shores of Lake Victoria, even though both of these trips are to Kenya.

Once the information is obtained, preventive advice and immunizations are provided. Cost-benefit analyses have been performed for some travel vaccines, and, in most cases, the risk of acquiring illness during travel is so low that the cost to prevent one case of vaccine-preventable illness is often not justified on a per-person basis.[16–19] Therefore, it is important for the travel medicine provider to develop a detailed risk profile and to administer vaccines when they are indicated, rather than just give shots for a particular destination without appropriate consideration.[6,20,21] Although many travelers access the clinic because of their desire to receive shots, the risks of vaccine-preventable disease are generally far less than those of travelers' diarrhea, respiratory illness, or accidents and injuries.[22–24] Education and counseling must be the cornerstones of care, particularly since the practice of travel medicine is entirely preventive. This should prompt the specialist to spend a significant portion of the visit on advice as an effective way to educate patients for the prevention of travel-related illness.[17,25]

Advice may be given in verbal, written, or audiovisual formats. The most important aspect is to provide it in a consistent, clear, and straightforward fashion, preferably in multiple formats. It is expected that this will enhance the likelihood that the traveler will comply with preventive measures and, therefore, remain healthy on his/her trip.[26–28] Clear advice on malaria chemoprophylaxis, as an example, has been shown to improve the compliance with antimalarials by travelers[9,24,29] and is cost effective.[17]

Prior to giving vaccines, the patient should review precautions and side effects and then sign a consent form. Each vaccine administered should be recorded in the travel chart and in the traveler's International Certificate of Vaccination provided by either Canada or the United States. Vaccination records should include the type of vaccine, date of administration, manufacturer, lot number, site of administration, and signature of administrator. This will make it possible to review the vaccine if a patient experiences side effects or if the manufacturer recalls a particular lot number. Significant side effects should be reported via the Vaccine Adverse Events Reporting System (VAERS) in the United States (800-822-7967) and to the local public health unit in Canada (further information for Canada can be obtained in the *Compendium of Pharmaceuticals and Specialists*) for reporting in their Vaccine Associated Adverse Event Surveillance System (VAAESS).

In order to establish uniformity of decisions and advice, protocols may be established for each clinic. Although general guidelines exist for vaccines and there is detailed information on the prevention of certain illnesses overseas, the actual decision making of who receives which vaccine remains open to debate and opinion. If a clinic develops guidelines, they may lead to consistency between advisors and actions.

Permanent records should be maintained so that they can be referred to in the case of vaccination complications or if the traveler loses the certificate of vaccination or returns for health advice prior to a second, third, or subsequent trip. Some primary care physicians who refer patients to the clinic will want a copy of the vaccinations administered. Many clinics also maintain an electronic database, which can aid in reviewing trends and the epidemiology of a clinic population.

CLINIC CHARGES

The charges and reimbursement for travel medicine services vary considerably within the United States and Canada. In Canada, the travel visit and vaccines are usually not covered by provincial health plans. Private insurance companies throughout North America will often not pay for what they consider to be optional vaccines that are not cost effective. In addition, if there is reimbursement, the amount may vary considerably depending on the carrier and the geographic region. Thus, most travelers will be expected to pay for the cost of vaccines themselves. In 1999, U.S. Medicare will only reimburse for hepatitis B, influenza, pneumococcal, tetanus, and rabies vaccines. The reimbursement for other vaccines, as examples, may range from $34 to $68 among four carriers for meningococcal vaccine (purchase cost $55), and from $35 to $63 for yellow fever vaccine (purchase cost $55), with one carrier not covering it. In spite of this, it is reasonable to submit the charges to private insurance if the patient has that type of coverage. The clinic will then need to decide if it will accept the carrier's reimbursement level if it is less than the vaccine charge or require the patient to pay the difference.

Most clinics add a professional consultation fee that also may not be covered. In the United States, each vaccine and travel consultation is given both a procedural code (Current Procedural Terminology, CPT) and a diagnosis code (International Classification of Diseases, ICD-9). These codes for vaccines are listed in Table 10.2–7. Consultation visit codes (CPT) may be 99201 through 99205 for new patients and 99211-99215 for established patients, depending on the level of service. The ICD-9 code for a consultation without complaint or sickness is V65.8.

CHALLENGES TO TRAVEL CLINICS

In the survey of clinics worldwide, 10 issues comprised over 80% of all problems encountered by the services.[1] They are listed in Table 10.2–8. These issues fall into two main categories: travel clinic structure and administration issues and patient education issues. Staffing and space, dealing with telephone calls, and insurance coverage can all be handled with proper planning. If demand is sufficient, then increased staffing may be financially possible. An automated telephone advice service may be an option for handling telephone calls; however, both the CDC and the LCDC have fax information services (see Appendix). Therefore, the investment in such an information service by an individual clinic may be neither cost effective nor necessary. An approach to handling telephone calls is to have them triaged between those that are only requesting an appointment and those requesting advice. The appointment calls can be sent immediately to

Table 10.2–7.   CODING FOR VACCINATION CHARGES

VACCINE	ICD-9	CPT
Arthropod-borne (Lyme)	V05.1	90665
Cholera	V03.0	90725
Influenza	V04.8	90658
Japanese encephalitis	V05.0	90735
Measles, mumps, and rubella	V06.4	90707
Other specific bacterial disease	V03.89	
Meningococcal		90733
Pneumococcal		90732
Other specific viral disease	V05.8	
Polio	V04.0	
Inactivated		90713
Rabies	V04.5	
Intradermal		90676
Intramuscular		90675
Tetanus-diphtheria	V06.5	90718
Typhoid	V03.1	
Whole cell, inactivated		90692
ViCPS		90691
Viral hepatitis	V05.4	
Hepatitis A		90632
Hepatitis B		90746
Varicella	V05.4	90716
Yellow fever	V04.4	90717

ICD-9 = International Classification of Diseases, CPT = Current Procedural Terminology.

Table 10.2–8.   PROBLEMS ENCOUNTERED IN TRAVEL CLINICS*

Insufficient space, time, and staff to meet demands
Travelers presenting with a short time interval before departure
Telephone calls for advice
Need for standardized, up-to-date advice for clinic personnel
Conflicting and unreliable advice given to travelers by groups outside of travel clinics
Patient concern about the cost of service and vaccines
Difficulty in assessing patient compliance with and understanding of recommendations
Difficulty in accessing new medications and vaccines
Failure of insurance carriers to pay for services
Travelers having preconceived ideas about their needs

*These 10 comments comprised 82% of the total comments received. From Hill and Behrens.[1]

a scheduler, and a message can be taken for the calls requesting information or advice. The travel specialist can then set aside a portion of each day to return the calls so that they do not disrupt the flow of the clinic.

On the patient education side, it is important to initially present to the patient what can be expected from the visit. If the information is gathered and advice and recommendations presented in a clear and orderly fashion, most patients will agree with the recommendations even if they differ from those the patients received from outside sources or formulated on their own. Ultimately, however, it is the traveler who has the responsibility for his/her own health and decision making, and it is the role of the travel medicine specialist to inform and educate.

REFERENCES

1. Hill DR, Behrens RH. A survey of travel clinics throughout the world. J Travel Med 1996;3:46–51.
2. Committee to Advise on Tropical Medicine and Travel (CATMAT). Guidelines for the practice of travel medicine. An Advisory Committee Statement (ACS). Can Commun Dis Rep 1999;25:1–60.
3. Hill DR. Pre-travel health, immunization status and demographics of travel of individuals visiting a travel medicine service. Am J Trop Med Hyg 1991;45:263–270.
4. Blair DC. A week in the life of a travel clinic. Clin Microbiol Rev 1997;10:650–673.
5. Scoville SL, Bryan JP, Tribble D, et al. Epidemiology, preventive services, and illnesses of international travelers. Mil Med 1997;162:172–178.
6. Sloan DSG. Travel medicine and general practice: a suitable case for audit? BMJ 1993;307:615–617.
7. Carroll B, Behrens RH, Crichton D. Primary health care needs for travel medicine training in Britain. J Travel Med 1998;5:3–6.
8. Gardner TB, Hill DR. Knowledge of travel medicine providers: analysis from a continuing education course. J Travel Med 1999;6:66–70.
9. Lobel HO, Campbell CC, Pappaioanou M, Huong AY. Use of prophylaxis for malaria by American travelers to Africa and Haiti. JAMA 1987;257:2626–2627.

10. Keystone JS, Lawee D, McIntyre L, Spence H. Counseling travelers about malaria chemoprophylaxis. Can Med Assoc J 1984;131:715–716.
11. Demeter SJ. An evaluation of sources of information in health and travel. Can J Public Health 1989;80:20–22.
12. Keystone JS, Dismukes R, Sawyer L, Kozarsky PE. Inadequacies in health recommendations provided for international travelers by North American travel health advisors. J Travel Med 1994;1:72–78.
13. International Society of Travel Medicine, North American Charter for Travel Health. A consensus statement on providing travel health advice. http://www.istm.org/consensus.html. October 22, 1996.
14. Centers for Disease Control and Prevention. Health information for international travel, 1999–2000. Atlanta: U.S. Department of Health and Human Services, 1999.
15. Centers for Disease Control and Prevention. Summary of health information for international travel, DHHS publication no. 396. Atlanta: U.S. Department of Health and Human Services, 2000.
16. MacPherson DW, Tonkin M. Cholera vaccination: a decision analysis. Can Med Assoc J 1992;146:1947–1952.
17. Behrens RH, Roberts JA. Is travel prophylaxis worth while? Economic appraisal of prophylactic measures against malaria, hepatitis A, and typhoid in travellers. BMJ 1994;309:918–922.
18. Bryan JP, Nelson M. Testing for antibody to hepatitis A to decrease the cost of hepatitis A prophylaxis with immune globulin or hepatitis A vaccines. Arch Intern Med 1994;154:663–668.
19. Gray GC, Rodier GR. Prevaccination screening for citizens of the United States living abroad who are at risk for hepatitis A. Clin Infect Dis 1994;19:225–226.
20. Steffen R, Lobel HO. Epidemiologic basis for the practice of travel medicine. J Wilderness Med 1994;5:56–66.
21. Wilson ME. Critical evaluation of vaccines for travelers. J Travel Med 1995;2:239–243.
22. Reid D, Dewar RD, Fallon RJ, et al. Infection and travel: the experience of package tourists and other travellers. J Infect 1980;2:365–370.
23. Steffen R, Rickenbach M, Wilhelm U, et al. Health problems after travel to developing countries. J Infect Dis 1987;156:84–91.
24. Hill DR. The health of a large cohort of Americans traveling to developing countries. J Travel Med 2000;7:in press.
25. Genton B, Behrens RH. Specialized travel consultation. Part II: acquiring knowledge. J Travel Med 1994;1:13–15.
26. Packman CJ. A survey of notified travel-associated infections: implications for travel health advice. J Public Health Med 1995;17:217–222.
27. Reed JM, McIntosh IB, Powers K. Travel illness and the family practitioner: a retrospective assessment of travel-induced illness in general practice and the effect of a travel illness clinic. J Travel Med 1994;1:192–198.
28. McIntosh IB, Reed JM, Power KG. Traveler's diarrhea and the effect of pretravel health advice in general practice. Br J Gen Pract 1997;47:71–75.
29. Phillips-Howard PA, Blaze M, Hurn M, Bradley DJ. Malaria prophylaxis: survey of the response of British travellers to prophylactic advice. BMJ 1986;293:932–934.

APPENDIX

Internet Sites for Locating a Travel Clinic

Worldwide
American Society of Tropical Medicine and Hygiene: www.astmh.org
International Society of Travel Medicine: www.istm.org

Canada
Laboratory Centre for Disease Control—Travel Medicine Program: www.hc-sc.gc.ca/hpb/lcdc/osh/travel/clinic_e.html
Canadian Society for International Health: www.csih.org/trav_inf.html

Internet Resource Sites for Travel Clinics

World Health Organization: www.who.org

United States
Centers for Disease Control Travel Information: www.cdc.gov/travel/travel.html
Morbidity Mortality Weekly Report: www2.cdc.gov/mmwr/

Canada
Laboratory Centre for Disease Control—Travel Medicine Program: www.hc-sc.gc.ca/hpb/lcdc/osh/tmp_e.html
Committee to Advise on Tropical Medicine and Travel: www.hc-sc.gc.ca/hpb/lcdc/osh/reccom_e.html#catmat
Canada Communicable Disease Report: www.hc-sc.gc.ca/hpb/lcdc/publicat/ccdr

Fax Information Services for the Traveler

United States CDC: 888-232-3299
Canada's LCDR FAXLINK: 613-941-3900

Chapter 11

ENVIRONMENTAL DEGRADATION: MEDICAL IMPACT ON TOURISM AND TROPICAL MEDICINE

LEONARD C. MARCUS

This chapter addresses the impact of human degradation of the environment on tropical medicine and the health of tourists, a small part of an environmental health crisis. Human behavior affects the climate and the quantity and quality of food, water, and air profoundly, threatening life on earth in many ways.

POPULATION EXPLOSION

Human population is increasing at an unprecedented rate. World population was approximately one-quarter billion around 44 BC (assassination of Julius Caesar, which reduced the population by one), one half billion around 1492, 1 billion around 1776, and 2 billion around 1945. Current global population is about 5.5 billion and is expected to reach 9 billion by 2032.[1] As population grows, it becomes more difficult to provide supporting resources and infrastructure needed for public health. Tourists demand disproportionate support in food, housing, and other amenities.

The population explosion is greatest in developing countries where the disparity between resources provided to the local population and to tourists is most apparent. This can lead to hostility and crime against tourists. This threat might be reduced if enough income generated from tourism is put into the local economy to benefit the general population.

Demand for food parallels population growth. Most of the land suitable for agriculture has been tilled. Deforestation to develop new farmland is often counterproductive because of resultant soil erosion. It is estimated that 6 billion tons of topsoil are lost annually in India.[2] Health risks associated with deforestation include mud slides and severe floods.

As natural areas are developed, tourist pressure increases on remaining pristine areas, so, without proper management, they undergo degradation from excessive visitation, putting more pressure on the decreasingly available sites. Concentrating more tourists into fewer areas stresses their carrying capacity and infrastructure, increasing the risks of vehicular accidents on land, on water, and in the air and of infectious disease (e.g., from person-to-person transmission and from sewage-transmitted infections).

TOURIST INDUSTRY AND ENVIRONMENTALISM

The World Tourism Organization and the World Travel and Tourism Council recognize the threat of environmental degradation to global ecology and economics and support sustainable development of tourism. The Rio Declaration on Environment and Development[3] stated these principles:

- Travel and tourism should assist people in leading healthy and productive lives in harmony with nature; contribute to the conservation, protection, and restoration of the earth's ecosystem; be based on sustainable patterns of production and consumption; and use its capacity to create employment for women and indigenous peoples.
- Peace, development, and environmental protection are interdependent.
- Protectionism in trade, travel, and tourism services should be halted or reversed.
- Environmental protection should constitute an integral part of the tourism development process.
- Tourism development issues should be handled with the participation of concerned citizens, with planning decisions being adopted at the local level.
- Nations shall warn one another of natural disasters that could affect tourists or tourist areas.
- Tourism development should recognize and support the identity, culture, and interests of indigenous peoples.
- International laws protecting the environment should be respected by the travel and tourism industry.

The 10 priority areas for action by the industry are waste minimization, reuse, and recycling; energy efficiency, conservation, and management; management of fresh water resources; waste water management; hazardous substances; transport; land use planning and management; involving staff, customers, and communities in environmental issues; design for sustainability; and partnerships for sustainable development.

GLOBAL WARMING

Global warming results from accumulation of greenhouse gases such as carbon dioxide, water vapor, and methane, largely as the result of burning fossil fuels. These gases trap heat, blocking its radiation from earth. Atmospheric CO_2 has risen 25% since the industrial revolution and continues to rise at a rate faster than at any time in the past 160,000 years. The 1990s have been the warmest decade on record, and it is predicted that this warming trend will continue. Warming of oceans results in increased evaporation and precipitation, severe storms, and flash floods. Warming trends, especially at night and during winter, and increased precipitation favor outbreaks of arthropod, rodent, and water-borne diseases.[3]

Global warming could cause melting of glaciers and a concomitant rise in sea level, resulting in coastal flooding. One-third of the world's population lives within 60 kilometers of a sea coast,[1] so there would be mass migration inland. Any such population shift carries the risk of introducing infections from carrier (relatively immune) populations to susceptible ones. Massive migration stresses available food supply, sewage treatment, medical facilities, transportation, economics, and other organized aspects of society. Coastal tourist sites would suffer, but problems of tourists would pale compared to those faced by the general public.

Global warming will not occur in a smooth, predictable fashion.[4] It is likely to be characterized by periods of drought in some areas, flooding in others, and violent storms, such as occurred during the 1998 hurricane season, one of the most destructive on record. Besides the immediate threats to physical safety posed by these weather changes, water-, insect-, and rodent-borne epidemics often follow floods.[3]

Increasing temperatures will alter the distribution of flora and fauna. Some tropical vectors of disease are likely to move into currently temperate regions as they warm up.[5,6] Some tropical diseases may become endemic in the developed countries of Europe and North America. Marine-related diseases, including harmful algal blooms and cholera, are also increasing in incidence and geographic distribution.[7]

AIR POLLUTION

Smog causes significant morbidity and mortality.[8] Travelers to Los Angeles, Mexico City, and the heavily air-polluted cities of China and Southeast Asia often suffer significant respiratory problems, especially if they have cardiac or pulmonary diseases such as congestive heart failure, asthma, bronchitis, or emphysema. Such patients should avoid areas of heavy air pollution or stay indoors, preferably in air-conditioned quarters, and minimize exercise on smoggy days. They should have pretravel evaluation of their medical condition, be properly medicated, and carry an adequate supply of medicine.

OZONE DEPLETION AND ULTRAVIOLET RADIATION

Ozone depletion from the stratosphere results from release of chlorinated fluorohydrocarbons (CFCs) found in aerosols and refrigerants.[9] In 1978, CFC use was banned in the United States and in 1996 it was banned globally. The ozone layer shields against penetration of ultraviolet (UV) light. The increasing UV radiation of the earth, most severe in the Southern Hemisphere, has resulted in a dramatic increase in skin cancer, including melanoma, which has risen by 3% to 7% every year since the 1960s.[10]

Ultraviolet radiation modifies the activity of Langerhans' cells, the primary antigen-presenting cells in the epidermis. It also suppresses T lymphocytes and alters cytokine secretion, thus inducing immunosuppressive effects systemically and in the skin.[11] People should use protective clothing and sunscreens to reduce sun exposure.

CONSERVATION OF FRESH WATER

Tourists should be advised not to waste water. Resorts and hotels should provide tourists with the option of reusing towels and bed linen without daily laundering. Composting rather than flush toilets should be installed whenever possible.

CHEMICAL POLLUTANTS

Where chemical pollution of drinking water is a known problem, the traveler should use good bottled beverages or pass water through activated carbon or, preferably, reverse osmosis filters. Avoiding chemical pollutants in food and water is much more difficult than avoiding microbial pollution. There may be significant risk in countries with little regulatory control over pollutants, including developing countries racing to industrialize.

The toxic effects of chemical pollutants depend on the chemical(s) involved, the amount, route, and duration of exposure and health of the individual, including age, sex, pregnancy, and current illnesses. The effects may be subtle or dramatic, mild or severe. Diagnosis is often difficult because patients may not be aware of exposures, clinicians may not think of toxic problems, and toxicologic laboratory support may not be readily available. Toxicologic problems should be considered in individuals with unusual dermatologic, neurologic, or gastrointestinal symptoms not otherwise explained, especially if they have impaired renal or hepatic function. Pollutants may impair immunity and endocrine function.[12]

DAMS

Dams have considerable ecologic effects. They can alter the epidemiology of vector-borne diseases. For example, damming a swift stream may destroy the breeding area of black flies (Simulium damnosum), which transmit oncho-cerciasis, but the resulting lake could favor the spread of certain mosquito-borne diseases. The building of the Aswan Dam on the Nile River in Egypt markedly reduced urinary schistosomiasis (*Schistosoma haematobium*) but increased colonic schistosomiasis (*S. mansoni*) because of opposite effects on the intermediate snail hosts of these parasites.[13]

BIODIVERSITY LOSS

We are currently experiencing the greatest loss of plant and animal species since the decline of the dinosaurs. The greatest cause of this wave of extinction is loss of habitat. The greatest biodiversity is in rain forests, which are being destroyed at a rate of 1.5 acres per second.

Selective harvesting of trees can be sustainable and support indigenous people. Clear cutting provides a quick, unsustainable profit for a few landholders. As roads are cut into forests and trees are cut around them, the remaining trees form isolated islands that shrink because of more logging or from dehydration, which is maximal at the edge of the woods. Forests depend on rain, which they help perpetuate by transpiration from the leaves. This normal cycle is replaced by a vicious cycle with deforestation: fewer trees pump less water into the air, so there is less rain; trees dry up, weaken, and die, leaving fewer trees, less recycling of rain water, etc.

Although certain temperate forests depend on fire for self-renewal, fire is intensely destructive in rain forests. Fires, deliberately set in the rain forests of southern Mexico and in Indonesia in the late 1990s, caused widespread severe respiratory disease. Problems with visibility caused airplane crashes and car accidents thousands of miles from the conflagrations. The fires caused a drop in tourism and severe economic loss.

The greatest concentration of marine life is found in coral reefs, which are rapidly being destroyed through pollution, dredging, destructive fishing practices, etc.[14,15] As a result, thousands of marine species are in danger of extinction.

Seven hundred thirty-four species of fish, 124 amphibians, 253 reptiles, 1,107 birds, and 1,096 mammals were listed as vulnerable to or in immediate danger of extinction in 1996.[16] Many endangered species are predators, such as bears, felids, canids, avian raptors (hawks, owls, eagles), crocodilians, and snakes. Their loss increases the risk of rodent-borne illnesses such as leptospirosis, hantaviruses, and various viral hemorrhagic fevers. Likewise, the loss of frogs, toads, and other insectivores increases the risk of insect-borne diseases. Biodiversity loss also results in economic loss as tourists go elsewhere to fish, hunt, or view wildlife.

Many medicines come from natural sources (e.g., various antibiotics from molds, digitalis from foxglove, vincristine from periwinkle plants, tamoxifen from the Pacific yew, etc.). Plants from tropical forests and marine life from coral reefs are particularly likely sources of new medications but are being destroyed at a rate faster than they can be studied.[17] The loss includes potential therapy for tropical diseases.

Practitioners of travel medicine should encourage responsible ecotourism, for example, by distributing brochures about regulations against trade or importation of endangered species or their products, such as provided by the World Wildlife Fund and Environment Canada. Tourists who collect or damage artifacts, minerals, plants, and animals can cause significant harm to their destination site.

CONCLUSION

Tourists want to visit places with favorable weather, air, and water quality and attractive flora and fauna. The higher the economic level of their trip, the greater the accommodations and infrastructural support required. This may deflect transportation systems, food and water supply, area available for food production, and medical care away from poorer, local people.

Tourists suffer from degradation of the environment, including exposure to pesticides, smog, and other pollutants, and to weather fluctuations caused by global warming. They are subject to changing patterns of vector-borne diseases, which are influenced by global warming, agricultural practices, habitat alteration, and destruction of predators. Thus, the health of tourists and the environment is reciprocally linked.

Control of major environmental problems depends on industrial and governmental action. Medical personnel should familiarize themselves with medical aspects of environmental degradation and become involved with these issues politically and scientifically. Practitioners of travel medicine should teach patients about the illnesses associated with environmental degradation and how to avoid contributing to or suffering from them, and they should be prepared to diagnose and treat these conditions.

REFERENCES

1. Gore A. Earth in the balance. New York: Houghton Mifflin, 1992.
2. Agenda 21 for Sustainable Development. United Nations Commission on Sustainable Development, 1992.
3. Epstein PR, ed. Extreme weather events: the health and economic consequences of the 1997/1998 El Nino and La Nina. Boston: Center for Health and the Global Environment, Harvard Medical School, 1999.
4. Maskell K, Mintzer IM, Callander BA. Basic science of climate change. Lancet 1993;342:1027–1031.
5. Patz VA, Epstein PR, Burke TA, et al. Global climate change and emerging infectious diseases. JAMA 1996;275:217–223.
6. Epstein PR, Diaz HF, Elias S, et al. Biological and physical signs of climate change: focus on mosquito-borne disease. Bull Am Meteorol Soc 1998;78:409–417.
7. Health Ecological and Economic Dimensions of Global Change (HEED). Marine ecosystems: emerging diseases as indicators of change. Boston: Center for Health and the Global Environment, Harvard Medical School, 1998.

8. Dockery DW, Pope CA, Xu X, et al. An association between air pollution and mortality in six U.S. cities. N Engl J Med 1993;329:1753–1759.

9. Molina MJ, Rowland FS. Stratospheric sink for chlorofluoromethanes, chlorine atom catalyzes destruction of ozone. Nature 1974;249:810–814.

10. Armstrong BK, Kricker A. How much melanoma is caused by sun exposure? Melanoma Res 1993;3:395–401.

11. Jeevan A, Kripke ML. Ozone depletion and the immune system. Lancet 1993;342:1159–1160.

12. Colburn T, Dumanoski D, Myers JP. Our stolen future. New York: Dutton, 1996.

13. El-Sayed HF, Rizkalla NH, Mehanna S, et al. Prevalence and epidemiology of *Schistosoma mansoni* and *S. haematobium* infection in two areas of Egypt recently reclaimed from the desert. Am J Trop Med Hyg 1985;52:194–198.

14. Richmond RH. Coral reefs: present problems and future concerns resulting from anthropogenic disturbance. American Zoologist 1993;33:524–536.

15. Wilkinson CR. Coral reefs of the world are facing widespread devastation: can we prevent this through sustainable management practices? In: Proceedings of the 7th International Coral Reef Symposium 1992;1:11–21.

16. Baillie J, Groombridge B, eds. 1996 IUCN Red List of Threatened Animals. Gland, Switzerland: World Conservation Union, 1996.

17. Chivian E. Species extinction and biodiversity loss: the implications for human health. In: Chivian E, McCally M, Hu H, et al., eds. Critical condition. Human health and the environment. Cambridge, MA: MIT Press, 1993:193–224.

Chapter 12

RISK TO TRAVELERS BY REGION AND ENVIRONMENTAL FACTORS

12.1 NORTHERN AFRICA

REMON R. ABU-ELYAZEED

Algeria, Egypt, Libyan Arab Jamahiriya, Morocco, and Tunisia are characterized by a generally fertile coastal area and a desert hinterland with oases that are often foci of infections.

Food- and water-borne diseases are the primary cause of illness in travelers. Diarrhea affects up to 50% of all travelers. Enterotoxigenic *Escherichia coli* is the most common causative agent of travelers' diarrhea (TD), a syndrome characterized by a twofold or greater increase in the frequency of unformed bowel movements. Contaminated food and drinks are the sources for the introduction of infection into the body. Other causes of TD in this region include *Salmonella, Shigella, Campylobacter, Giardia lamblia, Cryptosporidium,* and *Entamoeba histolytica.* Hepatitis A and E occur throughout the area. With the exception of Tunisia, typhoid fever is prevalent in the region. Brucellosis is common in some areas, resulting from consumption of sheep or goat dairy products. Alimentery helminthic infections are also common. Although a common problem in the past, cholera now occurs only sporadically. Since 1990, no cases of cholera have been reported from the region. Schistosomiasis, a parasitic infection resulting from wading or swimming in water infested with the organism, is very prevalent in the Nile valley of Egypt. Focal cases of the disease in other countries in the area have been reported. Poliomyelitis, highly endemic in the region in the past, has been controlled due to successful eradication efforts with viral transmission interrupted in most of the region. Only 14 cases of poliomyelitis have been reported from Egypt in 1997 and no cases have been reported from Algeria, Libyan Arab Jamahiriya, Morocco, or Tunisia since 1992.

Arthropod-borne diseases are unlikely to be a major problem to travelers to this area. A limited risk for malaria exists in certain parts of Algeria (Sahara Region), Egypt (Faiyoum oases only), Libyan Arab Jamahirya, and Morocco. There is no risk of malaria for travelers visiting the major tourist area in North Africa including Nile cruises. Dengue fever, filariasis, leishmaniasis, relapsing fever, Rift Valley fever, sandfly fever, typhus, and West Nile fever also occur in this region, but the risk to travelers is low.

Other hazards include injuries, heat, dust, and animal-associated hazards. The major causes of serious disability or loss of life in travelers are injuries, not infections. Motor vehicle crashes are common and result from a variety of factors, including inadequate roadway design, hazardous conditions, lack of appropriate vehicles and vehicle maintenance, inattention to pedestrians, and unskilled drivers. A traffic accident in an area that is not well served medically is more likely to be fatal.

Heat, both directly and indirectly, is responsible for some diseases and can give rise to serious skin conditions. Excessive heat and humidity, alone or in conjunction with vigorous activity, may lead to heat exhaustion due to salt and water deficiency. Heatstroke, a more serious condition, may occur due to insensible loss of fluid in the dry desert environment. The ultraviolet rays of the sun can cause severe and very debilitating sunburn in lighter-skinned persons. Dermatophytoses (athlete's foot) are often made worse by warm and humid conditions.

Breathing and swallowing dust when traveling, especially on unpaved roads or in arid areas, may be followed by nausea and malaise and may increase susceptibility to infection of the upper respiratory tract.

Animal-associated hazards including rabies and bites from snakes and scorpions are relatively rare. However, when camping or staying in rustic or primitive accommodations, they present a risk.

BIBLIOGRAPHY

World Health Organization. International travel and health: vaccination requirements and health advice. Geneva: WHO, 1998.

Centers for Disease Control. Health information for international travel 1996–97. Atlanta: U.S. Department of Health and Human Services, 1997.

12.2 SUB-SAHARAN AFRICA

ALAIN R. BOUCKENOOGHE

Sub-Saharan Africa (which includes Angola, Benin, Burkina Faso, Burundi, Cameroon, Cape Verde, Central African Republic, Chad, Comoros, Congo-Brazzaville, Côte d'Ivoire, Democratic Republic of the Congo, Djibouti, Equatorial Guinea, Eritrea, Ethiopia, Gabon, The Gambia, Ghana, Guinea, Guinea-Bissau, Kenya, Liberia, Madagascar, Malawi, Mali, Mauritania, Mauritius, Mozambique, Niger, Nigeria, Réunion, Rwanda, Sao Tome and Principe, Senegal, Seychelles, Sierra Leone, Somalia, Sudan, Togo, Uganda, Tanzania, Zambia, and Zimbabwe) lies entirely within the tropics and has a vegetation that varies from tropical rain forests in the west and center to wooded steppes in the east, and from the Sahel desert of the north through the dry Sudan savannas to the moist orchard savanna and woodlands in the equatorial regions.

Many of the diseases listed below occur in localized foci and are often confined to rural areas. This, combined with the geographic remoteness and the precarious condition of the health infrastructure in many countries in this region, is a particular challenge to travelers in those rural areas, emphasizing the importance of good travel preparation, prophylaxis, carriage of self-treatment kits, and consideration of evacuation plans.

Arthropod-borne diseases are a major health problem to the traveler. Malaria occurs throughout the area, except at over 2,000 meters altitude, and has also not been reported recently from Réunion and the Seychelles. *Plasmodium falciparum* is predominant, whereas *P. vivax* is very rare. *P. ovale* is uncommon outside West Africa but *P. malariae* is found throughout. Filariasis is widespread with *Wuchereria bancrofti* and *Mansonella perstans* existing in about all countries, whereas *Loa loa* is seen mainly in West and Central Africa. Despite intensive efforts by the Onchocerciasis Control Programme since the early 1970s, onchocerciasis (river blindness) has endemic foci in all of the countries listed except the island countries of the Atlantic (but it is present on the island of Bioko) and Indian Oceans, the greater part of Kenya, Djibouti, Mauritania, Mozambique, Somalia, Zambia, and Zimbabwe. Visceral leishmaniasis, mainly by *L. donovani*, and the cutaneous form, mainly by *L. major* and *L. aethiopica*, are found more often in the drier areas with epidemics of visceral leishmaniasis in Southern Sudan and the borders of Kenya, Somalia, and Ethiopia. African sleeping sickness (human trypanosomiasis) is reported from all countries except Djibouti, Eritrea, Somalia, Mauritania, The Gambia, and the island countries. The risk to travelers is particularly high in rural areas of Southern Sudan, Northern Angola, the Democratic Republic of the Congo, and Uganda. Lice-borne *Borrelia recurrentis* and tick-borne *B. duttoni* relapsing fever occur, as do flea-borne *Rickettsia typhi* and tick-borne *R. conorii* typhus. *R. prowazekii* is endemic in the cooler mountainous regions with occasional epidemic spread. Human ehrlichiosis has not been reported. Plague is reported consistently from those countries where persistence of plague in wild rodents forms natural endemic foci. Tungiasis and myiasis are widespread. Many arboviral diseases transmitted by mosquitoes, ticks, and sandflies are found throughout and only some of the more common ones are mentioned. Among flaviviridae, yellow fever occurs periodically in unvaccinated populations mainly in tropical forest areas of Africa; dengue, but not dengue hemorrhagic fever, has been documented. The more common alphaviridae are chikungunya, which is widespread, and o'nyong-nyong, which is mainly in Uganda and neighboring areas. Rift Valley fever causes occasional epidemics. Other hemorrhagic fevers include Crimean-Congo hemorrhagic fever, which is transmitted by a tick, Lassa fever and Hantaan, which are acquired through indirect contact with rodents, and rarely Marburg and Ebola, with no evident reservoir or vector. Lassa fever is confined to West Africa but other arenaviridae are found throughout the region, causing significant mortality.

Food- and water-borne diseases are highly endemic. Invasive enteritis such as shigella, salmonella, campylobacter, and amoeba infections and noninvasive diarrheal diseases such as cholera, enterotoxigenic *Escherichia coli,* and other pathogenic *E. coli* are widespread. There were recent outbreaks of *E. coli* 0157 in East Africa. *Cryptosporidium* and other coccidia are common, and so is *Giardia.* Intestinal tape- and roundworms are hyperendemic. Dracunculiasis (Guinea worm) was prevalent in West Africa but has reduced significantly and is now a target for eradication. Hepatitis A, E, and D are endemic. Paragonimiasis (lung fluke) has been reported from Cameroon and Nigeria. Echinococcosis is prevalent in all animal-breeding areas. Poliomyelitis, endemic in most countries, is declining. Schistosomiasis is omnipresent on the mainland.

Hepatitis B is hyperendemic. HIV-1 and -2 have high prevalence with an increasing epidemic of tuberculosis. Trachoma remains a serious public health problem. Cyclic meningococcal meningitis epidemics are found during the dry season in the "meningitis belt" of the Sahel from Sudan to The Gambia. Anthrax and brucellosis are found in many foci. Leptospirosis is widespread and rabies common.

Other hazards include snakebites. Motor vehicle accidents are the main cause of death to travelers.

BIBLIOGRAPHY

Jelinek T, Bluml A, Loscher T, Nothdurft. Assessing the incidence of infection with *Plasmodium falciparum* among international travelers. Am J Trop Med Hyg 1998;59(1):35–37.

Kachur SP, Reller ME, Barber AM, et al. Malaria surveillance—United States, 1994. MMWR CDC Surveill Summ 1997;46(5):1–18.

Smith DH, Pepin J, Stich AH. Human African trypanosomiasis: an emerging public health crisis. Br Med Bull 1998;54:341–355.

Day JH, Grant AD, Doherty JF, et al. Schistosomiasis in travellers from sub-Saharan Africa. BMJ 1996;313:268–269.

Brouqui P, Harle JR, Delmont J, et al. African tick-bite fever. An imported spotless rickettsiosis. Arch Intern Med 1997;157: 119–124.

Raoult D, Ndihokubwayo JB, Tissot-Dupont H, et al. Outbreak of epidemic typhus associated with trench fever in Burundi. Lancet 1998;352:353–358.

12.3 SOUTHERN AFRICA

JOHN A. FREAN

The region of Southern Africa region comprises Botswana, Lesotho, Namibia, Saint Helena, South Africa, and Swaziland and varies physically from the Namib and Kalahari deserts to fertile plateaus and plains and to the more temperate climate of the southern coast. These countries are on the verge of becoming poliomyelitis free and the risk of this disease is now low. As far as other diseases are concerned, the risks posed by them are discussed below according to the category of traveler.

BUSINESS TRAVELERS

After crime and motor vehicle accidents, food- and water-borne disease is probably the most significant danger for business travelers. Municipal water supplies are generally safe to drink in South Africa but it is not safe to assume that this applies across the whole region. Sexually transmitted infections, including HIV, are common. Malaria risk is absent or minimal in large cities in this region; for travelers outside cities, the highest risk is during summer months (October-May) in the far northern and eastern parts of South Africa, eastern Swaziland, northern Botswana, and northern Namibia.

ROUTINE TOURISTS

Risks for tourists are the same as for business travelers, except that visits to the region's game reserves result in exposure to malaria, tickbite fever, and arbovirus infections (including Crimean-Congo hemorrhagic fever, Rift Valley fever, West Nile fever, and others) and a higher risk of food and water-borne disease. Swimming in fresh water carries the risk of schistosomiasis over much of the region, apart from the Free State and the Northern and Western Cape Provinces of South Africa and Lesotho. Extremely high temperatures occur in summer in northern Namibia and Botswana.

ADVENTURE TOURISTS (RIVER RAFTERS, BACKPACKERS, OVERLAND TRAVELERS)

This category of traveler is likely to be exposed to higher risks of arthropod-borne disease, especially malaria, tickbite fever, and arbovirus infections. Tick-borne relapsing fever and trypanosomiasis occur in northern Botswana (Okavango swamps) and in northern Namibia (Kavango and Caprivi regions). There is a plague focus in Ovambo in Namibia. There may be exposure to snakebites (neuro-, cyto-, and hemotoxic) and scorpion stings. River rafters are at risk for schistosomiasis, giardiasis, cryptosporidiosis, hepatitis A and E, amebiasis, and bacterial intestinal pathogens. Wild animal (crocodile, hippopotamus) attacks are potential dangers in some rivers. Wildlife rabies is endemic in this region, but there is also a canine rabies epidemic in Kwazulu-Natal in South Africa, which originated in Mozambique and which is spreading southward.

SPECIAL INTEREST TRAVELERS (SCIENTISTS, DOCTORS, NATURALISTS)

This category of traveler, depending on the nature of the special interest and the duration of visit, may be exposed to additional risks. Doctors who work in the region are likely to be exposed to hepatitis B and HIV, among other infectious diseases; naturalists may be at higher risk for anthrax (endemic in Etosha Game Reserve in Namibia), rabies, tickbite fever, plague, or other arthropod-borne diseases, snakebites, or injuries from wild animals. Certain travelers may be at high risk for sexually transmitted diseases including HIV.

BIBLIOGRAPHY

Thurston H, Stuart J, McDonnell B, et al. Fresh orange juice implicated in an outbreak of *Shigella flexneri* among visitors to a South African game reserve. J Infect 1998;36:350.

Swanepoel R, Barnard BJH, Meredith CD, et al. Rabies in southern Africa. Onderstepoort J Vet Res 1993;60:325–346.

Stanek G. Borreliosis and travel medicine. J Travel Med 1995;2: 244–251.

Mabey D. Sex and travel. Br J Hosp Med 1995;54:264–275.

Hargarten SW. Injury prevention: a crucial aspect of travel medicine. J Travel Med 1994;1:48–50.

12.4 NORTH AMERICA

JOAN L. WILLIAMS

North America includes Bermuda, Canada, Greenland, St. Pierre and Miquelon, and the United States of America (including Hawaii). The incidence of communicable diseases in North America is unlikely to be any greater, and perhaps less, than that found in the international traveler's home country.

In 1994, an international commission certified North America to be free of wild poliovirus. In the United States, proof of immunization against diphtheria, measles, poliomyelitis, and rubella is required for entry into school. In addition, most states also require immunization against hepatitis B, mumps, pertussis, and tetanus.

However, infectious diseases do occur, and travelers to specific regions must be aware of their risk factors, which are determined by the area to which they travel, the time of year, and the recreational activities in which they participate.

ARTHROPOD-BORNE DISEASES

Tick-borne diseases are the most common arthropod-borne diseases in North America. Risk is highest for persons who work or recreate in wooded areas (camping, hunting, hiking, fishing, landscaping, forestry, wildlife or parks management) from late spring (May) until September, or until the temperature drops below 45°F.

Lyme disease is reported in 44 states but predominantly occurs in three distinct geographic regions: the northeast (Maine, Massachusetts, Connecticut, Rhode Island, New York, New Jersey, Maryland, Pennsylvania, and Delaware), which reports about 90% of the total cases, the Midwest (Wisconsin and Minnesota), and the west coast (California and Orgegon). The deer tick is the carrier in the northeast and Midwest and the western deer tick is the carrier along the west coast.

Rocky Mountain spotted fever (RMSF) occurs in the Rocky Mountain states (Colorado and Wyoming), but the incidence is highest in the southeast and south central U.S., with the majority of cases reported from Oklahoma and North Carolina. RMSF is transmitted by the Rocky Mountain wood tick in the west and the American dog tick in the east.

Ehrlichiosis is manifested in humans as two separate infections: human monocytic ehrlichiosis (HME) and human granulocytic ehrlichiosis (HGE). Both infections have similar symptoms but vary in their geographic distribution. HME, transmitted by the Lone Star tick, occurs throughout the southeastern states, with the highest density in the Ozark mountain area (Arkansas) and in the mid-Atlantic states. HGE, transmitted by the deer tick and possibly the American dog tick, has been reported in Minnesota, Wisconsin, Massachusetts, Connecticut, Rhode Island, New York, Pennsylvania, Maryland, Florida, Arkansas, and California.

Tularemia, like HME, is spread by the Lone Star tick and occurs in the U.S. and Canada.

Relapsing fever, transmitted by a tick with the same name, occurs west of the Mississippi River and specifically in the mountain areas of the western U.S.

Mosquito-borne diseases occur sporadically and, unless there is an outbreak, they pose a low risk to the tourist.

Dengue fever has reportedly been acquired in Laredo, Texas, and along the Texas-Mexico border. It is spread by the female *Aedes aegypti* mosquito, which bites in the morning after daybreak and in the late afternoon before dark. However, on overcast days, in shady areas, and indoors, the mosquito bites all day.

Viral encephalitis occurs and is associated with specific species of mosquitoes or ticks and specific ecologic systems. Therefore, there is a geographic and seasonal limitation to each disease. California encephalitis virus occurs annually in the Midwestern states (Ohio, Wisconsin, Minnesota, Illinois, Indiana, and Iowa). Clinical disease is most prevalent in children < 15 years of age. Outbreaks due to other arboviruses (St. Louis, Western equine, and Eastern equine encephalitis) vary markedly each year.

Leishmaniasis has been reported in Texas and Oklahoma. Sandflies are the vector and are commonly found in rodent burrows or on the perimeter of forested areas.

In the summer of 1999, more than 30 cases, including 4 deaths, of West Nile fever occurred in the New York City area. The initial case(s) was believed to be carried by mosquitoes aboard an airliner from western Africa.

OTHER ARTHROPOD-BORNE DISEASE

Plague rarely and sporadically occurs in the southwest U.S., and the risk to tourists is extremely low. Infected fleas transmit the disease. Plague vaccine is no longer manufactured.

FOOD- AND WATER-BORNE DISEASES

There is a very low risk of these diseases to the healthy tourist. Tap water is potable throughout the region. The risk of acquiring food- and water-borne diseases can be attributed to several factors. First, there is an ever-increaseing number of people who eat in fast-food restaurants and salad bars, and 80% of outbreaks in the U.S. occur in persons eating outside the home. Second, there has been a significant change in eating behaviors. Trends are for a greater intake of fresh and raw fruits and vegetables. Third, there is an increase in the susceptible population of immunosuppressed persons. These include persons of advanced age, on cancer chemotherapy, or with organ transplants and HIV disease. Fourth, North American travelers may acquire intestinal illnesses abroad, carry them home, and infect close personal contacts.

In the U.S., there have been cases of, and fatalities from, food- and water-borne illnesses. In 1993, a multistate, northwestern regional outbreak of *Escherichia coli* 0157:H7 was linked to eating improperly cooked hamburger meat at a fast-food restaurant chain. Consumption of raw or inadequately cooked eggs remains the leading cause of *Salmonella* sp outbreaks. *Campylobacter* sp infections are sporadically acquired from eating inadequately cooked chicken, raw milk, or raw eggs, and Guillain-Barré syndrome has been reported as a serious sequelae. Norwalk virus, *Vibrio* sp, and hepatitis A have been acquired from eating raw shellfish (oysters, shrimp, and crab) harvested from the warm waters along the Gulf Coast (Texas and Louisiana). Persons with underlying liver disease are more susceptible to these illnesses, and *Vibrio* sp. infections are often fatal. Ciguatera poisoning can result from eating reef fish (amberjack, barracuda, grouper, and red snapper) in Hawaii and Florida. The highest risk season is February to September, and the ciguatoxin is heat stable; therefore, it is not destroyed by cooking the fish. Outbreaks of parasitic diseases also occur. *Giardia lamblia* is the most prevalent enteric parasite in the U.S. and Canada. Infection occurs after ingesting the cysts via water or food and person-to-person contact. Consumption of cold surface water (mountain streams and wells) contaminated by beavers is a common source of infection. Outbreaks have occurred in the mountainous regions of the northeast, the northwest, and the Rocky Mountain states in the U.S. and in British Columbia, Canada. Person-to-person transmission is known to occur in sexually active male homosexuals and persons with inadequate fecal-oral hygiene such as those in daycare centers and custodial institutions. Cyclospora outbreaks have also occurred in the U.S. after eating raspberries imported from Guatemala. In Canada, the North American liver fluke is present in fish (longnose sucker, yellow perch, brook trout, and fallfish).

OTHER DISEASES

Influenza occurs annually from November to April in all areas.

Hepatitis B is endemic in the Inuit population of northern Canada and the Alaskan Eskimos. Persons anticipating sexual contact with persons in known risk groups are advised to be immunized.

Rabies occurs in bats in the U.S., Canada, and Greenland. In the U.S., there is a need for increased precautions due to the presence of rabies in raccoons, foxes, skunks, and groundhogs in the mid-Atlantic states (Delaware, Maryland, New Jersey, New York, Pennsylvania, Virginia, West Virginia, and Washington, DC). Arctic and red fox carry rabies in Alaska and Canada.

Hantavirus pulmonary syndrome has been reported in 24 states and Canada. The highest incidence in the U.S. occurs in New Mexico, Arizona, and California and is contracted by inhaling aerosolized rodent (deer or white-footed mouse) urine or excreta.

Leptospirosis associated with recreational activities in freshwater streams is reported from Hawaii.

Respiratory-acquired fungal diseases occur in the U.S. Histoplasmosis is endemic in the Missouri and Mississippi River Valley area, and coccidioidomycosis can be acquired in the southwestern U.S., particularly Arizona and California.

Tuberculosis occurs throughout the region, particularly in the larger cities.

PRECAUTIONS

- In Bermuda, the source of the water supply is rainwater stored in cisterns; therefore, the potential for water contamination exists.
- Persons with environmental allergies are at risk in urban and rural locations.
- Poison ivy and poison oak are present.
- Portuguese man-of-war is prevalent in the waters off Bermuda. Their stings produce serious, but not fatal, illness.

BIBLIOGRAPHY

Altekruse SF, Cohen ML, Swerdlow DL. Emerging foodborne diseases. CDC 1997;3:285–293.

Centers for Disease Control and Prevention. Health information for international travel. Atlanta: U.S. Department of Health and Human Services, 1999.

Johnson RT. Acute encephalitis. Clin Infect Dis 1996;123:219–226.

Khan AS, Khabbaz RF, Armstrong LR, et al. Hantavirus pulmonary syndrome: the first 100 U.S. cases. J Infect Dis 1996;173:1297–1303.

Mandell GL, Bennett JE, Dolin R. Principles and practice of infectious diseases. 5th Ed. Philadelphia: Churchill Livingstone, 2000.

Peters CJ, Khan AS, Zaki SR. Hantivirus in the United States. Arch Intern Med 1996;156:705–706.

Plotkin SA. Rabies. Clin Infect Dis 2000;30:4–12.

Powers JH, Scheld WM. Human ehrlichiosos: the newest tick-borne disease. Contemp Intern Med 1996;8(7):68–78.

Tauxe RV. Emerging foodborne diseases: evolving public health challenge. CDC 1997;3:425–434.

Thorner AR, Walker DH, Petri WA Jr. Rocky mountain spotted fever. Clin Infect Dis 1998;27:1353–1360.

Travax® Software. Milwaukee, WI: Shoreland, Inc., Jan. 21, 2000.

12.5 MAINLAND MIDDLE AMERICA

PABLO C. OKHUYSEN

The topography of Mainland Middle America (Belize, Costa Rica, El Salvador, Guatemala, Honduras, Mexico, Nicaragua, and Panama) includes arid areas in Northern Mexico and tropical rain forests in the South. The central plateaus and highland valleys generated by the region's extensive mountain ranges have a pleasant year-round temperature.

ARTHROPOD-BORNE DISEASES

Malaria is present in all countries of the region; rates of transmission vary according to the country of destination from 1 to 17 per 100,000 inhabitants and are the highest in Belize and Nicaragua. In general, travel to the coastal areas and the lowlands has the highest risk. Malaria transmission does not occur in highland valleys above 1,500 ft. Malaria is present in the nonurbanized coastal areas of Mexico, with a sharp increase in the Oaxacan Coast. *Plasmodium vivax* accounts for the vast majority of cases in Mainland Middle America. *Plasmodium falciparum* accounts for only 3% to 5% of cases. All travelers should follow protective measures. Chloroquine remains the prophylactic drug of choice for malarial prevention except for Eastern Panama, where chloroquine resistance is present east of the Canal. For that region, mefloquine or doxycycline should be used. Dengue fever, both classic and hemorrhagic, also occurs, particularly in Honduras, El Salvador, and Nicaragua. Recent outbreaks with some fatalities have been reported in Honduras and Nicaragua. Increased incidence has also been noted in Northeast and Northwest Mexico. Visceral leishmaniasis occurs in El Salvador, Guatemala, Honduras, and Southern Mexico, whereas cutaneous and mucocutaneous leishmaniasis occurs in all regions. Bancroftian filariasis is limited to Costa Rica. American trypanosomiasis (Chagas' disease) and onchocerciasis (river blindness) are present in localized rural foci in Central Mexico, Guatemala, and El Salvador. Venezuelan equine encephalitis is present in all regions.

FOOD- AND WATER-BORNE DISEASES

Enteric infections due to water- and food-borne pathogens are common in this region. Travelers' diarrhea is mostly due to enterotoxigenic *E. coli* and *Shigella* sp. For travelers with more prolonged stays or rural travel, the risk of typhoid fever increases. Cholera, amoebiasis, bacillary dysentery, and infection with *Giardia intestinalis* are also common in the resident population but are responsible for relatively few cases in travelers. Hepatitis A is endemic in the region and outbreaks of hepatitis E have been reported in Central Mexico. Helminthic infections are common, particularly with *Ascaris, Strongiloides, Enterobious,* and *Taenia* sp. Water should be consumed after boiling for 1 minute or only if bottled. Although the incidence of multiresistant *Shigella* type I has increased, quinolones remain effective as empiric therapy for travelers' diarrhea.

Because of the disruption of land transportation after Hurricane Mitch, regions of Honduras, El Salvador, and Guatemala have had shortages of food, medicine, and other supplies. Flooding has interrupted and/or polluted drinking water supplies. This and the lack of regular electrical flow for refrigeration have increased the incidence of food- and water-borne infections. Leptospirosis has been a problem in Nicaragua and Honduras for some years, with a recent re-emergence.

OTHER DISEASES

Because few individuals vaccinate their pets, rabies is present in the region. Rabies in bats is also common. Preexposure vaccination should be considered in those staying for more than 30 days or those who anticipate animal contact or are engaged in spelunking. Poliomyelitis has been eradicated in the Americas and polio booster vaccinations for travelers to the region are no longer needed. Altitude in Mexico City, Guadalajara, and Guatemala City may cause temporary fatigue, insomnia, nausea, headache, and dyspnea. In addition, volcanic activity in the Popocateptl (located 38 miles southeast of Mexico City) threatens a considerable number of villages and contributes to the worsening of the air quality of the city.

CRIME AND SECURITY

In recent years, crime against foreigners has increased in the region particularly in Mexico, Guatemala, and El Salvador. In Mexico, violence against foreigners has reached a critical state. Of particular note are bus, taxicab, and automated teller associated assaults. Travelers to Mainland Middle America should be encouraged not to travel alone, to leave valuable possessions in a hotel safe, and to avoid travel on highways after dark. Although civil wars in Nicaragua, El Salvador, and Guatemala have officially ended, crimes continue to be caused by armed groups.

BIBLIOGRAPHY

Centers for Disease Control and Prevention. Outbreak of leptospirosis among white-water rafters—Costa Rica, 1996. JAMA 1997;278:808–809.

Gubler DJ. Dengue and dengue hemorrhagic fever. Clin Microbiol Rev 1998;11:480–496.

Malaria in the Americas, 1996. Epidemiol Bull 1997;18:1–8.

Mintz ED, Weber JT, Guris D, et al. An outbreak of Brainerd diarrhea among travelers to the Galapagos Islands. J Infect Dis 1998;177:1041–1045.

12.6 CARIBBEAN MIDDLE AMERICA

DEANNA ASHLEY

The Caribbean Middle America region is made up of a number of islands (English speaking: Antigua and Barbuda, Bahamas, Barbados, British and U.S. Virgin Islands, Cayman Islands, Dominica, Grenada, Jamaica, Montserrat, St. Kitts and Nevis, St. Lucia, St. Vincent and the Grenadines, Trinidad and Tobago, and Turks and Caicos Islands; Spanish speaking: Cuba, Dominican Republic, Puerto Rico; Dutch speaking: Aruba, Netherlands Antilles; French speaking: Guadeloupe, Haiti, Martinique).

Many of the islands are mountainous with peaks 1,000 to 2,500 m high and ranging in size between <30.2 m² and >10,000 m², the archipelago of the Republic of Cuba being the largest. The chain of islands in the eastern Caribbean from St. Kitts in the north through to St. Vincent and the Grenadines in the south is part of a volcanic chain, with the volcano of the Soufriere Hills in Montserrat having a prolonged phase of eruption since July 1995 that continues to date. All of these islands have a tropical climate with periods of heavy rainfall. During the months of June to November, the region is subject at times to very heavy rainfall, storms, and hurricanes with wind speeds ranging from 60 to 150 mph.

Disease risks vary from country to country and in general reflect the level of socioeconomic development and the social inequities in each country.

Most of the islands have good health status, as evidenced by greater than 80% of the population with access to safe drinking water and basic sanitation and life expectancy of 70 years or greater.

VECTOR-BORNE DISEASES

Malaria-active transmission still exists in Haiti and the Dominican Republic, where *Plasmodium falciparum* was the main cause of infection but was not resistant to chloroquine. In the other islands, the vector for malaria transmission exists, but local transmission has not occurred in over three decades.

Dengue is now endemic in all of the islands in the area, with outbreaks occurring during the past 5 years in Cuba, Puerto Rico, and Jamaica. The first major outbreak of dengue hemorrhagic fever occurred in Cuba in 1981, with subsequent cases occurring in Cuba, Puerto Rico, and Jamaica in 1997 and 1998. Cases of dengue hemorrhagic fever were also reported during these outbreaks.

FOOD- AND WATER-BORNE DISEASES

Diarrhea affecting travelers to this region occurs in 15% to as high as 40% of visitors. Enterotoxigenic *Escherichia coli* has been identified as the main cause of this illness. Other organisms associated with this disease have been *Shigella* and *Salmonella*. Outbreaks of food-borne illness occur from time to time in all of the islands, with *Salmonella, Shigella*, and *Staphylococcus* sp being the most common organisms associated with these outbreaks.

Entamoeba histolytic and hepatitis A are also responsible for some illness in the region. Cholera has not been reported from any island in the region for over 50 years.

HIV/SEXUALLY TRANSMITTED DISEASES

Reported annual AIDS incidence rates within the region are relatively high, ranging from <50 to >1,250 per million population (1996). Heterosexual spread is the main mode of transmission. In the region, the prevalence of HIV infection among women receiving ANC ranges from <1% to 7%, whereas among sex workers the rate is between 3% and 25% (1993). The prevalence of sexually transmitted diseases ranges from 5% to >14% (1993).

The highest rates for tuberculosis exist in the Dominican Republic and Haiti, with high associated co-infection with HIV (incidence rate of >40 per 100,000), whereas within the other Caribbean islands, rates range from 5 to 35/100,000 population.

LEGIONELLA PNEUMOPHILA (LEGIONNAIRES' DISEASE)

In the Caribbean, a few cases of legionnaires' disease have been identified in travelers returning from Bahamas, Barbados, Cuba, and the Dominican Republic. The most recent were three cases reported from Antigua in 1996.

OTHER COMMUNICABLE DISEASES

Massive immunization efforts within the Caribbean region over the past decade supported by the Pan American Health Organization have led to eradication of the wild poliovirus and the elimination of measles. There have been no confirmed cases of poliomyelitis or measles occurring in this region for over 3 years.

Resurgence of rubella occurred in the region in 1995, with the resulting increase in the number of infants born with congenital rubella syndrome. In April 1998, the Caribbean Community established the goal of eliminating rubella by the year 2000, and mass immunization campaigns are now being undertaken in the region to achieve this goal.

BIBLIOGRAPHY

Caribbean Regional Epidemiology Centre. Communicable diseases feedback reports. Port of Spain: Pan American Health Organization, 1997 and 1998.

Caribbean Epidemiology Centre. Travel associated legionnaires disease. EPI News 1996;2(3):6–7.

Cholera situation in the Americas. Report 17. Washington, DC: PAHO, 1995.

Lewis M, Irons B, Carrasco F, et al. The burden of congenital rubella syndrome in the English-speaking Carribean. In:

Abstracts of the XIII meeting of the Technical Advisory Group on Vaccine Preventable Diseases. Washington, DC: Pan American Health Organization, 1999:43–45.

Measles elimination in the Americas. JAMA 1996;275:224.

Pan American Health Organization. Health in the Americas. Vols. 1 and 11, Washington, DC: PAHO, 1998.

Pan American Health Organization. The impact of the Expanded Program on Immunization and the Polio Eradication Initiative on Health Systems in the Americas. Final report of the Taylor Commission. Washington, DC: PAHO, 1995.

12.7 TROPICAL SOUTH AMERICA

JAVIER A. ADACHI

Tropical South America is a region that includes 10 different countries (Bolivia, Brazil, Colombia, Ecuador, French Guiana—including Guadeloupe and Martinique—Guyana, Paraguay, Suriname, and Venezuela), from the Pacific Coast to the Atlantic Coast, passing through the high Andean peaks and the Amazon basin, the largest rain forest of the world. Because of its great variety of natural wonders and its rich cultural history, this area of the world attracts a huge amount of tourists each year, especially from industrialized countries. Some of them also enjoy and experience ecologic and adventure tourism. Spanish is the official language in most of the countries, except for Brazil (where Portuguese is the official language), French Guiana (French), Guyana (English), and Suriname (Dutch). All of the countries are considered to be in the group of developing countries, and they share (in different degrees) common problems in public health that are present in countries with a lack of adequate economic resources, such as deficiencies in water supply and basic sanitation services, and an adequate system to register reportable cases.

A wide variety of infectious and tropical diseases are prevalent in this area of the world, and the risk of their acquisition depends on the region that the tourist is visiting (Table 12.7–1), time of exposure, and care and behavior about food and personal hygiene.

The following are some of the numerous communicable diseases that are important causes of illness in these countries, for their own population and for tourists in general:

- **Vector-Borne Diseases.** Malaria, American trypanosomiasis (Chagas' disease) and new-world leishmaniasis affect people in all 10 countries. Onchocerciasis occurs in Brazil, Ecuador, and Venezuela. Filariasis is reported in Brazil, Guyana, Peru, and Suriname. Plague occurs in Bolivia, Brazil, Ecuador, and Peru. Yellow fever, dengue, and viral encephalitis have been reported in all countries, except Paraguay. Bartonellosis (Oroya fever or Carrión's disease) occurs in Bolivia, Colombia, Ecuador, and Peru. Typhus has been found in Colombia and Peru.
- **Food- and Water-Borne Diseases.** Bacterial (e.g., enterotoxigenic *Escherichia coli*, *Vibrio cholerae*), viral (e.g., rotavirus), and parasitic diarrheal diseases (amebiasis, helminthic diseases), as well as hepatitis A, are common in all of the areas. Paragonimiasis is found in Ecuador, Peru, and Venezuela. Since 1991, when the epidemic of cholera started in Peru, there have been reported autochthonous cases of cholera in all countries.
- **Zoonoses.** Brucellosis has been commonly reported, echinococcosis occurs in Bolivia, Brazil, Colombia, Ecuador, and Peru, and rabies has been reported from many countries.
- **Chronic Communicable Diseases.** Tuberculosis is found in all countries and leprosy is endemic in the Amazon basin.
- **AIDS.** AIDS has been reported in all 10 countries, with a high incidence in Brazil. Because sexual transmission predominates, it is highly recommended that travelers avoid sexual promiscuity and engage only in protected sex.
- **Other Diseases.** Rodent-borne arenavirus hemorrhagic fever is found in Bolivia and Venezuela, whereas rodent-borne pulmonary syndrome occurs in Brazil and Paraguay. Hepatitis B and delta are highly endemic in the Amazon rain forest. Snakes, leeches, and spiders are hazardous in the same rain forest.
- **Accidents and Violence.** Violence in general is a serious public health problem in all countries (especially in Colombia and Peru), whereas accidents are one of the main reasons for hospitalization throughout this region.

Table 12.7-1. PREVALENT INFECTIOUS DISEASES IN THE DIFFERENT COUNTRIES OF THE TROPICAL SOUTH AMERICA REGION

COUNTRY	INFECTIOUS DISEASES
Bolivia	Malaria, trypanosomiasis, leishmaniasis, Bolivian hemorrhagic fever, yellow fever, dengue, plague, measles, hepatitis A and B, AIDS, cholera and other diarrheal diseases, fasciolasis, cysticercosis, rabies, brucellosis, bartonellosis, echinococcosis, tuberculosis, and leprosy
Brazil	Malaria, trypanosomiasis, leishmaniasis, yellow fever, dengue, schistosomiasis, plague, AIDS, hepatitis B and delta, filariasis, onchocerciasis, cholera and other diarrheal diseases, rabies, leptospirosis, cysticercosis, meningococcal meningitis, hantavirus infection, purpuric fever caused by *Haemophilus aegyptius,* tuberculosis, and leprosy
Colombia	Malaria, trypanosomiasis, leishmaniasis, yellow fever, dengue, Venezuelan equine encephalitis, typhus, AIDS, hepatitis B, cholera and other diarrheal diseases, rabies, echinococcosis, bartonellosis, tuberculosis, and leprosy
Ecuador	Malaria, trypanosomiasis, leishmaniasis, yellow fever, dengue, onchocerciasis, plague, AIDS, rabies, cholera and other diarrheal diseases, cysticercosis, echinococcosis, paragonimiasis, brucellosis, bartonellosis, tuberculosis, and leprosy
French Guiana	Malaria, trypanosomiasis, yellow fever, dengue, AIDS, cholera and other diarrheal diseases, schistosomiasis, leptospirosis, tuberculosis, and leprosy
Guyana	Malaria, cholera and other diarrheal diseases, Venezuelan equine encephalitis, AIDS, tuberculosis, and leprosy
Paraguay	Malaria, trypanosomiasis, leishmaniasis, dengue, AIDS, cholera and other diarrheal diseases, hantavirus infection, tuberculosis, and leprosy
Peru	Malaria, trypanosomiasis, leishmaniasis, yellow fever, dengue, plague, hepatitis A, B, and delta, AIDS, cholera and other diarrheal diseases, rabies, brucellosis, bartonellosis, leptospirosis, plague, typhus, echinococcosis, cysticercosis, strongyloidiasis, fasciolasis, paragonimiasis, tuberculosis, and leprosy
Suriname	Malaria, dengue, yellow fever, schistosomiasis, leptospirosis, AIDS, cholera and other diarrheal diseases, filariasis, tuberculosis, and leprosy
Venezuela	Malaria, trypanosomiasis, leishmaniasis, yellow fever, dengue, onchocerciasis, schistosomiasis, plague, AIDS, cholera and other diarrheal diseases, rabies, paragonimiasis, Venezuelan equine fever and Venezuelan hemorrhagic fever, tuberculosis, and leprosy

RECOMMENDED READINGS

Pan-American Health Organization. Health in the Americas. Washington, DC: PAHO, 1998.

World Health Organization. International travel and health. Geneva: WHO, 2000.

12.8 TEMPERATE SOUTH AMERICA

JUAN PABLO CAEIRO

This region includes Argentina, Chile, the Falkland Islands (Malvinas), and Uruguay. The mainland ranges from the Mediterranean climatic area of the western coastal strip over the Andes divide to the steppes and desert of Patagonia in the south and to the prairies of the northeast.

The arthropod-borne diseases are relatively unimportant except for the occurrence of American trypanosomiasis (Chagas' disease). Outbreaks of malaria occur in northwestern Argentina (on the border with Bolivia and Paraguay). Cutaneous leishmaniasis are reported from the northeastern part of the country. Recently, dengue has reappeared mainly in the provinces of Salta and Misiones in nothern Argentina.

There is no risk of malaria in Chile, Uruguay, and in the Falkland Islands. Travelers to rural northern Argentina should take chloroquine to prevent malaria.

There is no requirement for yellow fever vaccination certificate in this region, and vaccination is advised only if you are visiting outside urban areas in Argentina.

Of the food- and water-borne diseases, gastroenteritis (mainly salmonellosis) is relatively common in Argentina, especially in suburban areas and among children below the age of 5 years. Some cases of cholera were reported in Argentina and Chile in 1996. Enterohemorrhagic *Escherichia coli* is endemic to Buenos Aires, Argentina, where hemolytic uremic syndrome (HUS) is a common cause of acute renal failure in children. Both *E.*

coli strains 0157:H7 and non-0157:H7 have been associated with diarrhea and HUS in Argentina.

The highest risk for travelers' diarrhea is in Chile, whereas in Argentina and Uruguay, the risk is low. Typhoid fever is not very common in Argentina but hepatitis A and intestinal parasitosis are widespread, the latter especially in the coastal region. Taeniasis (tapeworm), typhoid fever, and viral hepatitis are reported from the other countries.

Echinococcosis (hydatid disease) can be found in rural areas of the three countries, mainly in southern Chile and Argentina. There is an extremely low risk for tourists.

Trichinosis is prevalent in Uruguay; therefore, raw or poorly cooked meats should be avoided.

Anthrax is an occupational hazard in the three mainland countries. Meningococcal meningitis occurs in the form of epidemic outbreaks in Chile. Rodent-borne Hantavirus pulmonary syndrome has been identified in the north-central and southwestern regions of Argentina, in Uruguay, and in Chile.

An investigation of an outbreak of Hantavirus pulmonary syndrome due to Andes virus in southwestern Argentina provided the first reliable evidence of nosocomial and person-to-person transmission of a Hantavirus.

Argentine hemorrhagic fever, caused by the arena virus Junin, is endemic in a well-defined area of north-central Argentina. Most infections occur in agricultural workers. Recently, an effective, attenuated vaccine has been shown to prevent this illness.

Coccidiodomycosis, discovered by Alejandro Posadas in Buenos Aires in 1892, is endemic in the central arid areas of the south zone (Patagonia) and in the province of Catamarca in northern Argentina.

Automobile accidents are a substantial cause of injury among travelers to this region, so people should walk and drive defensively.

BIBLIOGRAPHY

Centers for Disease Control and Prevention. Hantavirus pulmonary syndrome in Chile—1997. MMWR Morb Mortal Wkly Rep 1997;46:949–951.

Enria D, Padula P, Segura EL, et al. Hantavirus pulmonary syndrome in Argentina: possibility of person to person transmission. Medicina (B Aires) 1996;566:709–711.

Istúriz RE, Gotuzzo E. Diseases of Latin America. Infect Dis Clin North Am 1994;8:1–269.

Lopez EL, Diaz M, Grinstein S, et al. Hemolytic uremic syndrome and diarrhea in Argentine children: the role of Shiga-like toxins. J Infect Dis 1989;160:469–475.

Rivas M, Balbi L, Miliwebsky, et al. Sindrome urémico hemolítico en niños de Mendoza, Argentina: asociación con la infección por *Escherichia coli* productor de toxina Shiga. Medicina (B Aires) 1998;58:1–7.

Wells RM, Sosa Estani S, Yadon ZE, et al. An unusual hantavirus outbreak in southern Argentina: person-to-person transmission? Emerg Infect Dis 1997;3:171–174.

12.9 EAST ASIA

ANTHONY JOHNSON HEDLEY AND ABU SALEH M. ABDULLAH

East Asia embraces China (including Hong Kong Special Administrative Region [SAR]), the Democratic People's Republic of Korea, Japan, Macao, Mongolia, and the Republic of Korea. The area includes the high mountain complexes, the desert and the steppes of the west, and the various forest zones of the east, down to the subtropical forests of the southeast.

Arthropod-borne diseases are an important cause of morbidity throughout the area. Malaria, principally *Plasmodium falciparum* and *P. vivax,* is endemic in many parts of the rural areas of China, and in recent years cases have also been reported from the Korean peninsula. Imported cases have occurred in the Hong Kong SAR and Japan. Although reduced in distribution and prevalence, bancroftian and brugian filariasis are still reported in southern China. A resurgence of visceral leishmaniasis is occurring in rural areas of China. Cutaneous leishmaniasis has been reported recently from Xinjiang, Uygur Autonomous Region. Plague has been reported in both China and Mongolia, and bubonic plague is more common in summer and autumn months. Rodent-borne hemorrhagic fever with renal syndrome caused by Hantavirus is endemic in China and Korea, and epidemics of dengue fever may occur in some countries. Japanese B encephalitis is prevalent in the rural areas of most of the countries in this area (especially China, Japan, and Korea). It occurs during summer and autumn in the temperate region. The principal vector is the Culicine (Culex tritaenorhyncus) mosquito. Mite-borne or scrub typhus may be found in scrub areas in southern China, certain river valleys in Japan, and in the Republic of Korea. A tick-borne infection, Russian spring-summer encephalitis, which is closely related to tick-borne encephalitis and is transmitted by Ixodes persulcatus ticks, may occur in China, Korea, and Japan.

Food- and water-borne diseases such as the diarrheal diseases and hepatitis are common in most countries. Cholera and typhoid fever may occur in the rural areas of

China and the Korean peninsula, and imported cases have been reported in Japan and Hong Kong SAR. Epidemics of cholera and typhoid fever may be frequent during the rainy season or after flooding. Cholera outbreaks have occurred in the Hong Kong SAR from unscrupulous use of harbour water in restaurant fish tanks. Hepatitis A outbreaks are common in almost every country and population immunity is declining. The prevalence rate of hepatitis A antibody in China among subjects aged 1 to 59 years is about 81% and over 70% among subjects older than 30 years in the Hong Kong SAR. Hepatitis E is prevalent in northwestern and northeastern parts of China (overall prevalence of hepatitis E antibody is 17% in China), with a few reported cases in Macao and Hong Kong SAR. Clonorchiasis (oriental liver fluke) and paragonimiasis (oriental lung fluke) are reported in China, Japan, Macao, and the Republic of Korea and fasciolopsiasis (giant intestinal fluke) in China. Brucellosis occurs in China.

A positive hepatitis B carrier state (prevalence rate is about 10% in China and Hong Kong SAR) is highly endemic in this region, and hepatitis C is also reported in some countries (prevalence rate of hepatitis C antibody is 3% in China and 0.2%–0.3% in the Hong Kong SAR). The present endemic area of schistosomiasis (bilharziasis) is the central Chang Jiang (Yangtze) river basin in China; active foci no longer exist in Japan. Poliomyelitis eradication activities have rapidly reduced poliovirus transmission and surveillance shows that this has been interrupted in China since 1994; Mongolia no longer reports cases. Trachoma and leptospirosis occur in China. Rabies is endemic in some countries. Outbreaks of meningococcal meningitis occur in Mongolia. Intestinal parasitic infections such as ascariasis, hookworm, trichuriasis, amebiasis, and giardiasis may occur in the rural areas where environmental hygiene and sanitation are inadequate. Human immunodeficiency virus infection is becoming an important sexually transmitted disease in this region and the incidence of infection is escalating in many countries. The estimated reported adult prevalence rate is about 0.06% in China (Hong Kong SAR 0.08%) and about 0.01% in other countries in the East Asia region. Dramatic increases in commercial sex including child prostitution and unsafe sex are associated with these trends.

Besides snakebites and leeches, other health risks to this region are environmental and social hazards and include altitude, cultural and sociopolitical factors, and natural disasters.

BIBLIOGRAPHY

Centres for Disease Control and Prevention. Recommendations for prevention and control of hepatitis C virus (HCV) infection and HCV-related chronic disease. MMWR Morb Mortal Wkly Rep 1998;47(RR-19):1–39.

Hitchcock M, King VT, Parnwell MJ. Tourism in Southeast Asia. London: Routledge, 1993.

Phoon WO, Chen PC. Textbook of community medicine in Southeast Asia. Chichester: John Wiley, 1986.

World Health Organization. International travel and health: vaccination requirements and health advice. Geneva: WHO, 1995.

12.10 EASTERN SOUTH ASIA

KEE-TAI GOH

From the tropical rain and monsoon forests of the northwest, Eastern South Asia extends through the savanna and the dry tropical forests of the Indochina peninsular to the tropical rain and monsoon forests of the islands bordering the South China Sea. The area includes Brunei Darussalam, Cambodia, Indonesia, Lao People's Democratic Republic, Malaysia, Myanmar, The Philippines, Singapore, Thailand, and Vietnam.

Arthropod-borne diseases are an important cause of morbidity and mortality throughout the area. Malaria and filariasis are endemic in many parts of the rural areas of all countries or areas, except for Brunei Darussalam and Singapore, which have been certified free from indigenous malaria by the World Health Organization. Multidrug-resistant falciparum malaria is prevalent in the border areas of Cambodia/Myanmar/Thailand. Foci of chloroquine-resistant vivax malaria have emerged in Indonesia (Irian Jaya, Lombok, Sulawesi, Nias Island, West Kalimantan), Thailand, Myanmar, Cambodia, and Vietnam. There has been a resurgence of dengue and dengue hemorrhagic fever in all of the countries in the region, with epidemics occurring in both urban and rural areas, except for Brunei Darussalam, where normally only imported cases occur.[1] Transmission of Japanese encephalitis occurs in most rural agricultural areas with rice cultivation and pig farming. Singapore has eradicated the disease by phasing out pig farming and instituting systematic mosquito control measures.[2] Plague foci exist in Myanmar and Vietnam, and mite-borne or scrub typhus has been reported in deforested areas in most countries.

Food- and water-borne diseases such as cholera and other watery diarrheas, amebic and bacillary dysentery, enteric fevers (typhoid and paratyphoid), and hepatitis A and E are common. Water-borne outbreaks of cholera and hepatitis E may occur in areas with poor environmental hygiene and sanitation. Among helminthic infections, fasciolopsiasis (giant intestinal fluke) may be acquired in most countries in the area; clonorchiasis (oriental liver fluke) in the Indochina peninsula; opisthorchiasis (cat liver fluke) in the Indochina peninsula, the Philippines, and Thailand; and paragonimiasis (oriental liver fluke) in most countries.

Sexually transmitted diseases, including AIDS, are common. Hepatitis B ranges from intermediate to high endemicity. In countries where hepatitis B vaccination is routinely carried out, the hepatitis B carrier rates in children have been declining.[3] The prevalence of hepatitis C varies from area to area. Poliovirus transmission appeared to have been interrupted in the region, including the Mekong delta area in Cambodia and southern Vietnam, Lao People's Democratic Republic, Indonesia, and Myanmar. Tuberculosis is prevalent in both urban and rural areas. Other childhood vaccine-preventable diseases such as pertussis, measles, and diphtheria continue to occur in areas where the vaccination coverage is low. Epi-

demics of acute hemorrhagic conjunctivitis caused by coxsackievirus A_{24} variant and enterovirus 70 appear periodically. Trachoma exists in Indonesia, Myanmar, Thailand, and Vietnam. Schistosomiasis (bilharziasis) is endemic in the southern Philippines and in central Sulawesi (Indonesia) and occurs in the Mekong delta in Vietnam. Melioidosis occurs sporadically in rural areas throughout the region and is highly endemic in northeastern Thailand.

Other hazards include rabies, snake bites, and leeches.

REFERENCES

1. Goh KT. Dengue in Southeast Asia. JAMA (Southeast Asia) 1998;14:5–6.
2. Goh KT. Vaccines for Japanese encephalitis. Lancet 1996; 348:340.
3. Goh KT. Hepatitis B immunisation in Singapore. Lancet 1996;348:1385–1386.

12.11 MIDDLE SOUTH ASIA

SANTANU CHATTERJEE

Arthropod-borne diseases are endemic in this region (which includes Afghanistan, Armenia, Azerbaijan, Bangladesh, Bhutan, Georgia, India, Islamic Republic of Iran, Kazakstan, Kyrgyzstan, Maldives, Nepal, Pakistan, Sri Lanka, Tajikstan, Turkmenistan, and Uzbekistan). Malaria is reported from most areas of Middle South Asia except Georgia, Kazakstan, Kyrgyzstan, Maldives, Turkmenistan, and Uzbekistan.[1] Risk is high throughout the Indian subcontinent in both rural and urban areas, especially during and immediately after the monsoon season. Incidence of *Plasmodium falciparum* is increasing and chloroquine resistance is reported from many parts. The eastern areas of Bangladesh, the southern districts of Bhutan and Nepal, the southern borders of Tajikstan, especially around the region of Khatlon Oblast, and Afghanistan have reported increasing incidence of *P. falciparum* infection.[2] A recent upsurge of vivax malaria was observed in the eastern districts of Armenia with seasonal peaks during summer and the southern parts of Azerbaijan.[3] Filariasis is common in the southern delta area of Bangladesh, southeastern coastal regions of peninsular India, and the southwestern coastal belt of Sri Lanka. Sandfly fever is on the rise and a sharp increase in visceral leishmaniasis has been noted in the eastern districts of Bangladesh, the northern plains of India adjoining Nepal, and in the Baltistan region of Northern Pak-

istan. Cutaneous leishmaniasis occurs in Afghanistan, India (Rajasthan), the Islamic Republic of Iran, and Pakistan. There are very small isolated foci of cutaneous and visceral leishmaniasis in Azerbaijan, Kyrgyzstan, Tajikstan, and Uzbekistan. Natural foci of plague exists in India and Kazakstan. An outbreak of plague occurred in India in 1994.[4] Tick-borne relapsing fever and typhus occur in Afghanistan and India. Dengue hemorrhagic fever occurs in eastern and northern parts of India and to a lesser extent in Sri Lanka. Recent outbreaks of dengue fever have been reported from Bangladesh, India, Pakistan, and Sri Lanka.[5] A major dengue epidemic occurred in India (New Delhi) in 1996.[6] Japanese encephalitis is endemic in the low-lying eastern areas of Nepal, the eastern and northeastern parts of India, and Sri Lanka.[7] Sporadic outbreaks occur in the Kerala state of Southern India during the rainy season. Crimean-Congo hemorrhagic fever exists in the western areas of this region.

Food- and water-borne diseases are common throughout the region, particularly cholera and other watery diarrheas, the dysenteries, typhoid, hepatitis A and E, and helminthic infections. A novel serotype of *Vibrio cholerae,* designated *V. cholerae* serotype 0139 (synonym Bengal), was responsible for many outbreaks in 1992, but this has since declined in intensity and *V. cholerae El Tor* is now the predominant strain.[8] Hepatitis E is the major etiologic agent for sporadic acute viral hepatitis in this region, and large epidemics periodically occur in the Indian subcontinent.[9] Amebiasis is endemic in certain areas with up to 50% of the population being affected in India.[10] Giardiasis is an important cause of chronic diarrhea, particularly in the long-term, budget traveler.[11] Prevalence of helminthic infestations varies from 5% to 76% in certain areas.[12] Brucellosis and echinococcus (hydatid diseases) are common in many countries in this region.

Hepatitis B is endemic. The national average hepatitis B carrier rate in India is 4.7%.[13] Long-stay visitors and occupational groups like volunteer staff doing medical social work are at increased risk. An isolated focus of urinary schistosomiasis (bilharziasis) persists in the southwestern region of the Islamic Republic of Iran. Occasional outbreaks of meningococcal meningitis are reported from Nepal, although risk to travelers is low. Poliomyelitis is on the decline in this region but should still be considered a risk to visitors, especially for those intending to visit the Indian subcontinent. Trachoma is common in Afghanistan, northern parts of India, Islamic Republic of Iran, Nepal, and Pakistan. Ear and superficial skin infections are common among visitors to Maldives and other beach destinations in this region.[14] Diphtheria outbreaks are reported from Azerbaijan, Georgia, Kazakstan, Kyrgyzstan, Tajikstan, Turkmenistan, and Uzbekistan. Human rabies is a major hazard in most areas in this region. In the Indian subcontinent, the annual incidence of known human cases are estimated to be around 30,000, whereas 500,000 receive postexposure treatment every year.[15] Among the sexually transmitted diseases, hepatitis B and HIV pose the highest risk for the traveler.[16] HIV is a major public health problem, especially in the Indian subcontinent, where transmission patterns show a preponderance of heterosexual spread.[17]

REFERENCES

1. World Health Organization. International travel and health: vaccination requirements and health advice. Geneva: WHO, 1998:43–52.
2. Pitt S, Pearcy BE, Stevens RH, et al. War in Tajikstan and reemergence of *Plasmodium falciparum*. Lancet 1998;352:1279.
3. Davidiants V, Mannrikian M, Sayadian G, et al. Epidemic malaria transmission— Armenia 1997. MMWR Morb Mortal Wkly Rep 1998;47:526–528.
4. Panda SK, Nanda SK, Ghosh A, et al. The 1994 plague epidemic of India: molecular diagnosis and characteristics of *Yersinia pestis* isolates from Surat and Beed. Curr Sci 1996;71:794–799.
5. Halstead SB. The twentieth century dengue pandemic: need for surveillance and research. World Health Stat Q 1992;45:292–298.
6. Ramji S. Dengue strikes Delhi. Indian J Pediatr 1996;33:978.
7. Centers for Disease Control and Prevention. Inactivated Japanese encephalitis virus vaccine. Recommendations of the Advisory Committee on Immunization Practice (ACIP). MMWR Morb Mortal Wkly Rep 1993;42(No RR–1):1–15.
8. Sundaram SP, Revathi J, Elango V, et al. Aetiology of cholera in Tamil Nadu: recent observations. Trans R Soc Trop Hyg 1998;92:164–165.
9. Panda SK, Acharya SK. Hepatitis E virus infection: where are we? Natl Med J India 1998;11:56–58.
10. Ravdin JI. Amoebiasis. Clin Infect Dis 1995;20:1453–1464.
11. Gray SF, Rouse AR. Giardiasis—a cause of travelers' diarrhoea. CDR Review 1992;2:45–47.
12. Ananthakrishnan S, Nalini P, Pani SP. Intestinal geohelminthiasis in the developing world. Natl Med J India 1997;10:67–71.
13. Thyagarajan SP, Jayaram S, Mohanavalli B. Prevalence of HBV in the general population of India. In: Sarin SK, Singhal AK, eds. Hepatitis B in India: problems and prevention. New Delhi: CBS, 1996:5–16.
14. Plentz R. Nontropical and noninfectious diseases among travellers in a tropical area during a five year period (1986–1990). In: Lobel HO, Steffen R, Kozarsky RE, eds. Travel medicine 2. Proceedings of the Second Conference on International Travel Medicine. Atlanta: International Society of Travel Medicine, 1992:77.
15. Sehgal S, Bhattacharya D, Bhardwaj M. Longitudinal studies in innocuity, safety and efficacy of human anti-rabies vaccine in an endemic country—India [abstract 6.06]. Proceedings of the International Rabies Meeting, Pasteur Institute, Paris, March 13–14, 1997.
16. De Schryver, Meheus A. International travel and STD. World Health Stat Q 1989;42:90–99.
17. Pais P. HIV and India: looking into the abyss. Trop Med Int Health 1996;1:295–304.

12.12 WESTERN SOUTH ASIA

ADEL SULAIMAN

Western South Asia (Bahrain, Cyprus, Iraq, Jordan, Kuwait, Lebanon, Oman, Qatar, Saudi Arabia, Syrian Arab Republic, Turkey, the United Arab Emirates, and Yemen) ranges from the mountains and steppes of the northwest to the large deserts and dry tropical scrub of the south.

The arthropod-borne diseases, except for malaria in certain areas, are not a major hazard for the traveler.

Malaria does not exist in Kuwait and no longer occurs in Bahrain, Cyprus, Israel, Jordan, Lebanon, or Qatar. Its incidence in the Syrian Arab Republic and United Arab Emirates is low, but elsewhere it is endemic in certain rural areas. Chloroquine-resistant malaria does occur in Oman. Cutaneous leishmaniasis is reported throughout the area; visceral leishmaniasis, although rare throughout most of the areas, is common in central Iraq, in the southwest of Saudi Arabia, in the northwest of the Syrian Arab Republic, in Turkey (southeast Anatolia only), and in the west of Yemen. Murine and tick-borne typhus can occur in certain countries. Tick-borne relapsing fever and sandfly fever may occur. Crimean-Congo hemorrhagic fever has been reported from Iraq, United Arab Emirates, and Oman. Limited foci of onchocerciasis are reported from Yemen.

The food- and water-borne diseases are, however, a major hazard in most countries in the area. Diarrheal diseases due to enterotoxigenic *Escherichia coli*, *Salmonella*, and *Shigella* are a constant threat, especially in light of increasing resistance of the enteric pathogens in the area to antibiotics. Cholera has been reported recently in Iraq (53 cases in 1998). The typhoid fevers and hepatitis A exist in all countries. Dracunculiasis occurs in isolated foci in Yemen. Taeniasis (tapeworm) is reported from many countries in the area. Brucellosis is reported from most countries and there are foci of echinococcosis (hydatid disease).

Hepatitis B is endemic. With improved testing, the prevalence of hepatitis C is increasing. Hepatitis E is a potential hazard in areas with large populations of guest workers who originate from countries in which hepatitis E has caused epidemic disease. Sexually transmitted diseases are a worldwide hazard and strict precautions are as necessary in Western South Asia as elsewhere. Schistosomiasis (bilharziasis) occurs in Iraq, Saudi Arabia, the Syrian Arab Republic, and Yemen. The risk of poliovirus infection is low in most countries in the area, with the exception of Yemen. Iraq reported 24 cases of confirmed polio in 1996. It is unclear how the recent conflicts involving Iraq would affect the incidence of communicable diseases in the country. Trachoma and animal rabies are found in many of the countries. Endemic nonvenereal syphilis, or bejel, occurs in some parts of Saudi Arabia, Iraq, and Jordan. The greatest hazards to pilgrims to Mecca and Medina are heat and water depletion if the period of Hajj (Muslim pilgrimage) coincides with the hot season.

BIBLIOGRAPHY

Centers for Disease Control. Global cholera update. 1998 notifications as of 30 November 1998.

Centers for Disease Control. Health information for travelers to the Middle East.

Olfield III, et al. Endemic infectious diseases of the Middle East. Rev Inf Dis 1991;13(Suppl 3):S199–S217.

Wild poliovirus transmission in bordering areas of Iran, Iraq, Syria, and Turkey, 1997–June 1998. MMWR Morb Mortal Wkly Rep 1998;47:588–592.

12.13 NORTHERN EUROPE

JONATHAN H. COSSAR

The area encompassed by these countries (Belarus, Belgium, Czech Republic, Denmark with Faroe Islands, Estonia, Finland, Germany, Iceland, Ireland, Latvia, Lithuania, Luxembourg, Netherlands, Norway, Poland, Republic of Moldova, Russian Federation, Slovakia, Sweden, Ukraine, the United Kingdom with the Channel Islands and the Isle of Man) extends from the broadleaf forests and the plains of the west to the boreal and mixed forest to be found as far east as the Pacific Ocean. Travelers should be up to date with the immunization schedule for their home country including poliomyelitis, diphtheria, and tetanus. The incidence of communicable diseases in most parts of the area is such that they are unlikely to prove a hazard to the international traveler greater than that found in his or her own country. Health risks in the region are greater in the more recent democracies (Belarus, Czech Republic, Estonia, Latvia, Lithuania, Poland, Republic of Moldova, Russian Federation, Slovakia, Ukraine) predominantly on the eastern margins of the area. Long-stay expatriates, teachers, and health care workers to these countries should ensure protection to tuberculosis and hepatitis B, be aware of the risk of sexually transmitted diseases and HIV infection, and consider typhoid protection if unable to ensure good quality local food and water. Awareness of the risks from road traffic accidents and workplace accidents is also important; for example, over 1.3 million European Union citizens died as a result of an unintentional injury between 1984 and 1993.[1]

Rabies is endemic in wild animals (particularly foxes, >50% of total) in rural areas of northern Europe.[2] With the exceptions of Albania, Austria, Finland, Greece, Iceland, Ireland, Italy, Macedonia, Norway, Portugal, the mainland and islands of Spain, Sweden, United Kingdom, Channel Islands, and the Isle of Man, rabies protection should be considered for those having regular contact with animals such as veterinarians, particularly in the more remote areas or if going to be more than 24 hours away from a source of vaccine.

Otherwise, in most of the areas very few precautions are required.

Of the arthropod-borne diseases, there are very small foci of tick-borne typhus in east and central Siberia. Tick-borne encephalitis, for which a vaccine exists, and Lyme disease (new vaccine available in the U.S. from December 1998)[3] may occur throughout forested areas where vector ticks are found. The season of highest risk for the former is spring to early summer but for the latter also extends through to the autumn. Campers, walkers, ramblers, orienteers, and long-stay residents are at most risk of exposure to bites, particularly when wearing short sleeves and shorts. Rodent-borne hemorrhagic fever with renal syndrome is now recognized as occurring at low endemic levels in this area.

The food- and water-borne diseases reported—other than the ubiquitous diarrheal diseases—are taeniasis (tapeworm) and trichinellosis in parts of northern Europe and diphyllobothriasis (fish tapeworm) from the freshwater fish around the Baltic Sea area. *Fasciola hepatica* infection can occur. Hepatitis A, giardiasis, and amebiasis occur in the Eastern European countries (Belarus, Czech Republic, Estonia, Latvia, Lithuania, Poland, Republic of Moldova, Russian Federation, Slovakia, Ukraine). The incidence of certain food-borne diseases

(e.g., salmonellosis and campylobacteriosis) is increasing significantly in some countries.[4]

All endemic countries in the area are now making intense efforts to eradicate poliomyelitis. Within the Russian Federation, poliovirus transmission remains a possibility only in the area of Chechenia. The annual total of human cases rarely reaches double figures; the Russian Federation has the highest number. In recent years, Belarus, the Russian Federation, and Ukraine have experienced extensive epidemics of diphtheria. Diphtheria cases, mostly imported from these three countries, have also been reported from neighboring countries: Estonia, Finland, Latvia, Lithuania, Poland, and the Republic of Moldova. Both sporadic cases and clusters of *Legionella* infection occur throughout the area, in keeping with the ubiquitous nature of the organism.

Extreme cold in winter is a climatic hazard in parts of northern Europe.

REFERENCES

1. Eurorisc (European Review of Injury Surveillance and Control). Newsletter 3, Glasgow, 1998.
2. World Health Organization. Rabies bulletin Europe 1/98. Geneva: WHO, July 1998.
3. International Society of Travel Medicine. NewsShare, Glasgow, 1st Quarter, 1999.
4. World Health Organization. International travel and health. Geneva: WHO, 1998.

12.14 SOUTHERN EUROPE

WALTER PASINI

Southern Europe (Albania, Andorra, Bosnia and Herzegovina, Bulgaria, Croatia, France, Gibraltar, Greece, Hungary, Italy, Liechtenstein, Malta, Monaco, Portugal [with the Azores and Madeira], Romania, San Marino, Slovenia, Spain [with the Canary Islands], Switzerland, the Former Yugoslav Republic of Macedonia, and Yugoslavia) extends from the broadleaf forests in the northwest and the mountains of the Alps to the prairies and in the south and southeast the scrub vegetation of the Mediterranean.

Among the arthropod-borne diseases, sporadic cases of murine and tick-borne typhus and mosquito-borne West Nile fever occur in some countries bordering the Mediterranean littoral. Both cutaneous and visceral leishmanias and sandfly fever are also reported from this area. Leishmania/HIV coinfections have been notified from France, Italy, Portugal, and Spain. Tick-borne encephalitis (TBE), for which a vaccine exists, is common in Austria, Hun-

gary, and northern Yugoslavia. It occurs at a lower frequency in Bulgaria, Romania, and France. Serologic evidence for TBE infection, as well as sporadic cases, has been reported from Albania, Greece, and Italy. Lyme disease and rodent-borne hemorrhagic fever with renal syndrone may occur in the eastern and southern parts of the area.

Malaria is frequently reported as an imported disease from travelers of the industrialized countries of the region coming mainly from sub-Saharan Africa.

The food- and water-borne diseases—bacillary dysentery and other diarrheas, typhoid fever—are more common in the summer and autumn months, with a high incidence in the southeastern and southwestern parts of the area. Brucellosis can occur in the extreme southwest and southeast and echinococcosis (hydatid disease) in the southeast. *Fasciola hepatica* infection has been reported from different countries in this area. Hepatitis A occurs in the Eastern European countries. The incidence of certain food-borne diseases (e.g., salmonellosis and campylobacteriosis) is increasing significantly in some countries.

AIDS

In the industrialized countries of the region, the availability of antiretroviral therapy has continued to reduce progression to AIDS, deaths, and mother-to-child transmission of HIV. In most of these countries, however, the number of new HIV infections has remained relatively constant in recent years. As of November 2, 1999, the cumulative numbers of reported AIDS cases were the following: Spain, 54,964; France, 49,421; Italy, 44,516; Switzerland, 6,641; Portugal, 6,020; Romania, 5,928; Greece, 1,964; Austria, 1,915; Yugoslavia, 806; Hungary, 328; Croatia, 144; Slovenia, 81; Bulgaria, 60; Malta, 47; Monaco, 40; Macedonia, 29; Bosnia and Herzegovina, 17; San Marino, 14; and Albania, 11. It is probably that the cases reported by eastern countries could be underreported. Analysis of HIV incidence by age group and gender shows that in the younger age groups, more women than men are affected. This calls for specific strategies to protect women from infections, in particular through sex education and empowerment of girls and women.

OTHER SEXUALLY TRANSMITTED DISEASES

In previous decades, the European region experienced a steady decrease in the incidence of the main sexually transmitted diseases such as syphilis and gonorrhea. More recently, the new epidemic of syphilis occurred in the Russian Federation and in the New Independent States, and also involved some countries of Southern Europe. Trichomoniasis, genital warts, herpes infection, chlamydial genital infections, and other STDs are reported in all of the countries.

HEPATITIS B

Most countries of Northern and Western Europe have a very low prevalence of hepatitis B virus infection, with less than 0.5% of the population being surface antigen carriers; incidence rates, too, are very low. Hepatitis B is endemic in the southern part of Eastern Europe (Albania, Bulgaria, Romania, and Yugoslavia). In these countries, all modes of hepatitis B transmission are found including child-to-child transmission, nosocomial infection of health care personnel and patients through unsafe injection and sterilization procedures, unsafe blood products, and traditional medical and cosmetic skin-piercing procedures, as well as through percutaneous drug use and sexual transmission.

OTHER DISEASES

Poliomyelitis elimination in the region is part of the global eradication initiative and entails strategies of high routine immunization coverage, supplementary mass immunization, and enhanced surveillance. All countries in Southern Europe, where poliomyelitis was, until recently, endemic, are conducting eradication activities, and the risk of infection in most countries is very low. However, a large poliomyelitis outbreak occurred in 1996 in Albania affecting Yugoslavia (Serbia and Montenegro) and Greece (due to imported type 1 poliovirus); it had been interrupted by the end of 1996.

The resurgence of tuberculosis (TB) is a challenging problem in the region. The previous downward trend in western countries is now leveling off or being slightly reversed. The spread of *Mycobacterium tuberculosis* resistant to antimicrobial chemotherapy is worsening the situation. The resurgence is linked to HIV infection, substance abuse, and immigration. Furthermore, some countries are not systematically following the World Health Organization's guidelines for the diagnosis and treatment of TB, particularly the directly observed treatment, short-course strategy.

Rabies in animals exists in most of the southern countries of the region except Albania, Gibraltar, Greece, Italy, Malta, Monaco, the former Yugoslav Republic of Macedonia, Portugal, and Spain, except Ceuta/Melilla.

Haemophilus influenzae type B, with meningitis, epiglottitis, and pneumonia as the most serious manifestations, is still a widespread disease. With the implementation of routine immunization in early infancy and childhood, several states of the region have dramatically reduced the occurrence of invasive disease.

BIBLIOGRAPHY

Centers for Disease Control and Prevention. Health information for international travel, 1999–2000. Atlanta: Department of Health and Human Services, 2000.

World Health Organization. International travel and health: vaccination requirements and health advice. Geneva: WHO, 1999.

World Health Organization, Regional Office for Europe. Country highlights, 1997. Copenhagen: WHO, 1997.

World Health Organization. Weekly Epidemiological Records, 1998–1999. Geneva.

12.15 PACIFIC ISLANDS

TILMAN A. RUFF

The Pacific Island countries and areas are spread over an enormous expanse of ocean, with the larger mountainous islands of Melanesia in the west giving way to smaller volcanic and coral atoll islands in the north and east. Levels of infrastructure and hygiene and sanitation vary widely. Infectious disease risks are described in Table 12.15–1.

Noninfectious marine hazards include ciguatera fish poisoning, which is highly prevalent, especially in Polynesian and Micronesian areas; a variety of toxic animals, including sea snakes; and coral injuries.

REFERENCES

1. World Health Organization. International travel and health. Geneva: WHO, 1998.
2. Mackenzie JS, Broom AK, Hall RA, et al. Arboviruses in the Australian region, 1990 to 1998. Commun Dis Intell 1998; 22:93–100.

Table 12.15–1.   SELECTED INFECTIOUS DISEASES—PACIFIC ISLANDS

Vector-borne diseases	
Malaria	Endemic only in Melanesian countries—Papua New Guinea (PNG), Solomon Islands, and Vanuatu[1]; both *P. falciparum* (often resistant to choloroquine and pyrimethamine-sulfadoxine) and *P. vivax*. Incidence is high (holoendemic) in PNG and Solomons. *P. vivax* resistant to chloroquine described in PNG and Solomons but no cases reported in travelers. *P. vivax* Chesson strain (relatively primaquine resistant) widespread.
Dengue	Periodic epidemics, generally every 3–5 years, sometimes with hemorrhagic cases
Murray Valley encephalitis	Occurs in PNG lowlands
Japanese encephalitis	Self-limited epidemics described in Guam and Saipan (Northern Mariana Islands). Recently shown to be endemic in Western Province of PNG; probably spreading.[2]
Typhus	Predominantly scrub typhus (*Orientia tsutsugamushi*) in Melanesia
Filariasis	Diurnally periodic *Wuchereria bancrofti* widespread, varying prevalence
Ross River virus	Reported in PNG and Solomon Islands. Large, self-limited epidemic in other islands, particularly Fiji, in 1979–1980 with over 50,000 reported cases, almost certainly triggered by a viremic traveler from Australia.[2]
Enteric infections	Diarrheal diseases (occasionally including cholera, especially in Micronesia), typhoid and common helminths are widespread with variable prevalence. Hepatitis A generally common. Eosinphilic meningitis due to *Angiostrongylus cantonensis* seen in travelers. No poliomyelitis cases reported for over 5 years.[1] Pigbel (necrotizing enterocolitis due to *Clostridium perfringens* type C) is common in the PNG highlands, where it is targeted by immunization.
Other infections	
Hepatitis B	Hyperendemic throughout the region, with population carrier rates of up to 30%. Variable prevalence of hepatitis D—high in some islands.

12.16 AUSTRALIA, NEW ZEALAND, AND ANTARCTICA

TILMAN A. RUFF

The climate and terrain in this region vary enormously, from tropical, through desert, to Mediterranean and temperate in Australia; from subtropical to temperate in New Zealand; and from subpolar to freezing polar in Antarctica. Except in Australian Aboriginal communities, where many infections typically seen in developing countries are still prevalent, travelers will generally not be at greater risk of communicable diseases than in their country of origin.[1]

However, a number of diseases are endemic in specific regions, particularly tropical Australia, which covers 40% of the continent (Table 12.16–1). As elsewhere, new infections and changing epidemiology of known infec-

Table 12.16–1.   SELECTED INFECTIOUS DISEASES—AUSTRALIA

Vector-borne diseases	
Malaria	Last indigenous case 1962
	Periodic introduced cases in Torres Strait Islands and North Queensland
	Area N of latitude 19° S malaria receptive
Dengue	Spread of *Aedes aegypti* and increasingly frequent epidemics of dengue in north Queensland since 1981–1982[2]
Australian encephalitis	Mostly due to flaviviruses Murray Valley encephalitis and, occasionally, Kunjin viruses. Endemic in Kimberley region of Western Australia and adjacent Northern Territory (NT).[1]
Japanese encephalitis	1995 outbreak with subsequent ongoing transmission in Torres Strait Islands and human and animal infections on mainland Australia in 1998.[3] Significant potential to spread more widely.[2]
Ross River virus (RRV), Barmah Forest virus	These alphaviruses cause fever, rash, and polyarthritis. RRV is most common documented arboviral infection. Both are widespread.[2]
Rickettsial infections	All three groups of rickettsial diseases occur[4]: (1) scrub typhus (*Orienta tsutsugamushi*) is found in Queensland, NT, and Kimberley region; (2) spotted fever group (SFG): Queensland tick typhus (*Rickettsia australis*) along whole eastern seaboard, Flinders Island Spotted Fever *(Rickettsia honei)* in Flinders Island off southern Australia, and an unidentified SFG infection in Tasmania; (3) endemic (murine) typhus *(R. typhi)* is found in scattered foci in Queensland, South and Western Australia. Q fever *(Coxiella burnetii)* is widespread.
Other infections	
Melioidosis	Infection with *Burkholderia pseudomallei* is an important cause of sepsis in northern Australia. Most common cause of fatal community-acquired bacteremic pneumonia in NT.
Recently described infections associated with reservoir in bats	Equine morbillivirus—2 human cases (1 fatal) in Queensland 1995.[4] Australian bat lyssavirus —1 fatal human case rabies-like encephalitis Queensland 1995[5]; preventable by rabies pre- or postexposure immunization.[6] New paramyxovirus ("Menangle" virus) associated with febrile rash illness, 1997.[7]

tions continue to be described. Global warming is expected to result in southward expansion of the range of a number of tropical infections.

Noninfectious hazards include venomous snakes, which are widespread (no snakes in New Zealand); saltwater crocodiles, which are found in northern Australia; box jellyfish (*Chironex fleckeri*), a summer (maximal December–March) hazard in tropical marine waters; and ciguatera fish poisoning, which is prevalent along much of the Queensland coast and in eastern Northern Territory.

REFERENCES

1. World Health Organization. International travel and health. Geneva: WHO, 1998.

2. Mackenzie JS, Broom AK, Hall RA, et al. Arboviruses in the Australian region, 1990 to 1998. Commun Dis Intell 1998;22:93–100.

3. Hanna JN, Ritchie SA, Phillips DA, et al. An outbreak of Japanese encephalitis in the Torres Strait, Australia, 1995. Med J Aust 1996;165:256–260.

4. Odorico DM, Graves SR, Currie B, et al. New *Orienta tsutsugamushi* strain from scrub typhus in Australia. Emerg Inf Dis 1998;4:641–644.

5. O'Sullivan JD, Allworth AM, Paterson DL, et al. Fatal encephalitis due to a novel paramyxovirus transmitted from horses. Lancet 1997;349:93–95.

6. Lyssavirus Expert Group. Prevention of human lyssavirus infection. Commun Dis Intell 1996;20:505–507.

7. Chant K, Chan R, Smith M, et al. Probable human infection with a newly described virus in the Family Paramyxoviridae. Emerg Infect Dis 1998;4:273–275.

Chapter 13

MEDICAL PROBLEMS OF HIGH ALTITUDE

PETER H. HACKETT AND DAVID R. MURDOCH

Due to modern modes of transportation and the explosion in adventure travel, millions are now visiting high-altitude areas throughout the world. In Colorado alone, there are estimated to be more than 20 million visitors each year who go to 2,500 m altitude or higher.[1] The Himalayan Kingdom of Nepal issues permits to over 100,000 trekkers each year, with most of these tourists ascending to over 3,000 m and many to over 5,000 m. Hundreds of thousands visit other high-altitude regions in Europe, Africa, South America, Asia, and North America annually (Figure 13–1). Few of these travelers have any knowledge of the special problems associated with high-altitude exposure. Increasingly, health care providers are being asked to give advice on the prevention and treatment of high-altitude medical problems, as well as the effect of high-altitude on preexisting illnesses (Table 13–1). Despite advances in this field, many travelers continue to become ill at high altitude and some die. Clearly, better education of the population at risk and of those advising them is essential. The travel medicine literature is starting to address the safety and hazards of high-altitude exposure, and responsible tour operators should be disseminating this information.

THE HIGH-ALTITUDE ENVIRONMENT

High altitude is a hypoxic environment. Since the concentration of oxygen in the troposphere remains constant at 21%, the partial pressure of oxygen decreases as a function of the barometric pressure (Figure 13–2). In Denver (1,610 m), air pressure is 17% less than sea level and therefore contains 17% less oxygen. The air of Aspen, Colorado (2,438 m) has 26% less oxygen, and the barometric pressure on top of Mount Everest is merely one-third that of sea level. Paul Bert, in his classic experiments of the late 19th century, showed that supplemental oxygen prevented symptoms of altitude illness during hypobaric exposure and concluded that hypoxia, not the hypobaria, was responsible for illness.[2]

For purposes of discussion, the range of high altitude may be divided based on physiologic effects. From 1,500 m to 3,500 m above sea level (4,900 ft to 11,500 ft) is considered *high altitude*; decreased exercise performance and increased ventilation (lower arterial P_{CO_2}) occur, without major impairment in arterial oxygen transport, although altitude illness is common with abrupt ascent to over 2,500 m (8,200 ft). *Very high altitude* encompasses the range of 3,500 m to 5,500 m (18,000 ft), where maximum arterial oxygen saturation falls to less than 90% ($PaO_2 < 60$ mm Hg), and extreme hypoxemia may occur during exercise, sleep, and altitude illness. Abrupt ascent to these altitudes may be dangerous; a period of acclimatization is required. *Extreme altitude,* over 5,500 m, is accompanied by severe hypoxemia and hypocapnea, and abrupt ascent precipitates illness in nearly all individuals. At this altitude, progressive physiologic deterioration eventually outstrips acclimatization, and permanent human habitation is impossible.

Although physiologic effects such as a decrease in arterial carbon dioxide pressure start as low as 1,500 m, medical problems resulting from high-altitude exposure generally occur above 2,500 m. The critical factor is the sleeping altitude, not the height to which one travels during the day. Hypoxic stress is greatest during the night because of lower ventilation during sleep, as well as periodic breathing, a common phenomenon above 2,500 m (Figure 13–3). A threshold for potentially serious altitude illness is a sleeping altitude of about 2,800 m. At this elevation, arterial oxygen pressure in healthy persons drops to less than 65 mm Hg, and arterial oxygen saturation will drop precipitously with any further decrease in P_{O_2}.

In addition to hypoxia, the high-altitude environment poses several other stresses. Adiabatic cooling rate is approximately 6.5°C per 1,000 m altitude gain, so that high-altitude areas are considerably colder. Ultraviolet (UV) penetration increases approximately 12% per 1,000 m,

Table 13–1. MEDICAL PROBLEMS OF HIGH ALTITUDE

ACUTE ILLNESS IN THE UNACCLIMATIZED	PROBLEMS POTENTIALLY AGGRAVATED BY ALTITUDE (PARTIAL LIST)
Acute mountain sickness	Hypertension
Cerebral edema	Arteriosclerotic heart disease
Pulmonary edema	Congestive heart failure
Peripheral edema	Chronic lung disease
Retinopathy	Arteriosclerotic
Thromboembolism	cerebrovascular disease
Sleep periodic breathing	Pulmonary hypertension
Disordered sleep	Disorders of pregnancy and childbirth
	Seizure disorders
	Sickle cell anemia
	Radial keratotomy

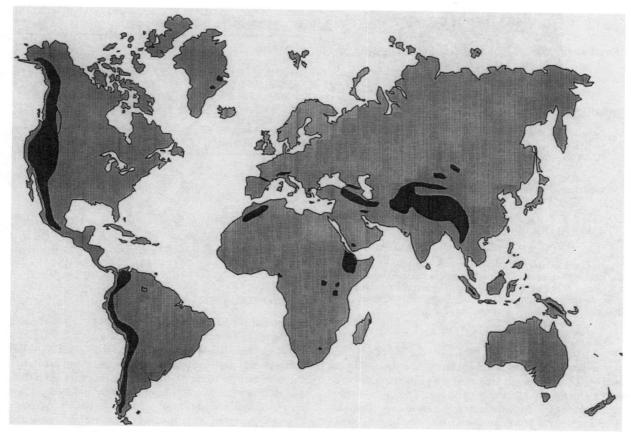

Figure 13–1.   World map showing inhabited areas over 2,500 m altitude.

making UV keratitis, sunburn, and other sun-related problems a much greater concern at high altitude. Mountainous terrain is often treacherous, and combined with the climatologic factors, problems such as trauma, frostbite, and hypothermia may result. Since barometric pressure falls in a curvilinear function with increasing altitude, gases expand, increasing intestinal gas, and trapped gas can cause dental pain, fractured fillings, and dysbaric problems such as barotitis media and barosinusitis.

ACCLIMATIZATION

Persons rendered acutely hypoxic become dizzy, faint, and rapidly unconscious if hypoxic stress is sufficient. These same individuals, given days to weeks to develop the exact same degree of hypoxia, are able to function quite well. Although the fundamental process of this acclimatization takes place in the metabolic machinery of cells and mitochondria, acute "struggle" responses are critical while allowing the cells time to adjust.

VENTILATION

Defense of alveolar P_{O_2} through increased ventilation is the primary initial adaptation. The hypoxic ventilatory response (HVR) is a function of the carotid body, which senses a decrease in arterial oxygenation and inputs to the central respiratory center in the medulla to increase ventilation. The HVR is thought to be genetically determined so, to a large extent, how quickly one acclimatizes to altitude is inherited. Respiratory depressants will impair acclimatization, and stimulants may improve the ventila-

Figure 13–2.   Increasing altitude results in a fall of inspired PO_2 (P_IO_2), arterial PO_2 (PaO_2), and arterial oxygen saturation ($SaO_2\%$). Note: (1) the difference between inspired and arterial PO_2 narrows at high altitude due to increased ventilation; (2) $SaO_2\%$ is well maintained while awake until over 3,000 m. (From Hackett et al.[31])

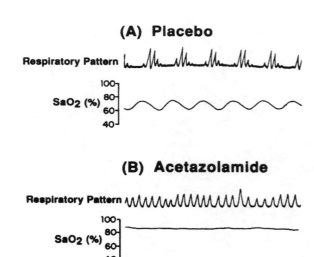

Figure 13–3. Respiratory patterns and arterial oxygen saturation (SaO$_2$%) with placebo and acetazolamide in two sleep studies of a subject at 4,300 m. Note the pattern of hyperpnea followed by apnea during placebo treatment that is attenuated with acetazolamide. (Adapted from Hackett and Roach.[15])

Table 13–2. BLOOD GASES AT VARIOUS ALTITUDES

ALTITUDE	PaO$_2$	SaO$_2$	PaCO$_2$
Sea level	90–95	96	40
1,524 m (5000 ft)	75–81	95	35
2,286 m (7,500 ft)	69–74	92–93	31–33
4,572 m (15,000 ft)	48–53	86	25
6,096 m (20,000 ft)	37–45	76	20
7,620 m (25,000 ft)	32–39	68	13
8,848 m (29,029 ft)	26–33	58	9.5–13.8

Source: Hackett et al.[31]

tory response. Alcohol and respiratory depressants should thus be avoided during the ventilatory acclimatization of the first few days of altitude exposure. The initial hyperventilation is quickly attenuated by respiratory alkalosis, which acts as a brake on the respiratory center. Renal excretion of bicarbonate then compensates for the respiratory alkalosis, pH returns toward normal (but never reaches normal), and ventilation continues to increase. This process of maximizing ventilation, termed "ventilatory acclimatization," culminates after 4 to 7 days at a given altitude. After this time, altitude illness is unlikely at the same altitude, but each step increase to a higher altitude brings a renewed risk of altitude illness. With continuing ascent, the central chemoreceptors reset to progressively lower Pco$_2$ values, and the completeness of acclimatization can be gauged by the arterial Pco$_2$. Acetazolamide, which forces a bicarbonate diuresis, greatly facilitates this process. An appreciation of the "normal" values for blood gases and acid-base status with acclimatization at various altitudes indicates the extreme hypoxemia that can be tolerated via the process of acclimatization (Table 13–2).

BLOOD

Viault first observed the hematopoietic response to altitude in 1890. We now know that within 2 hours of ascent to altitude, erythropoeitin is increased in plasma and over days to weeks results in increased red cell mass. This adaptation has no importance during initial acclimatization, but when excessive, results in marked polycythemia (hemoglobin > 20 g/dL). A corollary is that people with moderate anemia seem to acclimatize without problems. Shifts in the oxyhemoglobin dissociation curve are thought to be minimal in vivo at altitude since the increase in 2,3 diphosphoglycerate (DPG), which is proportional

to the severity of hypoxia and shifts the curve to the right, is offset by the alkalosis, which shifts the curve to the left. Naturally occurring left-shifted hemoglobin is an advantage at altitude.

FLUID BALANCE

Peripheral venous constriction on ascent to altitude causes an increase in central blood volume, which triggers baroreceptors to suppress antidiuretic hormone (ADH) and aldosterone and induce a diuresis. Combined with the bicarbonate diuresis from the respiratory alkalosis, this results in decreased plasma volume and hyperosmolality (serum osmolality of 290–300), which the body appears to permit by a reset of the osmol center of the brain. Clinically, diuresis and hemoconcentration is a healthy response; altitude illness is associated with antidiuresis and fluid retention. The benefit of this relative dehydration may be to ameliorate brain swelling (see Acute Mountain Sickness).

CARDIOVASCULAR

Stroke volume is decreased initially because of the decreased plasma volume, and an increased heart rate maintains cardiac output. Maximum exercising heart rate declines at altitude proportional to the decrease in Vo$_2$ max. Cardiac muscle in healthy persons is able to withstand extreme levels of hypoxemia (PaO$_2$ < 30 mm Hg) without evidence of ST segment changes or ischemic events. Blood pressure is mildly elevated on ascent secondary to increased sympathetic tone.

The pulmonary circulation constricts with exposure to hypoxia. This is an advantage during regional alveolar hypoxia, such as pneumonia, but is a disadvantage during the global hypoxia of altitude exposure. As a result, pulmonary pressure increases. The degree of hypertension is quite variable, and those with a hyperreactive response are much more susceptible to high-altitude pulmonary edema.

Cerebral blood flow increases on ascent to altitude (despite the hypocapnic alkalosis), which increases oxygen delivery to the brain. This response, however, is limited by the increase in cerebral blood volume, which may increase intracranial pressure and produce and/or aggravate symptoms of altitude illness.

EFFECTS ON EXERCISE

One of the more dramatic effects of ascent to altitude is a reduction in exercise performance. Maximum oxygen consumption decreases approximately 10% for each 1,000-m altitude gain above 1,500 m. This does not recover appreciably with acclimatization, although submaximal endurance markedly increases after 10 days. Consequently, it is nearly impossible to train at altitude with the same intensity as at sea level. Athletes who train at sea level are at a distinct disadvantage when competing at high altitude. Records for endurance-type events are always better at low altitude, and a period of adequate acclimatization is necessary to maximize performance before an event at high altitude. On the other hand, high-altitude exposure, by increasing hemoglobin concentration, benefits performance at low altitude. Unacclimatized travelers need to reduce their usual sea level pace according to comfort and plan more frequent rests at high altitude.

HIGH-ALTITUDE SYNDROMES

High-altitude syndromes of primary concern are those problems attributed directly to hypobaric hypoxia: acute hypoxia, acute mountain sickness (AMS), high-altitude pulmonary edema (HAPE), high-altitude cerebral edema (HACE), retinopathy, peripheral edema, sleeping problems, and a group of neurologic syndromes. Other syndromes, not necessarily related to hypoxia, include thromboembolic events (which may be attributable to dehydration, prolonged incapacitation, polycythemia, and cold), high-altitude pharyngitis and bronchitis, and UV keratitis. Although the different hypoxic clinical syndromes overlap, all share a fundamental mechanism, are seen in the same setting of rapid ascent in unacclimatized persons, and respond to the same essential therapy: descent and/or oxygen.

ACUTE HYPOXIA

The syndrome of acute hypoxia occurs in the setting of sudden and severe hypoxic insult, such as accidental decompression of a pressurized aircraft cabin, or a failed oxygen system in a pilot or high-altitude mountaineer. Sudden overexertion precipitating arterial desaturation, acute onset of pulmonary edema, carbon monoxide poisoning, and sleep apnea may result in relatively acute hypoxia as well. Unacclimatized persons become unconscious at an arterial oxygen saturation of 50% to 60%, an arterial Po_2 of less than about 30 mm Hg, or a jugular venous Po_2 less than 15 mm Hg. Acute hypoxia is reversed by immediate administration of oxygen, rapid descent, and/or correction of the underlying cause such as removal of the carbon monoxide source or repair of the oxygen delivery system. Symptoms of acute hypoxia reflect the sensitivity of the central nervous system (CNS) to this insult: dizziness, lightheadedness, and dimmed vision progressing to loss of consciousness. Hyperventilation has been shown to increase the time of useful consciousness during acute alveolar hypoxia.

ACUTE MOUNTAIN SICKNESS

INCIDENCE

AMS is the most common and benign of the high-altitude illnesses. Incidence varies depending on rate of ascent and altitude attained (Table 13–3). In medium-altitude ski resorts, the incidence ranges from 10% at 2,300 m to 40% at 3,000 m.[3] On Mount Rainier, 70% of mountaineers develop some degree of AMS because of the very rapid ascent (sea level to 4,500 m in less than 36 hours),[4] whereas 84% of travelers flying directly from Kathmandu (1,300 m) to Hotel Everest View in Nepal (3,860 m) develop AMS.[5] High incidences of AMS would also be expected among tourists to popular high-altitude destinations such as Lhasa (3,658 m), La Paz (3,625 m), and Cuzco (3,415 m). Persons living in intermediate altitudes such as Denver are much less likely to become ill because they are partially acclimatized. In general, the susceptibility to mountain sickness is reproducible in a given individual, with some being relatively resistant and others being particularly susceptible. Men and women are equally affected, as are children. Concomitant respiratory infection may be a risk factor. Contrary to popular

Table 13–3. INCIDENCE OF ALTITUDE ILLNESS IN VARIOUS GROUPS

STUDY GROUP	NUMBER AT RISK PER YEAR	SLEEPING ALTITUDE (m)	MAXIMUM ALTITUDE REACHED (m)	AVERAGE TIME TO ASCEND (days)*	AMS (%)	HAPE AND/OR HACE† (%)
Western United States visitors	40 million	2,100 2,800 3,000	3,500	1–2	12–25 15–30 42	0.01
Mount Everest trekkers	10,000	3,000 to 5,000	5,500	1–2 (fly-in) 10–13 (walk-in)	47 23	1.6 0.05
Mount Rainier climbers	9,000	3,000	4,392	1–2	67	NA
Indian soldiers	Unknown	3,000–5,500	5,500	1–2	NA	2.3–15.5

*Days to sleeping altitude from low altitude.
†HAPE = high-altitude pulmonary edema; HACE = high-altitude cerebral edema; NA = reliable estimate not available.
Adapted from Hackett et al.[31]

opinion, there is no relationship between susceptibility to AMS and physical fitness.

CLINICAL PRESENTATION

The diagnosis of AMS is based on the setting, symptoms, and physical findings. The setting is rapid ascent of an unacclimatized person to 2,000 m (6,600 ft) or higher. One to 6 hours later, but sometimes delayed for a day or more (and especially after a night's sleep), the typical symptoms of AMS develop. Headache is the most common, is usually described as bifrontal, and is worsened with bending over and Valsalva maneuver. Gastrointestinal symptoms include anorexia, nausea, and sometimes vomiting, and the chief constitutional symptoms are lassitude and weakness. The syndrome very much resembles an alcohol hangover, or even a viral syndrome, but myalgias and fever are absent. The person with AMS is often irritable and wants to be left alone. Sleepiness and a deep inner chill are also common. If the illness progresses, the headache becomes more severe, and vomiting, oliguria, and increased dyspnea develop. Lassitude may progress to the victim requiring assistance for eating and dressing. The most severe form of mountain sickness, HACE, is heralded by onset of ataxia and altered level of consciousness; coma may ensue within 12 hours if treatment is delayed.

Physical findings in mild AMS are nonspecific. Heart rate and blood pressure are usually within the normal range, although postural hypotension may be present. Localized rales may be detected. Slight fever is common, especially in the presence of pulmonary edema. Fundoscopy reveals venous tortuosity and dilatation, and retinal hemorrhages are common over 5,000 m or in those with pulmonary and cerebral edema. Fluid retention is a hallmark of AMS, which contrasts with the usual diuresis of acclimatization. It may result in peripheral edema, which occurs especially on the face and is particularly common in women. The differential diagnosis of AMS also includes hypothermia, carbon monoxide poisoning, pulmonary or CNS infection, dehydration, and exhaustion.

The natural history of the illness varies with altitude and other factors. A recent study at 2,700 m in Colorado showed a range in the duration of symptoms from 6 hours to 94 hours, with a mean of 15 hours, despite the fact that half of those with symptoms self-medicated.[6] In contrast, Indian soldiers airlifted to over 5,000 m had illness that persisted for weeks and even months in 15%.[7] Although generally benign, resolving with improved acclimatization at a given altitude, AMS will sometimes progress to its most severe, life-threatening form, HACE. Eight percent of those with AMS at 4,243 m (14,000 ft) in Nepal developed cerebral and/or pulmonary edema.[8] The hallmark of progression to HACE is truncal ataxia and altered mental status. If untreated, progressive neurologic deterioration is characterized by stupor, coma, and then death, all of which may develop within 8 to 24 hours after onset of ataxia and mental status changes. HACE is discussed in detail below.

PATHOPHYSIOLOGY

AMS is due to hypobaric hypoxia, but the exact sequence of events leading to illness is unclear. Figure 13–4 offers a schema for the pathophysiology. The symptoms indicate a neurologic etiology, and elevated cerebrospinal fluid pressure and scans confirming cerebral edema have been obtained in persons with severe AMS. Whether the more common mild illness of headache, anorexia, and malaise is due to mild cerebral edema has yet to be confirmed but seems likely. Two types of cerebral edema have been proposed. One is cytotoxic edema, due to failure of the sodium-potassium pump with subsequent intracellular accumulation of sodium and water. The other is a vasogenic edema, due to a leaky blood-brain barrier (see High-Altitude Cerebral Edema).

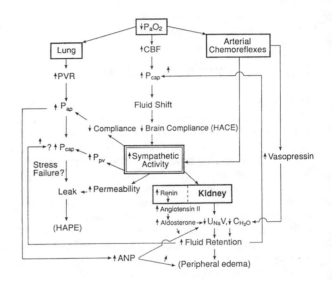

Figure 13–4. Pathophysiology of altitude illnesses. Central role of elevated sympathetic activity in the edemas of altitude: hypoxemia (PaO₂) elevates cerebral blood flow (CBF), which, in turn, raises cerebral capillary hydrostatic pressure (Pcap) such that a transcapillary fluid shift occurs. The resulting high-altitude cerebral edema (or AMS) reduces brain compliance. Elevated intracranial pressure and distortion of CNS structures provokes elevation of peripheral sympathetic activity above levels normally produced by stimulation of peripheral chemoreflexes. Hypoxia raises pulmonary vascular resistance, which raises pulmonary artery pressure (Pap). Elevated sympathetic activity to the lungs decreases compliance of pulmonary arteries and provokes pulmonary venous constriction and increased capillary permeability. The precise influence of hypoxic pulmonary vascular responses combined with increased pulmonary sympathetic activity on pulmonary hydrostatic pressure is unclear. The relative importance of pulmonary capillary stress failure is uncertain. Only small elevations of Pcap are required to cause large fluid fluxes if permeability is increased such that HAPE occurs. Increased sympathetic activity is associated with a neurogenic antinatriuresis such that fluid retention and peripheral edema occur. Increased aldosterone from sympathetic stimulation of renin or from adrenocorticotropic hormone and increased vasopressin from stimulation of chemoreflexes add to the tubular alpha-adrenergic antinatriuresis and opposes natriuretic effects from atrial natriuretic peptide (ANP) released by elevated central blood volume. However, ANP could contribute to peripheral edema, HAPE, or HACE. Renal fluid retention contributes to elevated Pcap in lung, brain and peripheral tissues. (From Krasney.[34])

No direct evidence for cytotoxic edema in humans at altitude has been reported. However, a large shift of fluid into the total intracellular space, presumably including the brain, has been demonstrated to take place over the first 3 days at altitude, at a time when AMS occurs. The time required for fluid shift and overhydration of the brain might explain the delay in onset of symptoms that distinguishes AMS from acute hypoxia. In support of the vasogenic theory, white-matter brain edema on magnetic resonance imaging was recently demonstrated in persons with HACE[9] and may also occur in AMS. The leaky blood-brain barrier is due either to loss of autoregulation and overperfusion or to hypoxia-induced increased permeability. The fact that steroids so effectively treat AMS[10] also supports the notion of vasogenic edema, since this is the only type of cerebral edema responsive to steroids. Further research is likely to reveal that brain swelling is due to both cytotoxic and vasogenic mechanisms.

The cerebral edema, interstitial pulmonary edema, peripheral edema, and the antidiuresis observed in AMS all point to an abnormality of water handling by the body. The mechanism is thought to be increased aldosterone and ADH, in contrast to the "normal" ADH and aldosterone suppression at high altitude and usual diuresis,[11] and an increase in atrial natriuretic peptide (ANP) that increases vascular permeability. A decrease in glomerular filtration has also been observed. The effectiveness of diuretics in prevention and treatment of AMS reinforces the importance of fluid retention in the pathophysiology.

Relative hypoventilation due to a sluggish hypoxic ventilatory response is a characteristic of AMS susceptibles and has been linked to fluid retention.[12] Hypoventilation, of course, results in greater hypoxic stress and is equivalent to being at a higher altitude. Higher Pco_2 and lower Po_2 also increase cerebral blood flow and aggravate brain swelling. Less hypocapnia may also reduce the stimulus for bicarbonate diuresis and aggravate fluid retention.

PREVENTION

Graded ascent with adequate time for acclimatization is the best prevention. A recommendation for those visiting resorts in the western United States is to spend a night at an intermediate altitude of 1,500 m to 2,000 m (Denver or Salt Lake City) before sleeping at altitudes above 2,500 m (8,200 ft). Mountaineers and trekkers should avoid abrupt ascent to sleeping altitudes over 3,000 m and then allow 2 nights for each 1,000-m altitude gain in camp altitude, starting at 3,000 m. There is considerable interpersonal variation in speed of acclimatization such that fast acclimatizers may find this recommendation too slow. Regardless, it is essential that those with symptoms of AMS should not ascend further until the symptoms have disappeared. Destinations such as Cuzco, Lhasa, and La Paz are serviced by aircraft, which transport travelers much too abruptly for adequate acclimatization. In such situations, it is critical to allow an acclimatization period on arrival before proceeding higher. Acetazolamide is a useful prophylactic agent for those with a past history of AMS or for unavoidable abrupt ascent without acclimatization stages. The drug acts by inhibiting the enzyme

carbonic anhydrase, slowing the hydration of carbon dioxide to hydrogen and bicarbonate ions. In the kidney, acetazolamide reduces reabsorption of bicarbonate, causing a bicarbonate diuresis and metabolic acidosis, which stimulates ventilation. The drug essentially mimics the process of ventilatory acclimatization. As a result, arterial Po_2 is higher, and sleep oxygenation remains high and stable, without periods of apnea (see Figure 13–3). Because of its diuretic action, it counteracts the fluid retention of AMS. Dosage regimens vary, but the standard recommendation is 250 mg twice daily. Although anecdotal reports suggest that 125 mg twice daily can be effective, this has yet to be confirmed in clinical trials. A slow-release formulation of acetazolamide, 500 mg per 24 hours, is a convenient alternative regimen. Acetazolamide should be started 24 hours before the ascent and continued for the first 2 days at altitude. The medication can then be discontinued and started again if illness develops. Since the drug acts by improving acclimatization, fear of masking serious illness is unwarranted.

Common side effects of acetazolamide include peripheral paresthesiae and sometimes nausea or drowsiness. The usual precautions of sulfa drugs apply to acetazolamide because of the sulfhydryl moiety. Since the drug inhibits the instant hydration of CO_2 on the tongue, the carbon dioxide in carbonated beverages can be tasted, ruining the flavor of beer and other drinks. An alternative for those allergic to sulfa is dexamethasone 4 mg every 12 hours starting the day of ascent and continuing for the first 2 days at altitude. Prophylactic use of aspirin is also useful in preventing high-altitude headache.[13]

Other ways that may enhance acclimatization and prevent AMS are to avoid overexertion the first 2 days at altitude, to avoid alcohol, to consciously increase breathing, and to perform mild exercise. Diminishing salt intake may also be helpful. A diet high in carbohydrates (>70% of calories) has been shown to reduce symptoms of mountain sickness by 30%.

TREATMENT (TABLE 13–4)

Descent and Oxygen The goals of treatment of AMS are to prevent progression, abort the illness, and improve acclimatization. Early diagnosis is essential. The initial clinical presentation does not predict eventual severity, and all persons with AMS must be carefully observed for progression. The three principles of treatment are to (1) not proceed to a higher sleeping altitude in the presence of symptoms, (2) descend if symptoms do not abate or become worse despite treatment, and (3) descend and/or treat immediately in the presence of a change in consciousness, ataxia, or pulmonary edema. Mild AMS is self-limited and generally improves with an extra 12 to 36 hours of acclimatization if ascent is halted. Descent is the definitive treatment for all forms of altitude illness, although it is not always an option nor always necessary. Remarkably, a drop in altitude of only 500 to 1,000 m is usually promptly effective. Evacuation to a hospital or to sea level is unnecessary except in the most severe cases. To simulate descent, portable hyperbaric chambers

Table 13–4.   SUGGESTED TREATMENT OF
HIGH-ALTITUDE ILLNESS

Mild acute mountain sickness
  Stop ascent
  Descend to lower altitude or acclimatize at same altitude
  Acetazolamide 125–250 mg bid to speed acclimatization
  Symptomatic treatment as necessary with analgesics and
  antiemetics

Moderate acute mountain sickness
  Immediate descent for worsening symptoms
  Low-flow oxygen if available
  Acetazolamide 125–250 mg bid and/or dexamethasone 4 mg q6h
  Hyperbaric therapy

High-altitude cerebral edema
  Immediate descent or evacuation
  Oxygen 2–4 L/min
  Dexamethasone 8 mg PO, IM, or IV, then 4 mg q6h
  Hyperbaric therapy if cannot descend

High-altitude pulmonary edema
  Immediate descent or evacuation
  Oxygen 4 L/min
  Nifedipine 10 mg PO, then 30 mg extended release q12h if no
    oxygen or descent
  Hyperbaric therapy if cannot descend
  Minimize exertion and keep warm

Periodic breathing
  Acetazolamide 125 mg QHS PRN

are being used in various locations to treat AMS (Figure 13–5). The patient is inserted into the fabric chamber and a pressure of about 14 kPa (2 psi) is achieved by means of a manual or automated pump. At an altitude of 3,900 m, the pressure is equivalent to a drop in altitude of 1,700 m. A valve system and continuous pumping creates sufficient ventilation to avoid CO_2 accumulation or O_2 depletion.

Oxygen effectively relieves symptoms but is often unavailable in the field and is generally reserved for mod-

erate to severe AMS in order to conserve supplies. Oxygen promptly relieves headache, dizziness, and most other symptoms, although ataxia may resolve more slowly. Nocturnal low-flow oxygen (0.5 to 1 liter per minute) is particularly helpful and efficient. The combination of oxygen and descent provides optimal therapy, especially in more severe cases.

Medical Therapy   Pharmacologic treatment offers an alternative to descent or oxygen in mild to moderately severe AMS. Although acetazolamide has been widely used empirically for treatment of AMS, controlled studies have been hindered by the reluctance of ill persons to enrol in placebo trials. One recent study confirmed its usefulness in treatment in a small number of patients.[14] The usual dose regimen is 250 mg two or three times daily, and treatment should be continued until symptoms of AMS resolve. The drug can be restarted if symptoms return. Since acetazolamide acts by improving acclimatization, fear of masking serious illness is unwarranted.

Symptomatic treatment of AMS is sometimes sufficient.[15] Aspirin 650 mg, ibuprofen 600 to 800 mg, or acetaminophen 650 to 1,000 mg (with or without codeine) can be given for headache. Prochlorperazine, 5 to 10 mg IM, is useful for nausea and vomiting and has the advantage of augmenting the hypoxic ventilatory response.

Dexamethasone, 4 mg PO, IM, or IV every 6 hours, is quite effective therapy for AMS but is best reserved for moderate to severe AMS, since it may be associated with significant side effects and does not aid acclimatization, sometimes resulting in rebound symptoms when discontinued.[16,17] The mechanism of action of dexamethasone might be to reduce vasogenic edema by decreasing permeability of the blood-brain barrier. The use of acetazolamide to speed acclimatization and a brief course of dexamethasone to treat illness can be a useful combination. The use of diuretics is reasonable because of the fluid retention associated with AMS. Furosemide 20 to 40 mg every 12 hours until improved was reported effective by the Indian Army,[7] although other investigators have not been enthusiastic about its use because of concerns of potential hypovolemia, hypotension, and incapacitation.

HIGH-ALTITUDE CEREBRAL EDEMA

HACE is defined clinically as the presence of progressive neurologic deterioration in someone with AMS or HAPE. It is characterized by altered mental status, ataxia, stupor, and progression to coma if untreated. Headache, nausea, and vomiting are not always present. Because of raised intracranial pressure, focal neurologic signs such as third and sixth cranial nerve palsies may result from distortion of brain structures or by extra-axial compression. Truncal ataxia is an early sign and can be tested by asking the patient to walk heel to toe along a straight line. HACE is usually associated with pulmonary edema.

Pathologically, necropsies have described severe, diffuse cerebral edema with multiple small hemorrhages and sometimes thrombosis. Death is attributed to brain herni-

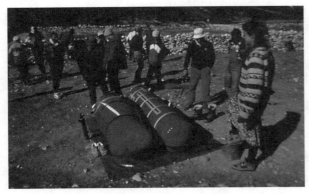

Figure 13–5.   A portable hyperbaric bag used for treatment of altitude illness. With a foot pump, a pressure of 2 psi is maintained, which is equivalent to a descent of over 1,500 m (5,000 ft). Copyright 1996. The Wilderness Medical Society, High Altitude Medicine, Slide Set. Reprinted with permission from the Wilderness Medical Society.

ation. (For pathophysiology, see Acute Mountain Sickness.)

The treatment of HACE is the same as for severe AMS: oxygen, descent, and steroids. Of these, descent is the highest priority. Acetazolamide may be an adjunct, but immediate reversal of the illness is the goal; improving acclimatization comes later. In acutely ill patients who cannot descend, the combination of steroids, supplemental oxygen, and a portable hyperbaric chamber is optimal therapy and should always be followed by descent when possible. Comatose patients require additional airway management, bladder drainage, and other coma care. For coma, the use of hyperventilation to decrease intracranial pressure is a reasonable approach, keeping in mind that the Pco_2 is already low and pH high in these individuals. Additional acute hyperventilation could produce cerebral ischemia; monitoring of arterial blood gases and, if available, cerebral blood velocities by transcranial Doppler may be advisable. Loop diuretics such as furosemide 40 to 80 mg or bumetanide 1 to 2 mg may help reduce brain overhydration, but hypoperfusion must be avoided. Hypertonic solutions of saline, mannitol, or urea have been used too infrequently to establish clinical guidelines. Coma may persist for days or even for weeks after evacuation to lower altitude, and the patient may still recover, sometimes with sequelae. A persistent comatose state is unusual, however, and mandates exclusion of other possible etiologies.

HIGH-ALTITUDE PULMONARY EDEMA

HAPE is the most lethal of the altitude illnesses. Since the condition is easily reversible with descent and/or oxygen, the cause of death is usually lack of early recognition, misdiagnosis, or inability to descend to a lower altitude. Few conditions are so rewarding to treat and so tragic in death.

EPIDEMIOLOGY

The incidence of HAPE varies from less than 1 in 10,000 skiers in Colorado, to 2% to 3% of climbers on Mount McKinley, and was reported as high as 15% in some regiments in the Indian Army who were airlifted to high altitude during the Indian/Chinese war. Women appear less susceptible than men. Risk factors include heavy exertion, rapid ascent, cold, excessive salt ingestion, use of sleeping medication, and a previous history indicating inherent individual susceptibility.

CLINICAL PRESENTATION

Early in the course of illness, when the edema is still interstitial or localized, the victim develops a dry cough, decreased exercise performance, dyspnea on exertion, increased recovery time from exercise, and localized rales, usually in the right mid-lung field. Late in the course of the illness, tachycardia, tachypnea, dyspnea at rest, marked weakness, productive cough, cyanosis, and more generalized rales develop. As hypoxemia worsens, consciousness becomes impaired. Victims usually become comatose and then die. Early diagnosis is critical, and decreased exercise performance and dry cough are enough to raise the suspicion of early pulmonary edema. The typical victim is strong and fit and may or may not have symptoms of AMS prior to onset of HAPE. The condition typically worsens at night and is most commonly noticed on the second night at a new altitude.[18] Fever up to 38.5°C is common, and tachycardia and tachypnea generally correlate with severity of illness. On cardiac auscultation, a prominent P2 and right ventricular heave may be appreciated. Electrocardiogram (EKG) generally reveals right axis deviation and a right ventricular strain pattern consistent with acute pulmonary hypertension. Chest x-ray findings progress from interstitial to localized alveolar to generalized alveolar infiltrates as the illness progresses from mild to severe.

PATHOPHYSIOLOGY

The exact cause of the edema is unclear. Being noncardiogenic, it falls into the same category as acute respiratory distress syndrome (ARDS), near-drowning, and neurogenic pulmonary edema. Catheter studies have revealed no element of left ventricular failure or elevated wedge pressure. Pulmonary hypertension is the sine qua non of the disorder. Since there is a high protein but reversible leak, it appears that high pressures are somehow transmitted to the microcirculation. Uneven hypoxic vasoconstriction on the arterial side has been postulated as causing unprotected, unconstricted areas to be exposed to high pressures and overperfusion, but pulmonary venoconstriction is also an attractive hypothesis, since this raises microvascular pressure. The reversibility of the phenomenon is remarkable and indicates a lack of any permanent architectural lung damage such as occurs in ARDS. On the capillary level, there may be stretching of cell junctions or pores in the endothelium when exposed to high pressures, with immediate cessation of the leak when pressures are normalized. Other factors known to contribute to pathogenesis include poor carotid body function (HVR), preexisting pulmonary hypertension, and an exaggerated pulmonary pressor response to hypoxia. Pulmonary hypertension, congenital pulmonary vascular abnormalities, and any significant compromise of the pulmonary circulation are contraindications to altitude exposure because of the danger of pulmonary edema.

TREATMENT

The key to successful treatment of HAPE is early recognition, since in its early stage it is easily reversible. Optimal therapy depends on the environmental setting, evacuation options, availability of oxygen or portable hyperbaric chambers, and ease of descent. Immediate descent is the treatment of choice. During descent, exertion by the victim must be minimized. Reports of victims dying during descent are probably related to overexertion offsetting the benefit of lower altitude. Supplementary oxygen provides excellent results and can actually completely resolve pulmonary edema without descent to a lower altitude but may require 36 to 72 hours to do so. Such quantities of oxygen are rarely available to trekking, mountaineering, and skiing groups but may be available at ski resorts or medical facilities. Oxygen immediately lowers pulmonary artery pressure and improves arterial oxygenation. Its use is life saving when descent is not an option; in such cases, rescue groups should make delivery of oxygen to the victim the highest priority. Bed rest may be adequate for very mild cases and bed rest with supplemental oxygen may suffice for moderate illness.

Since oxygen and descent are so effective, experience with drugs has been limited. Nifedipine, either 10 mg PO or 30 mg PO extended release, was reported to be of clinical benefit, to reduce pulmonary artery pressure by 30% to 50%, and to increase arterial oxygen saturation.[19,20] The mechanism is presumably lowering of pulmonary pressure, which reduces the gradient for flux of fluid across the membrane, and changing blood flow distribution in favor of flow to drier areas of the lung. Hypotension is a potential problem with nifedipine, and the results are not nearly as dramatic as with oxygen or descent, which still remain the treatments of choice. Deaths due to HAPE are generally due to misdiagnosis or inability to descend or give oxygen, usually in more remote areas such as the Andes or the Himalayas. However, deaths in well-populated ski areas near hospitals still occur because of lack of recognition of the seriousness of the problem by the patient or their family. Preventive education by the travel industry, the ski industry, and health practitioners could effectively reduce mortality and morbidity.

Hospitalization may be warranted for severe cases that do not respond immediately to descent, especially if cerebral edema is present. Intubation, high F_IO_2, and positive end-expiratory pressure are rarely required. Occasionally, pulmonary artery catheterization is useful to exclude a cardiac component to the edema in persons with heart disease. The patient with HAPE who does not make the usual rapid improvement should be evaluated for pulmonary emboli, mediastinal pulmonary artery obstruction, or other pulmonary circulatory abnormalities, such as congenital absence of a pulmonary artery.[1] Residua such as fibrosis and impaired pulmonary function tests have not been reported. An episode of HAPE is not a contraindication to subsequent ascent, but patients should be advised on staged ascent and acetazolamide prophylaxis, as well as recognition of early signs and symptoms.

Preventive measures for pulmonary edema are the same as for mountain sickness: gradual ascent allowing time for acclimatization, the appropriate use of acetazolamide if ascent must be rapid, mild physical activity the first 2 days at altitude, and avoidance of respiratory depressants. Persons with a past history of HAPE have demonstrated susceptibility and must take these precautionary measures, as well as be alert for the early symptoms and signs. Acetazolamide has empirically been effective in reducing recurrent pulmonary edema, and nifedipine has recently been proven to work for prophylaxis.[21]

SLEEP AT HIGH ALTITUDE

Insomnia is the single greatest malady of travelers to high altitude. Due to the effect of hypoxia on sleep stages, more time is spent awake, with a significant increase in arousals, but only slightly less REM time. The frequent arousals are a common source of complaints but are innocuous and improve with time at altitude. Some arousals are due to the typical periodic breathing (Cheyne-Stokes) in those sleeping above 2,700 m (9,000 ft): 6- to 12-second apneic pauses are interspersed with cycles of vigorous ventilation. Interestingly, the sleep periodic breathing has not been related to AMS. A low dose of acetazolamide (125 mg) a few hours before bedtime is quite effective in relieving periodic breathing and maintaining arterial oxygen saturation. High-altitude travelers should be warned of this phenomenon to allay panic and inappropriate concerns that it may be due to mountain sickness or pulmonary edema. The use of benzodiazepines to facilitate sleep at high altitude has been generally discouraged because of the theoretical risks of respiratory depression. Recent preliminary data suggest that short-acting benzodiazepines are actually associated with improved nocturnal oxygen saturation, but this will need to be confirmed.[22]

PERIPHERAL EDEMA

Swelling of the face and distal extremities is common at high altitude. Peripheral edema was reported in 18% of trekkers at 4,200 m in Nepal and was twice as likely in females; it was often associated with mountain sickness, but not always.[23] The presence of peripheral edema should raise suspicion of altitude illness and prompt a thorough examination for pulmonary and cerebral edema. The problem can be treated with diuretics but, if left untreated, will resolve spontaneously with descent. The mechanism is presumably similar to that of the fluid retention of AMS, but with edema formation peripherally rather than in the brain and lung.

HIGH-ALTITUDE RETINOPATHY

Retinal abnormalities described at high altitude include retinal edema, tortuosity and dilatation of retinal veins, disc hyperemia, retinal hemorrhages, and, rarely, cotton wool exudates. Retinal hemorrhages are asymptomatic, except for rarely occurring macula hemorrhages, and are not considered an indication for descent unless visual changes are present. They resolve spontaneously in 10 to 14 days. Hemorrhages are common above a sleeping altitude of 5,000 m and occur at lower altitudes in persons with altitude illness.

OTHER NEUROLOGIC SYNDROMES OF HIGH ALTITUDE

Until recently, most neurologic events at high altitude were attributed to HACE or AMS. Clearly, this has been a diagnostic oversimplification. Several other syndromes have now been described at high altitude, including altitude syncope, cerebrovascular spasm (migraine equivalent), cerebral arterial or venous thrombosis (infarct), transient ischemic attack, and cerebral hemorrhage. These syndromes are typically characterized by focal neurologic findings, more so than in cerebral edema. Differentiation in the field, however, may be impossible. The etiology of many focal neurologic events at high altitude remains obscure.

Other problems may be due to exacerbation or unmasking of underlying disease, such as previously asymptomatic brain tumors and epilepsy. Presumably, space-occupying lesions become symptomatic because of increased brain volume at altitude. Hyperventilation (hypocapnic alkalosis), which is commonly used to induce seizure activity on electroencephalogram, may explain unmasking of a seizure disorder at altitude, whereas changes in cerebral blood flow may exacerbate vascular lesions. Differentiation of the various neurologic syndromes may be impossible in the field, and treating as if cerebral edema were present is reasonable, with a rapid descent to lower altitude, oxygen and steroids, and evacuation to a hospital if symptoms persist despite treatment. Fortunately, focal neurologic signs usually resolve spontaneously and do not recur upon re-ascent. However, a thorough cerebrovascular evaluation before advising further altitude exposure may be prudent.

THROMBOSIS

Cerebral and peripheral venous thrombosis and pulmonary embolism have been reported at high altitude, especially after exposure to extreme altitudes (>5,500 m). Risk factors include polycythemia and increased blood viscosity, dehydration, cold, and inactivity (e.g., tent-bound in bad weather).

HIGH-ALTITUDE PHARYNGITIS AND BRONCHITIS

Most unacclimatized persons exercising at altitudes over 2,500 m develop a dry, hacking cough. With exposure to extreme altitudes for prolonged periods of time, a purulent bronchitis and a painful pharyngitis become nearly universal. Among trekkers to Mount Everest Base Camp, 42% developed cough (half of these producing sputum) and 39% had sore throat.[24] These problems may not be of an infectious nature; high volumes of dry, cold air through the lungs may induce respiratory heat loss and cause purulent secretions on that basis alone. Cough receptor sensitivity is increased after several days at high altitude,[25] and bronchospasm may also be triggered by respiratory heat loss. Severe coughing spasms can result in cough fracture of ribs.

Breathing of steam, hard candies or lozenges to increase salivation, and forced hydration may provide some benefit, as well as analgesics as necessary. A silk balaclava or similar material across the nose and mouth that is sufficiently porous to allow large-volume ventila-tion but trap some moisture and heat helps ameliorate these bothersome high-altitude conditions.

ULTRAVIOLET KERATITIS

UV keratitis, also known as snow blindness, is a particular problem at high altitude because of the increased solar radiation. The symptoms of this photokeratitis are severe pain, a foreign body or gritty sensation, photophobia, tearing, conjunctival erythema, chemosis, and eyelid swelling. The condition is generally self-limiting and heals within 24 hours but can be disabling. Systemic analgesics are usually necessary, and eye patches, if practical, will also help make the patient comfortable. Topical anesthetic agents should be avoided if possible, as they are toxic to corneal epithelium and will reduce awareness of further trauma. A person caught without sunglasses and exposed to snow and high elevations can fashion protection by cutting narrow horizontal slits in cardboard, foam, or any available material and fastening them in front of the eyes (Eskimo sunglasses).

CHILDREN AT HIGH ALTITUDE

Little information exists about altitude illness in children. Although it appears that susceptibility to AMS is similar to adults, the diagnosis of AMS may be more difficult to make in young children who may not be able to verbalize symptoms. Nonspecific signs such as food refusal, irritability, and excessive crying may be the only indication of the condition. If in doubt, altitude illness should be assumed. Treatment of altitude illness in children follows the same principles as adults, with appropriate pediatric doses of drugs (acetazolamide 5 mg/kg/d in divided doses every 8 to 12 hours; dexamethasone 0.15 mg/kg every 6 hours).

CONDITIONS AGGRAVATED BY HIGH ALTITUDE

Persons with heart, lung, or blood diseases should exercise special care at high altitude since they have less efficient means of using oxygen from the air than healthy persons. Although individuals with one of these underlying conditions may be able to function satisfactorily at sea level, the rarefied atmosphere at altitudes 1,500 m and higher might produce difficulties. Emphysema, lung abscess, tuberculosis, pulmonary fibrosis, pneumothorax, congestive heart failure, recent heart attack, congenital or rheumatic valvular heart disease, and chronic anemia such as sickle cell anemia are some of the conditions in which high altitude might be harmful.

CHRONIC LUNG DISEASE

People with chronic obstructive pulmonary disease (COPD) who ascend to altitude often report increased dyspnea and reduced exercise ability. Obviously, any person who is hypoxic at sea level will be more hypoxic at altitude and generally more symptomatic. However, persons with mild or moderate COPD have been shown to acclimatize well at moderate altitudes of 2,000 m to 2,500 m, in part because they are already partially acclimatized to hypoxia.[26] Persons with severe COPD may require supplemental oxygen at altitude, and persons already on home oxygen at sea level must increase the F_IO_2 on ascent to altitude. High altitude per se does not exacerbate asthma, and persons with chronic bronchospasm often report easier breathing at altitude due to lower air density and/or cleaner air. Peak flow meters (such as the Mini-Wright) have a tendency to under-read at altitude and can be misleading.[27] Those with COPD and asthma should optimize their pulmonary function before ascending to altitude and maintain their medications. Persons with lung disease (but with normal pulmonary circulation) have not been shown to be predisposed to any of the altitude illnesses.

CORONARY ARTERY DISEASE

What to advise patients with cardiovascular disease about altitude exposure is problematic. High altitude has been shown to be much less of a stress on the heart than exercise. Numerous EKG studies, echocardiograms, heart catheterizations, and exercise tests have failed to demonstrate cardiac ischemia or cardiac dysfunction in healthy persons at high altitude, even when arterial Po_2 was less than 30 mm Hg. Ascent to altitude has not been associated with increased risk of acute cardiac ischemic events even in those with arteriosclerotic heart disease. On the other hand, data are sparse, and most doctors advise coronary patients to avoid altitude because of the "conventional wisdom" that hypoxia must be bad for one's heart. Recent studies in patients with coronary artery disease performed in Vail showed earlier onset of angina compared to sea level but no impairment of ability to acclimatize to the altitude.[28] Others have found that patients post-coronary artery bypass have done quite well even up to altitudes of 5,550 m.[29] However, patients with congestive heart failure often decompensate at high altitude, apparently due to fluid retention and altered hemodynamics rather than ischemic decompensation of the myocardium. Although the available evidence suggests that altitude is generally safe for patients with coronary disease, more study is necessary to help clearly identify subcategories of cardiac patients that may be at increased risk.

HYPERTENSION

Hypertension is not a contraindication to altitude exposure. Numerous studies have shown a slight increase in blood pressure in normotensives on ascent, probably secondary to increased catecholamines. Limited studies of hypertensives have observed transient exacerbation that did not require extra treatment, but, again, further study is necessary.

SICKLE CELL DISEASE

Even the cabin altitude of pressurized aircraft may cause patients with hemoglobin sickle cell and sickle tha-

lassemia disease to have vaso-occlusive crisis. Ascent to high altitude is a contraindication for these patients. Sickle cell trait is not considered an increased risk, although splenic infarction syndrome has been reported in persons with this trait when exercising at altitude.

DIABETES MELLITUS

Diabetics may find that increased energy expenditure at altitude alters their carbohydrate and insulin requirements. Diabetic control may be further complicated by inaccurate and inconsistent performance of blood glucose meters above 2,000 m.[30]

PREGNANCY

Although women living permanently at high altitude have an increased risk of pregnancy complications such as low birth weight and neonatal hyperbilirubinemia, no data suggest that short visits to high altitude by lowlanders increase risk in pregnancy. On the other hand, few data are available. The normal Po_2 of the fetus is 29 to 33 mm Hg, and the mild maternal hypoxia induced by resort-type altitudes does not generate significantly greater hypoxic stress. However, given the general lack of information, it is probably prudent to advise pregnant women not to sleep over 3,000 m for a prolonged period of time, and they should probably avoid altitudes greater than 5,000 m.[31] Perhaps the greater concern when traveling to these locations is the remoteness from medical facilities should any of the common complications occur.

CONTRACEPTION

The risks, if any, from taking oral contraceptives at high altitude are unclear. Thrombosis is the main concern given other prothrombotic factors at altitude such as polycythemia and dehydration. However, there is currently no evidence to support this increased risk

RADIAL KERATOTOMY

Persons who have had radial keratotomy (RK) for refraction correction no longer have structurally normal corneas. Deep radial incisions have been made that interrupt stromal fibers in the area of the incision, allowing the central cornea to become flattened, improving far-sighted vision. On ascent to altitude, however, the swelling of the hypoxic cornea is not uniform after RK, with resultant flattening and significant visual changes.[32] The problem is likely to become worse with decreasing accommodation as one ages. In contrast, photorefractive keratectomy (PRK), a laser technique that shaves the anterior cornea uniformly without incisions, appears to cause no change in vision at high altitude.[33] For individuals who may travel to high altitude, PRK or laser in situ keratomileosis (LASIK) is preferable to RK for surgical correction of myopia. Those with past RK can correct their vision by bringing with them spectacles of increasing plus power.

SUMMARY

All travelers should have a basic understanding that ascent to altitude may be associated with certain health problems that can be life threatening, and that any illness at altitude should be suspected as being altitude illness unless clearly otherwise. Travelers may more easily remember that early AMS is almost exactly like an alcohol hangover. With the simple recommendation that ascent should be stopped if symptoms of AMS develop and descent should be initiated if the victim fails to improve or becomes worse, a number of lives can be saved each year. This advice, in conjunction with the proper use of medication, may allow large numbers of people to significantly reduce the morbidity from these problems and even continue with their planned travel.

Most patients with chronic illnesses can safely travel to modest altitudes, including those with coronary artery disease, COPD, and hypertension. Some may require supplemental oxygen; all should be informed about possible adverse events and appropriate preventive measures. The physician who cares for patients who wish to travel plays a very important role in their lives by helping them to improve their enjoyment and quality of life.

REFERENCES

1. Hackett PH, Roach RC. High-altitude medicine. In: Auerbach PA, ed. Wilderness medicine. St. Louis: Mosby, 1995:1–37.
2. Bert P. Barometric pressure. Bethesda, MD: Undersea Medical Society, 1978.
3. Honigman B, Theis MK, McLain J, et al. Acute mountain sickness in a general tourist population at moderate altitudes. Ann Intern Med 1993;118:587–592.
4. Ellsworth AJ, Larson EB, Strickland D. A randomized trial of dexamethasone and acetazolamide for acute mountain sickness prophylaxis. Am J Med 1987;83:1024–1030.
5. Murdoch DR. Altitude illness among tourists flying to 3740 meters elevation in the Nepal Himalaya. J Travel Med 1995; 2:255–256.
6. Dean AG, Yip R, Hoffman RE. High incidence of mild acute mountain sickness in conference attendees at 10,000 feet altitude. J Wilderness Med 1990;1:86–92.
7. Singh I, Khanna PK, Srivastava MC, et al. Acute mountain sickness. N Engl J Med 1969;280:175–184.
8. Hackett PH, Rennie ID, Levine HD. The incidence, importance, and prophylaxis of acute mountain sickness. Lancet 1976;2:1149–1154.
9. Hackett PH, Yarnell PR, Hill R, et al. High altitude cerebral edema evaluated with magnetic resonance imaging: clinical correlation and pathophysiology. JAMA 1998;280:1920–1925.
10. Ferrazzini G, Maggiorini M, Kriemler S, et al. Successful treatment of acute mountain sickness with dexamethasone. BMJ 1987;294:1380–1382.
11. Bärtsch P, Shaw S, Wiedmann P, et al. Aldosterone, antidiuretic hormone and atrial natriuretic peptide in acute mountain sickness. In: Sutton JR, Coates G, Houston CS, eds. Hypoxia and mountain medicine. Burlington, VT: Queen City, 1992: 73–81.
12. Hackett PH, Rennie ID, Hofmeister SE, et al. Fluid retention and relative hypoventilation in acute mountain sickness. Respiration 1982;43:321–329.
13. Burtscher M, Likar R, Nachbauer W, Philadelphy M. Aspirin for prophylaxis against headache at high altitudes: randomised, double blind, placebo controlled trial. BMJ 1998;316:1057–1058.
14. Grissom CK, Roach RC, Sarnquist FH, Hackett PH. Acetazolamide in the treatment of acute mountain sickness: clinical efficacy and effect on gas exchange. Ann Intern Med 1992; 116:461–465.
15. Hackett PH, Roach RC. Medical therapy of altitude illness. Ann Emerg Med 1987;16:980–986.
16. Levine BD, Yoshimura K, Kobayashi T, et al. Dexamethasone in the treatment of acute mountain sickness. N Engl J Med 1989;321:1707–1713.
17. Hackett PH, Roach RC, Wood RA, et al. Dexamethasone for prevention and treatment of acute mountain sickness. Aviat Space Environ Med 1988;59:950–954.
18. Hackett PH, Roach RC. High-altitude pulmonary edema. J Wilderness Med 1990;1:3–26.
19. Oelz O, Maggiorini M, Ritter M, et al. Nifedipine for high-altitude pulmonary edema. Lancet 1989;2:1241–1244.
20. Hackett PH, Roach RC, Hartig GS, et al. The effect of vasodilators on pulmonary hemodynamics in high-altitude pulmonary edema: a comparison. Intl J Sport Med 1992; 13(Suppl 1):S68–S70.
21. Bärtsch P, Maggiorini M, Ritter M, et al. Prevention of high-altitude pulmonary edema by nifedipine. N Engl J Med 1991; 325:1284–1289.
22. Dubowitz G. Effect of temazepam on oxygen saturation and sleep quality at high altitude: randomised placebo controlled crossover trial. BMJ 1998;316:587–589.
23. Hackett PH, Rennie ID. Rales, peripheral edema, retinal hemorrhage and acute mountain sickness. Am J Med 1979;67: 214–218.
24. Murdoch DR. Symptoms of infection and altitude illness among hikers in the Mount Everest region of Nepal. Aviat Space Environ Med 1995;66:148–151.
25. Barry PW, Mason NP, Riordan M, O'Callaghan C. Cough frequency and cough receptor sensitivity are increased in man at altitude. Clin Sci 1997;93:181–186.
26. Graham WG, Houston CS. Short-term adaptation to moderate altitude. Patients with chronic obstructive pulmonary disease. JAMA 1978;240:1491–1494.
27. Pollard AJ, Mason NP, Barry PW, et al. Effect of altitude on spirometry and the performance of peak flow meters. Thorax 1996;51:175–178.
28. Levine BD, deFilippi CR, Zuckerman JH. High-altitude exposure in the elderly: the Tenth Mountain Division study. Circulation 1997;96:1224–1232.
29. Hultgren HN. Effects of altitude upon cardiovascular diseases. J Wilderness Med 1992;3:301–308.
30. Gautier J-F, Duvallet A, Bigard AX, et al. Influence of simulated altitude on the performance of five blood glucose meters. Diabetes Care 1996;19:1430–1433.
31. Hackett PH, Roach RC, Sutton JR. Medical problems of high altitude. In: Auerbach PS, Geehr E, eds. Management of wilderness and environmental emergencies. St. Louis, MO: Mosby, 1988:1–34.
32. Mader TH, White LJ. Refractive changes at extreme altitude after radial keratotomy. Am J Ophthalmol 1995;119: 733–737.
33. Mader T, Blanton C, Gilbert B, et al. Refractive changes during 72-hour exposure to high altitude after refractive surgery. Ophthalmology 1996;103:1188–1195.
34. Krasney JA. A neurogenic basis for acute altitude illness. Med Sci Sport Exerc 1994;26:195–208.

Chapter 14
MARINE HAZARDS

JUDITH R. KLEIN AND PAUL S. AUERBACH

Marine organisms that are hazardous to humans are predominantly found in tropical and warm temperate oceans. The burgeoning interaction of people with the marine environment has inevitably increased the risks of related injury and illness. Marine hazards include animals that envenom; those that bite, puncture, or shock, but do not envenom; and those that are poisonous following ingestion.

ENVENOMATIONS

Most serious envenomations occur in Indo-Pacific and North American waters. Venoms often contain multiple heat- and gastric-labile polypeptides that bind specifically to receptors. They are delivered via venom glands that lie adjacent to spines or via coelenterate stinging organelles called cnidae.[1]

SPONGES

Sponges are generally stationary animals composed of horny, elastic exoskeletons. Within the exoskeleton are tiny spicules of calcium carbonate or silica. Sponges are frequently colonized by coelenterates; these secondary inhabitants are often responsible for "sponge diver's disease," a dermatitis that can cause local skin necrosis. Some sponges also produce crinotoxins.

Contact with sponges may produce either an allergic or an irritant dermatitis, or a combination of both. Allergic dermatitis likely occurs when the allergens enter through minor abrasions, such as when the sponge is handled without gloves. A few hours after contact, local itching and burning occur, which may progress to local joint swelling and soft-tissue edema. With extensive dermal contact, constitutional symptoms of fever, chills, malaise, dizziness, and nausea may occur. Untreated, mild reactions will subside in 3 to 7 days, but severe reactions may progress to erythema multiforme or an anaphylactoid reaction in 7 to 14 days. Irritant dermatitis occurs when the silica or calcium carbonate spicules with or without toxins become embedded in the skin. In severe cases, skin desquamation may occur in 10 days to 2 months.

Irritant and allergic dermatitis are difficult to differentiate clinically. Therefore, treatment should be initiated for both. Decontamination is the primary step. After gently drying the skin, embedded spicules should be removed with adhesive tape or a commercial facial peel. Gauze soaked in dilute (5%) acetic acid (vinegar) should be applied as soon as possible for 10 to 30 minutes and three to four times daily thereafter. Isopropyl alcohol may be applied if acetic acid is not available. Delayed or inadequate decontamination may result in excessive formation of bullae, which may become infected.

After decontamination, topical corticosteroids or mild emollient cream should be applied to the skin. Erythema multiforme and severe allergic reactions, including weeping, crusting, and vesiculation, may improve with systemic corticosteroids, such as prednisone (60–100 mg) tapered over 2 to 3 weeks.[1]

Clostridium tetani has been cultured from sea sponges. Therefore, appropriate tetanus immunization should be provided. Other significant infections may develop after sponge contact, making frequent follow-up wound checks important. Once infection occurs, the wound should be cultured and appropriate antibiotics prescribed.

COELENTERATES

Coelenterates are a diverse group of invertebrates. Those that are dangerous to humans possess venom-containing stinging cells, or nematocytes, and are called cnidaria. The cnidaria include the hydrozoans (e.g., fire coral, Portuguese man-of-war), scyphozoans (e.g., box jellyfish), and anthozoans (e.g., anemones). The nematocytes are located near the mouth or on the outer surface of the tentacles and are triggered by contact with the victim. Nematocysts are the envenoming structures within nematocytes.

Fire corals are not true corals. They are sessile bottom dwellers that assume upright club-shaped or branching structures (Figure 14–1) and attain heights of up to 2 meters. Tiny nematocyst-bearing tentacles protrude from their lime carbonate exoskeletons. Envenomation is common among unwary snorkelers and scuba divers, who frequently handle or lean upon these creatures. The Portuguese man-of-war lives on the ocean's surface. Nematocyst-bearing tentacles are suspended from a nitrogen- and carbon monoxide-filled floating sail and may reach 30 meters in length. Tentacles in larger species may carry more than 750,000 nematocysts each. Detached and fragmented tentacles retain their potency for many months.

The scyphozoans comprise the true jellyfish or medusae, free-swimming creatures that may cause mild to severe envenomations. One species, the box jellyfish (*Chironex fleckeri*), is reputed to be the most venomous sea creature and may cause death within 2 minutes of

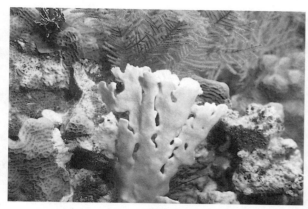

Figure 14–1. Fire coral is an extremely common stinging hazard in tropical oceans. (Photo by Paul Auerbach, M.D.)

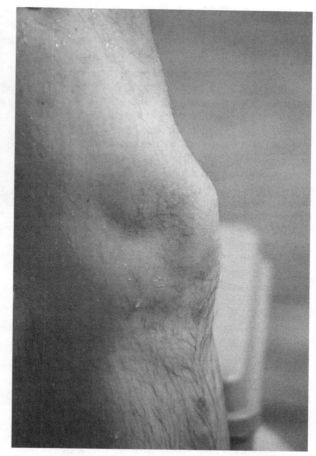

Figure 14–2. Knee of a diver demonstrates a hydroid sting. (Photo by Paul Auerbach, M.D.)

stinging. It is found in the quiet, shallow waters off the coast of northern Queensland, Australia.

Sea anemones, often found in tidal pools, are multicolored, flower-like, sessile animals with finger-like tentacles that produce a mild to moderate sting. Envenomation by anthozoans such as the sea anemone rarely cause fatality.

The severity of coelenterate envenomation is related to the species and season; number of nematocysts triggered; size of the animal; size, age, and health of the victim; and location and surface area of the sting. Mild envenomation causes an immediate stinging sensation and pruritus (Figure 14–2). The nematocysts may leave pathognomonic linear reddish-brown wheals or tentacle prints on the skin.[2] Local edema, desquamation, ulceration, and necrosis may develop with more severe envenomation. A systemic reaction may develop when a large number of nematocysts or a potent venom is involved; systemic symptoms may include nausea, vomiting, malaise, headache, vertigo, paralysis, hypotension, dysrhythmias, pulmonary edema, and coma. Death rarely ensues. Allergic reactions may play a significant role in human response to coelenterate envenomation.

Treatment of the dermatitis involves decontamination and pain control. The nematocysts should be removed immediately by rinsing the wound with seawater, not fresh water. Gentle fresh water application or rubbing the skin will activate the nematocysts, causing more envenomation. A forceful stream of freshwater, such as that applied from a high-volume showerhead, may dislodge tentacles and improve the situation. Visible tentacles should be removed with forceps or a gloved hand. Application of 5% acetic acid (vinegar) will inactivate the toxin. If the sting is from a box jellyfish (*Chironex fleckeri*), vinegar should be liberally applied before any attempt is made to remove the tentacles.[3] Following application of the vinegar, or in the event that vinegar is not available, the pressure-immobilization technique for venom sequestration should be applied. This consists of wrapping the limb with a crepe or elastic bandage tightly enough to occlude the superficial venous and lymphatic drainage, but not tightly enough to occlude the arterial circulation. Following the wrap, the limb is splinted or otherwise immobilized until the victim can be brought to definitive medical attention.

To treat the sting of other coelenterate species, if vinegar is not available, isopropyl alcohol, dilute ammonia, powdered or dissolved papain (e.g., meat tenderizer), or baking soda (sodium bicarbonate) may be used, with variable success. Remaining nematocysts can be removed by applying foaming (shaving) soap or cream and scraping the area with a razor. Local treatment may alleviate the pain, but intravenous opioid analgesia may be required.

Victims who exhibit a systemic reaction, the elderly, or the very young should be observed for at least 6 to 8 hours. Supportive treatment will be required for cardiovascular and respiratory collapse. Management of anaphylaxis should follow standard treatment protocols.

Following envenomation by the box jellyfish, *Chironex* antivenom (Commonwealth Serum Laboratories, Melbourne, Australia) should be administered as soon as possible. The antivenom should be repeated at 2- to 4-hour intervals until the dermatitis and systemic symptoms are no longer worsening.[4]

SEABATHER'S ERUPTION

Seabather's eruption, commonly misnomered "sea lice," is a dermatitis that results from contact with ocean water, especially in the Caribbean. The stinging creatures are commonly larvae of certain thimble jellyfishes, although multiple coelenterates may cause this syndrome.[5] Seabather's eruption occurs when larvae become trapped under swimwear, activating nematocysts; this results in a stinging sensation that is intensified with freshwater application.[6] The stinging may also occur on exposed skin in the open ocean or surf. Erythematous wheals, vesicles, or papules occur within a few minutes to 12 hours and may persist for 2 to 14 days. The rash is accompanied by intense pruritus. Other symptoms may include headache, chills, fatigue, vomiting, conjunctivitis, and urethritis. Fever is common in children with extensive eruptions.

A thorough soap and water scrub upon leaving the water and timely removal of contaminated swimwear provides some degree of prophylaxis. Once the stings have occurred, powdered or dissolved papain seems more effective as a topical decontaminant than vinegar. Pruritus is usually controlled with calamine lotion with 1% menthol. A topical steroid preparation may be beneficial, as the envenomation is superficial. More severe eruptions may be treated with an oral antihistamine or glucocorticoid.

SEA URCHINS

A sea urchin is a free-living echinoderm with a central body surrounded by a hard shell, from which spines (Figure 14–3) or triple-jawed seizing organs called pedicellariae protrude. Venom is located within the spines and pedicellariae. The spines are sharp and brittle; once embedded in flesh, they lodge deeply and are difficult to extract.

Envenomation immediately causes intense pain, rapidly followed by the appearance of erythema, edema, and local myalgias. If multiple spines penetrate the skin, systemic effects may occur, such as nausea, vomiting, abdominal pain, paresthesias, paralysis, hypotension, syncope, and respiratory compromise due to the presence of a neurotoxin within the venom. Delirium may also develop due to severe pain. Severe synovitis may develop if a spine enters a joint; peripheral neuropathy may occur if a spine contacts a nerve. Envenomation by pedicellariae produces a similar, although often more severe, clinical syndrome.

Immersion of the affected area in nonscalding hot water (up to 45°C or 113°F) for 30 to 90 minutes provides the most effective initial pain relief. Detached pedicellariae and spines must be removed to limit further envenomation. Pedicellariae may be removed by applying shaving foam followed by gentle scraping with a razor. Embedded spines are more difficult to remove as they are easily fractured. Delicate spines will often be absorbed in 2 to 3 weeks. However, if a spine is positioned in a weight-bearing location, intruding upon a bony joint, tendinous surface, or critical vascular or nerve structure, it may be advised to remove it. Thick spines must be removed to absolutely prevent infection, foreign body granuloma, and dermoid inclusion cyst formation. After removal of a spine, a black or purplish discoloration from the spine dye may persist for 48 hours. Spines should be removed with the aid of an operating microscope. Wounds should not be probed blindly. Soft-tissue density radiography or magnetic resonance imaging may help elucidate the presence and location of spines. A deep puncture wound is most likely to initiate a secondary infection and is an indication for prophylactic antibiotics. As with any other penetrating envenomation, appropriate tetanus prophylaxis should be administered.

STARFISH

Starfish are free-living stellate animals covered with thorny spines of calcium carbonate crystals. A slimy venomous material is produced in the epidermis and covers the spines. The crown-of-thorns starfish *Acanthaster planci* is a particularly venomous species found around the coral reefs of the Pacific and Indian Oceans, the Red Sea, the Gulf of California, and the Great Barrier Reef. Its venom-covered spines attain lengths of up to 6 cm and can easily penetrate diving gloves (Figure 14–4).

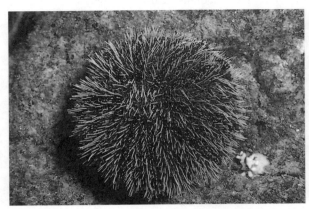

Figure 14–3. The spines of a sea urchin easily penetrate thin diving gloves. (Photo by Paul Auerbach, M.D.)

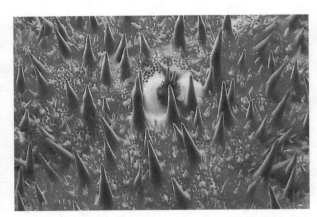

Figure 14–4. Crown-of-thorns sea star spines close up. (Photo by Paul Auerbach, M.D.)

Following penetration of the skin by the spines of *A. planci*, immediate pain, bleeding, and mild edema occur. The pain is generally moderate and lasts for 2 to 3 hours. Multiple puncture wounds may induce paresthesias, nausea, vomiting, lymphadenopathy, and paralysis. Granulomatous lesions may develop from retained spine fragments. Prolonged localized edema and pruritus may occur in previously sensitized victims.

Treatment for starfish envenomation is supportive. The wound should be immersed in nonscalding hot water (up to 45°C or 113°F) for 30 to 90 minutes or until there is adequate pain relief. The puncture wound should be irrigated and explored to remove any foreign material. Retained fragments are rare but may often be visualized with a soft-tissue radiograph or by a skilled ultrasonographer.

BRISTLEWORMS

Bristleworms are segmented marine worms encountered by divers mainly in Floridian and Caribbean waters. They are slow-moving animals found on coral, under rocks, or among sponges. When stimulated, the bristleworm's body contracts and its bristles become erect. The bristles detach easily and penetrate the skin of the unwary snorkeler or diver.

The sting causes an intense urticarial reaction, followed by local edema and papule formation. Although the pain lasts only a few hours, the urticaria may persist for 2 to 3 days.

Treatment consists of bristle removal and pain control. Large bristles should be removed with forceps. Smaller spines should be removed by drying the skin, then applying and removing adhesive tape, a thin layer of rubber cement, or a commercial facial peel. Pain may be alleviated by irrigating the affected area with 5% acetic acid (vinegar), powdered or dissolved papain, isopropyl alcohol, or dilute ammonia. Severe inflammatory reactions may respond to a topical or systemic corticosteroid.

CONE SHELLS

Cone shells are soft-bodied invertebrates of the phylum Mollusca with beautiful calcified shells. At least 18 of the more than 300 cone shell species are venomous, and many of these are found in Indo-Pacific waters.[1] Harpoon-like radular teeth are impregnated with venom and discharged into the curious victim via an extensible proboscis. The venom consists primarily of neurotoxins similar to tetrodotoxin and saxitoxin.

Most stings are on hands or fingers and are akin to bee stings. Localized burning or stinging may be followed by perioral and peripheral paresthesias, nausea, weakness, ataxia, bulbar dysfunction, and generalized muscular paralysis leading to respiratory failure.[2] The effects of a mild sting may disappear within a few hours, whereas a severe envenomation may take weeks to resolve.

Immediate treatment consists of pressure immobilization for venom containment. Less effective alternatives that have been mentioned are hot water soaks and administration of local anesthetic. With severe envenomation, treatment should focus on respiratory and cardiovascular supportive care. No antivenin exists for this envenomation.

OCTOPUS

Like cone shells, octopuses are also mollusks but lack calcified shells. The most dangerous species, the Australian blue-ringed octopus (*Octopus maculosus*) and the spotted octopus (*O. lunulata*), are smaller than 10 to 20 cm and found in tidal rock pools and other shallow waters. Bites are rare but can result in severe, even fatal, envenomations. Paralytic neurotoxins are excreted from salivary glands and are forcefully injected into victims via a powerful beak. One adult octopus may carry enough venom to paralyze 10 adults.

Most bites consist of puncture wounds on the hand due to gloveless handling. These are frequently unnoticed and only minimally painful. Within 10 to 15 minutes, facial numbess may progress to bulbar dysfunction, nausea, weakness, ataxia, and, ultimately, flaccid paralysis with respiratory failure. The victim may be alert despite complete paralysis.

Field therapy is the pressure immobilization technique. Treatment is supportive and recovery begins within 4 to 10 hours but may take up to 4 days. No antivenin exists for this envenomation.

STINGRAYS

Stingrays envenom more humans than does any other single variety of marine vertebrate. They are nonaggressive, however; most envenomations are due to careless handling or accidental stepping on the animal. Stingrays are usually found partially submerged in the sand or mud with only eyes, spiracles, and part of the caudal appendage ("tail") exposed. When provoked, the stingray's tail, which contains one to four venomous spines, whips upward and thrusts the spine(s) into the victim. The strike itself can cause a significant wound and associated bleeding. Secondary bacterial infection frequently occurs.

Stingray envenomation, which typically occurs in the lower extremity, immediately causes severe local pain and edema. The pain intensity peaks at 30 to 60 minutes and may last for 48 hours. The wound is initially cyanotic but rapidly becomes erythematous as hemorrhage and necrosis develop in fat and muscle. Systemic manifestations include nausea, vomiting, diarrhea, tachycardia, diaphoresis, headache, syncope, seizures, muscle cramps and fasciculations, paralysis, generalized edema, hypotension, arrhythmias, and death.

The goals of treatment are to provide effective pain relief, inactivate the venom, and prevent infection. Severe systemic effects require appropriate resuscitative intervention. The wound should be irrigated immediately. If sterile saline or water is not available, tap water can be used. Irrigation removes venom and foreign material and provides mild analgesia. Obvious retained integumentary sheath should be removed from the wound as it may continue to envenom. As soon as possible, the wound should be soaked in nonscalding hot water (45°C or 113°F) for 30 to 90 minutes. This may diminish the pain somewhat; however, addition of a local anesthetic or regional nerve block is often necessary. After soaking, thorough surgical exploration of significant wounds should be performed. The wound should then be packed with sterile gauze with planned delayed primary closure or sutured loosely around adequate drainage. Secondary bacterial infections frequently occur and prophylactic antibiotics (see below) are recommended for all but the most minor wounds. A victim should be observed for a minimum of 3 hours in case systemic effects develop.[7]

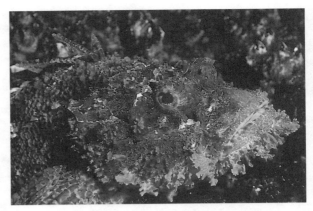

Figure 14–6. Scorpionfish. (Photo by Paul Auerbach, M.D.)

SCORPIONFISH, LIONFISH, AND STONEFISH

Scorpionfish, lionfish (or zebra fish), and stonefish belong to the family *Scorpaenidae*. They live in shallow, tropical, or temperate waters. Whereas lionfish are colorful coral reef fish (Figure 14–5), scorpionfish (Figure 14–6) and stonefish (Figure 14–7) are well-camouflaged bottom dwellers. Their dorsal, pelvic, and anal spines contain venom, which varies in potency depending on the species and the season. Stonefish venom is particularly potent and includes a toxin that causes paralysis of cardiac, smooth, and skeletal muscle.

Envenomation occurs when the unwary victim steps on or handles the fish. A puncture wound(s) results in immediate and intense pain lasting up to 12 hours. Local ischemia and cyanosis occur, while edema and erythema may spread to involve the entire limb. Systemic signs include nausea, vomiting, diarrhea, abdominal pain, arthralgias, fever, delirium (due to severe pain), seizures, paralysis, hypotension, bronchospasm, congestive heart failure, and, rarely, death (stonefish puncture) within 6 to 8 hours. Wounds frequently become infected and may take months to heal.

As soon as possible, the wound should be soaked in nonscalding hot water (45°C or 113°F) for 30 to 90 minutes. This may achieve partial pain relief. Addition of a local anesthetic or regional nerve block is often necessary. After soaking, the wound should be gently debrided and explored cautiously to remove any remaining spines. Prophylactic antibiotics are indicated. Stonefish antivenom (Commonwealth Serum Laboratories, Melbourne, Aus-

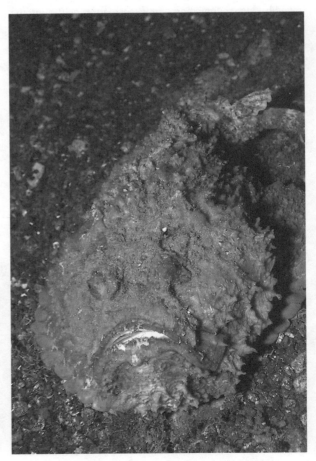

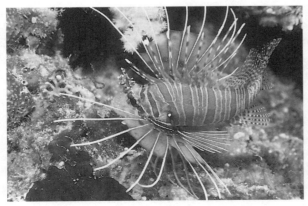

Figure 14–5. Lionfish. (Photo by Paul Auerbach, M.D.)

Figure 14–7. Stonefish. (Photo by Paul Auerbach, M.D.)

tralia) is recommended in a case of severe envenomation (marked pain, systemic symptoms, multiple punctures).

SEA SNAKES

There are at least 54 species of sea snakes, all of which are venomous. Although sea snakes are common in tropical waters, such as the Pacific and Indian Oceans, they are not found in the Atlantic Ocean or Caribbean Sea. Sea snakes are nonaggressive, with most attacks occurring in self-defense. Most bites (80%) do not result in significant envenomation because the fangs are short and easily dislodged from their sockets. The venom is more toxic than that found in most terrestrial snake venoms and contains neurotoxins and myotoxins.

The diagnosis of a sea snake bite is based on absence of pain at the puncture site, presence of small fang marks (usually 1 to 4, although occasionally up to 20), occurrence of the bite while in the water or handling a fishing net, development of characteristic symptoms, and identification of the snake.

The onset of symptoms varies from 5 minutes to 8 hours. After 30 to 60 minutes, a victim develops myalgias and stiffness, sialorrhea, and a "thick tongue." Within 3 to 6 hours, pain occurs with passive muscle movements, followed by ascending flaccid or spastic paralysis and possibly coma. Death may occur due to acute renal and respiratory failure. The mortality is 25% in victims who do not receive antivenom and 3% overall.

Treatment is similar to that for a terrestrial snake bite. To reduce the absorption of venom, the affected limb should be immobilized in a dependent position. A gauze pad should be placed over the fang marks and held firmly in place by a circumferential bandage that encompasses the entire extremity. The bandage should occlude lymphatic and venous circulation, but not arterial circulation, and should be kept in place until the victim can receive antivenom. If any sign of envenomation occurs, polyvalent sea snake antivenom, specific sea snake antivenom, or tiger snake antivenom should be administered. A victim may be discharged from medical care following 8 hours of observation if no systemic symptom has occurred.

BITES

Marine animals that bite but do not transfer any toxin to their victims are more widely dispersed than their venomous counterparts. They are often larger and more feared by human aquatic enthusiasts. Management of lacerations and punctures resulting from shark, barracuda, or eel bites can be very challenging as such wounds are often at high risk for infection.

SHARKS

Sharks, although typically nonaggressive animals, are implicated in 50 to 100 attacks on humans and 6 to 10 fatalities each year. Most commonly implicated in these attacks are the great white, tiger, bull, and oceanic white tip sharks. Great whites most commonly inhabit the warm waters of southern Australia, the east coast of South Africa, and cool, seal-populated waters of Northern California between Tomales Bay and Ano Nuevo (the infamous "Red Triangle"). The odds of being attacked by a shark along the North American coastline is less than 1 in 5 million.[1]

Sharks rely on an acute perception of movement and keen auditory and olfactory senses in hunting. Attacks on humans frequently occur at the surface within 100 feet of shore and are postulated to be the result of an unfortunate similiarity between the silhouette of a human on a surfboard and that of a sea lion. Most attacks are so-called "hit and runs," involving only single bites. However, initial "bumps" by the shark prior to biting may result in severe skin abrasions from placoid scales present on shark skin.

Lacerations resulting from shark bites are often severe because of the great force and tearing actions of shark jaws. Legs are most frequently bitten, followed by hands and arms. Thoracic or abdominal wounds may involve massive tissue loss. Hemorrhage and drowning lead to the deaths of 15% to 25% of shark attack victims.

Treatment, first and foremost, consists of management of hypovolemic shock. Compression and elevation of wounds and rapid fluid resuscitation are critical. Once victims are hemodynamically stable, wounds should be irrigated thoroughly, foreign bodies (teeth, seaweed, sand) removed, and devitalized tissue debrided in the emergency department or operating room. Wounds should be considered contaminated by bacteria, so tetanus prophylaxis and appropriate parenteral antibiotics (see below) should be administered. Wounds may either be closed loosely around multiple drains or packed open for delayed primary closure. Abrasions from shark "bumping" should be treated as second-degree burns.

BARRACUDA

Barracuda are more commonly observed by human divers than sharks and inhabit Atlantic, Caribbean, and Indo-Pacific waters. The great barracuda (*Sphyraena barracuda*) is the only species known to attack humans and may do so in turbid waters when attracted by shiny objects. It is a rapid swimmer with large, knife-like teeth.

Bites, although infrequent, result in straight or V-shaped lacerations in contrast to the crescent-shaped bite of the shark. Hemorrhage is moderate and crush injuries much less severe than with shark attack. Treatment is identical to that for a shark bite.

MORAY EELS

Moray eels are found in tropical, subtropical, and some temperate waters. They are powerful and potentially savage animals that live in holes, under coral, and in crevices. Most moray eels will avoid confrontation; however, if

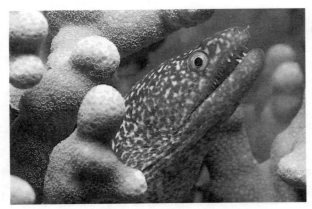

Figure 14–8. Moray eel. (Photo by Paul Auerbach, M.D.)

provoked or cornered, such as when a diver reaches into a cave, a moray eel will strike.

The moray's narrow, vice-like jaws (Figure 14–8) may inflict severe puncture wounds, crush injuries, and lacerations. Occasionally, the moray will not release the victim. Ripping a moray eel off the victim may worsen the injury.

If the eel remains attached to the victim, the jaws may need to be broken or the animal decapitated. The wound should be thoroughly irrigated and explored for retained teeth. Due to the high risk of infection, prophylactic antibiotics (see below) should be initiated; small puncture wounds should not be sutured.[8] If the wound is extensive or gaping, the edges may be loosely approximated, allowing adequate drainage.

MARINE BACTERIOLOGY AND ANTIBIOTICS

Wounds acquired in the marine environment become infected after penetration of the skin introduces pathogenic organisms and debris. Therefore, primary therapy of marine-acquired wounds includes copious irrigation and meticulous débridement. All foreign material and devitalized tissue should be removed. Complex wounds may require surgical exploration and repair. Primary closure of deep wounds increases the risk for infection and is usually contraindicated. Large or gaping wounds may be loosely sutured with adequate drainage.

Although infections are most commonly caused by *Staphylococcus* and *Streptococcus* species, *Vibrio* species and *Pseudomonas* are often implicated in severe soft-tissue infections.[8] Cellulitis caused by *Vibrio vulnificus*, although uncommon, has a 25% mortality rate in individuals with underlying chronic illness.[9]

Minor abrasions or lacerations usually do not require prophylactic antibiotics. However, a victim who is immunocompromised (e.g., leukemia, AIDS, or corticosteroid dependent), is chronically ill (e.g., diabetes or hemophilia), or has severe liver disease should receive ciprofloxacin, trimethoprim-sulfamethoxazole, or doxycycline.

A victim with a serious injury, such as a large laceration, deep puncture wound, or a retained foreign body, should receive prophylactic antibiotics. Recommended parenteral antibiotics include a third-generation cephalosporin (cefotaxime or ceftazidime), ciprofloxacin, an aminoglycoside, or trimethoprim-sulfamethoxazole. Imipenem-cilastatin should be reserved to treat established infections. Trimethoprim-sulfamethoxazole, ciprofloxacin, or doxycycline may be used for outpatient management of these injuries.

REFERENCES

1. Auerbach PS, Halstead BW. Hazardous aquatic life. In: Auerbach PS, Geehr EC, eds. Management of wilderness and environmental emergencies. 2nd Ed. St. Louis: Mosby, 1989: 933–1028.
2. Hawdon GM, Winkel KD. Venomous marine creatures. Aust Fam Phys 1997;26:1369–1374.
3. Pearn J. Sea, stingers, and surgeons: the surgeon's role in prevention, first aid, and management of marine envenomations. J Pediatr Surg 1995;30:105–110.
4. Burnett JW, Calton GJ. Jellyfish envenomation syndromes updated. Ann Emerg Med 1987;16:1000–1005.
5. Tomchik RS, Russell MT, Szmant AM, Black NA. Clinical perspectives on seabather's eruption, also known as "sea lice." JAMA 1993;269:1669–1672.
6. Freudenthal AR, Joseph PR. Seabather's eruption. N Engl J Med 1993;329:542–544.
7. Fenner PJ, Williamson JA, Skinner RA. Fatal and non-fatal stingray envenomation. Med J Aust 1989;151:621–625.
8. Erickson T, Vanden Hoek TL, Kuritza A, Leiken JB. Emergency management of moray eel bites. Ann Emerg Med 1992; 21:148–152.
9. Kumamoto KS, Vukich DJ. Clinical infections of *Vibrio vulnificus*: a case report and review of the literature. J Emerg Med 1998;16:61–66.

14.1 Diving-Related Health Problems

ERICH W. RUSSI

Scuba is an acronym for "self-contained underwater breathing apparatus." There are several ways one can go under water: breath-hold, helmet diving, submarine, etc. "Diving with scuba" means using an apparatus that is completely carried by the diver and not connected to the surface—hence self-contained. Scuba diving has become a worldwide recreational sport activity. The open-circuit scuba enables the diver to breathe high-pressure gas from a cylinder through a regulator, which reduces the inhaled gas to ambient pressure and allows exhalation into the water.

The rapidly changing ambient pressure under water may cause a variety of physiologic alterations. Given the popularity of scuba diving and the number of diving accidents, physicians should be aware of the specific hazards and medical conditions encountered under water.

BASIC PHYSICS

Since most diving-related complications are a consequence of the behavior of gases under changing conditions of pressures, it is appropriate to remember the two most relevant gas laws. Boyle's law states that at a constant temperature, the volume of gas varies inversely with the pressure applied ($P_1 \times V_1 = P_2 \times V_2$). The physiologic consequences of this law explain the pressure-related diving diseases, that is, barotrauma. Henry's law states that the amount of a given gas that will dissolve in a liquid at a given temperature is a function of the partial pressure of the gas in contact with the liquid and the solubility coefficient of the gas in that particular liquid. This law provides the explanation of decompression sickness and nitrogen narcosis.

DIVING-RELATED ACCIDENTS

Drowning is reported to be the most common cause of death among divers. Barotrauma is the most prevalent nonfatal complication encountered in scuba. While diving, unequal pressures may build up between some cavity of the body (e.g., the middle ear, the sinuses, the lungs, etc.) and the ambient air pressure. The consequences of barotrauma may range from mild discomfort in the affected region (e.g., ears, sinuses), to various levels of pain, to rupture of an organ, such as the tympanic membrane or a part of the lung. Escaped air can enter the pulmonary veins, from where it can travel to the arterial circulation. Arterial gas embolism as a complication of pulmonary barotrauma accounts for about 30% of recreational scuba diving fatalities. Bubbles may develop in the body of the diver whenever he ascends and is exposed to a reduction in environmental pressure (decompression). If symptoms occur, the condition is called decompression sickness (DCS). Nitrogen acts as a general anesthetic as

its partial pressure increases. The symptoms of nitrogen narcosis are similar to those of alcohol overdose.

BAROTRAUMA

Barotrauma refers to tissue injuries caused by a failure of a gas-containing body space to equalize its internal pressure to the corresponding changing ambient pressure. The risk of barotrauma is greatest near the water surface, when even a few meters of change in depths accompany large changes in gas volume. An overview on the different forms of barotrauma is presented in Table 14.1–1.

Barotrauma of the middle ear during descent is the most common disorder in diving. If a scuba diver descends and pressure across the tympanic membrane cannot be equalized over the eustachian tube due to faulty clearing technique or to infection of the upper respiratory tract, a sensation of pressure, followed by pain and hearing impairment, develops. With deeper descents, the ear drum may rupture. A reverse squeeze occurs when the diver ascends with a blocked eustachian tube, causing increased pressure and pain within the tympanic cavity.

Alternate vertigo is caused by an asymmetric increase in the pressure of the middle ear transferred to the labyrinth. The symptoms consist of nausea and disorientation.

Sinus barotrauma is a consequence of blockage of the sinus ostia and causes pain, most commonly over the frontal sinus.

Table 14.1–1. **DIVING-RELATED MEDICAL PROBLEMS**

Drowning, near-drowning
Barotrauma
  Barotrauma of descent
    Barotrauma to the middle ear
    Alternobaric vertigo
    Barodontalgia
  Barotrauma of ascent
    Reverse squeeze of the ear/sinus
    Alternobaric vertigo
    Pulmonary barotrauma and sequelae (e.g., pneumothorax, pneumomediastinum, arterial air embolism)
    Barodontalgia
    Gastrointestinal expansion distress
Decompression sickness
  Type I: localized joint pain ("the bends"; caisson disease), pruritus and skin rashes, localized swelling
  Type II: neurologic: usually damage to the spinal cord: paresthesias, paraparesis, paraplegia
Hazards of diving gases
  Nitrogen narcosis
  Oxygen toxicity: seizures

Divers breathing compressed gas while immersed at pressure are subject to the risk of pulmonary overinflation as pressure is reduced during ascent. Normally, intrapulmonary and environmental pressures are equalized by exhalation during ascent. The mechanism underlying pulmonary barotrauma (PBT) is believed to be the consequence of the following events: air, unable to escape through the airways, ruptures into the extra-alveolar tissues, where it spreads along the perivascular sheaths to cause mediastinal emphysema or pneumothorax. Arterial gas emboli occur if air ruptures into the pulmonary capillaries, arrives in the left heart, where gas buoyancy, in the diver who will be upright in ascent, directs the gas into the carotid arteries. Of itself, PBT may be only a minor problem, but the consequent complication of cerebral arterial gas embolism can be fatal. PBT may present with hemoptysis, chest discomfort, pneumothorax, mediastinal emphysema, or, at worst, tension pneumothorax. Symptoms of arterial gas embolism include unconsciousness, motor weakness or paralysis, somatosensory changes, visual disturbance, vertigo, or headache. The highest risk of PBT is considered to occur near the surface, where the rate of gas expansion is greatest. PBT occurs in the presence of two precipitating factors: breath-holding ascent and local air trapping. Breath-holding during ascent occurs in association with panic, buddy-breathing, and acute laryngospasm (aspiration of sea water). Local air trapping is the result of bronchoconstriction (asthma), mucous plugs (asthma, bronchitis), blebs or air-containing pulmonary cavities (pulmonary emphysema).

DECOMPRESSION SICKNESS

During diving, the tissues are loaded according to the increased ambient pressure with the inspired gases oxygen and nitrogen. Since nitrogen is not metabolized, its content in the tissues increases proportional to the ambient pressure. When the diver ascends, the ambient pressure decreases. When the sum of the gas tensions in the tissue exceeds the ambient pressure, supersaturation occurs. Under these conditions, free gas from the tissue forms bubbles that may rupture cell membranes and obstruct vessels leading to organ dysfunction. Patent foramen ovale (PFO) has been suggested as a risk factor for the occurrence of decompression sickness in divers. PFO is the result of an incomplete fusion of the two leaflets of the oval fossa after the reversal of the atrial pressures after birth. Patency of the foramen ovale is present in about 30% of the normal population. The suggested mechanism is paradoxical nitrogen bubble embolization after dives that would normally not lead to DCS (i.e., where the nitrogen bubbles would be "filtered out" by the lung vasculature). Several of the PFO studies in divers who suffered from DCS show a markedly increased prevalence of PFO. Given a high venous nitrogen bubble load, patency of the foramen ovale (PFO) can be the cause of paradoxical arterial nitrogen bubble emboli, thus leading to decompression illness. A rise in pulmonary artery pressure and retrograde rise in right atrial pressure due to pulmonary embolization of nitrogen bubbles might be responsible for a right-to-left blood shunt through a PFO. These arterial nitrogen bubbles would most likely migrate cephalad, thus causing high-spinal, cerebral, cerebellar, vestibular, or cochlear DCS symptoms.

DCS can be classified according to the organ or tissue affected. Furthermore, in order to differentiate cases in respect to prognosis and for standardization of therapy, DCS type I (mild) and type II (serious) may be distinguished (see Table 14.1–1). Type I comprises mild insult, such as localized joint pain ("the bends"), pruritus and skin rashes, pain, and localized edema. Type II includes neurologic deficits with eventual permanent injuries or death. Nervous system involvement is most commonly characterized by spinal cord damage. The spinal cord lesions present with paresthesias and numbness as well as paraparesis or paraplegia of the lower extremities involving bladder and bowel function.

NITROGEN NARCOSIS

Nitrogen in air acts as a general anesthetic as its partial pressure increases. The symptoms of nitrogen narcosis are similar to those of alcohol overdose ("martini" effect). They are characterized by intellectual impairment and by changes in behavior. Certain factors such as cold, stress, and heavy work may increase the possibility of nitrogen narcosis.

OXYGEN TOXICITY

Since the pressure of all inhaled gases increases with increasing depth, there is risk of inhaling too much oxygen and developing oxygen toxicity. This is unlikely to occur because the depth limit in recreational diving effectively limits length of exposure to oxygen concentrations that are not toxic for the central nervous system.

PREVENTION OF DIVING-RELATED COMPLICATIONS

BAROTRAUMA

Barotrauma of the Middle Ear   Ear pressure must be equalized during a dive. If this cannot be achieved, the dive must be stopped immediately. Problems can be avoided if diving is curtailed during a cold (e.g., due to blocked eustachian túbe). If pain persists, and hearing loss, loss of equilibrium, or bleeding occur, an ear, nose, and throat specialist should be consulted.

Pulmonary Barotraumas   Most PBT with arterial gas embolism are caused by breath-holding and/or a rapid or uncontrolled ascent in the water. Although PBT can occur during a normal ascent, it is a much less common occurence. The diver must breathe normally during free ascent with scuba such that air is vented properly until surfacing. In case of pneumothorax, the chest has to be drained by a chest tube. If neurologic deficits are present, the patient must be transported to the nearest recompression chamber in a comfortable horizontal position while breathing 100% oxygen.

DECOMPRESSION SICKNESS

Dive profiles may influence the likelihood of DCS. The deeper the dive and the more decompressions required, the higher the incidence of decompression sickness. Decompression sickness can be largely avoided if the rate of ascent is controlled by intermittent stops according to decompression tables. Adherence to appropriate decompression tables and dive computers reduces the risk of DCS but does not eliminate it entirely. Many cases of DCS have been reported in divers who have been decompressed in strict compliance with published tables. However, the risk for the occurrence of DCS increases under certain circumstances, which are listed in Table 14.1–2. Repeated dives or flying within a certain time after diving may also be a source of difficulty since after a dive, considerable quantities of nitrogen may remain in the tissues. Furthermore, some physiologic and environmental factors are believed to increase the likelihood or severity of DCS. Most of these influence the blood supply to tissues and therefore the speed of gas uptake or release. Such factors consist of exercise, low water temperature, female gender, and obesity. The risk for DCS can be reduced if the rate of ascent is controlled by intermittent stops according to decompression tables considering the above-mentioned cofactors. Although rapid decompression will predispose to DCS, a majority of divers who develop DCS have apparently complied with the decompression tables.

When neurologic symptoms are present, the patient should be transported, while breathing 100% oxygen and well hydrated, to the nearest recompression chamber under medical supervision.

NITROGEN NARCOSIS

This complication can be avoided by adhering to the international sport diving standards, which do not recommend diving beyond 30 meters. Experience and physical condition are vital factors to consider before attempting a deep dive, which should not be undertaken without an experienced and familiar partner. Alcohol, tranquilizers, and psychoactive drugs should be avoided.

The dive should be stopped at the onset of signs of nitrogen narcosis. The partner has to remain cool, control the situation, seize the patient from behind using water rescue training techniques, and return with him to the surface with all of the necessary decompression stops.

FLYING AFTER DIVING

Nitrogen may accumulate and form bubbles during the ascent if the next dive occurs within a short time frame or if the diver travels shortly thereafter in a commercial aircraft, which cruises at a usual cabin pressure (which corresponds to an altitude of up to 8,000 ft). Accordingly, the special aspects of repeated dives and of air travel after diving have to be taken into account by the diver.

Recreational divers frequently return home by airplane after diving holidays. The Divers Alert Network and other organizations have made general recommendations according to various diving activities (e.g., single dives, repetitive dives, decompression dives, etc.). The recommendations are guidelines and not dogma. After single dives per diving day, a minimum surface interval of 12 hours is recommended. After multiple dives for several days or dives that required decompression stops, an extended surface interval beyond 12 hours should be observed.

MEDICAL FITNESS FOR DIVING

Divers must have a reasonable level of fitness and must also be free of other limitations comprising safety in the underwater milieu. The underwater environment requires the diver to adapt to various specific changes, which are summarized in Table 14.1–3.

Table 14.1–4 summarizes conditions that are generally regarded as permanent contraindications for scuba diving. It is generally agreed that symptomatic asthma is a contraindication to diving because of limitation in exercise capacity and because uneven bronchoconstriction and mucus in the airways may trap air distally and lead to barotrauma of ascent. However, there is no unanimity about when or whether someone with asymptomatic asthma should dive. A conservative recommendation is that any person with asthma who experiences frequent exacerbation or continuously needs medication to control symptoms (i.e., with current asthma) should refrain from diving and that intending divers with a past history of asthma and asthmatic symptoms within the previous 5

Table 14.1–2. RISK FACTORS FOR DECOMPRESSION SICKNESS

Repetitive dives
Exceeding no-decompression limits
Diving on the edge of no-decompression limits
Flying after diving
Diving at altitude

Table 14.1–3. PHYSIOLOGIC CONSEQUENCES OF PARTICULAR ASPECTS OF THE UNDERWATER ENVIRONMENT

Difficulty in propulsion through the surrounding water
Rapid heat loss to water generally colder than body temperature
Breathing gas of increased density
Cardiovascular changes caused by immersion

Table 14.1–4. CONDITIONS REGARDED AS CONTRAINDICATIONS FOR SCUBA DIVING

Any significant exercise limiting problems (e.g., heart failure, pulmonary insufficiency, etc.)

History of spontaneous pneumothorax

Obstructive lung disease, particularly presence of nonventable air spaces (e.g., emphysema with bullae, blebs)

Other lung diseases (e.g., cryptogenic pulmonary fibrosis, pneumoconiosis, sarcoidosis with fibrosis, etc.)

Serious ear problems (e.g., permanent perforation of tympanic membrane; Meniere's disease)

Seizure disorders

years should be advised not to dive. However, in a recently published paper that reviewed the theoretical issues underlying the prohibition against scuba diving for asthmatic patients and critically examined relevant accident data, the authors concluded that "available data suggest asthmatic patients with normal airway function at rest, and with little airway reactivity in response to exercise or cold air inhalation, have a risk of pulmonary barotrauma similar to that of normal subjects."

SUGGESTED READINGS

Dick APK, Massey EW. Neurologic presentation of decompression sickness and air embolism in sport divers. Neurology 1985;35: 667–671.

Edmons C, Lowry C, Pennefather J. Diving and subaquatic medicine. 3rd Ed. Oxford: Butterworth-Heinemann, 1994.

Leitch DR, Green RD. Pulmonary barotrauma in divers and the treatment of cerebral arterial gas embolism. Aviat Space Environ Med 1986;57:931–938.

Martin L. Scuba diving explained. Flagstaff, AZ: Best, 1997.

Melamed Y, Shupak A, Bitterman H. Medical problems associated with underwater diving. N Engl J Med 1992;326:30–35.

Moon RE, Camporesi EM, Kisslo JA. Patent foramen ovale and decompression sickness in divers. Lancet 1989;11:513–514.

Neumann TS, Bove AA, O'Connor RD, Kelsen St. G. Asthma and diving. Ann Allergy 1994;73:344–350.

Russi EW. Diving and the risk of barotrauma. Thorax 1998; 53(Suppl 2):S20–S24.

Strauss RH. Diving medicine. State of the art. Am Rev Respir Med 1979;119:1001–1023.

Wilmshurst PT, Byrne JC, Webb-Peploe MM. Relation between interatrial shunts and decompression illness in divers. Lancet 1989;II:1302–1306.

WEB SITES

Professional Association of Diving Instructors: http://www.padi.com

Divers Alert Network (DAN): http://jshaldane.mc.duke.edu

Diving Medicine Online: http://w ww.gulftel.com/~scubadoc/

Undersea and Hyperbaric Medical Society: http://www.uhms.org/

Doc's Diving Medicine: http://weber.u.washington.edu/~ekay/

Diving and Hyperbaric Medicine Books: http://www.diveweb. com/best/Hyperbaric Oxygen

Therapy Information Center: http//www.marketnet.com/mktnet/ wound/hbo2.html

14.2 SEAFOOD INFECTION AND INTOXICATION

VERNON E. ANSDELL

Seafood is a very important cause of infection and intoxication worldwide. Even in developed countries, outbreaks are relatively common despite strict regulations covering fish and shellfish consumption. In developing countries, where regulations are often nonexistent or woefully inadequate, outbreaks of infection and intoxication are inevitably more frequent. The international traveler is at potentially high risk of illness and should be counseled carefully regarding the risk of eating fish and shellfish while traveling in developing countries. Unfortunately, most infections and toxins do not affect the appearance, smell, or taste of seafood and cannot be detected prior to consumption. At a minimum, all fish and shellfish should be adequately cooked, but even this precaution may not prevent illness since many toxins are heat stable. Table

14.2–1 summarizes some key guidelines that should be considered when counseling travelers regarding consumption of seafood in developing countries. Clinicians should always take a careful dietary history from returned travelers with relevant symptoms in order to avoid missing a diagnosis of seafood-related illness.

It is likely that seafood-related illness in international travelers will become increasingly common in the future. Important factors may include the increased numbers of travelers to developing countries and the increased popularity of adventurous eating involving seafood such as raw fish, sushi, and exotic species. Many outbreaks of shellfish poisoning are associated with algal or dinoflagellate blooms. Also known as "red tides," they are becoming more frequent in many areas as a result of fac-

Table 14.2–1. GUIDELINES FOR SEAFOOD INGESTION IN DEVELOPING COUNTRIES

PREVENTION GUIDE	COMMENT
Avoid raw or undercooked fish or shellfish	Increased risk of various bacterial, viral, and parasitic infections
Refrigerate fish promptly after capture (e.g., mahimahi, tuna, mackerel, amberjack)	Increased risk of scombroid poisoning
Avoid large (>6 lbs), carnivorous, reef fish (e.g., barracuda, grouper, moray eel, snapper, jack, seabass)	Increased risk of ciguatera poisoning
Avoid pufferfish (especially the ovaries, liver, intestines, and skin)	Increased risk of pufferfish (fugu) poisoning
Avoid shellfish associated with red tides (dinoflagellate blooms)	Increased risk of paralytic, neurotoxic, diarrheic, and amnesic shellfish poisoning
Immune compromised, alcoholics, and patients with chronic liver disease should avoid shellfish	Increased risk of life-threatening *Vibrio vulnificus* and *Vibrio parahemolyticus* infections
Children should avoid shellfish	Increased risk of *fatal* paralytic shellfish poisoning

tors that influence the marine environment such as ocean warming, coastal construction projects, fertilizer run-off, and increased sewage release associated with population growth.

SHELLFISH

Shellfish are a particulary important cause of infection and intoxication. Historically, raw or undercooked shellfish have been responsible for a wide range of viral and bacterial infections including hepatitis A, Norwalk virus, *Salmonella*, *Shigella*, and *Vibrio* species. In addition, ingestion of shellfish containing toxins produced by dinoflagellates and diatoms may result in important intoxications such as paralytic, neurotoxic, diarrheic, and amnesic shellfish poisoning.

Shellfish include mollusks and crustaceans. Mollusks can be divided into bivalves, which have two shells joined by a hinge (e.g., clams, oysters, mussels, cockles, and scallops), and gastropods, which have whorled snail-like shells (e.g., whelks and periwinkles). Bivalve mollusks are filter feeders that concentrate a wide range of microorganisms and toxins in the gills and intestines. As a result, some viruses may be concentrated 100-fold. Unfortunately for shellfish fanciers, the main edible portion of most bivalve mollusks is the alimentary tract. (Scallops are relatively safe since the adductor muscle is the main edible portion.) With the exception of scallops that tend to live and breed in deeper waters, all mollusks grow in and are harvested from inshore coastal waters, often near sewage outlets in developing countries.

Crustaceans (e.g., shrimps, crabs, lobsters, scampi, and crayfish) are mobile animals with hard, articulated

exoskeletons. They are not filter feeders but can acquire surface contamination with bacteria or viruses from polluted water or from improper handling after capture.

Attempts to guarantee the safety of shellfish destined for human consumption have proved very difficult. For example, monitoring the safety of shellfish grounds by measuring coliform counts does not give a reliable estimate of the level of viral contamination.[1] The risk of infection is often compounded by inadequate storage and preparation of shellfish. Freezing at temperatures of −5° to −17°C is not adequate to prevent transmission of certain viruses. Well-cooked shellfish often have a rubbery texture, and there is a tendency to undercook them. It has been shown that clams may open their shells within 1 minute of steaming, but it takes at least 6 minutes for internal temperature to reach adequate levels to kill.

INFECTIONS

BACTERIAL INFECTIONS

Seafood-related bacterial infection typically occurs as a result of either (a) organisms in the natural marine environment (e.g., *Vibrio* species, *Plesiomonas,* and *Aeromonas*) or (b) bacteria associated with fecal contamination (e.g., *Vibrio* species, *Salmonella, Shigella, Campylobacter, Yersinia, Listeria, Clostridium, Staphylococcus,* and *Escherichia coli*).

Vibrio cholerae infections are often related to consumption of fish or shellfish.[2] The organism has been shown to survive for many weeks in shellfish such as crabs and mollusks, despite refrigeration.[3] In the Pacific Islands and the Asian subcontinent, outbreaks of cholera have been caused by consumption of raw shrimp, raw fresh fish, salted raw fish, and cooked squid. In Europe, mussels, clams, and cockles have been responsible for several outbreaks, and cooked crabs caused a large outbreak in Guinea-Bissau. Inadequate cooking is often responsible for outbreaks of cholera, and one study clearly showed that crabs boiled for less than 10 minutes or steamed for less than 30 minutes still harbored live *V. cholerae*.[2]

In travelers, the risk of cholera appears to be very low. It was estimated at 0.2 per 100,000 air travelers returning to the United States from endemic countries.[4] Some of the highest rates have been reported in Japanese tourists (5 cases per 100,000 travelers from all destinations and 13 cases per 100,000 travelers from Bali)[5] and were thought to be due, in part, to increased consumption of raw seafood. The number of cases of cholera in travelers appears to be increasing, and several cases have been linked to consumption of seafood and the current outbreak in South America.[5,6] A large outbreak of cholera in travelers involved over 75 passengers who were served a seafood salad on a flight from Lima to Los Angeles.[4] In addition, crabs transported from Ecuador were responsible for two outbreaks of cholera in the United States. Ceviche is a very popular raw fish dish in many parts of Latin America but is considered high risk for several infections, including cholera. It is usually prepared with raw fish or shellfish marinated in lemon or lime juice.

Travelers to Latin America should probably avoid ceviche, although, theoretically, if the dish is prepared with an adequate amount of lemon or lime juice and marinated for a sufficient time, the risk of cholera should be very small.

Vibrio vulnificus infections result from consumption of raw or undercooked shellfish and fish or exposure of wounds to contaminated seawater. The organism is one of the most invasive and rapidly lethal human pathogens. In humans, it may cause a self-limited gastroenteritis, wound infections, or primary septicemia.

Wound infections and primary septicemia may be associated with mortality rates of up to 50%, especially in alcoholics or patients with chronic liver diseases[7,8] (e.g., hepatitis B, hepatitis C, cirrhosis, or hemochromatosis). Other predisposing factors for septicemia include diabetes, chronic renal insufficiency, immunosuppressive drugs, hematopoietic disorders, and conditions that reduce gastric acid such as gastrectomy and drugs such as histamine-2 antagonists and proton pump inhibitors).[9] Raw oysters are the most common source of infection,[8] but boiled shrimp, grilled crab, and deep fried fish[10,11] have also been responsible. In one study in Brazil, 12% of oysters tested were positive for *V. vulnificus*. The organism may survive freezing but is killed by adequate cooking. The risk for travelers to developing countries is uncertain, but individuals at increased risk of serious infection, especially those with alcoholism, chronic liver disease, and certain other chronic medical problems, should avoid shellfish, particularly oysters.

Vibrio parahemolyticus is distributed worldwide in both tropical and temperate inshore coastal and estuarine waters. Infection occurs after eating raw or inadequately cooked shellfish such as crabs, shrimps, lobster, and oysters[8] and is usually associated with factors such as improper refrigeration, inadequate cooking, cross-contamination with other seafood, and recontamination.[12] Infected shellfish may be very common, and in one study, 77% of oysters in Brazil had evidence of *V. parahemolyticus* infection. In immunocompetent individuals, *V. parahemolyticus* causes a mild to moderate gastroenteritis. More severe illness occurs in a number of chronic medical conditions including chronic liver disease, alcoholism, iron overload states, diabetes, hematologic malignancies, reduced gastric acid (gastrectomy, histamine-2 antagonists or proton pump inhibitors), or immune deficiency disorders.[8,11] The organism survives freezing but is killed by adequate cooking.

Plesiomonas and *Aeromonas* organisms have been responsible for seafood-related outbreaks of gastroenteritis in many parts of the world. A variety of seafood such as raw oysters, mussels, cuttlefish, and salt mackerel have been responsible. *Aeromonas* caused a particularly large outbreak of 472 cases of gastroenteritis following ingestion of frozen raw oysters.

Coastal marine waters may be contaminated by bacteria such as *Vibrios, Salmonella, Shigella, Campylobacter, Yersinia, Listeria, Clostridium, Staphylococcus,* and *E. coli* that are discharged in untreated or inadequately treated sewage. As a result, fish and shellfish become contaminated and may cause infection when eaten. Filter-feeding bivalve mollusks (e.g., oysters, cockles, mussels, and clams) concentrate microorganisms and are particularly likely to be responsible for infection.

Salmonella typhi infection related to seafood consumption is relatively common in developing countries, and nontyphoidal salmonellae (including *S. paratyphi* and *S. enteritidis*) have been responsible for many shellfish-related outbreaks worldwide. *Shigella* species have been implicated in several shellfish-related outbreaks, probably because the organism requires only a low infectious dose and survives for long periods in bivalves such as clams and oysters. In contrast, *Campylobacter* organisms survive poorly in salt water and are a rare cause of seafood-borne infections. *Yersinia enterocolitica* and *Listeria monocytogenes* are rare causes of seafood-related infection. These organisms are able to multiply at low temperatures, however, thereby increasing the potential for human illness from contaminated cold-stored or frozen seafood.

VIRAL INFECTIONS

Pathogenic viruses (e.g., hepatitis A, hepatitis E, Norwalk and other small round viruses, Coxsackie viruses, and rotavirus) may be introduced into the marine environment in untreated or inadequately treated sewage. Enteric viruses are more resistant than enteric bacteria to sewage treatment processes and may remain viable in seawater for many weeks or months. Filter-feeding bivalve mollusks are particularly likely to be responsible for viral infections because of their ability to retain filtered products in the gills and alimentary tract and accumulate them in the liver.

Adequate cooking is important to eliminate viruses and render shellfish safe for human consumption. For example, it is recommended that the internal temperature of mollusks must be maintained at 90°C for at least 90 seconds before consumption.

Hepatitis A virus can survive in seawater for up to 1 year, and shellfish can concentrate hepatitis A virus up to 15 times the level in the surrounding water. Numerous outbreaks of hepatitis A have been reported as a result of eating contaminated shellfish such as oysters, clams, cockles, and mussels. The largest reported outbreak occurred in Shanghai, China, in 1988 when almost 300,000 people developed hepatitis A after eating raw or inadequately cooked clams.[13] Hepatitis E is largely water borne, although some cases have been associated with shellfish ingestion.

Norwalk virus is the most common cause of acute gastroenteritis following shellfish consumption.[14] Multiple outbreaks have been reported, usually as a result of ingestion of inadequately cooked clams or oysters. Infection is prevented by adequately cooking shellfish (e.g., steaming for at least 4 to 6 minutes).

PARASITE INFECTIONS

Anisakiasis (Anisakidosis) Most seafood-related parasite infections in humans are the result of ingestion of freshwater fish rather than saltwater fish (e.g.,

Diphyllobothrium latum and *Gnathostoma spinigerum*). An important exception is anisakiasis (anisakidosis), which is caused by marine nematodes ("herring worms" or "cod worms") such as *Anisakis simplex, Anisakis physeteris,* and *Pseudoterranova decipiens.* Adult worms are found in large sea mammals (e.g., dolphins, whales, seals, and sea lions), and the infective, intermediate-stage larvae are found in seafood such as cod, sole, flounder, salmon, mackerel, red snapper, tuna, herring, octopus, and squid. Human infections occur after eating raw, undercooked, pickled, salted, or smoked fish or squid containing infective larvae. Anisakid larvae measure 25 to 30 mm × 0.5 to 0.7 mm and are often visible to the naked eye. Infection is particularly likely to occur after ingestion of seafood delicacies such as sashimi, sushi, sunomono, ceviche, oka, and poisson cru. Anisakiasis is most common in Pacific Ocean waters. In Japan, where raw seafood is very popular, over 2,000 cases are diagnosed every year.

Clinically, anisakiasis may present in several different forms depending on the location of the infective larvae (i.e., luminal, gastric, intestinal, or ectopic). Symptoms of anisakiasis may mimic a wide variety of gastrointestinal conditions including peptic ulcer, reflux esophagitis, carcinoma of the stomach, appendicitis, Crohn's disease, cholecystitis, ileus, intussusception, intestinal obstruction, peritonitis, pancreatitis, and carcinoma of the pancreas.

Luminal Anisakiasis. In this form, larvae are unable to penetrate the mucosal surface and are expelled by coughing, vomiting, or manual extraction from the oropharynx.

Gastric Anisakiasis. This is, by far, the most common clinical form of anisakiasis. Symptoms are caused by infective larvae burrowing into the gastric mucosa and often mimic an acute peptic ulcer. Patients typically present with acute, severe epigastric pain within 1 to 12 hours of eating infected fish or squid. Not infrequently, there may be nausea, vomiting, urticaria, or a low-grade fever. There may be leukocytosis, but eosinophilia is often absent in the early stages. Tests for fecal occult blood may be positive. The diagnosis of gastric anisakiasis is confirmed by identifying a larval worm embedded in the gastric mucosa during esophagogastroduodenoscopy. Local hemorrhage, extensive mucosal edema, or ulceration may be present. Larval worms may be outlined by contrast radiography. In addition, ultrasound or contrast radiography may demonstrate a characteristic focal edematous lesion. Treatment is by direct endoscopic removal of the larval worm since anthelminthic drugs appear to be ineffective. If the worm is not removed during the acute stage, chronic gastric anisakiasis may develop.

Intestinal Anisakasis. This form usually presents 1 to 7 days after infection and is often the result of larval invasion of the distal ileum. Symptoms may include lower abdominal pain, diarrhea, nausea, vomiting, and mild fever. Leukocytosis sometimes with eosinophilia may be present. Eosinophilic ascites is often found in this form of anisakiasis. Fecal occult blood tests may be positive. Contrast radiography or ultrasound may demonstrate thickened mucosa and luminal narrowing of the small intestine. Ultrasound may demonstrate ascites.

Ectopic Anisakiasis. This form of infection occurs when larvae are found outside of their usual location in the stomach or intestine. Possible ectopic sites include the peritoneal cavity, lymph nodes, liver, pancreas, ovaries, gallbladder, and pleural cavity. Symptoms are mild and nonspecific. Eosinophilia may be present. Serologic tests are often positive but are not readily available. The diagnosis is often made when larvae are found incidently during surgery.

Adequate cooking of fish will kill the larvae and prevent infection. Fish intended for raw consumption should be frozen to –20°C for at least 72 hours.

INTOXICATIONS

SCOMBROID

Scombroid is one of the most common fish poisonings and occurs worldwide in both temperate and tropical waters. The disease occurs after eating improperly refrigerated or preserved fish containing high levels of histamine[15] and often resembles a moderate to severe allergic reaction. Fish that cause scombroid include dark or red-muscled fish belonging to the family *Scombridae* such as albacore, bluefin and yellowfin tuna, mackerel, saury, skipjack, and bonito. Several nonscombroid fish may also be responsible including mahimahi (dolphinfish) (Figure 14.2–1), sardine, pilchard, anchovy, herring, bluefish, amberjack, and black marlin. Cases of fish poisoning closely resembling scombroid were described by Captain Edmund Fanning while sailing in the North Atlantic in 1797 (Figure 14.2–2).

Fish that cause scombroid have high levels of the amino acid histidine in the flesh. As a result of improper storage, histidine is converted to histamine and other scombrotoxins by bacteria with high histidine decarboxylase activity. These bacteria occur as normal surface flora or secondary contaminants and include *Morganella morganii, Klebsiella pneumoniae, E. coli, Aerobacter aerogenes,* and *Plesiomonas shigelloides.*

Conversion of histidine to histamine and other scombrotoxins occurs optimally at 20° to 30°C, and scombroid usually occurs in fish that have not been promptly refrigerated after capture. Histamine and other scombrotoxins are resistant to freezing, cooking, smoking, or canning.

Increased urinary histamine was demonstrated in patients with scombroid following an outbreak in a hospital cafeteria.[15] The precise role of histamine in scombroid is still unresolved, however, and other scombrotoxins may also be important. Most oral histamine is inactivated to N-acetylhistamine by intestinal bacteria, but it is postulated that other scombrotoxins may inhibit this process or may facilitate absorption of histamine from the gastrointestinal tract. As anticipated, patients taking drugs such as isoniazid that inhibit histamine metabolism are at increased risk of scombroid.

Symptoms of scombroid poisoning usually appear abruptly 10 to 60 minutes after eating contaminated fish,

Table 14.2–2.   SUMMARY OF SEAFOOD TOXINS

SYNDROME	TOXIN	ORIGIN OF TOXIN	SEAFOOD VEHICLE	GEOGRAPHIC DISTRIBUTION	TYPICAL SYMPTOMS
Scombroid	Histamine	Histidine converted to histamine by enzyme action	Inadequately refrigerated, histidine-rich fish (e.g., mahimahi, tuna, mackerel, skipjack)	Worldwide	Flushing, headache, nausea, vomiting, diarrhea, urticaria
Ciguatera	Ciguatoxin Maitotoxin	Dinoflagellates. *Gambierdiscus toxicus* and others	Large carnivorous tropical and subtropical reef fish (e.g., barracuda, grouper, moray eel, snapper, jack, seabass)	Tropical and subtropical waters between 35° north and 35° south. Most common in the Caribbean and South Pacific Islands.	Gastroenteritis followed by neurologic symptoms (e.g., dysesthesiae, temperature reversal, pruritus, weakness). Rarely, bradycardia and hypotension.
Pufferfish poisoning	Tetrodotoxin		Pufferfish, porcupine fish, and, rarely, ocean sunfish	Worldwide. Most common in Japan, Indo-Pacific Oceans.	Perioral paresthesiae, nausea, dizziness followed by weakness, numbness, slurred speech, incoordinatioin, respiratory failure
Paralytic shellfish poisoning	Saxitoxin	Dinoflagellates. *Alexandrium species* and others	Bivalve shellfish	Worldwide. Most common in temperate coastal waters.	Paresthesiae of face and limbs, gastroenteritis. Rarely, dysphonia, ataxia, weakness, respiratory failure.
Neurotoxic shellfish poisoning	Brevetoxins	Dinoflagellates. *Gymnodinium breve*	Bivalve shellfish	Rare. Gulf of Mexico and New Zealand.	Gastroenteritis and neurologic symptoms (e.g., paresthesiae, temperature reversal, vertigo, ataxia). Respiratory and eye irritation in the presence of aerosols.
Diarrheic shellfish poisoning	Okadaic acid and others	Dinoflagellates. *Dinophysis* species	Bivalve shellfish	Japan, Europe (France), Canada, New Zealand, and South America	Gastroenteritis
Amnesic shellfish poisoning	Domoic acid	Diatoms. *Pseudonitzschia* species	Mussels	Extremely rare—Northeast Canada only	Gastroenteritis followed by neurologic symptoms (e.g., amnesia, cognitive impairment, headache, seizures)

although they may appear within a few minutes of ingestion or be delayed for up to 8 hours. Untreated, symptoms typically last for an average of 4 hours but may persist for 24 hours. Symptoms often resemble an acute allergic reaction and are frequently misdiagnosed as an allergy to fish. Affected fish often have a peppery, sharp, metallic, or bitter taste but may be normal in taste and appearance. There are several characteristic symptoms of scombroid poisoning. Flushing of the skin resembling sunburn with a sharply demarcated edge confined to the face and upper body may be present. Pruritus is common, and there may be urticaria or angioneurotic edema. A throbbing headache is commonly present. Gastrointestinal symptoms include nausea, vomiting, abdominal cramps, and diarrhea. Other clinical features may include perioral paresthesiae, burning of the mouth and gums, conjunctival suffusion, palpitations, blurred vision, and diaphoresis. Scombroid is usually a benign, self-limited illness; rarely, however, it may produce a more serious illness with respiratory compromise, malignant arrythmias, and hypotension. Serious illness seems to be more likely in the elderly, asthmatics, or patients taking isoniazid or

monoamine oxidase inhibitors. Deaths are extremely rare, and none have been reported in recent years. Persons already taking antihistamines may be somewhat protected.

Diagnosis is usually made on clinical grounds. There may be a clustering of cases, which helps to exclude the possibility of fish allergy. If available, leftover fish should be frozen and the diagnosis confirmed by measuring histamine levels.

Treatment with histamine-1 antagonists (e.g., diphenhydramine) given orally or parenterally provides symptomatic relief. Newer, second-generation, nonsedating histamine-1 antagonists (e.g., astemizole) have not yet been proved to be as effective. Histamine-2 antagonists (e.g., cimetidine) given orally or parenterally may shorten the course of illness[16] and have been particularly useful in controlling headache.[16,17] A combination of histamine-1 and -2 antagonists may be particularly valuable but rarely may cause hypotension. Steroids have not been shown to be of any benefit. In severe scombroid poisoning intravenous fluids, inhaled bronchodilators, oxygen, and pressor agents may be indicated. If large quantities of conta-

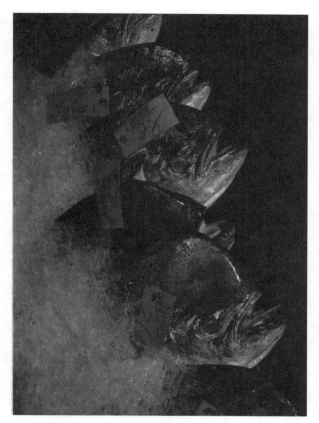

Figure 14.2–1. Mahimahi (dolphin fish), one of the most common causes of scombroid. Prompt refrigeration, using ice as shown here, will prevent poisoning. (Photo by David Ansdell.)

refrigeration until the fish is prepared for consumption. Fish kept at 15° to 20°C or less prior to cooking should be safe for consumption.

CIGUATERA

Ciguatera fish poisoning is one of the most common causes of marine poisoning, and over 50,000 new cases are estimated to occur worldwide each year.[18] It is widespread in tropical and subtropical waters between the latitudes of 35° north and 35° south and is particularly common in the Pacific and Indian Oceans and the Caribbean Sea. Most cases follow ingestion of coral reef fish containing potent toxins such as ciguatoxin or maitotoxin that originate in dinoflagellates found in coral reefs. Other toxins that may be involved include scaritoxin, okadaic acid, and palytoxin.[19,20] Average annual incidence rates for ciguatera fish poisoning vary from 5 to 50 per 100,000 in major endemic areas with rates of up to 500 per 100,000 or even higher in some areas of the South Pacific during certain years.[21,22]

The toxins that cause ciguatera poisoning originate from dinoflagellates such as *Gambierdiscus toxicus* that are found in tropical waters on the surface of certain seaweeds and adhering to dead coral surfaces. Dinoflagellates are ingested by herbivorous fish and the toxins are concentrated as they pass up the food chain to large (usually greater than 6 pounds) carnivorous fish and finally to humans[23] (Figure 14.2–3).

Ciguatoxin and maitotoxin are among the most lethal natural substances known[24] and may be concentrated up to 50 to 100 times in parts of the fish such as the liver, gas-

minated fish have been consumed within the previous hour, then gastric lavage or catharsis may be appropriate.

The most important preventive measure is to chill the fish promptly after capture and maintain adequate

During this period we caught, with hook and grains, as many of the Spanish mackerel, or bonetos, as were wished for; shoals of these fish, as well as the dolphin, being all around us;...On eating of the dolphin and mackerel, almost all on board were affected with a severe pain in the head, which shortly after was much inflamed; the eyes became red, and these distressing symptoms were attended with violent vomiting. Those who were thus affected, were evidently poisoned; the head and some of the limbs began also to swell, which swelling increased, until they had attained a most disagreeable form, having at the same time, a reddish cast over the head and limbs thus swollen... Whenever the fish, on being taken out of the water, was immediately cooked, and then eaten, no evil or unpleasant sensation was experienced;...

Figure 14.2–2. An account of apparent scombroid poisoning during Captain Edmund Fanning's voyage in the North Atlantic, 1797. From Fanning E. Voyages and discoveries in the South Seas, 1792–1832. New York: Dover, 1989.

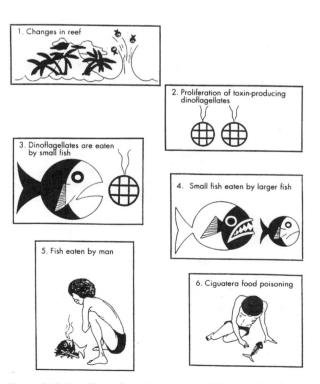

Figure 14.2–3. Chain of events in ciguatera fish poisoning. Copyright SPC, Secretariat of the Pacific Community (formerly South Pacific Commission), South Pacific Bulletin 3rd Quarter 1979.

trointestinal tract, roe, and head. The toxins do not affect the appearance, texture, smell, or taste of the affected fish and are not destroyed by gastric acid, cooking, canning, drying, freezing, smoking, salting, or pickling.

Over 400 species of fish have been implicated in ciguatera poisoning. They are mainly carnivorous reef fish such as grouper, snapper, barracuda, jacks, sea bass, and moray eels. Certain herbivorous or omnivorous reef fish such as surgeon fish and parrot fish may also be responsible.

Ciguatera-like illnesses were known in ancient Egypt. Some of the earliest recorded cases in travelers were in the crews sailing with European explorers such as Christopher Columbus and James Cook[25] (Figure 14.2–4). Captain Bligh and his followers apparently developed ciguatera poisoning after the historic mutiny aboard HMS Bounty. The name "ciguatera" was given by the Portuguese biologist Don Antonio Parra (ca. 1771). He used the term to describe fish poisoning that resembled poisoning from the turban shell snail known by Cuban natives as "cigua."

The onset of symptoms is usually within 1 to 3 hours of eating contaminated fish but may occur within 15 to 30 minutes or be delayed for up to 30 hours. Most symptoms resolve within 1 to 4 weeks. A wide range of symptoms has been reported, but, typically, there is an acute gastrointestinal illness followed by neurologic symptoms and, rarely, cardiovascular collapse. Gastrointestinal symptoms occur in 40% to 75% of cases and include diarrhea, nausea, vomiting, and abdominal pain. They usually occur 1 to 3 hours after eating affected fish and may last for 1 to 2 days. Neurologic symptoms tend to occur later and may be delayed for up to 72 hours. They may last for several months or even years. Neurologic symptoms include paresthesias involving the extremities, tongue, throat, and perioral area and paradoxical dysesthesias such as temperature reversal. Temperature reversal, where cold objects feel hot and hot objects feel cold, is very characteristic of ciguatera poisoning but not pathognomic

since it may also occur in neurotoxic shellfish poisoning. Another very characteristic symptom of ciguatera poisoning is pain in the teeth or a sensation that the teeth are numb or loose. This has been reported in about one-third of cases. Visual symptoms include blurred vision and transient blindness. Chronic neuropsychiatric symptoms may be very disabling and include malaise, depression, headaches, myalgias, and fatigue.[26]

Cardiac manifestations include bradycardia (possibly due to cholinesterase inhibition), tachycardia, and other arrhythmias.[22,27] Hypotension in the absence of hypovolemia may be due to the hypotensive properties of maitotoxin. Persistent symptomatic hypotension has been described and is probably due to an increase in parasympathetic tone and impaired sympathetic reflexes. Hypertension has also been described. The cardiac effects of ciguatera poisoning may be serious but usually resolve within 5 days of onset.

General symptoms include profound weakness, chills, sweating, arthralgias, myalgias, and a metallic taste in the mouth. Pruritus, particularly involving the palms and soles, occurs 2 to 5 days after ingestion of contaminated fish and has been reported in 5% to 89% of cases.[21] It is particularly common in New Caledonia where ciguatera poisoning is known as "la gratte" or "the itch." It seems to be more common in the Pacific than the Caribbean.[24]

Death is usually from respiratory or cardiac failure and is most common in those who have eaten parts of the fish known to contain high levels of toxin such as the liver, intestines, or roe.[28] Case fatality rate is usually from 0.1% to 1%, depending on geographic location.[21] A mortality rate of almost 20% was reported in one outbreak in Madagascar when over 500 people became ill after eating a shark.[29]

Disturbances to reef systems and the subsequent proliferation of toxic dinoflagellates have been shown to have an important impact on the incidence of ciguatera poisoning, although there is often a 6- to 12-month time lag. Reef systems may be disrupted by natural disasters such as hurricanes, tidal waves, heavy rains, and earthquakes or human activities such as underwater nuclear explosions, coastal construction projects, dredging, shipwrecks, or golf course run-off.

Several factors have been shown to influence the severity of ciguatera poisoning. These include the amount of fish eaten and consumption of parts known to contain high levels of toxin such as the head, liver, intestine, and roe or soup made from those parts. Previous exposure to ciguatera also increases the severity of poisoning, probably as a result of accumulation of toxin or immune sensitization.

Medical management is mainly symptomatic and supportive. If patients are seen within 3 hours of ingestion of contaminated fish, emetics such as ipecac or gastric lavage followed by activated charcoal may be indicated. In theory, antiemetics and antidiarrheals should be avoided because they may prolong toxin contact time. Bradycardia responds to atropine. Volume depletion and hypotension require intravenous fluids. Hypotension in the absence of volume depletion is treated with pressors such as dopamine or dobutamine. Intravenous calcium gluconate 10% can be used to treat the inhibited calcium uptake caused by ciguatoxin. Treatment of prolonged

The Night before we came out of Port two Red fish about the Size of large Bream and not unlike them were caught with hook and line of which Most of the officers and Some of the Petty officers dined the next day. In the Evening every one who had eat of these fish were seiz'd with Violant pains in the head and Limbs, so as to be unable to stand, together with a kind of Scorching heat all over the Skin, there remained no doubt but that it was occasioned by the fish being of a Poisoness nature and communicated its bad effects to every one who had the ill luck to eat of it even to the Dogs and Hogs, one of the latter died in about Sixteen hours after and a young dog soon after shared the same fate: and it was a week or ten days before all the gentlemen recovered.

Figure 14.2–4.   An account of apparent ciguatera poisoning during Captain James Cook's voyage in the South Pacific in 1774. From The journals of Captain James Cook on his voyage of the Resolution and Adventure 1772–1775. London: Hakluyt Society, 1982:469–470.

orthostatic hypotension may require sodium and fluid replacement, fludrocortisone acetate, and lower extremity support stockings. Lidocaine or mexilitene have been used to treat ventricular arrhythmias. Treatment options for specific symptoms include cyproheptadine or hydroxyzine for pruritus, acetaminophen or nifedipine for headache, and nonsteroidal anti-inflammatory agents for musculoskeletal pains. Amitriptyline appears to be effective in treating depression associated with ciguatera poisoning and may also be effective in treating other neuropsychiatric symptoms such as dysesthesias.[30] Chronic fatigue associated with ciguatera poisoning has been treated successfully with fluoxetine (Prozac).[31]

Intravenous mannitol (1g/kg over 30 minutes) may dramatically reduce the severity and duration of neurologic symptoms, particularly if given within the first 24 hours of poisoning.[32–34] Mannitol should be used with caution, however, and only after ensuring adequate hydration. The mechanism of action is unclear.

Travelers to endemic areas, particularly the Caribbean and Indo-Pacific regions, should be warned about the risk of ciguatera poisoning and should avoid or limit consumption of reef fish, particularly fish weighing over 6 pounds. The risk of ciguatera fish poisoning in travelers to an endemic area has been estimated at 300 in 10,000, which is similar to the risk of acquiring hepatitis A.[35] Particularly high-risk fish such as tropical moray eels or barracuda should never be eaten.[36] It is important to emphasize avoidance of parts of the fish known to contain large amounts of toxin such as the head, liver, intestine, and roe or soup made from these parts and consumption of larger reef fish weighing more than 6 pounds.

Radioimmune assays or enzyme-linked immunosorbent assays have been developed to investigate ciguatera poisoning. Hokama et al. at the University of Hawaii pioneered the use of immunochemical methods for detection of toxin.[37] A commercial immunoassay has recently become available for the identification of toxic fish (Cigua–check™, Oceanit Test Systems Inc., Honolulu). The test is easy to perform and very sensitive, but it is relatively expensive (cost approximately $5 [U.S.] per test). It will probably have limited value for travelers to endemic areas.

Any patient with a history of ciguatera poisoning should avoid consumption of reef fish, fish sauces, shellfish, alcoholic beverages, nuts, and nut oils since they may provoke recurrent symptoms. There are many misleading folklores that claim to predict the presence of

Table 14.2–3. **EXAMPLES OF MISLEADING FOLKLORES THAT CLAIM TO DETECT THE PRESENCE OF CIGUATOXIN**

A silver coin cooked with the fish will turn black

Tasting the slime from the fish's eye produces a tingling sensation

Grated coconut cooked under the fish will turn green

Rubbing fish liver on the gums will produce a tingling sensation

toxin (Table 14.2–3), and it is important to warn travelers that these are not reliable.

Diagnosis of ciguatera poisoning is usually made on clinical grounds. If a portion of the fish is still available, it should be frozen and, if possible, submitted to a laboratory that can test for presence of toxin.

In a survival situation, organ meat should be fed to susceptible animals such as dogs, cats, or mongooses. If the animals show no sign of illness, then the flesh of the fish should be safe for human consumption.

PUFFERFISH (FUGU) POISONING

Pufferfish or fugu poisoning occurs after ingestion of fish containing tetrodotoxin, a potent neurotoxin. Potentially toxic fish are distributed widely throughout the world and include pufferfish, porcupine fish, and ocean sunfish. The toxin is usually concentrated in the ovaries, liver, intestines, and skin of the fish. Pufferfish poisoning has been recognized since ancient Egyptian times. One of the earliest recorded outbreaks of pufferfish poisoning in travelers may have involved Captain Cook and members of his crew who became ill after eating pufferfish liver while sailing in the South Pacific during their second voyage around the world in 1774[38] (Figure 14.2–5).

Most cases of pufferfish poisoning occur in Japan where pufferfish or fugu is eaten as a very expensive and prized delicacy. The fugu is filleted, thinly sliced, and then arranged in traditional patterns such as a crane. The fugu experience is characterized by tingling of the lips and tongue, a sensation of generalized warmth and flushing, and a feeling of euphoria and exhilaration.[38,39] Over the 78-year period from 1886 to 1963 there were 6,386 cases of fugu poisoning in Japan with approximately 59%

This afternoon a fish being struck by one of the natives near the watering place, the Captain's clerk purchased it, and sent it to him after his return on board. It was of a new species, something like a sun-fish, with a large, long, ugly head. Having no suspicion of its being of a poisonous nature, they ordered it to be dressed for supper; but, very luckily, the operation of drawing and describing took up so much time that it was too late, so that only the liver and roe were dressed, of which the two Mr. Fortsters and the Captain did but taste. About three o'clock in the morning they all found themselves seized with an extraordinary weakness and numbness all over their limbs. The Captain had almost lost the sense of feeling; nor could he distinguish between light and heavy bodies, of such as he had strength to move; a quart pot full of water and a feather being the same in his hand. They each took an emetic, and after that a sweet, which gave them much relief. In the morning, one of the pigs which had eaten the entrails was found dead.

Figure 14.2–5. An account of apparent pufferfish poisoning during Captain James Cook's voyage in the South Pacific in 1774. From Forster JR. Resolution. In: Journal of Johann Rheinhold Forster, 1771–75. Vol. 4. London: Hakluyt Society, 1982:649–651.

mortality.[38,40] Increased awareness of fugu poisoning and strict regulation and training of licensed fugu chefs has resulted in far fewer cases and lower mortality in recent years. For example, in the 10-year period from 1967 to 1976, there were 1,105 cases and 372 deaths (34% mortality) and from 1983 to 1992 there were only 449 cases and 49 deaths (11% mortality).[39] Nowadays, all cooks and restaurants handling fugu must be licensed, and most cases of pufferfish poisoning occur in inexperienced fishermen who prepare their own food. In 1996, three cases of fugu poisoning occurred in San Diego in chefs who ate prepackaged, ready-to-eat fugu illegally imported from Japan.[41]

Tetrodotoxin is a heat-stable, water-soluble, nonprotein toxin that is 50 times more potent than strychnine. It acts by binding to sodium channels and blocking axonal nerve transmission and results in ascending paralysis and respiratory failure. In addition to pufferfish, porcupine fish, and ocean sunfish, tetrodotoxin has been found in a wide variety of other marine animals including the blue-ringed octopus, starfishes, flatworms, various crabs, and mollusks. It has also been found in frogs, newts, and salamanders.

Levels of toxin are highest in the ovaries, liver, intestine, and skin, but the body distribution of toxin may vary in different fish species. The toxin does not alter the taste or appearance of the fish. It is not destroyed or inactivated by cooking, canning, freezing, or smoking and, despite the fact that the toxin is water soluble, is very difficult to remove from the fish.

Symptoms of pufferfish poisoning may develop within a few minutes of ingestion of toxic fish or may be delayed for up to 4 hours or longer. Early onset of symptoms and ingestion of large amounts of toxin tend to be associated with more severe poisoning.[42] Initial symptoms include perioral paresthesiae and numbness, nausea, and dizziness.[43] There may be progression to more generalized paraesthesiae and numbness, dysarthria, ataxia, ascending paralysis, and a variety of other symptoms such as headache, hypersalivation, diaphoresis, vomiting, abdominal pain, and diarrhea. In the most severe cases, there is widespread paralysis, respiratory insufficiency, and cardiac involvement manifested by bradycardia and other arrhythmias and hypotension. Most deaths are due to respiratory failure and occur within the first 6 hours. The prognosis is usually excellent in patients who survive the first 24 hours.[44]

Diagnosis is made on clinical grounds. There is no specific antidote for tetrodotoxin and treatment is aimed at limiting absorption of toxin and treating the adverse effects. Absorption of toxin can be limited by gastric lavage, which is indicated if patients are seen within 3 hours of ingestion of toxic fish.[40] There is evidence that lavage using 2 liters of 2% $NaHCO_3$ followed by activated charcoal in 70% sorbitol may be beneficial. Emetics such as ipecac should be avoided because of the risk of aspiration. In severe cases, intravenous fluids, vasopressors, endotracheal intubation, and ventilatory support may be indicated.[39] Bradycardia may respond to atropine.[39] Edrophonium or neostigmine has been used successfully to treat muscle weakness.[43,45]

It is impossible to guarantee that fish are free from toxin, and travelers should be advised to avoid any potentially toxic fish even when prepared by trained chefs in licensed restaurants. In life-threatening (survival) situations, travelers should take advantage of the water-soluble properties of the toxin. Viscera and skin must not be eaten, and the muscle of the fish should be shredded into small pieces, kneaded, and soaked in water for at least 4 hours prior to consumption.

PARALYTIC SHELLFISH POISONING

Paralytic shellfish poisoning (PSP) has been recognized for over 200 years. The first recognized outbreak in travelers was in 1793 and was reported in Captain George Vancouver's "A Voyage of Discovery to the North Pacific Ocean and Round the World." PSP is the most common and most serious form of shellfish poisoning[46] and occurs after eating contaminated bivalve mollusks (clams, cockles, mussels, oysters, and scallops) containing saxitoxin and other potent neurotoxins produced by dinoflagellates (e.g., *Alexandrium* species). Rarely, PSP has been reported after eating other seafood such as chitons, certain species of crab, limpets, starfish, mackerel, and scad.[21] Saxitoxin, like ciguatoxin and tetrodotoxin, causes paralysis by blocking sodium channels in nerve cell membranes. It is 50 times more potent than curare. Saxitoxin and other toxins that cause PSP are heat stable and survive normal cooking procedures.

As in other forms of shellfish poisoning, outbreaks of PSP often follow dinoflagellate blooms. In the past, most cases of PSP occurred in cold, temperate waters above latitude 30°N and below latitude 30°S. Outbreaks in tropical and subtropical waters have become more frequent, however, with cases reported from countries such as Guatemala, El Salvador, Mexico, Thailand, Singapore, Malaysia, Papua New Guinea, India, and the Solomon Islands.

Symptoms of PSP may occur within 30 minutes of eating toxic shellfish but can be delayed for 3 hours or longer. Early symptoms include paresthesiae of the lips, tongue, and face and later the arms and legs. Affected persons may complain of a floating sensation.[38] Other symptoms may include headache, increased salivation, nausea, vomiting, and diarrhea. Hypertension may be an important finding. Severe cases are usually associated with ingestion of large doses of toxin and clinical features such as ataxia, dysphagia, and mental status changes. Flaccid paralysis and respiratory insufficiency occur in the most severe cases. Deaths are typically caused by respiratory failure and tend to occur within 12 hours of eating toxic shellfish. Recovery usually occurs within a week but may occasionally be prolonged for several weeks.

Case fatality rate averages 6% but ranges from 0% to 44%. Mortality is higher in children, who seem to be particularly sensitive to the effects of the toxin. The highest mortality rates tend to occur in areas with poor access to advanced life support.[47] This is a very important consideration for shellfish fanciers who are traveling in developing countries.

Diagnosis is usually made on clinical grounds. Creatine kinase levels may be elevated, and one study showed an increase in the MB fraction in the absence of myocardial damage.[48] The reasons for this observation were not clear. In special circumstances, the diagnosis can be confirmed by a standard mouse bioassay method.

Treatment is mainly symptomatic and supportive. Gastric lavage or use of a cathartic or enema may be indicated in certain situations.[38,43] Mechanical ventilation may be indicated if there is respiratory failure. Atropine should be avoided since saxitoxin and its derivatives may be anticholinergic.[49]

PSP can be prevented by avoiding potentially contaminated shellfish. This is particularly important in children who are at greater risk of fatal illness. It is important to emphasize that cooking will not destroy the toxin. Because of the lack of sophisticated medical facilities for resuscitation and mechanical ventilation, it is prudent for all travelers to developing countries to avoid potentially toxic shellfish.

NEUROTOXIC SHELLFISH POISONING

Neurotoxic shellfish poisoning (NSP) occurs after eating bivalve mollusks (e.g., oysters, clams, scallops, and mussels) contaminated by heat-stable brevotoxins produced by the marine dinoflagellate *Gymnodinium breve*. *G. breve* is an important cause of red tides and has been responsible for the deaths of large numbers of fish, sea birds, and marine mammals such as manatees.

NSP usually presents as a gastroenteritis accompanied by neurologic symptoms and often resembles mild paralytic shellfish poisoning or ciguatera poisoning. Inhalation of brevotoxins from the seaspray associated with a red tide may cause an acute respiratory illness often referred to as aerosolized red tide respiratory irritation (ARTRI).

NSP was first described on the west coast of Florida in 1844. Since then, it has been reported from the Gulf of Mexico, the east coast of Florida, the North Carolina coast, and New Zealand. It is expected to be reported from other areas of the world in the future.

Symptoms of NSP may develop within 15 minutes of ingestion of contaminated shellfish or be delayed for up to 18 hours. Gastrointestinal symptoms include abdominal pain, nausea, vomiting, and diarrhea. There may be myalgias and dizziness. Neurologic symptoms include circumoral paresthesias, paresthesias of the arms and legs, temperature reversal, vertigo, and ataxia. Symptoms may last for several hours or a few days. Symptoms of ARTRI occur almost immediately after exposure and include a nonproductive cough, wheezing, conjunctival irritation, and rhinorrhea. Asthmatics are particularly susceptible, and there is some anecdotal evidence of long-term pulmonary symptoms following ARTRI in the elderly or those with preexisting lung disease.

Treatment of NSP and ARTRI is symptomatic and supportive. Preventive measures include avoiding shellfish associated with red tides and limiting coastline exposure to red tides and aerosolized brevotoxins. Particle masks can be used to prevent inhalation of aerosolized toxins.

DIARRHEIC SHELLFISH POISONING

Diarrheic shellfish poisoning (DSP) results from ingestion of contaminated bivalve mollusks (clams, mussels, and scallops) containing okadaic acid and other toxins produced by various marine dinoflagellates (*Dinophysis fortii* or *Dinophysis acuminata*).

Historically, DSP was reported predominantly from Japan and European countries such as the Netherlands, Italy, and Spain. As a result of increased global spread of toxic dinoflagellates, however, outbreaks have recently been reported from Canada, South America, Australia, New Zealand, and Indonesia. As in other shellfish poisonings, outbreaks tend to follow red tides or dinoflagellate blooms. Okadaic acid triggers sodium release by intestinal cells and produces diarrhea. Symptoms usually appear 30 minutes to 6 hours after ingestion of contaminated shellfish, although onset may be delayed for up to 12 hours. Typically, symptoms last for up to 4 days and include diarrhea, abdominal cramps, nausea, vomiting, weakness, and chills. The severity of symptoms is usually related to the amount of toxin ingested. No fatalities have been reported. Diagnosis is usually made on clinical grounds and treatment is symptomatic and supportive.

AMNESIC SHELLFISH POISONING

Amnesic shellfish poisoning (ASP) is a recently described toxic encephalopathy. It was first identified in 1987 after an outbreak involving over 100 Canadians who had eaten mussels contaminated by domoic acid harvested off Prince Edward Island.[50] Domoic acid is a heat-stable toxin produced by diatoms such as *Nitzschia pungens*. High levels of toxin have been demonstrated in shellfish in areas such as the Pacific Northwest, the Gulf of Mexico, and off the west coast of Scotland, although no clinical cases have been reported from those areas.

In the Prince Edward Island outbreak, symptoms of ASP developed within 15 minutes to 38 hours (median 6 hours) of ingestion of contaminated mussels. Acute gastrointestinal symptoms were very common and included nausea, vomiting, abdominal cramps, and diarrhea.[50] Neurologic features occurred in over one-third of patients and included headaches, short-term memory loss, confusion, disorientation, dizziness, seizures, and coma.[50,51] Several patients developed long-term cognitive dysfunction.[51] There were four deaths, all in patients over 70 years of age.

Treatment for ASP is symptomatic and supportive. Potentially contaminated shellfish, particularly those associated with red tides, should never be eaten.

REFERENCES

1. DuPont HL. Consumption of raw shellfish — is the risk now unacceptable? N Engl J Med 1986;314:707–708.
2. Blake PA, Allegra DT, Snyder JD, et al. Cholera—a possible endemic focus in the United States. N Engl J Med 1980; 302:305–309.
3. De Paola A. *Vibrio cholerae* in marine foods and environmental waters: a literature review. J Food Sci 1981;46:66–70.

4. Swerdlow DL, Ries AA. Cholera in the Americas. Guidelines for the clinician. JAMA 1992;267:1495–1499.

5. Taylor DN, Rizzo J, Meza R, et al. Cholera among Americans living in Peru. Clin Infect Dis 1996;22:1108–1109.

6. Sanchez JL, Taylor DN. Cholera. Lancet 1997;349:1825–1830.

7. Hill MK, Sanders CV. Localized and systemic infection due to *Vibrio* species. Infect Dis Clin North Am 1987;1:687–707.

8. Desenclos JA, Klontz KC, Wolfe LE, Hoecherl S. The risk of *Vibrio* illness in the Florida raw oyster eating population, 1981–1988. Am J Epidemiol 1991;134:290–297.

9. Sacks-Berg A, Strampfer MJ, Cunha BA. *Vibrio vulnificus* bacteremia: report of a case and review of the literature. Heart Lung 1987;16:706–709.

10. Eng RHK, Chmel H, Smith SM, et al. Early diagnosis of overwhelming *Vibrio vulnificus* infections. South Med J 1988; 81:410–411.

11. Klontz KC, Lieb S, Schreiber M, et al. Syndromes of *Vibrio vulnificus* infections. Clinical and epidemiologic features in Florida cases, 1981–1987. Ann Intern Med 1988;109:318–323.

12. Hlady WG, Klontz KC. The epidemiology of *Vibrio* infections in Florida, 1981–1993. J Infect Dis 1986;173:1176–1183.

13. Halliday ML, Kang L, Zhou T, et al. An epidemic of hepatitis A attributable to the ingestion of raw clams in Shanghai, China. J Infect Dis 1991;164:852–859.

14. Fang G, Araujo V, Guerrant RL. Enteric infections associated with exposure to animals or animal products. Infect Dis Clin North Am 1991;5:681–701.

15. Morrow JD, Margolies GR, Rowland J, and Roberts II LJ. Evidence that histamine is the causative toxin of scombroid-fish poisoning. N Engl J Med 1991;324:716–720.

16. Auerbach PS. Persistent headache associated with scombroid poisoning: resolutin with oral cimetidine. J Wilderness Med 1990;1:279–283.

17. Blakesly M. Scombroid poisoning: prompt resolution of symptoms with cimetidine. Ann Emerg Med 1983;12:104–106.

18. Hughes JM, Merson MH. Fish and shellfish poisoning. N Engl J Med 1976;295:1117.

19. Kodama AM, Hokama Y, Yasumoto T, et al. Clinical and laboratory findings implicationg palytoxin as a cause of ciguatera poisoning due to *Decapterus macrosoma* (mackerel). Toxicon 1989;27:1051–1053.

20. Sims JK. A theoretical discourse on the pharmacology of toxic marine ingestions. Ann Emerg Med 1987;16:1006–1015.

21. Bagnis R, Kuberski T, Laugier S. Clinical observation on 3,009 cases of ciguatera (fish poisoning) in the South Pacific. Am J Trop Med Hyg 1979;28:1067–1073.

22. Morris JG, Lewin P, Hargrett NT, et al. Clinical features of ciguatera fish poisoning: a study of the disease in the US Virgin Islands. Arch Intern Med 1982;142:1090–1092.

23. Randall JE. A review of ciguatera, tropical fish poisoning, with a tentative explanation of its cause. Bull Mar Sci Gulf Carib 1958;8:236–267.

24. Swift AEB, Swift TR. Ciguatera. Clin Toxicol 1993;31:1.

25. Cook, J. A voyage towards the South Pole and round the world. Vol. 2. London: Strahan and Cadell, 1777.

26. Peam JH. Chronic fatigue syndrome: chronic ciguatera poisoning as a differential diagnosis. Med J Aust 1997;166: 309–310.

27. Engleberg NC, Barrett TJ, Fisher H, et al. Ciguatera food poisoning: major common source outbreak in the USVI. Ann Intern Med 1983;98:336–337.

28. Vernoux JP, Lahlou N, El Andaloussi SA, et al. A study of the distribution of ciguatoxin in individual Caribbean fish. Acta Tropica 1985;42:225.

29. Habermehl GG, Krebs HC, Rasoanaivo P, et al. Severe ciguatera poisoning in Madagascar: a case report. Toxicon 1994; 32:1539.

30. Davis RT, Villar LA. Symptomatic improvement with amitriptyline in ciguatera fish poisoning. N Engl J Med 1986;315:65.

31. Berlin RM, King SL, Blythe DG. Symptomatic improvement of chronic fatigue with fluoxetine in ciguatera fish poisoning. Med J Aust 1992;157:2131–2133.

32. Palafox NA, Jain LG, Pinano AZ, et al. Successful treatment of ciguatera food poisoning with IV mannitol. JAMA 1988;259:2740–2742.

33. Blythe DG, De Sylva DP, Fleming LE, et al. Clinical experience with IV mannitol in the treatment of ciguatera. Bull Soc Pathol Exot 1992;85:425.

34. Pearn JH. Ciguatera and mannitol: experience with a new treatment regimen. Med J Aust 1989;151:77.

35. Zlotnick BA, Hintx S, Park DL, et al. Ciguatera poisoning after ingestion of imported jellyfish: diagnostic application of serum immunoassay. Wilderness Environ Med 1995;6:288.

36. Lange WR, Snyder FR, Fudala PJ. Travel and ciguatera fish poisoning. Arch Intern Med 1992;152:2049–2053.

37. Hokama Y, Asahina AY, Shang ES, et al. Evaluation of the Hawaiian reef fishes with the solid phase immunobead assay. J Clin Lab Anal 1993;7:26.

38. Mills AR, Passmore R. Pelagic paralysis. Lancet 1988;331: 161–164.

39. Kaku N, Meier J. Clinical toxicology of animal venoms and poisons. New York: CRC Press, 1995.

40. Sims, JK. Pufferfish poisoning: emergency diagnosis and management of mild human tetrodotoxin. Ann Emerg Med1986; 15:1094–1098.

41. Centers for Disease Control and Prevention. Tetrodotoxin poisoning associated with eating puffer fish transported from Japan – California, 1996. MMWR Morb Mortal Wkly Rep 1996;45:389–391.

42. Harrison LJ. Poisonous marine morsels. J Fla Med Assoc 1991;78:219–221.

43. Eastaugh J, Shepherd S. Infectious and toxic syndromes from fish and shellfish consumption. A review. Arch Intern Med 1989;149:1735–1740.

44. Bower E, Hart R, Matthews P, Howden M. Nonprotein neurotoxins. Clin Toxicol 1981;18:813–863.

45. Chew SK, Chew LS, Wang KW, et al. Anticholinesterase drugs in the treatment of tetrodotoxin poisoning. Lancet 1984;2:108.

46. Smart D. Clinical toxicology of shellfish poisoning. In: Meier J, White J, eds. Handbook of clinical toxicology of animal venoms and poisons. New York: CRC Press, 1995:33–57.

47. Hartigan-Go K, Bateman DN. Red tide in the Philippines. Hum Exp Toxicol 1994;13:824.

48. Cheng H-S, Chua SO, Hung J-S, Yip K-K. Creatine kinase MB elevation in paralytic shellfish poisoning. Chest 1991;99: 1032–1033.

49. Sakamoto Y, Lockey RF, Krzanowski JJ. Shellfish and fish poisoning related to the toxic dinoflagellates. South Med J 1987;80:866–872.

50. Perl TM, Bedard L, Kosatsky T, et al. An outbreak of toxic encephalopathy caused by eating mussels contaminated with domoic acid. N Engl J Med 1990;322:1775–1780.

51. Teitelbaum JS, Zatorre RJ, Carpenter S, et al. Neurologic sequelae of domoic acid intoxication due to the ingestion of contaminated mussels. N Engl J Med 1990;322:1781.

Chapter 15

MEDICAL RISKS OF TEMPERATURE EXTREMES

ERIC L. WEISS

INTRODUCTION

International travel for business and recreation has seen a substantial recent increase, but perhaps more interesting has been the relative boom in "adventure travelers," those adrenaline-seeking travelers intentionally straying off the beaten path. In addition to being at increased risk for many of the maladies described elsewhere in this text, such travelers regularly expose themselves to environmental extremes, from the heat of the Serengeti safari to the cold of Glacier Bay. The following chapter will provide an overview of the medical risks of such environmental extremes.

HISTORY

Medical complications of hot or cold exposure have been described all the way back to biblical times. The groups most affected have historically been involved in the making of war. Roman armies suffered substantial losses from heat illness in 24 BC. More recently, Egypt lost 20,000 men to heatstroke during the 6-day war with Israel in 1967. In the United States, more than 4,000 people die from heatstroke each year. Heatstroke is also the second leading cause of death among young athletes in the U.S. On the cold front, military casualties are again the greatest. Hannibal lost nearly half of his troops to cold in crossing the Alps; Napoleon left France for Russia with 12,000 men during the winter of 1812 and returned 6 months later with only 350 effective soldiers. During times of peace, the population at risk for environmental illness is much smaller and consists primarily of those who are unintentionally without home or shelter and those who choose to travel to areas and situations of risk. Let us focus on this latter group.

PHYSICS

Simply stated, we become hot when we gain heat faster than we can lose it and become cold when we lose heat faster than we can gain (or produce) it. There is a finite amount of heat produced by our basal metabolic rate (BMR = 65 to 85 kcal/hour).[1] Moderate exercise (300 kcal/hour) or simply standing in the sun (150 kcal/hour) contributes to our heat load. Without any

mechanism to lose this heat, our bodies would warm at a rate of 1.1°C per hour for 4.5 hours until our core temperature reached 42°C, when oxidative phosphorylation is known to uncouple. There are four conventional mechanisms of heat transfer and an understanding of them will assist us in understanding the pathophysiology and treatment of heat- and cold-related illness.

Conduction is heat transfer between two bodies or surfaces in direct contact. Heat gain or loss by conduction can only take place when there is a temperature differential between the two surfaces. Conduction plays a relatively little role in heat transfer unless one is sitting on granite or lying on snow.

Convection is heat transfer from a surface to a gas or liquid caused by the movement of molecules. Note that heat exchange between your body and water is technically convection. Thermally neutral water is approximately 33°C (91.4°F). As water "conducts" heat 25 times greater than air, submersion in water any colder than this is a risk for hypothermia. Practically, significant risk begins in water colder than 25°C (77°F).

Radiation refers to the transfer of heat via electromagnetic waves. Most energy transfer is via thermal infrared radiation; however, on a bright sunny day, solar radiation can be significant (see above).

Evaporation (phase change) or evaporative cooling is our biggest defense against heat illness. When water changes state from liquid to gas, a significant amount of energy is transferred: each 1.7 mL of evaporated sweat allows the body to lose 1 kcal of heat. In a neutral environment, sweating does not occur, and evaporative losses (from the respiratory system) account for only 15% of the body's heat loss. However, as the ambient temperature approaches 35°C (84.5°F), and radiation can no longer effectively occur, evaporative heat loss becomes the body's sole mechanism for heat transfer. Note that high humidity will adversely affect the body's ability to lose heat by interfering with evaporation.

HEAT PHYSIOLOGY

Given this overview of the "physical" components of heat transfer, we need now consider the "physiology" of heat transfer in order to predict those at risk for heat illness and understand the theory behind the treatment of heat illness.

When a traveler from the temperate region to the Serengeti ventures out under the midday sun, his or her body will respond with several physiologic mechanisms for increasing heat loss. Superficial and deep thermal receptors relay information to the hypothalamus, which, in turn, mediates cutaneous vasodilatation and an increase in heart rate/stroke volume, bringing warm blood and hence heat to the skin surface.[2] In addition, our 2 to 3 million sweat glands (distributed in decreasing frequency over palms, soles, head, trunk, and extremities) begin contributing to evaporative heat loss. Note that the scalp, face, and upper torso are probably the most important areas for evaporative heat loss. Thus, wearing a hat or shirt has more implications than wearing long pants. It is important to note that there is a significant opportunity for improvement on this physiologic response via adaptation.

Heat adaptation can be an important step toward preventing heat-related illness. Educating travelers at risk should be part of every travel medicine consult. Although adaptation can occur with just simple exposure to hot environments (sun, sauna), maximal benefit requires exercise in the heat, preferably an hour a day, over a period of 8 to 10 days. If one is unable to find a suitably warm training environment, exercise alone will afford more than 50% of the adaptive benefit. In addition to positive effects on heart rate and stroke volume, adaptation causes the earlier onset of sweating and cutaneous vasodilatation via a lower core temperature trigger point, as well as the ability to sustain vigorous sweating for a more prolonged period of time. The peak sweat rate can be almost doubled to nearly 3 L/hour. More importantly, the ability of the sweat gland to resorb sodium is greatly increased, dropping sweat sodium concentrations from approximately 60 mEq/L to less than 10 mEq/L. This hypotonic sweat loss affords protection against dehydration through an earlier effect on increasing serum osmolarity and hence earlier sensation of thirst and an urge to drink. Regardless of sweat sodium concentration, it is well appreciated that by the time the exercising individual is thirsty, he/she is significantly dehydrated. It should also be noted that as easily as one can adapt to the heat, one can lose this adaptive advantage over a similar period of time.

HEAT ILLNESS RISK

The risk of heat illness can be significantly increased by situations that impede the mechanisms described above for normal heat transfer. Given that evaporation of sweat represents a principal heat defense, it should be no surprise that hot and humid environmental conditions are the most common heat illness risk factors. Other physical factors that increase risk include obesity, skin disorders that impede sweating (burns, scleroderma), and heavy clothing (firefighters, certain trade workers, selected athletes). Physiologic risks include the extremes of age (blunted thermoregulatory response), hyperthyroidism, and, notably, dehydration. Dehydration threatens the very mainstay of the host defense mechanism (sweating), but more importantly, dehydration can increase the activity of the cellular sodium pump, which can, in and of itself,

raise core temperatures by more than 2°C. Anticholinergic drugs, including over the counter antihistamines, can also significantly impede sweating. Other drugs of concern include beta-blockers (blunt cardiovascular response) and those drugs that can directly increase muscle activity or cause seizures (cocaine, amphetamines, PCP, and other stimulants).

HEAT ILLNESS PREVENTION

Take advantage of the human body's ability to adapt to heat stress! If you are a traveler from the temperate region to the tropics, give yourself adequate time for physical training. Fluid intake needs to be strongly stressed. Take rest breaks and drink cold, pleasantly flavored, dilute beverages. Note that most commercially available drinks contain too much sugar; dilute these by half or two-thirds. Wear light-colored, loose-fitting clothing. Hats are fine for sun protection but remember the significant role of scalp blood flow and sweat in the heat transfer process. Lastly, note that the standard "dry bulb" temperature is a poor predictor of heat illness as it does not take humidity into account. A "wet bulb globe temperature" is a much better predictor and is measured with a special thermometer able to account for both temperature and relative humidity.

HEAT ILLNESS

Although heat illnesses have conventionally been described as separate entities, it is important to understand that they all represent different stages along a heat illness continuum. Nowhere is this more important than in the usual academic arguments over "heat exhaustion" versus "heatstroke." In the search for an exact diagnosis, patient care is often delayed or, frankly, compromised. The potentially fatal nature of heat illness should never be forgotten.

HEAT SYNCOPE

An episode of fainting in an environment conducive to heat stress can be deemed "heat syncope" once the physician has eliminated other, more serious, diagnosis (seizure, arrhythmia, etc.). Heat syncope is felt to be secondary to a combination of dehydration and vasomotor instability. Core temperatures are always normal, and the patient responds well to a horizontal position and gentle fluid replacement.

HEAT CRAMPS

Heat cramps have been commonly described, particularly in workers subject to significant heat stress. Cramps involve skeletal muscle that has recently undergone several hours of sustained effort, often associated with the ingestion of large amounts of water. Given this combination, many argue for sodium/water imbalance or sodium transport effect as etiology, but this is still hotly debated.

Other authors suggest a direct spinal neural mechanism unrelated to biochemical changes in either the blood or skeletal muscle. It appears that acclimatized individuals are at much less risk. Treatment should not include "salt tablets" as they are a gastric irritant; rather, balanced salt solutions should be administered either by mouth or intravenously in more seriously affected individuals.

"PRICKLY HEAT"

Also known as *miliaria rubra* or heat rash, prickly heat is felt to be a result of plugged and infected sweat glands, perhaps with a particular species of coagulate-negative staphloccoci. Clinically, these appear as pruritic vesicles on an erythematous base. There is also some evidence to suggest that ultraviolet exposure and skin damage (sunburn) may contribute due to the separation of the superficial layers of skin ("peeling") and its effects on sweat gland duct function. Prevention should focus on wearing light, loosely fitting clothing and avoiding situations of prolonged sweating and excessive sun exposure. Talc or cornstarch powders should be avoided as they themselves can contribute to pore plugging. Topical antibacterials such as chlorhexadrine may be indicated. Oral antibiotics should be used for extensive or pustular involvement.

HEAT EDEMA

Lower extremity edema is commonly reported by unacclimatized individuals from the temperate region on arrival in the tropics. Pathophysiology is unclear but would seem to be due to a combination of vascular pooling and cutaneous vasodilatation. The important point to make is that these patients should rarely be treated with diuretics as this does little besides increase their risk for dehydration. Simple reassurance and elevation of the affected part should suffice.

HEAT EXHAUSTION

Again, it is important to point out that there is a substantial gray area between the diagnoses of "heat exhaustion" and "heatstroke." It is best to remember them as two points along a continuous line.

Heat exhaustion has also been termed "heat prostration" and represents the situation where the victim is beginning to feel the effects of his or her body's struggle to deal with heat stress. The victim's temperature is usually normal, but "technically" is always less than 41°C. Sweating is still intact and, more importantly, so is cerebral function. The victim is often dehydrated and complains of fatigue, nausea, weakness, vertigo, and occasionally muscle cramps. Salt and water deficits are usually mixed and in severe cases, checking the patient's electrolytes would be warranted. Treatment should focus on removing the victim from the heat, having him/her rest, and repleting his/her fluid deficit orally. Aggressive cooling methods (see below) should be instituted for anyone with temperatures of 40°C or more. Further heat stress should be avoided for at least 24 to 48 hours.

HEATSTROKE

Heatstroke is a true medical emergency.[3] Before aggressive treatment measures were used, the mortality from heatstroke exceeded 50%. The classic "triad" for a heatstroke diagnosis includes (1) temperature greater than 41°C, (2) central nervous system disturbance, and (3) cessation of sweating. Again, denying a patient aggressive treatment because he/she only has two of the three cardinal features can be a fatal mistake. Anyone with an elevated temperature and central nervous system changes mandates immediate therapy. Other causes of temperature elevation (infection, drug toxicity, thyroid storm) need also be considered. Markedly elevated hepatic transaminases are typical of heatstroke, however, other labs are rarely diagnostic.

Although the treatment is the same, there is some utility in defining two subcategories of heatstroke: "classic" heatstroke and "exertional" heatstroke. Classic heatstroke patients are typically elderly, chronically ill persons living in poorly ventilated housing. These patients have a more gradual onset of symptoms and have cessation of sweating 80% to 100% of the time. The more appropriate subcategory for the traveler is the patient with exertional heatstroke. This patient is usually young and healthy, exerts himself/herself in a hot environment, and suffers the relatively acute onset of delirium or coma. Prodromal symptoms may include weakness, dizziness, nausea, or vertigo (see heat exhaustion symptoms). It is important to note that sweating is still present in at least 50% of the cases of exertional heatstroke.

Heatstroke treatment focuses on patient stabilization, including airway control and IV access, and immediate cooling. Drawing on our understanding of the physics of heat transfer, one might predict that there are two principal methods for the rapid cooling of heatstroke patients.

1. *Ice Water Immersion.* Water transfers heat 25 times better than air. Immersing the victim in ice water has been shown to bring down core temperatures at a rate of 0.13°C to 0.16 °C/min. Another study showed equally good cooling rates using water at the more usable temperature of 15°C. This "cold" water was significantly easier for the health care team to work with than the "ice" water described above. Despite the excellent cooling rates, patient immersion carries some obvious disadvantages. Airway control and advanced life support activities are difficult to perform. Vomiting or diarrhea and the cold water itself can be a significant challenge to the health care team. An appropriate vessel is also not always available. There has also been debate that the cold water causes peripheral vasoconstriction and hence decreases heat transfer or, worse, can cause shivering, actually adding to the heat load. Clearly, if safe ice or cold water immersion is available to the heat stroke victim, it can be lifesaving; however, it is useful to know that another effective treatment modality is available if cold water is not.
2. *Evaporative Cooling.* Khogali and associates developed a "body cooling unit" in response to the need to treat numerous cases of heat illness during the annual

religious pilgrimage to Mecca.[4] The victim is suspended in a hammock-like net and sprayed with a mist of tepid water (warm enough to prevent cutaneous vasoconstriction). Warm air is then directed at the victim from all sides. This relatively available and user-friendly set-up has achieved reasonable cooling rates of 0.06°C to 0.31°C/min.

Ice water peritoneal lavage, gastric lavage, and rectal lavage have been used but offer no significant advantage. Cardiopulmonary bypass has been used in very selected cases. The traveler in the field should pursue aggressive evaporative cooling (see above), ice packs in the groin and axilla (near major vessels), and emergent transfer to a medical facility. Acetaminophen is ineffective and may worsen the likely already present hepatic damage. Alcohol sponge baths are never to be recommended because of the risk of alcohol toxicity.

COLD PHYSIOLOGY

The physics of heat transfer are the same regardless if one is in a hot or cold environment. The physiology, however, is different. Exposure to cold causes an initial increase in both heart and respiratory rate. Cold water immersion causes an initial gasp reflex followed by hyperventilation and a greater than 50% reduction in breath holding capability. Peripheral vasoconstriction is significant in an effort to reduce heat loss. With decreasing core temperature, heart and respiratory rate begin to fall. Below a core temperature of 32°C, one encounters many cardiac dysrhythmias. The PR and QRS intervals widen on ECG, and one may see a characteristic "J" or "Osborne" wave (a rounded "hump" immediately following the QRS, seen best in leads II and V6). At 25°C, ventricular fibrillation is common. Renal blood flow is also decreased; however, there is a commonly seen "cold diuresis," perhaps secondary to inhibition of antidiuretic hormone release or inhibition of renal tubular function. Cerebral function is also affected. Early symptoms include slurred speech, poor judgment, and ataxia. Stupor is usual at 32°C with coma following at 30°C.

Actual freezing of extremities is another hazard in temperatures below 0°C. Cutaneous sensation ceases at tissue temperatures of 10°C. It requires temperatures of below –4°C to actually freeze tissue due to the offsetting production of metabolic heat.

In contrast to the well-described ability to adapt to heat, there appears to be little, if any, physiologic ability to acclimatize to cold. It is clear that a hardy Eskimo "feels" the cold less than a more temperate colleague; however, the Eskimo will freeze just as fast as anyone else. "Adaptation" needs to be based on training, experience, and the avoidance of those behaviors known to increase the risk of cold illness.

COLD ILLNESS RISK

Situations that increase heat loss are a risk and are numerous. Cold water immersion, inadequate or damp clothing,

or wind exposure all are convective risks. Sunburn or alcohol use can cause increased peripheral blood flow to otherwise cool extremities. Alcohol is a much bigger risk as a modifier of common sense and good judgment. Decreased heat production is seen in the extremes of age (poor shivering), in various endocrinopathies (diabetes, hypothyroidism), and, arguably, in the very tired or very hungry.

COLD ILLNESS PREVENTION

As true adaptation is not an option, prevention depends on being smart. Physical fitness, adequate nutrition, and rest when appropriate only make sense. Wet clothing should be changed promptly. Dehydration is to be avoided. Heads and necks should be covered and tight-fitting clothing should be avoided. Alcohol causes peripheral vasodilatation and a misleading sensation of feeling "warm all over" as precious heat is radiated away. Tobacco causes vasoconstriction and an increased risk of extremity freezing (frostbite). Extremities should always be kept dry, mittens are better than gloves, and metal surfaces should never be touched with bare skin in extreme cold. Lastly, much of our perception of feeling warm or cold is based on peripheral temperature sensors rather than true core temperature. Warming the skin can give the perception that one is all "warmed up," even though core temperatures may still be low. Similarly, it is common for swimmers to feel subjectively colder standing wet in the breeze rather than in the water where the rate of heat loss is significantly greater. Take-away lessons: the "chilled" victim should not venture back out into the cold too soon, and if stuck in a survival situation in cold water, get physically out of the water as much as possible.

COLD ILLNESS

As is the case with heat illness, there are many shades of gray and overlap between the classically described diagnosis ascribed to cold exposure. Most victims of frostbite will simultaneously be victims of hypothermia and so on. The risks and preventive measures are much the same for all cold-related illness. Systemic cold illness is termed hypothermia. Peripheral or extremity cold illness can be further divided in freezing versus nonfreezing injury. Freezing injury is deemed frostbite. Nonfreezing injury has been called immersion foot or trench foot, if secondary to "wet" cold, or chilblains or pernio, if secondary to "dry" cold. Again, remember that there can be much overlap (and hence confusion) regarding extremity cold injury.

"IMMERSION FOOT"/TRENCH FOOT

Immersion foot is a nonfreezing injury secondary to exposure to "wet" cold. It is classically described in military situations where wet lower extremities are exposed, over hours to days, to temperatures of 0°C to 10°C. No ice crystals are formed, but neurovascular damage is sustained. Extremities are usually pale, swollen, and numb but may exhibit painful paresthesias and muscle cramping. Treatment should be much as described below for frostbite. Long-term sequelae are similar; however, overall prognosis is better than for frostbite injuries.

CHILBLAINS/PERNIO

Less severe than immersion foot, chilblains is a syndrome of erythema and tender blue plaques or nodules associated with burning paresthesias and intense pruritis after an exposure to "dry," nonfreezing cold. The skin lesions typically occur 12 to 14 hours after exposure. It is likely that chilblains and immersion foot share a common pathophysiology that includes sympathetic instability and some degree of microvascular injury. Treatment is supportive.

FROSTNIP

Even less severe is the diagnosis of "frostnip," which is very superficial and reversible ice crystal formation associated with intense vasoconstriction. No long-term tissue injury is described. Frostnip is perhaps best used as a barometer of being unprepared: those with any cold injury are clearly at risk for developing another.

FROSTBITE

Frostbite injury is secondary to true freezing as extremity temperature drops below 0°C. The "freezing injury cascade" has been described in four phases. The prefreeze stage occurs as tissue temperature drops to 5°C to 10°C. Sensation is abolished and blood vessels spasm and develop endothelial leak. Actual ice crystal formation occurs in the freeze-thaw stage as the skin temperature cools below −4°C. This is shortly followed by the vascular stasis phase, during which time it is believed that significant endothelial damage occurs. Ultimately, there is tissue death during the late ischemia phase. Note that the majority of injury is felt to be secondary to microvascular injury and subsequent ischemia rather than directly as a result of tissue ice crystal formation.

Initial frostbite symptoms include numbness and clumsiness. Victims complain that their extremities feel like a "piece of wood." Skin may appear yellowish white or mottled blue. The extremity will appear frozen regardless of the true depth of the frostbite injury. Early on, it is difficult to predict the actual extent of frostbite injury.

Perhaps the most important concept in the treatment of frostbite is that of not thawing and then refreezing the injured extremity. Refreezing will significantly worsen the existing microvascular injury. Do not attempt to thaw a frostbitten limb until you can ensure no further cold injury. It is preferable to walk on a frozen foot than risk the significantly worse outcome associated with refreezing. The frozen extremity should be splinted and wrapped loosely in dry dressings. Systemic hypothermia should be assumed and core temperatures should be elevated to at least 34°C before active frostbite treatment is begun.

Once in a safe environment, extremities should be thawed by rapid rewarming.[5] This is achieved by immersing the injured part in a circulating water bath at 40°C to 42°C. Higher temperatures may injure marginal tissues. Direct tissue massage should be avoided, but encourage active extremity movement. Rewarming takes 20 to 30 minutes and may be associated with significant pain. Parenteral narcotics may be indicated.

Blister treatment is controversial. In an effort to limit exposure to toxic arachidonic acid products, most authors will debride clear blisters and apply topical aloe vera (a thromboxane inhibitor). Hemorrhagic blisters should be left intact. Extremities should be dressed and elevated. Ibuprofen should be given to limit prostaglandin-induced injury and tetanus immunization status checked. Extremity edema progresses for 48 to 72 hours after rapid rewarming. It takes up to 90 days for final demarcation between viable and nonviable tissue to become evident. This has led to the surgical quip: "frostbite in January, amputation in July."

Many other therapies exist but are not well accepted or proven at this time. These include the use of peutoxifylline, low-molecular-weight dextran, heparin, intra-arterial reserpine, or sympathectomy. Hyperbaric oxygen therapy is also under renewed investigation. Similarly, several diagnostic adjuncts have been considered including angiography, triple-phase bone scan, magnetic resonance imaging, and magnetic resonance angiography.[6] None have consistently predicted degree of tissue involvement at the time of presentation.

Late sequelae to frostbite injury are common. In one series, 65% of military injuries had long-term residual symptoms.[7] Symptoms included, in decreasing order, excessive sweating, pain, coldness, numbness, abnormal skin color, and stiffness of the joints.

HYPOTHERMIA

It stands to reason that hypothermia accompanies most, if not all, of the above-mentioned cold injuries. It is also easily the most life threatening. Hypothermia is defined as a core temperature of less than 35°C (89.6°F).[8] Numerous different factors can contribute to the development of hypothermia including those that decrease heat production (endocrine disease, insufficient calories, or poor muscle mass), increase heat loss (cold water immersion, skin disorder including sunburn), or impair thermoregulation (drug abuse including alcohol, infection, and shock/trauma). The body has several defense mechanisms to combat core temperature drop. These include efforts at minimizing heat loss (peripheral vasoconstriction) and maximizing heat production (shivering). However, once core temperature drops below 31°C or 32 °C, shivering ceases, peripheral vasoconstriction is likely maximal, and the body becomes poikilothermic and will gradually cool to ambient temperature.

The victim of hypothermia will experience a predictable sequence of events as his/her core temperature drops. The severity of these events also helps grade the degree of hypothermia. "Mild" hypothermia is from 33°C to 35°C. Shivering thermogenesis is maximal, cold diuresis is evident, and ataxia and apathy may develop. Below 32°C, hypothermia should simply be considered "severe." Stupor is present at 32°C, coma at 30°C. Shivering ceases at 31°C, mandating the need for active rewarming as the victim is no longer able to effectively warm themselves. Atrial fibrillation is common at 32°C and the risk of ventricular fibrillation increases below 30°C. Note that defibrillation attempts rarely succeed below core temperatures of 30°C.

In the field, the mildly hypothermic victim should have wet clothing removed and be insulated to prevent further heat loss. Warm, sweet drinks may be given, but alcohol and caffeine (as well as tobacco) are to be discouraged. After transport to a warm, safe environment, the victim should be reminded that it takes many hours for the core temperature to fully correct: the sensation of being "warmed up" may be misleading.

Caring for the severely hypothermic victim is more demanding. Field management is usually complicated by environmental challenges to the would-be rescuers. Core temperature measurement is impractical, and it can be extremely difficult just to determine if the victim has any signs of life. Anticipate myocardial irritability and handle the victim *very gently*. Take at least a full minute to feel for pulses and "look, listen, and feel" for respiratory activity. If no signs of life are encountered, begin cardiopulmonary resuscitation (CPR). In order to allow time for ventricular filling, chest compression rates should be reduced (somewhere between half and normal rates) in proportion to the degree of hypothermia.[9] CPR should be begun even if it is anticipated that it will be interrupted (for extrication, evacuation, etc.). Intermittent flow may be adequate in the hypothermic state.

It is impossible to provide clinically significant "rewarming" in the field environment. Emphasis should be on gentle and timely evacuation and the *prevention of further heat loss*. Patients should be insulated against the four mechanisms of heat transfer. Most remember to minimize "evaporation" and "convection/radiation" by removing wet clothing and covering the victim with blankets, jackets, ensolite pads, or even newspaper. Many forget to consider true "conduction" by leaving the victim in contact with a cold surface. Insulate the victim completely! If available, heated, humidified oxygen and warmed IV fluids may be administered. Warm packs may also be placed in the axilla and groin. Be careful not to burn the patient.

True rewarming cannot be accomplished until the victim reaches a medical facility. In the emergency department, the core temperature should be measured to confirm hypothermia and a Doppler can be used to locate a pulse. A cardiac monitor should also be applied, using benzoin or even needle electrodes if necessary. Most severely hypothermic victims are also dehydrated. Warmed normal saline should be administered intravenously.

Warming modalities can be divided into those that are "passive" versus "active." Active rewarming is usually required for those victims with core temperatures below 32°C as their shivering mechanisms are extinguished and their normal metabolic heat production is significantly compromised. Active rewarming techniques can be further divided into those that are "external" versus "internal." Active external rewarming (AER) involves applying heat directly to the skin via heat lamps, hot water bottles, and heating blankets. Recently, excellent rewarming has been described using "forced air rewarming," where a

"hot air blanket" (Bain Hugger, Augustine Medical Inc., MN) is used to transfer heat to the patient. There are theoretical concerns that warming the extremities early will cause peripheral vasodilatation and shunting of cold, acidotic blood back to the core, thus causing core temperature "afterdrop" and perhaps precipitating cardiac arrhythmias. Thus, AER should be directed at the victim's trunk in the setting of mild hypothermia. In severe cases, truncal AER should be used in conjunction with more aggressive "internal" or core rewarming.

Active core rewarming (ACR) techniques range from being readily available and relatively noninvasive to the other extreme. ACR techniques to be used on all victims of hypothermia include the administration of warm (40°C to 45°C), humidified air, via endotracheal tube if necessary, and the use of warmed intravenous fluids. IV fluid bags may be heated in a microwave oven.[10] Gastrointestinal and bladder irrigation may also be used. A novel and noninvasive approach to improve access to cool core blood was recently described where hypothermic patients had a single forearm and hand wrapped in a specialized heating mitt and subjected to subatmospheric pressure, mechanically dilating hand vessels and significantly increasing heat transfer. More aggressive techniques include mediastinal irrigation, closed thoracic lavage, and peritoneal lavage. Cardiopulmonary bypass, perhaps the "gold standard" in ACR, can produce three to four times the heat transfer than the other ACR techniques.[11] Lastly, the use of microwave technology, or diathermy, has been reported both experimentally in the United States and clinically in the People's Republic of China.[12]

REFERENCES

1. Stewart CE. Preventing progression of heat injury. Emerg Med Rep 1987;8:16.
2. Gisolfi CV, Wenger CB. Temperature regulation during exercise, old concepts, new ideas. Exerc Sports Sci Rev 1984;12:339.
3. Costrini AM. Cardiovascular and metabolic manifestations of heatstroke and severe heat exhaustion. Am J Med 1979;66:296.
4. Khogali M, Weiner JS. Heat stroke, report on 18 cases. Lancet 1980;1:276.
5. McCauley RL. Frostbite injuries: a rational approach based on the pathophysiology. J Trauma 1983;23:143.
6. Mehta RC, Wilson RA. Frostbite injury, prediction of tissue viability with triple-phase bone scanning. Radiology 1989;170:511.
7. Taylor MS, Kulungowski MA, Hamelink JK. Frostbite injuries during winter maneuvers: a long-term disability. Mil Med 1989;154:411.
8. Danzl DF. Multicenter hypothermia survey. Ann Emerg Med 1987;16:1042.
9. Danzl DF. Blood flow during closed chest compression in hypothermic humans. J Wilderness Med 1991;7:12.
10. Werwath DL. Microwave ovens, a safe new method of warming crystalloids. Am Surg 984;50:656.
11. Deimi R, Hess W. Successful therapy of a cardiac arrest during accidental hypothermia using extracorporeal circulation. Anaesthesist 1992;41:93.
12. Zhong H, Qinyi S, Mingjlang S. Rewarming with microwave irradiation in severe cold injury syndrome. Chin Med J (Engl) 1980;93:19.

Chapter 16

DISEASES AND DISORDERS CAUSED BY THE SUN

DANIEL ANDRES DICESARE AND ADELAIDE A. HEBERT

INTRODUCTION

BENEFITS OF THE SUN

The sun has been a source of inspiration throughout the ages. Properties that make the sun invaluable for life on earth are obvious, such as light (visible radiation) and warmth (infrared radiation). With regard to human skin, ultraviolet radiation (UVR) from the sun has only one important physiologic role: the synthesis of vitamin D, vital for calcium homeostasis.[1,2] Only 10 to 15 minutes of natural sunlight two to three times a week is sufficient for adequate levels of vitamin D production.[1] In reviewing disorders caused by the sun, it is imperative that health care professionals have a basic understanding of the solar spectrum and how different environmental and individual skin characteristics influence sun exposure.

THE SOLAR SPECTRUM

The sun's radiation reaching the earth includes part of UVR 200 nm to 400 nm, visible light 400 nm to 760 nm, and infrared with wavelengths of 760 nm to 3,000 nm.

With regard to human health, the most damaging form of solar electromagnetic radiation is UVR. This portion of the solar spectrum can be further categorized according to the following wavelengths: UVA (320 to 400 nm), UVB (290 to 320), and UVC (200 to 290).[3] Although the intensity of erythema produced by UVR to human skin is variable, all ultraviolet wavelengths are capable of producing erythema.

UVB radiation from the sun is considered to be the most erythrogenic and carcinogenic since it delivers a high amount of energy to the superficial layers of the skin (stratum corneum and epidermis). UVB are the rays primarily responsible for suntanning, sunburning, and skin cancers.[1,4] UVB does not penetrate through glass and is most intense between the hours of 10:00 am and 4:00 pm.[5,6]

UVA delivers less energy to the skin than UVB and mainly produces a suntan rather than a sunburn.[4] However, UVA emitted by the sun remains fairly constant throughout the day, reaching the earth's surface at a rate of 10 to 100 times that of UVB.[1] The longer wavelengths of UVA penetrate more deeply into the skin, reaching the dermis and subcutaneous fat,[1,7] thus contributing to chronic skin injury. The role of UVA in photoaging and as a tumor promoter is now well established.[8]

UVC energy is mostly absorbed and filtered in the atmosphere and thus does not reach the earth's surface. UVC is used in germicidal lamps and mercury arc lamps.[4] Thus, UVC erythema results only from skin exposure to these artificial light sources.

ENVIRONMENTAL FACTORS

An important environmental factor, which offers a natural protection to human skin, is the atmospheric ozone layer. This atmospheric gas absorbs all of UVC, large amounts of UVB radiation, but little UVA radiation. The protective effect of ozone against UVB erythema (sunburn) is correlated to the time of sun exposure. At noon, the sun is approximately at a 90-degree angle to the earth's surface; thus, the sun's radiation passes through the least amount of ozone. In late afternoon (4:00 pm) or in early morning (10:00 am), when the angle of the sun is decreased in relation to the earth surface, solar radiation must pass through more ozone.[2,6] Protection of UVB from ozone is such that a fourfold increase in the time of sun exposure at 4:00 pm is needed to obtain an erythema similar to that obtained at noon.[2]

Altitude also influences exposure to UVR. At higher altitudes, there is a greater intensity of UVR, such that for every 1,000 feet above sea level, the UVR exposure increases by 4%.[1] Other environmental factors affecting UVR include pollutants, cloud cover, and snow. Cloud cover and pollutants mainly absorb infrared radiation (decreasing ambient temperature); however, they only scatter UVR and absorb little of it. Thus, on cloudy days, even though ambient temperature is cooler, large amounts of UVR still reach the earth, which can cause severe sunburn. Snow can reflect as much of 85% of UVB radiation.[2] This, coupled with high altitude, can lead to severe sunburn in snow skiers.

Other environmental factors such as wind, temperature, and humidity have been implicated in contributing to skin damage by UV radiation.[6]

INDIVIDUAL FACTORS

A patient's sensitivity to solar ultraviolet erythema is variable. This variability correlates with the patient's skin type (Table 16–1).

The importance of solar energy in human survival is undeniable; however, most evidence shows that sunlight

Table 16–1.   HUMAN SKIN TYPES

SKIN TYPE	REACTION TO SUNLIGHT	DESCRIPTION
I	Always burns, never tans	Pale, freckles, red or sandy hair
II	Always burns, tans minimally	Fair skin, blue eyes
III	Burns moderately, tans gradually	Dark-haired Caucasian
IV	Burns minimally, always tans	Olive skin, Mediterranean
V	Burns rarely, tans well	Indian, Latin American
VI	Never burns, dark pigmented tan	Very dark skin, Afro-Caribbean

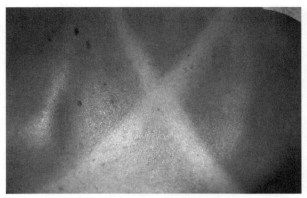

Figure 16–1.   Well-demarcated erythema on the back due to sunburn.

can cause acute and chronic skin disorders and/or aggravate many cutaneous disorders.[3,9–11] Prolonged and unprotected exposure to solar UV radiation can lead to sunburn, photoaging, and skin cancers and exacerbate photosensitive disorders. Proper use of protective clothing and sunscreens, behavior modification, and awareness of photosensitizing medications can prevent many of these short- and long-term damaging effects. This chapter will review the main diseases and disorders caused by the sun.

SUNBURN

Sunburn is an acute and transient cutaneous inflammation following exposure to UVR. Although some artificial sources of light emit UVR, sunlight remains the major source of all human UVR exposure.

ACUTE SUN INJURY

Since exaggerated sunburn response may be secondary to phototoxic drugs or systemic medical problems, a good medical history, a list of medications, and time of exposure to sunlight are imperative in evaluating patients presenting with sunburn.

Patients with acute sunburn usually present with tender, bright erythema on areas exposed to sunlight (Figure 16–1). Sunburn can also occur in areas covered with clothing, depending on the skin type of the patient, time of exposure, and type of clothing. In severe sunburn, patients may present with fever, weakness, and skin lesions that are edematous, painful, and blistering (Figure 16–2).

CHRONIC SUN INJURY

Repeated excessive exposure to sunlight over time can result in photoaging (dermatoheliosis) (Figure 16–3). Chronic sun exposure can cause coarse, wrinkled, and yellowish-colored skin. Photoaged skin can be irregularly pigmented, have telangiectasis, and be more prone to the development of tumors.

Specific disorders of chronic photodamage include:
Actinic/solar keratoses (AK). These are small (up to 1-cm diameter) rough-surfaced areas on sun-exposed areas of the skin (most commonly on dorsal area of the hands, face, and neck). AK have the potential of progressing to squamous cell carcinoma (SCC).

Actinic/solar elsatosis. The chronically sun-exposed skin in this condition is yellowish, thickened, and wrinkled.

Taking a few precautions can minimize much of the damage to the skin that occurs as a function of exposure to UVR. Preventive measures are the most effective, especially for people with skin types I and II. Sunscreens

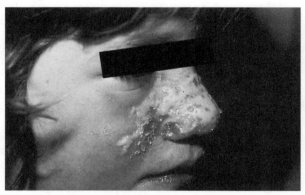

Figure 16–2.   Erythema, edema, and blister formation due to prolonged sun exposure in a fair-skinned child.

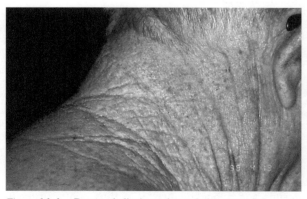

Figure 16–3.   Dermatoheliosis on the neck demonstrating waxy, yellow changes in the skin with wrinkling due to chronic sun exposure.

should be applied to all exposed areas, and photoprotective clothing should be worn. Physicians and pharmacists should provide patients with a list of medications with the potential of causing phototoxic reactions.

PHOTODRUG REACTIONS

Certain medications can make an individual more sensitive to the sun and can exacerbate the effects of UVR exposure. Physicians and health care providers should be aware of topical or systemic drugs that have the potential to cause photosensitivity. Drug-induced photosensitivity reactions are of two types: phototoxic and photoallergic.

Phototoxic drug reactions, more common than photoallergic reactions, are frequently referred to as an exaggerated sunburn. An acute phototoxic drug reaction usually presents hours after sunlight exposure and is characterized by erythema, with or without edema, and in severe reactions bullae and vesicles may be present. The reaction is limited to sun-exposed areas, such as the face, the "V" neck area of the chest (Figure 16–4), back of the neck, dorsal aspect of the hand, and anterior aspects of the legs. Chronic inflammatory skin changes such as scaling and lichenification may be seen after repeated exposure to sunlight with the phototoxic agent.[2]

Photoallergic drug reactions involve an immunologic response in which light causes a structural change in a drug or chemical so it acts as a hapten, which combines with proteins forming an antigen. Once the antigen is formed, specialized cells in the epidermis present the antigen to immunocompetent cells, leading to hypersensitivity.[12] Topically applied antimicrobials and fragrances are the most common cause of photoallergic drug reactions.[2] Acute photoallergic drug reactions are usually pruritic and eczematous, resembling allergic contact eczematous dermatitis. In chronic photoallergic drug reactions, the skin is scaly, pruritic, and lichenified, similar to the skin changes seen in chronic eczema (Figure 16–5). Distribution of the lesions is usually confined to sun-exposed areas; however, there might be spreading onto adjacent nonexposed skin. Thus, photoallergic reactions are not as well demarcated as phototoxic reactions.[13]

Table 16–2 provides a list of some of the most common drugs that can cause photosensitivity.

PHYTOPHOTODERMATITIS

Phytophotodermatitis (PPD) is a phototoxic reaction of the skin in which the photosensitizing chemical is contained in a plant, vegetable, or fruit. Psoralens contained in certain plants are the most common photoactive chemical causing PPD. Table 16–3 provides a list of common plants associated with PPD. Celery pickers, carrot processors, gardeners, people exposed to grassy meadows near beaches, and bartenders working with lemons or limes are at risk of developing PPD. In northern latitudes, PPD is seen mostly in the summertime; however, it is a year-round risk in tropical climates.

Clinical presentations usually resemble exaggerated sunburn on the areas of contact. Intense erythema and in severe cases even blistering can occur. Residual hyperpigmentation can result and may persist for months. The most common sites for PPD lesions are the arms, legs, and face. The lesions are usually scattered and limited to the areas of contact with the offending chemical (Figure 16–6). People using certain perfumes containing oil of bergamot (which contains 5-methoxypsoralen) may present with bizarre lesions such as erythematous or hyper-

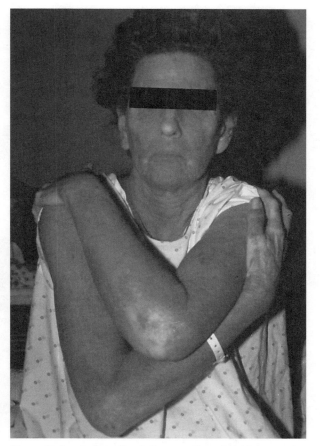

Figure 16–5. A photoallergic drug reaction mimicking extensive eczema.

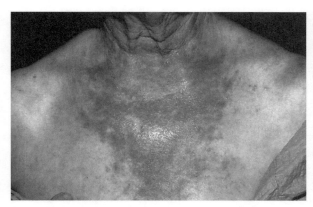

Figure 16–4. A phototoxic drug reaction with well-demarcated erythema and edema of the skin of the neck following sun exposure.

Table 16–2. SOME DRUGS AND CHEMICALS THAT CAN CAUSE PHOTOSENSITIVITY*

ANTIBIOTICS	NONSTEROIDAL ANTI-INFLAMMATORY DRUGS	ANTIHISTAMINES AND ANTITUSSIVES	CHEMOTHERAPEUTIC AGENTS
Ciprofloxacin	Benoxaprofen	Cyproheptadine	Decarbazine
Demeclocycline	Ibuprofen	Diphenhydramine	Fluorouracil
Doxycycline	Indomethacin	Promethazine	Methotrexate
Griseofulvin	Naproxen		Vinblastine
Minocycline	Piroxicam	**DIURETICS**	
Nalidixic acid	Sulindac		**FRAGRANCE CHEMICALS**
Norfloxacin		Chlorothiazide	
Ofloxacin	**CARDIOVASCULAR DRUGS**	Furosemide	Bergamot oil
Oxytetracycline		Hydrochlorothiazide	6-Methylcoumarin
Sulfonamides	Amiodarone		Musk ambrette
Tetracycline	Captopril	**ANTIPARASITIC DRUGS**	
Timethoprim	Nifedipine		
		Chloroquine	
		Quinine	
		Thiabendazole	

*Adapted from Drugs that cause photosensitivity. Med Lett Drugs Ther 1995;37:35–36.

pigmented whorls and streaks where the perfume was applied.

PPD is often a misdiagnosed condition that has been confused with cellulitis, lymphangitis, erythema mulitiforme, thrombocytopenic purpura, fungal infections, and even child abuse.[14–16] A careful history of exposure to certain plants and recognition of patterns on physical examination will aid in making the diagnosis.

Residual postinflammatory hyperpigmentation may persist for 2 to 3 months and usually resolves without intervention.

Prevention of PPD may be achieved by using sunscreens and educating patients about common plants (i.e., lemons, limes, etc.) that have been implicated in PPD.

Table 16–3. COMMON PLANTS ASSOCIATED WITH PHYTOPHOTODERMATITIS*

COMMON NAME	BOTANICAL NAME
Lemon	*Citrus limonum*
Lime	*Citrus acida*
Persian lime	*Citrus aurantifolia*
Bergamont	*Citrus bergamia*
Celery	*Apium graveolens*
Garden carrot	*Daucus sativa*
Wild carrot	*Daucas carota*
Parsley	*Petroselium sativum*
Parsnip	*Pastinaca sativa*
Fennel	*Foeniculum vulgare*
Dill	*Anethum graveolens*
Fig	*Ficus carica*
Buttercup	*Ranunculus spp*
Mustard	*Brassica spp*
Mustard	*Sinapis arevensis*

*Adapted from Anderson DN, Laude TA, Shalita AR. Phytophotodermatitis: an often misdiagnosed condition. J Clin Dermatol 1998;1(2):14–16.

MELASMA (CHLOASMA)

Melasma is an acquired hyperpigmentation of sun-exposed areas (mainly the face) and is exacerbated by sunlight. Melasma primarily affects women of child-bearing age and occasionally afflicts males (only 10% of cases are men).[13] The most common cause of melasma is pregnancy or the use of oral contraceptives. Lesions are usually symmetric light to dark brown macules and may occur in any sun-exposed area but typically involve the forehead, cheeks, and temple areas (Figure 16–7). The hyperpigmented lesions usually appear over a period of weeks after exposure to sunlight in the summer months.

POLYMORPHOUS LIGHT ERUPTION

Polymorphous light eruption (PMLE) is the most common of the idiopathic photosensitive disorders. This condition occurs in all races and skin colors but is more fre-

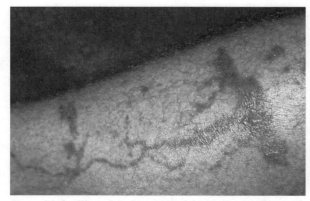

Figure 16–6. Phytophotodermatitis of the leg that developed following lemon juice dripping on the leg of a young woman at the beach.

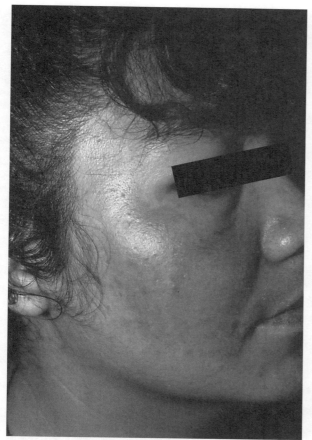

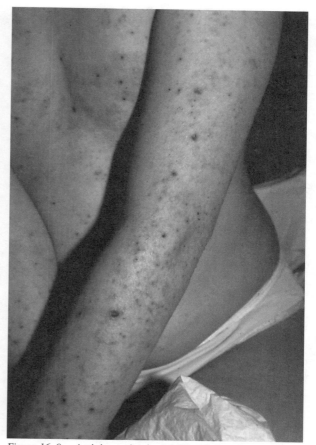

Figure 16–7.   Melasma of the face in a woman of child-bearing age.

Figure 16–9.   Actinic prurigo in a child with American-Indian heritage.

quently seen in skin types I, II, III, and IV (see Table 16–1). Females are affected more commonly, and the average age of onset is in the mid twenties. The various morphologic patterns of PMLE include small papulovesicles, eczematous lesions, large papules, edematous plaques, and erythematous macules. The most frequent morphologic presentations are the papular and papulovesicular eczematous eruptions[17] (Figure 16–8). Intense

itching is commonly present and may precede the onset of the eruption. Rubbing and scratching the eruptions may lead to lichenification.

PMLE is caused by sun exposure; thus, skin eruptions are usually limited to sun-exposed areas, such as the face, posterior neck, "V" pattern on the chest, and the limb extensor surfaces. Distribution of the lesions in PMLE is patchy and irregular and may involve areas covered by clothing. Typically, the skin eruption occurs within hours to 2 days after sun exposure and may resolve spontaneously in 1 to 2 weeks.

The diagnosis of PMLE is usually made from the clinical presentation, delayed onset of the eruption, and morphology of the lesions. However, it is important to rule out systemic lupus erythematous (SLE) in the differential diagnosis.

A hereditary type of PMLE, also known as actinic prurigo, occurs almost exclusively in American Indians (North and Central). In this group, the eruption usually appears in childhood.[13] Actinic prurigo is an autosomal dominant photodermatitis. The clinical presentation is that of both an acute and chronic, severely pruritic dermatitis (Figure 16–9). Chelitis of the lips may be the only presenting symptom in actinic prurigo.

Other rare idiopathic photosensitive disorders include chronic actinic dermatitis, which is a very severe

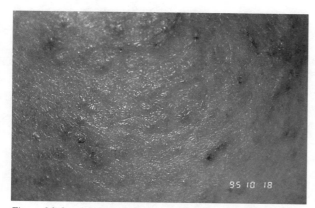

Figure 16–8.   A papulovesicular eruption of polymorphous light eruption on the neck and chest.

eczema occurring in elderly men in sun-exposed areas, and solar urticaria.[18]

SOLAR URTICARIA

Solar urticaria is a rare type of photosensitivity. Clinically, this condition is characterized by wheals, erythema, edema, and pruritus, which develop minutes after exposure to sunlight. The lesions usually disappear within 1 hour and resolve completely, without scarring. Some patients develop systemic symptoms such as nausea, anxiety, abdominal cramps, and headaches. Exposure to large surface areas can lead to a generalized urticaria and shock. Solar urticaria may persist for years but may resolve spontaneously.

The etiology of solar urticaria is unknown; however, some cases appear to be mediated by IgE (a type I immediate hypersensitivity reaction).

SYSTEMIC DISORDERS EXACERBATED BY THE SUN

Many diseases are photoaggravated by sunlight. This section will review only the more common disorders exacerbated by the sun, such as lupus erythematous (discoid LE and SLE), dermatomyositis, and herpes labialis. Table 16–4 provides a more extensive list of diseases exacerbated by the sun.

LUPUS ERYTHEMATOUS

LE may be divided for practical purposes into chronic cutaneous LE (also known as discoid lupus), subacute cutaneous LE, and SLE. Sunlight is also an important factor in some patients. The action spectrum of LE includes UVA and UVB. Ultraviolet light may precipitate both cutaneous and systemic symptoms of LE.[19]

Table 16–4. DISEASES EXACERBATED BY SUNLIGHT*

Acne vulgaris

Atopic dermatitis (eczema)

Bullous pemphigoid

Dermatomyositis

Erythema multiforme

Herpes simplex labialis

Lichen planus

Lupus erythematosus

Pemphigus vulgaris

Pellagra

Pseudoporphyria

Psoriasis

Rosacea

Seborrheic dermatitis

*Adapted from Harber LC, Brickers DR. Photosensitivity diseases: principles of diagnosis and treatment. 2nd Ed. Philadelphia: BC Decker, 1989:288.

Discoid LE (chronic cutaneous LE) is at one end of the LE disease spectrum; it is usually confined to the skin, and systemic involvement is not a feature. Female to male ratio is 2:1. Most of the patients have skin lesions on the head, scalp, face, and neck (Figure 16–10).

The differential diagnosis of discoid LE includes AK, plaque psoriasis, PMLE, lichen planus, tinea faciale, and SLE. Discoid lesions may be seen in up to 19% of patients with SLE.[20] Only 5% of discoid LE patients will develop SLE.[21]

At the other end of the spectrum, SLE affects not only the skin but, as its name implies, is a multisystem disease with the possibility of virtually all organ systems being affected. SLE has been associated with a number of immunologic abnormalities such as the production of autoantibodies, decreased levels of serum complement, and increased levels of circulating immune complexes. This disorder usually affects young adult females and is more common and more severe in blacks than in whites.

Dermatologic manifestations of SLE include a "butterfly" malar rash, discoid lesions, atrophic scarring, mucus membrane ulcers, periungual telangiectasia, alopecia, and photosensitivity. Abnormal skin reactions to sunlight must be considered mainly in SLE and in subacute cutaneous LE. Whereas sunlight aggravates only a few patients with discoid LE, approximately one-third of

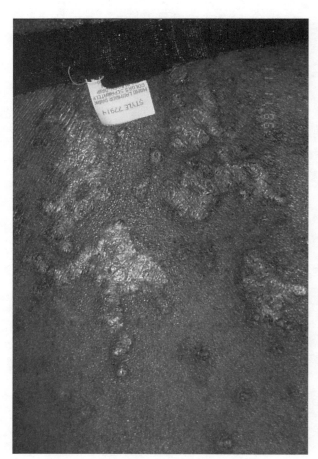

Figure 16–10. Lesions of discoid lupus erythematosus on the back.

patients with SLE have photosensitivity. Sunlight is a major environmental factor and is responsible for precipitating or aggravating SLE in about 30% to 50% of patients.

Between the ends of the spectrum of LE exists the subset of LE known as subacute cutaneaous LE. Patients with this type of LE have prominent photosensitivity with low incidence of renal or central nervous system involvement and only have mild systemic symptoms (i.e., joint pain, myalgias, fever, and malaise). Skin lesions of subacute cutaneous LE are usually widespread symmetric scaly annular reddish plaques on sun-exposed areas of the face, chest, back, and arms. The lesions resolve without scarring; however, residual hypopigmentation and telangiectasias may persist. Approximately 15% of patients with subacute cutaneous LE will develop SLE.[22]

Diagnosis of SLE and subacute LE is achieved by taking into consideration several criteria. The presenting clinical symptoms (American College of Rheumatology criteria), determination if visceral involvement, serologic studies (i.e., ANA, anti-dsDNA, anti-Sm, Anti-Ro/SSA antibodies), hematologic studies (leukopenia, thrombocytopenia, rheumatoid factor, etc.), and histopathology aid in the diagnosis.

DERMATOMYOSITIS

Dermatomyositis is a systemic autoimmune inflammatory disorder of the skin and skeletal muscle. This condition can occur at any age, most frequently presenting in the forties and fifties. Female to male ratio is 2:1. Patients with onset of dermatomyositis after the age of 50 have an increased risk of underlying malignant tumors such as gastrointestinal, lung, ovarian, uterine, and breast cancers.

Clinically, in a patient with dermatomyositis, skin involvement or muscle weakness may predominate. Patients may complain of symptoms of proximal muscle weakness (i.e., difficulty climbing stairs and raising arms over head) and/or of skin symptoms.

A cutaneous lesion characteristic of dermatomyositis is the erythematous streaky papules on the dorsal aspect of the hands known as Grotton's sign and Grotton's papules. Another hallmark lesion is known as "periorbital heliotrope." This is a flat reddish-purple erythema around the eyes usually associated with edema. Patients with dermatomyositis may also present with intense erythema on the forehead, malar area, "V" area of the chest, and neck. Patients with dermatomyositis may complain of intense itching, which can be disabling.

The cutaneous clinical symptoms of dermatomyositis can be precipitated or exacerbated by sunlight. The action spectrum includes both UVB and UVA. About half of patients with dermatomyositis experience photosensitivity.[23] The differential diagnosis in the early stages of cutaneous dermatomyositis should include contact dermatitis, atopic dermatitis, seborrheic dermatitis, and PMLE. In the later stages, the differential diagnosis includes SLE and drug reaction (i.e., hydroxyurea, penicillamine, etc.). Diagnosis is based on the presence of the characteristic skin lesions, proximal muscle weakness, and laboratory (i.e., elevated serum muscle enzymes) and magnetic resonance imaging findings.

HERPES SIMPLEX LABIALIS

Herpes labialis is a very common, self-limiting vesicular eruption on the lips and oral mucosa due to the infection with herpes simplex virus (HSV). There are two types of HSV. Type 1 usually affects facial and nongenital areas, and type 2 generally affects the genital area. The locations for each type are not absolute.

Herpes labialis is most commonly due to HSV type 1. Primary infection with HSV type 1 usually occurs in childhood and is often mild. Recurrent herpes lesions occur at the similar site of original inoculation. These recurrences are typically triggered by systemic stress (i.e., colds), local trauma, and sunlight.

Lesions of herpes infections are typically described as grouped vesicles with crusting on a 1- to 2-cm erythematous base (Figure 16–11). Lesions usually resolve within 2 weeks in immunocompetent patients.

Diagnosis can be made from clinical presentation and if necessary may be confirmed with a Tzanck smear of the fluid from a vesicle. Viral cultures may also be done to confirm diagnosis.

Sun protection may be achieved by the use of physical opaque sunblocks over the lips (i.e., zinc oxide).

SKIN CANCERS

SKIN CANCER FACTS

The incidence of skin cancers has been on the rise in most parts of the world for several decades.[12,13] Skin cancer is now the most common form of cancer in the United States. The three most common types of skin cancers are basal cell carcinoma (BCC), SCC (both classified as nonmelanoma skin cancers), and malignant melanoma. For the year 1999, the Centers for Disease Control estimates a combined 1 million new cases of BCC and SCC, and the American Cancer Society expects that about 44,200 new cases of malignant melanoma will be diagnosed. Estimates suggest that in 1999, a total of 9,200 deaths will occur secondary to skin cancers, 7,300 of these from malignant melanoma alone.[24,25]

Excessive exposure to UVR from the sun (including history of sunburns) is considered to be the most important risk factor in the development of skin cancers.

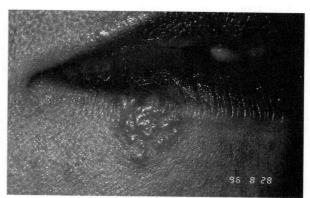

Figure 16–11.   Grouped vesicles on a red base in herpes labialis.

Approximately 90% of skin cancers occur on sun-exposed areas of the body.[2] Other risk factors for the development of skin tumors are listed on Table 16–5. A history of severe sunburn in childhood is an important risk factor in the development of malignant melanoma and BCC, whereas chronic exposure to the sun is a significant risk for SCC.

Most people receive more than 80% of their lifetime sunlight exposure by age 18 to 20, and the majority of sun-protective products are used by those greater than age 20.[1]

NONMELANOMA SKIN CANCERS

BCCs and SCCs (nonmelanoma skin cancers) occur predominantly among older patients of skin type I or II. Both of these skin cancers occur more frequently in males. Mortality rates are usually low if they are detected and treated early. However, these nonmelanoma skin cancers can lead to significant morbidity.

Basal Cell Carcinoma BCC is the most common type of skin cancer, typically occuring on sun-exposed areas (mainly face, neck, dorsum of the hands, and trunk) (Figure 16–12). BCC is a slow-growing tumor that rarely metastasizes. However, these tumors are locally invasive and if untreated may destroy underlying structures (i.e., cartilage, bone, and soft-tissue structures), causing disfigurement. Thus, BCC can invade deeply and cause serious problems in certain locations of the face such as around the eyes, nose, the inner canthus of the ear, and the temple.

Squamous Cell Carcinoma SCC is the second most common skin tumor in Caucasians. This is a malignant tumor derived from keratinocytes (skin and mucus membranes) and has the potential to metastasize. Chronic exposure to sunlight is by far the most common cause of SCC; thus, these tumors typically develop in sun-exposed areas (i.e., on the rim of the ear, the face, the lower lip, neck, forearms, and hands). SCC frequently develops from actinic (solar) keratosis (see chronic sun injury section for details on AK).

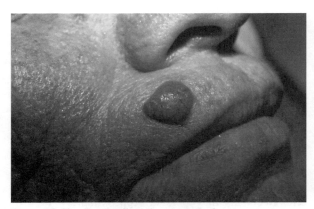

Figure 16–12. Basal cell carcinoma on the face.

Clinically, SCC may present as isolated or multiple lesions on sun-exposed areas. The lesion may appear as a red indurated nodule or scaly patch. Lesions are usually round or oval in shape and are often eroded, crusted, and ulcerated (Figure 16–13). SCC can develop into large masses and metastasize if left untreated. Thus, at time of presentation, patients should be examined for lymph node metastasis. If detected and treated early, SCC has a 95% cure rate.

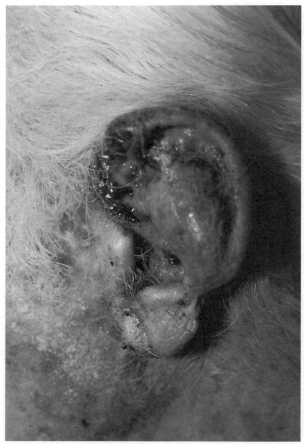

Figure 16–13. Ulcerated squamous cell carcinoma of the ear lobe.

Table 16–5. RISK FACTORS FOR SKIN CANCERS

RISK FACTORS FOR MELANOMA	RISK FACTORS FOR NON-MELANOMA SKIN CANCERS
Light skin color	Light skin color
Family history of melanoma	Family history of skin cancer
Personal history of melanoma	Personal history of skin cancer
Large number of moles	Chronic exposure to the sun (squamous cell carcinoma)
Presence of freckles	History of severe sunburns in childhood (basal cell carcinoma)
History of severe sunburns in childhood	

MALIGNANT MELANOMA

Melanoma is a tumor that originates from malignant transformation of melanocytes. The cutaneous lesions are characterized by irregularity in color, irregularity of the border of the lesion, and size of 6 mm or more (Figure 16–14). This form of cutaneous maligancy constitutes the most serious and lethal type of skin cancer. Although non-melanoma skin cancers occur more frequently, malignant melanoma is the most rapidly increasing form of cancer in the United States and is responsible for more than 75% of all skin cancer deaths.[24] The incidence rate of melanoma has increased about 4% per year from 5.7 per 100,000 in 1973 to 13.3 in 1995.[25]

The incidence of melanoma is about 10 times higher in Caucasians than in African Americans.[25] Many factors are involved in the development of malignant melanoma. (see Table 16–5). Of these, the role of sunlight exposure has been the most controversial. However, epidemiologic studies support the role of solar UVR exposure (in particular, severe sunburn in childhood) as a definite risk factor for malignant melanoma.[11,13,32]

SUN PROTECTION

TOPICAL SUNSCREENS

Sunscreens reduce the harmful effects of the sun by absorbing, reflecting, or scattering UVR, specifically UVB and/or UVA. Topical sunscreens are most commonly used and can be classified as chemical or physical.

Chemical Sunscreens   Most chemical sunscreens function by absorbing UVB (erythrogenic radiation), thus preventing sunburn while still allowing UVA to reach the skin and cause tanning. However, with increased awareness of the damaging effects of UVA radiation, broad spectrum chemical sunscreens have been developed to offer both UVB and UVA protection. Most chemical sunscreens are available in creams, lotions, or gels.

UVB Chemical Sunscreens. Chemical sunscreens that absorb only UVB include para-aminobenzoic acid (PABA) and its esters, salicylates and cinnamates.

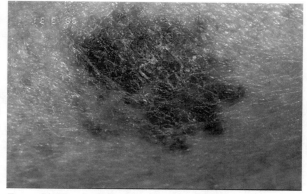

Figure 16–14.   A malignant melanoma of the upper back with irregularity in color and border.

For many years, PABA has been the primary active compound in chemical sunscreens.[7] PABA provides best protection in the UVB range of 260 to 313 nm and offers no UVA protection. PABA esters include padimate O and padimate A and offer UVB protection in the range of 290 to 315 nm. These PABA esters cause less contact dermatitis and do not stain clothing.[7,27] Pamidate A is the least allergenic of the PABA esters but can cause photo-contact dermatitis.[28]

Topical salicylates also only absorb UVB but are less likely than PABA to cause contact dermatitis. Another advantage of salicylates is that some can be easily added in cosmetic formulations.

The cinnamates also filter UVB, and although they cause fewer cases of dermatitis than PABA, they do cross-react with other chemicals, such as balsam of Peru.

UVA Chemical Sunscreens. UVA protection is easier to accomplish in the range of 320 to 340 than in the longer wavelengths of UVA (340 to 400 nm).[29]

UVA absorbers include the benzophenones (oxybenzone and dioxybenzone) and anthranilates. All of these offer weak UVB protection and thus must be used in combination with a UVB chemical sunscreen to provide adequate broad-spectrum photoprotection. The anthranilates absorb UVA in the range of 322 and 350. They are weak UVB absorbers and must also be used in combination with other UVB chemical sunscreens, such as cinnamates, to offer broad-spectrum protection from the sun.

Parsol 1789 (t-butyl methoxydibenzoylmethane), a newer UVA absorber, offers broad UVA protection in the range of 310 to 400 nm. Several new sunscreens combine Parsol 1789 or avobenzone with a good UVB-protective agent (i.e., pamidate O or one of the cinnamates) to provide excellent broad-spectrum sun protection.

Chemical sunscreens, for most individuals, provide adequate protection from the sun if used properly. However, chemical sunscreens do not offer total protection from sunlight. Patients that require total protection from solar UVR should avoid sun exposure and use physical sunscreen.

Physical Sunscreens   Physical sunscreens are thick pastes and creams that reflect, scatter, and form an opaque barrier to sunlight, thus blocking UVR and visible light (290 to 760) from the skin. Physical sunscreens include zinc oxide, titanium dioxide, kaolin talc, and magnesium silicate. The addition of coloring agents such as iron oxide (a visible light absorber) has been shown to greatly improve photoprotection and cosmetic appearance of physical sunblocks.[30]

Sunscreens should be used on a daily basis, even on cloudy or hazy days, for adequate photoprotection. Sunscreens should be applied 30 to 60 minutes prior to sunlight exposure. Care should be taken to apply sunscreen on all skin surfaces exposed to sunlight, including the tips of the ears, dorsum of hands, and feet. After swimming or intense sweating, reapplication of sunscreen is necessary to maintain protection from solar UVR. Habitual use of broad-spectrum sunscreens from an early age can prevent acute and chronic skin damage.

PHOTOPROTECTIVE CLOTHING

Topical sunscreens offer adequate photoprotection on sun-exposed areas; however, most people do not use sunscreens on nonexposed areas of their bodies when wearing clothing. The average cotton T-shirt only provides a sun protection factor (SPF) of 7, which is inadequate photoprotection.[31] Thus, clothing with adequate photoprotective properties should be worn when outdoors.

Photoprotective clothing provides a simple, practical, and medically safe means of significantly reducing UVR exposure and preventing skin damage. The photoprotective property of clothing depends mainly on the fabric content, weave, and color. Fabrics that are tightly woven are more effective in blocking sunlight than those with loose weave. Cotton fabrics tend to be more tightly woven and offer more protection against solar UVR than knitted polyester or nylon.[32]

White-colored fabrics of equal weave of colored fabrics allow more sunlight to penetrate and reach the skin surface. Thus, the presence of dyes increases photoprotection significantly. Clothing that is wet readily allows more transmission of UVR to reach the skin and offers less photoprotection. Thus, a wet white T-shirt an individual wears while swimming offers only minimal photoprotection.

Appropriate long-sleeved shirt, pants, 4-inch brim hats, sunglasses, and gloves can increase sun protection. Several companies (Solumbra by Sun Precautions, Tempe, Arizona, [800] 882-7860; www.Solumbra.com) manufacture lines of photoprotective clothing with SPF of greater than 30. This clothing is designed to provide complete and long-lasting protection from the sun without chemical additives. Photoprotective clothing is an underused important component of the overall strategy in sun protection.

CONCLUSIONS

The role of the sun in human survival is undeniable; however, solar UVR can cause a number of acute and chronic skin disorders and/or aggravate several photosensitive disorders among travelers. Knowledge of the solar spectrum and different diseases and disorders caused by the sun will aid health care providers in the proper history and work-up toward the proper diagnosis, prevention, and treatment.

Counseling travelers and patients in behavior modification and the proper use of sunscreens and outdoor clothing can prevent many of the short- and long-term damaging effects of the sun. Appropriate sun-protective measures should become a daily habit from an early age for all individuals. General health care providers should work closely with dermatologists to optimize prevention and treatment in photosensitive patients.

REFERENCES

1. Hebert AA. Photoprotection in children. Adv Dermatol 1993; 8:309–325.
2. Harber LC, Bickers DR. Photosensitivity diseases. Principles of diagnosis and treatment. 2nd Ed. Philadelphia: BC Decker, 1989.
3. Gasparro FP, Mitchnick M, Nash JF. A review of sunscreen safety and efficacy. Photochemi Photobiol 1998;68:243–256.
4. Pathak MA. Sunscreens: topical and systemic approaches for protection of human skin against harmful effects of solar radiation. J Am Acad Dermatol 1982;7:285–312.
5. Dobes WL. Public education: an approach. Skin cancer awareness project using the solar meter. J Am Acad Dermatol 1986;14:676–679.
6. Cavallo J, DeLeo VA. Sunburn. Dermatol Clin 1986;4:181–187.
7. Natow AJ. Sunscreens. Cutis 1986;38:157–158.
8. Matsui MS, DeLeo VA. Longwave ultraviolet radiation and promotion of skin cancer. Cancer Cells 1991;3:8–12.
9. Donawho C, Wolf P. Sunburn, Sunscreen and melanoma. Curr Opin Oncol 1996;8:159–166.
10. Marks R. An overview of skin cancers. Incidence and causation. Cancer 1995;75:607–612.
11. Katsambas A, Nicolaidov. Cutaneous malignant melanoma and sun exposure. Recent development and epidemiology. Arch Dermatol 1996;132:444–450.
12. Allen JE. Drug-induced photosensitivity. Clin Pharmacol 1993;12:580–586.
13. Fitzpatrick TB, Johnson RA, Polano MK, et al. Color atlas and synopsis of clinical dermatology. New York: McGraw-Hill, 1992.
14. Anderson DN, Laude TA, Shalita AR. Phytophotodermatitis. An often misdiagnosed condition. J Clin Dermatol 1998;1:14–16.
15. Barradell R, Addo A, McDonagh AJG, et al. Phytophotodermatitis mimicking child abuse. Eur J Pediatr 1993;291–292.
16. Goskowicz MO, Fredlander SF, Eichenfield LF. Phytophotodermatitis in San Diego County. Pediatrics 1993;31:828–830.
17. Epstein JH. Polymorphous light eruption. In: DeLeo VA, ed. Dermatologic clinics. Photosensitivity diseases. Vol. 4. Philadelphia: WB Saunders, 1986:243.
18. Murphy G. Photosensitive diseases. Ir Med J 1990;83:131–132.
19. Hymes SR, Jordan RJ, Arnett FC. Lupus erythematosus. In: DeLeo VA, ed. Dermatologic clinics. Photosensitivity diseases. Vol. 4. Philadelphia: WB Saunders, 1986:267–276.
20. Rothfield NF. Systemic lupus erythematous: clinical aspects and treatment. In: Macarthy DJ, ed. Arthritis and aligned conditions. Philadelphia: Lea & Febiger, 1985.
21. Gawkrodger DJ. Dermatology. An illustrated colour text. London: Churchill Livingstone, 1997.
22. Sontheimer RD. Lupus erythematous. In: Freedberg IM, eds. Fitzpatrick's dermatology in general medicine. Vol. 2. New York: McGraw-Hill, 1999:1993–2009.
23. Cheong WK, et al. Cutaneous photosensitivity in dermatomyositis. Br J Dermatol 1994;131:205–208.
24. Centers for Disease Control. Preventing skin cancer: the nation's most common cancer at a glance 1999. Available at: www.cdc.gov/nccdphp/dcpe/nscpep/skin.htm. U.S. Department of Health and Human Services, CDC, 1999.
25. American Cancer Society. Cancer facts and figures. Available at: www.cancer.org. 1999.
26. Wienstock MA. Controversies in the role of sunlight in the pathogenisis of cutaneous melanoma. Photoderm Photobiol 1996;63:406–410.
27. Taylor CR, Stern RS, Leydenm JJ, Gilchrest BA. Photoaging/photodamage and photoprotection. J Am Acad Dermatol 1990;22:1–15.
28. Camarasa JG, Serra-Baldrich E. Allergic contact dermatitis to sunscreens. Contact Dermatol 1986;15:253–254.

29. Roelandts R, Sohrabuand N, Garmyn M. Evaluating the UVA protection of sunscreens. J Am Acad Dermatol 1989;21:56–62.

30. Kaye ET, Levin JA, Blank IH, et al. Efficiency of opaque photoprotective agents in the visible light range. Arch Dermatol 1991;127:351–355.

31. Adam J. Sun-protective clothing. J Cutan Med Surg 1998;3: 50–53.

32. Welsh C, Diffey B. The protection against solar actinic radiation afforded by common clothing fabrics. Clin Exp Dermatol 1981;6:577–582.

Chapter 17

HOTEL SWIMMING POOL HYGIENE AND SAFETY

RODNEY Y. CARTWRIGHT

INTRODUCTION

Swimming pools are a major attraction in most holiday hotels. Many are no longer rectangular pools, shallow at one end and deep at the other, suitable more for competitive swimming rather than recreational activities. Interconnected pool complexes of different shapes and sizes with areas for water recreational activities, diving, or lounging at a waterside bar are now to be found. A children's pool separated from the main complex by a physical barrier is now an essential requirement. The pool acts as a magnet for children, especially at the very beginning of a holiday when they have little or no concept of potential hazards. Adults who do swim throughout the year will spend a considerable part of their holiday in or by the hotel pool. The swimming pool is a positive attraction yet at the same time can be a danger both from accidents and the transmission of infection. The hotelier needs to take appropriate action to reduce any risks.

Accident and illness statistics are difficult to obtain. Data collected by the U.K. Federation of Tour Operators representing the major operators in the U.K. indicate that pool-associated deaths account for nearly 10% of 300 accidental deaths in 64 million British package tourists between 1994 and 1998 inclusive. Individual factors vary but include unsupervised children, diving into shallow water, and alcohol-associated activities. Illness data are obtained primarily from outbreak reports depending largely on the surveillance systems in different countries. They will be considered under the specific infections below.

A safe pool requires both a good design and good management. It also requires common sense by the user—a factor frequently ignored and very difficult to influence. This chapter will consider some of the fundamental principles and various methods for ensuring microbiologic safety.

THE POOL

There is no such thing as a standard pool. Architects have designed pools as an integral attraction for a hotel. Pools are to be found in many different sizes and shapes and often in many different interconnected sections (Figure 17–1). They are, however, all basically a lined hole in the ground filled with water for recreational purposes. They may have features such as water flumes. The depth of a pool will vary according to the intended use, with most pools having varying depths. It is essential that the users are aware of the pool depth so that they can adjust their activities accordingly. Diving into shallow water is well recognized as a cause of spinal injury when the head strikes the bottom of the pool.[1,2] Conversely, a weak or nonswimmer will not wish to enter water that is deeper than can be safely managed.

Pool depth markings should be clear and unambiguous and given in feet and inches as well as the metric system. Frequently, they are painted on the edge of the pool and become worn and difficult to read, so regular inspection and repainting should be part of the standard planned preventive maintenance schedule. The use of different colors on the pool bottom can also be used to reinforce depth markings.

The pool surrounds should be of a non-slip material and there should be no unevenness or lips at the pool edge that may result in loss of balance or tripping by a pool user.

Bridges across pool areas should have appropriate fencing on each side to prevent children from falling in the water.

Children's areas or pools should be physically separated from adult areas. The water may be continuous with a main pool but a barrier should prevent young children from easily entering the main pool where they may be out of their depth. The children's pool should be clearly indicated.

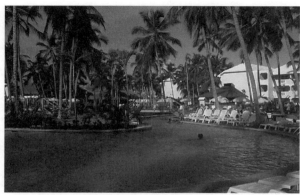

Figure 17–1. The pool as an integral attraction for a hotel. To view this figure in color, refer to CD-ROM.

The pool area should have clear signs in the appropriate languages indicating to guests the rules that should be followed to reduce any risks to pool users. These may include no running or horse play; ensuring children always have adult supervision; times when a lifeguard, if ever, is present; keeping glass away from the pool; not to use the pool if drinking alcohol or using medication that may impair judgment; using a shower before entering the pool; and diving only in designated areas.

A lifebelt should be clearly visible and easy to reach.

THE WATER

The water used in swimming pools may originate from a freshwater source or sea water from a nearby coastal inlet. Fresh water is the most common and is recirculated with appropriate filtration and disinfection with the aim of maintaining the microbiologic quality of the water at an acceptable level. It is essential that the quality of the water is maintained at all times when the pool is in use. This is ideally achieved by using a continuous, efficient automatic disinfectant dosing system. Periodic manual disinfectant dosing cannot be guaranteed to achieve consistent disinfection, especially when there are variable bather loads, yet this method is common in many hotels, even those with large pool complexes.

Pathogenic microbes can enter the pool in the source water but this is usually of minor consideration. The primary source of infecting organisms is the bathers themselves. Skin soilage will pass into the pool and children not infrequently have "an accident" in a pool. The residual disinfectant in the water should be able to inactivate such contaminants yet remain below the irritant level for pool users.

Chlorine is the most well-used disinfecting agent, although bromine-based compounds, chlorine dioxide, ozone, metallic ions (in particular, copper and silver), and polymeric biguanide have all been used. The system chosen must take into account the size, design, and use of the pool. The operation and maintenance of a chosen system are important. Hotels may be visited with state-of-the-art pool hygiene systems but no proper training for the staff and difficulties in obtaining appropriate chemicals and spare parts. The operation of a pool requires maintenance staff with an understanding of the processes they are managing. They must also understand the difficulties and potential dangers associated with the use of powerful disinfecting agents.

Initially, chlorine gas was used, but the danger associated with the use of the gas has led to replacement by sodium hypochlorite, solid calcium hypochlorite, and the chlorinated isocyanurates. They all result in the formation of hypochlorous acid and hypochlorite ions in the water. Both have disinfecting properties but the hypochlorous acid is stronger. Their formation is pH dependent, and the higher the pH level, the lower the level of hypochlorous acid. The optimal pH will vary with the disinfectant type but is usually in the range of 7.2 to 7.8. Lower pH values can be corrosive and irritating for swimmers' eyes. Bacteria and viruses are inactivated by chlorine but not *Cryp-tosporidium* oocysts, the removal of which requires efficient filtration. Chlorine will also react with ammonia present in pools from the decomposition of sweat and urine introduced by bathers. Continuous chlorination will usually ensure that the resulting chloramines are kept at acceptable levels, but complaints of eye irritation and chlorine odours should suggest that the process is not operating at an optimal level. This can be confirmed by measuring both the free and combined chlorine levels in the pool water. Regular water monitoring should be undertaken for all pools.

A not uncommon situation is the manual dosing of pool water once, or occasionally twice a day, with free chlorine measurements and sometime pH readings being taken shortly afterwards. Any question as to the chlorine profile during the day and with varying bather loads is usually met with a look of incomprehension, although an assurance is given that the pool is adequately disinfected and safe to use! In every pool treatment plant, there should be a written record of free chlorine levels and pH readings at least twice daily: one set of readings when the maximum chlorine level is expected and one set toward the end of maximum bather activity. For many hotels, this will mean 7 to 8 am and 3 to 4 pm with chlorine dosing early in the morning before the first set of readings. This assumes that there is no continuous dosing system with automatic chlorine level measurement. As a rule of thumb, free chlorine levels should be just above 1 mg/L (ppm) at all times.

Bromine using bromochlorodimethylhydatoin is used in some smaller pools, with hypobromous acid being the active disinfectant. As with chlorine-based disinfectants, bromine systems require careful control and monitoring.

The choice of the disinfectant depends on a number of factors including the properties of the raw water—in particular its hardness and alkalinity. The availability of the disinfecting agent is crucial and the ability of staff to operate the chosen system is fundamental. The Pool Water Guide of the U.K. Pool Water Treatment Advisory Group gives further information.[3]

Water filtration is part of all water treatment processes. The filters remove particulate matter including skin scales and hair. They maintain the clarity of the water, an important factor not only for aesthetic purposes but also for safety so that any bathers in difficulty under the water can be easily seen. Water turbidity is measured in nepholometric turbidity units, but, in practice, the ability to recognize the side of a coin lying at the bottom of the deep end in an undisturbed pool is an easy measurement. Filters for hotel pools should be sand filter and should be regularly backwashed with the backwash water going to waste. It is essential to maintain correct pressures and flow rates across filters and to check pressure differentials at intervals specified by the designers.

INFECTIONS ASSOCIATED WITH SWIMMING POOLS

This section summarizes the main infections that have been associated with hotel pools, which, in general, are preventable provided that the pool is maintained correctly.

The majority of infections will occur when disinfection levels are allowed to fall below the operating limits.

Superficial foot infections may well comprise the most common and least recognized swimming pool-associated infections. Bathers with athlete's foot (tinea pedis) or verrucae (plantar warts) can contaminate swimming pool surrounds and readily pass the infection to other bathers.[4–7]

Gastrointestinal infections may occur, but most reports are due to viral or parasitic causes with minimal bacterial outbreaks—a fact that probably reflects the general satisfactory level of disinfection. *Escherichia coli* O157 has, however, been associated with children's paddling pools and is a matter of particular concern because of the potentially serious nature of the infection.[8,9] Viral causes include echovirus,[10,11] enteroviruses,[12] and adenovirus. *Cryptosporidium* poses a more serious problem because of the resistance of oocysts to chlorine. There are now increasing numbers of well-documented outbreaks associated with swimming pool use.[13–17]

Swimmer's ear (otitis externa) is a well-recognized problem caused by wetting, dewaxing, and degreasing of the outer ear. This may result in an external ear infection, particularly with *Pseudomonas aeruginosa* from substandard pool water.[18]

Eye irritation and conjunctivitis are usually not of microbial origin but are due to chemical irritation and, in particular, excessive chloramine levels.

Diseases that cause particular concern and alarm are those due to HIV and hepatitis B virus. There is no published evidence that either of these viruses have been transmitted through swimming pool water. Both are susceptible to the principal disinfectants, apart from the dilution effect, and the recognized routes of spread being the sexual or parenteral route.

CONCLUSIONS

Safety and hygiene are essential elements for swimming pools, particularly those in hotels. Emphasis should be given to the proper maintenance of pools as this is essential to safeguard the health of guests. Infections can occur but rarely do, and when they do it is invariably due to a breakdown in the disinfection process. Hoteliers should be encouraged to maintain their pools at a demonstrable high standard, and this should be reinforced by inspectors from local public health departments. Further details on managing swimming pools can be found in an article by Dadswell[19] and the Pool Water Guide published by the U.K. Pool Water Treatment Advisory Group.[3]

REFERENCES

1. Blanksby BA, Wearne FK, Elliott BC, Blitvich JD. Aetiology and occurrence of diving injuries. A review of diving safety. Sports Med 1997;23:228–246.
2. DeVivo MJ, Sekar P. Prevention of spinal cord injuries that occur in swimming pools. Spinal Cord 1997;35:509–515.
3. Pool Water Treatment Advisory Group. Treatment and quality standards. London: PWTAG, 1999.
4. Bolanos B. Dermatophyte feet infection among students enrolled in swimming courses at a university pool. Bol Asoc Med P R 1991;83:181–184.
5. Attye A, Auger P, Joly J. Incidence of occult athlete's foot in swimmers. Eur J Epidemiol 1990;6:244–247.
6. Detandt M, Nolard N. Fungal contamination of the floors of swimming pools, particularly subtropical swimming paradises. Mycoses 1995;38:509–513.
7. Oren B, Wende SO. An outbreak of molluscum contagiosum in a kibbutz. Infection 1991;19:159–161.
8. Brewster DH, Brown MI, Robertson D, et al. An outbreak of *Escherichia coli* O157 associated with a children's paddling pool. Epidemiol Infect 1994;112:441–447.
9. Hildebrand JM, Maguire HC, Holliman RE, Kangesu E. An outbreak of *Escherichia coli* O157 infection linked to paddling pools. Commun Dis Rep CDR Rev 1996;6(2):R33–R36.
10. Papapetropoulou M, Vantarakis AC. Detection of adenovirus outbreak at a municipal swimming pool by nested PCR amplification. J Infect 1998;36:101–103.
11. Kee F, McElroy G, Stewart D, et al. A community outbreak of echovirus infection associated with an outdoor swimming pool. J Public Health Med 1994;16:145–148.
12. Lenaway DD, Brockmann R, Dolan GJ, Cruz-Uribe F. An outbreak of an enterovirus-like illness at a community wading pool: implications for public health inspection programs. Am J Public Health 1989;79:889–890.
13. Bell A, Guasparini R, Meeds D, et al. A swimming pool-associated outbreak of cryptosporidiosis in British Columbia. Can J Public Health 1993;84:334–337.
14. Joce RE, Bruce J, Kiely D, et al. An outbreak of cryptosporidiosis associated with a swimming pool. Epidemiol Infect 1991;107:497–508.
15. MacKenzie WR, Kazmierczak JJ, Davis JP. An outbreak of cryptosporidiosis associated with a resort swimming pool. Epidemiol Infect 1995;115:545–553.
16. McAnulty JM, Fleming DW, Gonzalez AH. A community-wide outbreak of cryptosporidiosis associated with swimming at a wave pool. JAMA 1994;272:1597–1600.
17. Sorvillo FJ, Fujioka K, Nahlen B, et al. Swimming-associated cryptosporidiosis. Am J Public Health 1992;82:742–744.
18. Seyfried PL, Fraser DJ. Pseudomonas aeruginosa in swimming pools related to the incidence of otitis externa infection. Health Lab Sci 1978;15:50–57.
19. Dadswell JV. Managing swimming, spa, and other pools to prevent infection. Commun Dis Rep CDR Rev 1996;6(2):R37–R40.

Chapter 18

THREATS OF SECURITY DURING INTERNATIONAL TRAVEL

PETER V. SAVAGE

For any traveler, concerns of health and security go hand in hand and should be included in preparations for foreign travel. On Copacabana Beach in Rio de Janeiro, a visitor unfamiliar with the environment is as much at risk for being mugged and robbed (and injured) as for being overexposed to the sun's rays.

Although it is not the duty of the travel medicine professional to know all of the security risks at their traveling client's destination, it is effective practice and good business to be aware of readily available security advisories that can reduce a client's exposure to security risks. Parents of an American student were most thankful to Maryland's Passport Health for including a State Department advisory on risks of road travel in Guatemala. The student did not go on a college-sponsored trip and was not on the bus carrying five fellow students who were raped by road bandits.

Other examples abound. Travelers may have had their hepatitis A and B vaccinations and their tetanus/diphtheria, and taken the proper malaria prophylaxis. However, if they land in the airport in Mexico City or Bogota, Columbia, take the wrong taxicab, and are held for ransom or robbed and left in their underclothes in a remote part of town, the shots will have availed them little. Since this security risk is well documented, a travel medicine professional can perform a service of real value—maybe even save someone's life—by making such information available to the traveler.

The purpose of this chapter is <u>not</u> to tell travel medicine professionals that they should become security specialists but to provide insight in the following ways:

1. Alert travelers to known security risks,
2. Show travelers how they can learn about risks ahead of time, and
3. Recommend means to plan for security risks and emergencies and deal with them.

There are four areas where travelers often fail to do their homework or plan for predictable problems on a trip, and where travel medicine professionals can offer constructive advice:

1. Travelers fail to gain advance intelligence about the health and security risks at their intended destination. In fact, they often fail to know what basic questions to ask about taxis, use of credit cards and teller machines, and street crime, to mention a few.
2. Travelers fail to put in one place, in an office or home file, basic documents that could be helpful if they have a crisis on their trip—if they are robbed or lose their passport, travelers' checks, or cash.
3. Travelers fail to develop a rudimentary plan or procedure if things go wrong during a trip. Is there insurance to cover a medical emergency requiring air evacuation? Who handles affairs at home if the traveler is incapacitated?
4. Travelers fail to consider what to carry on a trip that will enhance security, avoid problems, and, perhaps, make life more convenient and enjoyable such as a hideaway wallet for carrying a passport and money, a water filter for safe drinking water, and an inflatable pillow for comfortable sleep on an airplane.

In corporate security circles, these four elements, but especially the first (threat analysis) and the third (crisis management), form the basis of a crisis management plan (CMP). In the case of a "high-profile" traveler (e.g., Henry Kissinger or Oprah Winfrey), a team of professionals will have focused on every detail of the plan. As a travel medicine professional dealing with the traveler, your service is usually confined to the travel medicine and health part of the plan. In most cases, however, travelers coming for vaccinations and counseling at a travel clinic have not considered any of the elements of a plan in any systematic way, and your advice adds value to the service, perhaps even saving someone's life.

Recent changes have taken place in corporate approaches to comprehensive security planning for traveling executives. Organized and sometimes state-sponsored terrorism and movements of national liberation supported by the former Soviet Union resulted in corporate and free world government attention to and investment in comprehensive protective security measures. Kidnapping and assassination of corporate executives and government officials made corporate CMP mandatory and made protective security and kidnap and ransom insurance a priority. The disappearance of the Soviet Union, the change to a decentralized corporate management model, and the corporate emphasis on maintaining only profitable services have undone many of the CMPs designed to protect corporate travelers. Even corporate medical services and travel medicine are frequently outsourced. By reason of these changes, corporate travelers, as well as tourists, may arrive at a travel clinic with no notion of crisis management planning or the need for considering security and health risks inherent in foreign travel. These changes will generate new clients for travel clinics.

ADVANCE INTELLIGENCE

The example used in the following paragraphs is an American traveler, and the information resources are available through the U.S. State Department. In most cases, these resources are available for anyone calling from anywhere, and State Department travel advisories can be picked up on the Internet at http://travel.state.gov. Similarly, Centers for Disease Control (CDC) information is available at http://www.cdc.gov.

The responsibility of travel health professionals is to ensure that their traveling clients know that there may be security risks in addition to health risks and provide them, at the very least, with U.S. State Department travel advisories relating to their destination. This responsibility is not trivial or ancillary since there is a growing body of legal decisions affecting the professional. Both U.S. state and federal courts have held that travel agents and travel managers have a duty to provide the CDC and State Department advisories, which are readily available. Failure to honor this duty has resulted in liability when the client was not informed about the health risks of high-altitude travel in LaPaz, Bolivia, about prior incidents of street robberies in Jamaica, and about a series of highway robberies in Guatemala. Although there are no cases to date involving a travel clinic, there have been awards against corporations for incomplete advice given to corporate travelers resulting in the traveler contracting malaria. It is clear that the minimum requirement can be met by a travel clinic by subscribing to commercial reporting services, which regularly update CDC requirements and provide State Department travel advisories. State Department advisories are also available by telephone (202-647-5225), by fax (202-647-3000), or by Internet at http://travel.state.gov. Meeting these minimum requirements alone may not completely serve your traveling client.

It is not difficult for travel health professionals to inform their traveling clients—or distribute as a handout providing reliable information—about security conditions. Sources are free at the U.S. government and embassies, whereas private sources charge a fee for advisories. Both are outlined below.

Note that overseas embassies of most countries do provide information to their citizens about security conditions abroad, although they may not have a single officer designated to do this.

Following are instructions for a traveler to contact a regional security officer (RSO) at the U.S. embassy:

1. Telephone the State Department in Washington, DC (202-647-4000) and ask to be connected to the country desk covering the destination country.

2. Ask the country desk for the name and number of the RSO at the embassy.

3. Telephone the RSO during normal business hours in the destination country to ask questions about local security issues:

   - What cab to take from the airport.
   - Terrorist or street crime problems.
   - Local dress (especially for women).
   - Communication issues—telephone use and getting around town.
   - Use of credit cards and money machines, travelers' checks, credit cards, and foreign exchange.
   - Local food and water problems.
   - Recent incidents involving Americans or foreigners.

4. Information about the embassy RSO may be found on the Internet (ds.state.gov) under the heading "Key Officers of Foreign Posts." Some embassies have their own Web sites.

5. Technically, the RSO is responsible for U.S. citizens doing business abroad, whereas tourists are supposed to deal with the consular section. In this writer's experience, an RSO has never refused to supply security information to a caller from the U.S. or a local hotel.

6. In many cases where the traveler is not a U.S. citizen, the traveler is affiliated with an American corporation, religious institution, school, or faculty. The RSO's mission is to protect the security interests of American institutions and their employees. Non-American citizens on such missions can expect the same cooperation from the RSO as any American citizen.

If the U.S. embassy is closed or the RSO cannot be reached, a traveler might consider calling the American Chamber of Commerce affiliate in the destination country. The Chamber's telephone number in Washington, DC, is 202-463-5460 and the Web site is www.uschamber.org—international section for overseas affiliates. The overseas Chamber affiliate may be helpful or be able to refer the traveler to the local office of an American company. The travel medicine professional can provide his or her traveling client access to someone on location who can offer local security advice.

The American model for seeking advance information is not applicable for all travelers worldwide. Most embassies, however, have an officer—a minister counselor, consul, or attaché—who deals with embassy security or who maintains contact with local police so that their citizens can be protected if they are arrested or need help from the police. Swiss, Argentine, Lithuanian, German, Dutch, and Chinese embassies, for example, all have such staff in the U.S.A. Embassies are more likely to have such a service in countries where their visiting nationals or their personnel are at risk—the Turkish Embassy in France or Germany, for example.

The underlying idea is the same whenever a traveler from any nation is going to a destination that is unfamiliar and where the language is unknown to the traveler. A

THREATS OF SECURITY DURING INTERNATIONAL TRAVEL   135

Dutch traveler going to Brazil may seek out a Dutch Embassy officer, the representative of a Dutch shipping line, the KLM representative in Brazil, or a Dutch business executive who has offices in Brazil for advice on what problems he/she may face and should plan for.

Private security companies regularly supply subscribing multinational corporations and institutions with information about risks to their overseas personnel and assets. These companies use a combination of public and first-hand direct observation sources for reports. These reports, available for a fee, range from a summary of daily trouble spots to in-depth analysis of political, terrorist, and crime threats to foreign interests. When a travel medicine professional has a client who is planning a trip to a location in political or economic crisis, these security companies are a resource. Three of the companies in this field are listed below:

Air Security International
2925 Briarpark Drive, 7th Floor
Houston, TX 77042
Tel: +1-713-430-7300 or 800-503-5814
Fax: +1-713-430-7018
Web site: www.airsecurity.com (security program and/or world watch)

Parvus International/Armor Group
David G. Wiencek
1401 K Street NW, 10th Floor
Washington, DC 20005
Tel: +1-202-289-5600
Fax: +1-202-289-0210
E-mail: dwiencek@armorgroup.com
Web site: www.armorgroup.com

Control Risk Group
David Bittner
17499 Old Meadow Road, Suite 120
McLean, VA 22102
Tel: +1-703-893-0083
Fax: +1-703-893-8611
E-mail: davidbittner@control-risk.com
Web site: www.control-risk.com

TRAVELER'S OFFICE OR HOME DOCUMENTS FILE

A travel medicine professional can be of great assistance to a traveler by briefing him/her on or providing a printed list of documents to be kept at home or office during travels. These documents will be very important if a traveler has a mishap or becomes ill, injured, robbed, or imprisoned:

- A trip itinerary and schedule so that someone can find the traveler and note an unexpected absence.
- A photocopy of the traveler's airline ticket or, at least, telefax confirmation, so that a lost or stolen ticket can be replaced quickly or a reservation confirmed.
- A photocopy of the traveler's passport and visa papers.
- A record of the traveler's blood type and Rh factor.

- A list of any special health conditions or medical restrictions and drugs with generic names, telephone numbers of the traveler's doctor, and a copy of the health insurance ID card.
- An eyeglass prescription or spare set of glasses from which a new prescription could be derived and sent to the traveler.
- A photocopy of the traveler's International Certificate of Vaccination (yellow booklet) so that a doctor treating the traveler overseas can know the prior vaccinations if the original record is lost or stolen.
- A photocopy of traveler's checks—or a record of their numbers—and credit cards.
- A copy of your emergency medical assistance agreement (see Chapter 42.1 Medical Emergencies Abroad: Indications for and Logistics of Aeromedical Evacuation).
- If appropriate, a power of attorney over your affairs so that a spouse or designated person can provide assistance to the traveler during the trip by sending funds from your bank account or deal with the medical emergencies of an underage child.

If a traveler is going to a high-risk trouble spot—an oil worker going to Colombia or Yemen—this list might include a copy of a kidnapped ransom agreement, an emergency communications plan, and a list of people to contact in the company employing the traveler.

A PLAN WHEN THINGS GO WRONG

A travel medicine professional is not in a position to work through the possible personal and family needs of a traveler during a crisis of an unforeseen nature. It is important, however, that the traveler be aware of emergency medical assistance (see Chapter 42.1) so that an unexpected illness or injury can be managed by responsible medical personnel at a reasonable cost. It is also advisable for the traveler to plan in advance who is going to help from home if injured and in need of medical records or support. The travel clinic can assist a client by underscoring the importance of advance planning.

Some problems are predictable and solutions can be preplanned. A travel medicine specialist can aid in providing the necessary resources. For example, even in Europe, street crime (pickpockets, auto thieves) can be a threat, and single women can expect to be the target of unwanted attention. Several books dealing with these issues are:

The Art of Executive Protection, Robert L. Oatman, Noble House, Baltimore, MD (about $30). Available from R.L. Oatman and Associates. Tel: 410-494-1126; Fax: 410-494-1163. Although written for instruction to those protecting executives, Chapter 7 on international travel is helpful to all security-conscious travelers.
The Security Connection for Family Protection, Issy Boim, Air Security International, Houston, TX (about $30). Tel: 800-502-5814 or 713-430-7300; Fax: 713-430-7010.

The Safety Minute: 01, Robert L. Siciliano, Safety Zone Press, Boston, MA (about $15). Tel: 800-438-6223; Fax: 800-279-6393. P.O. Box 15145, Boston, MA 02215. Web site: www.safetyminute.com.

The Safe Travel Book, Peter Savage, Lexington Books (a bargain at $13.00). Tel: 800-462-6420; Fax: 800-338-4550. Also available at Passport Health: Toll Free 888-499-7277 and www.passporthealthusa.com.

ITEMS FOR TRAVELERS TO INCLUDE IN THEIR TRAVEL KITS

A travel medicine professional is well qualified to show a travel client what should be included in a first-aid kit. An outline of such needs is covered in Chapter 6 Pretravel Planning.

Practical items that can be essential for a traveler in distress include:

- A photocopy of your passport and two extra passport photos for ease of replacement at a U.S. embassy in case of loss or theft.
- An international driver's license—available for $5.00 at the American Automobile Association (AAA)—which serves as an identity document in place of a passport (except for crossing international borders).
- An International Certificate of Vaccination (yellow booklet), which shows the traveler's record of vaccinations with the correct international date sequence (day, month, year).
- A list of the traveler's medications, with generic names and dosages.
- A written description of any traveler's health problems translated into the languages of the countries to be visited.
- An extra set of eyeglasses (contact lenses).
- Automobile Rental Insurance Information: If you plan to rent a car abroad, learn in advance what insurance is required for that country and whether it can be covered by your credit card. Having to read or learn this in a foreign language at a hurried auto-rental counter is not advisable. Your AAA or auto insurance provider may help here. Also learn about the collision insurance waiver associated with your credit card if you want to avoid the sometimes very high prices charged by rental car services abroad. Some rentals will require a copy of the credit card's policy in writing. One good source is The Kremwel Holiday Autos (leasing agent in Europe for Renault and Peugot), Tel: 800-678-0678 or 914-835-5555, Fax: 914-835-5449.
- Proof of parentage/custody. A single parent escorting underage children may be required to show documen-

tation proving he/she is the parent of the child, a power of attorney from the other parent, or evidence of divorce or a death certificate of the other parent to verify legitimate custody of the child. These documents may have to be translated and certified by the embassy in the U.S. Women parents may be the subjects of closer scrutiny in Latin countries.

Again, the example used here is an American traveler. The practical items listed for a traveler in distress are also appropriate for a traveler of any nationality. For example, being a member of a national automobile club affiliated with the Alliance of International Tourism (based in Geneva, Switzerland) often entitles local club members to discounts with international affiliates anywhere.

There are several well-known travel supply catalogues to serve as guides to travelers and travel medicine professionals:

Medical and Security Items for Travel

Stuart Rose, MD's Travel Medicine, Inc. Free catalogue. 351 Pleasant Street, Suite 312, Northampton, MA 10160. Tel: 800-TRAV-MED; 413-584-0381; Web site: www.travmed.com.

Passport Health USA Catalogue of Travel Accessories. Toll Free tel: 888-499-PASS (7277); Web site: www.passporthealthusa.com.

Travel Catalogues

Magellan's Travel Supplies Catalogue. Tel: 800-962-4943; Fax: 800-962-4940; Web site: www.magellans.com.

Travel Smith, Outfitting Guide and Catalogue. Tel: 800-950-1600; Web site: www.travelsmith.com.

The reference books mentioned here under "A Plan When Things Go Wrong" also provide lists of items under categories of medicine, security, and convenience.

CONCLUSION

Unlike any provider of services, a travel medicine professional has an opportunity to enhance a traveler's awareness of health and security issues. In a certain sense, the traveler is seeking "bad news" when he/she comes to be vaccinated against disease. You have an opportunity to quantify the "bad news" and to educate your client about issues of health and security. Ignorance is the worst enemy of a safe trip, and your sensitivity to the full range of your client's needs translates into a safe trip and an appreciative client.

Chapter 19

EMERGING INFECTIOUS DISEASES AND TRAVEL

STEPHEN M. OSTROFF

One of the more notable features of the 20th century was the remarkable improvement in the health status of mankind. This improvement was especially notable in persons living in the developed countries of the world. In the United States, the average life expectancy in 1900 was 45 years. Today, life expectancy approaches 80 years, with comparable figures in most western European nations, Japan, Australia, and New Zealand.[1] A number of factors have contributed to the increased longevity. One of the most frequently cited has been the ability to treat and prevent serious infectious diseases. This has resulted from a combination of scientific and public health achievements, notably new technologies, including the recognition and development of antimicrobial agents, improvements in hygiene (especially in the areas of food, water, and waste management), and the delivery of effective and safe vaccines.[2] By the concerted application of these measures, smallpox was eradicated in the 1970s and poliomyelitis will soon meet a similar fate. Tuberculosis, the most common cause of death in the United States in 1900, was transformed into a highly treatable illness; today, only about 1,000 persons die from this disease each year in this country.[3]

Despite these impressive achievements, infectious diseases are far from vanquished. They remain well ahead of any other diagnosis as the developing world's most common cause of death (responsible for 35% of deaths), and even in developed countries, pathogens continue to produce substantial morbidity and mortality.[1] Some of the greatest infectious disease challenges ever to confront mankind occurred during the 20th century. One example is the 1918–1919 Spanish influenza epidemic, which is the largest recognized epidemic in human history, responsible for more than 20 million worldwide deaths.[4] The contemporary pandemic of HIV/AIDS, first recognized only 20 years ago, has resulted in more than 33 million infected persons and 14 million deaths.[5] On a global basis, AIDS is now the world's fourth leading cause of death, with the epidemic continuing to expand into new areas.[1] Although tuberculosis is no longer a major killer in developed countries, in the developing world there are still 1.5 million deaths annually.[1]

Emergence of infectious diseases also remains a significant concern. In the last 20 years alone, dozens of previously unrecognized infectious diseases have been recognized (Table 19–1), whereas others thought to be under control have become resurgent. Infectious agents have also been linked to chronic illnesses not previously believed to have an infectious etiology. Examples include the role of *Helicobacter pylori* in peptic ulcer disease and gastric carcinoma and the relationship between human papilloma virus and cervical cancer.[6,7] The recognition of new infectious diseases will certainly continue in the 21st century, since today, even when the best diagnostic technology is applied to common syndromes like pneumonia and diarrhea, the causative agent often cannot be identified.

In its landmark 1992 report, *Emerging Infections: Microbial Threats to Health in the United States,* the Institute of Medicine of the United States National Academy of Sciences identified several factors intimately linked to the emergence of infectious agents.[8] These include evolving human demographics (particularly population growth), human behavior, changing patterns of land use, technologic and industrial innovation, failure to effectively use proven public health interventions, and microbial adaptability. The Institute also recognized a strong linkage between global travel and commerce and disease emergence. This chapter explores the relationship between emerging diseases and travel.

RELATIONSHIP BETWEEN DISEASE EMERGENCE AND TRAVEL

There are several reasons that travel plays a significant role in the emergence of infectious diseases. Among the more important are the following:

- Individuals who travel may visit locations where they come in contact with microbes that are different from the ones at home. This happens when individuals travel from a developed region to a developing one and vice versa. There are more examples of the impact of travel from the developed to the developing countries than in the other direction.
- Travelers may serve as unwitting vectors transporting pathogens from one location to another, resulting in disease emergence, or recognition, far from its normal distribution.
- Travelers often tour in groups, meaning that many persons can be simultaneously exposed to an emerging

Table 19–1.   A SAMPLE OF EMERGING INFECTIOUS DISEASES IDENTIFIED SINCE 1975

YEAR	DISEASE OR PATHOGEN
1976	Legionnaires' disease Ebola hemorrhagic fever
1977	Cryptosporidiosis Hantaan virus (hantavirus)
1979	*Campylobacter* enteritis
1980	Human T lymphotropic virus I and II
1981	HIV/AIDS Toxic shock syndrome
1982	*Escherichia coli* O157:H7
1984	*Helicobacter pylori* Brazilian purpuric fever
1986	*Chlamydia pneumoniae* Ehrlichiosis Human herpesvirus 6 Cyclosporiasis
1989	Hepatitis C virus
1992	Cat scratch bacillus *Vibrio cholerae* O139
1993	Hantavirus pulmonary syndrome
1994	Human herpesvirus 8 (Kaposi's sarcoma virus) Hendra virus
1996	Pteropid bat virus (Australian lyssavirus) Variant Creutzfeldt-Jacob disease
1997	Avian influenza A (H5N1)
1999	Nipah virus Avian influenza A (H9N2)

pathogen with resultant outbreaks of disease. Such a situation can result in the first detection of a heretofore unrecognized problem.

• Some emerging diseases have a strong association with settings likely to be frequented by travelers (i.e., legionnaires' disease and hotels).

• Individuals often engage in activities that put them at higher risk of disease exposure during travel than they would routinely experience. Examples include risks associated with adventure and extreme travel, outdoor activities, food consumption, and sexual behavior.

• Mass population movements (i.e., refugee and humanitarian disasters) are unique travel situations that often are associated with disruption of public health services (vaccinations, safe water, inadequate waste disposal). Such circumstances are prime breeding grounds for infectious diseases, which can then rapidly spread.

Given these opportunities, it is little surprise that many prominent emerging infectious diseases have had important connections to travel. As the number of persons crossing international boundaries continues to rise, the role of travel in the spread of infectious diseases will probably grow in tandem.

EMERGING DISEASES ASSOCIATED WITH TRAVEL

LEGIONNAIRES' DISEASE

Legionnaires' disease is an example of an emerging infection that has had a strong relationship to travel. It was originally recognized in 1976 during an outbreak of illness at an American Legion convention in Philadelphia with 182 total cases and 29 fatalities. Illness was associated with persons visiting or staying at a specific hotel.[9] Since then, other outbreaks have been associated with hotels and tourist lodges, whirlpool spas on cruise ships, and other settings frequented by tourists[10–21] (Table 19–2). In addition, many sporadic cases of legionnaires' disease occur in persons who have been traveling during their incubation period. Surveillance data from England and Wales illustrate this relationship; among 226 legionnaires' disease cases reported in 1997, 50% were in persons who had traveled within the United Kingdom or abroad before the onset of illness.[22] It is unclear if the proportion of sporadic cases associated with travel is similar in other countries since the disease is not as thoroughly investigated there as in the United Kingdom.

There are several possible reasons why legionnaires' disease is so strongly linked to tourism. Disease occurs more frequently in older persons, particularly those with underlying pulmonary or cardiovascular disease. In developed countries, retirees have the time and resources to travel. They also often travel in groups, making clusters easier to spot. Some of the outbreaks in Table 19–2 occurred among retirees. Legionnaires' disease is considered an illness that has emerged due to 20th century technologic advances such as air conditioning and large-scale hot water supplies. Tourist destinations have many of the types of systems favored by *Legionella* sp, including cooling towers, whirlpool spas, and decorative fountains. Finally, within Europe, there is an organized system to investigate legionnaires' disease (the European Working Group on *Legionella* Infections) where the potential to spot outbreaks linked to travel is enhanced.

HUMAN IMMUNODEFICIENCY VIRUS

The origins and subsequent spread of the human immunodeficiency virus (HIV) are the subject of intensive scientific investigation and debate. Studies suggest that the virus originated in nonhuman primate species and then jumped species to humans in central Africa.[23,24] Spread from the initial foci occurred for many reasons, but among these, population movements and travel have played an important role. As one example, reports note that the virus spread along major trucking routes in Africa to towns and cities from the countryside.

Several foci with early high HIV/AIDS prevalence, such as the Caribbean and Thailand, have long been tourist destinations. Haiti was a major tourist destination in the 1970s, which may have facilitated movement of the virus from this location to North America. Studies have documented that by the early 1980s, Haiti already had a

Table 19–2.   A SAMPLE OF *LEGIONELLA* SP OUTBREAKS ASSOCIATED WITH TRAVEL/TOURISM

YEAR	LOCATION	SETTING/RISK FACTOR	NO. ILL	REFERENCE
1976	Philadelphia	Hotel convention/cooling tower(?)	182	9
1988	California	Hotel/decorative fountain	34	10
1986–1990	Ischia, Italy	Hotel/hot water supply	6	11
1987	Vermont	Tourist lodges/??	17	12
1992	Beijing	Hotel/water supply	5	13
1992	Orlando	Hotel/decorative fountain	5	14
1993	Spain	Hotel/water supply	5	15
1994	Atlantic	Cruise ship/whirlpool spa	50	16
1995	Sydney	Hotel/car park	28	17
1995	Turkey	Hotel/??	7	18
1997–1998	Spain	Hotel/??	3	19
1998	France	Multiple/??	6	20
1999	Amsterdam	Flower show/whirlpool spa	228	21

high prevalence of HIV infection.[25] Thailand may reflect a circumstance where tourists introduced the infection from other parts of the world. During the 1980s, when the country had little HIV infection, Thailand was a popular destination for "sex tourism." Infected tourists may have introduced the virus to Thai commercial sex workers as a result of this practice.[26] Now the country has among the highest number of HIV infections in Asia, although recent aggressive prevention campaigns appear to be having an effect.[27] In other locations such as Japan and the Middle East, early cases of HIV infections often occurred among persons who had been abroad to locations already affected by AIDS.

INFLUENZA

It remains unclear how influenza viruses move from one location to another. Hypotheses have involved spread via animal species (particularly birds) and movement due to environmental factors. However, there is growing evidence that travelers play an important role in the global spread of influenza.[28] In 1997, influenza A (H3N2/Sydney-like) was first recognized in North America among tourists on an autumn cruise in the Canadian maritime provinces and coastal New England.[29] This influenza A subtype quickly established itself in North America and became the predominant cause of influenza illness during the 1997–1998 season. In the summer of 1998 and again in 1999, influenza-like illness was recognized among tourists who were members of land-sea tours of Alaska and the Canadian Yukon.[30,31] In 1998, more than 2,199 cases of acute respiratory infection were recognized, with 71 cases of radiologically confirmed pneumonia and two deaths.[30] The median age of persons with pneumonia was 72 years, reflecting the high-risk elderly populations who participate in these cruises. In 1999, at least 428 illnesses were detected.[31] During both years, illness spread to crew members of the cruise ships, facilitating ongoing transmission from one cruise to the next. In many cases, illness was not noted until travelers had returned home, suggest-

ing that these persons could serve as vectors for influenza virus movement to many other locations. Since more than 70,000 persons participate in these tours each summer from around the world, the impact could be substantial.[30] Of note, summer influenza in Alaskan cruises had previously been reported during the 1980s.[32] During 1999, an outbreak of influenza was also noted on a Mediterranean cruise, suggesting that this phenomenon is not confined to North America.[33]

Influenza outbreaks have also been identified in other tourist and travel settings. In 1997, an outbreak of influenza A (H3N2) was reported among 81 adolescents who stayed in a crowded ski hostel in Austria; two students were hospitalized with pneumonia and one died.[34] A 1983 epidemic of influenza on the remote Pacific island of Niue was determined to have occurred when two travelers returning from New Zealand introduced the virus to the island.[35] In a 1993 survey, influenza-like illness was among the most common complaints in persons returning to Alaska from travel to the Russian Far East.[36]

Mobile military populations are another group of travelers who have been linked to the spread of influenza. Their role in the spread of the 1918–1919 Spanish influenza pandemic during World War I has been hypothesized.[37] In the 1980s, an outbreak of influenza at the Naval Air Station in Key West, Florida, was linked to an air squadron that had traveled to Puerto Rico.[38] In recognition of this phenomenon, the U.S. Air Force routinely monitors its globally distributed personnel for influenza viruses.[39] This system has demonstrated through the use of molecular techniques the movement of influenza virus subtypes from base to base.

Two human outbreaks of avian influenza have recently been recognized. Although neither has been travel associated, they are important to travelers' health because both occurred in Hong Kong, which is a major travel hub in Asia. The first outbreak occurred in 1997 and was due to influenza A (H5N1), a subtype not previously recognized to cause human illness.[40,41] A total of 18 human cases were recognized with 6 (33%) fatalities;

most illnesses were in children and young adults.[42] Human illness occurred coincident with circulation of the same virus in chickens, which developed fatal encephalitis when infected.[43] The outbreak was terminated in late 1997 with the slaughter of more than 1 million chickens in Hong Kong. No additional human cases of influenza A (H5N1) have been subsequently identified, and epidemiologic studies suggested that the virus was not spread from person to person.[44] Because of concerns that travelers could spread the virus to other locations with a resultant global pandemic, enhanced surveillance for avian influenza was established in other parts of Asia and North America with direct and indirect travel links to Hong Kong. Special advisories for travelers to Hong Kong were also issued.

In 1999, a second outbreak of avian influenza was identified in Hong Kong. This outbreak involved two children who were infected with influenza A (H9N2), a subtype also not previously associated with human illness.[45] Studies have suggested that internal genes of this virus are similar to those from the influenza A (H5N1) strain that produced disease in 1997.[46] The influenza A (H9N2) strain also circulated in poultry in Hong Kong and mainland China but did not produce fatal illness similar to the 1997 outbreak.

MALARIA

Malaria is among the leading global causes of infectious disease mortality, resulting in an estimated 1.1 million deaths in 1998.[1] The majority of these deaths occur in children under 5 years of age in Africa. Malaria has increased in both frequency and geographic range.[47–49] At the same time, drug-resistant forms of falciparum and vivax malaria have become significant problems. These factors have combined to make malaria one of the most problematic of all emerging infectious diseases.[50]

Malaria is also among the most common of the serious emerging infections associated with travel. During the period 1990–1995, in the United States a mean of 1,085 persons (range 910 to 1,275) was diagnosed with malaria per year.[51] These cases are almost evenly split between Americans who acquired malaria while visiting a malaria-endemic region (mean 530 persons per year) and foreigners from endemic areas who developed malaria while in the United States (mean 451 persons per year). Many of the remaining cases occurred in U.S. military personnel deployed overseas; similar problems occur among the military of other developed countries when they are deployed.[52] Vivax malaria accounted for 48% of cases diagnosed in the United States, whereas falciparum malaria accounted for 39%. The major source locations for U.S. malaria cases reported in 1995 is shown in Table 19–3. Many of these locations are not major tourist destinations. The reported illnesses are believed to occur among persons from these countries while visiting the United States and among immigrants from these countries who visit their home country and do not perceive a need to use preventive therapy.

Other developed countries also have high rates of malaria, particularly France, Germany, Italy, and the

Table 19–3. MAJOR SOURCE LOCATIONS FOR IMPORTED MALARIA AND PERCENTAGE OF CASES IN THE UNITED STATES, 1995[51]

VIVAX MALARIA (%)		FALCIPARUM MALARIA (%)	
India	39	Nigeria	35
Honduras	15	Ghana	13
Pakistan	7	Africa, unspecified	7
Central America, unspecified	6	Africa, western	4
Guatemala	3	Haiti	3

United Kingdom.[53] In these countries, the relative proportion of vivax to falciparum disease varies based on tourism and immigration patterns. However, falciparum malaria has been an increasing problem, with reported case-fatality rates as high as 3.6%.[53]

Although almost all cases of malaria recognized in nonendemic countries are linked to travel or residence in endemic parts of the world, autochthonous (locally acquired) cases do occur. These are cases reported in persons with no history of travel to endemic areas who have no other risk factors for malaria acquisition (i.e., blood transfusion). In the United States, since 1990 locally acquired vivax malaria has been reported in the states of California, Florida, Georgia, Michigan, New Jersey, New York, and Texas, whereas locally acquired falciparum malaria has been reported in New York and Virginia.[51,54–56] Autochthonous malaria has also been recognized in Europe.[57–59] The small number of recognized cases probably underestimates the frequency of indigenous transmission, since a diagnosis of malaria is less likely to be considered in persons without a relevant travel history. Even among travelers, malaria is both underdiagnosed and not reported to public health authorities. A survey of hospitals and laboratories in Michigan after the recognition of a locally acquired case showed that only 20% of other cases had been reported to the health department.[60] Although surveys in other areas have shown better reporting to health authorities, this suggests that thousands of malaria cases may occur annually in the United States.

There are several possible explanations for cases of indigenous malaria. One possibility is that while they are traveling, infected persons from endemic areas are bitten and then introduce the parasite into the local mosquito populations. The local mosquitoes become carriers and then transmit the organism to persons residing in the nonendemic area. In the United States, a number of the indigenous vivax malaria cases have occurred in rural areas when large numbers of migrant agricultural laborers from endemic regions were present. This scenario was thought to be the cause of an outbreak of malaria in southern California in 1986.[61] An alternative explanation is that carrier mosquitoes or their larvae travel by ship or plane with international cargo and then produce illness around international transit hubs. This phenomenon has been referred to as "airport malaria."[57–59] Since many currently nonendemic zones have had past problems with malaria, concerns have been expressed that continued introduction of malaria parasites could allow the disease to re-establish a foothold. This is of particular concern due to global warming and the potential for expanded ranges for host vector-mosquitoes during an era of de-emphasized vector control programs.

OTHER VECTOR-BORNE DISEASES

In addition to malaria, other emerging vector-borne diseases are of particular concern to travel medicine. These include dengue fever, yellow fever, and the viral encephalitides.

Over the last decade, the incidence and geographic extent of dengue fever has risen sharply.[62,63] Almost 100 million cases of dengue fever are estimated to occur annually. The World Health Organization (WHO) estimates that this infection was responsible for 140,000 deaths in 1997, making it among the top 10 worldwide causes of infectious disease mortality.[64] Global population movements have resulted in the cocirculation of all four dengue subtypes within many geographic areas. The repeated human infections that result are thought to be a risk factor for development of dengue hemorrhagic fever.[65] This complication of dengue infection has also risen sharply in recent years, particularly in the Americas.[62] Besides global population movement, other reasons for the rise in dengue fever include increasing urbanization in the tropical zones of the world and possibly climate change.[66,67] Urban sprawl is an important factor for dengue virus because the *Aedes* mosquito vectors thrive in an urban environment.

Dengue fever epidemics have swept a number of popular tourist destinations in Asia, the Pacific, the Caribbean, and South America. Among the locations affected in recent years are Singapore,[68] French Polynesia,[69] Cuba,[70] Puerto Rico,[71] and Rio de Janeiro.[72] Although the impact has been greatest among local populations in these places, tourists from developed countries have also been affected.[73-79] Dengue fever is estimated to occur in 1 of every 1,000 tourists who travel to an endemic area.[62] The sources for imported dengue among travelers vary by home country. Among Israeli, German, Norwegian, and British travelers, most acquired illness in Southeast Asia.[73,75-77] The largest proportion of tourists from southern France acquired illness in the French West Indies or French Guyana.[78] In the United States, between 1987 and 1993, an average of 20 laboratory-confirmed imported dengue fever cases were reported annually.[80] In recent years, this number has been higher, possibly due to increased dengue activity in the Caribbean and Central America; in 1995, there were 86 confirmed cases identified.[80] In 1996, a total of 43 cases were detected, with the largest proportion of confirmed cases linked to the Caribbean.[80]

Point source dengue outbreaks among travelers have also been recognized. In 1996, a group of United States tourists to the British Virgin Islands developed dengue fever when they returned home to Pennsylvania and Maryland[81] and a similar outbreak occurred among Canadian tourists to Barbardos in 1997–1998.[82] In 1995 and 1999, dengue outbreaks in Mexico spilled over into the Rio Grande valley of Texas, with resulting autochthonous transmission.[83] Dengue also poses significant risks to aid workers,[84] soldiers,[85,86] and others who spend extended periods in dengue-prone areas. Prevention of dengue fever in tourists is currently limited to measures that avoid mosquito exposure. Dengue vaccines are under evaluation but are unlikely to be available for several years.[87]

Yellow fever is another re-emerging vector-borne infection.[88] Significant increases in the incidence of yellow fever have occurred in South America and Africa,[88,89] despite the availability of an effective vaccine. Vaccination of travelers to affected areas has limited the risk of yellow fever among tourists, but recent fatal cases in Europe and North America among unvaccinated travelers suggest that renewed efforts are needed to ensure that travelers receive appropriate preventive measures. In 1997, a Tennessee resident became the first U.S. citizen diagnosed with yellow fever since the 1920s after vacationing in the Amazon basin.[90] In the same year, yellow fever was diagnosed in a traveler to Brazil after returning to France.[91] In 1999, fatal cases of yellow fever were diagnosed in a German traveler to Cote D'Ivoire and an American who acquired illness in Venezuela (unpublished data).

In 1999, two notable outbreaks of viral encephalitis were reported. In late 1998, an increased number of encephalitis cases was recognized in Malaysia. The outbreak was concentrated in rural areas with extensive pig farming and was initially reported as Japanese encephalitis. However, studies eventually identified a previously unrecognized paramyxovirus, which is now called Nipah virus.[92,93] This virus is related to Hendra virus, which was recognized in 1994 after an outbreak of pulmonary hemorrhage in thoroughbred horses and horse trainers in Australia.[94] In Malaysia, a total of 282 human cases of encephalitis were identified, with 77% of cases laboratory confirmed. A small number of cases was also reported from Singapore in slaughterhouse workers. There were a total of 108 deaths, producing a case-fatality rate of 38%. Indistinguishable viruses were isolated from humans and pigs, and epidemiologic findings suggested direct transmission to humans due to close contact rather than aerosol spread. There were no cases in tourists or other travelers, although the outbreak did have a significant impact on the tourist industry. Studies are under way to define the reservoir for Nipah virus. The related Hendra virus has been reported to have a natural reservoir in migratory fruit bats (*Pteropus* species).[94]

In 1999, the first recognized outbreak of West Nile encephalitis in the Western Hemisphere occurred in the New York City metropolitan area.[95-97] Previously, members of this virus family had been seen only in Europe, Asia, and Australia. A total of 62 cases of encephalitis with seven fatalities occurred. One of the fatal infections was in a 75-year-old man who had traveled from Toronto to New York City during his incubation period.[97] He became ill after returning to Canada and is the only travel-associated case. It is unclear how the virus migrated from its natural range to North America. Introduction through a traveler who was incubating the illness is one hypothesis, since high-titer viremia does occur with West Nile prior to the onset of symptoms. Since New York is a major international travel hub, this outbreak reinforces the fact that such locations are vulnerable to the introduction of nonendemic pathogens.

EMERGING DISEASES AND OUTDOOR ACTIVITIES

Certain emerging zoonotic and vector-borne diseases are linked to outdoor activities and thus pose a special risk for travelers. While on holiday, many travelers spend more time outdoors than when they are at home. This is especially true with adventure travelers.

One such disease is hantavirus pulmonary syndrome, which in 1993 was first recognized in the Americas when a cluster of cases occurred in the Four Corners region of the southwestern United States.[98] This illness is characterized by a nonspecific prodrome followed by the abrupt onset of fulminate pulmonary edema requiring intensive life support.[98] In some individuals, up to one liter of fluid has been removed from the respiratory tract per hour, leading to severe hemodynamic instability. Although the usual incubation period is 1 to 2 weeks, it can be as long as 6 weeks after exposure.

Through mid-1999, a total of 217 cases of hantavirus pulmonary syndrome have been diagnosed in 30 states.[99] Among these cases, 59% are male, and the median age is 37 years. The youngest person diagnosed with hantavirus pulmonary syndrome was a 10 year old, and the oldest case was in a 69 year old. Illness has also been reported from Canada[100] and from Argentina, Brazil, Chile, Paraguay, Peru, and Uruguay in South America.[101–6] At least nine hantaviruses associated with human disease

have been identified in North and South America since 1993; all are associated with high mortality[107] (Figure 19–1). The mortality rate for hantavirus pulmonary syndrome in the United States is 43%.

Human hantavirus infection occurs on exposure to persistently infected rodents that excrete the virus in urine, saliva, and feces. Human infection occurs via inhalation of these aerosolized excreta, although there is evidence for person-to-person transmission of the South American hantaviruses.[105,108,109] Rodents associated with hantavirus in the Americas generally inhabit rural areas. Persons engaged in outdoor rural activities, either because of their occupation or for leisure, have been disproportionately affected.[110–112] The occupational link is thought to partially explain the male preponderance seen in North America.[100]

Hantavirus pulmonary syndrome has been reported in association with outdoor recreational activities, such as camping and hiking.[113–115] Use of rural cabins, especially those that have been unoccupied for an extended period, appears to represent an especially high risk.[116,117] Rural outdoor activities have also been associated with Puumala hantavirus infection in northern Europe, where the disease is transmitted by the bank vole, which lives along stream beds and other areas frequented by outdoor enthusiasts.[118] Studies have shown that the risk for hantavirus infection is linked to a combination of prevalence of carriage in rodents and the density of the rodent population;[99,119] the latter fluctuates with environmental conditions.[120]

Hantavirus pulmonary syndrome outbreaks have occurred in popular tourist areas. In the United States, the initial outbreak occurred in the Four Corners area of the southwest and produced a major disruption in tourist activities. Other cases have occurred in the Sierra Nevada

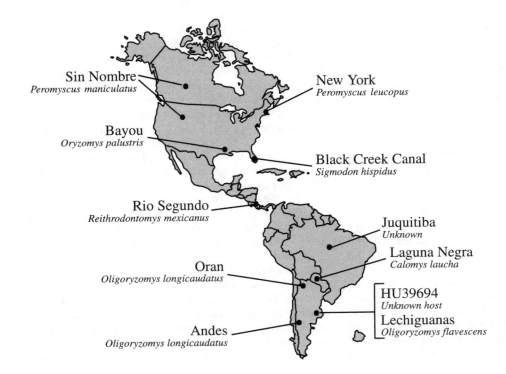

Figure 19–1. Hantavirus as associated with human disease identified in North and South America.

range of California. In Argentina, the first recognized cases were in El Bolson, an area adjacent to Andean ski resorts, and a case in Chile occurred in a traveler to Bolivia.[103] Since there is no vaccine or specific therapy for hantavirus infection, persons engaged in outdoor activities in hantavirus-endemic areas should be aware of appropriate measures to reduce their risk of exposure.[99,121]

Lyme disease and ehrlichiosis are two emerging tickborne infections that are also associated with outdoor activity. Lyme disease was first reported among Connecticut children in 1977[122] but has since been recognized to have a global distribution in temperate zones of the northern hemisphere.[123] The causative agents are *Borrelia* species that are transmitted by *Ixodes* species ticks. In the United States, the number of recognized cases of Lyme disease continues to increase. During 1992–1998, a total of 88,967 cases of Lyme disease were reported to public health authorities, with the annual number rising from 9,896 cases in 1992 to 16,802 cases in 1998 (Centers for Disease Control [CDC], unpublished data). Studies indicate that cases reported to public health authorities underestimate the incidence of disease by seven- to 12-fold,[124] suggesting that at least 100,000 cases occur in the United States annually. Disease is highly focused in the coastal northeastern states and the upper midwestern United States, where more than 90% of infections occur. It is unclear whether the increases are related to improved surveillance and reporting or represent increasing exposure and infection.[125] The geographic range of human illness has not changed significantly, but increasing case counts are seen in most reporting areas. It has been suggested that the increases may reflect changing demographic patterns with increased numbers of persons living in suburban and rural areas at higher risk for exposure.[126,127] Other studies find that the number of vector ticks has increased in areas of high disease prevalence.[128]

Major risk factors for Lyme disease include peridomestic activities such as gardening and clearing of underbrush in persons who live in rural areas.[125] However, hikers and campers are also at increased risk.[129] Thousands of cases of Lyme disease are diagnosed annually in the United States in persons who do not live in areas considered to be Lyme endemic (CDC, unpublished data). Whereas some of these cases are locally acquired in areas of low endemicity, others are related to travel to high-risk areas in the coastal northeast or upper Midwest during the warmer times of the year. The Advisory Committee on Immunization Practices recommends that persons who travel to such areas during the spring and summer transmission season and engage in outdoor activities consider vaccination against Lyme disease using the newly available outer surface protein A (Osp-A) vaccine.[130]

Human ehrlichiosis was first recognized in 1986 in a 51-year-old resident of Michigan who acquired his infection while traveling in Arkansas.[131] The causative organism was named *Ehrlichia chaffeensis* after Fort Chaffee, Arkansas, where the exposure occurred. Since 1986, several forms of ehrlichiosis have been identified. *E. chaffeensis* causes human monocytic ehrlichiosis, which mainly occurs in the southeastern United States.[132] In the

early 1990s, a second form of ehrlichiosis was described in the upper midwestern United States[133]; this form is called human granulocytic ehrlichiosis and the causative agent is similar to *E. phagocytophila*. In 1999, a third human form of ehrlichiosis was described in Missouri linked to infection with *E. ewingii*.[134] All three forms of disease are characterized by an undifferentiated flu-like illness with fever, chills, malaise, headache, nausea, and vomiting.[126,132,135] Leukopenia and thrombocytopenia are commonly seen laboratory abnormalities. Complications include shock, renal failure, and disseminated intravascular coagulation, and mortality rates up to 5% have been reported. The mortality rate appears to be higher for the granulocytic form of the disease than the monocytic form.[126] However, the nonspecific nature of ehrlichiosis suggests that many cases are not diagnosed, especially the milder forms of illness.[136]

Like Lyme disease, ehrlichiosis occurs mostly among persons in rural locations, the majority of whom report a tick exposure during the summer months.[137] In one study, 66% of patients resided in rural areas, with another 26% living in suburban areas.[137] A total of 75% of cases occurred in males, with a median age of 44 years. This age distribution is much higher than for Lyme disease, which is most common in children. In one outbreak of ehrlichiosis in Tennessee, golfing activities represented the major risk factor, and illness was more common in persons who were less skilled at the game as evidenced by higher scores.[138] The study found that chasing the ball into the rough was an independent risk factor for illness. Ehrlichiosis has also been seen in military personnel during outdoor training exercises.[139,140]

The tick vector for *E. chaffeensis* and *E. ewingii* is *Amblyomma americanum* (the Lone Star tick), whereas the human granulocytic ehrlichia agent is transmitted by *Ixodes* species. It is not uncommon to find *Ixodes* ticks that are co-infected with *Ehrlichia* sp and *Borrelia burdorferi*, and human co-infections appear to be common.[141–143] The geographic distribution of human granulocytic ehrlichiosis follows that of Lyme disease, and ehrlichiosis is increasingly recognized throughout Europe in areas with Lyme disease.[142–146] A case of ehrlichiosis has been diagnosed in a traveler to Mali,[147] and disease has been seen in Thailand.[148] Ehrlichiosis is readily treated with tetracycline derivatives, but there is no vaccine. Measures to reduce tick exposure are essential for persons who will travel to endemic areas.

VIRAL HEMORRHAGIC FEVERS

Marburg and Ebola viruses are the only two known members of the filovirus family. Both produce fulminant viral hemorrhagic fever with high mortality, and both have recently re-emerged in Africa. Although most disease occurs in rural zones of Africa, travel-associated illness has been reported for both viruses.

Marburg virus was first identified in 1967 when an outbreak occurred among persons who were harvesting kidneys from nonquarantined African green monkeys imported to Marburg, Germany, from Uganda.[149–151] Some of the materials from these monkeys were forwarded to Yugoslavia, where additional cases occurred. A total of 31 cases with 23% mortality were reported.

After this outbreak, only three additional episodes of Marburg hemorrhagic fever were identified involving six cases (three fatal). Travel played a prominent role in these cases. In 1975, an Australian student traveling through Africa was diagnosed with Marburg infection in South Africa.[152,153] He was thought to have acquired illness while touring Zimbabwe, where he had slept outdoors and in a house infested with bats. His traveling companion and a nurse in South Africa became secondarily infected. A 1980 case occurred in a French engineer who had traveled near Kitum cave in western Kenya, which was also the site of a later case in 1987.[151,154,155] One of the physicians caring for the 1980 case also became ill and died of Marburg infection. In 1991, a suspected Marburg case occurred in a Swedish student who traveled to Kenya to visit his parents and engaged in numerous outdoor activities while in Africa.[156] This represented the last suspected Marburg case until 1999, when an outbreak involving at least 70 persons (with almost 90% mortality) occurred among illegal gold miners in northeastern Democratic Republic of Congo.[157] In this outbreak, at least one case was retrospectively diagnosed in an individual with a compatible illness in 1994, and there is anecdotal evidence of repeated epidemics in the area over a period of years. Although extensive efforts to identify a natural reservoir associated with these cases have been conducted, to date these efforts have been unsuccessful.[151]

Ebola virus was first recognized in 1976 when large outbreaks occurred in Sudan and Zaire.[158,159] The Sudanese outbreak involved 284 (53% case fatality) and the Zaire outbreak involved 318 cases (79% case fatality). In 1979, a smaller outbreak involving 34 cases (65% case fatality) occurred in the same Sudanese village as the 1976 outbreak.[160] These outbreaks were characterized by person-to-person transmission through direct contact with body fluids, were focused in hospital settings, and involved extensive transmission among health care workers. Ebola virus was quiescent until the 1990s, but in recent years outbreaks and sporadic cases of illness have occurred in Cote D'Ivoire, Gabon, and Zaire (Democratic Republic of Congo), and a travel-associated case has been identified in South Africa.[161–163] The largest episode was in Kikwit, Zaire, and involved 315 cases (81% case-fatality rate).[163]

The case in Cote D'Ivoire occurred in a 34-year-old ethologist involved in long-term studies of chimpanzees in the Tai National Forest.[161] After performing a necropsy on one of the deceased chimpanzees, which was subsequently confirmed to be infected with Ebola virus,[164] the researcher became ill 8 days later and was evacuated to Switzerland, where she survived her illness. The South African cases involved a Gabonese physician who had been caring for persons with viral hemorrhagic fever in Libreville in 1996.[162] When he became ill in late October 1996, he traveled to Johannesburg for treatment, but the diagnosis of Ebola was not suspected by his caregivers. It was only diagnosed retrospectively when a nurse involved

in his care became ill and died from Ebola hemorrhagic fever 1 month later. Although this case illustrates the potential for spread of Ebola through infected travelers, no such cases have occurred in Europe or North America. However, in 1986, a case of Lassa fever (an arenavirus that causes hemorrhagic fever) was identified in an individual who had traveled to Nigeria to attend a funeral and did not become ill until he returned to his home in Chicago.[165] In that incident, there was no secondary transmission in the Chicago hospital.

More recently, three fatal cases of Lassa fever have been imported to Europe.[166,167] One involved a 23-year-old female traveling in Ghana, Burkina Faso, and Cote D'Ivoire in December 1999. All three of these countries have not previously been identified as Lassa endemic. Even though ill, she returned to Germany via Portugal and was transferred between hospitals before the cause of illness was determined. The second case involved a male British foreign aid worker in Sierra Leone, who returned to England in February 2000 upon becoming ill. The third case involved a Nigerian who worked for a multinational corporation and was thought to be ill with meningitis in March 2000. When he did not improve, he was transferred to Germany for further care and was diagnosed with Lassa fever. Investigation of all three cases demonstrated no secondary transmission to passengers of air flights or health care workers in European hospitals.

VACCINE-PREVENTABLE DISEASES

International travel has been an important aspect of two vaccine-preventable diseases, measles and diphtheria, which have re-emerged during the 1990s. Measles incidence worldwide has declined over the past decade, but this disease remains an important global cause of mortality and morbidity.[1] This disease has been targeted for global eradication, and the countries of the Western Hemisphere have been actively engaged in elimination efforts.[168] Significant declines in measles have occurred throughout the hemisphere. In the United States, only 100 measles cases were identified in 1998.[169] Of these 100 cases, 26 were internationally imported, and 45 others were importation associated. The remaining 29 could not be classified as imported cases, but studies of viruses from these cases suggest that they were linked to unrecognized international importation. The largest sources of importation were Asia (50%), followed by Africa (25%) and Europe (15%). In contrast, Europe was the largest source for imported cases to the United States during 1994–1997.[169] In a study of 16,000 adults diagnosed with measles in the United States between 1985 and 1995, a total of 289 (1.8%) were associated with international travel.[170] Studies of measles case sources for all imported cases between 1991 and 1994 showed the largest numbers of cases imported from Mexico (31% of cases), followed by Japan (5%) and Germany (5%).[171] However, based on travel patterns, the rate of measles importation per million travelers was highest for individuals from the Philippines (8.4 importations per million travelers), followed by India (6.6 cases per million travelers) and the former Soviet

Union (6.6 cases per million travelers). Because of the large number of travelers from Japan and Germany, the rates were lower (1.9 and 1.6 per million travelers, respectively).[171]

In 1996, only 2,109 measles cases were identified in the entire Western Hemisphere, and 29 of the 47 countries in the region reported no measles.[172] However, in 1997, a resurgence of the disease occurred, with over 27,000 cases reported.[172,173] Of these cases, 95% occurred in urban areas of Brazil, with a focus among young adult males who had migrated from rural areas of the country in search of work. Genomic sequencing of viruses from Brazil suggested that the outbreaks were related to importation of measles from western Europe. Most of the remaining cases were linked to an outbreak in western Canada, where studies also suggested that the virus was imported from Europe.[172] As large numbers of measles cases continue to occur in some developed and many developing countries, the risk for importation due to international travel will remain high even in countries with a strong control program.

Diphtheria is a disease that has been largely controlled in most developed countries. In the United States, a total of 41 cases were reported between 1980 and 1995, for an average incidence of < 3 cases per year.[174] Of cases with known importation status, 27% were known to result from importation, and all culture-confirmed cases after 1988 were known to have been imported. In the early 1990s, a large outbreak of diphtheria began in areas of the former Soviet Union.[175,176] By 1995, a total of 47,808 cases were reported in the former Soviet Union. At least 20 cases of diphtheria were also reported among travelers to or from this area to other parts of Europe.[175] These included two Americans who became ill in Russia but were treated in western Europe,[177] although none of the cases identified within the United States could be linked to the Russian epidemic. Multiple surveys have demonstrated low levels of diphtheria immunity in populations of western Europe and North America,[174,178] highlighting the need for booster immunization against diseases like diphtheria in persons who are traveling to high-risk areas.

MISCELLANEOUS EMERGING INFECTIONS

Cyclosporiasis   Human infections with *Cyclospora cayatenensis* were first described in 1977 in Papua New Guinea.[179] The causative agent was initially identified as a cyanobacterium but was recharacterized as a coccidian parasite in 1993.[180,181] The resultant disease, cyclosporiasis, is characterized by persistent watery diarrhea, bloating, fatigue, and weight loss and can be treated with sulfonamide antibiotics.[180] Several early studies identified cyclosporiasis as a major problem in travelers, particularly to locations such as Nepal and to tropical areas.[182,183] A study of international travelers in Germany identified cyclosporiasis in 1.1% of returnees; the countries of origin included Mexico, Guatemala, India, and Thailand.[184] Case-control studies among travelers and expatriates in Nepal identified contaminated water as a major source of infection.[185]

Beginning in 1996, recurrent outbreaks of cyclosporiasis were identified in North America.[186,187] A strong association was noted in both 1996 and 1997 with consumption of fresh raspberries originating in Guatemala. In 1997, an outbreak on a cruise ship leaving from Florida was linked to mesclun lettuce, but the source of the product could not be traced.[188] During 1996 and 1997, a total of 96 raspberry-associated clusters of cyclosporiasis involving 1,487 ill persons were reported. In 1997, 39% of the events occurred in restaurants, clubs, hotels, inns, or resorts.[187] Due to the nature of these events and the long incubation period for cyclosporiasis (up to 2 weeks), a number involved travelers who were not diagnosed until they had returned home, particularly between locations such as Florida and New York City.[189] In 1999, *Cyclospora* outbreaks have continued in association with resort destinations (CDC, unpublished data). This agent must therefore be considered in travelers to both developed and developing country settings.

Variant Creutzfeldt-Jacob Disease   In 1996, a previously unrecognized variant of Creutzfeldt-Jakob disease was identified in Great Britain.[190] This variant was notable for its more protracted course and the younger age distribution of patients, most of whom were under 40 years of age, when the classic form of the disease is uncommon. This variant form of Creutzfeldt-Jakob disease was subsequently linked to an epidemic of bovine spongiform encephalopathy in British cattle,[191,192] leading to widespread bans of British beef. Almost all cases of variant Creutzfeldt-Jakob disease have been identified in Great Britain, and none have been definitely linked to travel. However, concerns have been expressed about the potential for the disease, which can have an incubation period of decades, to appear in persons who traveled for extended periods in Great Britain in the 1980s and early 1990s and were exposed to British beef. In recognition of this concern, several countries have taken steps to ban blood donations from such persons. In 1999, the U.S. Food and Drug Administration recommended that persons who spent a cumulative period of more than 6 months in Great Britain after 1980 defer from donating blood; similar efforts are under way in Canada and Japan.[193]

SURVEILLANCE FOR EMERGING INFECTIONS RELATED TO TRAVEL

Protecting travelers from illness due to emerging infectious diseases during travel, and protecting the public from diseases imported by travelers, requires the existence of robust systems to monitor and respond to these disease threats. Whether the problem is leptospirosis associated with white water rafting in Central America,[194] schistosomiasis associated with Lake Malawi,[195] or Rift Valley fever in Egypt or Kenya,[196,197] travelers and the health providers who care for them pre- and post-travel must have reliable, up-to-date information about health risks and how to avoid them.

Global public health systems to monitor for emerging diseases do not currently exist, although substantial progress has been made in the last decade to improve surveillance and response capacity. In the United States, plans exist to improve local, state, and national capacity through the development of active surveillance sites, sentinel networks, and enhanced diagnostic capacity.[198] One sentinel network developed through this initiative (the GeoSentinel network of the International Society of Travel Medicine) specifically monitors trends in illness among travelers seeking pre-and post-travel advice through travel medicine providers.[199]

Travel health information is available through the Division of Quarantine of the CDC, including the annual Health Information for International Travel,[200] an Internet Web page that provides geography-specific information on health risks and current disease outbreaks (www.cdc.gov), and a fax line to access similar data (877-FYI-TRIP).

Outside the United States, efforts to improve disease surveillance and response are under way in several areas. The member states of the European Union have developed networks with common databases for a number of illnesses (including legionnaires' disease and food-borne illness) that have relevance to travelers' health.[201] In South America, there are initiatives in the Amazon basin and the Southern cone nations to build a common surveillance infrastructure to monitor emerging diseases. An emerging infectious diseases network has been established through the Asian Pacific Economic Cooperation.[202] Finally, the WHO's Programme on Communicable Diseases has made significant progress in building capacity to collect and disseminate timely data on disease outbreaks through their Internet site (www.who.ch).[203] The International Health Regulations are being revised and updated to prioritize syndrome-based outbreak reporting, which might signify the emergence of a new pathogen, and to reflect current trends in travel.[204]

Regardless of their sophistication, these systems can never guarantee that all emerging health problems in travelers will be recognized, diagnosed, and reported. Frontline clinicians must continue to contribute by taking an appropriate travel history, ordering necessary diagnostic tests, and reporting unusual cases to public health authorities. They must also be aware of emerging disease threats and ensure that their patients receive appropriate preventive measures, including vaccinations, prophylactic medications, and educational materials.

REFERENCES

1. World Health Organization. The world health report 1999: making a difference. Geneva: WHO, 1999.
2. Centers for Disease Control and Prevention. Ten great public health achievements—United States, 1900–1999. MMWR Morb Mortal Wkly Rep 1999;48:241–243.
3. Centers for Disease Control and Prevention. Reported tuberculosis in the United States, 1996. Washington, DC: U.S. Government Printing Office, 1997.
4. Taubenberger JK, Reid AH, Krafft AE, et al. Initial genetic characterization of the 1918 "Spanish" influenza virus. Science 1997;275:1793–1796.
5. Fauci AS. The AIDS epidemic—considerations for the 21st century. N Engl J Med 1999;341:1046–1050.
6. Blaser MJ. *Helicobacter pylori* and gastric disease. BMJ 1998;316:1507–1510.
7. Franco EL, Rohan TE, Villa LL. Epidemiologic evidence and human papilloma virus infection as a necessary cause of cervical cancer. J Natl Cancer Inst 1999;91:506–511.
8. Lederberg J, Shope RE, Oaks SC, eds. Emerging infections: microbial threats to health in the United States. Washington, DC: National Academy Press, 1992.
9. Fraser DW, Tsai TR, Orenstein W, et al. Legionnaires' disease: description of an epidemic of pneumonia. N Engl J Med 1977;297:1189–1197.
10. Fenstersheib MD, Miller M, Diggins C, et al. Outbreak of Pontiac fever due to *Legionella anisa*. Lancet 1990;336:35–37.
11. Castellani Pastoris M, Benedetti P, Greco D, et al. Six cases of travel-associated legionnaires' disease in Ischia involving four countries. Infection 1992;20:73–77.
12. Mamolen M, Breiman RF, Barbaree JM, et al. Use of multiple molecular subtyping techniques to investigate a legionnaires' disease outbreak due to identical strains at two tourist lodges. J Clin Microbiol 1993;31:2584–2588.
13. Deng C. A report on investigation of an outbreak of legionnaires' disease in a hotel in Beijing. Chung Hua Liu Hsing Ping Hsueh Tsa Chih 1993;14:78–80.
14. Hlady WG, Mullen RC, Mintz CS, et al. Outbreak of legionnaires' disease linked to a decorative fountain by molecular epidemiology. Am J Epidemiol 1993;138:555–562.
15. Joseph C, Morgan D, Birtles R, et al. An international investigation of an outbreak of legionnaires' disease among UK and French tourists. Eur J Epidemiol 1996;12:215–219.
16. Jernigan DB, Hofmann J, Cetron MS, et al. Outbreak of legionnaires' disease among cruise ship passengers exposed to a contaminated whirlpool spa. Lancet 1996;347:494–499.
17. Bell JC, Jorm LR, Williamson M, et al. Legionellosis linked with a hotel car park—how many were infected? Epidemiol Infect 1996;116:185–192.
18. Public Health Laboratory Service Communicable Disease Surveillance Centre. Cluster of cases of legionnaires' disease associated with travel to Turkey. Commun Dis Rep 1995;5:175.
19. Public Health Laboratory Service Communicable Disease Surveillance Centre. A cluster of cases of legionnaires' disease associated with a hotel in Spain. Commun Dis Rep 1998;8:29.
20. Public Health Laboratory Service Communicable Disease Surveillance Centre. Legionnaires' disease among travellers to France, June 1998. Commun Dis Rep 1998;8:245.
21. Public Health Laboratory Service Communicable Disease Surveillance Centre. Legionnaires' disease-outbreak in the Netherlands. Commun Dis Rep 1999;9:123.
22. Joseph CA, Harrison TG, Ilijic-Car D, Bartlett CL. Legionnaires' disease in residents of England and Wales, 1997. Commun Dis Public Health 1998;1:252–258.
23. Gao F, Bailes E, Robertson DL, et al. Origin of HIV-1 in the chimpanze Pan troglodytes troglodytes. Nature 1999;397:436–441.
24. Weiss R, Wrangham RW. From Pan to pandemic. Nature 1999;397:385–386.
25. Pape J, Liautaud B, Thomas F, et al. Characteristics of the acquired immunodeficiency syndrome (AIDS) in Haiti. N Engl J Med 1983;309:945–950.
26. Weniger BG. Limpakarnjanarat K, Ungchusak K, et al. The epidemiology of HIV infection and AIDS in Thailand. AIDS 1991;5(Suppl 2):S71–S85.

27. Piot P. Learning from success: global priorities for HIV prevention: Thomas Parran Award lecture. Sex Transm Dis 1999; 26:244–249.

28. Bonabeau E, Toubiana L, Flahault A. The geographical spread of influenza. Proc R Soc Lond B Biol Sci 1998;265:2421–2425.

29. Centers for Disease Control and Prevention. Update: influenza activity—United States, 1997–98 season. MMWR Morb Mortal Wkly Rep 1997;46:1094–1098.

30. Centers for Disease Control and Prevention. Update: outbreak of influenza A infection—Alaska and the Yukon Territory, July-August 1998. MMWR Morb Mortal Wkly Rep 1998; 47:685–688.

31. Centers for Disease Control and Prevention. Outbreak of influenza A infection among travelers—Alaska and the Yukon Territory, May–June 1999. MMWR Morb Mortal Wkly Rep 1999;48:545–546, 555.

32. Centers for Disease Control and Prevention. Outbreak of influenza-like illness in a tour group—Alaska. MMWR Morb Mortal Wkly Rep 1987;36:697–698, 704.

33. Public Health Laboratory Service. Influenza on a cruise ship in the Mediterranean. Commun Dis Rep CDR Wkly 1999; 9:209, 212.

34. Lyytikainen O, Hoffmann E, Timm H, et al. Influenza A outbreak among adolescents in a ski hostel. Eur J Clin Microbiol Infect Dis 1998;17:128–130.

35. Taylor R, Nemaia H, Tukuitonga C, et al. An epidemic of influenza in the population of Niue. J Med Virol 1985; 16:127–136.

36. Beller M, Schloss M. Self-reported illness among travelers to the Russian Far East. Public Health Rep 1993;108:645–649.

37. Crosby AW. America's forgotten pandemic: the influenza of 1918. Cambridge, UK: Cambridge University Press, 1989.

38. Klontz KC, Hynes NA, Gunn RA, et al. An outbreak of influenza A/Taiwan/1/86 (H1N1) infections at a naval base and its association with airplane travel. Am J Epidemiol 1989;129:341–348.

39. Williams RJ, Cox NJ, Regnary HL, et al. Meeting the challenge of emerging pathogens: the role of the United States Air Force in global influenza surveillance. Mil Med 1997; 162:82–86.

40. Subbarao K, Klimov A, Katz J, et al. Characterization of an avian influenza A (H5N1) virus isolated from a child with a fatal respiratory illness. Science 1998;279:393–396.

41. Claas ECJ, Osterhaus ADME, van Beek R, et al. Human influenza A (H5N1) virus related to a highly pathogenic avian influenza virus. Lancet 1998;351:472–477.

42. Yuen KY, Chan PKS, Peiris M, et al. Clinical features and rapid viral diagnosis of human disease associated with avian influenza A (H5N1) virus. Lancet 1998;351:467–471.

43. Suarez DL, Perdue ML, Cox N, et al. Comparisons of highly virulent H5N1 influenza A viruses isolated from humans and chickens from Hong Kong. J Virol 1998;72:6678–6688.

44. Mounts AW, Kwong H, Izurieta HS, et al. Case-control study of risk factors for avian influenza A (H5N1) disease, Hong Kong, 1997. J Infect Dis 1999;180:505–508.

45. Public Health Laboratory Service. Avian strain of influenza A virus isolated from humans in Hong Kong. Commun Dis Rep CDR Wkly 1999;9:131, 134.

46. Guan Y, Shortridge KF, Krauss S, Webster RG. Molecular characterization of H9N2 influenza viruses: were they the donors of the "internal" genes of H5N1 in Hong Kong? Proc Natl Acad Sci U S A 1999;96:9363–9367.

47. Nchinda TC. Malaria: a reemerging disease in Africa. Emerg Infect Dis 1998;4:398–403.

48. Malakooti MA, Biomndo K, Shanks GD. Reemergence of epidemic malaria in the highlands of western Kenya. Emerg Infect Dis 1998;4:671–676.

49. Aramburu Guarda J, Ramal Asayag C, Witzig R. Malaria reemergence in the Peruvian Amazon region. Emerg Infect Dis 1999;5:209–215.

50. Krogstad DJ. Malaria as a reemerging disease. Epidemiol Rev 1996;18:77–89.

51. Williams HA, Roberts J, Kachur SP, et al. Malaria surveillance—United States, 1995. MMWR Morb Mortal Wkly Rep 1999;48(SS-1):1–23.

52. Miller SA, Bergman BP, Croft AM. Epidemiology of malaria in the British Army from 1982–1996. J R Army Med Corps 1999;145:20–22.

53. Muentener P, Schlagenhauf P, Steffen R. Imported malaria (1985–95): trends and perspectives. Bull WHO 1999;77: 560–566.

54. Kachur SP, Reller ME, Barber AM, et al. Malaria surveillance—United States, 1994. MMWR Morb Mortal Wkly Rep 1997;46(SS-5):1–18.

55. Layton M, Parise ME, Campbell CC, et al. Mosquito-transmitted malaria in New York City, 1993. Lancet 1995;346: 729–731.

56. Centers for Disease Control and Prevention. Probable locally acquired mosquito-transmitted *Plasmodium vivax* infection—Georgia, 1996. MMWR Morb Mortal Wkly Rep 1996; 46:264–267.

57. Castelli F, Cligaris S, Matteelli A, et al. "Baggage malaria" in Italy: cryptic malaria explained? Trans R Soc Trop Med Hyg 1993;87:394.

58. Isaacson M. Airport malaria: a review. Bull WHO 1989;67: 737–743.

59. Mantel CF, Klose C, Scheurer S, et al. *Plasmodium falciparum* malaria acquired in Berlin, Germany. Lancet 1995; 346:320–321.

60. Centers for Disease Control and Prevention. Mosquito-transmitted malaria—Michigan, 1995. MMWR Morb Mortal Wkly Rep 1996;45:398–400.

61. Maldonado YA, Nahlen BL, Roberto RR, et al. Transmission of *Plasmodium vivax* malaria in San Diego County, California, 1986. Am J Trop Med Hyg 1990;42:3–9.

62. Rigau-Perez JG, Clark GG, Gubler DJ, et al. Dengue and dengue haemorrhagic fever. Lancet 1998;352:971–977.

63. Gubler DJ. Dengue and dengue hemorrhagic fever. Clin Microbiol Rev 1998;11:480–496.

64. World Health Organization. The world health report, 1998. Geneva: WHO, 1998.

65. Burke DS, Nisalak A, Johnson DE, et al. A prospective study of dengue infections in Bangkok. Am J Trop Med Hyg 1988;38:172–180.

66. Jetten TH, Focks DA. Potential changes in the distribution of dengue transmission under climate warming. Am J Trop Med Hyg 1997;57:285–297.

67. Patz JA, Martens WJM, Focks DA, Jetten TH. Dengue fever epidemic potential as projected by general circulation models of global climate change. Environ Health Perspect 1998; 106:147–153.

68. Goh KT. Dengue—a re-emerging disease in Singapore. Ann Acad Med Singapore 1997;26:664–670.

69. Desparis X, Murgue B, Roche C, et al. Changing clinical and biological manifestations of dengue during the dengue-2 epidemic in French Polynesia in 1996/97—description and analysis in a prospective study. Trop Med Int Health 1998; 3:859–865.

70. Kouri G, Guzman MG, Valdes L, et al. Reemergence of dengue in Cuba: a 1997 epidemic in Santiago de Cuba. Emerg Infect Dis 1998;4:89–92.

71. Centers for Disease Control and Prevention. Dengue outbreak associated with multiple serotypes—Puerto Rico, 1998. MMWR Morb Mortal Wkly Rep 1998;47:952–956.

72. Nogueira RM, Miagostovich MP, Schatzmayr HG, et al. Dengue in the State of Rio de Janeiro, Brazil, 1986–1998. Mem Inst Oswaldo Cruz 1999;94:297–304.

73. Schwartz E, Mendelson E, Sidi Y. Dengue fever among travelers. Am J Med 1996;101:516–520.

74. Lopez-Velez R, Perez-Casas C, Vorndam AV, Rigau J. Dengue in Spanish travelers returning from the tropics. Eur J Clin Microbiol Infect Dis 1996;15:823–826.

75. Jensenius M, Gundersen SG, Vene S, Bruu AL. Dengue fever imported to Norway. Serologically confirmed cases 1991–96. Tidsskr Nor Laegeforen 1997;117:4230–4233.

76. Schwartz TF, Jager G, Gilch S. Imported dengue virus infections in German tourists. Zentralbl Bakteriol 1995; 282:533–536.

77. Shirtliffe P, Cameron E, Nicholson KG, Wiselka MJ. Don't forget dengue: clinical features of dengue fever in returning travellers. J R Coll Phys Lond 1998;32:235–237.

78. Badiaga S, Delmont J, Brouqui P, et al. Imported dengue: study of 44 cases observed from 1994 to 1997 in nine university hospital centers. Pathol Biol (Paris) 1999;47:539–542.

79. Teichmann D, Rogler G, Grobusch MP, et al. Imported dengue virus type 2 infection acquired during an outbreak in India. Eur J Clin Microbiol Infect Dis 1999;18:310–312.

80. Centers for Disease Control and Prevention. Imported dengue—United States, 1996. MMWR Morb Mortal Wkly Rep 1998; 47:544–547.

81. Karp BE. Dengue fever: a risk to travelers. Maryland Med J 1997;46:299–302.

82. Laboratory Centre for Disease Control. A point source dengue outbreak in Canadian tourists in Barbados. Can Commun Dis Rep 1998;24:161–164.

83. Rawlings JA, Hendricks KA, Burgess CR, et al. Dengue surveillance in Texas, 1995. Am J Trop Med Hyg 1998;59:95–99.

84. Eisenhut M, Schwarz TF, Hegenscheid B. Seroprevalence of dengue, chikungunya and Sindbis virus infections in German aid workers. Infection 1999;27:82–85.

85. Gambel JM, Drabick JJ, Swalko MA, et al. Dengue among United Nations mission in Haiti personnel, 1995: implications for preventive medicine. Mil Med 1999;164:300–302.

86. Trofa AF, DeFraites RF, Smoak BL, et al. Dengue fever in US military personnel in Haiti. JAMA 1997;277:1546–1548.

87. Chambers TJ, Tsai TF, Pervokov Y, Monath TP. Vaccine development against dengue and Japanese encephalitis: report of a World Health Organization meeting. Vaccine 1997;15: 1494–1502.

88. Robertson SE, Hull BP, Tomori O, et al. Yellow fever: a decade of reemergence. JAMA 1996;276:1157–1162.

89. Sanders EJ, Marfin AA, Tukei PM, et al. First recorded outbreak of yellow fever in Kenya, 1992–1993. I. Epidemiologic investigations. Am J Trop Med Hyg 1998;59:644–649.

90. McFarland JM, Baddour LM, Nelsen JE, et al. Imported yellow fever in a United States citizen. Clin Infect Dis 1997; 25:1143–1147.

91. Deubel V, Huerre M, Cathomas G, et al. Molecular detection and characterization of yellow fever virus in blood and liver specimens of a non-vaccinated fatal human case. J Med Virol 1997;53:212–217.

92. Chua KB, Bellini WJ, Rota PA, et al. Nipah virus: a recently emergent deadly paramyxovirus. Science 2000;288:1432–1435.

93. Goh KJ, Tan CT, Chew NK, et al. Clinical features of Nipah virus encephalitis among pig farmers in Malaysia. N Engl J Med 2000;342:1229–1235.

94. Mackenzie JS. Emerging viral diseases: an Australian perspective. Emerg Infect Dis 1999;5:1–8.

95. Centers for Disease Control and Prevention. Update: West Nile-like viral encephalitis—New York, 1999. MMWR Morb Mortal Wkly Rep 1999;48:890–892.

96. Briese T, Jia XY, Huang C, et al. Identification of a Kunjin/West Nile-like flavivirus in brains of patients with New York encephalitis. Lancet 1999;354:1261–1262.

97. Centers for Disease Control and Prevention. Update: West Nile virus encephalitis—New York, 1999. MMWR Morb Mortal Wkly Rep 1999;48:944–946, 955.

98. Duchin JS, Koster FT, Peters CJ, et al. Hantavirus pulmonary syndrome: a clinical description of 17 patients with a newly recognized disease. N Engl J Med 1994;330:949–955.

99. Centers for Disease Control and Prevention. Update: Hantavirus pulmonary syndrome—United States, 1999. MMWR Morb Mortal Wkly Rep 1999;48:521–525.

100. Werker DH, Artsob H. Of mice and mostly men—hantavirus pulmonary syndrome. Can Med Assoc J 1998;158:912–913.

101. Williams RJ, Bryan RT, Mills JN, et al. An outbreak of hantavirus pulmonary syndrome in western Paraguay. Am J Trop Med Hyg 1997;57:274–282.

102. Da Silva MV, Vasconcelos MJ, Hidalgo NT, et al. Hantavirus pulmonary syndrome. Report of the first three cases in Sao Paulo, Brazil. Rev Inst Med Trop Sao Paulo 1997;39:231–234.

103. Espinoza R, Vial P, Noriega LM, et al. Hantavirus pulmonary syndrome in a Chilean patient with recent travel in Bolivia. Emerg Infect Dis 1998;4:93–95.

104. Levis S, Morzunov SP, Rowe JE, et al. Genetic diversity and epidemiology of hantaviruses in Argentina. J Infect Dis 1998;177:529–538.

105. Toro J, Vega JD, Khan AS, et al. An outbreak of hantavirus pulmonary syndrome, Chile, 1997. Emerg Infect Dis 1998; 4:687–694.

106. Powers AM, Mercer DR, Watts DM, et al. Isolation and genetic characterization of a hantavirus (*Bunyaviridae*: hantavirus) from a rodent, *Oligoryzomys microtis* (muridae) collected in northeastern Peru. Am J Trop Med Hyg 1999; 61:92–98.

107. Monroe MC, Morzunov SP, Johnson AM, et al. Genetic diversity and distribution of Peromyscus-borne hantaviruses in North America. Emerg Infect Dis 1999;5:75–86.

108. Wells RM, Sosa Estani S, Yadon ZE, et al. An unusual outbreak in southern Argentina: person-to-person transmission? Emerg Infect Dis 1997;3:171–174.

109. Padula PJ, Edelstein A, Miguel SD, et al. Hantavirus pulmonary syndrome outbreak in Argentina: molecular evidence for person-to-person transmission of Andes virus. Virology 1998;241:323–330.

110. Jay M, Hjelle B, Davis R, et al. Occupational exposure leading to hantavirus pulmonary syndrome in a utility company employee. Clin Infect Dis 1996;22:841–844.

111. Khan AS, Spiropoulou CF, Morzunov S, et al. Fatal illness associated with a new hantavirus in Louisiana. J Med Virol 1995;46:281–286.

112. Rodriguez-Moran P, Kelly C, Williams TM, Hjelle B. Hantavirus infection in the Four Corners region of USA in 1998. Lancet 1998;352:1353.

113. Flood J, Mintz L, Jay M, et al. Hantavirus infection following wilderness camping in Washington State and northeastern California. West J Med 1995;163:162–164.

114. Khan AS, Ksiazek TG, Zaki SR, et al. Fatal hantavirus pulmonary syndrome in an adolescent. Pediatrics 1995;95: 276–280.

115. Centers for Disease Control and Prevention. Hantavirus pulmonary syndrome—Virginia, 1993. MMWR Morb Mortal Wkly Rep 1994;43:876–877.

116. Frampton JW, Lanser S, Nichols CR, Ettestad PJ. Sin Nombre virus infection in 1959. Lancet 1995;346:781–782.

117. Armstrong LR, Zaki SR, Goldoft MJ, et al. Hantavirus pulmonary syndrome associated with entering or cleaning rarely used, rodent-infested structures. J Infect Dis 1995;172:1166.

118. Clement J, Heyman P, McKenna P, et al. The hantaviruses of Europe: from the bedside to the bench. Emerg Infect Dis 1997;3:205–211.

119. Childs JE, Krebs JW, Ksiazek TG, et al. A household based case-control study of risk factors associated with hantavirus pulmonary syndrome in the southwestern United States. Am J Trop Med Hyg 1995;52:393–397.

120. Mills JN, Yates TL, Ksiazek TG, et al. Long-term studies of hantavirus reservoir populations in the southwestern United States: rationale, potential, and methods. Emerg Infect Dis 1999;5:95–101.

121. Centers for Disease Control. Hantavirus infection—southwestern United States: interim recommendations for risk reduction, 1993. MMWR Morb Mortal Wkly Rep 1993; 42(RR-11):1–13.

122. Steere AC, Malawista SE, Snyderman DR, et al. Lyme arthritis: an epidemic of oligoarticular arthritis in children and adults in three Connecticut communities. Arthritis Rheum 1977;20:7–17.

123. Barbour AG. Fall and rise of Lyme disease and other *Ixodes* tick-borne infections in North America and Europe. Br Med Bull 1998;54:647–658.

124. Meek JI, Roberts CL, Smith EV Jr, Cartter ML. Underreporting of Lyme disease by Connecticut physicians, 1992. J Public Health Manage Pract 1996;2:61–65.

125. Orloski KA, Campbell GL, Genese CA, et al. Emergence of Lyme disease in Hunterdon County, New Jersey, 1993: a case-control study of risk factors and evaluation of reporting practices. Am J Epidemiol 1998;147:391–397.

126. Walker DH, Barbour AG, Oliver JH, et al. Emerging bacterial zoonotic and vector-borne diseases: ecological and epidemiological factors. JAMA 1996;275:463–469.

127. Cromley EK, Cartter ML, Mrozinski RD, Ertel SH. Residential setting as a risk factor for Lyme disease in a hyperendemic area. Am J Epidemiol 1998;147:472–477.

128. Stafford KC 3rd, Cartter ML, Magnarelli LA, et al. Temporal correlations between tick abundance and prevalence of ticks infected with *Borrelia burgdorferi* and increasing incidence of Lyme disease. J Clin Microbiol 1998;36:1240–1244.

129. Strickland GT, Trivedi L, Watkins S, et al. Cluster of Lyme disease at a summer camp in Kent County, Maryland. Emerg Infect Dis 1996;2:44–46.

130. Centers for Disease Control and Prevention. Recommendations for the use of the Lyme disease vaccine. Recommendations of the Advisory Committee on Immunization Practices (ACIP). MMWR Morb Mortal Wkly Rep 1998;48(RR-7): 1–24.

131. Maeda K, Markowitz N, Hawley RC, et al. Human infection with *Ehrlichia canis*, a leucocytic rickettsia. N Engl J Med 1987;316:853–856.

132. Fritz CL, Glaser CA. Ehrlichiosis. Infect Dis Clin North Am 1998;12:123–136.

133. Bakken JS, Dumler JS, Chen S-M, et al. Human granulocytic ehrlichiosis in the upper Midwest United States: a new species emerging? JAMA 1994;272:212–218.

134. Buller RS, Arens M, Hmiel SP, et al. *Ehrlichia ewingii*, a newly recognized agent of human ehrlichiosis. N Engl J Med 1999;341:148–155.

135. Dumler JS, Bakken JS. Human ehrlichioses: newly recognized infections transmitted by ticks. Annu Rev Med 1998;49: 201–213.

136. Carpenter CF, Gandhi TK, Kong LK, et al. The incidence of ehrlichial and rickettsial infection in patients with unexplained fever and recent history of tick bite in central North Carolina. J Infect Dis 1999;180:900–903.

137. Fishbein DB, Dawson JE, Robinson LE. Human ehrlichiosis in the United States, 1985 to 1990. Ann Intern Med 1994; 120:736–743.

138. Standaert SM, Dawson JE, Schaffner W, et al. Ehrlichiosis in a golf-oriented retirement community. N Engl J Med 1995;333:420–425.

139. Petersen LR, Sawyer LA, Fishbein DB, et al. An outbreak of ehrlichiosis in members of an army reserve unit exposed to ticks. J Infect Dis 1989;159:562–568.

140. Yevich SJ, Sanchez JL, DeFraites RF, et al. Seroepidemiology of infections due to spotted fever group rickettsiae and Ehrlichia species in military personnel exposed in areas of the United States where such infections are endemic. J Infect Dis 1995;171:1266–1273.

141. Mitchell PD, Reed KD, Hofkes JM. Immunoserologic evidence of coinfection with *Borrelia burgdorferi*, *Babesia microti*, and human granulocytic *Ehrlichia* species in residents of Wisconsin and Minnesota. J Clin Microbiol 1996;34:724–727.

142. Bjoersdorff A, Brouqui P, Eliasson I, et al. Serological evidence of Ehrlichia infection in Swedish Lyme borreliosis patients. Scand J Infect Dis 1999;31:51–55.

143. Hunfeld KP, Brade V. Prevalence of antibodies against the human granulocytic ehrlichiosis agent in Lyme borreliosis patients from Germany. Eur J Clin Microbiol Infect Dis 1999;18:221–224.

144. Laferl H, Hogrefe W, Kock T, Pichler H. A further case of acute human granulocytic ehrlichiosis in Slovenia. Eur J Clin Microbiol Infect Dis 1999;18:385–386.

145. Nuti M, Serafini DA, Bassetti D, et al. Ehrlichia infection in Italy. Emerg Infect Dis 1998;4:663–665.

146. van Dobbenburgh A, van Dam AP, Fikrig E. Human granulocytic ehrlichiosis in western Europe. N Engl J Med 1999;340:1214–1216.

147. Uhaa IJ, MacLean JD, Greene CR, Fishbein DB. A case of human ehrlichiosis acquired in Mali: clinical and laboratory findings. Am J Trop Med Hyg 1992;46:161–164.

148. Heppner DG, Wongsrichanalai C, Walsh DS, et al. Human ehrlichiosis in Thailand. Lancet 1997;350:785–786.

149. Kissling RE, Murphy FA, Henderson BE. Marburg virus. Ann N Y Acad Sci 1970;174:932–945.

150. Slenczka WG. The Marburg virus outbreak of 1967 and subsequent episodes. Curr Top Microbiol Immunol 1999;235: 49–75.

151. Monath TP. Ecology of Marburg and Ebola viruses: speculations and directions for future research. J Infect Dis 1999;179(Suppl 1):S127–S138.

152. Gear JSS, Cassel GA, Gear AJ, et al. Outbreak of Marburg virus disease in Johannesburg. BMJ 1975;489–493.

153. Conrad JL, Isaacson M, Burnett Smith E, et al. Epidemiologic investigation of Marburg virus disease, southern Africa, 1975. Am J Trop Med Hyg 1978;27:1210–1215.

154. Smith DH, Johnson BK, Isaakson M, et al. Marburg-virus disease in Kenya. Lancet 1982;i:816–820.

155. Johnson ED, Johnson BK, Silverstein D, et al. Characterization of a new Marburg virus isolated from a 1987 fatal case in Kenya. Arch Virol 1996;11(Suppl):S101–S114.

156. Kenyon RH, Niklasson B, Jahrling PB, et al. Virologic investigation of a case of suspected haemorrhagic fever. Res Virol 1994;145:397–406.

157. Marburg Investigative Team. A community based outbreak of Marburg virus haemorrhagic fever in the Democratic Republic of Congo [abstract]. 4th Epiet Scientific Seminar, October 1999, Veyrier du Lac, France.

158. International Commission. Ebola haemorrhagic fever in Zaire, 1976. Bull World Health Org 1978;56:271–293.

159. WHO/International Study Team. Viral haemorrhagic fever in Sudan, 1976. Bull World Health Org 1978;56:247–269.

160. Baron R, McCormick J, Zubier O, et al. Ebola virus disease in southern Sudan: hospital dissemination in intrafamilial spread. Bull World Health Org 1983;61:997–1003.

161. Formenty P, Hatz C, LeGuenno B, et al. Human infection due to Ebola virus, subtype Cote D'Ivoire: clinical and biologic presentation. J Infect Dis 1999;179(Suppl 1):S48–S53.

162. Georges AJ, Leroy EM, Renaut AA, et al. Ebola hemorrhagic fever outbreaks in Gabon, 1994–1997: epidemiologic and health control issues. J Infect Dis 1999;179(Suppl 1):S65–S75.

163. Khan AS, Tshioko FK, Heymann DL, et al. The reemergence of Ebola hemorrhagic fever, Democratic Republic of the Congo, 1995. J Infect Dis 1999;179(Suppl 1):S76–S86.

164. Wyers M, Formenty P, Cherel Y, et al. Histopathological and immunohistochemical studies of lesions associated with Ebola virus in a naturally infected chimpanzee. J Infect Dis 1999;179(Suppl 1):S54–S59.

165. Holmes GP, McCormick JB, Trock SC, et al. Lassa fever in the United States: investigation of a case and new guidelines for management. N Engl J Med 1990;323:1120–1123.

166. World Health Organization. Lassa fever, case imported to Germany. Wkly Epidemiol Rec 2000;75:17–18.

167. Public Health Laboratory Service. Lassa fever imported to England. Commun Dis Rep Wkly 2000;10:99.

168. Centers for Disease Control and Prevention. Measles eradication: recommendations from a meeting co-sponsored by the World Health Organization, the Pan American Health Organization, and CDC. MMWR Morb Mortal Wkly Rep 1997;46 (RR-11):1–20.

169. Centers for Disease Control and Prevention. Epidemiology of measles—United States, 1998. MMWR Morb Mortal Wkly Rep 1999;48:749–753.

170. Miller M, Williams WW, Redd SC. Measles among adults, United States, 1985–1995. Am J Prev Med 1999;17:114–119.

171. Vitek CR, Redd SC, Redd SB, Hadler SC. Trends in importation of measles to the United States, 1986–1994. JAMA 1997;277:1952–1956.

172. Centers for Disease Control and Prevention. Progress toward elimination of measles from the Americas. MMWR Morb Mortal Wkly Rep 1998;47:189–193.

173. de Quadros CA, Hersh BS, Noguiera AC, et al. Measles eradication: experience in the Americas. Bull World Health Org 1998;76(Suppl 2):S47–S52.

174. Bisgard KM, Hardy IR, Popovic T, et al. Respiratory diphtheria in the United States, 1980 through 1995. Am J Public Health 1998;88:787–791.

175. Hardy IR, Dittmann S, Sutter RW. Current situation and control strategies for resurgence of diphtheria in newly independent states of the former Soviet Union. Lancet 1996; 347:1739–1744.

176. Vitek CR, Wharton M. Diphtheria in the former Soviet Union: reemergence of a pandemic disease. Emerg Infect Dis 1998; 4:539–550.

177. Centers for Disease Control. Diphtheria acquired by US citizens in the Russian Federation and Ukraine—1994. MMWR Morb Mortal Wkly Rep 1995;44:237–244.

178. Eskola J, Lumio J, Vuopio-Varkila J. Resurgent diphtheria— are we safe? Br Med Bull 1998;54:635–645.

179. Ashford RW. Occurrence of an undescribed coccidian in man in Papua New Guinea. Ann Trop Med Parasitol 1979;73: 497–500.

180. Soave R, Herwaldt BL, Relman DA. Cyclospora. Infect Dis Clin North Am 1998;12:1–12.

181. Ortega YR, Sterling CR, Gilman RH, et al. Cyclospora species—a new protozoan pathogen of humans. N Engl J Med 1993;328:1308–1312.

182. Shlim DR, Cohen MT, Eaton M, et al. An alga-like organism associated with an outbreak of prolonged diarrhea among foreigners in Nepal. Am J Trop Med Hyg 1991;45:383–389.

183. Himy O, Villard O, Kremer M. Cyclosporidia: a general review. J Travel Med 1995;2:33–36.

184. Jelinek T, Lotze M, Eichenlaub S, et al. Prevalence of infection with *Cryptosporidium parvum* and *Cyclospora cayetanensis* among international travelers. Gut 1997;41:801–804.

185. Hoge C, Shlim D, Rajah R, et al. Epidemiology of diarrhoeal illness associated with coccidian-like organisms among travelers and foreign residents in Nepal. Lancet 1993;341: 1308–1312.

186. Herwaldt BL, Ackers ML. An outbreak in 1996 of cyclosporiasis associated with imported raspberries. The Cyclospora Working Group. N Engl J Med 1997;336:1548–1556.

187. Herwaldt BL, Beach MJ. The return of Cyclospora in 1997: another outbreak of cyclosporiasis in North America associated with imported raspberries. The Cyclospora Working Group. Ann Intern Med 1999;130:210–220.

188. Centers for Disease Control and Prevention. Update: outbreaks of cyclosporiasis—United States and Canada, 1997. MMWR Morb Mortal Wkly Rep 1997;46:521–523.

189. Koumans EH, Katz DJ, Malecki JM, et al. An outbreak of cyclosporiasis in Florida in 1995: a harbinger of multistate outbreaks in 1996 and 1997. Am J Trop Med Hyg 1998;59: 235–242.

190. Will RG, Ironside JW, Zeidler M, et al. A new variant of Creutzfeldt-Jakob disease in the UK. Lancet 1996;347: 921–925.

191. Bruce ME, Will RG, Ironside JW, et al. Transmissions to mice indicate that 'new variant' CJD is caused by the BSE agent. Nature 1997;389:498–501.

192. Patterson WJ, Painter MJ. Bovine spongiform encephalopathy and new variant Creuzfeldt-Jakob disease: an overview. Commun Dis Public Health 1999;2:5–13.

193. Ramsay S, Birchard K, Watts J. Variant CJD fears prompt growing number of countries to ban British blood donations. Lancet 1999;354:754.

194. Centers for Disease Control and Prevention. Outbreak of leptospirosis among white-water rafters—Costa Rica, 1996. MMWR Morb Mortal Wkly Rep 1997;46:577–579.

195. Cetron MS, Chitsulo L, Sullivan JJ, et al. Schistosomiasis in Lake Malawi. Lancet 1996;348:1274–1278.

196. Arthur RR, el-Sharkawy MS, Cope SE, et al. Recurrence of Rift Valley fever in Egypt. Lancet 1993;342:1149–1150.

197. Centers for Disease Control and Prevention. Rift Valley fever—East Africa, 1997–1998. MMWR Morb Mortal Wkly Rep 1998;47:261–264.

198. Centers for Disease Control and Prevention. Preventing emerging infectious diseases: a strategy for the 21st century. Washington, DC: Department of Health and Human Services, 1998.

199. Freedman DO, Kozarsky PE, Weld LH, Cetron MS. GeoSentinel: the global emerging infections sentinel network of the International Society of Travel Medicine. J Travel Med 1999;6:94–98.

200. Centers for Disease Control and Prevention. Health Information for International Travel 1999–2000. Atlanta: Department of Health and Human Services, 1999.

201. Giesecke J, Weinberg J. A European centre for infectious disease? Lancet 1998;352:1308.

202. Kimball AM, Horwitch CA, O'Carroll PW, et al. The Asian Pacific Economic Cooperation Emerging Infections Network. Am J Prev Med 1999;17:156–158.

203. Heymann D, Dzenowagis J. Commentary: emerging and other communicable diseases. Bull World Health Org 1998;76: 545–547.

204. World Health Organization. Revision of the international health regulations. Wkly Epidemiol Rec 1999;74:252–253.

Chapter 20

TRAVELERS' DIARRHEA

20.1 EPIDEMIOLOGY AND CLINICAL ASPECTS

HEIKKI PELTOLA AND SHERWOOD L. GORBACH

"Travel broadens the mind, as it loosens the bowels."[1] This commentary on travelers' diarrhea (TD), although droll, should not disguise the fact that it is a serious concern, not only for the hapless traveler but for the tourist industry in general. Several prospective studies have shown that approximately 40% of the 20 million people traveling each year from industrialized countries to developing countries experience this scourge (Table 20.1–1).

Although virtually nobody dies from TD, and fewer than 1% are admitted to a hospital, every third person stricken with TD is confined to bed and 40% change their itinerary.[2–4] Several days of a trip can be wasted by this illness, a significant part of a vacation or of a business trip.

TD has a major impact on international tourism by lost revenues. Even the reputation of TD is enough to discourage tourists from risking a trip to a high-frequency area. Sadly, it is the developing countries that have the greatest need for foreign currency that lose the most tourists from fears of intestinal disruptions.

DEFINITION

Any bowel movement that fits the shape of the container is considered diarrhea. Although this working description serves well in the field, a more precise definition is required in order to compare findings by different investigations.

Most studies define TD as the passage of three or more loose stools in a 24-hour period in association with at least one of the following symptoms or signs of enteric disease: nausea, vomiting, abdominal cramps, fever, fecal urgency, tenesmus, or the passage of bloody or mucoid stools.[5] This definition has been modified in some studies to require either four or more loose stools in a 24-hour period or three or more loose stools in an 8-hour period with at least one of the additional symptoms or signs listed above (Table 20.1–2).[6] This refined definition takes into account the variable spectrum of TD.

Data on the appropriateness of the current definition derive from an analysis of U.S. adult travelers to Guadalajara, Mexico.[5] If diarrhea was mild, that is, one or two loose stools per 24 hours and one symptom of enteric disease, 60% of affected persons did well by the second day,

and only 22% continued to have mild diarrhea. Of these, one-quarter (6% of the original patients with mild TD) continued to have diarrhea over the subsequent 2 days. As the etiology was essentially the same in patients with mild or severe TD, the results suggest that travelers with mild TD are advised to wait before instituting therapy until at least three unformed stools are passed during 24 hours.

HISTORY

Various types of gastroenteritis have afflicted conquering armies, missionaries, sojourning merchants, diplomats, foreign office officials, people watchers, curio collectors, and itinerant scholars from time immemorial. During the current era, the tradition of TD continues, whether the trip is for pleasure or for a serious mission. During Operation Desert Shield, no less than 57% of American soldiers experienced TD at least once and 32% more often.[7] In another report of British troops flown out for immediate service overseas,[8] a 30% attack rate was observed. Most field commanders would agree that acute intestinal urges can seriously compromise combat readiness in a war zone.

Table 20.1–1. CURRENT DEFINITION OF TRAVELERS' DIARRHEA

1. ≥ 4 loose stools in a 24-hour period
    or
   ≥ 3 loose stools in an 8-hour period
    and
2. At least one of the following
   symptoms or signs of enteric disease:

	ESTIMATED FREQUENCY (%)
Nausea	10–70
Vomiting	10
Cramps	60
Fever	10–30
Fecal urgency	≈100
Abdominal pain or tenesmus	80
Bloody or mucoid stools	10

Table 20.1–2.   TRAVELERS' DIARRHEA

A DISEASE WITH NUMEROUS MONIKERS

Aden gut	Malta dog
Aztec two-step	Montezuma's revenge
Backdoor sprint	Passion
Bali Bali	Poonah pooh
Basra belly	Rangoon runs
Canary disease	Rome runs
Casablanca crud	San Franciscitis
Coeliac flux	Squitter
Delhi belly	Summer complaint
Emporiatic enteritis	Tokyo trots
GI's	Tourist trot
Greek gallop	Trotsky's
Gyppy (Egyptian) tummy	Travelers' diarrhea
Ho Chi Minhs	Turista
Hong Kong dog	Turkey trots
Maladie de la Mer Rouge	Zermattitis

Descriptions of TD are found from the Bible and other ancient sources. Consider this lamentation in Psalm 22, which is cited as an early description of TD: "I am poured out like water, and all my bones are out of joint, my heart is like wax; it is melted in the midst of my bowels, my strength is dried up like a potsherd." Over the centuries, when long-distance journeys were conducted mainly by sea, ship surgeons were specialists in TD. At the present time, tour guides and hotel concierges are called upon to organize consultations with local physicians, who regard TD as a major source of patients.

No other disease has attracted so many colorful monikers as TD: 32 are listed in Table 20.1–3. TD has been ascribed to spicy foods, change in the water, too much noonday sun, general vicissitudes of travel, or inhaled particles of sand. This list betrays a general theme: in the literature

Table 20.1–3.   GENERAL FEATURES OF TRAVELERS' DIARRHEA

Number one health problem in international tourism in terms of frequency and economic impact

Incidence depends on country of origin and destination: 20%–60% among travelers in Africa and Latin America, less than 10% in North America, Middle and South Europe, and Australia

Young adults (20–29 years) and small children have the highest incidence

No influence of gender

Onset of disease usually during the first week abroad; over 90% of cases occur before the end of the second week

In principle, many cases are preventable by precautions regarding food and drink, but great motivational problems exist

Several drug alternatives for treatment and prophylaxis

Recommendations: "Boil it, cook it, peel it - or forget it." Do not use routine antimicrobial prophylaxis, but start antimicrobial drugs and/or other agents when symptoms develop.

of travel, TD is mostly experienced during trips to exotic destinations, which are off the usual tourist routes. With the advent of modern transportation, TD is now associated with any trip to a developing country that has compromised sanitation and substandard food-handling facilities.

Serious scientific investigation of TD commenced during World War II. In 1943, Bulmer[9] observed in a military hospital in Egypt that the incidence of all diarrheal diseases declined with increasing length of service. This finding suggested the development of some immunity to TD. The same observation was made among U.S. Forces in the Middle East: the annual diarrhea rate per thousand decreased each year of service from 196, 170, 115, to 69.[8] Interestingly, African-American troops experienced less diarrheal disease than Caucasians.

In the 1950s, Ben Kean and his collaborators carried out extensive research on TD, and he is credited with establishing the scientific foundation on which subsequent research was based. The first study focused on the potential role of protozoa in the etiology of TD among American students visiting Europe.[10] Around 50% of nearly 600 participants developed diarrhea, but the 4% prevalence of *Entamoeba histolytica* in stool was the same on leaving and returning to the United States. There were no significant changes in the prevalence of other protozoa as well.

American tourists to Mexico and Hawaii were then investigated.[11] Although the two destinations had more or less similar climates, the incidence of TD among 1,265 tourists to Mexico was 33% versus 7.7% among those visiting Hawaii. This observation failed to support the view that climate is a significant factor in TD.

The hypothesis that TD could be an infectious disease inspired several studies in which antimicrobial agents were used to prevent the illness. In general,[12,13] although not invariably,[14] the experience was promising. Streptotriad, a tablet containing streptomycin, sulphadimidine, sulphathiazole, and sulphadiazine, was so effective that TD was proclaimed not to be a problem among the British Olympic teams in Rome in 1960 and Mexico City in 1968. It was proclaimed that "the UK deserved a special *no diarrhea* Gold medal!"[8]

Against the hypothesis of TD being an infectious disease contracted by the oral route was the experience that alimentary hygiene, no matter how rigorous, could not prevent all cases.

ETIOLOGY

An infectious etiology for TD was finally confirmed in the 1970s. Although suggested by Kean and collaborators,[12,15] the classic study was that of Rowe et al.[16] in which 540 British soldiers sent to Aden were investigated. Within the first 2 weeks, 7% of soldiers were stricken with TD; in 54%, a new *Escherichia coli*, serotype 0148K/H28, was isolated. This serotype was found in none of the healthy controls. This same *E. coli* strain was isolated from one of their laboratory technicians who developed diarrhea after handling the specimens, thereby establishing a causal connection with this organism. Some years later, the British finding was confirmed in American travelers.[17-19] Later studies have shown that *E. coli*, especially enterotoxigenic *E. coli* (ETEC), comprising several serotypes,[20] is the major cause of TD. ETEC is also a common pathogen among children in the endemic areas.[21] Indeed, it has been suggested that the magnitude of the TD problem locally can be estimated by studying the etiology of bacterial diarrhea in resident children.[22] Other etiologic agents include various pathogenic bacteria, protozoa, and viruses but very seldom helminths (Table 20.1-4).

A review of more than 20 reports on travelers to Mexico and other parts of Latin America, Asia, and Africa has shown that geographic differences exist among the culprits of TD (Table 20.1-5). In Latin America, for example, the median isolation rate of ETEC is about 40% (range 17% to 70%), whereas only 16% of TD in Asia (range 6% to 37%) is due to ETEC.[23]

Moreover, the causes of TD are not the same throughout the year. During the winter, Finnish tourists to Morocco developed *Campylobacter jejuni* in 46% of the bacteriologically confirmed cases, whereas ETEC took only the third place (14%) after *Salmonella* (16%) (Figure 20.1-1).[24] Not more than 15% of the study participants came down with illness. In contrast, one-third of such tourists developed TD in the fall. ETEC was the leading agent during this season, responsible for 56% of the cases, followed by *Salmonella* (44%). *Campylobacter* caused TD significantly more often in winter than in fall and ETEC and *Salmonella* significantly more often in fall than in winter. The differences are not explained by technical factors since the same laboratory was established locally in both seasons. It is possible that the difference in mean temperature played a role since campylobacteriacae survive better in cool circumstances.[25] This hypothesis is supported by observations of rotavirus diarrhea, which is a friend of cooler months and is more common in winter.

The Finnish experience agrees with that of other studies performed in Africa[26-28] in which ETEC was

responsible for only 36% of TD cases. Similarly, an investigation of TD in Thailand[29] found ETEC to be in third place (6%) after *Campylobacter* (41%) and *Salmonella* (18%). It seems that ETEC is a more common cause of TD in the New World than in Africa or Asia. If so, this has important implications for the development of appropriate antimicrobial drugs and vaccines for TD.

Vibrio cholerae is not an important agent in TD. There are very few descriptions of cholera as a cause of diarrhea in travelers.[30] Other vibrios, for example, *V. para-*

Table 20.1–4.   CAUSES OF TRAVELERS' DIARRHEA

ETIOLOGY	PERCENT ISOLATION
Bacteria	50–75
Escherichia coli	5–70
Enterotoxigenic (ETEC)	5–70
Enteroadhesive	?
Enteroinvasive	?
Campylobacter spp	0–30
Salmonella spp	0–15
Shigella	0–15
Aeromonas	0–10
Plesiomonas	0–5
Other	0–5
Protozoa	0–5
Giardia lamblia	0–5
Entamoeba histolytica	0–5
Cryptosporidium spp	?
*Cyclospora cayetanensis**	?
Viruses	0–20
Rotavirus	0–20
Calicivirus	0–10
Enteroviruses	?
No pathogen isolated	10–40

*Known as coccidian, cyanobacterium-like bodies or blue-green algae.

Table 20.1–5.   GEOGRAPHIC DISTRIBUTION OF PATHOGENS IN TRAVELERS' DIARRHEA

ORGANISM	LATIN AMERICA[18,42,62-67] (%)	ASIA[68-73] (%)	AFRICA[24,65,68,74,75] (%)	MIDDLE EAST[6,76] (%)
Enterotoxigenic *E. coli* (ETEC)	17–70	6–37	8–42	29–33
Enteroinvasive *E. coli*	2–7	2–3	0–2	1
Other *E. coli* (EPEC, EAEC, EHEC)	5–15	1	2–7	NA
Shigella spp	2–30	0–17	0–9	8–26
Salmonella spp	1–16	1–33	4–25	2
Camplylobacter jejuni	1–5	9–39	1–28	1–2
Aeromonas spp	1–5	1–57	0–9	1
Plesiomonas shigelloides	0–6	3–13	3–5	1
Vibrio cholerae non-O1	0–2	1–7	0–4	2
Yersinia spp	NA	0–3	NA	1
Rotavirus	0–6	1–8	0–36	NA
Entamoeba histolytica	NA	5–11	2–9	NA
Giardia lamblia	1–2	1–12	0–1	NA
Cryptosporidium	NA	1–5	2	NA
No pathogen identified	24–62	10–56	15–53	50–51

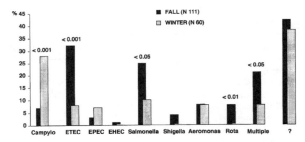

Figure 20.1–1. Bacteriologically proven etiology among Finnish tourists to Morocco in fall and winter 1989–1990. (Data from reference 24.) Significant differences indicate seasonal variation. The same individual could have more than one pathogen.

haemolyticus and *V. vulnificus,* can cause serious disease, especially in high-risk groups. Many patients with liver disease have died in the Gulf Coast states in the United States after eating raw oysters contaminated by *V. vulnificus.*[31]

Enteric pathogens other than bacteria are generally less important as a cause of TD. In some parts of the world, protozoa such as *Giardia*[32] or *Cryptosporidia,*[33,34] and during epidemic seasons, viruses such as rotavirus,[35] may be responsible for a considerable portion of TD cases.

A major problem in the interpretation of etiologic studies is that no pathogen has been identified in more than 40% of the cases, despite careful laboratory methodology. To add to the confusion, there is also a high incidence of mixed infections in which two or more pathogens are isolated from the initial stool specimen.

When no pathogen is identified by standard methods in TD, it is possible that known enteropathogens escape detection. Other potential pathogens should also be considered in such cases, for example, *Campylobacter upsaliensis* and *Campylobacter butzleri* among bacteria and astrovirus and coronaviruses, all of which can sometimes cause diarrhea in travelers. Processing several stool specimens per patient is likely to uncover more pathogens in cases of TD. Entirely new pathogens are also possible. A recent example is the coccidian or cyanobacterium-like protozoa with a proposed name *Cyclospora cayetanensis*[36] that causes severe TD in Nepal and elsewhere.[37]

It has been suggested that TD is caused by changes in normal flora without the introduction of enteric pathogens. There is a potential role for change in diet, excessive alcohol consumption, menstruation, or other factors that may induce gastrointestinal disturbances. It should not be forgotten, however, that the documented beneficial effect of prophylactic agents directed against bacterial pathogens in approximately 90% of recipients argues strongly that the majority of cases of TD are of bacterial origin.

PATHOGENESIS

The single most important etiologic agent is ETEC,[38–40] which excretes heat-labile toxin (LT), heat-stable toxin (ST), or both. Two types of genetic elements, usually plas-

mids, are required for pathogenicity in ETEC. The first type encodes for fimbria or some other structure on the outer membrane, which allows the bacterium to attach to the intestinal mucosa. The other type encodes for production of toxin.

The pathogenesis of LT-toxin producing ETEC and that of *V. cholerae* is similar, although not identical (Figure 20.1–2).[41] ETEC or *V. cholerae* colonizes the intestinal mucosa and produces toxin, causing watery diarrhea. LT, like cholera toxin, attaches to the GM_1 ganglioside of the epithelial cell, followed by release of the A-subunit of the toxin hexamer. The A-subunit penetrates the epithelial cell and stimulates adenyl cyclase, which increases concentrations of cyclic adenosine monophosphate (cAMP). The result is that the sodium-potassium pump function is disturbed and sodium is excreted actively into the lumen, along with transfer of water. Since reabsorption is less active, the patient develops diarrhea. ST toxins have a different chemical structure; instead of adenyl cyclase, they simulate guanylate cyclase.

The clinical picture caused by LT and ST toxins is similar, although ST toxin causes more vomiting and less diarrhea. The main site of activity in LT disease is the small intestine, whereas in ST disease both the small intestine and colon are involved. The clinical picture is not necessarily more severe when both LT and ST toxins are produced.

EPIDEMIOLOGY

COUNTRY OF ORIGIN AND DESTINATION

The risk factors associated with TD have been investigated adequately in only a few populations. The data are derived from studies of United States (mostly young) adult visitors to Mexico[6,10,11,17–19] and, to a lesser extent, other countries.[26–29] Among Europeans, Swiss and German,[2,42,43] Austrian,[44] British,[9,13,16,45–47] and Finnish travelers[3,24,32,33,48,49] have been studied most extensively.

An early clue that the geographic origin of the visitor could play a role in the incidence of TD came from an observation of political observers sent to Lebanon by the United Nations in 1958.[50] These officials were healthy

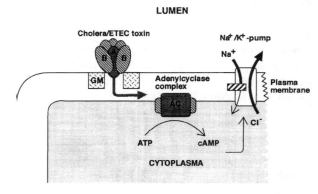

Figure 20.1–2. Activity of ETEC (LT and ST) toxins in the gastrointestinal epithelial cell mimics closely that of cholera toxin.

20- to 50-year-old men, 40% of whom fell ill if their home country was in Europe compared to 10% if the observers were from Asia or South America. Similar observations were made at international congresses in Teheran[51] and Mexico City,[19,52] where the intestinal well-being of the visitor was directly related to the country of origin. Again, Europeans and North Americans experienced more gastrointestinal distress than those from Asia, Africa, and South America.

A retrospective survey of almost 20,000 tourists, mostly from Switzerland and Germany, has produced many important findings on TD (Figure 20.1–3).[43] Over 30% of the travelers developed TD during their trip (mean length of the journey was 2 to 3 weeks). More than 80% of the respondents went on a vacation trip, so-called package tourism. This distribution accurately reflects the type of journey of the traveling public to the tropics and subtropics. Since the reporting rate was 82%, the data appear to be representative, although they probably underestimate more than exaggerate the reality.

When the destination was the United States or Canada, the risk of TD for a European was less than 5%; in contrast, TD rates of 25% to 30% occurred in trips to Latin America, up to 40% to Central Africa, and around 25% to Southeast Asia.

Great variations in the incidence of TD were observed in a more circumscribed geographic area when Finnish tourists traveled to the Mediterranean area and the Canary Islands.[3] On average, 18% of these Finnish travelers developed TD, but the incidence ranged from 10% or less in inland Spain and the Canary Islands to about 40% in Morocco. For others on a world tour and a West African cruise, the incidence was also 40% (Figure 20.1–4). These figures were higher than for a trip to Thailand, which was the only Asian country studied. The combined 34% incidence of TD in Egypt, Tunisia, and Morocco was significantly higher ($p < .001$) than the 5% to 10% incidence in mainland Spain or her islands.

On the basis of these studies, the world map can be divided into three major zones with regard to the incidence of TD for a traveler departing from the United States, Canada, Europe, and other industrialized areas.

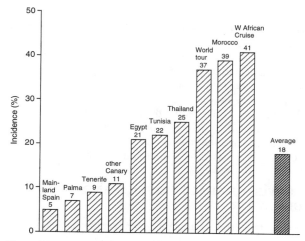

Figure 20.1–4. Increasing incidence of travelers' diarrhea among Finnish tourists (N = 2665) to destinations around the Mediterranean as compared to Thailand and a world tour. (Data from reference 3.)

The risk of TD is 7% or less when the destination is Middle Europe, the United States, Canada, Australia, or New Zealand. It increases to 20% when the destination is Southern Europe, Israel, Japan, South Africa, or certain Caribbean Islands. The highest incidence of TD, varying from 20% to 50%, prevails in trips to Africa, Latin America, the Middle East, and most parts of Asia.[2]

When a study team accompanies travelers on a journey, higher incidence rates are obtained from such prospective surveys than from retrospective questionnaires upon return: 53% in Latin America, 54% in Asia, and 54% in Africa, using the prospective study design.[23]

Previous visits to an endemic area have little influence on TD rates.[43,53] In the European series,[43] some protection from developing TD was associated with prior experience in developing countries, but the actual incidence rates were very close, 29.1% versus 32.3%. It seems that immunity gained by prior exposures to the causative agents of TD is of marginal value.

AGE AND GENDER

Most surveys of TD have concentrated on adult travelers. It appears that gender does not play a significant role in vulnerability to TD.[2,3,14,43] With regard to age, an observation from the 1950s[10] suggested that young adults are most prone to TD. This finding has been confirmed by several investigators, although not by all.[53] Beside the epidemiologic implications, it suggests a role for host factors in the pathogenesis of TD.

In the Swiss analysis,[43] there was a significant ($p < .0001$) difference between the 20- to 29-year-old versus older age groups. This finding has three possible explanations: young people are more liberal or experimental in their alimentary habits, their food consumption is greater, or they have less immunologic experience with the agents of TD than older people. Each of these factors could predispose younger people to infections of the gastrointestinal tract.

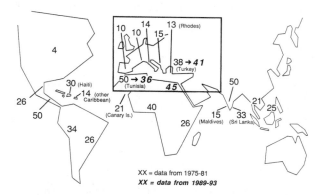

Figure 20.1–3. Incidence in percent of travelers' diarrhea within 2 weeks among 17,000 tourists from Middle Europe to various destinations. (Data from reference 43.)

In accordance with the general susceptibility of younger travelers, it appears that small children are even more vulnerable. In a retrospective Swiss survey[54] of children and adolescents, most with a destination in Latin America or Africa, TD occurred within 2 weeks in 40%, 9%, 22%, and 36% in the age groups of 0 to 2 years, 3 to 6 years, 7 to 14 years, and 15 to 20 years, respectively (Figure 20.1–5). Thereafter the incidence declined to 23% at the age of 70 years and more. Children of 3 to 6 years seemed to have the lowest risk of TD; this observation, however, was based on a small number (N = 47).

TRAVEL CHARACTERISTICS AND BEHAVIOR

It would be expected that the less adventurous the journey and the better the hotel, the lower the risk of TD. Although an upscale lifestyle should receive its just rewards, such is not the case. Indeed, it has been stated, ironically, that the more the traveler tries to avoid TD, the more likely he or she will fall victim to it.[2] This retrospective study suffered from having recall bias. High-standard hotels are not necessarily safer in terms of TD than low-priced hotels.[43] This is explained by the fact that salads, for example, are equally difficult to sterilize no matter how many stars the hotel carries in the gourmet guide book. The guest in a luxury hotel assumes unwarranted protection from TD in such surroundings. This is one of the illusions of the travel industry. The risk of TD in luxurious circumstances was manifest among travelers participating in a pricey West African cruise (see Figure 20.1–4).[3] Not less than 41% developed TD, a figure higher than that among tourists in mainland North Africa.

At least five studies[19,43,49,52,54] have addressed the question of whether the risk of TD could be reduced by consuming only foods and drinks that are generally considered safe: freshly prepared and steaming hot food, boiled or bottled drinks, dry bread, or peeled fruits. Except for one report,[42] the message is generally the same: dietary self-control is of little value in preventing TD. The principal problem is not the inability of dietary restrictions to prevent infection but the lack of motivation on the part of the traveler. Not more than 2% of the Swiss[42] and 5% of the Finnish travelers[49] were ready to adhere strictly to the accepted recommendations. No doubt, a high-quality water supply has a favorable effect on the risk of TD, as confirmed by studies of British tourists to Spain (Figure 20.1–6).[55]

Total nihilism is not justified, however. The adventurous travel style is not only associated with a higher risk of TD,[43,56] it has also been related to second attacks and multiple episodes of TD,[56] which are not common in the regular course of this disease. In addition, eating food from street vendors has been associated with an increased risk of TD,[57] where microbial contamination of food and beverage items is high.[58] Some investigators have been able to connect TD with risky foods such as steak tartare, raw oysters, puddings, and sandwiches with mixed fillings.[59] These associations were not generally observed among the Finnish tourists, although TD caused by *Campylobacter* sp was more common among those who had eaten steak tartare or salads.[60] It is also important to recommend dietary precautions in order to prevent other food- and water-borne infections, such as typhoid fever, brucellosis, polio, and bovine tuberculosis.

CLINICAL DISEASE

SYMPTOMS AND SIGNS

TD is easy to diagnose clinically: abrupt loose or watery bowel movement that forces the sufferer to seek relief immediately. The urgency can be so strong that fecal incontinence may occur. The following excerpt from Kean's classic article[15] captures the plight of the stricken traveler: "At 4 am he awakened with a start, desperately aware that he was about to move his bowels. He traversed the bed-to-bathroom distance in what must have been record time, and relieved himself of a totally watery bowel movement which was accompanied by slight 'transverse colon' cramps. The patient returned to bed in a stunned state, only to discover that no sooner had he arrived than he was constrained to leave again, with uncustomary alacrity. This stacatto ballet continued at 15-minute intervals with the patient exhibiting progressive weakness, profound malaise, increasingly severe cramps, almost constant nausea, and several episodes of vomiting."

TD does not begin right after arrival but toward the end of the first week in the endemic area.[2,60] Over 90% of

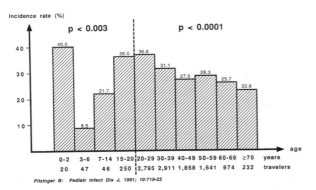

Figure 20.1–5. The risk of travelers' diarrhea in children less than 3 years of age. (Data from reference 53.)

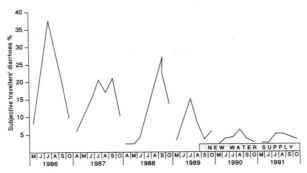

Figure 20.1–6.   Incidence of diarrhea among British tourists to Salou, Spain, before and after a new municipal water supply was installed. (Data from reference 55.)

the cases occur within 2 weeks. Most people have four to five loose stools a day, but at least 20% pass up to 20 watery motions over a 24-hour period.

Many symptoms and signs occur in the course of this disease. [5,44,60,61] Besides watery stools, fecal urgency and abdominal pain or tenesmus are experienced by almost all persons and cramps by more than half (see Table 20.1–2). Low-grade fever is found frequently, and it seems to be more common in cases with an identified pathogen occurring in 37% versus 18% in patients with no identified pathogen.[60] Mucus and blood are not seen in a typical case but are found more often in children with TD.[54] Headache, myalgia, and other general signs and symptoms are also common complaints.[60] The occurrence of nausea varies.

From a practical point of view, it is important to distinguish persons with potentially dangerous TD from those with the usual, milder presentation. Certain observations can be helpful. When TD presents with fever or with mucoid and/or bloody bowel movements, the condition is more severe. In Morocco,[60] where enteric pathogens were identified in 60% of TD cases, there was no difference in the groups with a positive culture in terms of onset of illness or the median frequency of stools during the first 24 hours; however, on the second and third days, the group with documented etiology experienced more diarrheal symptoms and excreted watery stools more frequently: 55% versus 28% in those without documented etiology. Diarrhea and the associated symptoms of nausea, abdominal pains, and, sometimes, fever lasted longer in patients with proven etiology than without.

Regarding the specific pathogens, TD caused by *Campylobacter* spp or *Shigella* tends to persist longer. In contrast, ETEC causes milder disease. Whether TD is caused by a single pathogen or several pathogens does not play a role in the type of symptoms or signs.

The average duration of TD in untreated subjects is 3 to 5 days, but the disease may persist throughout the stay.[2,3,5,61] Illness lasts more than 1 week in 8% to 15% of TD sufferers, and 2% develop chronic diarrhea lasting a month or more.[5]

Small children are more prone to severe and long-lasting illness. Limited data indicate that TD in children can persist for at least 3 weeks and can produce multiple relapses.[54]

Recovery from acute disease is likely to be shorter when the etiology cannot be identified. In one study,[60] TD persisted for 4 days or more in 50% when the pathogen was identified, whereas it abated within 2 days in 50% when the etiology was unconfirmed.

It is possible that a portion of TD without proven etiology is not caused by an infectious agent but rather by dietary indispositions related to chemical additives, heavy metals, or food intolerance. High intakes of fatty foods or alcohol can cause loose bowel movements in some individuals.

CONSEQUENCES OF TD

The observations that 20% to 30% of TD cases are confined to bed and 40% change their schedule due to TD[2,3,5,43] indicate that the disease is a major problem among travelers and can destroy a journey that is supposed to be recreational. Although local physicians are consulted frequently and medications are often prescribed, less than 1% of TD cases are referred to hospital. Reports of death are exceedingly rare. The average cost of a bout of TD was estimated to be $116.50 considering cost of medication and missed activites.

An epidemic can break out among a group of tourists and fatalities occur. The causative agent, however, is not a usual one of TD. Such was the case in an outbreak of *Salmonella typhimurium* among tourists in the Canary Islands in 1976 and in the cholera outbreak aboard a commercial airplane in 1992.[30] For most travelers, TD is an inconvenient and unwelcome interlude to their trip, which can be shortened with appropriate therapy.

REFERENCES

1. Gorbach SL. Travelers' diarrhea. In: Gorbach SL, Bartlett JG, Blacklow NR, eds. Infectious diseases. Philadelphia: WB Saunders, 1992:622–628.
2. Steffen R, van der Linde F, Gyr K, Schar M. Epidemiology of diarrhea in travelers. JAMA 1983;249:1176–1180.
3. Peltola H, Kyronseppä H, Hölsä P. Trips to the South—a health hazard. Morbidity of Finnish travellers. Scand J Infect Dis 1983;15:375–381.
4. Gorbach SL. Bacterial diarrhoea and its treatment. Lancet 1987;2:1378–1382.
5. Ericsson CD, Dupont HL. Travelers' diarrhea: approaches to prevention and treatment. Clin Infect Dis 1993;16:616–624.
6. DuPont HL, Ericsson CD, Mathewson JJ, et al. Oral aztreonam, a poorly absorbed yet effective therapy for bacterial diarrhea in US travelers to Mexico. JAMA 1992;267:1932–1935.
7. Hyams KC, Bourgeois AL, Merrell BR, et al. Diarrheal disease during Operation Desert Shield. N Engl J Med 1991;325:1423–1428.
8. Turner AC. Travellers diarrhoea. Ann Soc Belg Med Trop 1979;59:109–115.
9. Bulmer E. A survey of tropical diseases as seen in the Middle East. Trans R Soc Trop Med Hyg 1944;37:225–242.
10. Kean BH, Smillie WG. Intestinal protozoa of American travelers returning to the United States from Mexico. AMA Arch Ind Health 1958;18:148.
11. Kean BH, Waters SR. Incidence of diarrhea in travelers returning to the U.S. from Europe. AMA Arch Ind Health 1958;18:148.
12. Kean BH, Schaffner W, Brennan RW, Waters SR. The diarrhea of travelers. V. Prophylaxis with phthalylsulfathiazole and neomycin sulfate. JAMA 1962;180:367.
13. Turner AC. Traveller's diarrhoea: a survey of symptoms, occurrence, and possible prophylaxis. BMJ 1967;4:653–654.
14. Kean BH, Waters SR. The diarrhea of travelers. Drug prophylaxis in Mexico. N Engl J Med 1959;216:71–74.
15. Kean BH. The diarrhea of travelers to Mexico: summary of a five-year study. Ann Intern Med 1963;59:605.
16. Rowe B, Taylor J, Bettelheim KA. An investigation of traveller's diarrhoea. Lancet 1970;1:1–5.
17. Shore EG, Dean AG, Holik KJ, Davis BR. Enterotoxin-producing Escherichia coli and diarrheal disease in adult travelers: a prospective study. J Infect Dis 1974;129:577–582.
18. Gorbach SL, Kean BH, Evans DG, et al. Travelers' diarrhea and toxigenic Escherichia coli. N Engl J Med 1975;292:933–936.

19. Merson MH, Morris GK, Sack DA, et al. Travelers' diarrhea in Mexico. A prospective study of physicians and family members attending a congress. N Engl J Med 1976;294:1299–1305.

20. Levine MM. *Escherichia coli* that cause diarrhea: enterotoxigenic, enteropathogenic, enteroinvasive, enterohemorrhagic, and enteroadherent. J Infect Dis 1987;155:377–389.

21. Black RE, Merson MH, Huq I, et al. Incidence and severity of rotavirus and *Escherichia coli* diarrhoea in rural Bangladesh. Implications for vaccine development. Lancet 1981;1:141–143.

22. Sack RB. Treatment and prevention of travelers' diarrhea. In: Holmgren J, Lindberg A, Mollby R, eds. Development of vaccines and drugs against diarrhea. Lund, Sweden: Studentlitteratur, 1986:289–301.

23. Black RE. Epidemiology of travelers' diarrhea and relative importance of various pathogens. Rev Infect Dis 1990; 12(Suppl 1):S73–S79.

24. Mattila L, Siitonen A, Kyronseppä H, et al. Seasonal variation in etiology of travelers' diarrhea. Finnish-Moroccan Study Group. J Infect Dis 1992;165:385–388.

25. Shane SM, Montrose MS. The occurrence and significance of *Campylobacter jejuni* in man and animals. Vet Res Commun 1985;9:167–198.

26. Sack DA, Kaminsky DC, Sack RB, et al. Enterotoxigenic *Escherichia coli* diarrhea of travelers: a prospective study of American Peace Corps volunteers. Johns Hopkins Med J 1977;141:63–70.

27. Sack DA, Kaminsky DC, Sack RB, et al. Prophylactic doxycycline for travelers' diarrhea: results of a prospective double-blind study of Peace Corps volunteers in Kenya. N Engl J Med 1978;298:758–763.

28. Sack RB, Froehlich JL, Zulich AW, et al. Prophylactic doxycycline for travelers' diarrhea: results of a prospective double-blind study of Peace Corps volunteers in Morocco. Gastroenterology 1979;76:1368–1373.

29. Petruccelli BP, Murphy GS, Sanchez JL, et al. Treatment of traveler's diarrhea with ciprofloxacin and loperamide. J Infect Dis 1992;165:557–560.

30. Mascola L, Tormey M, Ewert D, et al. Cholera associated with an international airline flight. MMWR Morb Mortal Wkly Rep 1992;41:134–135.

31. Anonymous. *Vibrio vulnificus* infections associated with raw oyster consumption—Florida, 1981–1992. MMWR Morb Mortal Wkly Rep 1993;42: 405–407.

32. Hardie RM, Wall PG, Gott P, Bardhan M, Bartlett CLR. Infectious diarrhea in tourists staying in a resort hotel. Emerg Infect Dis 1999;5:168–171.

33. Jokipii L, Pohjola S, Jokipii AM. Cryptosporidiosis associated with traveling and giardiasis. Gastroenterology 1985; 89:838–842.

34. Gatti S, Cevini C, Bruno A, et al. Cryptosporidiosis in tourists returning from Egypt and the Island of Mauritius [letter]. Clin Infect Dis 1993;16:344.

35. Vollet JJ, Ericsson CD, Gibson G, et al. Human rotavirus in an adult population with travelers' diarrhea and its relationship to the location of food consumption. J Med Virol 1979;4:81–87.

36. Bendall RP, Lucas S, Moody A, et al. Diarrhoea associated with cyanobacterium-like bodies: a new coccidian enteritis of man. Lancet 1993;341:590–592.

37. Hoge CW, Shlim DR, Rajah R, et al. Epidemiology of diarrhoeal illness associated with coccidian-like organism among travellers and foreign residents in Nepal. Lancet 1993; 341:1175–1179.

38. Holmgren J, Svennerholm AM. Mechanisms of disease and immunity in cholera: a review. J Infect Dis 1977;136(Suppl): S105–S112.

39. Rowland HA. The pathogenesis of diarrhoea. Trans R Soc Trop Med Hyg 1978;72:289–302.

40. Field M, Rao MC, Chang EB. Intestinal electrolyte transport and diarrheal disease. N Engl J Med 1989;321:879–883.

41. Clements JD, Finkelstein RA. Demonstration of shared and unique immunological determinants in enterotoxins from *Vibrio cholerae* and *Escherichia coli*. Infect Immun 1978; 22:709–713.

42. Kozicki M, Steffen R, Schar M. 'Boil it, cook it, peel it or forget it': does this rule prevent travellers' diarrhoea? Int J Epidemiol 1985;14:169–172.

43. Steffen R. Epidemiologic studies of travelers' diarrhea, severe gastrointestinal infections, and cholera. Rev Infect Dis 1986;8(Suppl 2):S122–S130.

44. Kollaritsch H. Traveller's diarrhea among Austrian tourists in warm climate countries: I. Epidemiology. Eur J Epidemiol 1989;5:74–81.

45. Reid D, Dewar RD, Fallon RJ, et al. Infection and travel: the experience of package tourists and other travellers. J Infect 1980;2:365–370.

46. Cossar JH, Dewar RD, Reid D, Grist NR. Travel and health: illness associated with winter package holidays. J R Coll Gen Pract 1983;33:642–645.

47. Cartwright RY. Epidemiology of travellers' diarrhoea in British package holiday tourists. PHLS Microbiol Dig 1992;9:121–124.

48. Peltola H, Siitonen A, Kyronseppä H, et al. Prevention of travellers' diarrhoea by oral B-subunit/whole-cell cholera vaccine. Lancet 1991;338:1285–1289.

49. Mattila L, Siitonen A, Kyronseppä H, et al. Risk behaviour for traveler's diarrhea among Finnish travelers. J Travel Med 1995;2:77–84.

50. Haneveld D. Some epidemiological aspects of "travellers diarrhoea" in the Lebanon. Trop Geogr Med 1960;12:339–344.

51. Kean BH. Turista in Teheran. Travellers' diarrhoea at the 8th International Congresses of Tropical Medicine and Malaria. Lancet 1969;2:583–584.

52. Loewenstein MS, Balows A, Gangarosa EJ. Turista at an international congress in Mexico. Lancet 1973;1:529–531.

53. Ryder RW, Oquist CA, Greenberg H, et al. Travelers' diarrhea in Panamanian tourists in Mexico. J Infect Dis 1981;144: 442–448.

54. Pitzinger B, Steffen R, Tschopp A. Incidence and clinical features of traveler's diarrhea in infants and children. Pediatr Infect Dis J 1991;10:719–723.

55. Cartwright RY. Travellers' diarrhoea. Br Med Bull 1993;49: 348–362.

56. Bryant HE, Csokonay WM, Love M, Love EJ. Self-reported illness and risk behaviours amongst Canadian travellers while abroad. Can J Public Health 1991;82:316–319.

57. Tjoa WS, DuPont HL, Sullivan P, et al. Location of food consumption and travelers' diarrhea. Am J Epidemiol 1977; 106:61–66.

58. Sobel J, Mahon B, Mendoza CE, et al. Reduction of fecal contamination of street-vended beverages in Guatemala by a simple system for water purification and storage, hand washing, and beverage storage. Am J Trop Med Hyg 1998;59:380–387.

59. Kollaritsch H. Traveller's diarrhea among Austrian tourists to warm climate countries: II. Clinical features. Eur J Epidemiol 1989;5:355–362.

60. Mattila L. Clinical features and duration of travelers' diarrhea in relation to its etiology. Clin Infect Dis 1994;19:728–734.

61. DuPont HL, Galindo E, Evans DG, et al. Prevention of travelers' diarrhea with trimethoprim-sulfamethoxazole and trimethoprim alone. Gastroenterology 1983;84:75–80.

62. Mathewson JJ, Johnson PC, Dupont HL, et al. A newly recognized cause of travelers' diarrhea: enteroadherent *Escherichia coli*. J Infect Dis 1985;151:471–475.

63. DuPont HL, Reves RR, Galindo E, et al. Treatment of travelers' diarrhea with trimethoprim/sulfamethoxazole and with trimethoprim alone. N Engl J Med 1982;307:841–844.

64. Steffen R, Mathewson JJ, Ericsson CD, et al. Travelers' diarrhea in West Africa and Mexico: fecal transport systems and liquid bismuth subsalicylate for self-therapy. J Infect Dis 1988;157:1008–1013.

65. Wanger AR, Murray BE, Echeverria P, et al. Enteroinvasive *Escherichia coli* in travelers with diarrhea. J Infect Dis 1988;158:640–642.

66. DuPont HL, Ericsson CD, Mathewson JJ, et al. Zaldaride maleate, an intestinal calmodulin inhibitor, in the therapy of travelers' diarrhea. Gastroenterology 1993;104:709–715.

67. Bourgeois AL, Gardiner CH, Thornton SA, et al. Etiology of acute diarrhea among United States military personnel deployed to South America and west Africa. Am J Trop Med Hyg 1993;48:243–248.

68. Echeverria P, Blacklow NR, Sanford LB, Cukor GG. Travelers' diarrhea among American Peace Corps volunteers in rural Thailand. J Infect Dis 1981;143:767–771.

69. Speelman P, Struelens MJ, Sanyal SC, Glass RI. Detection of *Campylobacter jejuni* and other potential pathogens in travellers' diarrhoea in Bangladesh. Scand J Gastroenterol Suppl 1983;84:19–23.

70. Taylor DN, Echeverria P, Blaser MJ, et al. Polymicrobial aetiology of travellers' diarrhoea. Lancet 1985;1:381–383.

71. Taylor DN, Houston R, Shlim DR, et al. Etiology of diarrhea among travelers and foreign residents in Nepal. JAMA 1988;260:1245–1248.

72. Ahren CM, Jertborn M, Herclik L, et al. Infection with bacterial enteropathogens in Swedish travellers to South-East Asia—a prospective study. Epidemiol Infect 1990; 105:325–333.

73. Steffen R, Jori R, DuPont HL, et al. Fleroxacin, a long-acting fluoroquinolone, as effective therapy for travelers' diarrhea. Rev Infect Dis 1989;11:S1154–S1155.

74. Steffen R, Jori R, DuPont HL, et al. Efficacy and toxicity of fleroxacin in the treatment of travelers' diarrhea. Am J Med 1993;94:182S–186S

75. Haberberger Jr RL, Mikhail IA, Burans JP, et al. Travelers' diarrhea among United States military personnel during joint American-Egyptian armed forces exercises in Cairo, Egypt. Mil Med 1991;156:27–30.

76. Steffen R, Colland F, Tornieporth N, et al. Epidemiology, etiology, and impact of traveler's diarrhea in Jamaica. 1999;281: 811–817.

20.2 PREVENTION OF TRAVELERS' DIARRHEA: RISK AVOIDANCE AND CHEMOPROPHYLAXIS

CHARLES D. ERICSSON AND LEENA MATTILA

Travelers' diarrhea is a syndrome caused by many enteropathogens. Preliminary approaches to immunologic protection against the most common cause of travelers' diarrhea, enterotoxigenic *Escherichia coli* (ETEC), have been promising. However, vaccinees will still remain at risk for many other causative agents of travelers' diarrhea. Prevention of travelers' diarrhea must be weighted against highly efficacious treatment. Such treatment now results in upwards of 60% of ill persons passing no unformed stools after the first dose of therapy and over 90% becoming well within 24 hours.[1–3]

Prevention includes minimizing risks of developing diarrhea by careful selection of food and water, chemoprophylactic agents such as bismuth subsalicylate (BSS) or antimicrobial agents, boosting colonization resistance by taking *Lactobacillus* preparations, and avoidance of travel.

In the final analysis, prevention modalities in the control of travelers' diarrhea will not be necessary when host countries improve standards of public health and resorts within a developing country insist on their own hygienic controls.

RISK AVOIDANCE AND EDUCATION

ISSUES FAVORING EDUCATION

In developing countries, opportunities for breaks in the food hygiene chain are numerous. Moreover, public health services are often limited in developing countries. For this reason, knowledgeable officials are unable to inspect and guarantee the hygienic condition of all food establishments

Even though indirect transmission is probably the main route, direct person-to-person spread may also occur with some of these agents. For example, low infectious dose pathogens, such as *Rotavirus* or *Shigella*, may spread person to person by hands or by swallowing water while swimming. Contaminated food is the most important vehicle for transmission of all of the main travelers' diarrhea pathogens, especially those with a high infectious dose. In addition, water-borne gastroenteritis due to enterotoxigenic *Escherichia coli*, *Salmonella* spp, *Campylobacter* spp, or *Giardia lamblia* have been documented. Fecal-oral spread of gastrointestinal infections can occur by contact with fingers or lips or by contaminated utensils, kettles, porous wooden cutting surfaces, or dish towels

High numbers of enteropathogenic organisms have been found in foods associated with high attack rates of travelers' diarrhea. Flies are plentiful in open-air markets and have been incriminated in the transmission of *Shigella*.[4] The surfaces of fresh fruits and vegetables should be considered contaminated. Raw dishes such as ceviche and sashimi are popular but are a risk for infection with hepatitis A or *Vibrio* spp. Reheating food that was cross-contaminated but not stored at refrigeration temperatures can lead to enteric syndromes such as staphylococcal food poisoning due to heat-stable toxin. Temperatures about 160°F (71°C) are required to reliably kill microorganisms in food.[5] Food at this temperature is too hot to eat without first letting it cool.

Water and ice made from untreated water can be contaminated with enteric viruses, fecal coliforms, parasites such as *Giardia and Cryptosporidium,* and occasionally classic bacterial organisms such as *Salmonella typhi.* Water appears to be important in the transmission of wintertime diarrhea in locations such as inland Mexico. During winter in these locations, bacterial enteropathogens are much less frequently isolated than in the summer. Jugs of water found in hotel rooms should be assumed to contain tap water. Large bottles of water that are delivered to homes are usually safe, but the reusable bottles might not be cleaned sufficiently and are sometimes even filled with tap water. Clay filters do not reliably remove microorganisms and cysts from water.

Cholera is an emotionally charged issue that can be used to secure the attention of clients during pretravel education. Risk of cholera is very low for most travelers but higher in those who live or work in conditions of abject poverty. If travelers elect to take chemoprophylaxis, they are well advised to learn about food and water and to practice caution in their eating habits. In one study when travelers took prophylactic BSS, they were more protected from disease when they also exercised care in where they ate.[6]

On the other hand, some studies of the effect of dietary self-restrictions on the incidence of diarrhea have demonstrated no or only limited benefit of education.[7,8] Perhaps educators have not been creative enough in their choice of methods and the tools they used. Furthermore, they may not have spent enough time with the traveler. On the other hand, who pays for the extra time and effort required for better education? In centrally and cost-regulated systems, the provider may be reluctant to provide much more for travelers' diarrhea than a prescription for self-therapy.

APPROACH TO EDUCATION

Whether professional time is spent with travelers or educational pamphlets are supplied or recommended, certain principles should be stressed.

Food Persons living for a while in a country usually know about safe restaurants, and this advice should be heeded. Simple principles of food hygiene must be understood. "Heat kills germs" is a helpful learning tool. A nuance that sometimes escapes the traveler is that food should be thoroughly cooked. This is especially true of minced meat that can still harbor enteric pathogens if its center is not thoroughly cooked. "Dry things are safe" is advice that is grounded in the observation that most microorganisms require a moist environment to multiply. The phrase "think twice before anything raw enters your mouth" helps the traveler remember to avoid raw vegetables, especially salads, and raw seafood such as shellfish. "Items that can be peeled are safe." Travelers might worry about cutting open a melon because the knife might have carried exterior enteric organisms onto the interior fruit that is eaten. This is technically true, but the number of organisms is probably low. The principle taught should be to minimize risks and not to eliminate them entirely. Cleaning and soaking vegetables can be accomplished safely if the traveler has access to a kitchen with a reliable water source. However, this is frequently not the case for short-term travelers for whom the advice must ideally be no salads, cold sauces, cold desserts, and any similar cool, moist food item. Table 20.2–1 lists common foods, beverages, and culinary practices by their probable safety category.

Water Short-term travelers are wise to drink water from well-labeled, sealed containers. Bottled water, particularly carbonated water, and other beverages are usually safe. For trekkers and others needing to purify surface water for drinking, several approaches are feasible. Rather than boiling water for a full 5 to 10 minutes, which is the conservative recommendation, water can be effectively sterilized by bringing it to a roiling boil for 1 minute, then covering the pot and allowing it to cool to room temperature. The option of boiling is often limited by the availability of fuel. Iodine tablets or liquid can be used to disinfect water. Successful iodine disinfection depends on first filtering water of particulate matter and then exposing the clarified water to iodine for enough time, at the specified ambient temperature (e.g., 20 minutes at room temperature). Chlorine is not a satisfactory disinfectant; *Giardia and Cryptosporidium* can still be transmitted in chlorinated water. Newer technology employs silver, iodine resins, or reverse osmosis. These technologies appear to yield water that is safe even from virus contamination. However, most commercially available filters (0.2 μ) cannot reliably remove viruses if used without another modality like iodine or silver.

When ice is made from tap water, it should be avoided even when used in alcoholic beverages. This is because the alcohol kills the enteropathogens too slowly to be helpful during the time a traveler normally imbibes an alcoholic beverage.[9] Machine-made ice that comes in a labeled plastic container is probably safe.

General Hygiene Since fecal organisms cause travelers' diarrhea, travelers are well advised to wash and

Table 20.2–1.   RELATIVE SAFETY OF FOOD, BEVERAGES, AND CULINARY PRACTICES

	SAFE		PROBABLY SAFE	UNSAFE	
Food	Piping hot		Dry	Cold salads	Some cold desserts
	Peeled fruit		Jelly/syrup	Sauces	Fresh soft cheese
	Processed/packaged		Washed vegetables	Hamburgers	Raspberries/strawberries
	Cooked vegetables			Unpeeled fruit	
Beverages	Irradiated milk		Fresh citrus juices	Tap water	Alcohol and chipped ice
	Boiled water		Packaged ice	Uncarbonated, bottled fruit juices	Unpasteurized milk or butter*
	Iodized water		Bottled water	Chipped ice	
	Carbonated				
Dietary practices	Careful		Recommended restaurants	Adventuresome	Buffet food at room temperature
	Consider heat of food		Judicious alcohol	Vendors	Excessive alcohol

*Also *Brucella* risk.

dry hands frequently during a trip, especially after using public or shared toilets. Since soap and running water might not be available in some locations, travelers are wise to carry facial tissues for wiping after defecation and prepackaged moistened "wash-towelettes" or tubes of alcohol gel as a means for washing hands

NATURAL IMMUNITY

Persons indigenous to developing countries have immunity to a number of enteric pathogens, especially ETEC. Although they continue to be exposed and become transiently colonized, they no longer develop ETEC disease. Expatriates, long-term travelers, or frequent travelers are probably best served by not taking prophylaxis and by not treating mild diarrhea with an antimicrobial agent. Mild diarrhea that is characterized by passage of only one or two loose stools per 24 hours is quite short-lived, lasting on average only 1 to 2 days.[10] Not treating mild diarrhea predictably might promote the development of natural immunity.

CHEMOPROPHYLAXIS

ISSUES FAVORING CHEMOPROPHYLAXIS

Certain antibacterial agents afford up to 90%, and BSS about 65%, protection against TD.[3] *Lactobacillus* preparations have also been used to prevent diarrhea. Used as drugs, they promote colonization resistance and prevent the growth of potential enteropathogens to the level of an effective pathogenic inoculum. Studies of earlier *Lactobacillus* preparations have proven largely ineffective in preventing travelers' diarrhea. *Lactobacillus* GG, a colonizer isolated from humans, has shown modest utility in the prevention of travelers' diarrhea.[11,12] Lactobacilli that have been genetically engineered to be avid colonizers

might prove to be even more efficacious than *Lactobacillus* GG.

The Consensus Development Conference (CDC) in 1985 decided not to recommend chemoprophylaxis with either BSS or antimicrobial agents.[13] Approaching the problem as public health policy, they reasoned that the travelers' diarrhea was self-limiting and not life-threatening. As a consequence, adverse drug reactions of chemoprophylactic agents and the possibility that patients might abuse over-the-counter medications recommended against chemoprophylaxis. Recent recommendations have focused on a balanced risk-benefit assessment achieved by discussion with the traveler.[14,15] Factors to consider include the traveler's health status, the importance of the trip, the traveler's wishes, and the willingness of the traveler to follow guidelines on food and beverage selection.

Chemoprophylaxis probably should be offered to "at-risk hosts." For other travelers, we suggest that chemoprophylaxis be discussed only if the client raises the issue. The provider should probably steer most travelers to use empiric self-treatment rather than chemoprophylaxis.

The risk status of the host and the criticality of a trip should be used to decide whether to give BSS or an antimicrobial agent as chemoprophylaxis. Antimicrobial agents are recommended by some for travelers at highest risk for diarrhea or at known special risk for the consequences of diarrhea. Antimicrobial agents should be considered for subjects with decreased gastric acidity (whether inherently present or due to use of potent, long-acting H_2 blockers or proton pump inhibitors) and those with immunodeficiency (e.g., HIV infection). Antimicrobial prophylaxis should be considered also for those with underlying inflammatory bowel disease such as Crohn's disease or ulcerative colitis and for those with underlying medical illness, in whom an episode of diarrhea might precipitate a decompensation in their medical condition. Travelers known to be positive for human leukocyte antigen HLA-B27 should probably receive antimicrobial prophylaxis with a fluoroquinolone.

This is to lessen the risk of reactive arthritis by preventing infection by *Shigella, Salmonella,* and *Campylobacter.* Children less than 6 years of age are at greater risk than older children, probably because young children frequently put their environment in their mouth. Nevertheless, pediatricians generally avoid chemoprophylaxis in children and favor educating parents.[16]

CHEMOPROPHYLACTIC AGENTS

The currently recommended chemoprophylactic agents and their doses in adults are listed in Table 20.2–2. Chemoprophylaxis is not recommended for children. Any prophylactic agent should be started on the day of travel and continued daily for 2 days after leaving the at-risk region. This approach, although inadequately studied, helps to guarantee that the traveler is protected against airline food that might be contaminated. In addition, it effectively treats recently ingested enteric pathogens. Prophylactic agents have been studied for periods as long as 3 weeks, during which they appear to be safe. Chemoprophylaxis cannot be recommended for periods longer than 3 weeks because the potential for adverse reactions is unknown. Furthermore, longer-term travelers should be allowed to develop natural immunity.

Doxycycline is not listed in Table 20.2–2, because resistance to it is found in most parts of the world and limits its value. In addition, a specific recommendation for *Lactobacillus* has not been made because most preparations are still poorly studied. Furthermore, activated charcoal cannot be recommended as a prophylactic agent due to its lack of efficacy.

Bismuth Subsalicylate   A number of studies have confirmed the effectiveness of BSS-containing products in the prophylaxis of travelers' diarrhea.[17,18] The product appears to be most efficacious when given four times a day. The likelihood is that BSS must be ingested simultaneously with contaminated food or beverages to achieve the maximal antimicrobial effect of BSS. When the same total dose that provided 65% protection was taken in

two divided doses instead of four, protection decreased to 40%.

Travelers should not take therapeutic doses of "aspirin" when they take BSS because of the risk of salicylate poisoning. The use of BSS is best avoided by persons needing anticoagulation. This is because of the possibility of its interaction with warfarin. To avoid the distressing black tongue, travelers are asked to brush their teeth and tongue after the nighttime BSS dose and then rinse thoroughly.

Antimicrobials   When antimicrobial agents like fluoroquinolones are uniformly active against enteropathogens and when they are taken as a single dose daily, they predictably provide up to 90% protection.[19] Smaller doses might be sufficient but have not been adequately studied. In the author's experience (CDE), taking one dose of an antimicrobial agent only after ingesting a suspect meal is an effective approach to preventing diarrhea; however, this concept needs to be studied before a recommendation can be made.

ARGUMENTS AGAINST CHEMOPROPHYLAXIS

Adverse Reactions   Potential adverse drug reactions of chemoprophylactic agents are probably the strongest argument against routine prophylaxis for travelers' diarrhea (Table 20.2–3). Among the millions of travelers each year, serious and life-threatening reactions to chemoprophylaxis are likely to occur and a few might even die.

Use of BSS can lead to tinnitus even when the blood salicylate level is within the therapeutic range. Furthermore, black stools and tongue can occur as a result of the dissociation of BSS and subsequent formation of pigmented bismuth salts. Both conditions are harmless; however, the uninformed traveler might seek medical attention for presumed melena. Use of other bismuth salts (e.g., subgallate and subnitrate) can lead to a high bismuth blood level and serious adverse reaction (e.g., encephalo-

Table 20.2–2.   AGENTS RECOMMENDED FOR THE PREVENTION OF TRAVELERS' DIARRHEA

AGENT	% PROTECTION	DOSING REGIMEN	COMMENTS
Bismuth subsalicylate preparations	~65	Two 262 mg tablets chewed 4 times a day	Rinse mouth to avoid black tongue; do not use therapeutic doses of aspirin simultaneously
Trimethoprim-sulfamethoxazole	~70–80*	One double-strength tablet daily	Rising resistance worldwide
Fluoroquinolones	~90		Reserve for self-therapy
Norfloxacin		400 mg daily	
Ciprofloxacin		500 mg daily	
Ofloxacin		200–300 mg daily	
Levofloxacin		500 mg daily	

*In areas where *Campylobacter* is prevalent (e.g., Southeast Asia), protection can be predicted to be even lower.

Table 20.2–3.   CONSIDERATION OF ADVERSE REACTIONS IN THE CHOICE OF AGENTS FOR THE PREVENTION OF TRAVELERS' DIARRHEA

	FLUOROQUINOLONE (%)	BISMUTH SUBSALICYLATE (%)
Major side effects	0.01	0
Minor side effects	3	1
Protection against diarrhea	~90*	~65

*Efficacy for trimethoprim-sulfamethoxazole is lower.

pathy). Adverse drug reactions involving the central nervous system with BSS are otherwise exceedingly rare and have not been reported in healthy travelers using the product for less than 3 weeks.

Adverse reactions of other antimicrobial agents such as trimethoprim-sulfamethoxazole, doxycycline, or fluoroquinolones are more frequent and severe compared to those with BSS. These reactions include transient rashes such as sun sensitivity rash, vaginal candidiasis, and, ironically, gastrointestinal upset. Severe reactions may also occur, and these comprise anaphylaxis, death, and conditions such as Stevens-Johnson syndrome that are felt to occur in as many as 1 in 10,000 persons exposed to sulfonamide-containing products.[20]

Antimicrobial agents change the intestinal flora. Furthermore, changes in the anaerobic flora may cause long-term alterations in the metabolism of bile acids and pancreatic enzymes, although clinical effects are unknown. Overgrowth of *Clostridium difficile* with the subsequent development of colitis can rarely occur among travelers taking an antimicrobial agent for chemoprophylaxis. Antibiotic-associated colitis should enter into the decision-making evaluation process of diarrhea occurring despite antimicrobial agent prophylaxis.

To minimize potential adverse reactions, some practitioners advise taking *Lactobacillus* preparations along with antimicrobial agents. Although this practice is safe, its usefulness is uncertain. Women who know they develop *Candida* vaginitis easily should be prepared to treat themselves against such an outbreak.

Antimicrobial Resistance   In the past decade, a high level of bacterial resistance to commonly used antibiotics such as doxycycline and trimethoprim-sulfamethoxazole has been demonstrated in various parts of the world. Quinolone resistance has also been increasing both in the developed and the developing world due to wide use of these drugs. However, antimicrobial resistance occurs more frequently in developing countries. A major reason for this might be the widespread use of subtherapeutic doses of antimicrobial agents in countries where the drugs can be bought without prescription and are used indiscriminately. Compared to the effects of the abuse by indigenous populations of developing countries, the contribution to the local bacterial ecology by travelers must be miniscule.

The antimicrobial agent, which has the least antimicrobial resistance, is predictably the best antimicrobial for prophylaxis and therapy. Quinolones, for instance, might be the best for therapy, whereas trimethoprim-sulfamethoxazole might be preferred for prophylaxis despite its higher level of resistance and less protective benefit.[21]

The use of antimicrobial agents, especially those with anti-anaerobe activity, can even promote the development of infection by certain enteropathogens, namely, *Salmonella* and *Campylobacter*. The mechanism for this is not entirely clear but might include decreasing colonization resistance in the gut lumen and the in vivo development of resistance to that antimicrobial agent.

Costs   A classic comparison of the costs of chemoprophylaxis compared with the costs of self-treatment of diarrhea concluded that chemoprophylaxis was more cost effective for short-term travel.[20] The greatest costs were due to lost vacation time and the amortized costs of travel. Since the publication of that study, self-therapy with loperamide and an antimicrobial has proven so effective that lost vacation time due to diarrhea is minimal. Presently, self-therapy is usually cost beneficial when compared with prophylaxis. Future use of vaccines that protect against *E. coli*-mediated diarrhea will lessen the overall risk of travelers' diarrhea and make self-treatment of diarrhea even more appealing.

Complacency   The recommended antimicrobial agents do not protect against parasitic or viral disease, which together can account for over 10% of travelers' diarrhea. Routine use of chemoprophylaxis might engender complacency in eating habits and thereby cause a relative rise in the incidence of parasitic and viral diseases.

Interference with Malaria Prophylaxis   BSS is known to interfere with the absorption of doxycycline.[22] Regular use of BSS might lower circulating doxycycline blood levels and thereby increase the risk of malaria. If the two agents are ever used together, their administration should be separated by at least 2 hours.

IMMUNOLOGIC PROTECTION

Efficacious vaccines have been developed for cholera and typhoid (Chapter 22). However, both diseases are rare among travelers. A B-subunit whole cholera vaccine significantly protects against enterotoxigenic *E. coli* (ETEC) disease; however, this protection is considerably less than that achieved by antimicrobial agents. In one study, vaccine protection extended to some non-ETEC strains as well.[23] Vaccines directed specifically at ETEC and their colonization fimbriae promise to afford better protection. Development is ongoing. An effective ETEC vaccine is still unlikely to prevent more than about 50% of travelers' diarrhea. Vaccines against other enteropathogens such as *Shigella* are in early development.

Table 20.2–4. APPROACH TO PREVENTION OF TRAVELERS' DIARRHEA

Educate about risk factors

Vaccinate long-term or repeated short-term travelers

Typhoid vaccine

Other vaccines like newer cholera and *Shigella* vaccines as they become available

Chemoprophylaxis:

Physician initiated because of at-risk host or critical trip:

• Consider antimicrobial or BSS

Client initiated because of perceived critical trip:

• Consider BSS, possibly antimicrobial

Client initiated because of adventuresome eating habits, unwillingness to restrict diet, or preference for chemoprophylaxis:

• Consider BSS

Arm traveler with self-therapy medications

Loperamide

Fluoroquinolone

Bovine immunoglobulins from the colostrum of immunized cows have been shown to be effective in preventing disease by specific ETEC challenge strains. However, commercial development of this approach to passive immunity has not materialized. Furthermore, because of the large number of causes of travelers' diarrhea, immunologic protection is unlikely to supplant chemoprophylaxis or self-therapy in the immediate future.

As a rule, immunologic protection is preferred over chemoprophylaxis or empirical therapy. As enteric vaccines become available, the issue will likely be the cost of preventing a proportion of travelers' diarrhea. Travelers will still need to carry self-therapy medicines for treatment of any illness caused by enteropathogens that are not covered by the vaccine.

ALGORITHMIC APPROACH TO PREVENTION

The authors' consensus approach to diarrhea prevention is shown in Table 20.2–4. Providers must decide for themselves how comprehensively to provide education about risk factors. Providers must also decide whether they will raise the issue of chemoprophylaxis with all travelers, with at-risk travelers, or not at all or will respond only when asked. The authors' approach is to raise the issue with hosts who are at risk and when the itinerary seems overtly critical. For all other travelers, we prefer empirical self-therapy, although we realize that some providers might prefer to offer prophylaxis to all travelers. We feel that the critical issue is that the traveler be fully informed of the risks and benefits including the option of self-therapy.

REFERENCES

1. Ericsson CD, DuPont HL. Travelers' diarrhea: approaches to prevention and treatment. Clin Infect Dis 1993;16:616–626.
2. Ericsson CD, Nicholls-Vasquez I, DuPont HL, et al. Optimal dosing of trimethoprim/sulfamethoxazole when used with loperamide to treat travelers' diarrhea. Antimicrob Agents Chemother 1992;36:2821–2824.
3. DuPont HL, Ericsson CD. Prevention and treatment of travelers' diarrhea. N Engl J Med 1993;328:1821–1827.
4. Watt J, Lindsay D. Diarrheal disease control studies. 1. Effect of fly control in a high morbidity area. Public Health Rep 1948;63:1319.
5. Bandres JC, Mathewson JJ, DuPont HL. Heat susceptibility of bacterial enteropathogens: implications for the prevention of travelers' diarrhea. Arch Intern Med 1988;148:2261–2263.
6. Ericsson CD, Pickering LK, Sullivan P, et al. The role of location of food consumption in the prevention of travelers' diarrhea in Mexico. Gastroenterology 1980;79:812–816.
7. Kozicki M, Steffen R, Schär M. "Boil it, cook it, peel it or forget it:" does this rule prevent travellers' diarrhoea? Int J Epidemiol 1985;14:169–172.
8. Mattila L, Siitonen A, Kyrönseppä H. et al. Risk behavior for travelers' diarrhea among Finnish travelers. J Travel Med 1995;2:77–84.
9. Dickens DL, DuPont HL, Johnson PC. Survival of bacterial enteropathogens in the ice of popular drinks. JAMA 1985;253:3141–3143.
10. Ericsson CD, DuPont HL, Mathewson JJ. Epidemiologic observations of diarrhea developing in U.S. and Mexican students in Guadalajara, Mexico. J Travel Med 1995;2:6–10.
11. Hilton E, Kolakowski P, Singer C, Smith M. Efficacy of *Lactobacillus* GG as a diarrheal preventive in travelers. J Travel Med 1997;4:41–43.
12. DuPont HL. *Lactobacillus* GG in prevention of travelers' diarrhea: an encouraging first step. J Travel Med 1997;4:1–2.
13. Gorbach SL, Edelman R, eds. Travelers' diarrhea: National Institutes of Health Consensus Development Conference. Rev Infect Dis 1986;8:(Suppl 2):S109–S233.
14. DuPont HL, Khan FM. Travelers' diarrhea: epidemiology, microbiology, prevention, and therapy. J Travel Med 1994;1:84–93.
15. Ericsson CD, Kass R, Steffen R. Chemoprophylaxis for travelers' diarrhea: consensus. J Travel Med 1994;1:221–225.
16. Hayani KC, Ericsson CD, Pickering LK. Prevention and treatment of diarrhea in the traveling child. Semin Pediatr Infect Dis 1992;3:22–32.
17. DuPont HL, Ericsson CD, Johnson PC, et al. Prevention of travelers' diarrhea by the tablet formulation of bismuth subsalicylate. JAMA 1987;257:1347–1350.
18. Steffen R, DuPont HL, Heusser R, et al. Prevention of travelers' diarrhea by the tablet form of bismuth subsalicylate. Antimicrob Agents Chemother 1986;29:625–629.
19. Heck JE, Staneck JL, Cohen MB, et al. Prevention of travelers' diarrhea: ciprofloxacin versus trimethoprim/sulfamethoxazole in adult volunteers working in Latin America and the Caribbean. J Travel Med 1994;1:36–42.
20. Reves RR, Johnson PC, Ericsson CD, et al. A cost effectiveness comparison of the use of antimicrobial agents for treatment or prophylaxis of travelers' diarrhea. Arch Intern Med 1981;148:2421–2427.
21. Taylor DN. Quinolones as chemoprophylactic agents for travelers' diarrhea. J Travel Med 1994;1:119–121.
22. Ericsson CD, Feldman S, Pickering LK, et al. Influence of subsalicylate bismuth on absorption of doxycycline. JAMA 1982;247:2266–2267.
23. Peltola H, Siitonen A, Kyrönseppä H, et al. Prevention of travellers' diarrhoea by oral B-subunit/whole cell cholera vaccine. Lancet 1991;338:1285–1289.

20.3 TREATMENT OF TRAVELERS' DIARRHEA

GERALD S. MURPHY, BRUNO P. PETRUCCELLI, HERWIG KOLLARITSCH, AND DAVID N. TAYLOR

INTRODUCTION

Diarrhea is the most common health problem encountered by travelers, affecting 20% to 50% of those going to developing tropical and subtropical lands.[1-4] Travelers' diarrhea (TD) commonly lasts 3 to 5 days, and 90% of cases have resolved after 1 week.[1] Although generally a self-limited illness, TD can ruin a vacation or business trip. Many travelers are concerned about this and desire to know how to prevent or treat the condition. The most important risk factors for TD are difficult to modify. These include younger age, duration of stay, eating in restaurants, and the season during which travel takes place.[1,3,5] Studies of tourists have shown that dietary restriction is not associated with a lower incidence of TD.[1] This may be because it is difficult to completely avoid contaminated food and drink.[2] Given that most TD cannot be prevented, it is prudent to discuss treatment options with prospective travelers.

Kean noted in his classic studies on TD in the 1950s that persons who received oral neomycin during travel had a lower likelihood of developing TD than persons who did not receive antibiotics.[6] This observation suggested that bacterial pathogens caused TD, but antimicrobial treatment of TD did not become widespread until the early 1970s. During that decade, it became clear that enterotoxigenic *Escherichia coli* (ETEC) was a predominant cause of TD in much of the developing world.[7,8] The discovery of ETEC initiated 20 years of research and debate on the management of TD. During this period, antimotility, antisecretory, and adsorbent compounds were compared to each other and to antibiotic therapy. During the 1980s and early 1990s, fluoroquinolone (FQ) antibiotics proved that a single agent could effectively treat ETEC and most other causes of TD. Studies in the past decade have shown that the combination of an antibiotic to which the etiologic organism is susceptible plus the antimotility agent, loperamide, can reduce most cases of TD to just a few hours of discomfort. Travelers who have suffered for days with intestinal cramps or spent much of their vacation time touring restrooms in developing countries would gladly spend a few dollars to reduce their illness from days to hours. With the advent of this simple and highly effective therapy, self-administered treatment has become the preferred course for travelers going to the developing world.[2,4]

This chapter reviews the medications available to treat TD, discusses the common syndromes of TD, and gives a general approach to the patient. It updates resistance data on the most important bacteria, gives brief advice on the special issues of pediatric, pregnant, and immunocompromised travelers, and ends with suggestions for pretravel counseling about self-administered, standby therapy.

NONSPECIFIC THERAPEUTIC AGENTS

ORAL REHYDRATION AND DIETARY RECOMMENDATIONS

Although diarrheal illnesses are leading causes of infant mortality worldwide, diarrhea is rarely life threatening in travelers. Nevertheless, rehydration and restoration of normal electrolyte concentrations are important components of TD therapy.[4] The essential ingredients for effective oral rehydration are potable water, a glucose source, sodium and potassium ions, and either bicarbonate or citrate (Table 20.3–1). The net absorption of water and sodium is ensured by the cotransport effect of glucose and aided by the hypotonicity of the oral solution.[9] As long as excessive intake of salts relative to water is avoided, a careful titration of the above ingredients is unnecessary for the majority of TD cases in adults and children over the age of 2 years. Thus, emphasis should be placed on drinking solutions that are found palatable and contain some replacement salts and glucose. Fruit juices or soft drinks plus saltine crackers are usually sufficient. Caffeine should probably be minimized due to its diuretic effect.

The proportion of ingredients, including potassium and chloride, is particularly important for treating TD in children under 2 years of age. For these patients, fruit juices and soft drinks do not provide adequate electrolytes relative to their high sugar content. Prepared ingredients in the correct proportions are available commercially as solutions or as powders for reconstitution.[10] Alternatively, a rehydration solution can be made up from basic ingredients as outlined in Table 20.3–2.

Oral rehydration does not decrease the amount and duration of diarrhea and is perceived by many as counterintuitive.[11] Thirst may be an inadequate indicator of fluid requirements during an episode of diarrhea. For these reasons, patients may need encouragement to drink fluids. Severe cases of secretory diarrhea, or diarrhea associated with persistent vomiting, may require parenteral rehydration. The emergency treatment of life-threatening dehydration should follow appropriate guidelines for intravenous fluid resuscitation to replace gastrointestinal and insensible losses.[12]

Although feeding may appear to exacerbate diarrhea, continued feeding is not associated with adverse outcomes in infants and children.[13] In malnourished populations, feeding children during diarrhea reduces weight loss from repeated bouts of infection.[14] There are insufficient data to know whether temporary lactose intolerance or fat malabsorption is a significant factor in TD.

Table 20.3–1. ELECTROLYTES IN DIARRHEAL STOOL AND REPLACEMENT FLUIDS

	NA (MMOL/L)	K (MMOL/L)	BASE* (MMOL/L)	OSMOLALITY (MMOL/L)	CARBOHYDRATE† (GRAMS/L)
Normal plasma[12]	142	4.5	25		
Diarrheal stools[12]					
Children, nonspecific	56	25	15–30		
Child, cholera	100	25	35		
Adult, cholera	140	15	45		
Oral rehydration solutions[10]					
ORS (WHO formula) Jianas Bros.	90	20	30	310	20
CeraLyte-90 (Cera, powder)	90	20	30	260	40
Rehydralyte (Ross, liquid)	75	20	30	310	25
Maintenance					
CeraLyte-70 (Cera, powder)	70	20	30	220	40
Infalyte (Mead Johnson, powder)	50	25	50	200	30
Pedialyte (Ross, liquid)	45	20	30	250	25
Gatorade	25	8			40
Cola	2	<1	13		108
Apple juice	1	32			122
Orange juice	<1	54			109

*Bicarbonate or citrate.
† All glucose except CeraLyte, which uses rice-based carbohydrates.
  Adapted from Greenough,[10] Avery and Snyder,[11] and Backer.[12]

ANTIMOTILITY AGENTS

Several products besides antibiotics and oral rehydration salts are marketed for the relief of diarrhea. Some of these, along with their active ingredients, are listed in Table 20.3–3. The most useful are probably the antimotility agents derived from opium alkaloids. They relieve cramping by inhibiting intestinal smooth muscle contraction. The delay in transit time permits increased reabsorption of water and electrolytes. The opium alkaloids, morphine (tincture of opium, paregoric) and codeine, are effective in the short-term treatment of diarrhea but have narcotic effects and can induce drug dependence. Synthetic opioids with enhanced gut specificity became available in the late 1970s. These agents, diphenoxylate (a component of Lomotil) and loperamide (Imodium), produce only rare and mild occurrences of central nervous system side effects (e.g., drowsiness, dizziness, headache). Undesired enteric effects are also rare and include intestinal distention and obstruction; these are mainly risks to patients with ulcerative colitis or pseudomembranous colitis or children under the age of 5 years.[15]

For nonspecific therapy of TD, loperamide is currently the drug with the best safety and effectiveness.[16] Loperamide reduces the frequency and duration of diarrhea and relieves abdominal symptoms, compared to placebo.[17–19] Loperamide is more gut specific than diphe-

Table 20.3–2. HOMEMADE ORAL ELECTROLYTE SOLUTIONS: INGREDIENTS/LITER OF WATER

	COMPONENTS			
	SODIUM CHLORIDE	POTASSIUM CHLORIDE	SODIUM BICARBONATE	GLUCOSE
Recipe 1				
Mass	3.5 g	1.5 g	2.5 g	40 g
Household product	Table salt	Cream of tartar	Baking soda	Sugar
Kitchen measure	½ tsp	4 tsp	½ tsp	4 tbs
Recipe 2				
Drink alternately A then B.				
	A) 8 oz fruit juice + 1 pinch of salt + ½ tsp honey or corn syrup			
	B) 8 oz water + ¼ tsp baking soda			

Modified from Backer.[12]

Table 20.3–3. NONANTIBIOTIC AGENTS FOR TREATMENT OF DIARRHEA

Attapulgite (Diasorb, Donnagel)

Kaolin and pectin (Kaopectate)

Bismuth subsalicylate (Pepto-Bismol)*

Loperamide (Imodium)

Diphenoxylate-atropine (Lomotil)

Probiotic agents†

    Saccharomyces cervisiae or *boulardii* (Perenterol)

    Streptococcus faecium SF68 (Bioflorin)

    Lactobacillus acidophilus preparations

*Not available in Europe.
†Only available in some European countries.

noxylate and may also have antisecretory effects.[20] Loperamide does not potentiate the depressant effects of alcohol and barbiturates but may cause constipation. It has been rarely associated with necrotizing enterocolitis in children and is not recommended for childhood diarrhea.[21]

The combination of loperamide and antibiotic therapy often resolves symptoms in just a few hours.[22–25] Although antibiotics kill bacteria quickly, enterotoxins are still bound to enterocytes and continue to exert their effects until the gut endothelial cells are replaced, which takes about 24 to 36 hours. The antimotility agent reduces symptoms during this initial period before enterocytes with bound toxin are shed.

Antimotility agents have generally been discouraged in dysentery, based on a study in 1973 where Lomotil (diphenoxylate-atropine) was shown to prolong carriage of *Shigella* and decrease the effectiveness of the antibiotic oxolinic acid.[26] However, loperamide appears to be safer than Lomotil, even when given without an antimicrobial.[27–29] There was no significant prolongation of disease in students traveling in Latin America who developed shigellosis and took loperamide.[17] In practice, many patients are given the combination of an antibiotic and loperamide empirically, before the etiology of TD is known. To test the safety and efficacy of this in shigellosis, a recent double-blind, placebo-controlled trial looked at ciprofloxacin plus loperamide compared to ciprofloxacin alone for the treatment of dysentery caused by *Shigella* in Thai adults.[30] No adverse effects were seen in the combination therapy, and this group recovered faster, with fewer stools, than the group receiving the antibiotic alone. This was predominantly an outpatient study; there was only one case of dysentery caused by *Shigella dysenteriae* type 1, perhaps the most virulent strain, and no subjects under the age of 14 were enrolled. Therefore, these results should not be extrapolated to severely ill patients or to children. Most authorities would still not recommend loperamide when dysentery is apparent, but the above study gives some reassurance that if TD is caused by *Shigella*, the addition of loperamide is not likely to be harmful.

ANTISECRETORY COMPOUNDS

Enterotoxins, such as heat-labile (LT) and heat-stable (ST) toxins of ETEC and cholera toxin (CT), bind to enterocytes in the small intestine to produce secretion of fluid and electrolytes after stimulation of cyclic nucleotides. The balance between absorption and secretion of ions is thus disturbed. Even after the organisms are killed, these toxins continue to exert their effects. Investigations are ongoing to find clinically effective antisecretory compounds. An oral drug that could inhibit toxin-mediated secretion would be very helpful, if well tolerated.

One of the most promising antisecretory agents under study is zaldaride maleate, a benzimidazole that inhibits intestinal calmodulin. In a clinical trial among United States students who acquired TD in Mexico, zaldaride 20 mg, four times daily for 2 days, reduced the duration of diarrhea from 42 to 20 hours.[31] Reduction in stools was observed for persons who were infected with a variety of organisms. In a blinded, placebo-controlled comparison, zaldaride was better than placebo but not as effective as loperamide in reducing number of stools and shortening the time to cure.[32] The benefit of loperamide was greater during the first 24 hours, suggesting that the loperamide loading dose may have given an advantage over zaldaride. This was confirmed in a more recent study wherein the 2-day zaldaride regimen was initiated with a 40-mg loading dose, resulting in equivalent efficacy to loperamide.[33]

Other antisecretory compounds have been tried in experimental settings. Octreotide, a long-acting analogue of somatostatin, was recently tested in cholera patients with acute secretory diarrhea.[34] Octreotide, given with intravenous fluid replacement and ofloxacin, reduced the mean duration of diarrhea and the total volume of diarrhea. Granisetron, a 5-hydroxytryptamine receptor antagonist, was tested for its ability to block CT-induced enteric secretion in a human model.[35] Granisetron reversed CT-induced net water secretion, suggesting that highly selective agents such as granisetron targeted at the pathophysiologic processes that drive secretion could lead to useful treatments in the future.

BISMUTH SUBSALICYLATE

Bismuth subsalicylate (BSS; Pepto-Bismol) exhibits properties of antibacterial, anti-inflammatory, antisecretory, and adsorbent products. A toxin-binding mechanism has been shown for BSS using *Vibrio cholerae* and ETEC toxins.[36] BSS also acts directly as an antibacterial agent,[37] has anti-inflammatory and antisecretory effects through inhibition of prostaglandin synthesis,[38] and has decreased the symptoms of viral diarrhea.[39] A therapeutic dose of BSS is 30 mL (two tablets) orally every 30 minutes for eight doses—a large amount to take if nauseous. Side effects of BSS include black tongue, reversible tinnitus, and decreased absorption of antibiotics taken within 6 hours of taking BSS. The salicylate component is absorbed. Although not as effective as antibiotics, BSS has shown sufficient efficacy to warrant its use as a preventive measure for TD and for consideration as a treatment alternative to antibiotic therapy.[17,40–45]

ADSORBENTS AND HYDROPHILIC AGENTS

Several products are marketed for the treatment of diarrhea that may be categorized as adsorbents or hydrophilic agents. These substances are not absorbed by the intestinal mucosa, so there are few systemic side effects. Adsorbents are thought to act by binding toxins, bacteria, and viruses within the intestinal lumen or by protecting the mucosa. Except for attapulgite and polycarbophil, there are insufficient data to conclude that these compounds are effective.[46] Attapulgite is a magnesium aluminum silicate that absorbs up to eight times its weight in water. This renders the stools more formed, but the resulting net loss of water and electrolytes is as great or greater than untreated diarrhea.[47,48] In a comparison of efficacy, attapulgite was not as effective as loperamide.[44] A similar problem occurs with hydrophilic agents such as polycarbophil, methylcellulose, and psyllium products, which, due to their bulk-forming properties, are marketed as treatments for both constipation and diarrhea. Pectin, a fruit extract containing polygalacturonic acid, forms a colloid when added to some adsorbents. Neither the modes of action nor the clinical efficacies are proven for the silicate clays, hydrophilic agents, or pectin. They may provide an indirect sense of relief by making stools feel more formed, but in general have very little value[49] and should be considered obsolete.

WINE

In an effort to explain the popular reputation of wine as a digestive aid and anecdotal reports of wine preventing enteric infections, red and white wine were recently compared to BSS, ethanol, and water for ability to kill *E. coli*, *Shigella*, and *Salmonella* in vitro.[50] Undiluted wine and BSS were both effective in reducing the number of viable organisms, reducing counts by 10^5 to 10^6 after 20 to 30 minutes. Ethanol and tequila had a much more modest antibacterial effect. When the solutions were diluted, wine was much more effective in decreasing bacterial counts than BSS. The effect of the wine was not accounted for by ethanol alone. The clinical relevance of this observation is unknown, and there is no evidence that wine drinkers are at less risk than are other travelers.

BIOTHERAPEUTIC AGENTS

The intestinal lumen is a microscopic ecosystem, with beneficial, commensal, and pathogenic species in equilibrium. Broad-spectrum antibiotics disturb the balance of intestinal flora, sometimes leading to antibiotic-associated diarrhea and *Clostridium difficile*-associated disease (CDAD), including diarrhea and colitis. There is an effort to find living organisms that may be added to the intestinal microflora to inhibit enteric pathogens. These agents, called biotherapeutic agents or probiotics, have recently been reviewed.[51] *Lactobacillus* GG demonstrated no significant preventive effect on TD in an open-label study of 756 Finnish tourists traveling to Turkey.[52] A blinded, controlled study of the nonpathogenic yeast *Saccharomyces*

boulardii reduced diarrhea rates from 39% to 29% in Austrian travelers who received 1 g/d of active yeast.[53] Unfortunately, bacterial etiologies were not available in these studies. Treatment studies in TD are lacking, but *Lactobacillus* GG and *Saccharomyces boulardii* have been tried to treat CDAD with mixed results.[54] The spent culture supernatant of human *Lactobacillus acidophilus* strain LB demonstrated an antibacterial activity in vitro against several enteric pathogens, including *Salmonella typhimurium*, *Shigella flexneri*, and *E. coli*.[55] Biotherapeutic agents may offer an alternative approach to prevention and treatment of enteric infections, but they need to be characterized with toxicity and pharmacokinetic studies similar to those used for medications and must be tested in blinded, placebo-controlled trials.

ANTIBIOTIC THERAPY

PENICILLINS

Ampicillin is less useful as a presumptive treatment for TD due to widespread bacterial resistance; however, it is useful in TD where the pathogen is known to be susceptible.

TETRACYCLINES

Tetracyclines, including doxycycline, used to be effective in treating TD, but widespread resistance has reduced their effectiveness.[56,57] In Thailand, U.S. Forces taking doxycycline as malaria prophylaxis experienced high rates of TD caused by tetracycline-resistant organisms.[58] Doxycycline, given 100 mg twice daily, is better tolerated than tetracycline, which requires four times daily dosing. Doxycycline may be taken with food, which helps reduce gastritis. Tetracyclines, including doxycycline, should be avoided in children under the age of 8 years and in pregnant women, due to staining of immature teeth. BSS reduces tetracycline absorption. Tetracyclines may be considered for treatment of TD when the organisms are known to be susceptible.

MACROLIDES AND AZALIDES

Erythromycin is a useful drug for treatment of susceptible *Campylobacter* infections; however, it is not ideal as presumptive therapy for TD because it does not have a sufficiently broad spectrum of activity against gram-negative organisms. *Campylobacter* are important causes of TD in various parts of the tropical developing world.[5,59,60] In Thailand, *Campylobacter* is a major cause of TD among Peace Corps volunteers[59] and is the predominant cause of diarrhea in U.S. Forces on exercises.[24] During the 1980s, erythromycin shortened the duration of excretion of *Campylobacter* from 16 to 2 days but often failed to shorten the illness.[61–63] Azithromycin is an azalide antibiotic related to the macrolides that has several fold more activity against enteric pathogens than erythromycin.[64,65] Azithromycin attains very high tissue levels, including in the intestinal mucosa, where levels are sustained for 35 to 40 hours. It appears to have fewer gastrointestinal side effects than erythromycin and has recently proven useful in treating *Campylobacter* infections resistant to FQ.[66]

TRIMETHOPRIM AND SULFAMETHOXAZOLE

Trimethoprim alone was effective in the early 1980s for treatment of TD,[67,68] but resistance developed rapidly.[69] The combination of trimethoprim 160 mg plus sulfamethoxazole 800 mg (TMP-SMX, co-trimoxazole, Bactrim, Septra), taken twice daily for 5 days, decreases the severity and duration of illness,[67] an outcome that is even further improved by the simultaneous use of loperamide.[22] Table 20.3–4 summarizes the results of several placebo-controlled trials of TMP-SMX as presumptive treatment for acute infectious diarrhea.[22,67,70–72] Three-day and single-dose regimens produced results similar to 5-day regimens.

In nonsulfa-allergic patients, TMP-SMX is better tolerated than erythromycin or tetracycline and may be used in children. Resistance to TMP-SMX is increasing,[73] but it remains effective against ETEC in central Mexico.[74] Before using TMP-SMX, practitioners should review regional susceptibility information. TMP-SMX is not effective for *Campylobacter* or the nontyphoidal *Salmonellae*. Side effects include hypersensitivity reactions with fever and rash, headaches, and depression. The sulfa component may trigger asthma in susceptible individuals. TMP-SMX prolongs prothrombin times in patients taking warfarin and may increase phenytoin levels. It increases the hypoglycemic effect of sulfonylureas, the antifolate effect of methotrexate, and the hematopoetic toxicity of azathioprine but decreases cyclosporine levels. TMP-SMX is contraindicated in patients with megaloblastic anemia.

FLUOROQUINOLONES

The FQs have simplified treatment of TD by providing a safe and effective self-treatment for adult travelers. They have an excellent safety profile and a wide spectrum of coverage for enteric pathogens.[75,76] FQs rarely cause antibiotic-induced colitis, possibly because they lack anaerobic activity. More than 90% of the intestinal flora by weight is anaerobic, and leaving these organisms undisturbed may reduce the incidence of antibiotic-associated diarrhea and CDAD. FQs are well absorbed after oral administration, reach peak tissue levels quickly, and are cleared slowly enough to allow twice-daily dosing or even single-dose therapy.[77] Selection for resistant bacterial strains primarily depends on nonplasmid-transferable mutations, which are very rare (10^{-9}).[78] Table 20.3–5 summarizes the results of several placebo-controlled trials of quinolones as presumptive treatment for acute infectious diarrhea.[70,72,79–84] On the third day after beginning therapy, groups receiving FQ have a recovery rate 20% to 40% higher than groups that did not receive antibiotics. There are good data to recommend ciprofloxacin, ofloxacin, and norfloxacin for the treatment of TD. Fewer data are available about enoxacin.[72]

The most common adverse reactions to FQs are nausea and headache. Less common side effects include restlessness, insomnia, and nightmares. Quinolone blood concentrations may be decreased when taken within 2 hours of antacids or sucralfate. Quinolone concentrations are increased after cimetidine. Patients on warfarin may experience prolonged prothrombin times.

NEWER AGENTS

Recently, new FQs have been licensed: levofloxacin, sparfloxacin, grepafloxacin, and trovafloxacin. They have increased activity against gram-positive bacteria, a characteristic not useful in treating TD. Trovafloxacin also has anaerobic activity, which may theoretically be a disadvantage in a TD drug. The toxicity profiles of these newer FQs have recently been reviewed.[85] Fleroxacin is a trifluoronated quinolone that is not licensed in the U.S. because of a high rate of adverse reactions. These drugs are somewhat more toxic than the commonly used FQs and confer no theoretic advantage for TD so are not recommended at this time.

Some have suggested that the newer FQs with activity against gram-positive pathogens could simplify the

Table 20.3–4.   CONTROLLED CLINICAL TRIALS OF TRIMETHOPRIM-SULFAMETHOXAZOLE (160/800 MG) FOR ACUTE INFECTIOUS DIARRHEA

REGIMEN	DIFFERENCE COMPARED TO PLACEBO ARM		N (DRUG, PLACEBO)	REFERENCE
	PERCENT DECREASE IN DURATION OF DIARRHEA	INCREASE IN % WELL AT 72 HOURS		
Twice daily for 5 days	75	41	59, 62	70
	68	61	37, 35	67
	6	16	43, 49	72
Twice daily for 3 days	38	22	45, 45	22
	35*	na	11, 19	71
	19	8	94, 97	72
Two doses once	52	30	44, 45	22

*Subjects with *Shigella* only.

Table 20.3–5.   CONTROLLED CLINICAL TRIALS OF FLUOROQUINOLONES FOR ACUTE INFECTIOUS DIARRHEA

DRUG	RE GIMEN (MG)	PERCENT DECREASE IN DURATION OF DIARRHEA	DIFFERENCE IN % WELL AT 72 HOURS	N (DRUG, PLACEBO)	REFERENCE
Ciprofloxacin	500 twice daily for 5 days	64	39	60, 62	70
		49	31	38, 38	79
	500 × 1 dose	54	14	45, 38	80
Norfloxacin	400 twice daily for 5 days	n/a	21	257, 254	81
	400 twice daily for 3 days	64	29	51, 55	82
		54	NA	10, 19	71
		27	36	46, 48	83
Ofloxacin	300 twice daily for 5 days	30	18*	66, 79	84
	300 twice daily for 3 days	50	26*	81, 79	84
Enoxacin	400 twice daily for 5 days	13	16	47, 49	72

*Measured at 48 hours.

traveler's first-aid kit by providing one drug to treat respiratory, skin, and enteric infections. However, this goes against the aim of selecting an antibiotic with the narrowest spectrum of activity to treat the given condition. Further, these drugs are more expensive and have more side effects than the first-generation FQs such as ciprofloxacin. Finally, these broader spectrum FQs have no greater activity against *Campylobacter* than ciprofloxacin. A preferred course is selection of a macrolide (erythromycin) or an azalide (azithromycin) as second antibiotic. These drugs cover many respiratory pathogens and many *Campylobacter* strains.

There is interest in finding agents that are poorly absorbed from the gut to treat TD. Rifaximin is a rifamycin derivative with broad-spectrum antibacterial properties that is poorly absorbed from the gut. Rifaximin was recently tested at doses of 200, 400, and 600 mg three times daily for treatment of TD in adults traveling in Mexico.[86] It compared favorably with TMP-SMX in duration of diarrhea, number of unformed stools passed, and eradication of enteric pathogens. Bicozamycin, another poorly absorbed antibacterial agent, shortened the time to last unformed stool from 64 hours to 28 hours in a recent study.[87] Oral aztreonam was shown to reduce diarrhea from 80 hours to 44 hours.[88] Further testing is required before the merits of these drugs for treatment of TD can be judged.

APPROACH TO THE PATIENT

TRAVELERS' DIARRHEA SYNDROMES

At the onset of illness, there is very little to differentiate the various bacterial causes of TD. As the illness evolves, it may produce primarily a secretory diarrhea or a more invasive illness with mucous and blood. If the syndrome persists longer than 2 weeks, it may be called persistent diarrhea. These syndromes are discussed in more detail below. During history taking, the practitioner needs to determine whether invasive illness is likely, if adequate

hydration is being maintained, and if evidence of more serious disease is present. Many diseases other than TD, such as malaria and viral hepatitis, may have diarrhea or abdominal discomfort as a component and should be ruled out.[89] In addition, shigellosis and other enteric diseases may present initially without diarrhea and mimic other febrile illnesses.

The practitioner should ascertain the duration of symptoms and whether the diarrhea is predominantly watery or contains mucous and blood. Bowel urgency is nearly universal, but severe cramping or abdominal pains should be noted. Treatments already taken should be recorded. It is important to determine whether the patient is able to orally hydrate or cannot keep up with losses due to persistent vomiting. Physical examination should note temperature, pulse, and whether orthostatic hypotension is present. Mental status, moistness of mucous membranes, and skin turgor should be assessed to get a better impression of hydration. Jaundice, rash, nuchal rigidity, and abdominal tenderness should be looked for as evidence of other, serious disease.

Laboratory testing will depend on history and examination. Acute diarrhea in a well-hydrated patient with no other symptoms or signs may be treated empirically without initial laboratory testing. In a patient with tachycardia, dry mucous membranes, or poor skin turgor, one may wish to perform a urine-specific gravity and consider intravenous rehydration or directly observed oral rehydration. Any ill-appearing patient or one with high fever or abdominal tenderness should be investigated more thoroughly with complete blood count, electrolytes, and liver function tests. In these cases, blood, stool, and urine cultures should be considered. Patients with prolonged diarrhea should probably undergo stool examination at the outset, as this is more likely to influence therapy.

SECRETORY DIARRHEA

When diarrhea is predominantly watery, without blood or mucous in the stools, and there is minimal or no fever, it is considered secretory. In travelers, the usual etiologic agents are bacterial, such as ETEC, but viruses such as rotavirus and caliciviruses (Norwalk virus and Norwalk-like agents) may also be causes. Cholera is a particularly severe form of secretory diarrhea, but cholera is rare in travelers to nonepidemic areas.[90] When cholera does occur in tourists, it is not as severe as in indigenous populations, probably because tourists tend to be well nourished. Secretory diarrhea typically runs a self-limited course, lasting between 3 and 5 days.[4] To shorten this course to 1 day, ciprofloxacin 500 mg is given every 12 hours until symptoms are relieved. Normally, this will only take one to two doses, especially if combined with loperamide. Rarely will more than 3 days of therapy be required. The other first-generation FQs, ofloxacin (300 mg) or norfloxacin (400 mg), may also be used. Loperamide 2 mg may be given orally as two caplets initially, followed by one caplet after each loose stool up to a maximum of eight doses (16 mg) per day. Most patients use less than eight doses. Patients should be cautioned not to overuse loperamide as this might result in constipation. Recommendations for children and pregnant patients are discussed below.

INVASIVE DIARRHEA

Dysentery is an illness characterized by diarrhea with blood or mucous. Commonly, there is fever, and patients may be ill appearing with evidence of systemic disease. Abdominal pain may be present and can mimic appendicitis. Severe cramping may cause misery for some patients. Systemic disease with minimal or no diarrhea may occur, even though the source of the infection is an enteric agent. Invasive diarrhea in travelers is commonly caused by *Shigella, Campylobacter,* and *Salmonella* species. Strains of *E. coli* may also cause invasive disease. Enteroinvasive *E. coli* (EIEC) produces disease by the same pathogenic mechanisms as *Shigella* and enterohemorrhagic *E. coli* (EHEC) may cause hemorrhagic colitis or hemolytic-uremic syndrome (HUS).

Antibiotics are very effective in reducing symptoms due to *Shigella, Campylobacter,* and EIEC. Because these are the most common causes of dysentery in travelers, empiric treatment is indicated. Ciprofloxacin 500 mg is given orally, every 12 hours, for 3 to 5 days. If the patient is seriously ill and unable to take oral medications, parenteral ciprofloxacin may be administered. Other first-generation FQs may be used, as described for secretory diarrhea. Although loperamide may be safe in mild cases,[30] antimotility agents in general are best avoided if there is blood or evidence of systemic illness.[4] *Salmonella* are less effectively treated, and *Salmonella* carriage in the stool may actually be prolonged by antibiotic therapy. If cultures are done and results indicate salmonellosis, antibiotic therapy may be stopped. There is no evidence that antibiotics shorten the disease due to EHEC or prevent HUS; therefore, antibiotics are not indicated in HUS.[91,92]

PERSISTENT DIARRHEA

About 10% of TD cases last longer than 2 weeks and may be described as persistent diarrhea.[93,94] The term chronic diarrhea is usually reserved for diarrhea lasting longer than a month. Chronic diarrhea occurs in less than 3% of all TD cases but ranks second among all travel-related illnesses in number of lost work days. Persistent diarrhea may be due to inadequately treated or resistant bacterial infections; however, as the time since onset increases, there is greater likelihood that the diarrhea may be due to protozoan infections, such as *Giardia, Entamoeba, Cryptosporidia,* or *Cyclospora.* Whenever antibacterial therapy has been used, practitioners should consider the possibility of CDAD. In many cases of prolonged diarrhea, the etiology remains unclear.

Although a trial of empiric therapy is often effective, it may be useful in persistent diarrhea to initiate a more extensive work-up so that data will be available if empiric therapy fails. Stools can be sent for occult blood examination, fresh microscopic examination for fecal leukocytes and amebic trophozoites, and concentration and staining for cysts. If patients have already failed antibiotic therapy, *C. difficile* toxin assay should be requested. If resistant organisms are suspected, cultures for enteric pathogens (typically *Shigella, Salmonella,* and *Campylobacter*) may be sent with requests for antibiotic susceptibilities. *Entamoeba* trophozoites are best seen in fresh stool, but cysts may be seen in preserved specimens.

Cyclospora have recently been noted to cause persistent, watery diarrhea in travelers and expatriates in Nepal[95,96] and children in Peru.[97] Initially called cyanobacterium-like bodies, they were first seen with the modified acid-fast stain used to identify *Cryptosporidium.*[98,99] This stain uses dimethyl sulfoxide and carbol fuchsin to produce brilliant pink to fuchsia oocysts, 8 to 9 mm in diameter (versus 4 to 5 μm for *Cryptosporidium* cysts). Once recognized, it was found that they could be seen in unstained wet mounts of infected stool where they appeared as nonrefractile, double-walled spheres. Observations made during sporulation and excystation and morphologic features placed the organisms in the coccidian genus *Cyclospora,* and it was named *Cyclospora cayetanensis.*[97] *Cyclospora* can be concentrated by centrifugation of formalin-ether preparations of stool or by sucrose flotation in Sheather's solution.[100] In addition, they show blue autofluorescence when examined with a fluorescent microscope fitted with a 365-nm excitation filter.[101] *Cyclospora* do not react with commercially available monoclonal antibodies prepared against *C. parvum* or against enzyme-linked immunosorbent assays (ELISAs) for *Cryptosporidium antigen.*[102] Examination for *Cyclospora* should now be routine when stools from travelers with persistent diarrhea are sent to the laboratory.[103]

When TD has persisted for less than 30 days, a course of antibacterial therapy may be tried. In cases where symptoms have lasted over 30 days or antibiotic treatment has failed, parasitic causes of illness are more likely; therefore, antiparasitic therapy may be worthwhile regardless of the laboratory findings. Tinidazole 2 g daily as a single dose for 3 days (not available in the U.S.) or metronidazole 750 mg three times daily for 10 days may be given to presumptively treat giardiasis.[104,105] Alternatively, if *Cyclospora*-induced diarrhea is considered likely, TMP-SMX twice daily for 7 days may be employed. *Cyclospora* responds to TMP-SMX, 160 mg trimethoprim/800 mg sulfamethoxazole (Septra DS) twice daily for 7 days.[106] In the first treatment trial in Nepal, 71% still had *Cyclospora* in their stools after 3 days, but only 6% excreted oocysts after 7 days, suggesting that the longer therapy is required. Guidelines for the evaluation and treatment of CDAD have recently been published.[54] Failure to make an infectious diagnosis and failure to respond to empiric therapy should prompt consideration of tropical sprue. Malabsorption due to this syndrome may be assessed with the D-xylose test. Occasionally, an episode of TD may trigger a prolonged bout of irritable bowel syndrome or uncover underlying chronic bowel disease.

EMERGING ANTIMICROBIAL RESISTANCE

The most effective antibiotics for the treatment of TD have been quinolones, which, during the first half of the 1990s, effectively treated nearly all *Shigella*-, *Campylobacter*-, and EIEC-induced dysentery. Unfortunately, antibiotic resistance has been spreading.[107,108]

Shigella have developed resistance to multiple antibiotics, including tetracycline, TMP-SMX, ampicillin, and nalidixic acid.[107] FQs, such as ciprofloxacin, are the most reliable drugs for the treatment of shigellosis.[109–111] A recent report of 675 TD patients seen in a travel medicine clinic in Spain reported that 10% of TD cases were due to *Shigella*.[112] Of these, approximately three-quarters were tetracycline resistant, and half were resistant to ampicillin and TMP-SMX. There have been isolated reports of FQ resistance in *Shigella*, but this problem is not yet widespread. Because of concerns regarding the use of FQs in children, several alternative therapies for childhood shigellosis have been tried. In Bangladesh, azithromycin (500 mg on study day 1 followed by 250 mg on days 2 to 4) compared favorably to ciprofloxacin for treatment of shigellosis in adults.[113] Pivmecillinam is used for treating shigellosis in children in Bangladesh.[114]

Erythromycin is the traditional treatment for *Campylobacter* infections, although resistance occurs.[115] With the development of FQs in the 1980s, there was one class of drugs that could treat *Campylobacter* and the other causes of TD. However, FQ resistance spread during the 1990s.[66,116,117] In Thailand, azithromycin (500 mg orally once daily for 3 days) was equivalent to ciprofloxacin in reducing diarrhea in U.S. Forces with TD caused by *Campylobacter*.[66] Azithromycin was superior to ciprofloxacin in decreasing the duration of *Campylobacter* excretion in this study where all *Campylobacter* were susceptible to azithromycin, but only half were susceptible to ciprofloxacin. Unfortunately, in vitro azithromycin resistance is already present in Thailand.[117]

TD occurring while on prophylaxis has not been well studied. One would expect that resistant organisms may be more likely. If prophylaxis was with other than a quinolone, then a quinolone may be tried. After quinolone prophylaxis, the course is unclear. If a second course of antibiotics fails, the patient should be treated as described above.

DURATION OF THERAPY

During the 1980s, treatment of TD with TMP-SMX twice daily for 5 days was shown to be better than placebo, shortening the time to last unformed stool from 93 to 29 hours.[67] When quinolone antibiotics became available, they proved as efficacious as TMP-SMX when used twice daily for 5 days.[70–72,118] Given the short times to cure seen with antibiotics, trials using twice-daily therapy for 3 days were conducted and proved successful.[22,71,72,82,84]

Several studies have shown single-dose therapy to be equivalent to 3- or 5- day courses for therapies using trimethoprim,[68] TMP-SMX,[22] TMP-SMX with loperamide,[22,119] FQs,[79,120] and FQs plus loperamide.[24,121] Single-dose ciprofloxacin was compared to placebo in adults in Belize where it reduced time to last liquid stool from 50 to 21 hours.[80] These reports indicate that single-dose quinolone or TMP-SMX therapy is effective in treating TD due to susceptible agents. When organisms are resistant to quinolones, additional days of therapy are not more effective than one. Single-dose therapy for TD has several potential benefits. Cost and side effects are reduced, compliance is improved, and convenience and safety make self-administered therapy practical. Although not accepted by all practitioners, it is reasonable to recommend a single dose of FQ or TMP-SMX or two doses, 12 hours apart, for secretory diarrhea or empiric therapy of TD. If symptoms persist past 24 hours, travelers may continue antibiotics until symptoms resolve or 3 days of therapy have been completed. Dysentery should probably still be treated for 3 to 5 days pending further data.

SPECIAL SITUATIONS

QUINOLONE USE IN CHILDREN

Quinolone antibiotics are not recommended in children under most circumstances due to the appearance of changes seen in the immature articular cartilage of weight-bearing joints in several animal species. However, data are accumulating that FQ antibiotics may be used with relative safety in children with serious infections. Ciprofloxacin has been used extensively in children with cystic fibrosis in developed nations and in children with gastrointestinal diseases in developing countries. A recent review reported a search of MEDLINE and 12 other databases for references to arthropathy or cartilage damage associated with quinolone use in children.[122] In 31 multipatient studies representing 7,045 children and adolescents who were treated with FQs and followed up for signs or symptoms of arthropathy, there were 10 reports of joint manifestations that occurred after treatment with quinolones. All symptoms resolved in nine cases. In a subanalysis, arthralgia occurred in 1.5% of 2,030 treatment courses. A judicious trial of ciprofloxacin suspension for shigellosis in Bangladesh revealed no significant differences in joint symptoms between the ciprofloxacin group and the pivmecillinam control.[114] From these studies, it appears that quinolone arthropathy as seen in juvenile animals is not convincingly seen in children and adolescents.

In 1995, a report of an International Society of Chemotherapy commission detailed indications for quinolone use in children.[123] Gastrointestinal infections with invasive and resistant organisms, including multidrug-resistant *Shigella* and *Salmonella*, were included in the list of indications. The benefit and safety of ciprofloxacin in treating children with invasive salmonellosis in rural Africa were reviewed recently, with further support for the judicious use of FQs in children with carefully defined diseases.[124] Although these recommendations were mainly concerned with treatment of epidemics in developing nations, practitioners in the developed world may consider quinolones, with the informed consent of the parents, in pediatric patients who have serious infections or who have failed conventional therapy. Quinolones should not be used as routine therapy for mild diseases in children. Risks and benefits need to be weighed and parents consulted when the use of quinolones is deemed indicated. At present, TMP-SMX remains the drug of choice for children with TD, although many authorities would allow a mild case to run its course. Alternative antibiotics such as furazolidone may be considered, but recent experience suggests limited effectiveness possibly due to increasing resistance.[125–127]

DIARRHEA IN THE PREGNANT TRAVELER

TD in pregnancy poses a more difficult situation. The effects of quinolones on human fetal cartilage development have not been well studied. On the other hand, *Campylobacter* infections may lead to fetal infection, premature labor, and abortion. Mild TD should probably be treated with rest and fluids. Moderate to severe TD can be treated with ampicillin or erythromycin, considered safe in pregnancy. Organisms resistant to these drugs but susceptible to quinolones will cause the practitioner and patient to weigh risks and benefits. There are not enough data in the literature to give more specific advice at this time.

DIARRHEA IN THE IMMUNOCOMPROMISED TRAVELER

Immunocompromised travelers are most likely to present with the same organisms that cause TD in travelers with normal immune systems. When immunodeficiency is profound, such as when CD4+ lymphocyte counts drop below 100/μL, travelers are more susceptible to systemic bacteremia and metastatic bacterial infections. In a recent study of HIV-infected patients with *Campylobacter* bacteremia, 42% had a travel history and the mortality was 33%.[128] The parasites *Cryptosporidium*, *Isospora*, *Entamoeba*, *Giardia*, *Microsporidia*, and *Strongyloides* are more common in these patients. In addition, *Mycobacterium avium-intracellulare*, cytomegalovirus, and numerous other viral infections cause diarrhea in patients with low CD4+ counts. CDAD may be more common due to the plethora of antibiotics taken by immunocompromised patients.

Persons undergoing chemotherapy, who are immunocompromised for a short time, may be placed on ciprofloxacin prophylaxis. For others, ciprofloxacin is still the first line of treatment for diarrhea acquired during travel.

The dictum that thorough laboratory investigations should be performed to identify the etiology of infections in immunocompromised patients probably applies here, and it would be prudent to send stool for culture and examination concurrent with beginning empiric therapy. An extensive evaluation is only required when initial therapy fails. A summary of therapies for infectious diarrhea in immunocompromised patients may be found in the Guidelines on Acute Infectious Diarrhea in Adults, recently approved by the American College of Gastroenterology.[111]

PRETRAVEL COUNSELING

During pretravel counseling for travelers headed to the developing world, the practitioner should spend some time describing what constitutes a treatable case of TD. One or two loose stools a day, due to a change in environment and diet, are not uncommon and usually resolve spontaneously in a day or two without treatment. Treatment should be suggested when four or more loose stools occur in a 24-hour period or any number of loose stools is associated with symptoms of fever, cramps, nausea, vomiting, blood, or mucous in stools. Patients traveling from industrialized countries to the developing world are currently advised to bring along medication for the self-treatment of TD.[2,4] Adult travelers can be given about six doses of ciprofloxacin, 500-mg tablets for a typical 2-week vacation. When TD occurs, they may take one tablet by mouth initially and another in 12 hours. Normally, they will be well after this, but if symptoms continue they may finish the 3-day course. Alternatively, equivalent regimens of ofloxacin or norfloxacin may be used. They may also be given about 16 doses of loperamide, 2-mg caplets. They are taken two caplets initially and one after each loose stool to a maximum of eight per day. It is wise to remind travelers that it is not desirable to totally prevent defecation because it may complicate the illness or lead to constipation. Loperamide is probably most useful in voluminous diarrhea or when the situation makes visits to the toilet awkward. For children who are not sulfa-allergic, parents may be given six doses of TMP-SMX and be informed about various methods for oral rehydration. Loperamide is not recommended in children. It is helpful to provide written instructions to travelers. Worry about diarrhea is a frequent concern of travelers attending travel clinics. Travelers should leave feeling that they have the knowledge and tools to handle most diarrhea that may develop during their trip.

ACKNOWLEDGMENT

The principal investigator and first author of this chapter is an employee of the U.S. Government, whose work is in the public domain.

REFERENCES

1. Steffen R, van der Linde F, Gyr K, Schar M. Epidemiology of diarrhea in travelers. JAMA 1983;249:1176–1180.

2. Gorbach SL, Carpenter C, Grayson R, et al. Consensus conference: travelers' diarrhea. JAMA 1985;253:2700-2704.

3. Steffen R. Epidemiologic studies of travelers' diarrhea, severe gastrointestinal infections, and cholera. Rev Infect Dis 1986;8(Suppl 2):S122–S130.

4. DuPont HL, Ericsson CD. Prevention and treatment of traveler's diarrhea. N Engl J Med 1993;328:1821–1827.

5. Hoge CW, Shlim DR, Echeverria P, et al. Epidemiology of diarrhea among expatriate residents living in a highly endemic environment. JAMA 1996;275:533–538.

6. Kean BH. The diarrhea of travelers to Mexico: summary of five-year study. Ann Intern Med 1963;59:605–614.

7. Sack RB, Gorbach SL, Banwell JG, et al. Enterotoxigenic *Escherichia coli* isolated from patients with severe cholera-like disease. J Infect Dis 1971;123:378–385.

8. Merson MH, Morris GK, Sack DA, et al. Travelers' diarrhea in Mexico: a prospective study of physicians and family members attending a congress. N Engl J Med 1976;294:1299–1305.

9. Thillainayagam AV, Hunt JB, Farthing MJG. Enhancing clinical efficacy of oral rehydration therapy: is low osmolality the key? Gastroenterology 1998;114:197–210.

10. Greenough WB. Oral rehydration therapy: something new, something old. Infect Dis Clin Pract 1998;7:97–100.

11. Avery ME, Snyder JD. Oral therapy for acute diarrhea: the underused simple solution. N Engl J Med 1990;323:891–894.

12. Backer HD. Infectious diarrhea from wilderness and foreign travel. In: Auerbach PS, Geehr EC, eds. Management of wilderness and environmental emergencies. 2nd Ed. St. Louis: CV Mosby, 1989.

13. DiJohn D, Levine MM. Treatment of diarrhea. Infect Dis Clin North Am 1988;2:719–745.

14. Mazumder RN, Hoque SS, Ashraf H, et al. Early feeding of an energy dense diet during acute shigellosis enhances growth in malnourished children. J Nutr 1997;127:51–54.

15. Palmer KR, Corbett CL, Holdsworth CD. Double-blind crossover study comparing loperamide codeine and diphenoxylate in the treatment of chronic diarrhea. Gastroenterology 1980;79:1272–1275.

16. Fletcher P, Steffen R, DuPont H. Benefit/risk considerations with respect to OTC-descheduling of loperamide. Drug Res 1995;45:608–613.

17. Johnson PC, Ericsson CD, DuPont HL, et al. Comparison of loperamide with bismuth subsalicylate for the treatment of acute travelers' diarrhea. JAMA 1986;255:757–760.

18. Van Loon FPL, Bennish ML, Speelman P, Butler C. Double blind trial of loperamide for treating acute watery diarrhoea in expatriates in Bangladesh. Gut 1989;30:492–495.

19. Ericsson CD, Johnson PC. Safety and efficacy of loperamide. Am J Med 1990;88:(Suppl 6A):10S–14S.

20. Guandalini S, Fasano A, Rao MC, et al. Effects of loperamide on intestinal ion transport. J Pediatr Gastroenterol Nutr 1984;3:593–601.

21. Chow CB, Li SH, Leung NK. Loperamide associated necrotising enterocolitis. Acta Paediatr Scand 1986;75:1034–1036.

22. Ericsson CD, DuPont HL, Mathewson JJ, et al. Treatment of traveler's diarrhea with sulfamethoxazole and trimethoprim and loperamide. JAMA 1990;263:257–261.

23. Taylor DN, Sanchez JL, Candler W, et al. Treatment of travelers' diarrhea: ciprofloxacin plus loperamide compared with ciprofloxacin alone: a placebo-controlled, randomized trial. Ann Intern Med 1991;114:731–734.

24. Petruccelli BP, Murphy GS, Sanchez JL, et al. Treatment of travelers' diarrhea with ciprofloxacin and loperamide. J Infect Dis 1992;165:557–560.

25. Ericsson CD, DuPont HL, Mathewson JJ. Single dose ofloxacin plus loperamide compared with single dose or three day ofloxacin in the treatment of traveler's diarrhea. J Travel Med 1997;4:3–7.

26. DuPont HL, Hornick RB. Adverse effect of Lomotil therapy in shigellosis. JAMA 1973;226:1525–1528.

27. Amery W, Duyck F, Polak J, van den Bouwhuysen G. A multicenter double-blind study in acute diarrhoea comparing loperamide (R18553) with two common antidiarrhoeal agents and a placebo. Curr Ther Res 1975;17:263–270.

28. Nelemans FA, Zelvelder WG. A double-blind placebo controlled trial of loperamide in acute diarrhea. J Drug Res 1976;2:54–59.

29. Cornett JWD, Aspeling RL, Mallegol D. A double-blind comparative evaluation of loperamide versus diphenoxylate with atropine in acute diarrhea. Curr Ther Res 1977;21:629–637.

30. Murphy GS, Bodhidatta L, Echeverria P, et al. Ciprofloxacin and loperamide in the treatment of bacillary dysentery. Ann Intern Med 1993;118:582–586.

31. DuPont HL, Ericsson DC, Mathewson JJ, et al. Zaldaride maleate, an intestinal calmodulin inhibitor, in the therapy of traveler' diarrhea. Gastroenterology 1993;104:709–715.

32. Okhuysen PC, DuPont HL, Ericsson CD, et al. Zaldaride maleate (a new calmodulin antagonist) versus loperamide in the treatment of traveler's diarrhea: randomized, placebo-controlled trial. Clin Infect Dis 1995;21:341–344.

33. Silberschmidt G, Schick MT, Steffen R, et al. Treatment of travellers' diarrhoea: zaldaride compared with loperamide and placebo. Eur J Gastroenterol Hepatol 1995;7:871–875.

34. Abbas Z, Moid I, Khan AH, et al. Efficacy of octreotide in diarrhoea due to *Vibrio cholerae*: a randomized, controlled trial. Ann Trop Med Parasitol 1996;90:507–513.

35. Turvill JL, Farthing MJG. Effect of granisetron on cholera toxin-induced enteric secretion. Lancet 1997;349:1293.

36. Ericsson CD, Tannenbaum C, Charles TT. Antisecretory and antiinflammatory properties of bismuth subsalicylate. Rev Infect Dis 1990;12(Suppl 1):S16–S20.

37. Cornick NA, Silva M, Gorbach SL. In vitro antibacterial activity of bismuth subsalicylate. Rev Infect Dis 1990;12(Suppl 1):S9–S10.

38. Gorbach SL. Bismuth therapy in gastrointestinal diseases. Gastroenterology 1990;99:863–875.

39. Steinhoff MC, Douglas RG, Greenberg HB, Callahan DR. Bismuth subsalicylate therapy of viral gastroenteritis. Gastroenterology 1980;78:1495–1499.

40. DuPont HL, Sullivan P, Pickering LK, et al. Symptomatic treatment of diarrhea with bismuth subsalicylate among students attending a Mexican university. Gastroenterology 1977;73:715–718.

41. Steffen R, Mathewson JJ, Ericsson CD, et al. Travelers' diarrhea in West Africa and in Mexico: fecal transport systems and liquid bismuth subsalicylate for self-therapy. J Infect Dis 1988;157:1008–1013.

42. Steffen R, Heusser R, Tschopp A, DuPont HL. Efficacy and side effects of six agents in the self-treatment of travelers' diarrhoea. Travel Med Int 1988;6:153–157.

43. DuPont HL, Sanchez JF, Ericsson CD, et al. Comparative efficacy of loperamide hydrochloride and bismuth subsalicylate in the management of acute diarrhea. Am J Med 1990;88(Suppl 6A):15S–19S.

44. DuPont HL, Ericsson CD, DuPont MW, et al. A randomized, open-label comparison of nonprescription loperamide and attapulgite in the symptomatic treatment of acute diarrhea. Am J Med 1990;88(Suppl 6A):20S–23S.

45. Steffen R. Worldwide efficacy of bismuth subsalicylate in the treatment of travelers' diarrhea. Rev Infect Dis 1990;12(Suppl 1):S80–S86.

46. Dukes GE. Over-the-counter antidiarrheal medications used for the self-treatment of acute nonspecific diarrhea. Am J Med 1990;88(Suppl 6A):24S–26S.

47. Portnoy BL, DuPont HL, Pruitt D, et al. Antidiarrheal agents in the treatment of acute diarrhea in children. JAMA 1976;236: 844–846.

48. Alestig K, Trollfors B, Stenqvist K. Acute non-specific diarrhea, studies on the use of charcoal, kaolin-pectin and diphenoxylate. Practitioner 1979;222:859–862.

49. Kollartisch HH, Kremsner P, Wiedermann G, Scheiner O. Prevention of traveler's diarrhoea: comparison of different non-antibiotic preparations. Travel Med Int 1989;6:9–17.

50. Weisse ME, Eberly B, Person DA. Wine as a digestive aid: comparative antimicrobial effects of bismuth salicylate and red and white wine. BMJ 1995;311:1657–1660.

51. Elmer GW, Surawicz CM, McFarland LV. Biotherapeutic agents: a neglected modality for the treatment and prevention of selected intestinal and vaginal infections. JAMA 1996; 275:870–876.

52. Oksanen PJ, Salminen S, Saxelin M, et al. Prevention of travelers' diarrhoea by *Lactobacillus* GG. Ann Med 1990; 22:53–56.

53. Kollaritsch H, Holst H, Grobara P, Wiedermann G. Prophylaxe der Reisediarrhoe mit Sacharomyces boulardii. Forschr Med 1993;111:153–156.

54. Fekety R. Guidelines for the diagnosis and management of *Clostridium difficile*-associated diarrhea and colitis. Am J Gastroenterol 1997;92:739–750.

55. Coconnier M, Lievin V, Bernet-Camard M, et al. Antibacterial effect of the adhering human *Lactobacillus acidophilus* strain LB. Antimicrob Agents Chemother 1997;41: 1046–1052.

56. Echeverria P, Verhaert L, Ulyangco CV, et al. Antimicrobial resistance and enterotoxin production among isolates of *Escherichia coli* in the Far East. Lancet 1978;2:589–592.

57. Santosham M, Sack RB, Froehlich J, et al. Biweekly prophylactic doxycycline for travelers' diarrhea. J Infect Dis 1981; 143:598–602.

58. Arthur JD, Echeverria P, Shanks GD, et al. A comparative study of gastrointestinal infections in United States soldiers receiving doxycycline or mefloquine for malaria prophylaxis. Am J Trop Med Hyg 1990;43:608–613.

59. Taylor DN, Echeverria P, Blaser MJ, et al. Polymicrobial aetiology of travellers' diarrhoea. Lancet 1985;1:381–383.

60. Mattila L, Siitonen A, Kyronseppa H, et al. Seasonal variation in etiology of travelers' diarrhea. J Infect Dis 1992;165: 385–388.

61. Robins-Browne RM, Mackenjee MKR, Bodasing MN, Coovadia HM. Treatment of *Campylobacter*-associated enteritis with erythromycin. Am J Dis Child 1983;137:282–285.

62. Nolan CM, Johnson KE, Coyle MB, Faler K. *Campylobacter jejuni* enteritis: efficacy of antimicrobial and antimotility drugs. Am J Gastroenterol 1983;78:621–626.

63. Salazar-Lindo E, Sack RB, Chea-Woo E, et al. Early treatment with erythromycin of *Campylobacter jejuni*-associated dysentery in children. J Pediatr 1986;109:355–360.

64. Jones K, Felmingham D, Ridgway G. In vitro activity of azithromycin (CP-62,993), a novel macrolide, against enteric pathogens. Drugs Exp Clin Res 1988;14:613–615.

65. Williams JD. Spectrum of activity of azithromycin. Eur J Clin Microbiol Infect Dis 1991;10:813–820.

66. Kuschner R, Trofa AF, Thomas RJ, et al. Use of azithromycin for the treatment of *Campylobacter* enteritis in travelers to Thailand, an area where ciprofloxacin resistance is prevalent. Clin Infect Dis 1995;21:536–541.

67. DuPont HL, Reves RR, Galindo E, et al. Treatment of travelers' diarrhea with trimethoprim/sulfamethoxazole and with trimethoprim alone. N Engl J Med 1982;307:841–844.

68. Oldfield EC, Bourgeois AL, Omar AK, Pazzaglia GL. Empirical treatment of *Shigella* dysentery with trimethoprim: five-

day course vs. single dose. Am J Trop Med Hyg 1987; 37:616–623.

69. Black RE, Levine MM, Clements ML, et al. Treatment of experimentally induced enterotoxigenic *Escherichia coli* diarrhea with trimethoprim, trimethoprim-sulfamethoxazole, or placebo. Rev Infect Dis 1982;4:540–545.

70. Ericsson CD, Johnson PC, DuPont HL, et al. Ciprofloxacin or trimethoprim-sulfamethoxazole as initial therapy for travelers' diarrhea. Ann Intern Med 1987;106:216–220.

71. Lolekha S, Patanacharoen S, Thanangkul B, Vibulbandhitkit S. Norfloxacin versus co-trimoxazole in the treatment of acute bacterial diarrhoea: a placebo controlled study. Scand J Infect Dis 1988;56(Suppl):35–45.

72. De la Cabada FJ, DuPont HL, Gyr K, Mathewson JJ. Antimicrobial therapy of bacterial diarrhea in adult residents of Mexico—lack of an effect. Digestion 1992;53:134–141.

73. Sack RB, Rahman M, Yunus M, Khan EH. Antimicrobial resistance in organisms causing diarrheal disease. Clin Infect Dis 1997;24(Suppl 1):S102–S105.

74. Bandres JC, Mathewson JJ, Ericcson CD, DuPont HL. Trimethoprim/sulfamethoxazole remains active against enterotoxigenic *Escherichia coli* and *Shigella* species in Guadalajara, Mexico. Am J Med Sci 1992;303:289–291.

75. Keusch GT. Antimicrobial therapy for enteric infections and typhoid fever: state of the art. Rev Infect Dis 1988;10(Suppl 1):S199–S205.

76. Halkin H. Adverse effects of fluoroquinolones. Rev Infect Dis 1988;10(Suppl 1):S258–S261.

77. Wise R, Griggs D, Andrews JM. Pharmacokinetics of the quinolones in volunteers: a proposed dosing schedule. Rev Infect Dis 1988;10(Suppl 1):S83–S89.

78. Munshi MH, Sack DA, Haider K, et al. Plasmid-mediated resistance to nalidixic acid in *Shigella dysenteriae* type 1. Lancet 1987;2:419–421.

79. Pichler HET, Diridl G, Stickler K, Wolf D. Clinical efficacy of ciprofloxacin compared with placebo in bacterial diarrhea. Am J Med 1987;82(Suppl 4A):329–332.

80. Salam I, Ketelaris P, Leigh-Smith S, Farthing MJG. Randomised trial of single-dose ciprofloxacin for travellers' diarrhoea. Lancet 1994;344:1537–1539.

81. Wistrom J, Jertborn M, Ekwall E, et al. Empiric treatment of acute diarrheal disease with norfloxacin: a randomized, placebo-controlled study. Ann Intern Med 1992;117:202–208.

82. Mattila L, Peltola H, Siitonen A, et al. Short-term treatment of traveler's diarrhea with norfloxacin: a double-blind, placebo-controlled study during two seasons. Clin Infect Dis 1993;17:779–782.

83. Wistrom J, Jertborn M, Hedstrom SA, et al. Short-term self-treatment of travellers' diarrhoea with norfloxacin: a placebo-controlled study. J Antimicrob Chemother 1989;23:905–913.

84. DuPont HL, Ericsson CD, Mathewson JJ, DuPont MW. Five versus three days of ofloxacin therapy for traveler's diarrhea: a placebo-controlled study. Antimicrob Agents Chemother 1992;36:87–91.

85. Lipsky BA, Baker CA. Fluoroquinolone toxicity profiles: a review focusing on newer agents. Clin Infect Dis 1999; 28:352–364.

86. DuPont HL, Ericsson CD, Mathewson JJ, et al. Rifaximin: a nonabsorbed antimicrobial in the therapy of travelers' diarrhea. Digestion 1998;59:708–714.

87. Ericsson CD, DuPont HL, Sullivan P, et al. Bicozamycin, a poorly absorbable antibiotic, effectively treats travelers' diarrhea. Ann Intern Med 1983;98:20–25.

88. DuPont HL, Ericsson CD, Mathewson JJ, et al. Oral aztreonam, a poorly absorbed yet effective therapy for bacterial diarrhea in US travelers to Mexico. JAMA 1992;267: 1932–1935.

89. Sharp TW, Thornton SA, Wallace MR, et al. Diarrheal disease among military personnel during Operation Restore Hope, Somalia, 1992–1993. Am J Trop Med Hyg 1995;52:188–193.

90. Taylor DN, Rizzo J, Meza R, et al. Cholera among Americans living in Peru. Clin Infect Dis 1996;22:1108–1109.

91. Boyce TG, Swerdlow DL, Griffin PM. *Escherichia coli* O157:H7 and the hemolytic-uremic syndrome. N Engl J Med 1995;333:364–368.

92. Su C, Brandt LJ. *Escherichia coli* O157:H7 infection in humans. Ann Intern Med 1995;123:698–714.

93. DuPont HL. Capsuto EG. Persistent diarrhea in travelers. Clin Infect Dis 1996;22:124–128.

94. Taylor DN, Connor BA, Shlim DR. Chronic diarrhea in the returned traveler. Med Clin North Am 1999;83:1033–1052.

95. Schlim DR, Cohen MT, Eaton M, et al. An alga-like organism associated with an outbreak of prolonged diarrhea among foreigners in Nepal. Am J Trop Med Hyg 1991;45:383–389.

96. Hoge CW, Shlim DR, Rajah R, et al. Epidemiology of diarrhoeal illness associated with coccidian-like organism among travellers and foreign residents in Nepal. Lancet 1993;341:1175–1179.

97. Ortega YR, Sterling CR, Gilman RH, et al. Cyclospora species—a new protozoan pathogen of humans. N Engl J Med 1993;328:1308–1312.

98. Bronsdon MA. Rapid dimethyl sulfoxide-modified acid-fast stain of *Cryptosporidium* oocysts in stool specimens. J Clin Microbiol 1984;19:952–953.

99. Pottz GE, Rampey JH, Benjamin F. A method for rapid staining of acid-fast bacteria in smears and sections of tissue. Am J Clin Pathol 1964;42:552–554.

100. Sheather AL. The detection of intestinal protozoa and mange parasites by a floatation technique. J Comp Pathol 1923;36:266–275.

101. Long EG, White EH, Carmichael WW, et al. Morphological and staining characteristics of a cyanobacterium-like organism associated with diarrhea. J Infect Dis 1991;164:199–202.

102. Soave R, Herwaldt BL, Relman DA. Cyclospora. Infect Dis Clin North Am 1998;12:1–12.

103. Berlin OGW, Novak SM, Porschen RK, et al. Recovery of *Cyclospora* organisms from patients with prolonged diarrhea. Clin Infect Dis 1994;18:606–609.

104. Speelman P. Single-dose tinidazole for the treatment of giardiasis. Antimicrob Agents Chemother 1985;27:227–229.

105. Zaat JOM, Mank TG, Assendelft WJJ. A systematic review on the treatment of giardiasis. Trop Med Intern Health 1997;2:63–82.

106. Hoge CW, Shlim DR, Ghimire M, et al. Placebo-controlled trial of co-trimoxazole for *Cyclospora* infections among travellers and foreign residents in Nepal. Lancet 1995;345:691–693.

107. Sack RB, Rahman M, Yunus M, Khan EH. Antimicrobial resistance in organisms causing diarrheal disease. Clin Infect Dis 1997;24(Suppl 1):S102–S105.

108. Hoge CW, Gambel JM, Srijan A, et al. Trends in antimicrobial resistance among diarrheal pathogens isolated in Thailand over 15 years. Clin Infect Dis 1998;26:341–345.

109. Bennish ML, Salam MA, Haider R, Barzar M. Therapy for shigellosis. II. Randomized, double-blind comparison of ciprofloxacin and ampicillin. J Infect Dis 1990;162:711–716.

110. Cheasty T, Skinner JA, Rowe B, Threlfall EJ. Increasing incidence of antibiotic resistance in shigellas from humans in England and Wales: recommendations for therapy. Microb Drug Resist 1998;4:57–60.

111. DuPont HL. The Practice Parameters Committee of the American College of Gastroenterology. Guidelines on acute infectious diarrhea in adults. Am J Gastroenterol 1997;92:1962–1975.

112. Vila J, Gascon J, Abdalla S, et al. Antimicrobial resistance of *Shigella* isolates causing traveler's diarrhea. Antimicrob Agents Chemother 1994;38:2668–2670.

113. Khan WA, Seas C, Dhar U, et al. Treatment of shigellosis: V. Comparison of azithromycin and ciprofloxacin: a double-blind, randomized, controlled trial. Ann Intern Med 1997;126:697–703.

114. Salam MA, Dhar U, Khan WA, Bennish ML. Randomised comparison of ciprofloxacin suspension and pivmecillinam for childhood shigellosis. Lancet 1998;352:522–527.

115. Taylor DN, Blaser MJ, Echeverria P, et al. Erythromycin-resistant *Campylobacter* infections in Thailand. Antimicrob Agents Chemother 1987;31:438–442.

116. Piddock LJ. Quinolone resistance and *Campylobacter* spp. J Antimicrob Chemother 1995;36:891–898.

117. Murphy GS, Echeverria P, Jackson LR, et al. Ciprofloxacin- and azithromycin-resistant *Campylobacter* causing traveler's diarrhea in U.S. troops deployed to Thailand in 1994. Clin Infect Dis 1996;22:868–869.

118. Thornton SA, Batchelor RA, Wignall SF, et al. Norfloxacin compared to trimethoprim/sulfamethoxazole for the treatment of travelers' diarrhea among U.S. military personnel deployed to South America and West Africa. Mil Med 1992;157:55–58.

119. Ericsson CD, Nicholls-Vasquez I, DuPont HL, Mathewson JJ. Optimal dosing of trimethoprim-sulfamethoxazole when used with loperamide to treat traveler's diarrhea. Antimicrob Agents Chemother 1992;36:2821–2824.

120. Bassily S, Hyams KC, El-Masry NA, et al. Short-course norfloxacin and trimethoprim-sulfamethoxazole treatment of shigellosis and salmonellosis in Egypt. Am J Trop Med Hyg 1994;51:219–223.

121. Ericsson C, DuPont H, Mathewson J. Single dose ofloxacin plus loperamide compared with single dose or three days of ofloxacin in the treatment of travelers' diarrhea. J Travel Med 1997;4:3–7.

122. Burkhardt JE, Walterspiel JN, Schaad UB. Quinolone arthropathy in animals versus children. Clin Infect Dis 1997;25:1196–1204.

123. Schaad UB, Salam MA, Aujard Y, et al. Use of fluoroquinolones in pediatrics: consensus report of an International Society of Chemotherapy commission. Pediatr Infect Dis J 1995;14:1–9.

124. Green S, Tillotson G. Use of ciprofloxacin in developing countries. Pediatr Infect Dis J 1997;16:150–159.

125. DuPont HL, Ericsson CD, Galindo E, et al. Furazolidone versus ampicillin in the treatment of travelers' diarrhea. Antimicrob Agents Chemother 1984;26:160–163.

126. Prado Camacho JL. A comparison of furazolidone and ampicillin in the treatment of invasive diarrhea. Scand J Gastroenterol 1989;169:54–59.

127. Rodriguez RS, Chavez AZ, Galindo E. A randomized, controlled, single-blind study comparing furazolidone with trimethoprim-sulfamethoxazole in the empirical treatment of acute invasive diarrhea. Scand J Gastroenterol Suppl 1989;169:47–53.

128. Tee W, Mijch A. *Campylobacter jejuni* bacteremia in human immunodeficiency virus (HIV)-infected and non-HIV-infected patients: comparison of clinical features and review. Clin Infect Dis 1998;26:91–96.

20.4 PERSISTENT TRAVELERS' DIARRHEA

BRADLEY A. CONNOR

Most cases of travelers' diarrhea are acute in nature and will resolve within a week of onset of symptoms. Travel medicine practitioners and others who care for returning travelers have increasingly recognized subacute or chronic diarrheal syndromes in some returning travelers. Some cases of travelers' diarrhea persist for weeks, months, or even years, and the importance of chronic diarrhea as a presenting complaint is now well established in the post-travel setting. There are limited data on the incidence, natural history, and predisposing factors for chronic travelers' diarrhea, and an analysis of this condition is hindered somewhat by lack of uniformity in defining the syndrome. Indeed, some cases of persistent travelers' diarrhea are cases in which the diarrhea itself is actually a small complaint, but associated gastrointestinal symptoms such as cramping, bloating, gaseousness, and rectal urgency may predominate. In some cases, extreme and debilitating fatigue may follow a bout of travelers' diarrhea. In other cases, a distinct change in bowel habits such as intractable constipation may also follow acute travelers' diarrhea.

In a recent review of three studies, it has been found that up to 3% of travelers have persistent diarrhea longer than 30 days, and it has been estimated that between 3% to 10% will have diarrhea longer than 2 weeks.[1-3] This chapter will focus on the evaluation and management of the patient with chronic travelers' diarrhea, defined as diarrhea lasting longer than 2 weeks, the onset of which began during or shortly after travel. As important as recognizing the etiologies of chronic travelers' diarrhea will be recognizing distinct clinical syndromes. A combination of an etiologic and syndromic approach to this problem will often be more helpful than one or the other exclusively. The etiologies of chronic travelers' diarrhea are primarily but not exclusively infectious in nature. Bacteria, the most common cause of acute travelers' diarrhea, may also cause chronic travelers' diarrhea. Likewise, parasites and, in some cases, viruses can cause prolonged symptoms as well. In some cases, treatment of acute travelers' diarrhea may lead to continuing diarrhea because of bacterial overgrowth syndromes (e.g., *Clostridium difficile*, small bowel overgrowth). In other cases, a bout of acute travelers' diarrhea will unmask an underlying gastrointestinal syndrome such as celiac disease, inflammatory bowel disease, or irritable bowel syndrome.

INFECTIOUS ETIOLOGIES OF CHRONIC TRAVELERS' DIARRHEA

BACTERIA

Travelers' diarrhea is usually caused by a bacterial agent such enterotoxigenic *Escherichia coli*, *Shigella*, *Salmonella*, or *Campylobacter*.[2,4] These bacteria may also lead to persistent symptoms in some individuals. After an initial resolution of the infection, a carrier state may ensue with recrudescence of symptoms days to weeks later. Both *Salmonella* and *Shigella* species have been known to behave in this manner. In some cases, there is slow resolution of the acute infection leading to damage to the intestinal mucosa, which may take days to weeks to repair even after clearance of the organism. An individual who reports relapsing diarrhea in the first few weeks following enteric bacterial infection may be suffering from this postinfective intestinal inflammation.

Infections due to diarrheagenic forms of *E. coli* and *Shigella* generally last less than a week, and excretion of the organisms is usually less than 2 weeks. The illness due to nontyphoidal *Salmonella* and *Campylobacter* is also generally short, but fecal excretion of the organism may continue for 4 to 6 weeks. A careful history may suggest that chronic diarrhea may be several unrelated episodes and that the current infection was acquired shortly before returning home. A history of fever and the presence of fecal leukocytes, blood, or mucous may suggest a missed bacterial infection. Treatment history may indicate that the infection was not treated or treated inappropriately. Stool culture with antimicrobial susceptibility testing is often helpful. *Yersinia enterocolitica* should be considered in travelers going to temperate climates but is very rare in travelers returning from the tropics. Recently, organisms such as enteroadherent *E. coli* have been associated with this syndrome of persistent diarrhea. Enteroadherent *E. coli* have been suggested as causes of chronic diarrhea in children in the developing world and in African patients with AIDS.[5-8] Two studies recently suggested the possible importance of this organism as a cause of travelers' diarrhea.[9,10] *Aeromonas* and *Plesiomonas* infections have been associated with chronic diarrhea in a few instances.[11,12]

ANAEROBIC BACTERIA

C. difficile is a bacterial organism that elicits at least two toxins.[13] *C. difficile* infections may be a cause of persistent diarrhea in returned travelers. There is usually a history of prior treatment of diarrheal episodes with antibiotics. In some cases, diarrhea from *C. difficile* may result from the use of antimalarial chemoprophylactic agents such as mefloquine, chloroquine, or doxycycline. A careful history of prior antibiotic use and medications used during travel is important in suggesting this diagnosis. An examination of stool for *C. difficile* toxin should be included as part of the work-up.

PARASITIC INFECTIONS

Parasitic infections probably represent the most common causes of chronic diarrhea in returning travelers. With symptoms continuing for more than 14 days, parasitic causes increase in likelihood. In travelers to Nepal, *Giardia* was detected in 10% of travelers with symptoms for less than 14 days and in 27% of those with symptoms for more than 14 days.[14,15] The four most common protozoal agents that must be considered are *Giardia lamblia*, *Entamoeba histolytica*, *Cryptosporidium parvum,* and *Cyclospora cayetanensis. Microsporidia* and *Dientamoeba fragilis* are rare causes of persistent low-grade gastrointestinal symptoms.

Giardiasis   *G. lamblia* is the most common protozoan infection of returning travelers. This infection often presents with a predominance of upper gastrointestinal symptoms including nausea, eructation, and bloating in addition to diarrhea.[16] Untreated infections can persist for months. Diagnosis is usually made by stool examination, but multiple careful examinations may be necessary to demonstrate the organism. Stool antigen test kits for *G. lamblia* are available, but there is little evidence to suggest that they actually increase the diagnosis rate beyond careful and repeated stool examinations.[17] An examination of the duodenal aspirate either at the time of an upper gastrointestinal endoscopy or by duodenal string test can also increase the likelihood of diagnosis.[18] As upper endoscopy is an invasive examination and duodenal string tests have fallen out of favor in recent years, empiric treatment is appropriate in the context of persistent symptoms compatible with a *Giardia* infection. In the United States, metronidazole 250 mg tid for 7 days is usually recommended but may require more than one course for cure. Outside of the United States, the most commonly used medication is tinidazole, which is taken as a single 2,000-mg dose daily for 2 days.[16] Cure rates approach 100% with any of these regimens, but recently metronidazole and tinidazole-resistant strains have been reported. Quinacrine 100 mg tid is effective at eradication of *Giardia* but is currently unavailable in the United States. Albendazole 400 mg qd for 7 days has high efficacy in treating *Giardia* infections as well and is now used as second-line therapy.[19]

INTESTINAL AMEBIASIS

E. histolytica may actually be a very uncommon cause of travelers' diarrhea, as it has now been recognized that there are two morphologically indistinguishable species: *E. histolytica*, the true pathogen, and *E. dispar*, a nonpathogenic look-alike.[20] *E. histolytica* is a pathogen with symptoms ranging from a mild, chronic infection to severe and even fatal colitis. *E. dispar* is a nonpathogen. The organisms cannot be distinguished microscopically but nonmicroscopic tests are being developed. *E. dispar* is the much more common organism, estimated to be 10 times more common than the pathogenic *E. histolytica*.[21] Currently, we can describe three different presentations of *E. histolytica/E. dispar* infection. It now appears that the asymptomatic cyst passer is most likely infected with *E. dispar* and no treatment is indicated. This patient may be picked up on routine stool screening or as part of the work-up for a chronic diarrhea this organism may be

found, confusing the diagnosis. As a patient who is ill with what was previously termed a nondysenteric amebiasis may actually have *E. dispar* infection or may truly have a lower grade *E. histolytica* infection, therapy is usually offered to this individual.[22,23] Patients with true nondysenteric amebiasis usually present with an alternating form of illness in which a day of crampy diarrhea is often followed by 1 or 2 days of no diarrhea or even constipation. This pattern becomes cyclical. Fatigue and weight loss may eventually bring the patient to medical attention. Amebic colitis, the third form of amebiasis, is extremely rare in travelers. Low-grade diarrhea may progress over a matter of days to severe bloody colitis with cramps and tenesmus. In these cases, the bloody stool will typically show *E. histolytica* trophozoites with ingested red blood cells. Treatment of nondysenteric and dysenteric amebiasis is the same if the person is not critically ill. In the United States, metronidazole 750 mg tid for 10 days is used followed by a luminal agent such as paramomycin 500 mg tid for 10 days or iodoquinol 650 mg tid for 20 days. Outside of the United States, tinidazole 2 g daily for 3 days is extremely effective and well tolerated, again followed by a luminal agent.

A historic footnote to the issue of amebiasis in the returning traveler is a syndrome known as postdysenteric colitis. This syndrome, first described in 1943, reports continuing symptoms following treatment of true amebic dysentery. Two varieties of this syndrome, a functional nonulcerative colitis similar to postinfective irritable bowel syndrome and an ulcerative post dysenteric colitis indistinguishable from inflammatory bowel disease, were described.[24,25] As this syndrome was first described more than 50 years ago, it is likely that other unknown (at the time) pathogens were responsible, especially for the ulcerative type. *C. difficile* colitis may present with gross sigmoidoscopic and histologic appearances indistinguishable from, for example, ulcerative colitis.

CYCLOSPORIASIS

C. cayetanensis is a coccidian protozoan parasite that has recently been described as responsible for chronic diarrheal syndrome.[26] It has been the cause of annual seasonal outbreaks of persistent diarrhea in travelers and expatriate residents in Nepal and Peru, and the distribution of this organism appears to be worldwide.[27] *Cyclospora* during the premonsoon season in Nepal may be responsible for one-third of all diarrheal illness.[14] Outbreaks have also occurred in North America associated with imported Guatemalan raspberries.[28] In the initial studies from Nepal and Peru, which predated effective antibiotic therapy, travelers who acquired *Cyclospora* were sick with persistent diarrhea for 6 or more weeks.[26] Upper gastrointestinal symptoms predominate, and anorexia, malabsorption, and weight loss are common.[29] Fatigue and anorexia are extremely predominant and may help distinguish *Cyclospora* infection from other pathogens. *Cyclospora* can be identified in concentrated stool both by plain wet mount and by modified acid-fast staining. The organism is 8 to 10 microns in diameter, making it approximately twice as large as *Cryptosporidium*.

Trimethoprim-sulfamethoxazole double strength bid for 7 days has been found to be effective therapy.[30] Some patients require a slightly longer course of therapy. Despite numerous clinical trials, no alternative therapy to this sulfa-containing antibiotic has been identified.

CRYPTOSPORIDIOSIS

This protozoan pathogen was first described in association with chronic diarrhea in HIV-infected individuals. A widespread water-borne outbreak in the United States in Milwaukee, Wisconsin, in 1993 affecting 400,000 individuals demonstrated the effects that this organism can have on the immunocompetent as well.[31] Cryptosporidiosis may be a cause of chronic diarrheal symptoms in returning travelers.[32] Treatment trials have been conflicting, but recently the use of paramomycin (Humatin) has been found to be effective in treating immunocompetent travelers with cryptosporidiosis.[33,34] In the immunocompetent, the illness is self-limited and symptoms resolve within 1 to 3 weeks.[35]

ISOSPORIASIS

Immunocompetent travelers have been described who have returned to the United States with *Isospora* infections acquired in the Caribbean, India, and Africa. A case of chronic diarrhea and crampy abdominal pain occurred in an American traveling for 5 weeks in West Africa.[36] Patients have been successfully treated with a 10-day course of trimethoprim-sulfamethoxazole double strength qid.[37]

DIENTAMOEBA FRAGILIS

Another parasite that has been reported in returning travelers with persistent symptoms has been *Dientamoeba fragilis*.[38] In most studies, this organism has been an uncommon etiology of chronic travelers' diarrhea. Effective therapy is available with either iodoquinol 650 mg tid for 20 days or tetracycline 500 mg qid for 10 days.

In cases where a microbial etiologic agent is not readily identified, approaching the patient's complaints by way of a syndromic approach allows both a systematic way of ruling out some of the less common causes, allows a double check on some of the etiologic agents that may have been missed during the initial diagnostic evaluation, and provides the framework for therapy, either pharmacotherapy or a combination of diet and other intervention (Table 20.4–1).

CHRONIC DIARRHEA WITHOUT AN IDENTIFIABLE ETIOLOGY

In some cases of persistent diarrhea, no microorganism is identified, yet both patient and physician alike are convinced that they are dealing with an infectious disease. Chronic diarrhea symptoms can sometimes be linked to a distinct outbreak and a measurable length of illness. Considering that over the past two decades, new and previ-

Table 20.4–1.   AN APPROACH TO CHRONIC TRAVELERS' DIARRHEA

Etiologic
  Bacteria
  Parasites
  Clostridium difficile

Syndromic
  Malabsorption (± weight loss)
    Acute (postinfective), temporary
      Disaccharidase deficiency
    Subacute/chronic
      Subclinical tropical malabsorption
      Parasites
      Tropical sprue
      Celiac disease
      Small bowel overgrowth

Associated gastrointestinal symptoms
  Postinfective irritable bowel syndrome

Weight loss (without malabsorption)
  HIV
  Malignancy

Hematochezia
  Infectious colitis
    Clostridium difficile
    Entamoeba histolytica
    Campylobacter jejuni
  Inflammatory bowel disease

ously unrecognized enteric pathogens have been identified, it is certainly possible that some patients are suffering from chronic diarrheal syndromes caused by previously unrecognized infectious agents. *Campylobacter jejuni*, for example, one of the most common causes of travelers' diarrhea worldwide, was only first recognized as a pathogen in 1978. *Cryptosporidium*, an agent in both sporadic and travelers' diarrhea, was only first described as a human pathogen in 1982, and *Cyclospora*, which seasonally may be one of the more common causes of travelers' diarrhea in certain regions, was unrecognized prior to 1991. In addition, new diagnostic techniques have increased our ability to identify microorganisms responsible for some well-known diseases such as Whipple's. New diagnostic technologies have allowed identification of infectious disease by ELISA, polymerase chain reaction, and other indirect methods. The example of Brainerd diarrhea leads one to believe that other etiologic agents remain to be discovered as the cause of persistent diarrhea.

BRAINERD DIARRHEA

In 1983, an outbreak of chronic diarrhea occurred in Brainerd, Minnesota. The illness was characterized by an acute onset of watery diarrhea associated with urgency, a failure to respond to antimicrobial agents, and a duration of 2 to 36 months. Unpastuerized milk from a local dairy was epidemiologically implicated; however, an etiologic agent was never found.[39] A total of six outbreaks of Brainerd diarrhea have occurred in the United States since its initial description, and in 1992 an outbreak occurred on a cruise ship in the Galapagos Islands, Ecuador.[40,41] In the first weeks of illness, patients described the sudden onset of frequent watery diarrhea followed by gas and abdominal cramps. In most patients, weight loss ensues, and the illness waxes and wanes with periods of partial remission followed by exacerbations of gradually decreasing severity. In the initial outbreak, after 1 year, 12% were normal, 40% were improved, and 48% still had persistent diarrhea. The illness ranged in duration from 7 months to more than 42 months. Colonic biopsy specimens showed a distinctive increase in colonic surface epithelial lymphocytes, but markers for lymphocytic and collagenous colitis were absent. Extensive microbiologic studies failed to associate the illness with any known bacterial or parasitic cause. It is possible that Brainerd diarrhea may account for a number of sporadic cases of chronic diarrhea in returning travelers.

MALABSORPTION

POSTINFECTIVE MALABSORPTION

A useful point of departure is to evaluate for the presence of malabsorption. In some cases, malabsorption may be a temporary postinfective phenomenon. An attack of acute infectious diarrhea may precipitate an intestinal disaccharidase deficiency. Lactase deficiency is most common, and patients will report an increase in symptoms when ingesting lactose-containing products such as milk, cheese, or ice cream. In some, a sucrase deficiency may result, and symptoms are worsened by fruits or preserves. This type of postinfective malabsorption is common with diarrhea of any etiology, is temporary, and usually subsides within a few days to weeks after clearance of the organism.[42,43] Symptoms of a postinfective malabsorption include an exacerbation of diarrhea, soft stool, abdominal cramps, pain, and gaseous distention.[44] In some, a temporary postinfective lactose intolerance becomes permanent. This, in fact, may be a genetically predisposed individual with subclinical lactose intolerance whose condition has been provoked by the acute episode of diarrhea.

SUBACUTE MALABSORPTION

Subacute malabsorption is sometimes seen following travel and a syndrome of subclinical tropical malabsorption has been described, usually in indigenous healthy persons in the tropics but also in expatriates and long-term travelers to these regions as well. Subclinical tropical malabsorption is a benign condition characterized by decreased absorption of D-xylose and glucose, mild changes in small bowel architecture, and a variably abnormal D-xylose test. The syndrome is seasonal and invari-

ably remits when the expatriate or traveler returns to his/her home temperate climate.[45,46]

CHRONIC MALABSORPTION

Chronic malabsorption may result from infections by certain parasites. The most common parasitic cause of malabsorption is *G. lamblia*. Other parasites associated with malabsorption include *C. cayatanensis*, *I. belli*, *Strongyloides stercoralis*, *Ascaris lumbricoides,* and *Capillaria philippinensis*.

TROPICAL SPRUE

Tropical sprue is intestinal malabsorption acquired in the tropics that is associated with fatigue, weight loss, and anorexia. Tropical sprue is characterized by continuing diarrhea and steatorrhea following an acute gastrointestinal infection. Variable small bowel architectural changes, namely, crypt hyperplasia and villous atrophy, are noted. This condition eventuates in nutritional deficiencies and weight loss and the intestinal abnormalities worsen unless specific treatment is instituted.[47] The condition is more common in long-stay travelers but may also affect short-term travelers.[48] It occurs in most areas of the tropics but is predominant in Asia and occurs less frequently in Africa. Cases are reported from parts of the Caribbean, the Indian subcontinent, and the Middle East.[49] Available evidence suggests that tropical sprue is an infectious disease that is precipitated by an acute infection and propagated by the persistent contamination of the small bowel by an enteric pathogen. This is suggested by the fact that this syndrome follows acute infectious diarrhea. There are seasonal and household epidemics, but, to date, no specific causative microorganism has been identified. Tropical sprue is successfully treated with tetracycline 250 mg qid and folate 5 mg qd. Treatment courses vary between 6 weeks and 3 months. If symptoms have been present for a long time, vitamin B_{12} deficiency is often present, and parenteral vitamin B_{12} replacement is recommended. Sometimes, a second course of tetracycline and folate may be necessary in patients with long-standing illness. There is some suggestion that antibiotic self-treatment for acute travelers' diarrhea may lessen the incidence of subsequent tropical sprue.

SMALL BOWEL OVERGROWTH SYNDROME

Occasionally, chronic malabsorption is seen following acute travelers' diarrhea because of changes in gastrointestinal motility. Stasis of the upper small bowel and consequent small bowel overgrowth may lead to malabsorption. This condition is treated with a broad-spectrum antibiotic.[50]

CELIAC SPRUE

Occasionally, chronic malabsorption is due to celiac sprue, a condition that is probably genetically predisposed prior to the onset of foreign travel and unmasked by an episode of travelers' diarrhea. Celiac sprue, or gluten-sensitive enteropathy, is suggested by evidence of malabsorption, moderately severe to severe crypt hyperplasia and villous atrophy on small bowel biopsy, and serologic confirmation by antigliadin and antiendomysial antibodies and/or a serum tissue transglutaminase elevation. Treatment is by avoidance of wheat- and gliadin-containing products.

CHRONIC DIARRHEA WITH ASSOCIATED GASTROINTESTINAL SYMPTOMS

Perhaps the most common diagnosis in returning travelers with chronic diarrhea is what has now become known as the postinfective irritable bowel syndrome. Persons with this disorder complain of intermittent diarrhea, soft stool, crampy abdominal pain, bloating, and gas.[51] Was the patient truly free of similar symptoms prior to travel and is now perhaps somewhat more aware, or is this actually the new onset of a new syndrome? The diagnosis is suggested by the lack of systemic symptoms and maintenance of normal weight. The postinfective irritable bowel syndrome may represent a primary alteration in gut motility or be secondary to or exacerbated by an acute enteric infection. In some patients with postinfective irritable bowel syndrome, diarrhea is not present, but instead abdominal bloating, gas, and even constipation may predominate. Some patients with this syndrome present with a constipation predominant syndrome and others with a chronic post-travel debilitating fatigue out of proportion to other symptoms.

CHRONIC DIARRHEA ASSOCIATED WITH WEIGHT LOSS

When weight loss is associated with symptoms and malabsorption has been ruled out, serious consideration must be given to other causes. There is the temptation when evaluating the returning traveler with chronic diarrhea to assume that the etiology is infectious in nature. Patients themselves are often convinced that they are harboring an undiagnosed parasite or microbe and sometimes have taken numerous courses of antibiotics in an attempt to rid themselves of the microorganism. In evaluating these patients, it is wise to consider possible causes of their symptoms other than infectious etiologies. In a retrospective review of 129 patients from 1978 to 1984 with bloody diarrhea acquired in or within 2 weeks of return from the tropics, a full 25% had either inflammatory bowel disease or colon cancer.[52] In an older individual, hemoccult testing and endoscopic evaluation may be warranted. Noninfectious causes of chronic diarrhea in addition to inflammatory bowel disease and colon cancer include metabolic disorders, electrolyte disturbances, medication ingestion (sometimes surreptitious), and even occult alcoholism. Chronic diarrhea may also be the result of opportunistic infection in the HIV-infected individual

and in some chronic diarrhea may be the presenting symptom of a previously undiagnosed HIV infection.

CHRONIC DIARRHEA WITH HEMATOCHEZIA OR OTHER SYSTEMIC SYMPTOMS

The presence of rectal bleeding implies a lesion of the lower gastrointestinal tract. Infectious colitis caused by *C. difficile*, *E. histolytica*, or *Campylobacter* may cause dysentery, tenesmus, and rectal bleeding. Inflammatory bowel disease, especially ulcerative proctocolitis or ulcerative colitis, may also present with rectal bleeding. The persistence of diarrheal symptoms in the returning traveler may be the unmasking of a previously asymptomatic gastrointestinal disorder. A syndrome of ulcerative colitis has been described in returning travelers that does not respond to antibiotic therapy and is indistinguishable from idiopathic inflammatory bowel disease.[53] Is this the unmasking of a previously asymptomatic ulcerative colitis in a genetically predisposed individual or the true consequence of an acute intestinal infection? Before corticosteroids are administered, one must rule out *E. histolytica* infection with multiple negative stools and an indirect hemagglutination assay. Treatment with agents used for inflammatory bowel disease such as mesalamine or corticosteroids either by enema or orally are highly efficacious in ameliorating symptoms. Crohn's disease has been reported in returning travelers, perhaps coincidentally and unrelated to travel.

DIAGNOSTIC EVALUATION AND TREATMENT OF CHRONIC TRAVELERS' DIARRHEA

An evaluation of the patient with chronic travelers' diarrhea begins with a directed history. What was the specific itinerary? When did the patient get sick? What was the nature of the acute illness? What medications were taken during the trip either before the acute illness or for treatment of travelers' diarrhea or other maladies? Was malaria chemoprophylaxis taken? Evaluating specific symptoms of the current illness can help localize the site of infection to either upper or lower intestine. This may be helpful in determining more common etiologic agents. Pathogens that cause predominance of upper gastrointestinal symptoms may make parasitic causes such as *Giardia* or *Cyclospora* more likely. Symptoms of dysentery or tenesmus might focus attention on predominantly colonic diseases. The tests that are most useful include stool microscopy with wet prep, trichrome, and modified acid-fast stains. A minimum of three stool specimens is often necessary to increase sensitivity of the stool ova and parasite examination. Stool culture and sensitivity and stools for *C. difficile* would be included among initial stool testing. Other diagnostic tests such as stool specimen for occult blood can be expected to be positive in many individuals with diarrhea, but in an older individual the strong presence of a hemoccult positive stool may direct endoscopic evaluation to rule out structural disease of the gastrointestinal tract.

Blood tests most helpful are a complete blood count with differential, especially looking for eosinophilia, which might raise the suspicion of a helminth infection. Other diagnostic serologies would include amebic serology and HIV antibody. When necessary, further blood testing for thyroid function, electrolytes, calcium, gastrin, 5HIAA, and formal lactose tolerance testing may be considered.

A urine D-xylose test is a simple way to rule out malabsorption. After drinking a 25-g bolus of D-xylose dissolved in a glass of water, patients are instructed to collect all urines for the next 5 hours, forcing themselves to empty their bladder at the 5-hour mark. Patients are instructed not to eat for the first hour after drinking the D-xylose. A normal result is excretion of 20% or 5 g of D-xylose in the 5-hour period.

Endoscopic evaluation, although not a first-line diagnostic test, should be considered for those in whom systemic disease is suspected or for those with more serious or severe symptoms. Upper gastrointestinal endoscopy with a duodenal aspirate (looking for parasites) and a small bowel biopsy may be helpful in diagnosing upper gastrointestinal causes of chronic diarrhea including tropical sprue and certain parasitic diseases. Examination of the lower gastrointestinal tract by way of flexible sigmoidoscopy or colonoscopy with biopsies can in some pinpoint the cause of symptoms.

Additional diagnostic tests might also serve the dual purpose of empiric therapy. A response to quinolone antibiotics or azithromycin might be therapeutic and diagnostic of bacterial disease. Treatment with trimethoprim-sulfamethoxazole in cases of suspected *Cyclospora* may be therapeutic as well. A course of a nitroimidazole such as metronidazole or tinidazole might be warranted for empiric therapy of suspected *Giardia* or *Amoeba* infection.

Some patients respond to elimination diets. A suggested approach would be initially lactose, fructose, glucose, and fat restricted, in that order.

Antispasmodics and medications commonly used to treat irritable bowel syndrome such as chlordiazepoxide, clinidium, and/or limbitrol might be helpful adjuncts to therapy.

Antidiarrheals such as loperamide or diphenoxalate, tincture of opium, and/or bismuth compounds may afford relief of symptoms. The judicious use of fiber in the form of psyllium or methyl cellulose might be useful as well. Probiotics such as *Lactobacillus* or *Saccharomyces boulardii* may ameliorate symptoms in certain individuals.[54]

In suspected cases of inflammatory bowel disease, medications commonly used for these conditions, mesalamine or corticosteroids, may be efficacious. Occasionally, digestive enzymes such as lactase or pancrease afford symptomatic relief.

In summary, many patients with acute travelers' diarrhea did not recover completely but developed one of several chronic diarrheal syndromes. In some patients, an episode of travelers' diarrhea seems to unmask a preexisting, underlying gastrointestinal disorder. Many patients with chronic diarrhea elude diagnosis, and treatment may be problematic. Questions that remain include the magnitude of the problem worldwide, the natural history of this disorder or disorders, any specific predisposing factors, and, of course, the role of new or unrecognized etiologic agents.

REFERENCES

1. Addiss DG, Tauxe RV, Bernard KW. Chronic diarrheal illness in U.S. Peace Corps volunteers. Int J Epidemiol 1990;19:217–218.
2. Steffen R, van der Linde F, Gyr K, Schar M. Epidemiology of diarrhea in travelers. JAMA 1983;249:1176–1180.
3. DuPont HL, Capsuto EG. Persistent diarrhea in travelers. Clin Infect Dis 1996;22:124–128.
4. Katelaris PH, Farthing MJ. Traveler's diarrhea: clinical presentation and prognosis. Chemotherapy 1995;41(Suppl 1):40.
5. Baqui AH, Sack RB, Black RE, et al. Enteropathogens associated with acute and persistent diarrhea in Bangladeshi children less than 5 years of ag. J Infect Dis 1992;166:792.
6. Bhan MK, Raj P, Levine MM, et al. Enteroaggregative *Escherichia coli* associated with persistent diarrhea in a cohort of rural children in India. J Infect Dis 1989;159:1061–1064.
7. Black RE. Persistent diarrhea in children of developing countries. Pediatr Infect Dis J 1993;12:751.
8. Mathewson JJ, Jiang ZD, Zumla A, et al. Hep-2 cell adherent *Escherichia coli* in patients with human immunodeficiency virus-associated diarrhea. J Infect Dis 1995;171:1636.
9. Cohen MB, Hawkins JA, Weckbach LS, et al. Colonization by enteroaggregative *Escherichia coli* in travelers with and without diarrhea. J Clin Microbiol 1993;31:351–353.
10. Gascôn J, Vargas M, Quinté L, et al. Enteroaggregative *Escherichia coli* strains as a cause of traveler's diarrhea: a case-control study. J Infect Dis 1998;177:1409–1412.
11. Rautelin H, Hanninen ML, Sivonen A, et al. Chronic diarrhea due to a single strain of *Aeromonas caviae*. Eur J Clin Microbiol Infect Dis 1995;14:51.
12. Rautelin H, Sivonen A, Kuikka A, et al. Enteric *Plesiomonas shigelloides* infections in Finnish patients. Scand J Infect Dis 1995;27:495.
13. Bartlett JG. Antibiotic-associated diarrhea. Clin Infect Dis 1992;15:573–579.
14. Hoge CW, Shlim DR, Echeverria P, et al. Epidemiology of diarrhea among expatriate residents living in a highly endemic environment. JAMA 1996;275:533–538.
15. Taylor DN, Houston R, Shlim DR, et al. Etiology of diarrhea among travelers and foreign residents in Nepal. JAMA 1988;260:1245–1248.
16. Wright SG, Tomkins AM, Ridley DS. Giardiasis: clinical and therapeutic aspects. Gut 1977;18:343–350.
17. Addis DG, Mathews HM, Stewart JM, et al. Evaluation of a commercially available enzyme-linked immunosorbent assay for *Giardia lamblia* antigen in stool. J Clin Microbiol 1991;29:1137.
18. Goka AK, Rolston DD, Mathan VI, et al. The relative merits of faecal and duodenal juice microscopy in the diagnosis of giardiasis. Trans R Soc Trop Med Hyg 1990;84:66.
19. Dutta Ak, Phadke MA, Bagade AC, et al. A randomised multicentre study to compare the safety and efficacy of albendazole and metronidazole in the treatment of giardiasis in children. Indian J Pediatr 1994;61:689.
20. Jackson TF. *Entamoeba histolytica* and *Entamoeba dispar* are distinct species; clinical, epidemiological and serological evidence. Int J Parasitol 1998;28:181.

21. Reed SL. Amebiasis: an update. Clin Infect Dis 1992; 14:385–391.

22. Anand AC, Reddy PS, Saiprasad GS, Kher SK. Does non-dysenteric intestinal amoebiasis exist? Lancet 1997;349:89–92.

23. Nanda R, Baveja U, Anand BS. *Entamoeba histolytica* cyst passers: clinical features and outcome in untreated subjects. Lancet 1984;1:301–303.

24. Stewart GT. Post-dysenteric colitis. BMJ 1950;1:405–408.

25. Fung WP, Monteiro EH, Ang HB, et al. Ulcerative postdysenteric colitis. Am J Gastroenterol 1972;57:341–348.

26. Hoge CW, Shlim DR, Rajah R, et al. Epidemiology of diarrheal illness associated with coccidian-like organism among travellers and foreign residents in Nepal. Lancet 1993; 341:1175–1178.

27. Connor BA, Cyclospora infection: a review. Ann Acad Med Singapore 1997;26:632–636.

28. Herwaldt BL, Ackers ML. An outbreak in 1996 of cyclosporiasis associated with imported raspberries. The Cyclospora Working Group. N Engl J Med 1997;336:1548.

29. Connor BA, Shlim DR, Scholes JV, et al. Pathologic changes in the small bowel in nine patients with diarrhea associated with a coccidia-like body. Ann Int Med 1993;119:377–382.

30. Hoge CW, Shlim DR, Ghimire M, et al. Placebo-controlled trial of co-trimoxazole for cyclospora infections among travellers and foreign residents in Nepal. Lancet 1995;345:691–693.

31. MacKenzie WR, Hoxie NJ, Proctor ME, et al. A massive outbreak in Milwaukee of cryptosporidium infection transmitted through the public water supply. N Engl J Med 1994;331:161.

32. Gatti S, Cevini C, Bruno A, et al. Cryptosporidiosis in tourists returning from Egypt and the island of Mauritius. Clin Infect Dis 1993;16:344–345.

33. Bissuel F, Cotte L, Rabodonirina M, et al. Paramomycin: an effective treatment for cryptosporidial diarrhea in patients with AIDS. Clin Infect Dis 1994;18:447.

34. Fichtenbaum CJ, Ritchie DJ, Powderly WG. Use of paramomycin for treatment of cryptosporidiosis in patients with AIDS. Clin Infect Dis 1993;16:298.

35. Jokipii AMM, Hemila M, Jokipii L. Prospective study of acquisition of *Cryptosporidium, Giardia lamblia* and gastrointestinal disease. Lancet 1985;1:487–489.

36. Shaffer N, Moore L. Correspondence—chronic travelers' diarrhea in a normal host due to *Isospora belli*. J Infect Dis 1989;159:596–597.

37. Ebrahimzadeh A, Bottone EJ. Persistent diarrhea caused by *Isospora belli*: therapeutic response to pyrimethamine and sulfadiazine. Diagn Microbiol Infect Dis 1996;26:87.

38. Cuffari C, Oligny L, Seidman EG. *Dientamoeba fragilis* masquerading as allergic colits. J Pediatr Gastroenterol Nutr 1998;26:16.

39. Osterholm MT, MacDonald KL, White KE, et al. An outbreak of a newly recognized chronic diarrhea syndrome associated with raw milk consumption. JAMA 1986;256:484–490.

40. Parsonnet J, Trock SC, Bopp CA, et al. Chronic diarrhea associated with drinking untreated water. Ann Intern Med 1989;110:985–991.

41. Mintz ED, Weber JT, Guris D, et al. An outbreak of Brainerd diarrhea among travelers to the Galapagos Islands. J Infect Dis 1998;177:1041.

42. Montgomery RD, Beale DJ, Sammons HG, Schneider R. Postinfective malabsorption: a sprue syndrome. BMJ 1973;2:265–268.

43. Greene HL, McCabe Dr, Merenstein GB. Protracted diarrhea and malnutrition in infancy: changes in intestinal morphology and disaccharidase activities during treatment with total intravenous nutrition or oral elemental diets. J Pediatrics 1975;87:695.

44. Bhutta ZA, Hendricks KM. Nutritional management of persistent diarrhea in childhood: a perspective from the developing world. J Pediatr Gastroenterol Nutr 1996;22:17.

45. Keusch GT. Subclinical malabsorption in Thailand. I. Intestinal absorption in Thai children. Am J Clin Nutr 1972;25:1062.

46. Keusch GT, Plaut AG, Troncale FJ. Subclinical malabsorption in Thailand. II. Intestinal absorption in American military and Peace Corps personnel. Am J Clin Nutr 1972;25:1067.

47. Cook GC. Aetiology and pathogenesis of postinfective tropical malabsorption (tropical sprue). Lancet 1984;1:721–723.

48. Tomkins AM, James WPT, Walters JH, Cole ACE. Malabsorption in overland travellers to India. BMJ 1974;3:380–384.

49. Klipstein FA. Tropical sprue in travelers and expatriates living abroad. Gastroenterology 1981;80:590–600.

50. Bhatnagar S. Bhan MK, George C, et al. Is small bowel bacterial overgrowth of pathogenic significance in persistent diarrhea? Acta Paediatr Suppl 1992;381:108.

51. McKendrick MW, Read NW. Irritable bowel syndrome—post salmonella infection. J Infection 1994;29:1–3.

52. Harries AD, Myers B, Cook, GC. Inflammatory bowel disease: a common cause of bloody diarrhoea in visitors to the tropics. BMJ 1985;291:1686–1687.

53. Schumacher G, Kollberg B, Ljungh A. Inflammatory bowel disease presenting as travellers' diarrhoea. Lancet 1993;341:241–242.

54. Kirchhelle A. Fruhwein N. Toburen D. Treatment of persistent diarrhea with *S. boulardii* in returning travelers. Results of a prospective study. Fortschr Med 1996;114:136.

Chapter 21

MALARIA

21.1 MALARIA EPIDEMIOLOGY

HANS O. LOBEL AND S. PATRICK KACHUR

INTRODUCTION

Each year, some 25 to 30 million travelers from nontropical countries visit malaria-endemic countries, and up to 30,000 North American and European travelers contract malaria annually.[1] Worldwide, an estimated 300 to 500 million clinical cases of malaria occur each year, and more than 90% of the 1.5 to 2.0 million deaths attributed to malaria each year occur in African children.[2] Malaria poses a serious health problem not only for short-term travelers but especially for individuals deployed on humanitarian and military missions, missionaries, Peace Corps volunteers, and other expatriates living in malarious areas.

Malaria transmission occurs primarily in tropical and subtropical regions in sub-Saharan Africa, Central and South America, the Caribbean island of Hispaniola, the Middle East, the Indian subcontinent, Southeast Asia, and Oceania (Figure 21.1–1). In areas where malaria occurs, however, there is considerable variation in the intensity of transmission and risk of malaria infection. Malaria transmission occurs in urban areas in sub-Saharan Africa and the Indian subcontinent.

AGENT AND LIFE CYCLE

In humans, malaria infection is caused by one or more of four species of intracellular protozoan parasite. *Plasmodium falciparum*, *P. vivax*, *P. ovale*, and *P. malariae* differ in geographic distribution, microscopic appearance, clinical features, and immunogenic potential (Table 21.1–1). Although *P. vivax* infections are more commonly reported, worldwide *P. falciparum* malaria represents the most serious public health problem because of its tendency toward severe or fatal infections.

LIFE CYCLE

Although there are important differences between them, the four human malarias share a common life cycle. Malaria infection begins when an infective female mosquito injects *Plasmodium* sp sporozoites into the blood stream while feeding (Figure 21.1–2). The sporozoites circulate only momentarily; those that survive host immune defenses infect cells of the liver parenchyma. There they undergo

asexual reproduction (exoerythrocytic schizogony), producing hepatic schizonts. In 6 to 14 days, these schizonts mature and rupture, releasing merozoites into the blood stream. Merozoites then invade red blood cells (RBCs) where they undergo a second phase of asexual reproduction (erythrocytic schizogony), developing into rings, trophozoites, and, finally, erythrocytic schizonts. Once mature, the infected RBCs rupture, releasing still more merozoites into the blood stream and starting another cycle of asexual development and multiplication. Clinical symptoms are associated with the rupture of erythrocytic schizonts and usually develop after several cycles of erythrocytic schizogony. The classic clinical presentation of periodic fever occurs when the cycles of erythrocytic schizogony are synchronized. Malaria parasites continue to proliferate until (1) immune responses eliminate the infection, (2) effective antimalarial drugs kill all of the erythrocytic parasites, or (3) the host dies from the infection.

Eventually, some merozoites develop into sexual forms called gametocytes. Both male and female gametocytes circulate without causing symptoms and can be ingested by a mosquito during a subsequent blood meal. Sexual reproduction occurs within the mosquito, resulting in sporozoites in the salivary glands. The life cycle starts again when the infective mosquito bites another human. The mosquito is essential to the development of the malaria parasite and its transmission. The sporogonic cycle—the period of time between ingestion of gametocytes and becoming infective to humans—varies among

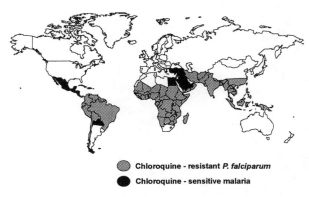

⬤ Chloroquine - resistant *P. falciparum*

● Chloroquine - sensitive malaria

Figure 21.1–1. Malaria-endemic areas of the world.

Table 21.1–1.   CHARACTERISTICS OF THE FOUR SPECIES OF HUMAN MALARIA

	P. FALCIPARUM	P. VIVAX	P. OVALE	P. MALARIAE
Exoerythrocytic cycle	6–7 days	6–8 days	9 days	14–16 days
Prepatent period	9–10 days	11–13 days	10–14 days	15–16 day
Incubation period (mean)	9–14 (12) days	12–17 (15) days to 6–12 months	16–18 (17) days or longer	18–40 (28) days or longer
Severity of primary attack	Severe	Mild to severe	Severe	Severe
Duration of primary attack*	16–36 hours or longer	8–12 hours	8–12 hours	8–10 hours
Duration of untreated infection*	1–2 years	1.5–5 years	1.5–5 years	3–50 years
Relapse	No	Yes	Yes	No
CNS complications*	Frequent	Infrequent	Infrequent	Infrequent
Anemia*	Frequent	Common	Infrequent	Infrequent
Renal insufficiency*	Common	Infrequent	Infrequent	Infrequent
Effects on pregnancy*	Frequent	Infrequent	Unknown	Unknown
Hypoglycemia	Frequent	Unknown	Unknown	Unknown

*Influenced by immunity. Documentation of complications for species other than *P. falciparum* is limited. Adapted from Bruce-Chwatt LJ. Essential malariology. 2nd Ed. New York: John Wiley and Sons, 1985:32.

the different species of parasite and anopheline vectors and can be affected by environmental conditions as well.

The timing of events in the life cycle of malaria parasites and the number of merozoites produced from each schizont differ among the four *Plasmodium* species that infect humans. Additionally, *P. vivax* and *P. ovale* can produce a dormant form (hypnozoites) that can persist in the liver for months up to 3 or 4 years, causing periodic relapses of parasitemia and illness (see Table 21.1–1). Hypnozoites result only from primary sporozoite inoculation in mosquito-borne infections. Although *P. falciparum* and *P. malariae* do not form hypnozoites, infection with these parasites can persist in the blood at subpatent or undetectable levels after resolution of symptoms. This very low-level parasitemia can result in recrudescence of clinical disease. Except in partially immune persons, *P. falciparum* rarely recrudesces more than several months after initial infection. However, recrudescent *P. malariae* infections can occur 40 years or longer after infection.

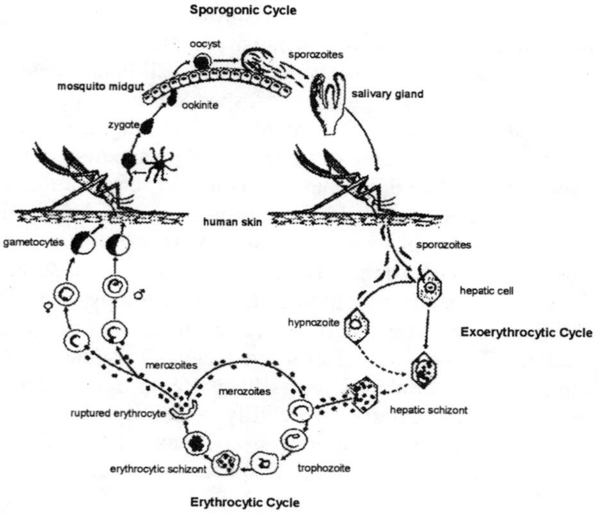

CLINICAL FEATURES AND DIAGNOSIS

Patients with malaria can present with a wide variety of symptoms and a broad spectrum of severity depending upon such factors as the infecting species and level of acquired immunity in the host.

CLINICAL PRESENTATION

Typical symptoms among nonimmune individuals with malaria include fever, chills, myalgias and arthralgias, headache, diarrhea, vomiting, and other nonspecific signs. Splenomegaly, anemia, thrombocytopenia, pulmonary or renal dysfunction, and neurologic findings may also be present. When synchronous infections (occurring when a majority of schizonts rupture at the same time) develop, each species of *Plasmodium* causes a characteristic pattern of periodic fever. The paroxysms of *P. vivax* and *P. ovale* malaria classically occur every 48 hours, whereas those of *P. malariae* occur every 72 hours. However, the classic presentation with predictably recurring fever and chills is highly variable and may not be present at all. This is particularly true early in the course of an illness, when the patient is taking medications that have antipyretic or antimalarial activity or when partial immunity exists. *P. falciparum* infections can feature a daily or irregular pattern of symptoms.

SEVERE OR COMPLICATED INFECTIONS

Uncomplicated malaria infection can progress to severe disease or death within hours. The potential for severe and

Figure 21.1–2. The malaria life cycle. Adapted from Oaks SC, Mitchell VS, Pearson GW, Carpenter CCJ, eds. Malaria obstacles and opportunities. Washington, DC: National Academy Press, 1991.

complicated illness is particularly ominous in patients with high levels of parasitemia and without partial immunity from prior exposure to malaria infection. *P. falciparum* is the major cause of severe disease and death; severe or fatal malaria rarely results from infections with *P. vivax*, *P. ovale*, and *P. malariae* unless there is another contributing cause of death or co-infection with *P. falciparum*. An extremely rare exception is splenic rupture, which can occur with acute nonfalciparum malaria.

Neurologic manifestations are the best known potentially fatal complication in nonimmune persons. Malaria with central nervous system (CNS) symptoms can progress from fever with subtle mental status changes to coma and death within hours. Cerebral malaria is defined as unarousable coma not attributable to any other cause in a patient infected with *P. falciparum*. Other acute complications include renal failure (especially in nonimmune adults), hemolytic anemia, hypoglycemia, metabolic acidosis, disseminated intravascular coagulation, shock, and acute pulmonary edema (particularly in nonimmune adults).

Falciparum malaria can also have devastating effects during pregnancy. In nonimmune women, acute malaria during pregnancy can be more severe than malaria in nonpregnant women and carries a high risk of maternal and fetal death if not treated promptly and adequately.

PATHOPHYSIOLOGY

The usual incubation period from infective mosquito bite to onset of symptoms ranges from 9 to 30 days, depending on the species of parasite (see Table 21.1–1), host immune status, infecting dose, and use of antimalarial drugs. The clinical symptoms associated with malaria infection are caused by a complex interplay between the parasite and the host immune response. Symptoms are associated with the asexual erythrocytic stage parasites. Exoerythrocytic forms (sporozoites, exoerythrocytic schizonts, and hypnozoites) and gametocytes do not cause clinical symptoms.

In general, higher levels of parasitemia are associated with clinical symptoms in partially immune populations and with severe or complicated disease in nonimmune persons. Almost all instances of severe or fatal malaria are caused by *P. falciparum* infections. This tendency has been linked to several peculiar features of falciparum parasites. First of all, exoerythrocytic and erythrocytic schizonts of *P. falciparum* release larger numbers of merozoites when they rupture, resulting in a more rapid rate of increasing parasitemia. *P. falciparum* is also able to infect both mature and immature red blood cells RBCs. In contrast, *P. vivax* and *P. ovale*, which cause milder clinical presentations, selectively infect immature RBCs and reticulocytes. Erythrocytes infected with *P. falciparum* adhere to the vascular endothelium of postcapillary venules. Several antigens that may mediate this property—adherence factors—have been characterized and implicated in severe or complicated malaria.

The host response to malaria infection also contributes substantially to the pathogenesis of the disease. Several specific mediators have been suggested both for uncomplicated infections and for severe and complicated malaria.[3] Malaria fever appears to arise from cytokines released by host mononuclear cells when erythrocytic schizonts rupture. Elevated levels of tumor necrosis factor alpha have been detected in patients during malaria fever[4-6] and immediately preceding paroxysms of *P. vivax* infection.[7] Elevated levels of other cytokines, including interferon-γ and interleukins-1 and 6 have also been described and may contribute to fever in malaria infection.[6,8]

Although the occurrence of severe and complicated malaria remains unpredictable and incompletely understood, it appears that both direct and immunologic effects play important roles in each of the major complications. Cerebral malaria appears to be caused partly by direct processes—such as the tendency for parasitized erythrocytes to sludge in capillaries and venules of the CNS, reduced deformability of infected RBCs, or adherence of infected cells to vascular endothelium and noninfected erythrocytes—and partly by immunologic responses—such as complement activation, immune complex-mediated vasculitis, cytokine release, and nitric oxide. Likewise, malaria-related anemia may evolve from direct effects—such as lysing of infected cells or their removal by the spleen—and immunologic effects—including inhibition of erythropoiesis, immune-mediated removal of noninfected RBCs, and autoantibodies to RBC antigens.[9]

DIAGNOSTIC TESTS

The diagnosis of malaria must be considered in all febrile patients who have traveled to or lived in malaria-endemic areas or who have received blood products, tissues, or organs from persons who have been to such areas. Direct microscopic examination of intracellular parasites on stained blood films is the standard for definitive diagnosis in nearly all settings. However, several other approaches exist or are in development, which may be appropriate under special conditions.

Although reliable diagnosis cannot be made on the basis of signs and symptoms alone, presumptive clinical diagnosis is the only realistic option in much of the malaria-endemic world because of the scarcity of resources and trained health personnel. Clinical diagnosis offers the advantages of ease, speed, and low cost. In areas where malaria is prevalent, clinical diagnosis usually results in all patients with fever and no apparent other cause being treated for malaria. However, clinical diagnosis of malaria can lead to ignoring other obvious and treatable causes of fever in a febrile patient.

A definitive diagnosis of malaria can be made by several approaches, including light microscopy, special staining, rapid antigen detection, and detection of parasite nucleic acid sequences. Definitive diagnosis can decrease the use of antimalarial drugs by patients not needing malaria therapy, improve the ability to identify patients in need of treatment for nonmalarial illnesses, and direct antimalarial therapy to specific species of malaria.

Simple light microscopic examination of stained blood films is the most widely practiced and useful method for definitive malaria diagnosis. With a minimum of equipment and recurring expense, fast and reliable diagnosis of malaria can be obtained even under the most difficult conditions. In areas where *P. falciparum* causes only a portion of malaria infections, microscopic diagnosis allows differentiation between species, a capability not possible at present with some of the newer technologies. Another advantage of this approach is that an experienced microscopist can also quantify the level of infection and distinguish clinically important asexual parasite stages (rings, trophozoites, and schizonts) from the sexual forms (gametocytes), which may persist without causing symptoms. This can be critical for determining whether a given treatment has been effective. Although several different stains can be used, Giemsa gives the best results. Specific disadvantages are that slide collection, staining, and reading can be time consuming and microscopists need to be trained and supervised to ensure consistent reliability. Although electricity is not needed as long as there is sunlight, the availability of electricity improves reliability and extends the hours during which diagnosis can be made available. Even when performed correctly, diagnosis by microscopy does have some important limitations. In nonimmune persons, symptoms may develop before there are detectable levels of parasitemia. For this reason, several blood smear examinations are needed to positively rule out a diagnosis of malaria in a symptomatic patient.

A modification of light microscopy, the quantitative buffy coat method (QBC™; Becton-Dickinson) was originally developed to screen large numbers of specimens for complete blood cell counts. Adapted for malaria diagnosis, the technique involves the use of a special fluorescent stain to highlight malaria parasites and centrifugation to concentrate parasites at a predictable location in a specially prepared capillary tube.[10] The advantages to QBC are that less training is required to operate the system and the test is quick. Field trials have shown that QBC may be marginally more sensitive than conventional microscopy under ideal conditions.[10-12] The disadvantages are that electricity is always required, special equipment and supplies are needed, and species-specific diagnosis is not reliable. These disadvantages generally prohibit the widespread use of QBC in many malaria-endemic countries.

A third diagnostic approach involves the rapid detection of parasite antigens, usually through enzyme-linked immunosorbent assay and radioimmunoassay techniques. Multiple experimental tests have been developed targeting a variety of parasite antigens.[13-15] One commercially available kit (ParaSight™-F,* Becton-Dickinson) detects the histidine-rich protein (HRP-II) of *P. falciparum*. Compared with light microscopy and QBC, this test yielded rapid and highly sensitive diagnosis of *P. falciparum* infection.[16,17] Advantages to this technology are that no special equipment is required, the test and reagents are stable at ambient temperatures, and no electricity is needed. The principal disadvantage is a high per-test cost.

---

*Use of trade names is for identification only and does not imply endorsement by the U.S. Public Health Service of the U.S. Department of Health and Human Services.

The test is specific for falciparum malaria and nonquantitative. Furthermore, detectable antigen can persist for 10 to 14 days after adequate treatment and cure, and the test cannot adequately distinguish a resolving infection from treatment failure due to antimalarial drug-resistant parasites. Although promising, this particular test cannot replace light microscopy, particularly in settings where infections with nonfalciparum species and asymptomatic parasitemias are prevalent.

Detection of parasite genetic material through polymerase chain reaction techniques has gained prominence as a research tool. It will almost certainly have a growing role in the diagnosis of malaria. Specific primers have been developed for each of the four species of human malaria. One important use of this new technology is in detecting mixed infections or differentiating between infecting species when microscopic examination is inconclusive.[18]

GEOGRAPHIC DISTRIBUTION

Figure 21.1–1 shows the areas of the world where malaria transmission occurs. The risk of malaria infection for travelers is high in sub-Saharan Africa, Papua New Guinea, the Solomon Islands, and Vanuatu. The risk is intermediate in the Indian subcontinent and Haiti and low in most of Southeast Asia, East Asia, and Central and South America. Information about the risk of infection in individual countries is provided in the World Health Organization's publication *International Travel and Health* and the Centers for Disease Control's publication *Health Information for International Travel*.

DISTRIBUTION OF FOUR *PLASMODIUM* SPECIES

Not all species of malaria are transmitted in all malarious areas. Although *P. falciparum* is transmitted in nearly all areas where malaria occurs, it accounts for over 90% of all malaria infections in sub-Saharan Africa and nearly 100% of infections in Haiti. *P. falciparum* causes two-thirds or more of malaria cases in Southeast Asia. *P. vivax* is only rarely transmitted in sub-Saharan Africa because most ethnic groups lack the RBC marker required for invasion by this parasite but predominates in Central America, most malarious areas of South America, and the Indian subcontinent. Recent reports have documented a resurgence of vivax malaria in the Central Asian republics of the former Soviet Union. *P. malariae* has a patchy distribution but may be transmitted in most of the malarious world. In contrast, *P. ovale* transmission is limited to tropical Africa and Papua New Guinea, although cases have also been reported from Vietnam.

DISTRIBUTION OF DRUG-RESISTANT STRAINS

Chloroquine-resistant *P. falciparum* (CRPF) was first recognized almost simultaneously in Thailand and South America in the late 1950s. CRPF was documented on the east coast of Africa in 1978. In the past 20 to 25 years,

CRPF has spread and intensified to the point that only Central America northwest of the Panama Canal, the island of Hispaniola (Haiti and the Dominican Republic), and limited regions of the Middle East remain free of chloroquine resistance. In all other endemic areas, malaria is, to varying extent, resistant to chloroquine. In some regions, chloroquine resistance has intensified to the point where chloroquine no longer has a significant effect on *P. falciparum* parasites and can no longer be relied on to provide effective treatment or prophylaxis. Finally, chloroquine-resistant *P. vivax* has emerged in South America, Southeast Asia, and the Indian subcontinent.

Drug resistance is not an all-or-nothing phenomenon. In any given area, a wide range of parasitologic responses can be found, from complete sensitivity to complete resistance. In parts of East Africa, resistance has intensified to the point where 80% to 90% of *P. falciparum* infections are moderately to highly resistant.

The problem of drug resistance is not limited to chloroquine. In parts of Southeast Asia, especially along the Thai-Cambodia and Thai-Myanmar borders, falciparum malaria has rapidly developed resistance to one compound after another. After chloroquine was abandoned as first-line therapy for malaria in Thailand in 1972 in preference to sulfadoxine-pyrimethamine, resistance to that drug developed and intensified. Currently, greater than 50% of *P. falciparum* infections show resistance to mefloquine (15 mg/kg) in some areas of Thailand. Cure rates were improved to 70% to 80% by increasing the dose of mefloquine to 25 mg/kg, but the incidence of side effects also increased. Increasing the dose of halofantrine from 24 mg/kg to 72 mg/kg over 72 hours improved cure rates from 65% to 99% but also increased the toxicity. Currently, multidrug-resistant malaria is being treated with a combination of mefloquine and artemisinin derivatives.

Drug resistance develops rapidly to dihydrofolate reductase inhibitors (such as pyrimethamine and proguanil) when used alone.[19] In Southeast Asia and South America, parasitologic response to quinine has been deteriorating.[20] Resistance to newer antimalarials, such as halofantrine, has been reported, especially in areas with established mefloquine resistance.

TRANSMISSION

Human malaria is transmitted by the bite of female mosquitoes belonging to the genus *Anopheles*. Of the 400 or so species of *Anopheles* in the world, approximately 60 are important vectors of malaria. However, a particular species of *Anopheles* may be an important vector in one area of the world and of little or no consequence in another. Table 21.1–2 lists several of the anophelines that have been incriminated as principal malaria vectors, their geographic distribution, and information on their susceptibility to malaria, preferred hosts, and breeding sites.

There are four stages in the mosquito life cycle: egg, larva, pupa, and adult. Eggs are deposited singly on water in suitable breeding sites where the developing embryo hatches as a larva after 2 or more days. At this stage, the mosquito undergoes a complete metamorphosis, emerging as an adult. The length of each developmental stage is temperature dependent. Generation times in the tropics can be as brief as 5 days. The lifespan of adults under natural conditions is difficult to determine but in the case of malaria vectors is clearly longer than the time required to become infective, probably 3 to 4 weeks.

Table 21.1–2.   FEATURES OF COMMON MALARIA VECTORS

SPECIES	DISTRIBUTION	SUSCEPTIBILITY TO MALARIA	HOST PREFERENCE	TYPICAL BREEDING SITES
An. albimanus	Western hemisphere from southeast Texas, Mexico, Central America to Ecuador, Venezuela, and Carribean	Low	Animal	Wide range from temporary collections of water to ponds, streams, and lakes
An. culicifacies	Indian subcontinent	Low	Animal	Sunlit collections of fresh water, including rice fields
An. darlingi	South America east of the Andes	Moderate	Human	Clear, fresh, partially shaded lagoons or marshes
An. dirus	Southeast Asian forests	High	Human	Shaded water collections
An. gambiae, An. funestus	Tropical Africa	High	Human	Fresh water collections exposed to sunlight
An. maculatus	Foothills of Southeast Asian countries and Indian subcontinent	Moderate	Human	Sunlit hilly streams
An. minimus	Southeast Asian hills	Moderate	Human	Margins of slow-moving sunlit streams
An. stephensi	Urban areas of the Indian subcontinent	Moderate	Human	Shaded wells, cisterns, cans, roof gutters

Differences in the behavior patterns of adult mosquitoes have a marked effect on their capacity to transmit malaria and on the choice of control methods used. Preferred time of biting, for example, can vary from daytime to late evening. The efficacy of many control measures varies depending on the mosquito activity cycle. For example, mosquito nets, an effective barrier to human-mosquito contact at night, probably have little effect on malaria transmission by daytime or outdoor biters.

CONCLUSION

It is likely that more travelers will be at risk of malaria in the future because of the expanding malaria problem and the rise in the number of travelers to areas with malaria. Use of effective prophylaxis will be increasingly important to prevent an increase in malaria morbidity and mortality among travelers.

REFERENCES

1. Lobel HO, Kozarsky PE. Update on prevention of malaria in travelers. JAMA 1997;278:1767–1771.
2. Kachur SP, Bloland PB. Malaria. In: Wallace RB, ed. Maxcy-Rosenau Textbook of public health and preventive medicine. 14th Ed. Norwalk, CT: Appleton and Lange, 1998:313–326.
3. Miller LH, Good MF, Milon G. Malaria pathogenesis. Science 1994;264:1878–1883.
4. Kwiatkowski D. Tumour necrosis factor, fever, and fatality in falciparum malaria. Immunol Lett 1990;25:213–216.
5. Grau GE, Taylor TE, Molyneux ME, et al. Tumor necrosis factor and disease severity in children with falciparum malaria. N Engl J Med 1989;320:1586–1591.
6. Kern P, Hemmer CJ, Van Damme J, et al. Elevated tumor necrosis factor alpha and interleukin-6 serum levels as markers for complicated *Plasmodium falciparum* malaria. Am J Med 1989;87:139–143.
7. Karunaweera ND, Grau GE, Gamage P, et al. Dynamics of fever and serum levels of tumour necrosis factor are closely associated during clincal paroxysms in *Plasmodium vivax* malaria. Proc Natl Acad Sci U S A 1992;89:3200–3203.
8. Kwiatkowski D, Hill AVS, Sambou I, et al. TNF concentration in fatal cerebral, nonfatal cerebral, and uncomplicated *Plasmodium falciparum* malaria. Lancet 1990;336:1201–1204.
9. Playfair JHL. The pathology of malaria: a possible target for immunisation? Immunol Lett 1994;43:83–86.
10. Spielman A, Perrone JB, Teklehaimanot A, et al. Malaria diagnosis by direct observation of centrifuged samples of blood. Am J Trop Med Hyg 1988;39:337–342.
11. Tharavanij S. New developments in malaria diagnostic techniques. Southeast Asian J Trop Med Public Health 1990;21(1):3–16.
12. Rickman LS, Long GW, Oberst R, et al. Rapid diagnosis of malaria by acridine orange staining of centrifuged parasites. Lancet 1989;1:68–71.
13. Mackey LJ, McGregor IA, Paounova N, Lambert PH. Diagnosis of *Plasmodium falciparum* infection in man: detection of parasite antigens by ELISA. Bull World Health Organ 1982;60:69–75.
14. Fortier B, Delplace J, Dubremetz F, et al. Enzyme immunoassay for detection of antigen in acute *Plasmodium falciparum* malaria. Eur J Clin Microbiol 1987;6:596–598.
15. Khusmith S, Tharavanij S, Kasemsuth R, et al. Two-site immunoradiometric assay for detection of *Plasmodium falciparum* antigen in blood using monoclonal and polyclonal antibodies. J Clin Microbiol 1987;25:1467–1471.
16. Shiff CJ, Premji Z, Minjas JN. The rapid manual ParaSight™-F. A new diagnostic tool for *Plasmodium falciparum* infection. Trans R Soc Trop Med Hyg 1993;87:646–648.
17. Uguen C, Rabodonirina M, De Pina JJ, et al. ParaSight™-F rapid manual diagnostic test of *Plasmodium falciparum* infection. Bull World Health Organ 1995;73:643–649.
18. Snounou G, Pinheiro L, Goncalves A, et al. The importance of sensitive detection of malaria parasites in the human and insect hosts in epidemiological studies, as shown by the analysis of field samples from Guinea Bissau. Trans R Soc Trop Med Hyg 1993;87:649–653.
19. Bjorkman A, Phillips-Howard PA. The epidemiology of drug-resistant malaria. Trans R Soc Trop Med Hyg 1990;84:177–180.
20. Bunnag D, Harinasuta T. Quinine and quinidine in malaria in Thailand. Acta Leidensia 1987;55:163–166.

21.2 PROTECTION AGAINST MOSQUITOES

ED W. CUPP

Mosquitoes (Order Diptera; Family Culicidae) are slender, delicate insects whose female adult stage routinely takes blood from humans and other animals as a source of nutrition and for reproduction. Among all medically important insects, this group is the most significant because of its ability to transmit a variety of human and animal pathogens. On a global basis, there are over 3,000 species of mosquitoes, and most (75%) are distributed throughout the humid tropical and subtropical life zones.[1,2]

Mosquitoes occupy a wide variety of habitats and can be found where standing water is available. Depending on the particular species, mosquito eggs may be deposited by the adult female onto the water's surface, in moist soil that will later be flooded, or in containers (natural or manmade) that eventually accumulate enough water to immerse the eggs. The larval stage ("wiggler") is an active, feeding stage that hatches from the egg and then passes through four developmental phases in the aquatic environment. The larva molts to the pupal stage ("tumbler"), and, after a brief time, the adults emerge and mate.

Inseminated female mosquitoes then search for blood, which serves primarily as a source of protein for ovarian development. Carbon dioxide and body odor, which are detected by sense receptors on the antennae and palps, serve as initial orientation cues, causing the females to fly upwind toward the source. At shorter range, visual stimuli (color, shape) and the convection currents of warm, moist air emanating from the host guide the mosquito.

Once a host has been found, the female mosquito inserts a set of thin, needle-like stylets into the skin. The stylets (n = 6) are held together as a single bundle ("fascicle") and, once introduced into the capillary bed of the host, allow the female mosquito to both secrete saliva into the feeding lesion and ingest blood at the same time. In *Aedes aegypti*, a relatively small mosquito, the fascicle is 0.2 millimeters in length and 50 micrometers in diameter. Mosquito saliva contains a variety of factors that prevent primary hemostasis (aggregation of blood platelets) and vasoconstriction. Some mosquitoes also possess powerful antithrombins to deter clot formation.

Only a small proportion of mosquito species has nuisance or medical value. However, certain species are efficient vectors of viruses, *Plasmodium* spp, and parasitic nematodes, and the physician/travel specialist should be aware of the more important taxa, their biting activity, and vector potential (Table 21.2–1).

Because of their broad biologic diversity and host specificity, mosquitoes exhibit different time periods of flight and host-seeking behavior, that is, activity may be diurnal, crepuscular (dawn or dusk), or nocturnal depending on the species. Heat and humidity are key factors that govern mosquito abundance and flight. Under normal circumstances, seasonal increases in rainfall and temperature usually contribute to increased densities of mosquito species. Accordingly, travelers should be aware that entering habitats producing mosquitoes during certain times of the year (spring/summer, "rainy" season, etc.) may result in higher than usual biting rates if no precautionary measures are taken. Thus, approaches for protection against bites may vary depending on season, geographic location, general habitat, and time of day.

The presence of common synanthropic species such as *Aedes aegypti*, *Culex quinquefasciatus,* or *Anopheles gambiae sensu stricto* is often tied to human activity, and population densities of these mosquitoes may be affected independently from the usual climatic factors. Urbanization, improper disposal of sewage and unwanted articles, irrigation, and development of artificial lakes and ponds are examples of nonclimatic factors that may contribute to increases in mosquito populations.

Protection from mosquito bites may employ one or more tactics, depending on the particular circumstances of the traveler. Here, a variety of measures are described, ranging from personal protection by use of repellents to security in domestic habitats. Depending on the intensity

Table 21.2–1.   GENERA OF COMMON MEDICALLY IMPORTANT MOSQUITOES IN THE WORLD

TAXON	MEDICAL IMPORTANCE	BEHAVIOR
Aedes spp	Vectors of arboviruses (dengue, yellow fever) and a human filarial nematode (*Wuchereria bancrofti*)	Typically bite during the day out of doors or indoors
Anopheles spp	Vectors of *Plasmodium* spp (malaria), arboviruses (e.g., o'nyong-nyong) and human filarial nematodes (*W. bancrofti, Brugia malayi, B. pahangi*)	Biting may be crepuscular or nocturnal; some species may blood feed during the day indoors in subdued light or outdoors in shade
Culex spp	Vectors of arboviruses causing encephalitis and human filarial nematodes (*W. bancrofti*)	Biting may be crepuscular, diurnal, or nocturnal. Some species may be highly pestiferous, biting at night.
Mansonia spp	Transmit human filarial nematodes (*B. malayi, W. bancrofti*) and may transmit arboviruses	Biting is nocturnal
Psorophora spp	Not medically important as vectors. May mechanically transmit *Dermatobia hominis* eggs/larvae (myiasis).	Typically bite during the day. Some species may be highly pestiferous.

of biting pressure, these methods may be employed singly or in combination.

Repellents applied directly to the skin serve as the first line of defense against mosquito bites.[3] To be effective, a repellent must be moderately volatile so that it offers protection at the skin-mosquito interface while also remaining on the skin in effective concentrations for reasonable periods of time following a single application. Environmental factors that commonly influence persistence include temperature (which increases sweating and also promotes volatility), moisture (rain, sweat), and wind. Skin-absorption characteristics are important as well since dermal and systemic toxicity may result if a chemical is too readily absorbed transdermally.[4]

Among repellents currently available, DEET (N,N-diethyl-3-methylbenzamide) is the most effective and has been used quite successfully for over 40 years. It possesses a number of favorable characteristics—efficacy against a wide variety of mosquito species (and other kinds of biting flies), persistence, acceptable mammalian toxicity—and when proper application is made, offers substantial personal protection. DEET-based repellents are available in a variety of formulations (lotions/creams, pump-spray liquids, sticks, etc.) with differing concentrations of the active ingredient. Current polymer-based formulations are most efficacious over time because of extended release of the active ingredient, thereby lessening the need for frequent application of more concentrated material.[5]

Selection of the proper concentration of DEET should be made with two general factors in mind: body size of the individual and degree of mosquito biting pressure. Under virtually all conditions, DEET is safe when applied as a topical repellent,[6] and DEET concentrations of 35% are normally sufficient to protect travelers from the bites of mosquitoes. However, although rare, neurologic problems have occurred in children when concentrations of DEET were quite high and/or application was repeated at too frequent intervals.[7,8] The American Academy of Pediatrics recommends a DEET concentration of 10% for children,[3] and the Environmental Protection Agency has released common sense guidelines for the safe use and proper application of repellents.[9] Specific formulations for children are available commercially.

Because of concerns regarding the possible toxicity of DEET and its strong properties as a solvent (DEET dissolves plastics, certain kinds of paints and varnishes, etc.), repellents employing essential plant oils as active ingredients are becoming increasingly popular as alternatives. However, although the insect repellent properties of certain plant products have been known for centuries, few rival DEET in efficacy and persistence against mosquitoes following a single application. The latter quality is a particular weakness of botanically based repellents, and attempts to develop more long-lasting formulations using polymer technology are under-way. Favorable results have been achieved using a time-released, 30% geraniol formulation. A lemon eucalyptus oil-based repellent (50% p-menthane-3,8 diol + isopulegol and citronellol as active ingredients—PMD) in a gel formulation has also proven as effective as DEET against several *Anopheles* spp in Africa following a single application.[10]

Proper clothing can also offer a high degree of personal protection from mosquito bites. Whenever possible, dark clothing should be avoided in favor of white or tan since many mosquito species are attracted to navy blue and black. Clothing should also cover most of the body (wear socks, long-sleeved shirts, long pants, hats) and prevent direct access to the skin.

Protective garments (shirts, pants, gaiters, hoods, boots) designed specifically to prevent the bites of insects such as mosquitoes are available commercially so that full body protection can be achieved where necessary. This type of clothing is made of a fine mesh cotton or polyester/cotton mixture to ensure air flow and comfort in a tropical/subtropical environment while preventing the bites of mosquitoes and related blood-sucking insects. As such, these garments offer an alternative to repellents applied directly to the arms, legs, neck, and face. The use of "mosquito boots" is another method that works specifically for mosquitoes that prefer to bite on the ankles and lower parts of the leg. These boots, which are lightweight leather and cover the foot, ankle, and lower calf of the leg, are usually worn in the evenings to avoid the bites of malarious mosquitoes such as *Anopheles gambiae* and *An. funestus* in Africa.

The application of permethrin (a pyrethroid insecticide [Permanone]) directly to clothing is another approach that works extremely well against mosquitoes and other biting arthropods. Permethrin is neurotoxic and repels mosquitoes by its very rapid "knock down" activity; in many situations, the mosquito is killed shortly after it has made contact with the treated clothing. Permethrin has a very favorable mammalian toxicity and persists in cloth for up to 2 weeks following a single treatment. It has also proven protective in outdoor situations when applied to tents.[11]

Indoor protection of travelers from mosquito bites can be achieved by the use of physical and chemical barriers. The selection of accommodations with adequate window screens is a requirement in tropical environments, particularly during the wet season of the year, because many species of mosquitoes rest out of doors but enter houses to bloodfeed. Others may rest indoors (under beds and sofas, in clothes closets, in showers, behind commodes, etc.) and then search for bloodmeals during the day (*Aedes* spp) or at night (*Anopheles* spp, *Culex* spp). An aerosolized space spray containing a pyrethroid or organophosphorus insecticide can be used to temporarily clear rooms of these types of mosquitoes and sanitize the area. Space sprays containing a carbamate insecticide (e.g., propoxur) are also effective and provide residual protection beyond that seen for pyrethroid or organophosphorus compounds by applying the material to mosquito resting places.

The use of mosquito coils containing an insecticide (usually a pyrethroid) is another approach to clear rooms of mosquitoes. These burn slowly to volatilize and release the insecticide into the air, thereby acting as a fumigant to kill resting mosquitoes. To achieve adequate protection, rooms should be closed to ensure saturation of all mosquito resting areas. A common strategy is to ignite the coil, leave the room, and return in 1 to 2 hours. Mosquito coils are inexpensive and easily portable by the traveler but do generate particles and gases that may affect persons with breathing problems. Care should be taken in this regard.

Protection by using bednets is highly recommended in the tropics where malaria and/or human filariasis are problems. These devices may already be in place in chosen accommodations or the traveler may carry a portable bednet (available commercially) to ensure ready availability. Regardless, bednets are a key feature of protection against bites by nocturnally active mosquitoes.

To be an effective barrier, the net should be intact with no holes or tears and should be tucked under the mattress to prevent movement during the night. The traveler should avoid sleeping next to the net since most mosquitoes will bloodfeed directly through the mesh if given the opportunity.

Bednets can be impregnated with insecticides to increase their effectiveness. Nets permeated with pyrethroids are effective against *Anopheles* spp (vectors of the etiologic agents of malaria and human filariasis) and *Culex quinquefasciatus* (a vector of *W. bancrofti*, the causative agent of human filariasis).[12] Several of these compounds (cyfluthrin @ 50 mg active ingredient per square meter, lambda-cyhalothrin @ 10 mg active ingredient per square meter, deltamethrin @ 3 mg per square meter) effectively repel mosquitoes for 6 to 15 months and may be lethal even when mosquitoes attempt to enter through tears in the net.

Table 21.2–2. RECOMMENDATIONS FOR PROTECTION FROM IMPORTANT MOSQUITO VECTORS

TAXON	RECOMMENDATION
Aedes aegypti, albopictus	Major vectors of arboviruses (e.g., *Ae. dengue*); actively bite during the day. Apply DEET during the day and use protective clothing or apply DEET and wear clothing treated with permethrin.
Anopheles gambiae, An. funestus	Common vectors of malaria and bancroftian filariasis in Africa that are nocturnally active. Apply DEET or PMD-based repellent, emphasizing treatment on the ankles and lower legs, shortly after dusk. Use a bednet (untreated or treated with a pyrethroid) when sleeping.
Culex quinque-fasciatus	Important vector of bancroftian filariasis and a major nuisance mosquito in the tropics. Nocturnally active, particularly late at night and in the early morning. Use a bednet (untreated or treated with a pyrethroid) when sleeping.

Using several of the more medically important species as examples, an integrated protection approach can be developed to protect the traveler in situations where mosquito-associated diseases occur. These are illustrated in Table 21.2–2, using the methods described above. Depending on the particular mosquito species and its habits, other examples can also be developed.

REFERENCES

1. Clements AN. The biology of mosquitoes. Vol. 1. Development, nutrition and reproduction. London: Chapman and Hall, 1992.
2. Clements AN. The biology of mosquitoes. Vol. 2. Sensory reception and behavior. Cary, NC: Oxford University Press, 1999.
3. Fradin MS. Mosquitoes and mosquito repellents: a clinician's guide. Ann Intern Med 1998;128:931–940.
4. Qiu H, Jun HW, McCall JW. Pharmacokinetics, formulations, and safety of insect repellent N,N-diethyl-3-methylbenzamide (DEET): a review. J Am Mosq Control Assoc 1998;14:12–27.
5. Kline DL, Schreck CE. Personal protection afforded by controlled-release topical repellents and permethrin-treated clothing against natural populations of *Aedes taeniorhynchus*. J Am Mosq Control Assoc 1989;5:77–80.
6. Goodyear L, Behrens RH. Short report: the safety and toxicity of insect repellents. Am J Trop Med Hyg 1998;59:323–324.
7. Roland EH, Jan JE, Rigg JM. Toxic encephalopathy in a child after brief exposure to insect repellents. Can Med Assoc J 1985;132:155–156.
8. Lipscomb JW, Kramer JE, Leiken JB. Seizure following brief exposure to the insect repellent N,N-diethyl-m-toluamide. Ann Emerg Med 1992;21:315–317.
9. Brown M, Hebert A. Insect repellents: an overview. J Am Acad Dermatol 1997;36(Part 1):243–249.
10. Trigg JK. Evaluation of a eucalyptus-based repellent against *Anopheles* spp. in Tanzania. J Am Mosq Control Assoc 1996; 12(Part 1):243–246.
11. Heal JD, Surgeoner GA, Lindsay LR. Permethrin as a tent treatment for protection against field populations of *Aedes* mosquitoes. J Am Mosq Control Assoc 1995;11:99–102.
12. Curtis CF, Myamba J, Wilkes TJ. Comparison of different insecticides and fabrics for anti-mosquito bednets and curtains. Med Vet Entomol 1996;10:1–11.

21.3 MALARIA PREVENTION

G. DENNIS SHANKS

INTRODUCTION

Malaria is one of the few common infectious diseases that can kill a tropical traveler. Because travelers to tropical Asia, the Amazon region of South America, and especially sub-Saharan Africa are often at risk of malaria infection, it is important to advise such travelers on the importance of malaria prevention. The basis of malaria prevention is twofold: avoidance of mosquitoes and chemoprophylaxis (drugs given to prevent symptomatic malaria). This section will deal primarily with chemoprophylaxis, but it is worth stating at the beginning that relatively easy (and usually underused) means of decreasing malaria infection risk exist in the form of insect repellents, window screens, and bednets.

Chemoprophylaxis is different from most therapeutic drug use. Instead of trying to treat an existing morbid condition, one is trying to maintain a healthy person in a risky environment. This requires chemoprophylaxis regimens to meet regulatory requirements and consumer expectations of very high effectiveness coupled with an extremely safe toxicity profile. This is particularly difficult within the usual restrictions of short-term travelers: quick departures, poor compliance, and distance from usual physician. Authoritative guides to malaria chemoprophylaxis are issued by various public health agencies but often cannot reflect the most recent developments.[1–3] Chemoprophylaxis can be quite successful in preventing disease and death due to malaria, but its rational use demands a thorough understanding of the possibilities and limitations of malaria chemoprophylaxis.[4]

APPROACH TO THE TROPICAL TRAVELER NEEDING CHEMOPROPHYLAXIS

A person expecting to travel to the tropics requires a medical history and review of current medication similar to any medical patient. Suggestions for appropriate questions to determine need for chemoprophylaxis include detailed travel itinerary, previous experience with antimalarial drugs, current medications that might interact or contraindicate certain drugs, concurrent medical problems or drug allergies, presence of any immunodeficiency, and, if female, reproductive status.

RISK TOLERANCE

Travelers accept additional risks inherent in leaving one's home. Zero-risk travel is not possible, just as all drugs carry a certain risk of adverse effects. Different travelers have different risk tolerances ranging from the adventure traveler hiking alone into unknown jungle to a businessman signing a contract in an airport lounge. Trying to understand the traveler's purpose and expectations is important to finding the appropriate regimen for prevention. No antimalarial drug is completely efficacious, just as no medication is completely free of adverse events. The travel physician's goal is to judge the malaria risk of his patient in conjunction with his likelihood of adverse events and tolerance of risk and then match the traveler with the appropriate chemoprophylaxis regimen.

ADVERSE EVENTS AND THEIR PERCEPTION

Humans only tolerate a limited amount of change. When this tolerance is exceeded during travel, various unwanted symptoms may impinge on the traveler's purpose. Given the large number of travelers, the frequency of chemoprophylaxis, the common occurrence of psychiatric conditions, and widespread publicity surrounding some antimalarial adverse events, it is not surprising that many travelers find ways to connect their symptoms with a pharmaceutical product. In randomized, blinded, placebo-controlled trials of prophylactic antimalarial drugs, as many symptoms are reported with placebo as with drug.[5,6] Except in unusual cases where the relationship between drug and adverse event is well established, it is nearly impossible to prove (or disprove) that a certain patient's symptoms are caused by a drug taken to prevent malaria. This situation can best be managed by the travel physician explaining to the patient the common adverse events expected with the regimen prescribed, how to minimize those symptoms, and when to stop a medication and seek medical advice. Medical advice received by some travelers and whom they choose to consult for health prevention information are often sadly lacking in quality. Simple explanations understandable to the traveler will greatly improve the chances that he/she will actually take the prevention regimen. If one finds a traveler unwilling to tolerate any adverse event risk, no matter how small, it is usually best to advise that he/she travel somewhere other than the tropics.

VERY HIGH- AND VERY LOW-RISK GROUPS

Generalizations can be made about malaria risk, but given the global resurgence of malaria and the inadequate surveillance systems in most countries, these can only be guidelines. The World Health Organization publishes lists of malaria risk by country that can usually be taken as accurate when the data were collected.[7] Travelers who should be regarded as having a high risk of malaria infection include most travelers to sub-Saharan Africa (especially West Africa), individuals whose work (entomologists, foresters) includes spending time in rural tropical areas especially at night, independent or "backpacker" travelers,[8] expatriates returning to the tropical country of their birth,[9] and individuals assisting during public health or humanitarian emergencies such as expatriate nongovernmental organization workers. Low-risk tropical travelers are typically going to the capital cities or major tourist destinations of Latin America or Asia, stay in upmarket hotels, travel on organized tours for 2 weeks or less, and spend most of their time in urban areas. Being high risk does not ensure malaria infection just as low-risk status does not guarantee lack of infection, but these generalities are useful in advising travelers.

COMPLIANCE

Investigation of returning travelers who develop malaria shows that the major reason for infection is failure to take chemoprophylaxis.[10] Failure to obtain pretravel advice, failure to take prescribed medication, termination of medication due to perceived drug-induced adverse events, or failure to continue medication after return from a malaria-endemic area are all common causes of chemoprophylactic failure. There are multiple reasons that might explain why persons fail to take chemoprophylaxis, but the basic problem is the difficulty of a healthy person understanding the need for ongoing medication to prevent a possible future infection. Various means have been tried to improve compliance, but the most effective is compulsory supervision of medication administration as practiced by disciplined military units. Lacking such draconian measures, other options that can be tried include carefully explaining the benefit of preventing a life-threatening infection to the traveler in order to convince him of its importance, special packaging material with separately identified pill holders or packets, associating medication administration with a common daily (or weekly) activity (such as tooth brushing), warning messages in airports, and distribution of malaria alerts through travel industry representatives. It is unclear if publicity surrounding deaths due to malaria increases compliance or if stories about drug-associated adverse events decreases compliance with chemoprophylaxis. The reality of the situation is, however, that the most important reason for poor effectiveness of malaria prophylaxis is failure to take the medication. New regimens that are simple and easy to administer are urgently needed in order to improve the effectiveness of malaria prevention.

PARTICULAR PROBLEMS AND UNKNOWNS

There are some situations and patients for which no simple answers exist. Certain groups of travelers have no obvious or even acceptable chemoprophylaxis regimen since the rise of chloroquine resistance has made malaria prevention increasingly difficult. Some suggestions for how to manage malaria prevention for children, pregnant women, and long-term travelers are included, but, in many cases, tropical travel for these groups involves increased risk of malaria infection due to imperfect or unavailable prevention regimens.

CHILDREN

Few antimalarial suspension formulations for children exist. Most antimalarial medications (chloroquine, proguanil, quinine) have very bitter tastes and any child will directly spit them out. Antimalarial tablets are not made for small children and, as such, dosing by breaking tablets is very problematic. Generally, the therapeutic margin of error is such that an approximate dosage can be managed (Table 21.3–1), but that still leaves hiding the crushed tablet in some food vehicle such as jam or sauce. Children (especially toddlers) can become very adept at refusing medication. The additional risk of malaria in children supposedly on adequate chemoprophylaxis is another variation of compliance failure when either frustrated parents or stubborn children do not manage to take the medication. Doxycycline, which is often a good alternative in areas

with multidrug-resistant falciparum malaria, cannot be given to children due to the propensity of the tetracyclines to stain growing teeth and bones in children less than 9 years old. Mefloquine is not officially approved for children <5 kg but some authorities have found no real reason not to give mefloquine weekly to very young children.[3]

PREGNANT WOMEN

Women who are or may become pregnant are of special concern since malaria in a pregnant woman can be very severe, threatening the lives of two persons. No drug can ever be said to be entirely safe in pregnancy. Some (particularly well-educated) women tend to overestimate the risk of drug-induced fetal malformations compared to risk of malaria during pregnancy. A pregnant traveler exposed to significant malaria transmission should be on chemoprophylaxis. Although unpopular, it is often wise to suggest that a pregnant traveler may not want to travel to a tropical area until after delivery.

It is generally accepted that chloroquine and/or proguanil can be safely given to pregnant women.[11] Mefloquine in the second half of pregnancy appears to be safe based on clinical trials on the Thai-Burmese border.[12] Mefloquine is not known to be a teratogenic risk during the first half of pregnancy, but this has never been proven.[13,14] Although antifolate drugs have been used for malaria treatment in Africa, pyrimethamine/sulfadoxine should not be used for malaria prevention in pregnant travelers.[15] Doxycycline has a known contraindication in that it is not given to young children or pregnant women due to the drug's ability to stain teeth and growing bones. If a woman who is taking doxycycline prophylaxis (or mefloquine for that matter) discovers that she has just become pregnant, it is sufficient to stop the drug and reassure the patient.

Table 21.3–1. DRUGS USED FOR THE PREVENTION OF MALARIA

DRUG	USAGE	ADULT DOSE	PEDIATRIC DOSE	NOTES
Chloroquine	Only in Middle East, Central America, Caribbean	300-mg base weekly	5-mg base/kg weekly	Bitter taste Start at least 2 weeks prior to travel Guard against accidental overdose
Proguanil combinations	Most popular in travelers from Britain and France	200 mg/day	<2 yr 50 mg 2–6 yr 100 mg 7–10 yr 150 mg	Apparently safe in pregnancy Used with chloroquine or antifolate High failure rates in Africa
Mefloquine	Usual recommendation for travelers to Africa	250 mg/week (1 tablet/week)	15–19 kg ¼ tablet 20–30 kg ½ tablet 31–40 kg ¾ tablet	Serious CNS adverse events rare (1:10,000) Many travelers report dysphoria >10 weeks before at steady-state drug concentrations
Doxycycline	Southeast Asia with areas of mefloquine resistance	100 mg/day	Not used in children <9 yr	Minor GI upset common Best taken with food Daily compliance very important
Primaquine	Eradicate liver stages of relapsing malaria	15- to 30-mg base/day for 2 weeks	0.5 mg/kg/day for 2 weeks; no liquid form	Not used in G6PD-deficient persons GI upset with higher doses Possible use for prophylaxis also?

CNS = central nervous system, GI = gastrointestinal, G6PD = glucose-6-phosphate dehydrogenase.

LONG-TERM TRAVELER

A common example of this group is expatriate managers who are assigned for business reasons to a malaria-endemic area for a year or more. These persons fall into a different category as their cumulative risk of malaria is often quite high, whereas their actual compliance with any chemoprophylaxis regimen is often quite low. Other long-term travelers who may be at considerably higher risk than most business expatriates are missionaries and Peace Corps or similar volunteers in rural areas. The psychology surrounding compliance is particularly difficult with long-term travelers as human nature tends to resist taking any chronic medication once the apparent threat (Well, I didn't get malaria last month, did I?) becomes the usual routine. Pretravel advice should focus on the availability of medical care at the destination and where the person will be sleeping and the importance of passive protective measures such as window screens. Some long-term travelers are really like frequent short-term travelers due to trips to endemic areas while spending the majority of their time in a low-risk area such as a capital city. It is often more practical to try to have the long-term traveler take prophylaxis when on trips to identifiably risky areas instead of trying (and failing) to maintain chemoprophylaxis for years on end.

IMMUNOCOMPROMISED TRAVELER

The most important patient to be aware of in this category is a person lacking a spleen. This part of the medical history can be missed if not directly asked as most splenectomies are done on young trauma victims and older travelers may not associate a long-past surgical procedure with malaria. Persons without spleens are no more susceptible to malaria than ordinary but if infected they are at very high risk of a fulminating infection. If a splenectomized traveler must go to a malaria-endemic area, great care must be taken to ensure that effective chemoprophylaxis is maintained.

Individuals living with HIV are a growing group of travelers who may also be at risk of malaria. Surprisingly, the rather severe cell-mediated immunity deficit seen in AIDS patients apparently does not predispose adults to more severe malaria infections.[16] AIDS patients are, however, usually on multiple other anti-infective medications, making the addition of yet another drug difficult. Although dapsone (often taken as PCP prophylaxis) has antimalarial activity, it cannot be depended on to protect a traveler. Travelers who are HIV infected should be given highly effective chemoprophylaxis, as their ability to tolerate a second life-threatening infection is unlikely to be great.

CURRENT REGIMENS FOR MALARIA CHEMOPROPHYLAXIS

See Table 21.3–1 for malaria chemoprophylaxis regimens. As a general rule, it is better to give antimalarial medications with a meal. Starting and stopping points for chemoprophylaxis are difficult to delineate but generally it is best to start at least a week prior to travel and to continue medication for a month after returning.

MEFLOQUINE

Mefloquine is the consensus choice for malaria chemoprophylaxis for short-term travelers to Africa. It is highly effective and generally well tolerated.[17] Contraindications to the use of mefloquine include a history of severe neuropsychiatric disease, especially seizures, and (by default) an unwillingness to take the drug. The latter is now very common following extensive publicity surrounding real or perceived adverse events associated with mefloquine. Those who cannot or refuse to take mefloquine should usually be assigned to doxycycline. In blinded, controlled trials, mefloquine has been shown to be safe, but rare (roughly 1:10,000), serious adverse events such as seizures and psychosis do occur.[17,18] It has been difficult to attribute any distinct adverse event(s) clearly to mefloquine during randomized, controlled studies.[5,6,19] Individuals whose lives would be threatened by even a rare seizure (such as aircraft pilots) should not generally be given mefloquine.

Many travelers have reported a vague dysphoria and sleep disturbances that many blame on mefloquine.[20] Although difficult to separate from other travel-related

Table 21.3–2.   PROBABLE FUTURE CHEMOPROPHYLACTIC AGENTS FOR MALARIA

DRUG	PROBABLE USAGE	NOTES
Azithromycin (Zithromax®)	Substitute for doxycycline	Unlikely to be highly effective in nonimmune individuals; must be taken daily
Primaquine	Short-term protection	Probable causal prophylactic (kills in liver) Not for use in G6PD deficient Not yet approved for malaria prevention
Atovaquone/proguanil (Malarone®)	Protection against multidrug-resistant falciparum malaria	Probable causal prophylactic (kills in liver) Currently licensed for treatment and prophylaxis in the U.S.A.
WR 238605 Tafenoquine	More effective, less toxic than primaquine	In early field trials Not for use in G6PD deficient Not available commercially

events, the adverse events associated with mefloquine have limited its use since many travelers now refuse to take it. An imperfect chemoprophylaxis that is actually taken is superior to one that is not taken at all, which makes the risk-benefit determination for short-term travelers to Africa more complex than one would expect. Current expert advice still favors the use of mefloquine despite the adverse publicity it has received.[2,21]

Mefloquine is given as a single tablet once a week. Although treatment regimens involving three to five times this amount often have gastrointestinal adverse events, the single weekly tablet is well tolerated. Mefloquine does not reach a steady-state blood concentration for many weeks following initiation of the drug.[5] Although a loading-dose regimen (one tablet per day for 3 days) has been field tested, for travelers it is best to start the medication 2 weeks prior to traveling if possible.[6]

Mefloquine can be used for expatriates under intense malaria exposure for extended periods of time.[22] Mefloquine should not be used in areas of known mefloquine resistance, which primarily involves forested areas of the Thai-Burmese and Thai-Cambodian border regions. Mefloquine prophylaxis failures are often detected many weeks to months following exposure due to the very long half-life of mefloquine.[23] Physicians seeing febrile post-travel patients should be aware that mefloquine resistance is not an absolute occurrence but may present as a suppressed infection weeks after travel with a very low (indeed undetectable) parasitemia. A careful medical history, physical examination, and repeated thick blood films are the best ways to rule out other possibilities in the extensive differential diagnosis of the returned traveler with fever.[24]

DOXYCYCLINE

Doxycycline is an antibiotic that is used to complete a cure of drug-resistant malaria, often in combination with quinine. It has also been found useful for chemoprophylaxis, particularly in Southeast Asia where mefloquine resistance leaves few available options.[25] In controlled field trials with closely monitored drug administration, daily doxycycline has been shown to be highly efficacious and safe in both Africa and Asia.[6,26]

Doxycycline for chemoprophylaxis has several problems that limit its use. One should not give it to young children or pregnant women. Vomiting may result if it is taken on an empty stomach. It is important to advise travelers to take doxycycline with a meal. Diarrhea and/or constipation are associated with chronic antibiotic use, but this is difficult to differentiate from changes in gut flora due to traveling. Sun sensitization can occur, and warnings against excessive ultraviolet light exposure are appropriate. Although doxycycline appears to have some effect against the liver stages of the parasite, this causal prophylactic effect cannot be relied on.[27] Therefore, doxycycline should be taken while in an endemic area and for 1 month following. An attempt to eliminate continuing the drug after leaving an endemic area and deal with relapsing malaria by adding daily primaquine was not encouraging when tried in Papua New Guinea.[28] Doxycycline,

like other current chemoprophylaxis regimens, should be continued for 1 month after leaving the endemic area. Doxycycline is very effective, but this is dependent on compliance with the daily regimen. The actual effectiveness of doxycycline is approximately equal to the rate of compliance. Doxycycline's inferior performance compared to mefloquine during military operations in Somalia was almost certainly due to the difference between daily and weekly regimen compliance.[29]

CHLOROQUINE/PROGUANIL

Chloroquine alone and proguanil alone are chemoprophylactic regimens that have been overcome by the march of drug resistance. Since both drugs are popular and well tolerated,[20] it was thought rational to combine the two. Unlike some drug combinations, there is no evidence of synergistic activity between the two components of chloroquine/proguanil. One is combining two partially effective drugs with the hope of achieving adequate protection.[30] For travelers going to areas without intense transmission, the combination usually works well,[31] but it must be considered of inferior efficacy compared to mefloquine or doxycycline.

Compliance is also a problem with this combination as chloroquine is taken weekly (except in France where 100 mg 6 of 7 days per week is used) and proguanil daily. Deaths have resulted from travelers who were confused as to the proper regimen and took daily chloroquine instead of daily proguanil. Careful and detailed patient instructions are important if one elects to prescribe chloroquine/proguanil. Some of this problem can be eliminated by the use of a combination tablet that has recently become available.[32] A similar (but different) drug called chlorproguanil has been used in tropical Africa and does seem to be reasonably interchangeable with proguanil.[33] Earlier attempts to use chlorproguanil as a weekly version of proguanil were not successful.

EXTINCT REGIMENS FOR MALARIA PREVENTION

Some drugs have been tried for malaria prevention and found to have serious problems usually in the form of unacceptable toxicity. The following drugs or drug combinations should not be used for the prevention of malaria.

AMODIAQUINE

Although still used for treatment, chronic use has resulted in granulocytopenia and hepatitis.

SULFADOXINE/PYRIMETHAMINE (FANSIDAR®, HOFFMAN LAROCHE)

Long-acting sulfa drugs can cause severe cutaneous reactions and have led to the abandonment of this combination for chemoprophylaxis.

MALOPRIM®

Pyrimethamine/dapsone (Maloprim®, Glaxo-Wellcome) is no longer used for chemoprophylaxis due to agranulocytosis seen when two tablets per week were taken.

QUININE

Although still a mainstay for the treatment of the hospitalized malaria patient, chronic suppression of malaria using daily quinine should not be used as it appears to predispose persons to blackwater fever.[34]

HALOFANTRINE

Generally, halofantrine is a very well-tolerated drug when used to treat malaria. Due to its highly variable bioavailability, however, some persons can experience acute fatal cardiac dysrhythmias.[35] Despite halofantrine's investigational use in a postexposure,[36] halofantrine should not be used to prevent malaria infection.

POSSIBLE FUTURE REGIMENS FOR MALARIA CHEMOPROPHYLAXIS

See Table 21.3–2 for future chemoprophylactic possibilities.

AZITHROMYCIN

Azithromycin (Zithromax®, Pfizer) is an antibiotic related to erythromycin with very good tissue penetration. It was thought that azithromycin's ability to kill liver stages of the malaria parasite might result in true causal prophylaxis and allow the discontinuation of drug on leaving an endemic area. Unfortunately, human challenge trials did not support this supposition.[37] Field trials of azithromycin for trachoma did indicate a significant antimalarial effect.[38] If weekly azithromycin could have been used, there, would have been a significant advantage over doxycycline; however, this was not true.[26] Field trials in Kenya indicated that daily azithromycin was required and that doxycycline appeared to be more efficacious. Subsequent trials in Asia have confirmed azithromycin's suboptimal efficacy. In light of its expense, it is unlikely that azithromycin will ever be used commonly for malaria prevention.

PRIMAQUINE

Primaquine is the only currently available drug that can reliably kill liver stages of malaria. Primaquine has been used for postexposure treatment of travelers who have been intensively exposed to relapsing malaria in order to eliminate residual liver parasites; however, this appears to be less effective in some areas such as Somalia.[39] Human malaria challenge data from the 1950s suggested that primaquine could be used as a causal prophylactic agent, which would be of considerable interest for very short-stay travelers. A daily regimen of primaquine has been used to prevent both falciparum and vivax malaria in Southeast Asia.[40] This has subsequently been confirmed by a larger field trial on the island of New Guinea.[41] Primaquine is not currently approved by any drug registration authority for malaria prophylaxis, but this may change in the near future. Primaquine should not be routinely used in glucose-6-phosphate dehydrogenase (G6PD)-deficient individuals due to the risk of hemolysis.

ATOVAQUONE/PROGUANIL

Atovaquone/proguanil (Malarone, Glaxo-Wellcome) is a new antimalarial drug combination that has particular usefulness for the treatment of multidrug-resistant falciparum malaria.[42] Because both components are individually very safe medications, atovaquone/proguanil seemed to be a very good potential chemoprophylactic drug. Field trials in Kenya that have subsequently been confirmed in South Africa and Zambia indicated that a fixed-combination tablet (250 mg atovaquone/100 mg proguanil) provided extremely effective and safe prevention of malaria infection for adults(Shanks, 1998).[43]

In Gabon, a similar study using a quarter-strength pediatric tablet was also very effective and safe in children.[44] Preliminary data indicate that atovaquone/proguanil may be causally prophylactic, but this has yet to be confirmed with field studies. Because of its efficacy against very drug-resistant forms of malaria and its excellent safety profile, atovaquone/proguanil is expected to be a very useful new chemoprophylactic once it is approved for use.

WR 238605

WR 238605 (also known as Tafenoquine) is a long-acting primaquine analogue that appears to be more effective and less toxic than primaquine.[44] Initial human challenge trials indicated that it could prevent malaria with its long half-life, indicating that no more frequent than weekly dosage would be required.(Brueckner, 1998).[46] Field trials in Kenya showed that when given to G6PD normal adults, WR 238605 was very effective and well tolerated (Shanks, unpublished). A short-course regimen of 400-mg base given three times over 3 days was able to prevent malaria very effectively for >100 days. If this finding can be confirmed in individuals with less than solid immunity to malaria, then it may be possible to protect most travelers with a course of medication that could be directly administered prior to travel. G6PD testing will remain necessary prior to any drug administration due to WR 238605's ability to cause severe hemolysis if given to G6PD persons.

CONCLUSION

Travelers to the tropics can be protected from malaria. Prevention currently depends on the judicious use of antimalarial drugs in conjunction with mosquito avoidance measures. A careful understanding of what protection benefits are expected compared to what adverse event risks are assumed is necessary in order to optimally advise travelers. The rise of drug resistance has made chemoprophylaxis decisions much more finely balanced than when chloroquine was universally effective. The popularization of tropical travel along with a much quicker response to legal sanctions when adverse events arise has further complicated chemoprophylaxis for malaria. No certain choice exists for several at-risk groups such as pregnant women or children. For the usual adult traveler who will be exposed to malaria, one uses mefloquine; if that is not advisable, the second choice is doxycycline.

Other, possibly better, drugs are in advanced stages of either field testing or the registration process. If we cannot improve on the current record of drug resistance, it is likely that these new medications will become useless in less time than it took to develop them. The malaria parasite is a clever and adaptive enemy that has managed to co-evolve with humans for a very long time. One should not suppose that any new drug or intervention against malaria will simply solve the complex problem of how to prevent malaria in travelers, but there are reasons to be optimistic. Malaria is not now regarded just as a problem for armies and development agencies. Tropical travelers are providing the stimulus to seek and obtain new weapons against malaria, if we can but use them wisely.

ACKNOWLEDGMENT

The author of this chapter is an employee of the U.S. Government, whose work is in the public domain.

REFERENCES

1. Committee to Advise on Tropical Medicine and Travel. Canadian recommendations for the prevention and treatment of malaria among international travellers. Nat Med 1996;2:204–208.
2. Bradley DJ, Warhurst DC. Guidelines for the prevention of malaria in travellers from the United Kingdom. PHLS Malaria Reference Laboratory, London School of Hygiene and Tropical Medicine. Commun Dis Rep. CDR Rev 1997;7:R137–152.
3. Centers for Disease Control and Prevention. Health information for international travel 1999–2000. U.S. Goverment Printing Office: Washington, DC, 1999.
4. Lobel HO, Kozarsky PE. Update on prevention of malaria for travelers. JAMA 1997;278:1767–1771.
5. Boudreau E, Schuster B, Sanchez J, et al. Tolerability of prophylactic Lariam regimens. Trop Med Parasitol 1993;44:257–265.
6. Ohrt C, Richie TL, Widjaja H, et al. Mefloquine compared with doxycycline for the prophylaxis of malaria in Indonesian soldiers. A randomized, double-blind, placebo-controlled trial. Ann Intern Med 1997;126:963–972.
7. World malaria situation in 1994. Part I. Population at risk. Wkly Epidemiol Rec 1997;72:269–274.
8. Behrens RH, Curtis CF. Malaria in travellers: epidemiology and prevention. Br Med Bull 1993;49:363–381.
9. Lackritz EM, Lobel HO, Howell BJ, et al. Imported Plasmodium falciparum malaria in American travelers to Africa. Implications for prevention strategies. JAMA 1991;265:383–385.
10. Gyorkos TW, Svenson JE, Maclean JD, et al. Compliance with antimalarial chemoprophylaxis and the subsequent development of malaria: a matched case-control study. Am J Trop Med Hyg 1995;53:511–517.
11. Phillips Howard PA, Wood D. The safety of antimalarial drugs in pregnancy. Drug Saf 1996;14:131–145.
12. Nosten F, ter KF, Maelankiri L, et al. Mefloquine prophylaxis prevents malaria during pregnancy: a double-blind, placebo-controlled study. J Infect Dis 1994;169:595-603.
13. Smoak BL, Writer JV, Keep LW, et al. The effects of inadvertent exposure of mefloquine chemoprophylaxis on pregnancy outcomes and infants of US Army servicewomen. J Infect Dis 1997;176:831–833.
14. Vanhauwere B, Maradit H, Kerr L. Post-marketing surveillance of prophylactic mefloquine (Lariam) use in pregnancy. Am J Trop Med Hyg 1998;58:17–21.
15. Steketee RW, Wirima JJ, Campbell CC. Developing effective strategies for malaria prevention programs for pregnant African women. Eur J Clin Chem Clin Biochem 1996;34:17–22.
16. Bloland PB, Wirima JJ, Steketee RW, et al. Maternal HIV infection and infant mortality in Malawi: evidence for increased mortality due to placental malaria infection. AIDS 1995;9:721–726.
17. Steffen R, Fuchs E, Schildknecht J, et al. Mefloquine compared with other malaria chemoprophylactic regimens in tourists visiting east Africa. Lancet 1993;341:1299–1303.
18. Croft A, Garner P. Mefloquine to prevent malaria: a systematic review of trials. BMJ 1997;315:1412–1416.
19. Schlagenhauf P, Lobel H, Steffen R, et al. Tolerance of mefloquine by SwissAir trainee pilots. Am J Trop Med Hyg 1997;56:235–240.
20. Barrett PJ, Emmins PD, Clarke PD, Bradley DJ. Comparison of adverse events associated with use of mefloquine and combination of chloroquine and proguanil as antimalarial prophylaxis: postal and telephone survey of travellers. BMJ 1996;313:525–528.
21. Winstanley P. Mefloquine: the benefits outweigh the risks. Br J Clin Pharmacol 1996;42:411–413.
22. Lobel HO, Miani M, Eng T, et al. Long-term malaria prophylaxis with weekly mefloquine. Lancet 1993;341:848–851.
23. Hopperus Buma AP, van Thiel PP, Lobel HO, et al. Long-term malaria chemoprophylaxis with mefloquine in Dutch marines in Cambodia. J Infect Dis 1996;173:1506–1509.
24. Svenson JE, Gyorkos TW, MacLean JD. Diagnosis of malaria in the febrile traveler. Am J Trop Med Hyg 1995;53:518–521.
25. Shanks GD, Roessler P, Edstein MD, Rieckmann KH. Doxycycline for malaria prophylaxis in Australian soldiers deployed to United Nations missions in Somalia and Cambodia. Proc Natl Acad Sci U S A 1995;92:11294–11298.
26. Andersen SL, Oloo AJ, Gordon DM, et al. Successful double-blinded, randomized, placebo-controlled field trial of azithromycin and doxycycline as prophylaxis for malaria in western Kenya. Clin Infect Dis 1998;26:146–150.
27. Shmuklarsky MJ, Boudreau EF, Pang LW, et al. Failure of doxycycline as a causal prophylactic agent against Plasmodium falciparum malaria in healthy nonimmune volunteers. Ann Intern Med 1994;120:294–299.
28. Shanks GD, Barnett A, Edstein MD, Rieckmann KH. Effectiveness of doxycycline combined with primaquine for malaria prophylaxis. Med J Aust 1995;162:306–307, 309–310.
29. Sanchez JL, DeFraites RF, Sharp TW, Hanson RK. Mefloquine or doxycycline prophylaxis in US troops in Somalia [letter]. Lancet 1993;341:1021–1022.
30. Garin D, Lamarque D, Ringwald P, et al. Efficacy of chloroquine-proguanil chemoprophylaxis against malaria in the Central African Republic. Trans R Soc Trop Med Hyg 1993;87:304–305.
31. Carme B, Peguet C, Nevez G. Compliance with and tolerance of mefloquine and chloroquine + proguanil malaria chemoprophylaxis in French short-term travellers to sub-Saharan Africa. Trop Med Int Health 1997;2:953–956.
32. Touze JE, Keundjian A, Fusai T, Doury JC. Human pharmacokinetics of chloroquine and proguanil delivered in a single

capsule for malaria chemoprophylaxis. Trop Med Parasitol 1995;46:158–160.

33. Nevill CG, Lury JD, Mosobo MK, et al. Daily chlorproguanil is an effective alternative to daily proguanil in the prevention of *Plasmodium falciparum* malaria in Kenya. Trans R Soc Trop Med Hyg 1994;88:319–320.

34. Tran TH, Day NP, Ly VC, et al. Blackwater fever in southern Vietnam: a prospective descriptive study of 50 cases. Clin Infect Dis 1996;23:1274–1281.

35. Nosten F, ter Kuile FO, Luxemburger C, et al. Cardiac effects of antimalarial treatment with halofantrine. Lancet 1993;341:1054–1056.

36. Shanks GD, Edstein MD, Kereu RK, et al. Postexposure administration of halofantrine for the prevention of malaria. Clin Infect Dis 1993;17:628–631.

37. Anderson SL, Berman J, Kuschner R, et al. Prophylaxis of *Plasmodium falciparum* malaria with azithromycin administered to volunteers. Ann Intern Med 1995;123:771–773.

38. Sadiq ST, Glasgow KW, Drakeley CJ, et al. Effects of azithromycin on malariometric indices in The Gambia. Lancet 1995;346:881–882.

39. Smoak BL, DeFraites RF, Magill AJ, et al. *Plasmodium vivax* infections in U.S. Army troops: failure of primaquine to prevent relapse in studies from Somalia. Am J Trop Med Hyg 1997;56:231–234.

40. Baird JK, Fryauff DJ, Basri H, et al. Primaquine for prophylaxis against malaria among nonimmune transmigrants in Irian Jaya, Indonesia. Am J Trop Med Hyg 1995;52:479–484.

41. Fryauff DJ, Baird JK, Basri H, et al. Randomised placebo-controlled trial of primaquine for prophylaxis of falciparum and vivax malaria. Lancet 1995;346:1190–1193.

42. Looareesuwan S, Viravan C, Webster HK, et al. Clinical studies of atovaquone, alone or in combination with other antimalarial drugs, for treatment of acute uncomplicated malaria in Thailand. Am J Trop Med Hyg 1996;54:62–66.

43. Shanks GD, Gordom DM, Klotz F, et al. Efficacy and safety of atovaquone/proguanil as suppressive prophylaxis for Plasmodium falciparum. Clin Infect Dis 1998;27:494–499.

44. Lell B, Luckner D, Ndjave M, et al. Randomised placebo-controlled study of atovaquone plus proguanil for malaria prophylaxis in children. Lancet 1998;351:709–713.

45. Peters W, Robinson BL, Milhous WK. The chemotherapy of rodent malaria. LI. Studies on a new 8-aminoquinoline, WR 238,605. Ann Trop Med Parasitol 1993;87:547–552.

46. Brueckner RP, Lasseter KC, Lin ET, et al. First time-in-humans safety and pharmacokinetics of WR 238605, a new antimallarial. Am J Trop Med Hyg 1998;58:645–649.

21.4 MALARIA TREATMENT

CHRISTOPHER J.M. WHITTY AND JAMES J. MWENEUANYA

INTRODUCTION

Malaria is the most common life-threatening infection acquired by travelers to tropical countries. Chemoprophylaxis reduces the risk of infection but does not remove it; thus, all critically ill patients within 12 months of returning from a malarious area must have malaria excluded, even if they took chemoprophylaxis. Prophylaxis reduces the chances of a traveler having malaria but may delay presentation. Malaria should also be considered in fever not due to other causes months or years after traveling to an area where *Plasmodium vivax* or *P. ovale* infections are common, as relapses due to liver hypnozoites occur long after initial exposure.

PRESENTATION

The clinical presentation of malaria is typically nonspecific with fever, headache, and rigors, but nothing should put clinicians off considering the diagnosis. Children may present with fits without a clear preceding history of fever. The most experienced tropical physician cannot be certain of the diagnosis or exclude it by history or examination. Nonclassic presentations including bloody diarrhea, malaise without fever, jaundice, or prolonged weight loss are not uncommon. There are no specific findings on examination, although splenomegaly is suggestive. The only safe way to approach malaria is to consider the diagnosis in any patient who is unwell and has recently returned from the tropics and then perform a diagnostic test (ideally, blood film for malaria). Other laboratory tests may be important in the management of patients with severe malaria but do not help in diagnosis. Full blood count will usually show low platelet count, but this is not invariable, and the degree of thrombopenia does not correlate well with disease severity. White cell count may be raised, and this should not put clinicians off the diagnosis. All blood indices may, however, be normal.

DIAGNOSTIC TESTS

There are several methods available for diagnosis of falciparum malaria, and a slightly smaller number for the other malaria species. New methods are currently being assessed, but no method has yet been demonstrated to be superior to the traditional method of light microscopy of thick and thin films in clinical practice.

Direct microscopy remains the gold standard for malaria diagnosis. Giemsa- or Field-stained thin and thick blood films enable the *Plasmodium* species and parasitemia to be determined with a high degree of accuracy by skilled microscopists.[1] The sensitivity of detection by the thick blood film is approximately 0.0001 parasites per 100 red cells. The newer methods discussed below are useful as an adjunct to direct microscopy, especially for those who are not regularly examining malaria films, but are not a substitute.

Fluorescence microscopy uses acridine orange dye, which selectively targets parasite DNA and has been incorporated into a commercial test (QBC II). This is as sensitive as thick films, although parasitemia estimation is unreliable.[2] It has the disadvantage of needing a trained microscopist to perform the test and requires a UV microscope.

HRP-2 antigen capture assays provide a qualitative method that uses a monoclonal antibody to a water-soluble protein of malaria parasites. It may show a positive result before and after that seen by microscopy.[3] It is an easy test to perform and does not need trained staff. It is useful in detecting *P. falciparum* in mixed infections, but the test is species specific: a *P. falciparum* HRP-2 antigen capture test will not detect other species of malaria. HRP-2 antigen tests are generally available for *P. falciparum* and on limited commercial release for *P. vivax* at the time of writing. The disadvantage of this technique is that it will miss other species of malaria and can provide no quantitative estimation of the parasitemia, which is important in management.[4]

NEW TECHNIQUES

Each *Plasmodium* sp produces lactate dehydrogenase (LDH) specific to the species. Monoclonal antibodies to these are undergoing field trials as a diagnostic tool. Each *Plasmodium* species produces a LDH specific to the species, and monoclonal antibodies against these have been incorporated in a capture technique.[5] This offers the possibility of being able to produce dipsticks that can reliably identify each species, although it is unlikely that an estimate of parasitemia will ever be available with this method.

Ribosomal DNA polymerase chain reaction has now progressed to sensitive detection and speciation of *Plasmodium* sp.[6] It is not currently suitable for clinical diagnosis of malaria as it is too slow and has no real practical advantages over microscopy (parasitemia estimation is crude, parasite staging impossible, and both false positives and false negatives occur). It is, however, valuable as a research tool.

NONFALCIPARUM (BENIGN) MALARIAS

Provided that a skilled microscopist is sure that a patient has one of the nonfalciparum malarias (vivax, ovale, and malariae) without mixed infection, the initial management is currently straightforward. Where the microscopist examining a film is unsure of the species, it should be treated as falciparum. Some microscopists examining blood films in nonendemic countries have limited practice in speciation, and in this situation, if the clinical presentation fits falciparum infection better, it is often wise for films to be re-examined or an alternative diagnostic method used. Three presentations should always raise the possibility that falciparum malaria is present. Critically ill patients are far more likely to have falciparum malaria than one on the benign forms. Patients returned from sub-Saharan Africa have an over 95% chance of malaria being

either pure falciparum infection or mixed infection. Any blood film with parasitemias over 1% or multiply infected cells is almost certainly falciparum.

With these caveats, it is safe to treat nonfalciparum malaria as an outpatient. Even untreated, these forms of malaria have a negligible mortality: only profound anemia commonly causes problems in otherwise healthy individuals, and this should be excluded with a full blood count. Almost all vivax malaria and all malariae and ovale malaria are fully chloroquine sensitive (1998). Early reports of chloroquine-resistant vivax malaria have come out of Papua New Guinea, Indonesia, and the Pacific Islands,[7] and possibly from India. Not all of these are entirely reliable. Chloroquine-resistant vivax is, however, rare even in these areas, and no reliable reports of chloroquine-resistant strains of ovale and malariae have been published at the time of writing. There is currently no reason not to use chloroquine as the first-line treatment in nonfalciparum malaria.

Chloroquine should be given at a total dose of 25 mg base/kg in divided doses, usually 10 mg/kg followed by 5 mg/kg at 8, 24, and 48 hours. In average-sized adults, this is usually given as 600-mg base, followed by three doses of 300 mg. Shorter dosing schedules are probably equally effective.[8] Chloroquine is well tolerated and rapidly effective in all sensitive strains of malaria. Persisting symptoms at the end of a course of treatment should raise the possibility that there is either an additional infection or (rarely) a resistant strain. A blood film should be repeated. Side effects are rare with chloroquine at treatment doses. Apart from occasional drug rashes, the main problems are pruritis in up to 50% of black-skinned individuals. Occasional transient neuropsychiatric reactions have been reported.

Vivax and ovale malaria lay down dormant forms of the parasite (hypnozoites) in the liver. Chloroquine has little or no effect on these and needs to be followed by a second drug to effect radical cure and prevent relapses weeks or months later. Currently, the only licensed drug for this is primaquine. Traditionally, this was given at 0.25 mg/kg for 14 days (an adult daily dose of 15 mg/day), but partial resistance seems to be widespread in Oceania and Southeast Asia and appearing elsewhere, so doubling this to 15 mg bd for 14 days in adults is sensible in travelers from these areas and probably advisable generally. Primaquine is contraindicated in pregnancy, and the newborn and pregnant women should be given a prophylactic course of weekly chloroquine (safe in pregnancy) at least until delivery, and ideally until the end of breast-feeding, followed by radical cure with primaquine. Primaquine is an oxidant drug and can cause hemolysis (occasionally serious hemolysis) in those with glucose-6-phosphate dehydrogenase (G6PD) deficiency. This should be routinely screened for before patients are prescribed primaquine, and, if present, current guidelines consulted. In mild G6PD deficiency, a weekly schedule may be appropriate, but this depends on current sensitivities.

In the currently rare cases of true chloroquine-resistant vivax malaria, all of the drugs used for treatment of *P. falciparum* malaria will cure the disease, although usually more slowly than chloroquine in sensitive strains.

Quinine, qinghaosu derivatives, and mefloquine are all reasonable choices; doses are as for *P. falciparum* below.

INITIAL ASSESSMENT OF THE PATIENT WITH FALCIPARUM MALARIA

It is easy to underestimate severity in falciparum malaria. The parasite goes through a repeating cycle of development and reproduction, and it is only at certain points of the cycle that significant pathologic damage occurs. This makes assessment much more difficult than for other infections. A patient can appear clinically well and then deteriorate rapidly despite adequate treatment as parasites mature. A low parasite count does not mean that the infection is trivial, and many of the complications of malaria can occur after all parasites have been cleared from the peripheral blood.

Any or all of the signs or test results in Table 21.4–1 indicate a complicated case of malaria that will need intensive monitoring and treatment. Rapid deterioration is likely.[9]

Where neurologic signs or coma are present, hypoglycemia should be immediately excluded, since both severe malaria and antimalarial drugs cause hypoglycemia. Pregnant women are at particular risk.

In the absence of these, other factors indicate a potentially complicated case:

* pregnancy,
* hyperpyrexia (>39°C),
* parasite count > 2%, and
* mature parasites (schizonts or late trophozoites) on the blood film.

TREATMENT

CHEMOTHERAPY OF *P. FALCIPARUM* MALARIA

Severe and Potentially Complicated Malaria
The key to treating both complicated and uncomplicated malaria is to give the patient effective antimalarial drugs

Table 21.4–1. SEVERE OR POTENTIALLY COMPLICATED MALARIA (WHO, 1990)

Reduction in conscious level
Neurologic signs or fits
Renal impairment (creatinine >250) or oliguria
Shock or hypotension
Parasite count >5% on blood film
Anemia (hematocrit <15%)
Signs of bleeding or disseminated intravascular coagulation
Jaundice
Pulmonary edema, hypoxia, or acidosis
Hypoglycemia (glucose <2.2 mmol/L)

as soon as the diagnosis is made. In cases of severe *P. falciparum* malaria, the choice is limited by the need to use parenteral drugs[9] (see below).

Parenteral quinine is the current gold standard for treating severe malaria in Europe and should be used in all cases except where there is a high chance of quinine resistance. Significant quinine resistance is currently limited to a very restricted geographic area (see below). In the U.S.A., parenteral quinine is not available, and quinidine should be substituted. Quinidine is a slightly more active antimalarial but has a four times greater effect on the heart. Both quinine and quinidine can cause arrhythmias and should never be given as bolus injections. Quinidine should be administered with ECG monitoring; if the QT interval is prolonged by more than 25%, stop the infusion. Both quinine and quinidine can cause hypoglycemia by direct stimulation of the pancreas.[10]

Quinine doses are usually started with a loading dose in severe cases of malaria. The two most commonly used regimens are 20-mg quinine dihydrochloride salt/kg over 4 hours in 5% dextrose or 0.9% sodium chloride[11] or 7-mg salt/kg infused over 30 minutes, followed by 10 mg/kg over 4 hours.[12]

A maintenance dose of 10 mg/kg every 8 to 12 hours should follow. This should be given by infusion over 4 hours. In children from quinine-sensitive areas, the frequency of infusion can be dropped to 12 hourly. Cinchonism (ringing in the ears, deafness, and vertigo) is not an indication to stop therapy. The therapeutic range for quinine has not been defined, but plasma concentrations between 8 and 15 mg/L (18 to 30 mmol/L) are safe and effective. Trough quinine levels should be checked after the third parenteral dose where available.

The quinidine loading dose is 10 mg base/kg infused over 1 hour, followed by 1.2 mg/kg per hour (0.02 mg/kg/min). The therapeutic range has not been determined, but plasma concentrations of 5 to 8 mg/L are considered effective and are usually safe. If plasma concentration monitoring is not available, consider reducing the dose of quinidine by a third on day 3 of treatment.

Once patients have begun to respond to treatment, they can be converted to oral therapy if tolerated. They should continue on quinine or quinidine until asexual parasites are eliminated from the peripheral blood. They should then have a second-line drug such as sulfadoxine-pyrimethamine (Fansidar) once, or doxycycline for 7 days to eliminate any residual parasites. Tetracyclines are contraindicated in children under 12 years old.

A summary of possible chemotherapy options is given in Table 21.4–2.

Uncomplicated *P. falciparum* Malaria The choice of possible treatments in uncomplicated malaria is wide, and patients can almost always be treated with oral drugs. Because it is extremely easy to underestimate malaria, admitting patients with *P. falciparum* is advisable. Chloroquine resistance is now so widespread that it is not advised unless there are no other antimalarials in stock where it can be used as a holding maneuver, as most parasite strains will have limited chloroquine sensitivity. In some areas of North America and Europe, getting antimalarials

Table 21.4–2. WIDELY USED REGIMES IN THE CHEMOTHERAPY OF SEVERE OR POTENTIALLY COMPLICATED MALARIA

	INITIAL DOSE	SUBSEQUENT DOSES
Quinine	20 mg salt/kg IV over 4 hours	10 mg salt/kg over 2–8 hours, every 8 hours
Quinidine (ECG monitoring advised)	10 mg base/kg IV over 1 hour	0.02 mg base/kg/min
Artemether (intramuscular)	3.2 mg/kg stat IM	1.6 mg/kg every 24 hours IM
Artesunate	2 mg/kg stat (IV/IM)	1 mg/kg at 12 hours then 1 mg/kg daily

other than chloroquine can take time, and it is a lot better than nothing while waiting for better drugs to arrive.

The choice of other antimalarials in uncomplicated malaria is guided primarily by side effects of the drugs, availability, and cost. Oral quinine, halofantrine, mefloquine, artemether derivatives, and atovaquone-proguanil are all highly effective antimalarials at present in most parts of the world and particularly in strains from Africa, where the majority of *P. falciparum* originates. As a general rule, it is advisable when treating nonimmune individuals to use a first-line drug and follow it with a second-line drug (usually doxycycline or sulfadoxine-pyrimethamine). Some possible treatment regimes are outlined in Table 21.4–3. The limitations of the various regimes below are a guide, but not exhaustive, and those unfamiliar with the drugs should consult the manufacturers' data sheets.

The most widely used regime outside Asia, and the one these authors would recommend, is oral quinine until the parasites are cleared from the circulation (assessed by daily blood films), and then either sulphadoxine/pyrimethamine as a single dose or a week of doxycycline. If it is impossible to do daily films, 5 days of treatment with quinine and then the second-line drug is probably the best option. In adults, the usual dose of oral quinine is 600 mg three times a day, but if cinchonism (a reversible ringing in the ears, deafness, and nausea) becomes a real problem and the patient's malaria seems to be improving, dropping to 600 mg twice daily is usually effective. Oral quinine used in therapeutic doses is safe, although unpleasant to take. Because of possible interactions potentiating severe arrhythmias with halofantrine, an alternative to quinine should be sought if halofantrine has been taken recently. Quinine should be used with caution after a treatment dose of mefloquine.

Oral artemether and other artemisinine derivatives are also safe. They must always be taken with a second-line drug or relapse rates on monotherapy are unacceptably high. It is likely that this class of drugs will take over from quinine as the first-line treatment of choice for malaria early in the 21st century.

Halofantrine is generally well tolerated in nonsevere malaria, but there is a small but real risk of sudden arrhythmias and death, and for this reason it is rarely used in most countries. The combination of halofantrine and quinine and halofantrine and mefloquine is particularly dangerous as these drugs can potentiate one another's arrhythmogenic properties.

Mefloquine used in treatment doses is also generally well tolerated, but there seems to be a small but real increase in neuropsychiatric reactions (occasionally severe) and of the postmalaria neurologic syndromes in patients treated with mefloquine, and it is seldom used for treatment outside the United States.

Early experience of treating with atovaquone-proguanil suggests that it is well tolerated, but insufficient numbers have been treated for rare but important side effects to emerge (as happened with halofantrine and mefloquine), and it is probably best reserved for quinine-resistant strains.

Chemotherapy in Multidrug-Resistant *falciparum* Clinically important quinine-resistant malaria is rare at present. It is currently (1998) a clinical problem in a very restricted area of Southeast Asia. Patients who come from the Thai-Burmese or Thai-Cambodian borders should be considered potentially to have quinine resistance, and in these, either supplementary or alternative drugs should be given. Resistance patterns change rapidly, and up-to-date information about resistance patterns should be sought in these patients. Only artemisinine (qinghaosu) derivatives can reliably take the place of quinine for parenteral treatment. The alternatives are:

- artesunate (as sodium artesunate) diluted in 5- to 10-mL 5% dextrose by intravenous or intramuscular injection (initial dose of 2.4 mg/kg, then 1.2 mg/kg at 12 and 24 hours and daily thereafter).
- artemether by intramuscular injection (initial dose of 3.2 mg/kg, followed by 1.6 mg/kg daily).

Table 21.4–3. POSSIBLE CHEMOTHERAPY REGIMES IN NON-SEVERE MALARIA

	ALL PATIENTS	ADDITIONAL TREATMENT IN NONIMMUNES
Quinine sulphate	600 mg three times a day until parasites clear (or 5 days)	Sulphadoxine-pyrimethamine 3 tablets single dose at end of quinine or doxycycline 100 mg a day for a week
Mefloquine	15 mg base/kg one dose	10 mg/kg 8–12 hours later
Halofantrine	8 mg/kg three times at 6- to 8-hour intervals	Repeat after a week
Oral artesunate	4 mg/kg daily for 3 days, then mefloquine 15 mg/kg or doxycycline 100 mg/day	

Both should be followed by a second-line drug. Reports of increased incidence of neurotoxicity with mefloquine make other choices of second-line drugs such as doxycycline more attractive.

Where artemisinine derivatives are not available, combined therapy with quinine or quinidine (as above) with doxycycline up to 3 mg/kg/day will reduce failure rates in quinine resistance.

In milder cases of quinine-resistant malaria, a variety of oral combinations are worth considering. Up-to-date information is essential, but the following combinations are worth considering:

- atovaquone + pyrimethamine (Malarone) for 3 days. This is currently highly effective, but a single mutation confers resistance, so when resistance comes, it will spread fast.
- quinine + doxycycline, followed by a further second-line drug. The advantage of this option is that most hospitals will have the drugs, although it can no longer be considered reliable in strains from Southeast Asia.
- an artesunate combined with another drug (e.g., coartemether). Artesunates should never be used as monotherapy as relapse rates are unacceptably high even in fully sensitive strains.
- halofantrine. Multidrug-resistant strains in Southeast Asia are usually resistant to halofantrine, but currently African strains seldom are. However, the undoubted efficacy of halofantrine as an antimalarial has to be set against the significant risks of cardiotoxicity.[13]

Sulphadoxine-pyrimethamine (Fansidar) resistance is spreading rapidly in Africa, and it is likely that during the lifetime of this textbook, it will no longer be an appropriate second-line drug in malaria acquired in most parts of the world.

GENERAL MANAGEMENT

The key points in management are outlined in Table 21.4–4, but general medical care is also important. Patients should be monitored for clinical and parasitologic response to treatment. Rises of parasite count up to 12 hours after instituting treatment may be due to the natural parasite cycle and should not be taken as evidence of treatment failure. There should be a fall of greater than 75% by 48 hours; if there is not, resistant malaria is likely, and treatment should be altered. Conventional clinical measures of response are time to recovery of consciousness, time to fever falling below 37.5°C, and time to parasite count falling by 50%, 90%, and 100%.

Fluid balance, renal function, and respiratory function should be monitored closely. Both renal and pulmonary function can deteriorate despite a parasitologic and clinical response to treatment.

In adults, optimizing fluid balance is the most difficult part of supportive care. Patients with severe malaria are often dehydrated and require initial rehydration. They may also require blood transfusion. Overhydration is easy, with potentially fatal results. The pulmonary complica-

Table 21.4–4. KEY POINTS IN THE MANAGEMENT OF MALARIA

Falciparum malaria is a common cause of severe illness in patients returned from the tropics.

Thick and thin blood films remain the diagnostic method of choice.

Severe malaria can occur even with low parasite counts.

Quinine, quinidine, or the artemisinine derivatives are the drugs of choice in severe malaria.

The most urgent priority is giving adequate antimalarial drugs. Debates about route of administration or exchange transfusion should not be allowed to delay this.

Renal failure, respiratory problems, and multiorgan failure can occur after parasites have all been cleared from the blood.

Children are at particular risk from anemia, which should be treated early.

Pregnant women are at particular risk, especially of hypoglycemia.

tions of malaria have a mortality of around 50% in intensive care units, and these may be precipitated by overvigorous hydration. The renal failure seen in malaria is almost always due to the sequestration of parasites in the kidney. Repeated fluid challenges to try to improve renal function are therefore inappropriate and constitute one of the most common avoidable errors in management of severe malaria.

Apart from antimalarial drugs and caution with fluids in adults, spotting and treating the complications of severe malaria early is the key to good management. No trials of potentially disease-modifying drugs (such as anti-tumor necrosis factor) have demonstrated any reduction in mortality or complications to date.[14]

COMPLICATIONS OF FALCIPARUM MALARIA

Cerebral Malaria Technically, cerebral malaria is unrousable coma without fits in the preceding 30 minutes with no cause except for malaria. Hypoglycemia should always be excluded. Mortality from cerebral malaria can be up to 30% even with ideal treatment. Despite this, adult patients who survive seldom have significant neurologic sequelae. In practice, any reduction in conscious level or neurologic signs in the context of malaria are significant, and patients should ideally be nursed in a high-dependency unit.

Adults. Trials have shown that prophylactic intramuscular phenobarbitone improves outcome in cerebral malaria; where this is not available, it is likely that other anticonvulsants given prophylactically help. Fits occur commonly in cerebral malaria and should be treated like any other. There is no contraindication to using benzodiazepines. The role of cerebral edema in the pathology of cerebral malaria is unclear, but it has been clearly demonstrated that steroids and mannitol have no place in the management of adult cases of cerebral malaria. There is no indication for routine lumbar puncture or computed tomography scanning in adult cerebral malaria, except where coexisting meningitis is suspected.

Children. Cerebral malaria is a common complication in children. Early treatment with effective antimalarials remains the priority. Early reports of trials suggest that prophylactic phenobarbitone is not helpful in children (1999), and fits should be managed as they occur. Lumbar puncture remains controversial, as malaria and meningitis may coexist in children, especially those who have been living in endemic areas. Some reports suggest that children with cerebral malaria may have raised intracranial pressure and that lumbar puncture should be deferred until there is clinical improvement,[15] but other studies have failed to confirm this. If lumbar puncture is not performed, antibiotics to cover bacterial meningitis are advisable.

Renal Problems   *Adults.*   Renal failure is one of the common causes of death in severe falciparum malaria. This can occur acutely or after the patient seems to have begun to recover. Hemofiltration and dialysis should be started early in renal impairment due to malaria, as this probably improves outcome, although there are currently no good trials to prove this. Extreme caution should be used to avoid overhydration. Quinine and quinidine are metabolized in the liver, so dosage seldom has to be adjusted for at least the first 3 days of treatment when patients are in renal failure. Where facilities to monitor drug levels are not available, it is conventional to reduce dosage by a third on day 3. Dialysis marginally reduces quinine levels. Certain antimalarial second-line drugs are best avoided in renal failure, in particular, Fansidar. Doxycycline is probably the second-line drug of choice, at a reduced dose of 100 mg a day.

"Blackwater fever," an old term mainly used for patients with black urine secondary to intravascular hemolysis, should be treated like any other malaria. It is sometimes triggered by antimalarial drugs, especially in cases of G6PD deficiency, but the risks of stopping treatment are almost always greater than those of the hemolysis itself.

Children.   The renal problems seen in adults are almost never seen in children, and monitoring creatinine is not routinely necessary.

Pulmonary Complications   *Adults.*   Pulmonary involvement in malaria is very serious, with a high mortality even with intensive care. Fluid overload should be excluded with the help of a Swan-Ganz catheter and, if present, corrected with diuretics. In severe cases, however, it may be caused by a form of adult respiratory distress syndrome. Apart from optimizing the fluid balance and giving high-flow oxygen and ventilatory support, no specific treatment has been shown to help.

Children.   Breathing difficulty has been shown to be a poor prognostic indicator in children. In most cases, it is, however, not due to pulmonary edema and is most usually associated with anemia, lactic acidosis, or both.[16] In these cases, transfusion is the most important therapeutic maneuver, but in the absence of safe blood being instantly available, vigorous fluid replacement is helpful.[17]

Hyperparasitemia   *Adults.*   The exact role of exchange blood transfusion where high parasite loads are present is controversial.[18] Exchange transfusion involves substituting unparasitized donated blood for the heavily parasitized blood of the patient. At parasitemias of less than 5%, it is not indicated. At parasitemias of greater than 10%, it has a place in certain cases where complications are present. At confirmed parasitemias of over 20%, it is very likely to be indicated. It should never be performed without close nursing and medical supervision to balance blood coming out with blood going in. Laboratory errors in estimation of parasitemias (by up to 10 times) are not uncommon, with overestimation more likely than underestimation. It is therefore advisable to have high parasitemias checked by a reference laboratory.

Children.   There is no good evidence supporting exchange transfusion in children. Children with hyperparasitemia will almost invariably become profoundly anemic, however, and early transfusion should be anticipated.

Anemia   Profound anemia is common in severe malaria, especially where there has been a prolonged history. Parasitized cells are broken down, and the parasite suppresses hemopoiesis, so there is seldom a reticulocytosis.

Adults.   Transfusion is usually indicated at hemoglobins of below 5 g/dL. Low platelets are almost invariable in malaria and require no specific treatment unless bleeding occurs. There is no association between platelet count and severity.

Children.   Anemia is the most common life-threatening complication in children under 2 years old and common in all children. There is a clear indication to transfuse at hemoglobins below 5 g/dL, but in any child with hyperparasitemia, respiratory distress, or heart failure, much earlier transfusion is advisable.

Disseminated Intravascular Coagulation   This is a rare but serious complication of severe malaria. It can present with profuse bleeding into the gut. Since almost all patients with DIC and malaria will already be anemic, blood transfusion is usually indicated. The role of heparin, fresh frozen plasma, and other treatments is no more clearly worked out than in other causes of DIC. It is probably a less common complication in children than in adults.

Shock (Algid Malaria)   Shock in malaria is often associated with coexisting sepsis, and all patients with this complication should receive broad-spectrum antibiotics with good gram-negative cover. Otherwise, treatment is supportive. Malaria has surprisingly little direct effect on cardiac function. In children, shocked patients are often anemic.

Pregnancy   Pregnant women who contract malaria are at significantly increased risk. Even women who are largely immune to malaria can become seriously ill during pregnancy. Quinine remains the antimalarial drug of choice but can induce premature labor, and hypoglycemia is a serious problem. There are currently no formal safety studies of artesunate derivatives in pregnancy, but extensive use worldwide has demonstrated no serious problems, and it is probably safe. Doxycycline is generally contraindicated. Fansidar should be used with caution and always given with a folate supplement. Pregnant women should have their treatment extended at least 48 hours beyond the point where they become parasite free on blood film and treated for a minimum of a week if no second-line agent is used. Recrudescence can occur more than a month after adequate treatment of pregnant women.

Anemia and hypoglycemia are common in pregnancy. Risk of abortion is increased, and congenital malaria is well recognized when malaria occurs near term, although more common in vivax cases. Low birthweight babies are common after malaria in pregnancy.

REFERENCES

1. Fleck SH, Moody AH. Diagnostic techniques in medical parasitology. 11th Ed. Cambridge, UK: Butterworth-Heinemann, 1993.
2. Moody AH, Hunt-Cooke A, Chiodini PL. Experiences with the Becton Dickinson QBC II centrifugal haematology analyser for heamatoparasites. Trans R Soc Trop Med 1993;84:782.
3. Swift CJ, Premji Z, Minjas JN. The rapid manual Para Sight F test. A new diagnostic tool for *Plasmodium falciparum* infection. Trans R Soc Trop Med 1993;87:646–648.
4. Chiodini PL. Non-microscopic methods for diagnosis of malaria. Lancet 1998;351:80–81.
5. Makler MT, Hinrichs DJ. Measurement of the lactate dehydrogenase activity of *Plasmodium falciparum* as an assessment of parasitaemia. Am J Trop Med Hyg 1993;48:205–210.
6. Snounou G, Viriyakosol S, Ping Zhu X, et al. High sensitivity of detection of human malaria parasites by the use of nested polymerase chain reaction. Mol Biochem Parasitol 1993;347:1511–1514.
7. Baird K, Basuru H, Purnomo, et al. Resistance to chloroquine by *Plasmodium vivax* in Irian Jaya, Indonesia. Am J Trop Med 1991;44:547–552.
8. Pussard E, Lepers JP, Clavier F, et al. Efficacy of a loading dose of oral chloroquine in a 36-hour treatment schedule for uncomplicated *Plasmodium falciparum* malaria. Antimicrob Agents Chemother 1991;35:406–409.
9. World Health Organisation. Severe and complicated malaria. Trans R Soc Trop Med Hyg 1990;84(Suppl 2):1–65.
10. White NJ. The treatment of malaria. N Engl J Med 1996;335:800–806.
11. White NJ, Warrell DA, Chathavanich P, et al. Severe hypoglycaemia and hyperinsulinemia in falciparum malaria. N Engl J Med 1983;309:61–66.
12. White NJ, Looreesuwan S, Warrell DA, et al. Quinine loading dose in cerebral malaria. Am J Trop Med Hyg 1993;32:1–5.
13. Davis TME, Supranaranond W, Pukrittayakamee S, et al. A safe and effective consecutive-infusion regimen for rapid quinine loading in severe falciparum malaria. J Infect Dis 1990;161:1305–1308.
14. Hien TT, White NJ. Qinghaosu. Lancet 1993;341:603–608.
15. Nosten F, ter Kuile FO, Luxemburger C, et al. Cardiac effects of antimalarial treatment with halofantrine. Lancet 1993;341:1054–1056.
16. White NJ. Not much progress in treatment of cerebral malaria. Lancet 1998;352:594–595.
17. Newton CR, Kirkham FJ, Winstanley PA, Pasvol G, et al. Intracranial pressure in African children with cerebral malaria. Lancet 1991;337:573–576.
18. English M, Muambi B, Mithani S, Marsh K. Lactic acidosis and oxygen debt in African children with severe anaemia. Q J Med 1997;90:563–569.
19. English M, Waruiru C, Marsh K. Transfusion for respiratory distress in life-threatening childhood malaria. Am J Trop Med Hyg 1996;55:525–530.
20. Wilkinson RJ, Brown JL, Pasvol G, et al. Severe falciparum malaria: predicting the effect of exchange transfusion. Q J Med 1994;87:553–557.

21.5 MALARIA: EMERGENCY SELF-TREATMENT BY TRAVELERS

PATRICIA SCHLAGENHAUF AND PENELOPE A. PHILLIPS-HOWARD

INTRODUCTION

Self-treatment of malaria on the basis of indicative symptoms is by no means a modern concept. Indeed, this response to fevers preceded the identification of plasmodia and the science of malariology. Cinchona bark was the 17th-century febrifuge, and the Chinese medicinal herb qinghaosu (*Artemisia annua L*) was even recommended for the treatment of fevers in a 341 AD pharmacopeia of emergency prescriptions.[1]

THE STRATEGY

DEFINITION, RATIONALE, AND GUIDELINES FOR USE

Standby treatment (SBT) is described by the World Health Organization (WHO) as the self-administration of antimalarial drugs when malaria is suspected and prompt medical attention is unavailable within 24 hours of the onset of symptoms.[2] Presumptive self-treatment is thus only indicated in emergency situations and must be followed by medical consultation as soon as possible.

The rationale for SBT is based on a risk-benefit analysis. Prophylactic drugs have traditionally been recommended to those at risk of acquiring malaria. The goal of prophylaxis is to prevent symptomatic malarial infection, a practice, however, that carries a risk of adverse events (AEs) estimated to occur at the rate of between 12% and 30%.[3] Most of these events are mild, but serious adverse events have been reported. The risk of actually acquiring malaria varies from a high of 8% per month in the Solomon Islands, to 2.4% in West Africa, to a markedly lower incidence in South and Central America (0.05% and 0.01%, respectively). These figures show that a risk-benefit analysis (AE versus avoided infections) is necessary for travelers minimally exposed to malaria infection. For low-risk, malaria-endemic areas of Asia and South America, the risk of toxicity from chemoprophylactic drugs actually outweighs the benefit of avoided infection, and here SBT offers an alternative option. Furthermore, it is recognized that no antimalarial prophylactic regimen gives complete protection, and this is especially true in areas of high transmission of resistant *Plasmodium falciparum*. Additional protection against breakthrough malaria can be afforded by the availability of a standby therapy. Thus, SBT has a place both for use alone and/or in combination with a chemoprophylactic regimen.

CRITERIA FOR RECOMMENDING SBT

A traveler visiting a malaria-endemic area, once only, for less than 1 week, does not require SBT. Other factors relevant to deciding on the need for standby medication include frequent or long-duration travel, the intended prophylactic cover, the risk of falciparum malaria, and the probable access to prompt diagnosis and treatment. Optimal chemoprophylactic regimens may not be chosen because of drug intolerance, concomitant use of interacting medications, or other contraindications. No chemoprophylactic regimen may be advised for travelers who intend to visit resorts or cities without malaria risk; in these situations, deviations from the itinerary can place them at risk, and standby therapy may be warranted. In summary, SBT may be required by travelers who:

- use suboptimal or no chemoprophylaxis and who may visit a remote malarious area far from health service facilities;
- have changing itineraries and possibly visit foci of multidrug resistance not adequately covered by their prophylactic regimen;
- have contraindications to priority antimalarials and are therefore prescribed suboptimal or no chemoprophylaxis;
- are abroad for many months and who, due to high exposure and poor compliance, are at high risk of infection (e.g., backpackers);
- frequently travel to malarious areas for short periods (aircrews,[4] business persons).

Individually targeted information on SBT is needed for expatriates, young children, pregnant women, and travelers with chronic illnesses.

GUIDELINES FOR USE OF SBT

The traveler should be provided with simple written guidelines to guide him or her in the use of SBT. The following sequence can be suggested:

1. The traveler is unwell with fever (>37.5°C) and/or other symptoms such as malaise, headache, myalgia, gastrointestinal tract symptoms, or shivering.
2. Medical attention is unavailable within 24 hours of onset of symptoms.
3. A minimal period of at least 6 days has elapsed since entering the malaria-endemic area.
4. The traveler reduces fever (with tepid sponging and paracetamol), which reduces the incidence of vomiting.
5. The SBT is administered with adequate fluids.
6. The traveler seeks medical attention at the first opportunity.

The traveler should be aware that the symptoms of malaria may often be mild, and, in some cases, fever is absent. The WHO emphasizes that the important factors determining the survival of patients with falciparum malaria are early diagnosis and appropriate treatment. It should be stressed that malarial symptoms often occur after leaving endemic areas and that malaria must be considered in the differential diagnosis of any fever in someone who has visited a malaria-endemic area within the past year. If use of SBT is necessary, the traveler should be aware of the need to seek medical attention as soon as possible to check the presumptive diagnosis and receive further advice and/or treatment.

International opinions differ on the role of presumptive treatment as shown by varying Swiss,[5] U.K.,[6] and CDC[7] guidelines. The WHO recommends the use of several agents as possible SBT (Table 25.1–1). Halofantrine is no longer recommended by the WHO for this indication and is for use under medical supervision only.

AVAILABLE OPTIONS FOR SBT

THERAPEUTIC EFFICACY AND TOXICITY OF SBT

Available data suggest good to excellent effectiveness for the agents currently recommended. It is, however, unclear how closely the therapeutic potency of malarial treatments for semi-immune populations can be correlated with the potency of similar regimens used by nonimmune subjects, but, in many cases, this is currently the only available information on which to base recommendations. Generalizations are further complicated by the evolution and changing epidemiology of drug-resistant strains. Areas of multidrug resistance pose a particular problem for SBT. Regions such as the northwestern (Myanmar) and eastern (Cambodia) border regions of Thailand are

Table 21.5–1.   AVAILABLE OPTIONS FOR SBT

GENERIC NAME(S)	TRADE NAME(S)	AMOUNT PER DOSAGE FORM	SBT DOSAGE REGIMEN (ADULT)*
Chloroquine	Aralen, Avlochlor, Nivaquine, Resochin	(Tablet) 100 or 150 mg (base) Syrups available	600 mg on days 1 and 2, followed by 300 mg on day 3
Sulphadoxine/pyrimethamine	Fansidar	(Tablet) 500 mg/25 mg	Three tablets in a single dose
Sulphadoxine/pyrimethamine/ mefloquine	Fansimef	(Tablet) 500 mg/25 mg/250 mg	Three tablets in a single dose
Sulphalene/pyrimethamine	Metakelfin	(Tablet) 500 mg/25 mg	Three tablets in a single dose
Mefloquine	Lariam, Mephaquin	(Tablet) 250 mg (US 228 mg)	5–6 tablets in divided doses[†] depending on body weight
Quinine (sulphate, bisulphate, dihydrochloride, hydrochloride)		(Tablet) 300 mg (salt)	600 mg (2 tablets) t.i.d. for 7 days (a total of 42 tablets)
Halofantrine (no longer on WHO recommended list)	Halfan	(Tablet) 250 mg (Suspension) Halfan S 100 mg/5 mL	500 mg (2 tablets) every 6 hours (total of 6 tablets), a second treatment dose should be administered 7 days later

*For children's fractions, see WHO yellow booklet.
[†]Manufacturer: 25 mg/kg for nonimmunes. WHO 15 mg/kg except for Thai borders then 25 mg/kg.

areas of multi-drug resistance that however, lie off the usual tourist trail. Travelers to areas of multi-drug resistance must be aware that the use of their emergency malarial treatment in such areas will most likely act as a short-term febrifuge and symptoms suppressant rather than a total cure, and that prompt medical attention is imperative.

Adverse events also pose a problem as the use of SBT may expose persons to a significant drug risk, and this is a major factor in the treatment of "possible" malarias. With mefloquine, serious neurotoxicity is approximately 60 times more probable after treatment than with prophylactic use of the agent.[8] Halofantrine has been associated with fatal electrocardiographic changes, namely, prolongation of the QT_c interval.[9]

Chloroquine   Chloroquine was the favored treatment for susceptible malaria; however, now only *P. malariae* and *P. ovale* remain fully sensitive to chloroquine. Resistant *P. vivax* have been reported.[10, 11] The use of chloroquine as a possible SBT is currently limited due to widespread chloroquine-resistant *P. falciparum* (CRPF). It has been reported that over 90% of isolates in some parts of Southeast Asia are now resistant to chloroquine. The drug, however, remains effective on Hispaniola, in Central America, and in the Near East.

Quinine   Quinine is effective against most chloroquine-resistant *P. falciparum*, although the sensitivity to this agent is also diminishing in certain areas, notably Thailand and Vietnam. Quinine is associated with a spectrum of AEs including nausea, vomiting, headache, tinnitus, and cardiovascular side effects This factor, together with its complicated dosage regimen, detracts from its usefulness as a SBT agent. Combination-treatment regimens of quinine plus tetracycline have proven successful in areas of quinine resistance, but the complexity of such

a combination regimen over a prolonged period (7 days) makes this a questionable option for SBT due to projected poor compliance. This treatment option is rather for malaria cases under a physician's supervision. On the plus side, quinine is a SBT agent that is considered safe for pregnant women,[2,8] who should nevertheless seek urgent medical attention for all febrile episodes.

Antifolate/Sulpha Drug Combinations (Fansidar, Metakelfin)   The problem of resistance has been further compounded by the increasing prevalence of parasites resistant to the antifolate and sulpha drug combinations particularly in Southeast Asia (especially Thailand and Myanmar) and in South America (Amazon Basin). The pyrimethamine/sulphadoxine (Fansidar) combination remains effective in parts of Africa (especially West Africa) and Southern Asia. In persons without known intolerance to sulphonamides, the risk of severe cutaneous side effects (Stevens-Johnson syndrome and toxic epidermal necrolysis) with SBT appears to be lower than that reported for systematic repetitive dosage in a prophylactic setting. However, at least one serious adverse event has been reported after SBT with Fansidar.[12]

Mefloquine   Multidrug-resistant strains remain largely sensitive to mefloquine except for the notorious border regions of Thailand, which contain the most drug-resistant parasites in the world, with mefloquine cure rates of only 41%[13] and lower. In vitro studies in both West Africa and Southeast Asia indicated the presence of resistant parasites prior to use of the drug in those particular areas, suggesting that emerging resistance will be a function of drug pressure. Despite the threat of the relentless rise in resistance, mefloquine satisfies many of the criteria required for standby treatment with a relatively simple dosage regimen over a short time period. Use of the split dosage should reduce the incidence of adverse events, especially vomiting, which occurs frequently at the levels used for therapy. Adverse events have been observed, especially nausea and dizziness, and cases of neuropsychiatric disturbances have been reported including sporadic episodes of seizures, hallucinations, depression, or acute psychosis. Although the incidence of serious neuropsychiatric events in a prophylactic setting is relatively rare, neurotoxicity appears more probable after treatment (1/216) than with prophylactic use of mefloquine.[5] The mechanism for serious neurotoxicity is unknown and may be dose related,[14] although serious AEs have occurred at relatively low plasma mefloquine concentrations. The drug has a long and variable mean terminal half-life with interindividual variation ranging from 6 to 33 days; thus, for those using mefloquine prophylaxis, malaria treatment with mefloquine or quinine should only be administered under close medical supervision due to the possibility of added toxicity. There are promising reports of the use of an oral mefloquine-artesunate combination treatment, and this may be a future possibility for the traveler. Luxemburger et al.[15] compared the therapeutic efficacy and toxicity of a combination of low-dose mefloquine (15 mg/kg) plus artesunate (10 mg/kg) with the standard 25 mg/kg mefloquine dose in 552 patients with uncomplicated falciparum malaria on the Thai-Burmese border and found that the combination gave faster clinical and parasitologic responses and prevented early treatment failure.

One central issue for clarification regarding mefloquine is the currently used SBT dose. The manufacturer cites therapeutic dosages for mefloquine (as Lariam) relative to body weight and immune status with nonimmunes over 45 kg to receive a total of 1,250- to 1,500-mg mefloquine (i.e., 20 to 25 mg/kg), whereas semi-immune persons of the same weight can be treated with a lower dose 750 to 1,000 mg (i.e., 15 mg/kg). For nonimmune adult travelers, the curative dose (total 6 tablets in one day) can be split into three doses at 6- to 8-hour intervals (e.g., 3 + 2 + 1 or 2 + 2 + 2) with the objective of reducing the incidence or severity of adverse events. More data are required, especially with regard to compliance with the split dose used in a SBT setting. The WHO[2] recommends a total mefloquine dose of 15 mg/kg or 1,000 mg (whichever is lower) except in Thai border areas of multidrug resistance, where a total dose of 25 mg/kg (or 1,500 mg) is recommended as an initial dose of 15 mg/kg followed 6 to 8 hours later by 10 mg/kg.

Fansimef This is a triple combination MSP (tablets containing mefloquine 250 mg/sulphadoxine 500 mg/pyrimethamine 25mg), which was developed to delay development of mefloquine resistance,[16] a strategy that did not hinder the emergence of resistant strains. The WHO does not include Fansimef in its list of recommended SBTs due to the concern that Fansidar added to mefloquine increases the risk of toxicity with little benefit.

Halofantrine Clinical trials have confirmed the efficacy of this phenanthrene methanol in the treatment of falciparum malaria in areas of chloroquine and sulphonamide/pyrimethamine resistance. In eastern areas of Thailand, the efficacy of halofantrine is quite low (29%). Some failures of halofantrine have been attributed to its poor and variable absorption. The efficacy and tolerability of this agent have also been assessed in the treatment of acute malaria in returned nonimmune travelers,[17] where malaria was imported from areas with drug-resistant falciparum parasites, mainly from Africa. The breakthrough rate after the recommended single dose was 12%, but an efficacy rate of 100% was observed in patients (n = 29) who received an additional therapeutic dose 1 week after the initial treatment. Only mild AEs were observed in this study. Other reported AEs include a transient rise in liver enzymes, cough, minor gastrointestinal tract symptoms, headache, occasional pruritus, and rash.[18] There is, however, considerable anxiety regarding the arrhythmogenic potential of this agent, which can be fatal. Eight patients are known to have experienced cardiac arrest with six deaths,[6] and no recently published update on fatalities is available. Halofantrine is no longer recommended by the WHO for self-treatment as a result of the reports describing prolongation of the QT_c intervals and ventricular dysrhythmias in susceptible individuals. These changes may be accentuated if halofantrine is taken with other antimalarial drugs that can decrease myocardial conduction.[2,6] Nevertheless, some countries continue to recommend halofantrine as a SBT when other agents are contraindicated but only for those persons known to have a normal QT_c interval. A recent paper suggests that pretreatment ECGs are poorly predictive of QT_c lengthening during therapy,[19] and the role and value of premedication ECG testing require clarification.

The manufacturer has expanded the list of contraindications to include a personal or familiy history of heart disease that causes QT interval prolongation, concurrent use of medication that may lengthen the interval, electrolyte imbalance, and thiamine deficiency. Halofantrine should not be given with food and the dose should not exceed 24 mg/kg given as 8 mg/kg for three doses at 6-hour intervals.

Artemisinin Derivatives The herb (wormwood) has been used in Chinese traditional medicine for over 2,000 years. Artemisinin is a compound with a peculiar structure, low toxicity, and high efficacy even in severe chloroquine-resistant *P. falciparum* malaria. This important antimalarial group (includes artemether, arteether, and artesunate) is available in several dosage forms including artesunate in tablet form. One disadvantage is a commonly reported recrudescence that can be avoided by combining the drug with a longer acting antimalarial. As previously mentioned, a single day's treatment with artesunate augments the antimalarial efficacy of mefloquine[15] and provides a rapid initial therapeutic response followed by the sustained action of the longer acting mefloquine. These agents are generally well tolerated, but there are worries regarding the neurotoxicity observed in animal studies.[20] The practical implications of use of these agents alone or in combination were, until recently, limited to use in endemic populations as the artemisinin derivatives needed to meet stringent Western safety standards before approval. In early 1999, a new oral fixed tablet combination containing artemether was registered in Switzerland for treatment and SBT of acute, uncomplicated *P. falciparum* or mixed malarial infections (see New Combinations).

Primaquine and the Radical Cure   To achieve a radical cure (i.e., elimination of exoerythrocytic stages of *P. vivax and P. ovale* only), a follow-up course of primaquine is necessary (contraindicated in persons with a G6PD deficiency). Presumptive use of primaquine by travelers is rarely indicated for regular travelers but could be considered for such groups as volunteers and missionaries returning home after extensive periods of exposure in areas where *P. vivax* and *P. ovale* are endemic or may be indicated for refugee groups.[21]

In summary, there are, theoretically, several available medications that could be used as presumptive treatment in emergency situations. The choice of SBT will depend on the expected parasite type and level of drug resistance, the traveler's medical history, the availability of medication in the country of prescription, the prophylactic agent used (if applicable), and, finally, the ease of administration of the SBT.

The range of options available are outlined in Table 25.1–1. Ideally, a SBT should be easily administered to ensure correct dosage and compliance, and here the simple therapy regimens have the advantage of easy administration.

SBT—USE IN CHILDREN

Infants and young children are at special risk of malaria and should avoid endemic areas, especially where CRPF is widespread. Screening with impregnated nets should be performed meticulously and prophylaxis administered if appropriate. In cases of fever, every attempt must be made to seek prompt medical attention. Recommendations regarding pediatric doses for SBT are particularly difficult to formulate, and the practical administration is further complicated by a paucity of pediatric formulations. Chloroquine is available in syrup form and halofantrine as the suspension (Halfan S). Otherwise, appropriate fractions of antimalarials can be crushed and powdered onto jam. The WHO[2] provides a table of approximate fractions of antimalarial dosages for children.

EXPERIENCE TO DATE WITH SBT

AIRCREWS

This group of frequently exposed travelers has provided data on the use of emergency presumptive therapy. Continuous chemoprophylaxis was optional for Swissair crews after 1985 and a therapeutic approach was favored for all tropical Swissair stations in the Far East and South America and for brief exposure in tropical Africa. Personnel carried Fansimef, later Lariam, as standby therapy for emergencies. After an almost total adoption of the treatment dose recommendation, there was no significant increase in the number of malaria cases, and standby medication was used by only 1% per year.[4]

TRAVELERS

The use of SBT by travelers has been reviewed.[22] In earlier studies, some 4% of travelers to East Africa used their standby medication where the attack rate is 0.2% to 1.5%, which would suggest a 2.5- to 20-fold overuse of SBT. Conversely, when a SBT strategy rather than prophylaxis was recommended for travelers to areas of low transmission such as Thailand, only a small number, <1%, used the standby medication.[23] This latter study examined the use of SBT in a cohort of 1,187 travelers who were prepared to self-treat malarial symptoms. Illness (fever as the main indicator) was reported by 10.4% of the group, and six persons actually used the SBT carried but only one of the six had a proven malaria. The characteristics of these SBT users including differential diagnoses are outlined in Table 21.5–2. A 1993 German study[24] followed up 3,434 travelers to areas of varying risk and showed a similar low use of SBT (1.4%), indicating that overuse of SBT is not a major problem in travelers.

IMPORTED MALARIA DATA

With regard to data on imported malaria cases as shown in Figure 21.5–1, the change of strategy from chemoprophylaxis to SBT for Swiss travelers to Thailand, starting in 1989, did not result in an increased incidence of imported malaria.

NEGATIVE FEATURES OF SBT

There are few data regarding the efficacy of SBT agents in the presence of resistant parasites, and carriage of SBT should not lead to a false sense of security as demonstrated by the failure of self-treatment using the presumptive oral therapy (pyrimethamine/sulphadoxine) reported in United States travelers returning from Kenya.[25] Travelers must be aware that use of SBT is an interim solution only and that prompt medical advice is essential even after a therapy has been successfully administered.

Travelers' knowledge and behavior remain major stumbling blocks, and many individuals, despite being made aware of the urgency of malarial treatment, choose to wait for their symptoms to resolve spontaneously rather than seek prompt medical attention as demonstrated in the Zurich study,[23] where two-thirds of those ill failed to seek immediate medical attention. This problem was further emphasized in an earlier U.K. survey,[26] where over 23% of respondents would have acted inappropriately if they experienced symptoms resembling malaria by taking extra prophylactic pills or by going to bed until symptoms resolved.

The main problem inherent in the SBT strategy is, however, the wide range of clinical presentations of malaria that complicate the self-diagnosis and can lead to over- or underuse of the medication with a poor proba-

Table 21.5–2   CHARACTERISTICS OF SBT USERS (N = 6) IN THE ZURICH STUDY (N = 1,187)[23]

USER	AGE	SEX	COUNTRY OF USE	SYMPTOMS	ONSET OF SYMPTOMS	M.D. CONSULTED	DIAGNOSIS	FEVER CLEARANCE
1	26	F	Columbia	Fever Headache Myalgia Diarrhea Vomiting	Day 17	Out of reach	Gastritis	3 days
2	38	M	Switzerland Returned from Malaysia	Fever Headache Chills Myalgia	Day 24	Yes	Malaria (microscopic confirmation)	3 days
3	28	F	Hong Kong on arrival from Indonesia	Fever Headache Chills Myalgia	Day 20	Yes	Viral infection	2 days
4	58	M	Switzerland on return from Indonesia	Fever Diarrhea Vomiting	>Day 7	Yes	Amebiasis	2 days
5	28	M	Sarawak (Malaysia)	Fever Shivering Myalgia Headache Diarrhea Vomiting	Day 17	Yes (2x M.D.)	Viral fever (dengue fever)	1 day
6	29	F	Nepal	Fever Diarrhea Headache Vomiting Shivering Myalgia	Day 6	Yes	Viral infection	1 day

bility of correct use of the SBT. Nothdurft et al.[24] found significant *P. falciparum* antibody levels in only 4 of 37 (10.4%) treatment users. Furthermore, data on the problems and frequency of treatment failures and nonmalarial fevers are lacking, and it is also unclear how nonimmunes will respond to therapy as most studies to date have been with semi-immune populations, and toxicity and efficacy profiles may differ.

NEW COMBINATIONS

Two new combination treatments have been registered in Europe: Malarone® and Riamet®. These therapies will undoubtedly play a major role in the treatment of malaria in endemic populations. The role of these agents as standby emergency treatment in nonimmune travelers remains to be determined and data are required for this indication.

MALARONE® (ATOVAQUONE 250 MG/PROGUANIL 100 MG)

The fixed-combination Malarone® (formerly BW566C) has been recently approved in several European countries for the treatment of acute, uncomplicated falciparum malaria in adults and children weighing > 10 kg. Each

tablet contains atovaquone 250 mg and proguanil hydrochloride 100 mg. The SBT dosage is divided over 3 days (Table 21.5–3), and the medication should be administered with food to increase absorption and bioavailability. The components of the medication work synergistically, and although early clinical studies (in the U.K., Thailand, and Zambia) with atovaquone monotherapy showed high rates of recrudescence, the combination with proguanil led to significantly improved cure rates[27] and was shown to be more effective than mefloquine in areas of multidrug resistance. A review of the safety data of the combination shows good tolerability compared to other antimalarials. AEs can be attributed to single entities or to the combination, and the most frequently reported events from clinical studies include headache (17% to 37%), nausea and vomiting (16% to 27%), and diarrhea (14% to 16%). In phase III studies with children, the most frequently reported events were coughing, headache, vomiting, abdominal pain, and anorexia. Serious adverse events reported include anaphylactic shock, seizures in two patients with a prior history of epilepsy, and a severe hemolytic episode in a G6PD-deficient individual. A recent review of 10 open-label clinical trials concluded that the atovaquone/proguanil combination is safe and effective for the treatment of malaria.[28] Further studies of the efficacy and tolerability of this combination in nonimmune travelers are required.

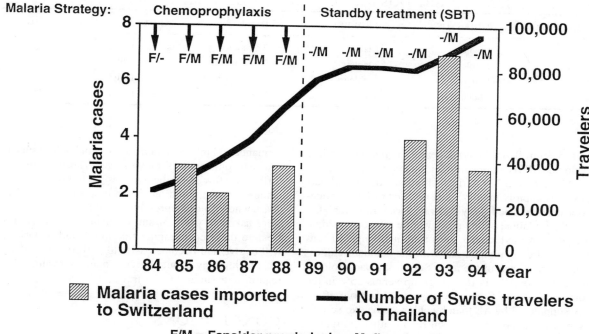

Figure 21.5–1. The figure indicates by bar the number of reported cases of malaria in Switzerland imported from Thailand from 1984 through 1994. In the autumn of 1988, standby treatment was recommended rather than chemoprophylaxis for Swiss travelers to normal tourist areas of Thailand. No significant increase in the number of cases occurred with the changeover in recommendation.

RIAMET® (ARTEMETHER 20 MG/LUMEFANTRINE 120 MG)

The second new oral fixed tablet combination, Riamet® (formerly CGP56697) or coartemether), was registered recently in Switzerland for treatment and standby emergency treatment of acute, uncomplicated *P. falciparum* or mixed malarial infections in adults and children. This new treatment is a fixed combination (1:6) of artemether (A), a derivative of artemisinin and lumefantrine (L) (formerly benflumetol), a synthetic racemic fluorene derivative of the aminoalcohol class, as potentiation between these drugs was observed in combination experiments. The recommended SBT dosage is an intensive 3-day administration

Table 21.5–3. MALARONE® SBT DOSAGE FOR NONIMMUNE TRAVELERS

WEIGHT (KG)	DAY 1	DAY 2	DAY 3	TOTAL
11–20	1 tablet	1 tablet	1 tablet	3
21–30	2 tablets	2 tablets	2 tablets	6
31–40	3 tablets	3 tablets	3 tablets	9
>40	4 tablets	4 tablets	4 tablets	12

(Table 21.5–4) and should be administered with food. Artemether is rapidly absorbed (C_{max}: 2 hours) and eliminated ($t_{1/2}$: 2 hours), and results in rapid and considerable reduction in parasite biomass and resolution of malaria symptoms, whereas L (C_{max}: 6 to 8 hours, $t_{1/2}$: 2 to 3 days) with delayed absorption and slower clearance eliminates residual parasites in a "mopping up" process. The efficacy of the combination is therefore dependent on the number of parasites remaining after artemether has been eliminated and the duration for which lumefantrine plasma concentrations exceed the minimum inhibitory concentration. Dose finding studies have indicated an efficacy >95% with a four-dose regimen in China and India but only 76.5% in Thailand,[29] where a six-dose regimen was subsequently tested with cure rates of 98%,[30] which is similar to cure rates observed with the current mefloquine/artesunate standard regimen. The efficacy and tolerability of the artemether-lumefantrine combination (4 × 4 regimen) compared to halofantrine was evaluated in travelers returning to the Netherlands and France. The recrudescence rate with the AL regimen was found to be unacceptably high (18%), and the investigators proposed a six-dose regimen over a 3-day period.[31] Clinical experience to date indicates rapid fever and parasite clearance, high cure rates, and reduced gametocyte carriage rates. In a ran-

Table 21.5–4.   RIAMET® SBT DOSAGE FOR NONIMMUNE TRAVELERS

WEIGHT (KG)	0 (DIAGNOSIS)	8 HOURS	DAY 2	DAY 3	TOTAL
10–<15 kg	1 tablet	1 tablet	2x 1 tablet	2x 1 tablet	6
15–<25 kg	2 tablets	2 tablets	2x 2 tablets	2x 2 tablets	12
25–<35 kg	3 tablets	3 tablets	2x 3 tablets	2x 3 tablets	18
Adult	4 tablets	4 tablets	2x 4 tablets	2x 4 tablets	24

domized controlled trial of AL versus the pyrimethamine/sulfadoxine (P/S) combination for the treatment of uncomplicated malaria in 287 African children, AL cleared parasites more rapidly than P/S and resulted in fewer gametocyte carriers. The 15-day cure rate was, however, higher with P/S, explained by the prophylactic effect of residual P/S levels.[32] A randomized, open trial involving 260 Tanzanian children compared AL with the standard chloroquine regimen used in the area. Seven-day parasitologic cure rates were 94% in the AL group versus 35% in the chloroquine group. Gametocytes were also more effectively suppressed by AL than by chloroquine. No serious drug-related adverse events occurred in either group, and there was no significant difference in symptom reporting. Drug-related adverse events included rashes (AL 3.8% versus CHL 3.9%) and pruritus (AL 0.8% versus CHL 6.2%).[33] Other reports indicate that the most commonly reported AEs include headache, dizziness, insomnia, abdominal pain, and anorexia. One area for particular scrutiny with this new combination is the cardiac effects of AL, particularly the prolongation of the QT_c interval as L has a similar chemical structure to halofantrine (both are classified as aminoalcohols). One randomized, double-blind, two-way crossover study has assessed the cardiac effects of AL and halofantrine in 14 healthy male subjects after single oral doses of the respective antimalarial were administered with a high-fat meal. No QT_c interval prolongation was observed with AL (480:80 mg), whereas halofantrine (500 mg) caused a significant increase in QT_c interval in all subjects.[34] This finding was confirmed in a prospective electrocardiographic study where no evidence of cardiotoxicity was observed in 150 patients treated with artemether-lumefantrine.[35]

USE OF DIAGNOSTICS

The use of a malaria diagnostic as an adjunct to the SBT strategy may be an attainable objective as previously proposed by Schlagenhauf et al.[23] Such a development would enable the traveler to test a blood droplet for malarial infection. Two recent studies have examined the feasibility of the use of the malaria rapid tests ParaSight F and MalaQuick (ICT) by travelers,[36,37] with the objective of assessing whether travelers can perform such a test and interpret test results. Test performance was often poor. More importantly, both tests were associated with high levels of false-negative interpretations, especially at low parasitemias commonly encountered in travelers, and the authors concluded that technical improvements in performance and interpretation are essential before such tests can be recommended for lay persons. These findings were further reinforced by the poor results in both test performance and interpretation shown in a study on the Kenya coast where tourists presenting with malaria symptoms were asked to perform and evaluate the malaria test.[38] Despite these encouraging findings, rapid malaria tests will evolve and become easier to perform and interpret. This technology should be continuously evaluated with regard to its suitability for travelers.

CONCLUSIONS

SBT is an option for clearly defined situations, whereas prophylaxis remains the safest choice for most travelers to areas of high transmission when the stay in a malarial area is longer than 1 week. Care should be taken in recommending a SBT strategy and antimosquito measures should be stressed. Concise advice is necessary for travelers stressing the importance of medical consultation at the first sign of illness. Travelers' behavior and the difficulty of defining simple diagnostic guidelines are delimiting factors in this strategy. To choose a suitable SBT agent, the following must be considered: level of malaria transmission at the destination, type and intensity of resistance, efficacy and toxicity of available options, prophylactic agent used (if applicable), and ease of administration of the standby therapy. Of the available WHO-approved agents, chloroquine is preferred in the limited geographic areas where this agent is still effective; otherwise, mefloquine appears to offer a good solution except for foci of multidrug resistance and for individuals with predisposing contraindications. Halofantrine is for use under medical supervision only. The future points to the newer combination therapies, assuming that experience in nonimmunes is favorable and possible provision of a simple diagnostic that would mitigate the most negative aspect of the SBT strategy, namely, the self-diagnosis of malaria.

REFERENCES

1. Hien TT, White NJ. Qinghaosu. Lancet 1993;341:603–608.
2. World Health Organization. Health risks and their avoidance. In: International travel and health 1999. Geneva: WHO, 1999.
3. Steffen R, Behrens RH. Travellers' malaria. Parasitol Today 1992;8:61–6.
4. Steffen R, Holdener F, Wyss R, Nurminen L. Malaria prophylaxis and self-therapy in airline crew. Aviat Space Environ Med 1990;II:942–945.

5. Schlagenhauf P, Hatz C, and le Groupe suisse de travail pour les conseils médicaux aux voyageurs. Traitement de secours antipaludique: actualisation 1997. Méd Hyg 1997;55: 1126–1127.

6. Bradley DJ, Warhurst DC. Guidelines for the prevention of malaria in travellers from the United Kingdom. Commun Dis Rep 1997;7:137–152.

7. Centers for Disease Control and Prevention. Health information for international travel 1996–97. Atlanta: Department of Health and Human Services, 1997.

8. Weinke T, Trautmann M, Held T, et al. Neuropsychiatric side effects after the use of mefloquine. Am J Trop Med Hyg 1991; 45:86–91

9. World Health Organization. Drug alert: halofantrine. Wkly Epidemiol Rec 1993;68:268–270.

10. Rieckmann KH, Davis DR, Hutton DC. *Plasmodium vivax* resistant to chloroquine? Lancet 1989;2:1183–1184.

11. Murphy GS, Basri H, et al. Vivax malaria resistant to treatment and prophylaxis with chloroquine. Lancet 1993;341:96–100.

12. Phillips-Howard PA, Behrens RH, Dunlop J. Stevens-Johnson syndrome due to pyrimethamine/sulphadoxine during presumptive self-therapy of malaria [letter]. Lancet 1989;9:803–804.

13. Fontanet AL, Johnson BD, Walker AM, et al. High prevalence of mefloquine resistant falciparum malaria in eastern Thailand. Bull WHO 1993;71:377–383.

14. ter Kuile FO, Luxemburger C, Nosten F, et al. Serious neuropsychiatric adverse events following mefloquine treatment: evidence for a dose relationship? Ph.D. thesis, 1994, University of Amsterdam.

15. Luxemburger C, ter Kuile FO, Nosten F, et al. Single day mefloquine-artesunate combination in the treatment of multidrug-resistant falciparum malaria.Trans R Soc Trop Med Hyg 1994;88:213–217.

16. Merkli B, Richle R, Peters W. The inhibitory effect of a drug combination on the development of mefloquine resistance in *Plasmodium berghei*. Ann Trop Med Parasitol 1980;74:1–9.

17. Weinke T, Loscher T, Fleischer K, et al. The efficacy of halofantrine in the treatment of acute malaria in non-immune travellers. Am J Trop Med Hyg 1992;47:1–5.

18. Bryson H, Goa K. Halofantrine: review of its antimalarial activity, pharmacokinetic properties and therapeutic potential. Drugs 1992;43:236–258.

19. Matson PA, Luby SP, Redd SC, et al. Cardiac effects of standard-dose halofantrine therapy. Am J Trop Med Hyg 1996;54:229–231.

20. Brewer TG, Grate SJ, Peggins JO, et al. Fatal neurotoxicity of arteether and artemether. Am J Trop Med Hyg 1994;51:251–259.

21. Grimmond TR, Cameron AS. Primaquine-chloroquine prophylaxis against malaria in Southeast Asian refugees entering S. Australia. Med J Aust 1984;140:322–325.

22. Schlagenhauf P, Steffen R. Stand-by treatment of malaria in travellers: a review. J Trop Med Hyg 1994;97:151–160.

23. Schlagenhauf P, Steffen R, Tschopp A, et al. Behavioural aspects of travellers in their use of malaria presumptive treatment. Bull WHO 1995;73:2:215–221.

24. Nothdurft HD, Jelinek T, Pechel SM, et al. Stand-by treatment of suspected malaria in travelers. Trop Med Parasitol 1995; 46:161–163.

25. Malaria in Travelers returning from Kenya: failure of self-treatment with pyrimethamine/sulfadoxine. MMWR Morb Mortal Wkly Rep 1989;38:363–364.

26. Behrens RH, Phillips-Howard PA. What do travellers know about malaria [letter]? Lancet 1989;1395.

27. Looareesuwan S, Viravan C, Webster HK, et al. Clinical studies of atovaquone alone or in combination with other antimalarial drugs for treatment of acute uncomplicated malaria in Thailand. Am J Trop Med Hyg 1996;54:62–66.

28. Kremsner PG, Looareesuwan S, Chulay JD. Atovaquone and proguanil hydrochloride for treatment of malaria. J Travel Med 1999;Suppl 1:S18–S20.

29. Gathmann I, Xiu-Quing J, Wright S, et al. Co-artemether: integrated summary of efficacy [abstract P30]. Clone Cure and Control, September 14–18, 1998, Liverpool, UK.

30. Van Vugt M, Looareesuwan S, Gathmann I, et al. A randomised trial of the six-dose regimen of artemether-benflumetol in comparasion with mefloquine-artesunate in the treatment of acute *Plasmodium falciparum* malaria [abstract P32]. Clone Cure and Control, September 14–18, 1998, Liverpool, UK.

31. Van Agtmael M, Bouchaud O, Malvy D, et al. The comparative efficacy and tolerability of CGP 56697 (artemether + lumefantrine) versus halofantrine in the treatment of uncomplicated falciparum malaria in travellers returning from the tropics to the Netherlands and France. Int J Antimicrob Agents 1999;12:159–169.

32. von Seidlein L, Jaffar S, Pinder M, et al. Treatment of African children with uncomplicated falciparum malaria with a new antimalarial drug, CGP 56697. J Infect Dis 1997;176: 1113–1116.

33. Hatz C, Abdulla S, Mull R, et al. Efficacy and safety of CGP 56697 (artemether and benflumetol) compared with chloroquine to treat falciparum malaria in Tanzanian children aged 1–5 years. Trop Med Int Health 1998;3:498–504.

34. Bindschedler M, Ezzet F, Degen P, Sioufi A. Comparison of the cardiac effects of the anti-malarials co-artemether and halofantrine in healthy subjects after single oral doses given with a high fat meal [abstract P29]. Clone Cure and Control, September 14–18, 1998, Liverpool, UK.

35. Van Vugt M, Ezzet F, Nosten F, et al. No evidence of cardiotoxicity during antimalarial treatment with artemether-lumefantrine. Am J Trop Med Hyg 1999;61:964–967.

36. Trachsler M, Schlagenhauf P, Steffen R. Feasibility of a rapid dipstick antigen-capture assay for self-testing of travellers' malaria. Trop Med Int Health 1999;4:442–447

37. Funk M, Schlagenhauf P, Tschopp A, Steffen R. ParaSight F versus MalaQuick™ (ICT) for self-diagnosis of travellers' malaria. Trans R Soc Trop Med Hyg 1999;93:268–272.

38. Jelinek T, Amsler L, Grobusch M. Self-use of rapid tests for malaria diagnosis by tourists. Lancet 1999;354:1609.

21.6 MALARIA VACCINES—CURRENT STATUS AND DEVELOPMENTS

MARCEL TANNER

FACTS AND ISSUES

Sir Ronald Ross gave the title "the solution of the great malaria problem" to his diary description of the discovery of the role of *Anopheles* mosquitoes in malaria transmission, but his most important discovery did not lead to the rapid solution he anticipated. The great hope for malaria control remains the development of a malaria vaccine, but despite great progress, we are still some way from having a vaccine that can be used in public health programs.

The impact of malaria is impressive when considering that half of the world's population is exposed, 300 to 500 million are infected every year, 200 to 300 million are diseased, and up to 1 million, mainly children, die each year of malaria.[1,2] These figures result in a global estimated burden of malaria of some 35 million disability adjusted life-years (DALYs)[3] of which 90% occurs in sub-Saharan Africa. The DALYs lost among travelers and short-term visitors to malarious areas only represent a minute fraction of this load; nevertheless, some 8,000 to 9,000 cases per year are imported into industrialized countries with a case-fatality rate ranging from 0% to 3.6%.[4]

Ever since the recognition of the mode of transmission, public health specialists and clinicians have developed and applied control strategies that are tailored to different endemic settings and situations. However, following initial successes, malaria control has become more difficult in recent years with declining interest in the industrialized world in diseases of the poor and the spread of resistance of the parasite to various drugs. Despite renewed national and international efforts within the World Health Organization's "Roll-Back-Malaria" program and successes recently observed with the promotion of insecticide-treated mosquito nets,[5,6] the availability of an effective vaccine against malaria would represent a major strengthening of any control strategy. However, malaria parasites are masterly in their survival strategies within their human and mosquito vector hosts. The life cycle is extremely complex, involving both intra- and extracellular compartments and with several different sexual and asexual developmental stages in both human and mosquito hosts. Four main observations justify the continued search for a malaria vaccine as a realistic option: (1) individuals living in endemic areas acquire immunity following continuous exposure (i.e., develop semi-immunity), (2) passive transfer experiments showed how immunoglobulins from semi-immune individuals could protect against clinical malaria,[7,8] (3) specific antibodies suppress growth and multiplication of malaria parasites in vitro, and (4) immunization with irradiated sporozoites of *Plasmodium falciparum* and *P. vivax* resulted in protective immunity in man.[9,10] Encouraged by these observations and experiments, malaria vaccine research has continued for decades.

Generally, three different stages of the parasite's life cycle are being targeted: (1) the infective sporozoite stages and the liver stages to prevent infection, (2) the sexual stages to block transmission, and (3) the asexual blood stages to prevent or reduce morbidity or mortality.

Laboratory research was particularly boosted by the possibility of cultivating *P. falciparum* in vitro from 1976 onward and has generated a very long list of potential vaccine candidates.[11,12] These comprise vaccine candidates of all possible types ranging from attenuated organisms, purified proteins, recombinant proteins, and synthetic peptides to naked parasite DNA. We will not list all of the candidates identified at the experimental level in this chapter but rather refer only to those vaccine candidates that have so far reached clinical trials.

Research on malaria vaccines faces a number of formidable and significant theoretical and practical challenges as summarized in Table 21.6–1. The theoretical difficulties are mainly based on the complexity of the parasite and its life cycle as well as their implications for the immune responses of the host. Despite a wealth of research on the immunology of malaria, there are still many open questions with regard to the dynamics of immunogenicity and immunodominance of conserved and variable malaria antigens and to what extent these key features govern morbidity patterns and the population structure.[13] Similarly, the careful and comprehensive analyses of the humoral and cellular immune responses of human trial volunteers has so far not revealed any significant association of immune indicators with clinical protection.[11,14] In addition, recent analyses of malaria parasite dynamics indicate that there is still much to be learned about semi-immunity and premunition in malaria.[15,16] The impressive growth of molecular techniques combined with the availability of well-documented population-based samples from long-term malaria control research and samples from phase III trials will certainly help to elucidate these questions.

The practical challenges are equally formidable and are mainly based on the fact that we lack surrogate measures of protection. Consequently, any potential vaccine candidate requires comprehensive clinical testing already at an early stage of development, a process that involves substantial costs. Given the lack of the surrogate measures, it is also very difficult to establish the criteria that lead from one clinical testing phase to the next one, particularly for the steps IIa to IIb and III. In addition, phase III testing of malaria vaccines is only possible under well-defined conditions relating to the malaria endemicity of the site, the local population's perceptions of malaria, and health systems and services factors.[5] Few places exist worldwide that satisfy these criteria, and great care is required when deciding to engage in the long (2 to 5

Table 21.6–1.   CHALLENGES IN MALARIA VACCINE DEVELOPMENT—FROM THE LABORATORY TO THE CLINICAL TRIAL LEVEL

THEORETICAL	PRACTICAL	ETHICAL
Genome is some 250× bigger than that of viruses or bacteria (> 6,000 genes)	Which type of vaccine and vaccine for whom?	What is the rationale for the clinical research?
Parasite uses intra- and extracellular compartments; leads to different disease patterns	Which stages of the cycle and which antigens should become targets—alone or combined?	Which are the ethical committees to be consulted and what is their competence?
Genetic polymorphism is substantial	Should—and how should—the antigens be combined?	What is the risk-benefit ratio of the trial and how to handle the differences of perception of the disease?
No sterile immunity can be observed in malaria among populations of endemic areas	Which adjuvant(s), delivery system should be used?	How to establish informed consent in the different endemic areas (i.e., the transcultural validity of concept of informed consent)
Mechanism of protection among semi-immune individuals is still not really known	How to combine a malaria vaccine with the schedules of EPI vaccines in endemic areas? Schedules and interactions.	How to choose placebos
Parasite with multiple strategies for evading host's immune defence mechanisms	No satisfactory animal model for human malaria species exists	How to deal with failure and with the risk that a vaccine trial may modify a given epidemiologic equilibrium
How to trigger effective, protective immune responses among infants	Who is ready to pay for vaccine research on a mid- to long-term basis?	How to ensure first benefit to the participating populations

years) process of phase III testing. All of these practical challenges are closely interrelated with ethical difficulties that require close attention. Clinical trials of malaria vaccines, in a situation where we lack the adequate animal models and surrogate measures of protection, have helped to readdress key ethical issues and represent an important contribution to the ongoing discussions on good epidemiologic practices as well as experiments involving human beings.

Finally, it is often underestimated that each strategic line of malaria vaccine research also has direct implications as to who could benefit from a particular type of vaccine. A vaccine whose target is the pre-erythrocytic stage of the parasite may be more useful for short-term visitors to endemic areas such as tourists, business travelers, and military personnel than for the populations in endemic areas themselves. The history of vaccine development has also demonstrated how the question of who will benefit is inherent in the choice of the vaccine targets and how research strategies are governed by the prevailing sociopolitical context. Consequently, and linked to very promising findings from rodent malaria models and particularly to the protective effect achieved by immunization with irradiated sporozoites,[9,10] the first malaria vaccine developments concentrated on the sporozoite and other pre-erythrocytic stages. However, recombinant and synthetic vaccine candidates derived from pre-erythrocytic stage antigens, in particular involving the repeat sequence of the circumsporozoite protein (CS protein), have not been protective in human phase IIa and IIb trials.[17–20] Thus, for a long time, there has been greater emphasis on the development of vaccines for short-term travelers rather than on the concept of vaccines that mimic the sta-

tus of semi-immunity, allowing infection but preventing morbidity. To date, the only asexual blood-stage vaccine to have undergone stage III trials is the synthetic peptide SPf66.[11,21,22]

CURRENT STATUS AND THE WAY FORWARD

Despite all efforts and achievements in research, we are currently still far from a malaria vaccine that can be applied either among short-term visitors or among residents of endemic areas. Table 21.6–2 summarizes the current status of clinical trials with different vaccine candidates. Only the multistage (sporozoite and asexual blood-stages), multicomponent, synthetic peptide vaccine SPf66[21] has undergone several and comprehensive phase III trials. The results of six double-blind, randomized, controlled trials—undertaken in areas of different malaria endemicity ranging from Latin America to Asia and Africa – revealed overall efficacy estimates of 23% (95% CI: 12 to 32) in reducing the incidence of the first and only attack of clinical *P. falciparum* malaria.[23] This review (within the Cochrane collaboration) concluded that this vaccine was safe and was the first to have reduced the risk of malaria among children living in endemic areas.

As the best use of a vaccine in Africa will be achieved if it can be delivered through the existing Expanded Programs of Immunization (EPI), a large phase III trial among infants, of SPf66 administered at 1, 2, and 7 months of age alongside the EPI vaccines, was undertaken in an area of high perennial transmission in Tanzania. While the vaccine was safe and did not modify the humoral

Table 21.6–2.   STATE OF CLINICAL TRIALS WITH DIFFERENT VACCINE TARGETS*

VACCINE TARGETS	TYPE[a]	CLINICAL TRIAL PHASES[b]				POTENTIAL FOR EFFECTIVE FUTURE APPLICATION[c]		KEY REFERENCES
		I	IIa	IIb	III	TRAVELERS	ENDEMIC AREAS	
Sporozoite stages								
Irradiated sporozoites	A	+	+	–	–	None	None	Clyde et al.,[9] Rieckmann et al.,[10]
CS proteins	R, D	+	+	+	–	High	Medium	Ballou et al.,[17] Herrington et al.,[18] Fries et al.,[19] Stuerchler et al.,[20] Wang et al.,[29]
CS proteins + TRAP	R	+	+	–	–	High	Medium-high	Stoute et al.,[25] Bojang et al.[26]
Hepatic stage in NYVAC-Pf7	D	+	+	–	–	Medium	Medium	Ockenhouse et al.[28]
Asexual blood stages								
MSP1+MSP2+RESA	R	+	+	+	–	Medium	High	Genton et al.[27]
AMA-1	R	+	–	–	–	?	?	
RAP-1	R	+	–	–	–	?	?	
Gametocyte stages								
Pfs-25 in NYVAC-Pf7	D	+	+	–	–	None (if alone)	Low (if alone)	Ockenhouse et al.[28]
Multiple stages								
Spf66	SP	+	+	+	+	None	None	Graves,[23] Acosta et al.[24]
NYVAC-Pf7	D	+	+	–	–	High	Medium	Ockenhouse et al.[28]

*The vaccines and vaccine candidates used were attenuated parasites, purified proteins, recombinant proteins, synthetic peptides, and DNA vaccines (for details, see respective references).
[a]Type of vaccine: A = attenuated organism, R = recombinant, SP = synthetic peptide, D = DNA vaccine.
[b]Summarizing if the vaccine(s) have been tested (+) or not (–) in the four trial phases, I, IIa, IIb, and III.
[c]Potential of the vaccine(s) at the practical level based on the results so far obtained and in view of further development of the vaccine. The assessment refers to application for endemic areas and for short-term visitors/travelers; four grades are used: no, low, medium, or high potential. Situations where predictions are not possible are marked with "?".

immune responses to EPI vaccines, it did not, however, reduce the risk of clinical malaria (vaccine efficacy: 2%; 95% CI: –16,16).[24] Consequently, and considering all other results of the comprehensive clinical testing, this vaccine, in its current alum-based formulation, does not appear to have a role in malaria control in sub-Saharan Africa. Although these results are disappointing for malaria vaccine development, the comprehensive testing of a vaccine has not only provided insight at the immunologic or molecular level. The experience with SPf66 has greatly enriched our understanding of the steps, criteria, and prerequisites of clinical tests with malaria vaccines.[5] In addition, it may provide the basis for future developments with synthetic peptides.

At present, we are left with three important field programs testing malaria vaccine:

1. Phase IIa and IIb—testing of the recombinant pre-erythrocytic vaccine RTS,S/SBAS2[25] has not only shown its potency in inducing effective cellular and humoral immune responses but also promising efficacy against artificial challenges[25] and in natural challenge experiments.[26] The recently completed phase IIb study among male adults in The Gambia showed an efficacy of 65% (95% CI: 38, 80) during the first 2 months and 16% (95% CI: –16, 39) during the full trial period against clinical episodes.[26]

2. Of equal interest are the most recent data from the phase IIb combination B (recombinant vaccine candidate with three merozoite antigens: MSP1+MSP2+RESA) vaccine trial in Papua New Guinea[27] among

118 school-aged children. In one subgroup, combination B showed an efficacy of 62% (95% CI: 13, 84) in reducing parasite density, the primary endpoint tested in this trial.

3. Finally, the development of DNA vaccines merits careful attention. Substantial new developments can be expected in this field as a result of the completion of the malaria genome project within the next few years.

The first trial with a DNA vaccine against malaria (NYVAC-Pf7) was a multicomponent, multistage vaccine comprising seven genes of *P. falciparum* (sporozoite-stage: CS, SSP2/TRAP; liver stage: LSA1; asexual blood-stage: MSP1, AMA1, SERA; sexual stage: Pfs25). These were combined and administered within an attenuated vaccinia virus as "vehicle" but did not result in any significant protection against malaria episodes. However, in phase IIa studies, there was some delay in the onset of parasitemia among vaccinated individuals when compared to controls.[28]

In a different series of trials, following experiments in rodent and monkey models, phase I trials with DNA vaccines involving genes from pre-erythrocytic parasite stages are in progress.[29] Phase II trials will only be started once the comprehensive evaluation of the phase I trials is completed.

This line of research is certainly only at its inception, and there is hope that major achievements will be made within the next decade. The advantages of DNA vaccines are manifold: (1) antigens expressed in their native forms can lead to improved processing by the immune system;

(2) cytotoxic T-cell responses may be induced and antigen-specific CD8[+] T cells enhanced; (3) the vaccines are easy to produce, purify, modify, and to combine; (4) they may induce long-term immunity; and (5) they may require only low numbers of doses. These advantages need to be contrasted with the potential disadvantages: (1) the introduction of foreign DNA may lead to its incorporation into host chromosomes and could create potential for transformation; (2) there is a possibility of incorporation into germ-line cells; (3) the introduction of foreign DNA could stimulate anti-DNA antibodies and thus autoimmune reactions; and (4) the persistent expression of antigens could lead to other unexpected consequences. Current vaccine development programs—not only in the field of malaria—are assessing these risks and weighing them against the potential benefits.

OUTLOOK AND PROSPECTS

The brief review of the evolution and status of malaria vaccine development at the clinical trial level has shown that we are still far from a malaria vaccine that will be available for short-term visitors traveling to, or populations living in, endemic areas. There are certainly very promising lines of development such as the recombinant pre-erythrocytic vaccine RTS,S/SBAS2,[25,26] the recombinant three-component blood-stage vaccine, (MSP1+MSP2+RESA),[27] and the DNA vaccine developments.[29] It is of particular importance that these lines of further development now include both vaccines that are suitable for the protection of short-term visitors/travelers by preventing infection and vaccines that would be highly suitable for the populations in endemic areas by preventing morbidity without affecting the development of semi-immunity. With regard to the latter, carefully designed phase III trials will be necessary to optimize efficacy at the population level by assessing (1) the optimal age of vaccination and integration into schedules of EPI programs and (2) the duration of protection in relation to boosting by natural exposure.

The search for improved immunogenicity of a vaccine by optimal delivery through combinations with novel adjuvants[30] is another related and important area of further experimental and clinical research. The adjuvants SEPPIC Montanide ISA 720 used for the combination B trials[27,31] liposome-monophosphyryl lipid A,[19] and the saponins, notably QS21,[32] applied with RTS,S/SBAS2[25,26,33] (Lalvani and colleagues, 1999), and the use of immunopotentiating reconstituted influenza virosomes[34,35] represent powerful alternatives to the previously used alum.

While recognizing the important lines of future malaria vaccine developments, we should not refrain from exploring new vaccine candidates or from optimizing existing vaccines such as multicomponent, multistage synthetic peptide vaccines, based on the experience obtained with SPf66. In addition, molecular immunology, biology, and molecular epidemiology should become more strongly interlinked in order to exploit the data from phase II and III trials and from other long-term malaria control and prevention programs in the best possible way.

This will provide further insight into key questions of the parasite's population dynamics, its effect on the host's immune system, and the determinants of transmission and will, thus, create the basis for innovative steps in vaccine design and delivery for different target populations.

Developing malaria vaccines also challenges the prevailing concepts of vaccines and vaccine delivery. Although we commonly assume that a vaccine should reach efficacy levels of > 90%, any malaria vaccine with an efficacy > 50% might already be a highly cost-effective public health tool for many endemic areas. Given the complexity of the parasite's life cycle and the polymorphism of malaria parasites, it may be necessary to consider using a vaccine as a public health tool at lower efficacy levels, combined with other malaria control strategies. Recent calculations consider a hypothetical malaria vaccine that costs 1 to 7 U.S. dollars per child per year, with duration of protection of 1 to 5 years, distributed within the EPI program and reducing all-cause childhood mortality by ≥ 30%. The cost per DALY of such a vaccine is 1 to 14 U.S. dollars, which compares very well with the use of insecticide-treated bednets at 7 to 14 U.S. dollars per DALY.[12]

Malaria vaccines that reach efficacy levels of > 90% against infective and pre-erythrocytic stages might be of great interest for short-term visitors and travelers to endemic areas. Such vaccines may, however, not be optimal for the population living in endemic areas, as they will reduce the immunologic experience of these populations and thus the development of semi-immunity. On the other hand, vaccines with efficacy levels of > 90% against asexual blood stages may well mimic semi-immunity and are highly suitable for populations of endemic areas, but will not be feasible or acceptable for short-term visitors/travelers. As outlined above, the current developments—be they with recombinant, synthetic, or DNA vaccines—may achieve the compromise of a multiantigen and multistage vaccine, highly effective for most target groups. Such a vaccine will be a major contribution to effective malaria control, if integrated with the currently available strategies such as (1) chemoprophylaxis for short-term visitors/travelers or (2) prompt treatment at a peripheral level for people in endemic areas and (3) effective exposure prophylaxis and the use of insecticide-treated bednets. The development of a malaria vaccine remains a major challenge for the next decade, but the achievements to date suggest that an effective and affordable vaccine is a highly realistic target.

REFERENCES

1. Murray CJL, Lopez AD. Mortality by cause for eight regions of the world: global burden of disease study. Lancet 1997; 349:1269–1276.
2. Snow RW, Craig M, Deichmann U, Marsh K. Estimating mortality, morbidity and disability due to malaria among Africa's non-pregnant population. Bull World Health Org 1999;77:624–640.
3. World Bank. World development report 1993—investing in health. New York: Oxford University Press, 1993.

4. Muentener P, Schlagenhauf P, Steffen R. Imported malaria (1985–1995): trends and perspectives. Bull World Health Org 1999;77:560–566.

5. World Health Organization. Guidelines for the evaluation of *Plasmodium falciparum* vaccines in populations exposed to natural infection. Document TDR/PF/VAC/96. Geneva: WHO, 1996.

6. Lengeler C. Insecticide treated bednets and curtains for malaria control (a Cochrane review). In: The Cochrane Library, Issue 3, update software (CD-ROM version). Oxford, 1998.

7. Cohen S, McGregor IA, Carrington SP. Gammaglobulin and acquired immunity to human malaria. Nature 1961;192: 733–737.

8. McGregor IA. The passive transfer of human malaria immunity. Am J Trop Med Hyg 1964;13:237–239.

9. Clyde DF, Most H, McCarthy V, Vanderberg JP. Immunization of man against sporozoite-induced falciparum malaria. Am J Med Sci 1973;266:169–177.

10. Rieckmann K, Carson PE, Beaudoin RL. Sporozoite-induced immunity in man against an Ethiopian strain of *Plasmodium falciparum*. Trans R Soc Trop Med Hyg 1974;68:258–259.

11. Facer CA, Tanner M. Clinical trials of malaria vaccines: the pace quickens. Adv Parasitol 1997;39:1–68.

12. Engers HD, Godal T. Malaria vaccine development: current status. Parasitol Today 1998;14:56–64.

13. Gupta S, Anderson RM. Population structure of pathogens: the role of immune selection. Parasitol Today 1999;15:497–501.

14. Hoffmann SL. Malaria vaccine development—a multi-immune response approach. Washington, DC: ASM Press, 1996.

15. Tanner M, Beck H-P, Felger I, Smith T. The epidemiology of multiple *Plasmodium falciparum* infections: general introduction. Trans R Soc Trop Med Hyg 1999;93(Suppl 1):1–2.

16. Smith T, Felger I, Tanner M, Beck H-P. Premunition in *Plasmodium falciparum*: insights from the epidemiology of multiple infections. Trans R Soc Trop Med Hyg 1999;93(Suppl 1): 59–64.

17. Ballou WR, Hoffmann SL, Sherwood JA, et al. Safety and efficacy of a recombinant DNA *Plasmodium falciparum* sporozoite vaccine. Lancet 1987;i:1277–1281.

18. Herrington DA, Clyde DF, Losonsky G, et al. Safety and immunogenicity in man of a synthetic peptide malaria vaccine against *Plasmodium falciparum* sporozoites. Nature 1987;328: 257–259.

19. Fries LF, Gordon DM, Schneider I. Safety, immunogenicity and efficacy of a *Plasmodium falciparum* vaccine comprising a circumsporozoite protein repeat region peptide conjugated to *Pseudomonas aeruginosa* toxin A. Infect Immun 1992;60: 1834–1839.

20. Stuerchler D, Just M, Berger R, et al. Evaluation of 5.1 (NANP); a recombinant *Plasmodium falciparum* vaccine candidate in adults. Trop Geogr Med 1992;44:9–14.

21. Patarroyo ME, Amador R, Clavijo P, et al. A synthetic vaccine protects humans against challenge with asexual blood stages of *Plasmodium falciparum* malaria. Nature 1988;332:158–161.

22. Tanner M, Teuscher T, Alonso PL. SPf66—the first malaria vaccine. Parasitol Today 1995;11:10–13.

23. Graves P. Human malaria vaccines: In: Garner P, Gelband H, Olliario P, Salinas R, eds. Infectious diseases module of the Cochrane database systematic reviews Issue 1(4), update software (CD-ROM version, 3 June 1997) Oxford, 1997.

24. Acosta CJ, Galindo CM, Schellenberg D, et al. Evaluation of the SPf66 vaccine for malaria control when delivered through the EPI scheme in Tanzania. Trop Med Int Health 1999;4: 368–376.

25. Stoute JA, Shoui MD, Heppner DG, et al. Preliminary evaluation of recombinant circumsporozoite vaccine against *Plasmodium falciparum* malaria. N Engl J Med 1997;336:86–91.

26. Bojang KA, Milligan PJM, Pinder M, et al. Randomized controlled efficacy trial of RTS,S/SBAS2 malaria vaccine in semi-immune adult Gambian males [abstract 1064]. Proc Am Soc Trop Med Hyg,1999.

27. Genton B, Anders RF, Saul AJ, et al. Safety, immunogenicity and pilot-efficacy of a three-component blood-stage vaccine (MSP1, MSP2, RESA) against *Plasmodium falciparum* in Papua New Guinea children [abstract 1070]. Proc Am Soc Trop Med Hyg 1999.

28. Ockenhouse CF, Sun PF, Lanar DE, et al. Phase I/IIa safety, immunogenicity, and efficacy trial of NYVAC-Pf7, a pox-vectored, multiantigen, multistage vaccine candidate for *Plasmodium falciparum* malaria. J Infect Dis 1998;177: 1664–1673.

29. Wang R, Doolan DL, Le ThP, et al. Induction of antigen-specific cytotoxic T lymphocytes in humans by a malaria DNA vaccine. Science 1998;282:476–480.

30. Gupta RK, Siber GR. Adjuvants for human vaccines—current status, problems and future prospects. Vaccine 1995;13: 1263–1276.

31. Lawrence GW. Phase I trial in humans of an oil-based adjuvant SEPPIC Montanide ISA 720. Vaccine 1997;15:176–178.

32. Kensil CR, Patel U, Lennik M, Marciani D. Separation and characterisation of saponins with adjuvant activity from *Quillaja saponaria* Molina cortex. Immunology 1991;146: 431–437.

33. Lalvani A, Moris P, Voss G, et al. Potent induction of focused Th1-type cellular and humoral immune responses by RTS, S/SBAS2, a recombinant *Plasmodium falciparum* malaria vaccine. J Infect Dis 1999;180:1656–1664.

34. Glück R. Liposomal presentation of antigens for human vaccines. Pharm Biotechnol 1995;6:325–345.

35. Pöltl-Frank F, Zurbriggen R, Helg A, et al. Use of reconstituted influenza virus virosomes as an immunopotentiating delivery system for peptide-based vaccine. Clin Exp Immunol 1999;177:496–503.

Chapter 22

VACCINE PREVENTABLE DISEASES

22.1 THE COMMERCIALLY AVAILABLE VACCINES

GERHARD WIEDERMANN AND HERWIG KOLLARITSCH

ROUTINE VACCINES

TETANUS

Vaccines Tetanus toxoid vaccines may be applied as a monovalent vaccine or in combination with diphtheria or as a multivalent vaccine together with pertussis, Haemophilus influenzae b, poliomyelitis, and/or hepatitis B components for vaccination of infants. Immunizations of older children, adolescents, and adults, as well as booster vaccinations, are ideally being performed with vaccines containing diphtheria-tetanus vaccines. This kind of vaccine is also most often used in international travel.

Monovalent tetanus vaccines usually contain 40 IU toxoid per dose (0.5 mL). Sometimes, the toxoid concentration is defined as limes flocculation (Lf) units. There is, however, no constant relation between IU and Lf. Vaccines are usually adsorbed and contain 1.25 to 2 mg aluminum hydroxide, sometimes aluminum phosphate. Thimerosal or another mercury-containing preservative is added. In case of allergy against mercury-containing preservatives, either deep intramuscular injection or application of compounds containing quarternary ammonium bases (such as T-Immun; Baxter-Immuno, Deerfield, IL, U.S.A.) may be used. The latter formulation contains 80 instead of 40 IU toxoid. Diphtheria-tetanus combinations for infants up to 6 years of age usually contain 30 IU diphtheria toxoid and 40 IU tetanus toxoid; children from age 7 years onwards and adults should be given reduced doses of diphtheria toxoid to avoid local or rare systemic side effects associated with the higher dose of diphtheria toxoid.[1,2] Such vaccines contain 20, sometimes 40, IU tetanus toxoid, Al^{+++} salts, and mercury-containing preservatives. Examples are Di Te Anatoxal "Berna" for adults (Swiss Serum and Vaccine Institute [SSVI]) with 2 IU diphtheria and 40 IU tetanus toxoids, dT-reduct (Pasteur Mérieux Connaught, Lyon, France) with 2 IU diphtheria toxoid and ≥ 20 IU tetanus toxoid, Diphtavax (Pasteur Mérieux Connaught) with ≥ 2 IU diphtheria toxoid and ≥ 20 IU tetanus toxoid, and tetanus diphtheria toxoids for adults (Wyeth Lederle, St. Davis, Philadelphia, PA, U.S.A.) containing 2 Lf diphtheria toxoid and 5 Lf tetanus toxoid and Td pŭr (Chiron Behring, Marburg, Germany)

containing 2 IU diphtheria toxoid and at least 20 IU tetanus toxoid. If protection against tetanus is optimal but diphtheria protection suboptimal, a monovalent diphtheria vaccine may be used. Such a vaccine for use in adults contains 2 IU diphtheria toxoid/dose, a mercury-containing preservative, and is adsorbed to aluminum hydroxide (Diphtherie Adsorbat Vaccine "Behring" for adults, Chiron Behring).

Schedule A primary immunization consists of three doses: the first two doses are given 4 to 8 weeks apart and the third dose is given 6 to 12 months later. Schedules for primary vaccination of children may vary, however, according to different recommendations of national expert groups. The interval between the first two doses may be extended up to 5 years. If at least two primary doses are documented, the interval of the third dose from the last injection may be indefinite. After primary immunization, boosters are recommended at 10-year intervals or adjusted to antibody testing by ELISA. Theoretically, a level of 0.01 mIU/mL is protective; in practice, immunity is accepted with antibody levels of more than 0.1 mIU/mL. A booster dose may be considered after a 5-year interval from a previous dose if travel to an underdeveloped country is planned when postexposure treatment after so called "trivial" injuries may be limited or delayed.[3]

Tolerability[2] Minor local reactions after injection of tetanus toxoid may occur within 48 hours. Severe local reactions eventually accompanied by fever and malaise have been found to correlate with high antibody levels if too many immunizations have been performed (local Arthus phenomenon). The problems of high rates of severe local and systemic reactions noted in earlier studies with diphtheria toxoid have been alleviated by introduction of improved purifying methods, use of absorbed vaccines, and reduction of toxoid doses in children and adults (see Vaccines).

Evidence collected so far favors a causal relation between tetanus toxoid and Guillain-Barré syndrome (GBS). Because the conclusions are not based on controlled studies, no estimate of incidence or relative risk is available. It would seem to be low.[2] Similarly, evidence collected by the Institute of Medicine[2] favors a causal relation between tetanus vaccination and brachial neuritis in the order of 0.5 to 1 excess risks per 100,000 tetanus recipients. Although controlled studies are not available, a causal relation between tetanus toxoid (not diphtheria toxoid) and anaphylaxis is being considered; incidence and relative risk, however, seem to be low.

Immunogenicity and Efficacy   Tetanus and diphtheria toxoids are excellently immunogenic, and immunogenicity and efficacy are closely related; protective concentrations of tetanus antibodies are in the range of 0.01 IE/mL conferring a minimal protection, whereas good and safe protection may be expected at 0.1 IE/mL. Specific antibodies persist for 13 to 14 years in 96% of vaccinees.[4] In case of diphtheria antitoxic antibodies, a concentration of 0.01 to 0.1 IE/mL is partially protective; protection against disease is expected at levels of 0.1 IE/mL. Protection is estimated to last for at least 10 years.

POLIOMYELITIS

Vaccines   Two kinds of vaccines are available: live oral vaccines (OPV according to Sabin) or inactivated vaccines for parenteral injection (IPV according to Salk). One dose of OPV contains 1×10^6, 1×10^5, and 3.16×10^5 $TCID_{50}$ of types I, II, and III, respectively. Trace amounts of antibiotics (neomycin, framicetin [aminoglycosides], or polymyxin B [polypeptide]) are present as well as stabilizing or solubilizing substances. Inactivated vaccines are nowadays available as enhanced potency vaccines (eIPV). One dose contains 40, 8, and 32 D-antigenic units for types I, II, and III, respectively. Modern vaccines usually do not contain thimerosal as a preservative but do contain phenoxyethanol. Trace amounts of streptomycin, neomycin, and polymyxin are also present.

Schedule   Three options are possible for vaccination of children according to the U.S. Advisory Committee on Immunization Practices (ACIP)[5] (Table 22.1–1).

After the fourth administration of OPV, duration of protection is considered to be lifelong.[6] According to European standards, primary vaccination of children is performed at a minimal interval of 6 weeks, usually 2 to 3 in the first and 1 in the second year, but observation of a strict schedule is not necessary because further doses are not boosters but rather fill "vaccination gaps." Another

dose of vaccine is given in the tenth year of life or later,[4] in some countries at school entry, and another dose when leaving school, and eventually from then on every 10 years. Enhanced potency vaccines may be given similarly to the above-mentioned schedule or twice at an interval of 4 to 8 weeks and the third dose after 6 to 12 months.[4] No field trials are available to demonstrate duration of protection after application of eIPV. Revaccination with eIPV is recommended every 10 years.[4] After application of the lower dose, IPV revaccinations were recommended every 5 to 10 years.[66] Due to decreasing incidence of poliomyelitis caused by wild virus and relatively increasing incidence of vaccine-associated paralytic poliomyelitis (VAPP), vaccination schedules using IPV or a sequential immunization are being preferred in developed countries. Despite the adoption of sequential vaccination, some cases of VAPP might still occur, and only the exclusive use of IPV will completely eliminate VAPP. On the other hand, the superior gastrointestinal immunity conferred by OPV will reduce the risk that persons being exposed during travel might subsequently reintroduce wild poliovirus into a developed country. Similarly, for epidemiologic reasons, national immunization days in residual endemic areas are being performed with OPV. The IPV option is now preferred in the U.S. and many European countries.

Vaccination of adults is recommended according to the U.S. ACIP when a relatively high risk of exposure to poliovirus is anticipated. In European countries, regular revaccinations are advocated. Persons at risk include travelers to polio-endemic countries, members of specific population groups with disease caused by wild poliovirus, laboratory workers handling virus-contaminated material, health care workers, and unvaccinated adults whose children receive OPV.

For unvaccinated adults (over 18 years), administration of IPV is recommended because the risk of VAPP is higher in adults than in children.

Tolerability   The most important adverse event after administration of OPV is VAPP. In the U.S., the overall risk for VAPP is approximately 1 in 2.4 million distributed doses and 1 in 750,000 first doses of OPV. Immunodeficient persons and persons receiving immunosuppressive therapy should not receive OPV because their risk for VAPP is 3,200- to 6,800-fold greater than in immunocompetent persons.[5] In central Europe (Germany),[4] the risk of VAPP after OPV seems to be somewhat

Table 22.1–1.   OPTIONS FOR POLIOMYELITIS VACCINATION IN CHILDREN

	CHILDREN'S AGE			
Vaccination schedule*	2 months	4 months	12–18 months	4–6 years
Sequential IPV/OPV	IPV	IPV	OPV	OPV
OPV‡	OPV	OPV	OPV†	OPV
IPV	IPV	IPV	IPV	IPV

IPV = inactivated poliovirus vaccine; OPV = live oral poliovirus vaccine.
*The vaccination schedule for children is subject to different recommendations by national Advisory Committees on Immunization Practices.
†For children who receive only OPV, the third dose of OPV may be administered as early as 6 months of age.

smaller (1 in 4.4 million distributed doses). Type 3 is the most common cause of VAPP.

Immunogenicity and Efficacy After a complete primary vaccination series with OPV, seroconversion is 100% for types 1 and 2 and 87% for type 3.[4] Also, an intense intestinal immune response is induced. An extended field trial in the former U.S.S.R. demonstrated an excellent efficacy (polio incidence of 10.6×10^{-5} in 1958 was reduced to 0.1×10^{-5} in 1964). It seems that protection outlasts persistence of antibodies. Already, two doses of IPV may induce 90% to 100% seroconversion. An enteral immunity is induced to some extent.

VACCINES AGAINST HEPATITIS

HEPATITIS A

Several vaccines from different manufacturers are available for immunization against hepatitis A (Table 22.1–2). They include Havrix for children and adults with three doses and one dose + booster immunization schedules,[7–17] Avaxim one dose + booster schedule for adolescents and adults,[18–20] Vaqta one dose + booster schedule for children and for adults,[21–24] and Epaxal as one dose + booster application for adults and children.[25–28] All vaccines except Epaxal (virosome vaccine) are inactivated and $AL(OH)_3$ adsorbed whole virus vaccines.

Tolerability None of the vaccines mentioned induced severe side effects according to extended clinical trials. Interestingly, there was no relation between antigen content of a vaccine dose and frequency or intensity of signs or symptoms reported. Local reactions in particular were probably caused by the aluminum present in the vaccine. The local tolerability of a nonaluminum adsorbed virosome vaccine (Epaxal) proved to be particularly good.

Immunogenicity Four weeks after the first application of any of the vaccines mentioned, seroconversion rates were >90% as measured by ELISA. In travel medicine, the question could arise, however, how quickly after starting vaccination a state of protection could be achieved. It has been shown that with a two-dose primary vaccination, neutralizing antibodies were observed approximately 1 month after the second vaccination. After application of a single-dose inactivated vaccine, neutralizing antibodies were observed after 14 days in 54.2% and 61.7% of vaccinees, and after 1 month seroconversion was 100% resp., 94.1% in two groups of vaccinees. After a booster, antibodies persisted in the protective range for decades. After application of the virosome vaccine, neutralizing antibodies were observed in approximately 84% after 14 days. The examples demonstrate that one-dose inactivated vaccine samples could be preferred if a quick response is needed.

Efficacy According to one field trial in Thailand,[11] protective efficacy was 94% following two doses of hepatitis A vaccine, and cumulative efficacy, including the postbooster period, was 95%. Using a single-dose application in upstate New York,[23] the protection efficacy was 100% after day 21. The protection against clinical disease and infection after application of a virosome formulated hepatitis A vaccine in an endemic area in Nicaragua was 100%.

HEPATITIS B

All of the vaccines listed in Table 22.1–3 are recombinant yeast-derived vaccines. Plasma-derived vaccines have

Table 22.1–2. **VACCINES AGAINST HEPATITIS A**

VACCINE (MANUFACTURER)	CONTENT OF ONE DOSE*
Havrix 360 EU (SKB)†	0.5 mL, strain HM175, inactivated, 360 EU, 0.725 mg Al(OH)₃, phenoxyethanol as preservative
Havrix junior 720 EU (SKB)	0.5 mL, strain HM175, inactivated, 720 EU, sterile in injector; 0.725 mg Al(OH)₃, phenoxyethanol as preservative
Havrix 720 EU (SKB)†	1 mL, strain HM175, inactivated, 720 EU, phenoxyethanol as preservative, 1.45 mg Al(OH)₃
Havrix 1440 EU (SKB)	1 mL, strain HM175, inactivated, 1440 EU, phenoxyethanol as preservative, 1.45 mg Al(OH)₃, sterile in injector
Avaxim (Pasteur Mérieux Connaught)	0.5 mL, GBM strain inactivated, 160 RIA units, phenoxyethanol as preservative, 0.3 mg A2⁺⁺⁺
VAQTA adolescent formulation (MSD)	0.5 mL, strain CR326F inactivated, 25 U (approximately 25 ng viral capsid protein), 0.225 mg Al⁺⁺⁺
VAQTA adult formulation (MSD)	1 mL, strain CR326F inactivated, 50 units (approximately 50 ng viral capsid protein), 0.45 mg Al⁺⁺⁺
Epaxal (SSVI)	0.5 mL of strain RG-SB, inactivated 500 RIA units as virosomal preparation (10 µg phospholipids, thimerosal as preservative, no adjuvant)

*Antigenic units of different manufacturers are not comparable. †Production stopped.
SKB = SmithKline Beecham, MSD = Merck Sharpe and Dohme, SSVI = Swiss Serum and Vaccine Institute.
For application schedules, see Chapter 22.2 Principles and Practices of Immunoprophylaxis.

been shown to be safe and effective, and comparisons between the two vaccines revealed no substantial differences with respect to immunogenicity and tolerability. However, limitations exist for mass vaccination programs in terms of availability of HBV carrier plasma and the cost of vaccine production. The introduction of recombinant hepatitis B vaccines allowed mass production and decreased cost. Moreover, the dependence on blood products, which are always emotionally stigmatized to some extent, may be avoided. Since the World Health Organization (WHO) and Centers for Disease Control (CDC)[29] have recommended the elimination of hepatitis B through universal childhood vaccination, the immunization against hepatitis B appears to be of special interest also in travel medicine. Except for prophylactic purposes, hepatitis B vaccinations may be necessary in certain situations, and special vaccination schedules may be required for newborns of HBsAg-positive mothers and for immunodeficient or dialysis patients and nonresponders.

The CDC[30] recommends that infants born to HBsAg-positive mothers should receive 0.5 mL hepatitis B immunoglobulin within 12 hours of birth and either 5 μg Recombivax HB® or 10 μg Engerix B® within 12 hours of birth, a second dose at the age of 1 to 2 months, and a third dose at the age of 6 months. If the HBsAg status of the mother is unknown, application of immunoglobulin may be omitted. Advisory committees of other countries recommend application of at least 100 IU hepatitis B immunoglobulin and application of hepatitis B vaccine (childhood formulation) at 0, 1, 2, and 12 months to newborns of HBsAg-positive mothers. If vaccination is applied only after day 7, a second dose of immunoglobulin should be given after 6 weeks. With the latter immunization schedule (0, 1, 2, 12), the seroconversion rate may be somewhat higher within an early phase of immunization.[4]

The optimal procedure for vaccination of nonresponders is not well established.[31] It seems, however, that most of them are not absolute nonresponders but rather low responders. Nonresponse may have a genetic background and was found to be related to DR3, DR7, DQ2, or absence of A2 alleles. Procedures such as application of double doses, repetition of immunization course, or repetitive vaccinations have been recommended to overcome nonresponse, whereas the benefit of additional application of thymopectin or cytokines, such as interleukin-2 or interferon-α, is questionable or of limited use.[31] Differing reports exist with respect to intradermal application of a hepatitis B vaccine. Whereas the U.S. ACIP recommends that hepatitis B vaccine be administered intramuscularly,[32] observations have been reported in recent years that repeated intradermal doses of hepatitis B vaccine may provoke an immune response even in patients nonresponsive to double IM doses.[33] It has been shown, however, that repeated IM injections (every 2 months[34] or every 6 to 8 weeks up to 13 times[35]) may often finally also lead to an immune response. There are two views with respect to duration of immunity and necessity of revaccinations.[36] One calls for surveillance of antibody levels in vaccinated persons and reimmunization at a calculated time period or when the measured level of antibodies declines to a certain low level. The other view states that immunity does not depend on detectable circulating antibody but rather on the capability of memory cells to give an immediate anamnestic response upon contact with the virus. This latter view is in line with WHO and U.S. Public Health Service policy and does not pursue routine reimmunization once that seroconversion has taken place. Many epidemiologic observations speak in favor of this point of view, but there is certainly no harm from reimmunization for persons or inhabitants of countries whose resources permit reimmunizations. It should be noted, however, that the first option intends to prevent infection, whereas the second option just wants to prevent illness.

Tolerability The incidence of reported reactions varied widely (from 0% to 60%) in different studies, apparently due to the scrupulousness with which minor signs and symptoms were reported. Local reactions reported consisted mainly of mild soreness up to 48 hours, accompanied sometimes by erythema, rarely by swelling

Table 22.1–3. VACCINES AGAINST HEPATITIS B

VACCINE (MANUFACTURER)	CONTENT OF ONE DOSE	APPLICATION SCHEDULE*
Engerix B 10 μg, SKB	0.5 mL, 10 μg HBsAg, 0.475 mg algeldrate (=0.25 mg Al+++), thimerosal, in a one-dose injector	IM 0, 1, 6 (12) months for children and adolescents up to the finished 15th year or 0, 1, 2, 12 months
Engerix B 20 μg, SKB	1 mL, 20 μg HBsAg, 0.95 mg algeldrate (=0.5 mg Al+++), thimerosal, in a one-dose injector	IM 0, 1, 6 (12) months vaccination
Recombivax (HB-MSD)† GEN-HB-VAX (MSD)	1 mL, 10 μg HBsAg, 1.44 mg aluminum hydroxide (=0.5 mg aluminum) thimerosal as preservative	IM 0, 1, 6 (12) or 0, 1, 2, 12 months
GEN-Hevac (Pasteur Mérieux Connaught)	0.5 mL, 20 μg HBsAg and pre S2 proteins, 1.25 mg Al+++, no preservative	IM 0, 1, 6 or 0, 1, 2, 12 months

SKB = SmithKline Beecham, MSD = Merck Sharp and Dohme.
* Vaccination schedules in children and adolescents might vary according to different recommendations of national Advisory Committees on Immunization Practices.
† Pediatric formulation: 0.5 mL contains 2.5 μg HbsAg; adolescent formulation: 0.5 mL contains 5 μg HbsAg; adult formulation: 1.0 mL contains 10 μg HbsAg; dialysis formulation: 1.0 mL contains 40 μg HbsAg. Each dose contains thimerosal as preservative and 0.5 mg Al+++ as Al(OH)₃.
Vaccines containing pre S1 and pre S2 additionallly are Hepogene® (Medeva, London) and Viro Hep B Berna (Swiss Serum and Vaccine Institute, Bern, in preparation).

and induration, a very low total local symptom score reflecting only mild reactions. General reactions were rarely observed and mostly of a subjective nature, such as headache, dizziness, or fatigue and, in some studies, raised temperature. Symptoms were less common after the second and third vaccinations, and allergic responses or IgE formation against eventual yeast contaminants were not observed.[4,37–39]

Only recently, however, the French Ministry of Health announced the decision in 1998 to suspend routine hepatitis B immunizations in French schools while continuing immunization of infants and high-risk groups. This decision was due to pressure from fundamentalist antivaccine groups in connection with concerns that hepatitis B vaccination might be linked to development or flare-up of demyelinating diseases, such as multiple sclerosis. Recent publications of the WHO,[40,41] which are in line with previous findings of the Institute of Medicine,[2] counter these allegations by stating that after evaluation of all data known so far, there is no evidence of an association between hepatitis B virus infection and multiple sclerosis or other demyelinating diseases. Moreover, among more than 550 million individuals who have been immunized since 1982, no evidence of a causal association with multiple sclerosis or other demyelinating diseases has ever been demonstrated. WHO strongly recommends that all countries using hepatitis B vaccine in their national programs should continue to do so and that countries not yet using it should begin as soon as possible.

Immunogenicity   Approximately 95% of immunologically healthy young or middle-aged people produce specific and protective antibodies after the third vaccination.[4] Appearance of protective antibodies follows a more protracted course than appearance of antibodies after hepatitis A vaccination. Individual antibody titers after a full course of immunizations were more diverse than in the case of hepatitis A vaccination. Seroconversion rates are lower in older people, smokers, obese persons, dialysis patients, and persons with some kind of immunodeficiency. At least in these persons, antibody testing should be considered. Females have significantly higher titers than males and heterosexual males had higher titers than homosexual ones. So-called nonresponders are often only low responders.

Efficacy   An effectively performed immunization procedure protects against hepatitis B with all of its complications, especially chronic hepatitis, liver cirrhosis, and hepatocellular carcinoma, and against hepatitis D. Up to 1997, more than 85 countries have followed the recommendations of WHO and included hepatitis B vaccination in their national immunization programs. Reports of epidemiologic surveillance from different geographic areas are promising in that incidence of and complications from hepatitis B could be drastically decreased in several countries (Table 22.1–4).[42,43]

VACCINES AGAINST ENTERIC DISEASES

Vaccines against enteric diseases exist partly as candidate vaccines (such as new vaccines against typhoid fever, enterotoxigenic *Escherichia coli* (ETEC), *Shigella*, *Campylobacter*) and partly as already licensed vaccines. Already licensed enteric vaccines are available as vaccines against typhoid fever and cholera.

TYPHOID FEVER

Since inactivated whole-cell vaccines against typhoid fever are obsolete because of a relatively high number of side effects and only moderate protection, there are two vaccines in use at the present time: a live vaccine and a polysaccharide vaccine.

Live Oral Vaccine   The live oral vaccine is available as Vivotif (SSVI, Bern) or Typhoral L (SSVI, distributed by Chiron Behring) and contains the Ty21a strain with a galactose epimerase defect. It has been extensively tested in field trials by Levine et al.[44] One enteric coated capsule contains at least 10^9 lyophilized bacteria. After colonization of the gut, they quickly deteriorate because of their enzyme defect so that there is practically no noticeable excretion of bacteria.

Schedule.   Three to four capsules are applied orally every other day on an empty stomach at best 1 hour before breakfast. The application of four doses is standard in the U.S. and Canada because of better immunogenicity.[45] Recently, a liquid formulation has been developed and

Table 22.1–4.   COMBINED HEPATITIS A/B VACCINES

VACCINE (MANUFACTURER)	CONTENT OF ONE DOSE	APPLICATION SCHEDULE
TWINRIX for adults (SKB)	1 mL, 720 EU hepatitis A virus, 20 µg hepatitis B-virus antigen protein, adsorbed to 0.4 mg Al-phosphate, and 0.05 mg Al hydroxide, preservative = phenoxyethanol, formaldehyde, and traces of neomycin as residuals	IM 0, 1, 6 (12) months for adults and adolescents after 15th year of life
TWINRIX for children (SKB)	0.5 mL, 360 EU hepatitis A virus, 10 µg hepatitis B-virus antigen protein, adsorbed to 0.2 mg Al-phosphate, and 0.025 mg Al hydroxide, preservative = phenoxyethanol, formaldehyde, and traces of neomycin as residuals	0, 1, 6 (12) months for children and adolescents up to 15 years of age

SKD = SmithKline Beecham.

field tested. It has been shown to be significantly more effective than the enteric coated version in Chile but only slightly more so in Indonesia.[46, 47] One advantage of a liquid formulation, which is presently not generally available, could be that it should be readily administered to children 2 to 6 years old who often refuse to swallow capsules. The vaccination (with enteric coated capsules) is effective 7 days after the last dose.[1] Protection lasts for 1 to 3 years, and if four doses (U.S.) were given, probably up to 5 years.

Tolerability. The tolerability has been proven to be remarkably good in placebo-controlled trials.

Immunogenicity. In Chilean schoolchildren, three doses resulted in a 64% seroconversion[44]; in other trials, seroconversion rates between 55% and 86% were observed.[48]

Efficacy. The results of the first field trial in Alexandria with a 96% protection rate over an observation period of 3 years could never be repeated. Trials in Chile exhibited an efficacy of 67% for 3 years and 63% for 10 years; trials in Indonesia were less effective.[49] All of these trials were performed in endemic areas, whereas prospective efficacy trials in travelers were never performed. It is encouraging, however, that the immune response rate for healthy adult Europeans was comparable to that of residents of an endemic area.[44]

Polysaccharide Vaccine The polysaccharide vaccine Typhim Vi contains 25 µg of α1-4, 2-deoxy-2N-acetyl galacturonic acid prepared from *Salmonella typhi* strain Ty2 with phenol as preservative.

Schedule. The vaccine is applied as a one-dose intramuscular injection to children over 2 years and adults. The vaccination is effective after 10 days and the booster interval is 3 years.[1]

Tolerability. The tolerability is very good, with eventual preferentially mild local reactions and very rare general side effects (mild, up to approximately 1%).

Immunogenicity. The immunogenicity is characterized by a 95% to 100% seroconversion and an immune response for 3 years.[1,50]

Efficacy. Efficacy trials have been performed in Nepal[51] with a protection rate of 72% to 80% ($p = .72 - .8$) and in South Africa[52] with a protection rate of $p = .64$ to .81 depending on the control and verification methodology. Efficacy in travelers has not been assessed.

When deciding which vaccine should be given in which situation, it must be kept in mind that the Ty21a strain is sensitive to certain antibiotics (e.g., synthetic penicillin, cephalosporins, ciprofloxacin, tetracycline). It should not be given simultaneously with proguanil, which affects seroconversion as well as geometric mean titers (GMTs)[56]; mefloquine does not affect seroconversion, according to one report, however, GMT. Simultaneous application of both vaccines with yellow fever vaccine is possible, and the yellow fever immune response might even be enhanced to some extent by the polysaccharide vaccine. The Vi-polysaccharide vaccine is theoretically not effective against Vi-negative typhoid fever strains. Although such strains have been detected—for instance, in 8% of investigated strains in South Africa[53]—their pathogenicity has not been proven.

CHOLERA

As in the case of typhoid fever vaccines, inactivated whole-cell vaccines against cholera are obsolete nowadays due to their insufficient tolerability and efficacy. If cholera vaccines should be applied in certain situations, two vaccines are available: a live oral vaccine and an inactivated oral one.

Live Oral Vaccine (Orochol®, Mutacol®, SSVI) This vaccine contains a live attenuated recombinant CVD103HgR strain.[54] This strain has been derived from the Inaba 569B strain, of which the gene for subunit A, the toxic component of the choleratoxin, has been deleted and a mercury resistance gene introduced with the consequence that this strain is only short lived and does not contaminate the environment. Additionally, the HgR gene may, at least theoretically, lead to improvement of the antigen presentation. The vaccine strain is additionally tetracyclin resistant.

Schedule. One oral dose contains approximately 1×10^8 CFU, lyophilized in one sachet together with a sachet of lyophilized bicarbonate buffer. Both sachets are dissolved in water and applied on an empty stomach (1 hour before, 1 hour after application).

Tolerability. The tolerability is very good so that eventual gastrointestinal side effects are probably due mostly to the buffer.[55]

Immunogenicity. Ninety-two percent seroconversion[54] takes place against wild Inaba strains and is somewhat less against heterologous strains.

Efficacy. Protection rates have been studied preferentially in challenge studies. Overall, an 82% to 100% protection has been observed and 62% to 67% against El Tor strain.[54] Protection was far less in a field trial in Indonesia for unknown reasons.[82] Protection lasts approximately 2 years (unpublished data). No protection, however, is being induced against cholera 0139 or against travelers' diarrhea.

Interaction Studies.[48,56] Combined administration of Ty21a and CVD103HgR is possible without negatively influencing tolerability or immunogenicity; it may, however, even improve the GMT of vibriocidal antibodies for a certain period of time. Simultaneous application of chloroquine and CVD103HgR reduces significantly the seroconversion rate as well as the GMTs of vibriocidal antibodies; simultaneous application of mefloquine with this vaccine on the other hand reduces vibriocidal GMTs to some extent but not the seroconversion rate. Simultaneous application of yellow fever vacccine or OPV does not adversely affect the vibriocidal response or yellow fever antibodies; an influence on polio antibodies is very difficult to assess.

Inactivated Oral Vaccine An inactivated oral vaccine[57] is also available (Dukoral, Swedish Bacteriological Laboratory, SBL Vaccin) that consists of a recombinant subunit B (1 mg) of cholera toxin and 10^{11} whole cells of several cholera strains. Two oral doses are applied at an interval of 7, 14, or 28 to 42 days on an empty stomach together with bicarbonate buffer. An eventual booster dose may be given after 10 months.

Tolerability and Immunogenicity.   Phase I and II trials in Swedish, Bangladeshi, and American volunteers have shown that this vaccine is safe and immunogenic with >80% producing antitoxic and vibriocidal antibodies.[58]

Efficacy.   Trials in Bangladesh with a vaccine containing conventionally produced CTB exhibited a protection rate of 85% for 6 months and around 50% for 3 years.[59] A similar vaccine containing a recombinant subunit B exhibited an 86% protection against cholera but not against symptomless infection.[60] This vaccine, however, also has some influence on travelers' diarrhea, apparently by means of the admixture of the B subunit of cholera toxin, which has a high homology with the B subunit of the labile toxin of ETEC. In the meantime, the strategy has shifted more to the development of a vaccine against travelers' diarrhea, and phase II and III trials are presently under way testing a cholera subunit B ETEC (whole-cell) vaccine. Such a vaccine, however, has not yet been licensed.

ROTAVIRUSES

The development is based on the fact that approximately 125 million cases occur and more than 870,000 children under 5 years of age die annually from rotavirus infections in developing countries. Death rates in industrialized countries are much lower; nevertheless, more than 100,000 infants or young children are hospitalized annually only in the U.S. Up to 1997, the WHO endorsed the use of such a vaccine in industrialized countries as a first step toward global eradication. The vaccine Rotashield/Rotamune (Wyeth Lederle) is a rhesus-human reassortant tetravalent vaccine (RRV-TV). One dose of the lyophilized vaccine containing 4×10^5 PFU is resuspended in 3 mL of a sodium citrate sodium bicarbonate buffer. The suspension is administered orally three times at an interval of 3 to 4 weeks. Field trials in the U.S.[61] and Finland[62] exhibited good efficacy of 80% to 91% against severe cases, whereas other trials in developing countries (such as Peru and Brazil) produced only poor results. The design of these latter studies, however, and an inadequate dosing could have been responsible for these disappointing results. In a new very well-designed study in Venezuela,[63] it could be shown that incidence of severe diarrhea could be reduced by 88% by such a vaccine and dehydration by 75%.

TRAVEL VACCINES TO BE APPLIED ACCORDING TO THE EPIDEMIOLOGIC SITUATION

YELLOW FEVER

Vaccine   The vaccine contains attenuated virus strain 17D cultivated in leukosis-free chick embryos and may still contain trace amounts of egg albumin (cave allergy against chicken protein). One dose should contain at least 1,000 LD_{50} (mouse units). Expressed in plaque-forming units, there is an exact correlation in that $\log LD_{50}$ = (log pfu)-0.8. Usually, yellow fever vaccines are much higher concentrated (three to seven times). According to the *European Pharmacopeia*,[64] thermostability should be adjusted in such a way that after incubation of the freeze-dried vaccine at 37°C for 14 days, one human dose (0.5 mL) should contain not less than 10^3 mouse LD_{50}. The lyophilized vaccine should be kept at 2 to 8°C. The solvent must not be frozen but should be kept below 25°C. When reconstituted, the vaccine should be used within 1 hour.

YF-Vax (Pasteur Mérieux Connaught) contains not less than 5.04 log10 pfu, gelatine and sorbitol as stabilizers, and no antibiotics according to PDR98. Stamaril is a similar compound from Pasteur Mérieux Connaught licensed in France containing not less than 1,000 mouse LD_{50}/dose. Arilvax (Evans) contains not less than 1,000 LD_{50} and trace amounts of neomycin sulphate and polymyxin B sulphate. A yellow fever vaccine produced by the Robert Koch Institute (Berlin) contains 1.5×10^4 pfu. Everywhere yellow fever vaccines are supplied only to yellow fever vaccination centers approved by the WHO and authorized to issue valid International Certificates of Vaccination against yellow fever.

Schedule.   According to WHO,[1] the vaccination is valid after 10 days for 10 years. If the yellow fever vaccine is not given simultaneously with other live attenuated vaccines, an interval of 4 to 6 weeks should be observed to preceding vaccinations and of 2 weeks if the yellow fever vaccination precedes. Simultaneous or even combined administration of typhoid Vi polysaccharide vaccine may enhance antibody production against yellow fever[65]; simultaneous Ty21a oral vaccine administration has no influence on each other's antibody response.

Tolerability.   Persons allergic to chicken protein may be allergic to yellow fever vaccine. If necessary, intradermal skin testing under close medical supervision may be performed. If compliance with travel requirements rather than risk of infection is the only reason for immunization, a person hypersensitive to chicken protein may obtain a waiver letter from his/her physician stating that vaccination is contraindicated (contact the respective embassy). According to USP Dispensing Information (USPDI),[66] children of 9 months of age or older may receive the vaccination if indicated in an endemic area, children 6 to 9 months old should be vaccinated when travel to an endemic area with an ongoing yellow fever epidemic cannot be avoided, children 4 to 6 months only in high-risk situations, and infants under 4 months not at all because of the risk of encephalitis, although this is minimal. The yellow fever vaccine is contraindicated in people with immunodeficiency and should not be given for theoretical reasons in pregnant women, although birth defects and malformations have never been reported in such instances. In persons with asymptomatic HIV infection (CD_4 >400) who are at risk of exposure to the virus, the benefit of vaccination may outweigh its risk. Breast-feeding is no contraindication.

Immunogenicity and Efficacy.   Yellow fever vaccine induces protective antibodies >90%.[66]

MENINGOCOCCAL VACCINES

Vaccines   Menomune (Pasteur Mérieux Connaught) contains freeze-dried capsular polysaccharides of meningococci A, C, Y, and W135. After reconstitution, one dose (0.5 mL) contains 50 μg of each polysaccharide and, according to *Physicians' Desk Reference* and USPDI (1998), thimerosal as a preservative. In the new formulations of Menomune, however, thimerosal is no longer present. The product contains lactose as a stabilizer. A similar tetravalent product is Mencevax (SmithKline Beecham [SKB], Rixensart, Belgium), which is freeze dried and after reconstitution 0.5 mL also contains 50 μg of each of the four polysaccharides and no preservative. Mencevax A+C (SKB) is a bivalent product licensed in some countries. Another product licensed in France is Imovax Meningo A+C (Pasteur Mérieux Connaught), which is freeze dried and contains 50 μg of polysaccharides A and C and no preservative. The polysaccharides mentioned are not conjugated. There is no vaccine presently available containing capsular polysaccharide of serogroup B, which is not immunogenic, probably because it shares epitopes with brain antigens.

Schedule   Since the vaccines contain T-cell–independent antigens, one dose only is injected subcutaneously. Reconstituted vials should be used within 24 hours of reconstitution. The vaccine is not recommended for children up to 2 years because an inadequate antibody response is to be expected, although infants older than 6 months may produce antibodies to serogroup A.

Tolerability   Similarly to other inactivated vaccines, mild and transient local or general reactions might be observed in vaccinees. Anaphylactic reactions are extremely rare at a rate of less than 1×10^{-5}, possibly after incidental IV application, eventually as hyperergic reaction after revaccination.[67] After a vaccination campaign in children, transient peripheral neurologic symptoms were observed[4,67] at a rate of approximately 1 in 1,300, which were possibly causally related.

Immunogenicity   A study in adults showed seroconversion (more than fourfold rise in antibacterial antibody titer) in more than 90% to 95% of participants. In children, seroconversion rates of bactericidal antibodies to serogroups A, C, Y, and W135 were 72%, 58%, 90%, and 82%, respectively, and seroconversions as measured by Radio-Immune-Assay (RIA) were 99% for A and C, 97% for Y, and 89% for W135.[66]

Efficacy   Vaccination is effective after 15 days,[1] respectively 10 to 14 days.[66] Antibody decline is more rapid in infants than in adults. In children younger than 4 years, efficacy declined in one study from more than 90% to less than 10% after 3 years and in older children to 67% after 3 years. In adolescents and adults, protection persists presumably for 3 to 5 years.

RABIES VACCINES (TABLE 22.1–5)

Ragilvax (Biocine/Sclavo) is another human diploid cell vaccine (HDCV). Locally manufactured vaccines that are not internationally available are primary hamster kidney cell vaccine, which is produced exclusively in Russia and China, and brain tissue vaccines, which are no longer recommended by WHO such as Semple vaccine (prepared on sheep or goat brain in India and Asia) and Fuenzalida (prepared on suckling mouse brain) in Latin America and Fuenzalida-type vaccines in Vietnam.

Schedules (Pre-exposure)[68]   For pre-exposure vaccination, IM or ID application is possible. For vaccines not licensed in the U.S. but in other countries, usually the same recommendations are given.

Primary Vaccination.   One IM dose (1 mL) or one ID dose (0.1 mL) is applied on days 0, 7, and 21 or 28. Alternatively, a primary IM vaccination series at days 0, 28, and 56 might be given according to European recommendations if there is no urgent need for protection.[4] It has been shown that chloroquine phosphate interferes with the antibody response to HDCV given intradermally. Intramuscular application provides a sufficient margin of safety. Consequently, for persons receiving chloroquine and pre-exposure rabies prophylaxis by ID route, the vaccination series should be initiated at least 1 month before travel. Other antimalarials structurally related to chloroquine (f.i. mefloquine) have not been evaluated in this respect but it would seem prudent to follow similar guidelines. Antibody testing after a primary vaccination course is not necessary.

Boosters.   Pre-exposure booster doses are given according to risk category. Persons at highest risk (persons working with live rabies virus in laboratories or vaccine production facilities) should have serum samples tested for antibodies every 6 months and boosters given accordingly (serum titer at least 1:5 by Rapid Fluorescent Focus Inhibition Test [RFFIT].[68] Persons at frequent risk such as other rabies diagnostic workers, veterinarians and staff, wildlife and animal control officers in areas where rabies is epizootic, or travelers to endemic areas (>30 days) or living there should be tested serologically or receive boosters every 2 years (the first booster after 1 year according to European recommendations). Infrequent risk (but greater than in the population at large) is accepted in veterinarians, veterinary students, and wildlife workers in low-endemicity areas. They should receive only a primary vaccination. In the population at large (rare risk), no vaccination is necessary.

Postexposure Therapy of Previously Vaccinated Persons   Previously vaccinated persons, if exposed to rabies, should receive two IM doses at days 0 and 3.[68] According to another schedule,[69] one booster should be given if the person was exposed to rabies within 1 year after vaccination, two injections (on days 0, 3) if prevaccination took place 1 to 5 years before exposure, and three injections (on days 0, 3, 7) if previously vaccinated persons were exposed to rabies after 5 to 10 years.

Postexposure prophylaxis should be performed according to WHO[70,81] guidelines and is not discussed here.

Tolerability[4,68]   Mild local reactions might occur in approximately 20% or, according to other reports, in 30% to 40% of recipients, and rarely general reactions such as raises of temperature, headache, muscle aches, dizziness, or gastrointestinal side effects (in some reports 5% to 40% of recipients). An immune complex-like reaction occurs in approximately 6% of persons receiving HDCV 2 to 21 days after booster doses (urticaria, arthralgia, gastrointestinal symptoms, angioedema, or fever). Such a reaction might be due to betapropriolactone altered human albumin in the HDCV vaccine. Very rare cases of GBS have been reported. A causal relationship for other central and peripheral nervous system disorders has not been established.

Immunogenicity and Efficacy   The modern rabies vaccines (see Table 22.1–5) are comparable in immunogenicity and safety. Postexposure prophylaxis is 100% effective provided that the recommended regimen (inclusively wound treatment, passive and active immunization) has been carefully observed; breakthroughs are reported when parts of this regimen were omitted. A serum titer of 1:25 for complete neutralization in the RFFIT test (equivalent to approximately 0.5 IU) 2 to 4 weeks after pre- or postexposure treatment is acceptable.[68] Serologic testing is recommended for persons continously under high risk every 6 months. Even after ID pre-exposure prophylaxis, routine serologic testing to confirm a satisfactory antibody response is not considered to be necessary.[71]

JAPANESE ENCEPHALITIS VACCINES

JE-Vax (Biken), which may be purchased from Pasteur Mérieux Connaught, contains freeze-dried partially purified and inactivated Nakayama-NIH strain prepared from mouse brain. Thimerosal is added as a preservative, and the diluent (1 mL/dose) is sterile water. Each dose contains traces of gelatin and formaldehyde but less than 50 ng mouse brain protein. No basic myelin can be detected at the threshold level. The potency is adjusted to a reference vaccine. One dose is 1 mL; children 1 to 3 years old receive a 0.5 mL subcutaneous application.

Seiken (Denka Seiken) is licensed in Japan and may be imported from Denka Seiken Co., Ltd., Tokyo. The vaccine is also prepared from a suspension of mouse brain infected with the Beijing strain. Prior to a purification step by ultracentrifugation performed as with the above-mentioned vaccine, the crude virus suspension is treated with protamine sulphate. The liquid, colorless preparation also contains traces of gelatin and polysorbate as stabilizers and thimerosal as a preservative. One dose is 0.5 mL and 0.25 mL for children under 3 years, subcutaneous application. One vial contains two doses.

In China, an inactivated and an attenuated virus strain is being produced in tissue culture; however, these vaccines are presently not available in western countries.

Schedule   For the Biken vaccine, a dose of 1 mL (0.5 mL for children, 1 to 3 years old) administered subcutaneously on days 0 to 7 and 30 (if there are time constraints, on days 0, 7, 14) is recommended. If necessary, a booster may be administered after 2 years. The recommendations for the Denka Seiken vaccine are two subcutaneous injections of 0.5 mL (0.25 mL for children under

---

Table 22.1–5.   RABIES VACCINES

TRADEMARK	MANUFACTURER	CONTENT OF ONE DOSE
Lyssavac-N	Swiss Serum and Vaccine Institute	PDEV, 1 dose = 1 mL = 2.5 IU preservative = thimerosal, freeze dried, application IM, pre-exposure vaccination
Imovax-Rabies ID	Pasteur Mérieux Connaught	HDCV, 1 dose = 0.1 mL = 0.25 IU, no preservatives, no stabilizers, freeze dried, <22 µg neomycin, <15 mg human albumin for intradermal application only; only for pre-exposure vaccination
Imovax-Rabies IM	Pasteur Mérieux Connaught	HDCV, 1 dose = 1 mL = 2.5 IU, freeze dried, no preservative, no stabilizer, <150 µg neomycin, <100 mg human albumin, application IM for pre- and postexposure prophylaxis
Imovax-Rabies vero (formerly Verorab)	Pasteur Mérieux Connaught	PVRV, 1 dose = 0.5 mL = >2.5 IU, freeze dried, no preservative, traces of neomycin, application IM, pre- and postexposure prophylaxis
Rabipur	Chiron Behring	PCEC, 1 dose = 1 mL = >2.5 IU, no preservative, traces of neomycin, chlortetracyclin, amphotericin B, freeze dried, application IM for pre- and postexposure vaccination
Rabivac	Chiron Behring	HDCV, otherwise similar to Rabipur, application = interchangeable with Rabipur
Rabies vaccine adsorbed (RVA)	SmithKline Beecham	FRhl-2, 1 dose = 1 mL = ≥2.5 IU, not more than 2 mg aluminum phosphate, thimerosal as preservative, for IM application, pre- and postexposure vaccination

PDEV = purified duck embryo vaccine, HDCV = human diploid cell vaccine, Frhl-2 = diploid cell line from fetal rhesus lung cells, PVRV = purified vero cell rabies vaccine, PCEC = purified chick embryo cell vaccine.

3 years of age) at an interval of 1 to 4 weeks for primary vaccination. Boosters should be given after 1 year, at the first sign of a local epidemic, or every 4 to 5 years. According to WHO,[1] boosters are recommended after 1 to 4 years.

Tolerability[72,73,83,84]   Japanese encephalitis vaccination may be associated with local or usually mild systemic side effects. Redness, swelling, and tenderness were observed in <1% to 31% (at an average 20%) of vaccinees according to several reports. Systemic side effects were seen in approximately 10% of vaccinees— according to other reports less than that. Systemic side effects were fever, headache, rash, malaise, gastrointestinal symptoms, chills, myalgia, and dizziness. Neurologic events (peripheral neuropathy, encephalopathy) were originally described in Japan in about 1 to 2.3 per million vaccinees and a possibly related GBS was recorded in the U.S. Since 1989, a new pattern of adverse events has been reported among travelers. The reactions were characterized by urticaria, angioedema, sometimes respiratory distress, hypotension, and skin exanthemas. Reactions occurred within 3 days after the first dose, after 3 days to 2 weeks after the second, and rarely after the third dose. During a campaign of military personnel, one death was recorded 60 hours after a first dose; the causal relationship was not precisely established.

The incidence of these adverse events varies widely (50 to 104 × 10^{-4} in Australia and Canada, 15 to 62 × 10^{-4} in the U.S., 0.7 to 12 × 10^{-4} in Denmark, U.K., Sweden). The vaccine constituents responsible for these events have not been identified. Whether different incidence rates are due to different vaccine lots or to different susceptibilities of vaccinees in different geographic areas is unknown. Recent observations reported only rare and mild side effects.[83,84] Persons who are allergic to any of the vaccine constituents or have experienced allergic reactions after previous vaccinations should not receive this vaccine. Other precautions include pregnancy, nursing, convulsions, and immunodeficiency.

Immunogenicity and Efficacy[72]   A neutralizing antibody titer of 1:≥10 protected mice against challenge. The vaccine is excellently immunogenic and efficacious in endemic areas. A study performed in the United States, however, showed that only 77% of recipients of the Biken vaccine produced adequate neutralizing antibodies after two doses and after a third dose seroconversion was 99% to 100%.[74] A vaccine efficacy of 80% after two doses was observed in a field trial in Taiwan.[72]

TICK-BORNE ENCEPHALITIS

Vaccines   FSME-IMMUN Inject-Injector is manufactured by Baxter-Immuno. FSME stands for the German word *Frühsommermeningoencephalitis* (spring/summer meningoencephalitis). One dose of 0.5 mL contains 2.0 to 3.5 µg tick-borne encephalitis virus antigen adsorbed to 1 mg aluminum hydroxide, thimerosal as a preservative, traces of gentamycin and neomycin, and albumin as a sta-

bilizer. The virus is grown on chick embryo cells, inactivated by formaldehyde, and highly purified. FSME Immun was reformulated and was licensed anew in 1999. The new formulation no longer contains thimerosal. Encepur is manufactured by Chiron Behring. One dose (0.5 mL) contains 1.5 µg virus protein, 1 mg aluminum hydroxide, polygeline as stabilizer, no preservative, and traces of chlortetracycline, gentamycin, neomycin, and formaldehyde. For both FSME Immun and Encepur, vaccines for children with half of the dosage are in development.

Schedule   The immunization schedule of FSME Immun consists of three doses of FSME Immun given intramuscularly, 2 weeks to 3 months apart, and a third dose 9 to 12 months later.[75] In case of an imminent trip to an endemic area, the interval between the first two doses may even be shortened. Presently, booster doses are recommended at 3-year intervals. For Encepur, a schedule of 0, 7, and 21 days and a booster after 1 year (365 days) may be recommended as a quick immunization schedule. Boosters are recommended after 3 to 5 years.[76]

Tolerability[67,75,77]   Local reactions and general side effects (myalgia, arthralgia, gastrointestinal symptoms, or pyrexia) were observed. Fever reactions may be a bit more frequent in children, but after introduction of efficient purification procedures (continuous flow-zonal ultrazentrifugation), these adverse reactions have become very rare, especially after application of the Baxter-Immuno vaccine. Extremely rarely cases of neuritis of varying degree were observed.[4] Eventual meningeal symptoms were simulated by myalgias.[67] Causal relation to cases of encephalopathy could never be established. A contraindication for the vaccination is a history of anaphylactic reactions after the consumption of egg protein. However, after application of more than 30 million doses of the vaccine, no cases of shock were observed.[75]

Immunogenicity   After application of three vaccinations with FSME Immun, the seroconversion rate was 98% as measured by the hemagglutination inhibition test and 99.5% as measured by ELISA.[75] Even after the second dose, seroconversion rates of >90% can be expected. Age is not a critical factor with regard to seroconversion; the GMTs, however, are higher in children and young adults than in elderly people. Seroconversion rates after a third dose of Encepur were 100% in ELISA and the neutralization test and nearly 100% in the hemagglutination inhibition test.[76]

Efficacy[75]   The Baxter-Immuno product affords a high degree of protection that is more than 90% after two doses and 98% to 99% after three doses.

MEASLES-MUMPS-RUBELLA (MMR)

Vaccines   MMRII (measles, mumps, rubella vaccine live; Merck Sharpe and Dohme [MSD], West Point, VA) is a sterile, lyophilized preparation. When reconstituted, one dose (0.5 mL) contains 1,000 TCID_{50} of a more attenuated line of Enders' measles Edmonston strain grown on cell cultures of chick embryo, 20,000 $TCID_{50}$ of the Jeryl Lynn (B level) strain of mumps virus grown on chick embryo cell cultures, and 1,000 $TCID_{50}$ of the Wistar RA 27/3 strain of attenuated rubella virus grown in human diploid cell culture. Each dose also contains traces of neomycin and sorbitol as well as hydrolized gelatin as stabilizers. Priorix (measles, mumps, rubella vaccine live; SKB) is a sterile, lyophilized vaccine grown on chick embryo cells (measles, mumps) resp. human diploid cells (rubella). One dose (0.5 mL) of the reconstituted vaccine contains 1,000 $TCID_{50}$ hyperattenuated Schwarz measles virus strain, 5012 $TCID_{50}$ of RIT 4385 strain (a derivative of the Jeryl Lynn strain), and 1,000 $TCID_{50}$ of the RA27/3 rubella strain. One dose also contains traces of amino acids, lactose, mannitol, neomycinsulfate, and sorbitol. Triviraten Berna (SSVI) also contains 1,000 $TCID_{50}$ Edmonston Zagreb and Wistar RA 27/3 strain each and, instead of the Jeryl Lynn strain, the attenuated Rubini mumps virus (10,000 $TCID_{50}$). These viruses are grown on human diploid cells instead of chick embryo cells. Although the Rubini strain is less immunogenic than the Jeryl Lynn strain, and although there are reports on very rare meningitis-like side effects after its application, Triviraten may be considered in cases of severe anaphylaxis against egg protein.

Schedule   The vaccine is applied subcutaneously according to the strategies and recommendations of the national ACIPs of diverse countries. Irrespective of these strategies, younger children traveling to measles-endemic countries in the developing world where the risk of contracting measles is far greater than in the developed world should have protection against measles. Younger children should be given single measles antigen vaccine after the age of 6 months. These children should then be revaccinated with MMR at the age of 12 to 15 months. It has been reported that men and those born in 1957 or later in the U.S. were more likely to be seronegative for measles and mumps. This finding supports readministering MMR vaccine to young adult U.S. travelers.[3]

Tolerability[2,67,78]   Local reactions are very rare. Fever and a mild, transient rash may occur in 5% of vaccinees after the seventh day. Thrombocytopenia was observed at a rate of 1 in 30,000 to 50,000. Although eventual encephalopathy was reported in temporal association with vaccination, a causal relationship of vaccination with encephalitis, GBS, demyelinating diseases, or subacute sclerosing panencephalitis (SSPE) has never been established. On the contrary, the use of measles vaccine has even reduced the incidence rate of SSPE. Orchitis, peripheral neuropathy, and ocular palsy were very rarely described in temporal association with the vaccination. If arthralgia was observed in older women, it rarely interfered with normal activities. Evidence indicates that persons receiving MMR vaccine are not at risk if they have egg allergies that are not anaphylactic or anaphylactoid in nature.[78] Delayed-type allergic reactions (contact dermatitis) do not preclude vaccination.

Immunogenicity   According to USPDI,[66] application of MMR live vaccine to seronegative children 11 months to 7 years old induces hemagglutination-inhibiting (HI) antibodies against measles in 95%, mumps neutralizing antibodies in 96%, and rubella HI antibodies in 99%. The presence of the antibodies has been correlated with protection.

Efficacy   For blockade of transmission, a vaccination rate of 92% to 95% is necessary for measles and mumps and of 85% to 87% for rubella. In many European countries (such as Germany, Austria, France, Spain, Italy), vaccination rates are only suboptimal at the present time. New strategies are necessary and in progress.

BACILLE CALMETTE-GUÉRIN

Although tuberculosis is a potential hazard for visitors to developing countries, most experts advise against the use of bacille Calmette-Guérin (BCG) vaccine and prefer to rely on purified protein derivative skintest (Mantoux) for pre- and post-travel screening. If vaccination is considered for long-term residents, preferentially children, several vaccines are available with different numbers of particles of the bovine type of *Mycobacterium tuberculosis* derived from the parent strain (Pasteur 1173P2, Copenhagen, or Glaxo, New York, Tokyo, and Montreal).[79] The inoculation should be strictly intradermal; otherwise, skin necrosis might occur. Protection rates between 0% to 80% are reported, but apparently this vaccination protects not so much against infection but rather against more severe complications such as disseminated disease and tuberculosis meningitis.

Side Effects   After vaccination, a nodule develops at the infection site within a month, first red, then turning blue. The nodule sometimes turns into a weeping ulcerative lesion. The local reaction disappears after 2 to 5 months. More severe side effects are ascending lymphoadenitis (0.36% after receipt of the Glaxo strain, approximately 7.4% after application of the Pasteur strain). The incidence of suppurative lymphadenitis might change when one vaccine preparation was replaced by another in a community. Other side effects are BCG ostitis and osteomyelitis (1 in 80,000 to 0.6 in 1 million) and bacteremia (BCG sepsis) in cases of immunodeficiency (range in newborn between 0.1 case per million to 1 in 50,000 recipients). The development of new vaccines against tuberculosis is needed, and several candidate vaccines should be available for human testing within the next few years.[80]

REFERENCES

1. World Health Organization. International travel and health. Geneva: WHO, 1999.
2. Stratton KR, Howe CJ, Johnston RB Jr, eds., Vaccine Safety Committee, Division of Health Promotion and Disease Prevention, Institute of Medicine. Adverse events associated with

childhood vaccines: evidence bearing on causality. Washington, DC: National Academic Press, 1994.

3. Hilton E, Singer C, Kozarsky P, et al. Status of immunity to tetanus, measles, mumps, rubella and polio among US travellers. Ann Intern Med 1991;115:32–33.

4. Jilg W. Schutzimpfungen. Landsberg/Lech, Germany: ecomed, 1996.

5. Centers for Disease Control. Induction of a sequential vaccination schedule of inactivated poliovirus vaccine followed by oral poliovirus vaccine. Recommendations of the Advisory Committee on Immunization Practices (ACIP). Poliomyelitis prevention in the United States. MMWR Morb Mortal Wkly Rep 1997;46(RR-3):1–25.

6. Patriarca PA, Wright RF, John TJ. Factors affecting the immunogenicity of oral poliovirus vaccine in developing countries: review. Rev Infect Dis 1991;13:926–939.

7. André FE, Hepburn A, d'Hondt E. Inactivated candidate vaccines for hepatitis A. Progr Med Virol 1990;37:72–95.

8. Wiedermann G, Ambrosch F, Andreé FE, et al. Safety and immunogenicity of an inactivated hepatitis A candidate vaccine in healthy adult volunteers. Vaccine 1990;8:581–584.

9. Just M, Berger R. Reactogenicity and immunogenicity of inactivated hepatitis A vaccines. Vaccine 1992;10(Suppl 1):110–113.

10. Jilg W, Bittner R, Bock H, et al. Vaccination against hepatitis A: comparison of different short term immunization schedules. Vaccine 1992;10(Suppl 1):126–128.

11. Innis BL, Snitbhan R, Kunasol P, et al. Protection against hepatitis A by an inactivated vaccine. JAMA 1994;17:1328–1334.

12. Van Damme P, Mathei C, Thoelen S, et al. Single dose inactivated hepatitis A vaccine: rationale and clinical assessment of the safety and immunogenicity. J Med Virol 1994;44:435–441.

13. McMahon BJ, Williams J, Mayer J, et al. Control of an outbreak of hepatitis A in Alaska using an inactivated hepatitis A vaccine [abstract]. In: Rizzetto M, Parcell RH, Gerin JL, Verme G, eds. Viral hepatitis and liver disease. Turin: Edizione Minerva Medica, 1977:925–927

14. Príkazský V, Oleár V, Cernoch A, et al. Interruption of an outbreak of hepatitis A in two villages by vaccination. J Med Virol 1994;44:457–459.

15. Van Damme P, Thoelen S, Cramm H, et al. Inactivated hepatitis A vaccine: reactogenicity, immunogenicity and long term persistence. J Med Virol 1994;44:446–451.

16. Wiedermann G, Kundi M, Ambrosch F, et al. Inactivated hepatitis A vaccine: long term persistence. Vaccine 1997;15:612–615.

17. Wiedermann G, Kundi M, Ambrosch F, et al. Estimated persistence of anti HAV antibodies after single dose and booster hepatitis A vaccination (0-6 schedule). Acta Tropica 1998;69:121–125.

18. Garin D, Vidor E, Wallon M, et al. Good immunogenicity of GBM strain inactivated hepatitis A vaccine in healthy male adults. Vaccine 1995;13:220–224.

19. Goilav Ch, Zuckerman J, Lafrenz M, et al. Immunogenicity and safety of a new inactivated hepatitis A vaccine in a comparative study. J Med Virol 1995;46:287–292.

20. Zuckerman J, Huang M. A comparison of immunogenicity and safety following the use of Avaxim® or Havrix® 1440 as a booster for subjects primed 6 months previously with Havrix® 1440. Presented at the Fifth International Conference on Travel Medicine, Geneva, Switzerland, March 24–27, 1997.

21. Ellerbeck E, Lewis J, Midthun K, et al. Safety and immunogenicity of an inactivated hepatitis A virus vaccine. In: Hollinger FB, Lemon SM, Margolis HS, eds. Viral hepatitis and liver disease. Proceedings of the 1990 International Symposium on Viral Hepatitis and Liver Disease. Baltimore: William and Wilkins, 1991:91–93.

22. Block SL, Hedrick JA, Tyler RD, et al. Safety, tolerability and immunogenicity of a formalin inactivated hepatitis A vaccine in rural Kentucky children. Pediatr Infect Dis J 1992;12:976–980.

23. Werzberger A, Mensch B, Kuter B, et al. A controlled trial of a formalin-inactivated hepatitis A vaccine in healthy children. N Engl J Med 1992;327:453–457.

24. Nalin D, Brown L, Kuter B, et al. Inactivated hepatitis A vaccine in childhood: implications for disease control. Vaccine 1993;11(Suppl):15–17.

25. Just M, Berger R, Drechsler H, et al. A single vaccination with an inactivated hepatitis A liposome vaccine induces protective antibodies after only 2 weeks. Vaccine 1992;10:737–739.

26. Ambrosch F, Wiedermann G, Althaus B, et al. Immunogenicity and protectivity of a new liposomal hepatitis A vaccine. Vaccine 1997;15:1209–1214.

27. Glück R, Mischler R, Brantschen S, et al. Immunopotentiating reconstituted influenza virus virosome vaccine delivery system for immunization against hepatitis A. J Clin Invest 1992;90:2491–2495.

28. Mayorga O, Egger M, Zellmeyer M, et al. Efficacy of a virosome-formulated hepatitis A vaccine in an endemic region in Nicaragua: a randomized placebo-controlled trial. Presented at the 37th International Conference on Antimicrobial Agents and Chemotherapy, Toronto, Sept 28–Oct 1, 1997.

29. Centers for Disease Control. Hepatitis B virus: a comprehensive strategy for eliminating transmission in the United States through universal childhood vaccination. Recommendation of the Immunization Practices Advisory Committee (ACIP). MMWR Morb Mortal Wkly Rep 1991;40(RR-13):1–25.

30. Centers for Disease Control. Immunization of adolescents. Recommendations of the Advisory Committee on Immunization Practices, the American Academy of Pediatrics, the American Academy of Family Physicians and the American Medical Association. MMWR Morb Mortal Wkly Rep 1996;45(No RR-13, Suppl):1–16.

31. Zanolli R, Morgese G. Hepatitis B vaccine: current issues. Ann Pharmacother 1997;31:1059–1067.

32. Centers for Disease Control. Inadequate immune response among public safety workers receiving intradermal vaccination against hepatitis B. MMWR Morb Mortal Wkly Rep 1991;40:569–572.

33. Waite NM, Thomson LG, Goldstein MB. Successful vaccination with intradermal hepatitis B vaccine in hemodialysis patients previously non responsive to intramuscular hepatitis B vaccine. J Am Soc Nephrol 1995;5:1930–1934.

34. Clemens R, Sänger R, Kruppenbacher J, et al. Booster immunisation of low and non-responders after a standard three-dose hepatitis B vaccine schedule — results of a post marketing surveillance. Vaccine 1997;15:349–352.

35. Chriske HW, Bock HL, Clemens R. Immunantwort auf Nachimpfungen mit einer rekombinanten Hepatitis-B-Vakzine bei Low- und non-Respondern. Arbeitsmed Sozialmed Präventivmed 1990;25:421–422.

36. Hilleman M. Vaccine perspectives from the vantage of hepatitis B. Vaccine Res 1992;1:1–15.

37. André FE, Safary A. Summary of clinical findings on Engerix B, a genetically engineered yeast derived hepatitis B vaccine. Postgrad Med J 1987;63(Suppl 2):169–178.

38. Wiedermann G, Ambrosch F, Kremsner P, et al. Reactogenicity and immunogenicity of different lots of a yeast-derived hepatitis B vaccine. Postgrad Med J 1987;63(Suppl 2):109–113.

39. Jilg W, Deinhardt F. Results of immunisation with a recombinant yeast derived hepatitis B vaccine. J Infection 1986;13(Suppl):47–51.

40. World Health Organization. No scientific justification to suspend hepatitis B immunization. Press release, WHO/67 2 Oct 1998.

41. Lack of evidence that hepatitis B vaccine causes multiple sclerosis. Wkly Epidemiol Rec 1997;72:149–156.

42. The Viral Hepatitis Prevention Board. Universal HB immunization by 1997: where are we now? Viral Hepatitis, Fact Sheet 2, Jan 1998:1–6.

43. Chang MH, Chen ChJ, Lai MS, et al. Universal hepatitis B vaccination in Taiwan and the incidence of hepatocellular carcinoma. N Engl J Med 1997;336:1855–1859.

44. Levine MM, Ferrecio C, Black RE, et al. Chilean Typhoid Committee: progress in vaccines against typhoid fever. Rev Infect Dis 1989;11(Suppl):552–567.

45. Levine MM, Taylor DN, Ferrecio C, et al. Tyhpoid vaccines come of age. Pediatr Infect Dis 1989;8:374–381.

46. Levine MM, Ferrecio C, Cryz S, et al. Comparison of enteric coated capsules and liquid formulation of Ty21a typhoid vaccine in a randomized controlled field trial. Lancet 1990; 336:891–894.

47. Simanjuntac CH, Paleologo FP, Punjabi NH, et al. Oral immunisation against typhoid fever in Indonesia with Ty21a vaccine. Lancet 1991;338:1055–1059.

48. Cryz SJ Jr, Que JU, Levine MM, et al. Safety and immunogenicity of a live oral bivalent tyhoid fever (*Salmonella typhi* 21a)-cholera (*Vibrio cholerae* CVD103-HgR) vaccine in healthy adults. Infect Immun 1995;63:1336–1339.

49. Levine MM, Svennerholm AM. Future enteric vaccines. In: Dupont HL, Steffen R, eds. Textbook of travel medicine and health. Hamilton, ON: BC Decker, 1997:1969–1977.

50. Tacket CO, Levine MM, Robbins JB. Persistence of antibody titres three years after vaccination with Vi polysaccharide vaccine against typhoid fever. Vaccine 1988;6:307–308.

51. Acharya IL, Lowe CU, Thapa R, et al. Prevention of typhoid fever in Nepal with the Vi capsular polysaccharide of *Salmonella typhi*. N Engl J Med 1987;317:1101–1104.

52. Klugman KP, Gilbertson IT, Kvornhof HJ, et al. Protective activity of Vi capsular polysaccharide vaccine against typhoid fever. Lancet 1987;21:1165–1169.

53. Arya SC. Typhoid Vi vaccine and infection by Vi-negative strains of *S. typhi*. J Travel Med 1997;4:207.

54. Levine MM, Kaper JB. Live oral vaccines against cholera: an update. Vaccine 1993;11:207–212.

55. Wiedermann G, Kollaritsch H, Jeschko E, et al. Adverse events after oral vaccination against cholera with CVD 103-HgR. Wien Klin Wochenschr 1998;110:376–378.

56. Kollaritsch H, Que JU, Wiedermann G, et al. Safety and immunogenicity of live oral cholera and typhoid vaccines administered alone or in combination with antimalarial drugs, oral polio vaccine or yellow fever vaccine. J Infect Dis 1997;175:871–875.

57. Holmgren G, Osek G, Svennerholm AM. Protective oral cholera vaccine based on a combination of cholera subunit B and inactivated cholera vibrios. In: Wachsmuth IK, Blake PA, Olsvik O, eds. Vibrio cholera and cholera. 1st Ed. Washington, DC: American Society for Microbiology 1994:415–424.

58. Jertborn M, Svennerholm AM, Holmgren G. Safety and immunogenicity of an oral recombinant cholera B subunit whole cell vaccine in Swedish volunteers. Vaccine 1992;10: 130–132.

59. Clemens JD, Sack DA, Harus JR, et al. Field trial of cholera vaccines in Bangladesh: results from 3 year follow up. Lancet 1990;335:270–273.

60. Sanchez JL, Vasquez B, Begue QE, et al. Protection efficacy of oral whole-cell/recombinant-B-subunit cholera vaccine in Peruvian military recruits. Lancet 1994;344:1273–1276.

61. Rennels MB, Glass RI, Dennehy PH, et al. Safety and efficacy of high-dose rhesus-human reassortant rotavirus vaccines — report of the National Multicenter Trial. Pediatrics 1996;97: 7–13.

62. Vesikari T. Clinical experience with rotavirus vaccine in Finland. Presented at the 2nd Satellite Symposium of the 14th Annual Meeting of the European Society of Paediatric Infectious Diseases (ESPID) Elsinore, Denmark, June 18–21, 1996.

63. Pérez-Schael I, Guntinas MJ, Pérez M, et al. Efficacy of the rhesus-rotavirus-based quadrivalent vaccine in infants and young children in Venezuela. N Engl J Med 1997;337: 1181–1187.

64. Europäisches Arzneibuch. 3rd Ed. Stuttgart: Deutscher Apothekerverlag, 1997.

65. Ambrosch F, Fritzell B, Gregor J, et al. Study of tolerance and immunogenicity of combined/associated yellow fever 17D and Vi polysaccharide vaccines in adults. In: Lobel HO, Steffen R, Kozarsky PE, eds. Travel medicine 2. Proceedings of the Second Conference on International Travel Medicine, Atlanta, 1991. International Society of Travel Medicine, 144–145.

66. USPDI drug information for the health care professionals. 18th Ed. Taunton, MA: World Color Book Services, 1998.

67. Quast U, Thilo W, Fescharek R. Impfreaktionen. Stuttgart: Hippokrates, 1997.

68. Centers for Disease Control Recommendations of the Advisory Committee on Immunization Practices (ACIP): rabies prevention, United States. MMWR Morb Mortal Wkly Rep 1991;40(RR-3):1–19.

69. Gerstl F, Maurer W. Die Indikation zur postexpositionellen Tollwutprophylaxe. Österr Ärztezeitung 1991;46:26–36.

70. WHO Expert Committee on Rabies. Guide for post-exposure treatment. 8th report. WHO Technical Report Series 1992:824.

71. Centers for Disease Control Recommendations of the Advisory Committee on Immunization Practices (ACIP): supplementary statement on rabies vaccine and serological testing. MMWR Morb Mortal Wkly Rep 1981;30:535–536.

72. Centers for Disease Control Recommendations of the Advisory Committee on Immunization Practices (ACIP): inactivated Japanese encephalitis vaccine. MMWR Morb Mortal Wkly Rep 1993;40(RR-1):1–15.

73. Physicians' desk reference. 52nd Ed. Montvale, NJ: Medical Economics, 1998.

74. Poland JD, Cropp B, Craven RB, et al. Evaluation of the potency and safety of inactivated Japanese encephalitis vaccine in US inhabitants. J Infect Dis 1990;161:878–882.

75. Kunz Ch. Tick-borne encephalitis in Europe. Acta Leidensia 1992;60(2):1–14.

76. Harabacz I, Bock H, Jüngst CH, et al. A randomized phase II study of a new tick-borne encephalitis vaccine using three different doses and two immunization regimens. Vaccine 1992; 10:145–150.

77. von Hedenström M, Heberle U, Theobald K. Vaccination agaisnt tick-borne encephalitis (TBE): influence of simultaneous application of TBE immunoglobulin on seroconversion and rate of adverse events. Vaccine 1995;13:759–762.

78. James JM, Burks AW, Roberson PK, et al. Safe administration of measles vaccine to children allergic to eggs. N Engl J Med 1995;332:1262–1266.

79. Milstein JB, Gibson JJ. Quality control of BCG vaccine by WHO: a review of factors that may influence vaccine effectiveness and safety. Bull WHO 1990;68:93–108.

80. Development of new vaccines for tuberculosis. Recommendations of the Advisory Committee for the Elimination of

Tuberculosis (ACET). MMWR Morb Mortal Wkly Rep 1998; 47(RR13):1–6.

81. Centers for Disease Control. Human rabies prevention: United States, 1999. Recommendations of the Advisory Committee on Immunization Practices (ACIP). MMWR Morb Mortal Wkly Rep 1999;48(RR-1):1–21.

82. Richie E, Punjabi NH, Sidharta V, et al. Efficacy trial of single dose live oral cholera vaccine CVD 103-HgR in North Jakarta, Indonesia, a cholera endemic area. Vaccine 2000;18: 2399–2410.

83. Nothdurft HD, Jelinek T, Marschang A, et al. Adverse reactions to Japanese encephalitis vaccines. J Infect 1996;32:119–122.

84. Defraites RF, Gambel JM, Hoke CH. Japanese encephalitis vaccine (inactivated, Biken) in U.S. soldiers: immunogenicity and safety of vaccine administered in two dosing regimens. Am J Trop Med Hyg 1999;61:288–293.

22.2 PRINCIPLES AND PRACTICES OF IMMUNOPROPHYLAXIS

ELIZABETH D. BARNETT, MICHEL REY, AND ROBERT T. CHEN

INTRODUCTION

Immunizations are among the most cost-effective medical and public health interventions available. Appropriate immunizations prior to travel can reduce the risk of vaccine-preventable diseases for the individual traveler and may also reduce the risk of international transmission of these diseases. For diseases like poliomyelitis, measles, and diphtheria, which have been or are being eliminated from certain geographic regions, adequate immunization of travelers will also minimize the risk of importation and reintroduction of these diseases.

A consultation for health information prior to travel also presents the health provider with an opportunity to update the traveler's status for immunizations routinely recommended for the general population and to educate the traveler about other health risks that may be encountered, such as diarrhea and malaria, which are not vaccine preventable.

The risk to travelers of contracting diseases depends on destination, duration of the trip, and nature and conditions of travel. The vaccine-preventable disease most commonly contracted by travelers is hepatitis A, which may occur as frequently as 20 cases per 1,000 travelers per month for travelers who are exposed to conditions of poor hygiene. Diseases for which travelers are at low risk include paralytic polio, which is estimated to occur at a rate of 20 per million unimmunized travelers, and Japanese encephalitis, occurring at an estimated rate of less than 1 per million for the usual traveler.[1] Risk of specific diseases may be increased during periods when outbreaks of disease are occurring, such as with meningococcal disease in sub-Saharan Africa, diphtheria in the newly independent states of the former Soviet Union, and yellow fever in parts of Africa and South America. Health information for international travel is now available widely, via print and electronic media, targeted toward both the professional and the consumer. Patients, however, will continue to require advice from well-informed providers to make decisions about their individual risks of contracting disease and potential benefits from immunization based on their specific circumstances and itineraries.

Detailed information about disease epidemiology and vaccine characteristics is presented in other chapters. This chapter will focus on disease risk specific to travelers and considerations taken in choosing whether a traveler is a candidate for specific vaccines. Because national standards for licensure differ, not all of the vaccines are available in all countries. Similarly, recommended vaccine schedules may differ somewhat by manufacturer and by the national authority.

GENERAL CONSIDERATIONS

Several key factors should be considered when planning immunizations for individuals traveling abroad. These include:

1. The detailed itinerary, including countries and regions of travel (rural, urban, or jungle), mode of travel (air or ground), purpose of travel (work or pleasure), type of travel (luxury or adventure), conditions of living (exposure to insects, sanitation available, access to medical care, etc.), and length of stay.

2. A list of vaccinations officially required for entry into all countries on the traveler's itinerary. (Requirements may occasionally change due to local outbreaks and may be subject to interpretation by local border authorities.)

3. A list of vaccine-preventable diseases the traveler may encounter and against which he/she should be immunized. (Information about the risk of disease by

country or region is routinely summarized and published. The actual risk of some diseases to travelers may be so low as to raise questions about the cost effectiveness of some immunizations to both the traveler and to society.[2] Some travelers may request a fuller course of immunizations than perhaps necessary, psychologically and emotionally analogous to purchasing additional travel insurance. Conversely, some travelers may have limited financial resources and may request that travel medicine experts provide specific information about risks of diseases upon which decisions can be made about how to spend their travel vaccine finances. Counseling and assisting the patient on weighing the risks and benefits of immunizations are appropriate in both settings.)

4. A personal immunization history of routine and travel vaccines, including primary series and booster doses.

5. The traveler's medical history, including illnesses, chronic conditions, pregnancy, or medications that may impact on use of and response to vaccinations.

6. The amount of time available prior to departure. (Some vaccines may require multiple doses or may not be given simultaneously with others. A key aspect of the art of travel medicine lies in providing an optimal individualized program of immunizations for each traveler in the time available prior to departure.)

SOURCES OF INFORMATION ON INTERNATIONAL TRAVEL

Sources of up-to-date information about localized outbreaks and changing local requirements are necessary for travelers and individuals advising them and are available in many countries.[3–6] A comprehensive listing of these sources is available in Chapter 8.

Although many primary care providers can and do provide travel vaccines and immunizations, clinics and services specializing in travel medicine are available in the United States, Europe, and other areas. Many clinicians find it helpful to work closely with travel medicine specialists who routinely stock a complete array of travel-related vaccines and who have expertise in advising travelers and knowledge of current recommendations about travel advice and immunizations. Information about locating travel medicine services is available in Chapter 10.

IMMUNIZATION SCHEDULES

Vaccines are generally licensed after they have undergone rigorous phased clinical trials demonstrating their safety and efficacy. The recommendations and contraindications for their use are then developed and updated routinely by national health authorities based on a careful balancing of the benefits, costs, and risks.

Most vaccines require multiple doses in order to produce protective immunity. The usual timetable for administering multiple doses of vaccine may need to be modified for travelers who face imminent departures. The minimum age for initial vaccination and minimum inter-

val between vaccine doses are noted in appropriate sections of the text. Data on efficacy and duration of immunity are summarized in Chapter 22.1.

Because national standards for licensure differ, not all vaccines are available in all countries. Recommendations from national authorities and the manufacturer's package inserts should therefore be consulted for up-to-date information and details, especially side effects and contraindications.

SIMULTANEOUS ADMINISTRATION OF VACCINES, IMMUNOGLOBULINS, AND ANTIMALARIALS

Scheduling the number of vaccines that must be given in a short period of time prior to travel presents a challenge for the practitioner. Fortunately, most antigens can be given simultaneously without compromising efficacy and safety.[7] Inactivated vaccines have been shown not to interfere with the immune response to other inactivated vaccines or to live vaccines and can be given simultaneously or at any time before or after a live vaccine. Most live vaccines may also be administered simultaneously without adversely affecting immune response, with one exception. The antibody responses to parenteral cholera and yellow fever vaccines may be lowered if given simultaneously or within 3 weeks of each other. Unless there are time constraints, yellow fever and parenteral cholera vaccines are best given when separated by at least a 3-week interval. Other live vaccines not administered on the same day should be administered more than 30 days apart in order to avoid the theoretical possibility of impairment of immune response to both vaccines. The only exceptions are oral polio vaccine (OPV) and measles, mumps, and rubella (MMR) vaccine, which can be administered before, with, or after each other.

Some travelers will receive immune globulin for protection against hepatitis A. Antibody responses to live vaccines could be diminished if given simultaneously with immune globulin. In general, live vaccines should be given either 2 weeks before or a minimum of 6 weeks, and preferably 3 months, after immune globulin, with the following exception. Immune globulin has not been shown to interfere with response to either OPV, yellow fever vaccine, or oral typhoid vaccine.[8,9] If there are time constraints, live vaccines may be given at the same time, at a body site remote from the immune globulin, recognizing that vaccine-induced immunity may not be optimal. For individuals who receive immune globulin at higher doses, more time may be required between immune globulin and vaccine.[8,10]

Live vaccines may interfere with an individual's response to tuberculin testing. Testing should be done ideally either prior to the live vaccine administration or a minimum of 4 to 6 weeks later.

Side effects may be accentuated when multiple vaccines are given simultaneously. When multiple immunizations are needed, separating those known for causing the most adverse effects may be considered if this will not adversely affect compliance with the full series of immunizations. Patients may take acetaminophen in the office at the time of administration of vaccines.

EFFECT OF ANTIMALARIALS AND ANTIMICROBIAL AGENTS ON VACCINE RESPONSE

Antimalarials in the chloroquine/mefloquine family, when administered simultaneously with human diploid cell rabies vaccine and oral typhoid vaccine, may interfere with their immunogenicity. Antimicrobial agents taken concurrently with oral typhoid vaccine may interfere with vaccine response. Ideally, the complete course of four doses of oral typhoid vaccine should be taken before initiating antimalarials. If this is not possible, the schedule of alternate-day administration of the four oral typhoid vaccine capsules should be altered so that capsules of Ty21a oral typhoid vaccine are not taken on the day when the weekly dose of chloroquine or mefloquine is taken. Rabies human diploid cell vaccine (HDCV) should not be administered by the intradermal dose or route when antimalarials in the chloroquine/mefloquine family are used. Although chloroquine has been shown to inhibit the replication of yellow fever virus in vitro, it does not appear to affect adversely the antibody response to yellow fever vaccine in vivo.[11]

IMMUNIZATION FOR INDIVIDUALS WITH SPECIAL CONSIDERATIONS: ALTERED IMMUNOCOMPETENCE

Special considerations are needed in immunizing persons with altered immunocompetence (including those with malignancies, with congenital or acquired immune-deficiency states, or receiving therapy with steroids, antimetabolites, radiation, or alkylating agents) because of the risk of complications after administration of live bacterial or viral vaccines to such individuals. Detailed recommendations regarding immunization of immunocompromised individuals are published elsewhere; information specific to immunocompromised travelers is discussed here.[12,13]

Because of the risk to immunocompromised individuals of acquiring paralytic polio or the possibility of transmission of OPV organisms, inactivated polio vaccine (IPV) should be given instead to immunocompromised individuals and to those, especially children, living in households with immunocompromised individuals. Steroid therapy that is short term (<2 weeks) and low to moderate dose (<20 mg/day or, for children, <2 mg/kg/day of prednisone), long-term therapy that is given on alternate days, and intra-articular, bursal, or tendon injection of corticosteroids in usual doses are not contraindications to live vaccine administration. Individuals whose immunosuppressive therapy with steroids has been stopped for 1 month or who have not received chemotherapy for 3 or more months may also receive live vaccines.

Persons with HIV infection, including children, should receive routine immunizations on schedule, with the following exceptions. IPV should be substituted for OPV for both the immunocompromised individual and for family members. Varicella vaccine is contraindicated, and, until more information is available about use of the recently licensed rotavirus vaccine, this vaccine is contraindicated in immune-compromised children. MMR should be given to all asymptomatic HIV-infected individuals when indicated and may be considered for selected symptomatic individuals when the risk of exposure to measles is high, as measles infection may be severe in the immunocompromised.

Immune response to vaccines may be suboptimal in immunocompromised individuals and antibody levels may wane more rapidly.[14,15] Such individuals should be informed that they may continue to be at increased risk and to take whatever measures available to prevent exposures.

IMMUNIZATION DURING ACUTE ILLNESS

Minor illnesses need not be contraindications to immunization. It is prudent to defer administration of vaccines during moderate to severe fevers or other illnesses because of the possibility of diminished immune response, the superimposition of vaccine side effects on disease symptoms, and the potential difficulty of distinguishing between a vaccine adverse event and a symptom of the illness. Routine temperature measurement is not needed prior to vaccination for individuals who are well.

ROUTINE CHILDHOOD AND ADULT IMMUNIZATIONS AND MODIFICATIONS NEEDED FOR TRAVELERS

Routine childhood and adult immunizations should be brought up to date as part of preparation for international travel. Information is available from many sources about routine immunizations; readers are referred to country-specific schedules for this information. In the United States, a schedule of recommended routine childhood immunizations is published every 12 months,[16] and information about adolescent[17] and adult[18,19] immunization is widely available. Country-specific vaccination schedules are available widely through local and national health departments. Information about accelerated schedules, for travelers with imminent departures, and about catch-up immunization, for those who have missed routine immunizations, is also available.[8] Table 22.2–1 lists vaccines recommended routinely for adults and children in many parts of the world, with areas of the world of greatest risk and specific indications for travelers. Most diseases listed are prevalent worldwide, although the risks of contracting these diseases may vary markedly depending on travel destination.

VACCINES FOR TRAVEL: SELECTED ROUTINE IMMUNIZATION ESPECIALLY IMPORTANT FOR TRAVELERS

DIPHTHERIA

In the preimmunization era, diphtheria was a major killer. Beginning in 1990, a major resurgence occurred in the former Soviet Union, with cases seen in travelers.[20,21] Epidemics of diphtheria have occurred in Thailand, Algeria, and Ecuador.[22] Although the risk of diphtheria to the typical traveler is very small, it is known that immunity to disease has waned in some areas where diphtheria has been under control for many years. This has occurred because of both a decrease in natural disease and decreased vaccine coverage. In the United States, 20% to 60% of adults over the age of 20 are susceptible to diphtheria,[23,24] and in Western Europe, serologic surveys have shown immunity to diphtheria to be poor among adults, particularly women, as men may be given boosters during military service.[25] Resurgence of disease in areas where diphtheria has previously been well controlled, coupled with recent increases in migrant populations, may result in transmission of disease into populations where there are

Table 22.2–1. VACCINATIONS RECOMMENDED ROUTINELY FOR CHILDREN AND ADULTS WITH SPECIAL INDICATIONS FOR TRAVELERS

DISEASE	VACCINE	AGE GROUPS	GREATEST AREAS OF RISK	SPECIAL INDICATIONS
Diphtheria	DTaP, DTP, or DT Td Multiple combinations*	<7 yr ≥7 yr	Developing world; countries of former U.S.S.R.	
Tetanus	DTaP or DTP Td Multiple combinations*	<7 yr ≥7 yr	Worldwide	
Pertussis	DTaP or DTP Multiple combinations*	<7 yr	Worldwide circulation of organism	No vaccine available for ≥7 yr
Polio	IPV and/or OPV IPV only Multiple combinations*	<18 yr and previously vaccinated adults Unvaccinated adults and immunocompromised individuals; all U.S. individuals as of January 1, 2000	Most developing world except Americas	Extra dose of IPV or OPV if previously fully immunized for persons traveling to areas of risk
Measles	MMR, MR, M	All ages for susceptibles	Most of the world	2nd dose indicated if no prior history of 2 doses on or after first birthday. Most persons born prior to 1957 can be considered immune and do not need vaccination.
Mumps	MMR, MR, M	All ages for susceptibles	Most of the world	
Rubella	MMR or MR	All ages for susceptibles	Most of the world	
Haemophilus influenzae type b	Hib Multiple combinations*	<5 yr	Most of the world	
Hepatitis B	Hepatitis B	Routine childhood and adolescent; older ages with special risk	Most of the world (see Figure 22.2–1 for areas most at risk)	Stays of ≥6 mo in developing countries or with occupational or behavioral risk factors for disease
Tuberculosis	BCG	Routine childhood and adult in some countries	Developing world	See text
Varicella	Varicella	All ages for susceptibles	Most of the world	
Influenza	Influenza	1 dose annually for ≥65 yr. Also younger for individuals of any age with risk factors such as chronic cardiac or pulmonary disease.	Most of the world	Northern Hemisphere season Dec. through Mar.; Southern Hemisphere season Apr. through Sept.
Pneumococcal	Pneumococcal polysaccharide Pneumococcal conjugate	All adults ≥65 yr. Also for individuals of any age with risk factors such as chronic cardiac or pulmonary disease. All children <24 mo in some countries	Most of the world	

*Availability of combination vaccines may vary by country. Practitioners should check resources for vaccines available in their specific countries.

individuals at risk for diphtheria. Travelers to these areas may be at increased risk as well. The travel consultation is an opportunity to bring every individual up to date with diphtheria immunization; a booster dose of combined diphtheria-tetanus toxoids (Td) every 10 years is acceptable in most countries. Specific vaccine formulations containing diphtheria toxoid are discussed in detail in Chapter 22.1.

TETANUS

The travel consultation is an opportunity for updating tetanus immunization. Unimmunized adults require three doses, and others require boosters every 10 years (see Table 22.1–1).

PERTUSSIS

Pertussis continues to be a disease of worldwide importance, affecting more than 50 million people and resulting in more than 500,000 deaths, despite widespread availability of vaccine.[26] Attack rates of pertussis are directly related to use of vaccine; following declines in the use of vaccines in Japan, Sweden, and Britain, resurgence of disease was noted.[27] The increased increment of risk for pertussis due to international travel is unknown. Children should complete as much of a primary series as possible or be given any boosters due prior to international travel.[28] Primary immunization for individuals 7 years of age may begin in infants 4 weeks of age, with three doses of combined diphtheria, tetanus, and pertussis vaccine administered at 4- to 8-week intervals. A minimum of two doses of pertussis vaccine is needed to confer some protection. In certain countries, boosting doses are administered during the second year of life and also at primary school entry. Acellular pertussis vaccines, now marketed in many areas, hold promise for equivalent or better efficacy than whole-cell preparations, with fewer side effects. Although there is substantial interest in protecting adults, currently, adults are not candidates for pertussis vaccine.

POLIOMYELITIS VACCINE (ORAL POLIO VACCINE), INACTIVATED POLIO VACCINE

The last case of paralytic polio due to wild-type poliovirus occurred in the Americas in 1991, and the Western Hemisphere was declared polio-free in 1994.[29] The program for worldwide polio eradication is proceeding rapidly. There remain, however, areas of the world where polio occurs, mainly in sub-Saharan Africa and some parts of South Asia, and maintaining adequate levels of immunization against polio remains important for travelers to these areas. Risk for polio to the unimmunized traveler to developing countries where polio occurs has been estimated to be 0.002% for asymptomatic disease and 0.0001% for paralytic disease.[30] Two safe and immunogenic vaccines are available, the oral and the inactivated polio vaccines. In most countries, OPV is used in all infants and children <18 years old without contraindications (e.g., immunodeficiency in the recipient or their household members). IPV is preferred for inadequately

immunized adults. In some countries, IPV is used for everyone. In the United States, an all inactivated polio vaccine schedule became effective January 1, 2000. Until January 1, 2001, OPV would be acceptable in some limited circumstances including the situation of unvaccinated children traveling in less than 4 weeks to a polio-endemic area.[31]

Travelers who have not completed a primary series should do so prior to departure. If time is a limiting factor, at least one dose of vaccine should be given prior to travel, with the rest completed upon arrival at 4-week intervals. If an infant travels prior to 6 weeks of age, a dose of vaccine should be given but not counted as part of the primary series. Those who have completed their childhood series and are traveling to an endemic area should be given, once, a single additional dose of OPV/IPV.

MEASLES, MUMPS, AND RUBELLA VACCINE

Measles is a major cause of morbidity and mortality in many developing countries. Mumps can cause parotitis, orchitis, and meningoencephalitis. Rubella can cause congenital rubella syndrome when pregnant women are infected. All three diseases remain endemic or epidemic in most countries worldwide. Good protection is conferred by receipt of combination MMR vaccine, or, if not available, by the individual antigen vaccines. In most developed countries, MMR vaccine is administered to all children at 12 to 15 months of age; in many countries, a second dose is also administered at a later age. Most infants 6 months of age should remain protected by maternally derived antibodies. Children 6 to 11 months of age traveling to a high-incidence area should receive an additional dose of single measles antigen vaccine (or, if not available, MMR) prior to departure. Such children should continue MMR vaccinations per routine schedule either upon arrival or return. Adults born before 1957 are assumed to have natural immunity and usually do not need immunization. Younger adults traveling to endemic areas can receive a single dose of MMR vaccine, although two doses at least 28 days apart are preferable.

HAEMOPHILUS INFLUENZAE TYPE B CONJUGATE VACCINE

Haemophilus influenzae type b is a leading cause of bacterial meningitis and other invasive bacterial disease in children worldwide. *Haemophilus influenzae* type b conjugate vaccines (HbCVs) are licensed for use in infants. Routine vaccination is recommended beginning at 2 months of age for all infants but may begin as early as 6 weeks of age if necessary. The number and timing of remaining doses depend on the type of conjugate vaccine used. Children <15 months of age should receive at least two vaccine doses prior to travel at an interval as short as 4 weeks apart. If vaccination is started at >6 months of age, fewer doses may be required. If previously unvaccinated, children less than 15 months of age should receive ideally at least two vaccine doses at least 4 weeks apart prior to travel. Healthy children between 15 months and

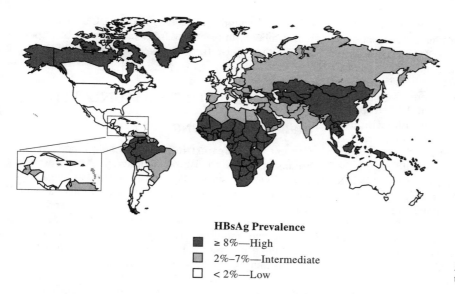

HBsAg Prevalence

- ◼ ≥ 8%—High
- ◼ 2%–7%—Intermediate
- ☐ < 2%—Low

Figure 22.2–1.   Geographic distribution of hepatitis B prevalence.[4]

5 years of age who have not been immunized previously need a single dose of vaccine.

HEPATITIS B VACCINE

Hepatitis B is one of the most common serious vaccine-preventable diseases to affect travelers. Worldwide prevalence of hepatitis B is shown in Figure 22.2–1. Risk of contracting hepatitis B is increased with longer length of stay, contact with population groups with high carrier rates of hepatitis B, occupations such as health care workers or laboratory workers, and behaviors such as injecting drug use and having multiple sex partners. For Swiss tourists traveling to developing countries, risk was reported to be 39/100,000 travelers for a stay of 1 month.[30] Long-term overseas workers are at greater risk; unimmunized U.S. missionaries serving in Africa were shown to have attack rates of 11% during the first 2 years of service and median annual attack rates of 1.2% over the next decade.[32] Professional workers in developing countries had a monthly incidence of symptomatic disease of 20 to 60/100,000.[33]

Consequences of hepatitis B virus (HBV) infection can range from asymptomatic illness to fulminant illness and death. Hepatitis B vaccine is safe and highly effective in preventing the acute and chronic consequences of HBV infection. Three intramuscular doses are required to produce a protective antibody response in more than 95% of infants, children, and adolescents and in more than 90% of healthy adults. In many countries, including the United States, routine infant immunization with hepatitis B vaccine is now recommended. Individuals without prior immunity to HBV, either from natural infection or vaccination, and who are traveling to areas of high HBV endemicity for 6 months should receive the three-dose series of vaccine. If insufficient time is available for three doses prior to travel, two doses given a minimum of 1 month apart may provide some protection. The risk of contracting HBV infection is likely to be low for most individuals traveling to endemic countries for less than 6 months. Immunization can be considered, however, for travelers who may have increased risk of exposure, such as health care workers, those who may have sexual contact with potentially infected individuals, individuals who might receive injections, and children who may have continuous close contact with local children who may have open skin lesions.

Demyelinating disease and autoimmune disorders have been reported after hepatitis B vaccination.[34] Epidemiologic studies are still needed, however, to assess whether these associations are causal, coincidental, or triggering of disease in genetically susceptible individuals.[35]

VARICELLA

Varicella vaccine has been incorporated into the schedule of routine childhood immunizations in the United States. Currently, risk of varicella to travelers may not be higher than risk at home, but this may change as vaccine coverage increases and opportunities for exposure decrease. Children should be brought up to date with varicella immunization during the visit for travel advice and immunization. Adults and children who have not been immunized previously can be asked about history of disease; some of these individuals may be candidates for serotesting prior to immunization, particularly those ≥13 years of age who will require two doses of vaccine for complete protection.

Vaccine is contraindicated in immunocompromised individuals and pregnant women, and specific guidelines should be consulted before immunizing individuals taking medications that alter immune function.[36]

BACILLE CALMETTE-GUÉRIN

Bacille Calmette-Guérin (BCG) is a live attenuated vaccine against tuberculosis (TB). It is a lyophilized preparation, which is injected by the intradermal route or multipuncture. It may be given simultaneously, at a separate site, with all other vaccines and immune globulin. Many

BCG vaccines are available throughout the world today. Community trials have reported vaccine efficacies ranging from 0% to 80% protection against TB, depending on vaccine strain and social, nutritional, and environmental characteristics of the test population.[37] Vaccine efficacy studies in newborns have reported protective efficacy against all forms of TB ranging from 17% to 90%, although protection against miliary, bone, or joint disease and tuberculous meningitis may be 75% or more.[38] A recent meta-analysis of 70 studies of BCG efficacy concluded that, on average, BCG vaccine could reduce the risk of tuberculosis by 50%.[39] In addition, BCG vaccination may provide some protection against leprosy.[40] In some countries, such as the United States, a program of surveillance using tuberculin skin testing and early identification and treatment of infected individuals is preferred over universal immunization with BCG.[41]

Estimates of risk for tuberculosis among travelers are difficult to obtain. Studies of military personnel who served during the war in Vietnam cite annual skin test conversion rates of 4.7%, compared with rates of 1% per year for Army personnel who remained in the U.S.[42] A study performed in California reported that tuberculin skin testing was 4.7 times more likely to be positive in children who had traveled outside the United States; it was also 2.4 times more likely to be positive in children who had a household visitor from countries having a high prevalence of tuberculosis.[43] Transmission of tuberculosis aboard commercial airplanes has been described.[44] The risk of acquiring infection in this manner is felt to be extremely low, and in one study risk of acquiring tuberculosis on an aircraft during the second half of 1994 was estimated to be 1 in every 9 million passengers, with 1 of every 26,000 passengers at risk for being exposed on the aircraft to an individual with active tuberculosis.[45] Risk to travelers is not felt to be high enough to warrant routine immunization of travelers. Health care providers may be asked to provide BCG immunization to individuals who will be living for extended periods of time where BCG vaccine is used routinely. BCG vaccination is not recommended as a routine strategy for TB control in the United States.[41] BCG might be considered, however, for individuals, especially children, who are to be long-term residents of areas where the incidence of disease is high (more than 30–40/100,000), and where occupation or living conditions may result in significant and unavoidable exposures to infected individuals. Because the protective effect of BCG has been confirmed mainly in children, it is unlikely that there would be many indications for BCG for adults who are traveling.

The major contraindication to immunization with BCG is congenital or acquired immunodeficiency because of the risk of dissemination of infection. Although BCG is contraindicated for individuals seropositive for HIV and symptomatic, it may be given to children who are HIV infected and asymptomatic, or whose status is unknown, in areas of the world where there is a high risk of TB.

BCG may be given to infants under 2 months of age without tuberculin skin testing if the infant is known not to have been exposed. Older individuals may be immunized following documentation of a negative tuberculin skin test. A major disadvantage of prior BCG vaccination is that tuberculin reactivity from vaccine may be impossible to distinguish from that produced by infection.

ROUTINE ADULT IMMUNIZATIONS

INFLUENZA VACCINE

Immunization against influenza is recommended for groups at increased risk of complications from disease and individuals, such as health care workers or household members, who might transmit disease to those at high risk. Individuals at greatest risk include persons ≥65 years of age and individuals of any age who are residents of chronic care facilities, have chronic pulmonary or cardiovascular disease, including asthma, are on long-term aspirin therapy, or have other chronic diseases putting them at risk for severe disease.[46] Influenza vaccine is underused in both adults and children who are candidates for vaccine.[47,48]

The risk of exposure to influenza during foreign travel is variable, depending on the season and destination. In the tropics, transmission occurs throughout the year, whereas peaks of transmission occur from December through March in the Northern Hemisphere and April through September in the Southern Hemisphere. Influenza vaccine is made by including strains thought most likely to cause disease in the next transmission season and is made available in the appropriate season. A visit for travel preparation is an opportunity to immunize individuals who are at risk and may not have been immunized previously. Recently, summer outbreaks of influenza in the Northern Hemisphere have highlighted the need for heightened surveillance for the role of influenza in outbreaks of respiratory disease and the role international travel may play in the spread of influenza.[49,50] Visitors from the tropics, where disease transmission occurs year round, and those who travel between Northern and Southern Hemispheres, which have opposite influenza seasons, are potential transmitters of influenza at times when local disease activity may be low.[51] Influenza vaccine should be offered to individuals at risk for influenza or its complications prior to travel if they were not immunized during the previous season or if they plan to travel to the tropics, travel with a large organized tour group at any time during the year, or travel to the opposite hemisphere during influenza season.[52]

Currently available influenza vaccine is an inactivated egg-grown preparation that usually produces high postvaccination antibody titers in most children and young adults. When there is good antigenic match between vaccine and circulating virus, influenza vaccine prevents illness in 70% to 90% of healthy individuals <65 years of age.[53] Children 12 years of age and under should receive only split virus vaccine (two doses of 0.25 mL IM for children 6 to 35 months of age, two doses of 0.5 mL IM for those 3 to 8 years, and one dose of 0.5 mL IM for those 9–12 years). Individuals over age 12 can receive whole or split virus vaccine, a single 0.5-mL dose given intramuscularly.

Adverse reactions to vaccination can include soreness at the vaccination site or one of two types of systemic reactions: fever, malaise, and myalgia, which begin 6 to 12 hours after immunization, or immediate reactions including hives, angioedema, wheezing, or anaphylaxis. Individuals with allergy to eggs should not be immunized without consulting a physician. A live attenuated, cold-adapted, trivalent intranasally administered influenza vaccine is being developed and holds promise for improving adherence to influenza vaccine recommendations.[54]

PNEUMOCOCCAL VACCINE

Disease caused by *Streptococcus pneumoniae*, including sepsis, pneumonia, and meningitis, occurs worldwide. The presence of penicillin-resistant strains of pneumococcus in many parts of the world provides further impetus to protect by immunization individuals susceptible to severe pneumococcal disease.

Pneumococcal vaccine is indicated currently for healthy adults ≥65 years of age, younger adults who have any chronic illness, such as cardiovascular or pulmonary disease, which may result in increased morbidity with respiratory infections, or individuals at increased risk of invasive pneumococcal disease, such as those with sickle cell anemia, functional or anatomic asplenia, nephrotic syndrome or chronic renal failure, immunosuppressive conditions, HIV infection, or cerebrospinal fluid leaks.[55] A recent study that demonstrated the efficacy of the vaccine in preventing invasive pneumococcal infections in immunocompetent patients with indications for its administration also suggested that the vaccine is currently underused in this group of patients.[56] The pretravel consultation is an opportunity to immunize individuals for whom the vaccine is indicated. Clinicians may also wish to consider immunization of individuals who will be traveling to areas where significant antibiotic resistance is present.

The currently available pneumococcal polysaccharide vaccine consists of purified capsular polysaccharide antigens of 23 pneumococcal serotypes. These serotypes cause 88% of cases of bacteremia and meningitis in adults and nearly 100% of cases of bacteremia and meningitis in children. Pneumococcal polysaccharide vaccine has limited immunogenicity in children younger than 2 years. In the United States, a 7-valent pneumococcal conjugate vaccine was licensed in February 2000 and is recommended routinely for all children under 24 months of age and for some children at high risk up to 59 months of age.[57] Children 2 years of age or older in other countries should be vaccinated with pneumococcal polysaccharide vaccine if they have any of the risk features previously mentioned. The dose of vaccine is 0.5 mL given subcutaneously or intramuscularly.

IMMUNIZATIONS FOR TRAVELERS

CHOLERA VACCINE

Cholera is a bacterial illness that may result in severe and life-threatening dehydration due to diarrhea and vomiting but is easily treatable with prompt rehydration. Currently, the world is in the midst of the seventh pandemic of cholera, which began in Asia in the early 1960s and spread to Africa, Europe, and Oceania and, in 1991, appeared in Peru and spread rapidly throughout Latin America. Cholera is caused by the bacterium *Vibrio cholerae* O1, transmitted through contaminated water and food. Recently, a new serogroup of *V. cholerae*, *V. cholerae* O139, has been implicated as the cause of epidemic disease in Bangladesh, India, and Thailand[58–61] and has caused infections in travelers.[59] Currently available vaccines that produce immunity to O1 strains, and natural immunity to the O1 type, are not protective against O139.[62]

The risk of cholera is very low for travelers; the disease is estimated to occur in 0.2 to 44 per 100,000 travelers.[63,64] Cholera surveillance data in the United States from 1992 to 1994 identified 160 cases of cholera; the estimated cholera rate among persons arriving in the U.S. from cholera-affected regions was 0.27 case per 100,000.[64] The mainstay of prevention of cholera is avoidance of high-risk foods, such as raw shellfish, and use of precautions when making other food selections. Unchlorinated water is also a common source of infection.

There are three vaccines against cholera available in different parts of the world. A parenteral, inactivated bacteria preparation that has been demonstrated to have an efficacy of 50% in reducing clinical illness in field trials in endemic areas is the only vaccine available in the United States. It does not prevent excretion of the *V. cholerae* bacteria or inapparent infection, and its protection lasts only 3 to 6 months, thereby limiting its public health value. A live vaccine prepared from a genetically engineered, attenuated *V. cholerae* O1 strain (CVD 103-HgR) is marketed in Europe, as well as an inactivated oral vaccine.

At this time, no country officially requires cholera vaccination as a condition of entry. Neither the World Health Organization (WHO) nor any country-specific immunization guidelines recommend routine immunization with cholera vaccine because of the low risk to travelers of contracting cholera, the ability to treat the disease effectively, and the limitations of most of the currently available vaccines.[66–69] Occasionally, some travelers report that they have been required to provide documentation of cholera immunization to obtain a visa; travelers to Mecca in particular have been faced with this issue. Occasionally, travel medicine providers may see the rare individual for whom vaccination is appropriate, such as someone who plans to work or live for extended periods of time in areas where cholera is highly endemic. Recommended vaccine schedules are available in Tables 22.2–2 and 22.2–3. If vaccine is to be given solely for the purpose of satisfying requirements of local authorities, a single dose is sufficient. Vaccination is not recommended for infants less than 6 months of age. Exclusive breastfeeding, or preparation of formula with boiled water, should be protective. Immunization is not recommended during pregnancy; specific safety information about use of cholera vaccine during pregnancy is not available. Side effects of the injectable vaccine include

Table 22.2–2.   CHOLERA VACCINES: INACTIVATED WHOLE CELL

DOSES	INTRADERMAL ROUTE*	SUBCUTANEOUS OR INTRAMUSCULAR ROUTE			COMMENTS
	≥5 YEARS OF AGE	6 MONTHS– 4 YEARS OF AGE	5–10 YEARS OF AGE	>10 YEARS OF AGE	
Primary series: 1 and 2	0.2 mL	0.2 mL	0.3 mL	0.5 mL	Give 1 week–1 month or more apart
Booster	0.2 mL	0.2 mL	0.3 mL	0.5 mL	1 dose every 6 months

*Higher levels of protection (antibody) may be achieved in children <5 years of age by the subcutaneous or intramuscular routes.

local pain and swelling, fever, and malaise and occur in 10% to 20% of vaccines.

Vaccination may provide a false sense of security to travelers, and vaccinated individuals should be advised specifically that the limited efficacy of the vaccine is easily overwhelmed and that the vaccine cannot substitute for other more effective prevention measures. Treatment of cholera is rapid replacement of fluids and electrolytes.[70] Prompt attention to fluid management during the recent outbreak in Peru resulted in a case fatality rate of less than 1%.

Antibody response to parenteral cholera and yellow fever vaccines may be impaired if these two vaccines are given simultaneously or separated by less than 3 weeks from each other; when possible, doses of these vaccines should be separated by at least 3 weeks. Live oral cholera vaccine may be given concurrently with oral typhoid, yellow fever, and oral polio vaccines.[71,72] Simultaneous administration of live oral cholera vaccine and the antimalarials mefloquine and chloroquine may adversely affect immune response to vaccine[68]; ideally, the vaccine series should be completed before beginning malaria prophylaxis with these agents.

HEPATITIS A VACCINE

Hepatitis A is one of the most common vaccine-preventable diseases to affect travelers. Prevalence of hepatitis A throughout the world is shown in Figure 22.2–2. For unimmunized short-term travelers to areas of hepatitis A endemicity, risk has been estimated to range from 3 to 109/1,000 travelers, for stays ranging from 2 weeks to 1 month.[73] For long-term travelers such as missionaries, attack rates were as high as 28% during the first 2 years of service.[74] Risk for disease depends on length of stay and conditions of travel, including frequency of exposure to contaminated food and water. Cases of hepatitis A, however, have been reported in tourists staying in luxury accommodation in countries where risk of hepatitis A is high.[75]

In developing countries, almost universal infection occurs during childhood, when the disease tends to be subclinical or mild. Older children and adults, however, may have greater morbidity, with more than 75% of adults developing symptomatic disease lasting 1 to 3 months. Mortality may be as high as 3% in the elderly or in individuals with underlying liver disease.[76] In many developed countries, the transmission of hepatitis A virus has declined significantly with improving hygiene and sanitation. Individuals born in Europe or North America since World War II have a low prevalence of immunity to hepatitis A. Rates of immunity are higher with increased age, history of jaundice, and birth or residence in a developing country. Up to 95% of individuals born and raised in developing countries with patterns of high endemicity for hepatitis A may be protected by naturally acquired antibody.[77]

Options for immunoprophylaxis of hepatitis A include intramuscular immunoglobulin and hepatitis A vaccine (Tables 22.2–4 and 22.2–5). Immune globulin was the mainstay of protection for many years and has been shown to be 85% to 90% protective. The major disadvantage of immune globulin is that it is short-acting and must be repeated for subsequent journeys or additional doses given during prolonged residence in endemic areas. Adverse events are rare, although the large volume required may result in local discomfort. One advantage of this preparation is that it may be given immediately prior to departure, and it is the only option for individuals with imminent departures (in < 2 weeks) and for children under 2 years of age.

Several vaccines for hepatitis A have been licensed in various countries throughout the world.[78,79] Hepatitis A vaccines have been demonstrated to be safe and immunogenic in adults and children 2 years of age and older.[72,80–86] Protective antibody levels developed in 94% to 100% of adults 1 month after the first dose, and individuals can be assumed to be protected 4 weeks after the first dose of vaccine. Few data are available about timing of appearance of neutralizing antibody. In a sample of vaccinated adults, neutralizing antibody was detected in 54% to 62% 14 days after the first dose and in 94% to 100% at 28 days after the dose.[87]

Table 22.2–3.   CHOLERA VACCINES: ORAL VACCINES

TYPE	DOSE	NUMBER OF DOSES	SCHEDULE	BOOSTER INTERVAL
Live	1 sachet	1	—	2 yr
Inactivated	1 sachet	2	0, 7–42 d	10 mo

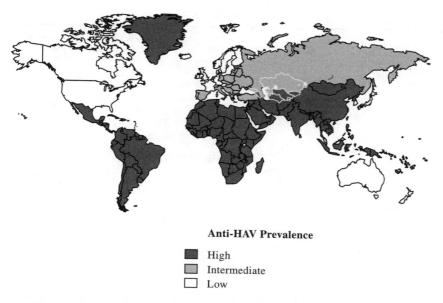

Anti-HAV Prevalence

■ High
▨ Intermediate
□ Low

Figure 22.2–2. Geographic distribution of HAV infection.[4]

Hepatitis A vaccine should be administered a minimum of 4 weeks prior to travel. Travelers departing in less than 2 weeks should receive immune globulin for immediate protection against hepatitis A. If long-term protection is desired, vaccine may be administered simultaneously, at a separate site. Use of vaccine in addition to immune globulin in this setting may be most cost effective when the traveler will be making five or more trips to hepatitis A endemic areas within the next 10 years.[88]

Few data are available regarding risk of hepatitis A in those immunized 2 to 4 weeks before departure. Although vaccine licensure information indicates that vaccines provide protection by 2 weeks after immunization, travelers to high-risk areas will be optimally protected by receiving immune globulin in addition to vaccine. A second dose of vaccine administered according to the appropriate schedule is necessary for long-term (up to 20 years) protection. All travelers should be advised about food and water precautions.

Hepatitis A vaccine is generally safe and well tolerated. When local reactions, such as soreness at the injection site, or general symptoms, such as fatigue or headache, occur, they are generally mild and short-lasting. Although

risk of vaccination during pregnancy should be low, risk of disease must be weighed against theoretical risk of immunization. Vaccine is inactivated and therefore may be used in immunocompromised individuals.

There are no specific contraindications to administering hepatitis A vaccines with other vaccines. Simultaneous administration of hepatitis A vaccine and diphtheria, oral and inactivated polio vaccines, tetanus, oral typhoid, cholera, Japanese encephalitis (JE), rabies, or yellow fever vaccines does not impair immune response to either vaccine or increase adverse events.[89] A recent study from Australia demonstrated safety of hepatitis A vaccine in HIV-infected men.[90]

Testing for susceptibility to hepatitis A before offering vaccine or immune globulin may be cost effective in specific situations. Candidates for testing may include individuals born during or before World War II in developed countries, individuals born and raised in areas of high endemicity,[77] and those with a history of jaundice. Other considerations include cost of testing compared with cost of immunization and ensuring that testing will not delay the ability to provide immunization if an individual is seronegative. It is estimated that if the cost of screening is one-third the cost of immunization and the

Table 22.2–4.   IMMUNE GLOBULIN FOR PROTECTION AGAINST VIRAL HEPATITIS A

| LENGTH OF STAY | BODY WEIGHT | | DOSE VOLUME† | COMMENTS |
	lb	kg*		
Short-term travel (<3 mo)	<50	<23	0.5 mL	Dose volume depends on body weight and length of stay
	50–100	23–45	1.0 mL	
	>100	>45	2.0 mL	
Long-term travel (3–5 mo)	<22	<10	0.5 mL	
	<50	<23	1.0 mL	
	50–100	23–45	2.5 mL	
	>100	>45	5.0 mL	

*kg = approximately 2.2 lbs.
† For intramuscular injection.

Table 22.2–5. RECOMMENDED DOSES OF HEPATITIS A VACCINES

VACCINE	GROUP	AGE (YR)	DOSE	VOLUME	NUMBER OF DOSES	SCHEDULE (MO)[†]
HAVRIX™ (SmithKline Beecham Biologicals)	Children and adolescents*	2–18	720 EL.U.	0.5 mL	2	0, 6–12
	Adults	>18	1,440 EL.U.	1.0 mL	2	0, 6–12
VAQTA™ (Merck and Co.)	Children and adolescents	2–17	25 U	0.5 mL	2	0, 6–18
	Adults	>17	50 U	1.0 mL	2	0, 6
AVAXIM™ (Pasteur Mérieux Connaught)	Adults	≥16	160 U	0.5 mL	2	0, 6–18

*An alternate formulation and schedule (three doses) is available for children and adolescents and consists of 360 EL.U. per 0.5-mL dose at 0, 1, and 6–12 months of age.
EL.U. = ELISA units, U = units.
[†]0 months represents timing of the initial dose; subsequent numbers represent months after the initial dose.

individual's likelihood of immunity is greater than 33%, testing should be cost effective.[91]

JAPANESE B ENCEPHALITIS VACCINE

JE is a mosquito-borne arboviral infection that affects primarily school-aged children and the elderly, with high fatality and frequent permanent neurologic sequelae.[92] Over 10,000 cases are reported annually from China, and major outbreaks have occurred in northeastern India and Southeast Asia. Thousands of cases occur annually in northern Thailand, and JE is also recognized in Nepal, Bangladesh, Sri Lanka, Hong Kong, Korea, Japan, Taiwan, the Philippines, Japan, and eastern Russia.[93] Risk to travelers is low, with estimates of risk ranging from <1 per million to 1 in 500 per month of exposure in rural endemic areas. Most travelers have no natural immunity to the disease. Although risk is highest for individuals who travel during the high transmission season and remain in endemic areas for extended periods of time, cases have occurred in short-stay tourists.[94–96]

The principal vector of transmission of JE is the mosquito *Culex triataeniorhynchus*, which bites primarily from dusk to dawn.[97] Transmission occurs during the summer and early fall in temperate regions. In subtropical and tropical areas, transmission fluctuates depending upon factors affecting the presence of the mosquito vector and their vertebrate hosts, such as rainfall, patterns of irrigation, and climatic conditions. Transmission may vary from season to season and from 1 year to the next. For detailed information about risk of JE by country, region, and season, see Table 25.1–3 and Figure 25.1–2. The risk to travelers of acquiring JE depends on length of residence in an endemic area, nature of the individual's activities, season of travel, and local conditions affecting transmission in the area at the time of travel.

The currently available JE vaccine is a purified, inactivated, mouse-brain–derived preparation. Early field trials revealed a vaccine efficacy of 80% to 91% for a two-dose schedule.[98–100] A single dose of vaccine had no demonstrable efficacy. A recent study in U.S. travelers demonstrated a seroconversion (reciprocal neutralizing antibody titer of ≥8–10) of 77%, with only 29% of vaccines maintaining adequate antibody levels 6 to 12 months after two doses. A third dose of vaccine given 6 to 12 months after the primary series resulted in development of titers ≥16 in all vaccines.[101] Therefore, current recommendations in the United States call for a three-dose schedule, with 1.0 mL of vaccine administered subcutaneously on days 0, 7, and 30.[98] An abbreviated schedule of three doses given on days 0, 7, and 14 may be used for travelers with imminent departure dates. Children from 1 to 3 years should receive 0.5 mL instead of the 1.0-mL dose. No data are available on safety or immunogenicity for children less than 1 year of age, and wherever possible, vaccination should be delayed until an infant is more than 1 year of age. A booster dose of 1.0 mL is recommended after 3 years; the full duration of protection of the three-dose schedule is unknown. A vaccine licensed in Japan is available in a two-dose schedule. Schedules for administration of vaccine are noted in Table 22.2–6.

JE vaccine is recommended for individuals who plan to reside in endemic or epidemic areas of JE transmission and for travelers who plan to spend a month or more in areas where transmission is known to occur, especially if travel to rural areas will occur. Individual circumstances, however, should be taken into account when making the decision to immunize. Travelers who plan to visit farms or rural or remote areas or who plan extensive outdoor activities may be at increased risk and may be offered vac-

Table 22.2–6. JAPANESE ENCEPHALITIS VACCINE

DOSES	SUBCUTANEOUS ROUTE		COMMENTS
	1–2 YR OF AGE	≥3 YRS OF AGE	
Primary series 1, 2, and 3	0.5 mL	1.0 mL	Days 0, 7, 30
Booster*	—	1.0 mL	1 dose at ≥36 mo

*In vaccinees who have completed a three-dose primary series, the full duration of protection is unknown; therefore, definitive recommendations cannot be given.

cine. Travelers whose itineraries include mainly urban areas and who will stay in facilities with adequate screens or air conditioning will be at lowest risk. All travelers should be offered information about personal protective measures against mosquito bites such as permethrin-impregnated bed nets, insect repellents, insecticide sprays, wearing protective clothing, and avoiding exposure to mosquitoes by remaining in screened or air-conditioned areas from dusk through the night.

Generalized urticaria and angioedema have occurred within minutes to as long as 2 weeks after vaccination (median 2 days) in approximately 1 in 1,000 vaccines. Individuals with a history of allergic disorders may have a higher risk for developing adverse reactions to JE vaccine. Epinephrine and other equipment to treat anaphylaxis should be available, and vaccinees should be observed for 30 minutes after immunization and warned of the possibility of such a reaction occurring in the 2 weeks after immunization. Vaccinees experiencing an allergic reaction should not receive further doses. Other adverse reactions to vaccine may include tenderness, erythema, or swelling at the injection site, headache, dizziness, fatigue, nausea, chills, fever, or lower back pain.

Individuals with hypersensitivity to mouse-derived vaccines or to thimerosal should not be vaccinated with JE vaccine. A single small study of immunization of children with underlying diseases did not demonstrate a changed pattern of adverse events or immune response after immunization.[102]

Limited data suggest that safety and efficacy of JE vaccine are not compromised by the simultaneous administration of DTP vaccine. No data are available about the effect on JE vaccine safety or efficacy with concurrent administration of other vaccines, antimalarial drugs, or other biologics.

MENINGOCOCCAL VACCINE

Disease caused by the bacterium *Neisseria meningitidis* is endemic throughout the world. Recurrent epidemics occur in the meningitis belt of sub-Saharan Africa, extending from Mauritania to Ethiopia, particularly during the dry season from December to June (Figure 22.2–3). Isolated outbreaks have been described in Mecca, Saudi Arabia, Nepal, and other areas. Risk to travelers is low, estimated to be 0.4 per million travelers per month for a stay in a developing country and up to 2,000/million in pilgrims to Mecca.[103] Outbreaks have occurred involving travelers, and travelers have become carriers of disease. American pilgrims who returned from Mecca, Saudi Arabia, following an epidemic of Group A meningococcal disease in 1987 were more than 11 times as likely to carry the organism back to their home countries as travelers returning from other parts of Saudi Arabia.[104] In 2000, the largest recorded outbreak of serogroup W-135 meningococcal disease occurred in Saudi Arabian nationals and pilgrims returning from the Hajj in Mecca and their close contacts.[105] Vaccination against meningococcal disease is required for pilgrims to Mecca, Saudi Arabia, on the annual Hajj, but most countries use a bivalent A and C vaccine. Individuals who will be traveling to countries within the meningitis belt of sub-Saharan Africa and who will have contact with the local population (individuals visiting friends and relatives, health care workers, long-term travelers such as missionaries and volunteer workers) are at higher risk and should be offered vaccine, especially during times when epidemics are occurring. Individuals who will travel to these areas and stay in tourist accommodations with little contact with the local population are at low risk.

Serogroup A is the most common cause of epidemics in the world, although serogroups B and C can also cause epidemic disease. The currently available vaccines are divalent or quadrivalent preparations consisting of purified capsular polysaccharides of serogroups A and C or A, C, Y, and W-135, which induce serogroup-specific immunity. The dose of vaccine is 0.5 cc given subcutaneously.

Duration of immunity, although not precisely known, appears to be at least 3 years in those vaccinated after age

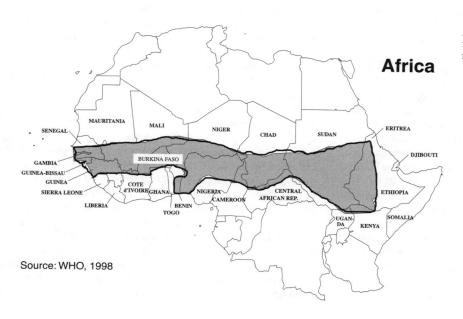

Figure 22.2–3. Areas with frequent epidemics of meningococcal meningitis.[4]

Source: WHO, 1998

4. Serogroup A polysaccharide vaccine has not been shown to be effective in children less than 3 months of age and may be only partially effective in infants between 3 and 11 months of age. Children less than 2 years old are not protected against serogroup C with polysaccharide vaccine. Children as young as 3 months of age can receive the polysaccharide vaccine if traveling to areas of epidemic meningococcal disease. Revaccination may be indicated for children immunized before 4 years of age after 2 to 3 years, particularly if they remain at high risk.

Meningococcal protein-conjugate vaccines, which would be immunogenic in infants, have shown promise in safety and efficacy studies in the Gambia.[106] A group C meningococcal polysaccharide conjugate vaccine was licensed recently in the U.K. The serogroup B polysaccharide is poorly immunogenic in humans, although outer membrane protein-based vaccines against serogroup B meningococcal disease are under investigation and have shown promise in field trials in Brazil and Norway.[107,108]

Adverse reactions are infrequent and mild, usually localized erythema lasting 1 to 2 days. Up to 2% of young children will develop transient fever after immunization. Safety of meningococcal vaccines during pregnancy has not been established. When considering immunization during pregnancy, the theoretical risk of immunization must be balanced against risk of contracting the disease.

RABIES VACCINE

The risk of rabies is highest for international travelers in areas of the world where dog rabies remains highly endemic, such as most developing countries of Africa and Asia and many parts of Central and South America.[109] A retrospective study of dog bites and licks experienced by travelers to Thailand suggests that these are experienced by about 10% of travelers during an average stay of 17 days.[110] Risk for travelers in this area may be significant, as up to 6.8% of street dogs in Thailand have been shown to carry the rabies virus.[111] Areas of the world that are rabies-free are noted in Table 22.2–7; travelers should be informed about risk of rabies in the region to which they will travel and advised to avoid contact with animals that could be rabies carriers, especially dogs, but including cats, skunks, raccoons, and bats.

Many products are available worldwide for pre-exposure prophylaxis of rabies; these are described in detail in Chapter 22.1. In addition, rabies immunoglobulin preparations provide passive immune protection of short duration. Vaccines may be used to provide pre-exposure prophylaxis (termed prophylaxis rather than immunization to emphasize that receiving this product before exposure does not obviate the need for treatment if an exposure occurs) or postexposure prophylaxis. Travelers who will be visiting areas where rabies is enzootic and where immediate access to appropriate medical care including biologics is limited are candidates for pre-exposure prophylaxis.[112]

Dosing recommendations for pre-exposure prophylaxis with rabies vaccines are noted in Table 22.2–8. In some countries, central nervous system- or brain tissue-derived vaccines are available but are not recommended due to uncertain immunogenicity and a high rate of seri-

Table 22.2–7 COUNTRIES REPORTING NO CASES OF RABIES

REGION	COUNTRIES
Africa	Cape Verde, Libya,* Mauritius,* Reunion, Seychelles*
Americas	
North	Bermuda, St. Pierre and Miquelon
Caribbean	Antigua and Barbuda, Aruba, Bahamas, Barbados, Cayman Islands, Guadeloupe, Jamaica, Martinique, Netherlands Antilles (Bonaire, Curaçao, Saba, Sint Maarten, and St. Eustatius), St. Christopher (St. Kitts) and Nevis, St. Martin, St. Vincent and Grenadines, Virgin Islands (U.K. and U.S.)
South	Uruguay
Asia	Bahrain, Brunei, Hong Kong, Japan, Kuwait, Malaysia (Malaysia-Sabah*), Maldives, Qatar, Singapore, Taiwan
Europe	Albania, Cyprus, Denmark, Faroe Islands, Finland, Gibraltar, Greece, Iceland, Ireland, Isle of Man, Italy, Jersey, Macedonia, Malta, Monaco, Norway (mainland), Portugal, Spain (except Ceuta/Melilla), Sweden, U.K.
Oceania	American Samoa, Australia, Cook Islands, Fiji, French Polynesia, Guam, Indonesia (with exception of Java, Kalimantan, Sumatra, and Sulawesi), Kiribati, New Caledonia, New Zealand, Niue, Papua New Guinea, Solomon Islands, Tonga, Vanuatu
	Most of Pacific Oceania is "rabies-free." For information on specific islands not listed above, contact the Centers for Disease Control and Prevention, Division of Quarantine.

The listed countries and political units reported that rabies was not present during 1996–1997. Bat rabies exists in some areas that are free of terrestrial rabies.
*Countries whose classifications may be considered provisional.
Sources: (1) World Health Organization: World Survey of Rabies 32, (for 1996); Division of Emerging and Other Communicable Diseases, WHO, Geneva, 1998; (2) WHO Collaborating Centre for Rabies Surveillance and Research: Rabies Bulletin Europe, 1997;21(4); and (3) Pan American Health Organization. Epidemiological surveillance of rabies in the Americas, 1997;29(1–33).[4]

ous adverse reactions.[113] These preparations are not regarded as safe or effective; individuals who may have received these products should be considered unimmunized for the purposes of planning a postexposure prophylaxis regimen. In general, pre-exposure immunization consists of three 1.0 mL IM doses of either product, given on days 0, 7, and 21 or 28. Some European schedules allow longer intervals between doses if desired. HDCV, but not rabies vaccine absorbed (RVA), may also be given by the intradermal route (0.1 mL ID on days 0, 7, and 21 or 28). Because of decreased antibody response to primary rabies immunization when given concurrently with chloroquine used for malaria prophylaxis,[114] the three doses of rabies vaccine should be completed prior to initiating malaria prophylaxis with chloroquine or mefloquine. If this is not possible, the IM route of administration should be used for the rabies vaccine. The dose of vaccine is the same for children and adults. Receipt of pre-exposure prophylaxis does not obviate the need for postexposure prophylaxis in the event of an animal bite, although the number of injections are reduced and there is no need for rabies immune globulin (RIG).

Table 22.2–8.   RABIES PRE-EXPOSURE PROPHYLAXIS SCHEDULE

TYPE OF VACCINATION	ROUTE	REGIMEN
Primary	Intramuscular	HDCV, PCEC, or RVA; 1.0 mL (deltoid area), one each on days 0,* 7, and 21 or 28
	Intradermal	HDCV; 0.1 mL, one each on days 0, 7, and 21 or 28
Booster	Intramuscular	HDCV, PCEC, or RVA; 1.0 mL (deltoid area), day 0 only
	Intradermal	HDCV; 1.0 mL, day 0 only

HDCV = human diploid cell vaccine, PCEC = purified chick embryo cell vaccine, RVA = rabies vaccine adsorbed.
*Day 0 is the day the first dose of vaccine is administered.

Postexposure prophylaxis should begin with immediate, thorough cleansing of any animal bite with soap and water. If available, a povidone-iodine solution or other virucidal agent should be used to irrigate the wound. Individuals previously vaccinated should receive two IM 1.0-mL doses of HDCV or RVA, one each on days 0 and 3. Individuals who have received pre-exposure prophylaxis should not be given RIG. Individuals not previously immunized should receive RIG, 20 IU/kg body weight and, if anatomically feasible, the full dose infiltrated around the wound(s); any remaining volume should then be given IM at a site distant from vaccine administration. Five 1.0-mL IM doses of vaccine are given, one each on days 0, 3, 7, 14, and 28. For adults, vaccine doses should be given only in the deltoid region; in children, the anterolateral thigh is acceptable. Vaccine should never be given in the gluteal area.

Although adverse reactions after vaccination with HDCV or RVA occur less frequently than with earlier products, local reactions (pain, erythema, swelling, or itching) are reported frequently. Systemic symptoms (headache, nausea, abdominal pain, muscle aches, and dizziness) have been reported in 5% to 40% of recipients. Approximately 6% of recipients will experience an immune complex-like reaction characterized by urticaria, pruritis, and malaise.[112] Once started, postexposure prophylaxis should not be interrupted or discontinued because of local or mild systemic reactions to vaccine.

Immunosuppressive illnesses, steroids, or other immunosuppressive agents, as well as antimalarials, may interfere with adequate immune response to vaccine. Pregnancy is not a contraindication to postexposure prophylaxis with rabies vaccine, and no harmful effects to the fetus from immunization have been noted. If risk of exposure is high, pre-exposure prophylaxis may be offered.[115] Immunosuppressive agents should not be administered during postexposure prophylaxis unless essential. When rabies vaccine is administered to immunosuppressed individuals or those taking immunosuppressive agents, a serum sample should be tested for adequate antibody response.

TICK-BORNE ENCEPHALITIS

Tick-borne encephalitis (TBE) is a viral central nervous system infection transmitted by the bite of the tick vector *Ixodes ricinus* or by unpasteurized dairy products from infected animals. It occurs in Russia and other countries of the former Soviet Union, as well as most countries in Europe, especially Austria, the Czech Republic, Slovakia, Germany, Hungary, Poland, Switzerland, and northern Yugoslavia. It has not been reported from Portugal, Belgium, the Netherlands, and Luxembourg.[116] Risk depends on season of travel, exposure to forested areas, and tick activity, with highest transmission occurring from May to June and September to October. Risk may be focused in circumscribed areas within countries. Risk to travelers who do not visit forested areas or consume unpasteurized dairy products is low. A study of American members of a military unit that lived and trained in a highly endemic area found an infection rate of 0.9/1,000/month of exposure.[117]

Vaccine against TBE is available in many countries in Europe (although not in the United States) and is recommended for high-risk individuals (such as forestry workers) and others who plan extended travels through endemic areas. Protection against tick bites may be provided by wearing protective clothing and using insect repellents containing DEET.

Vaccine is given in a three-dose series, with the first two injections 2 weeks to 3 months apart and a third dose 9 to 12 months later. Boosters are recommended at 3-year intervals. Side effects of vaccine include local and mild systemic reactions. Individuals with egg allergy should not receive this vaccine.

TYPHOID VACCINE

Typhoid fever occurs in all parts of the world, but especially where poor sanitary conditions are found. It is estimated that more than 60% of the world's cases occur in Asia and about 35% in Africa. The majority of cases in developed countries are acquired abroad.[118] In the United States, 62% of cases reported between 1975 and 1984 occurred in international travelers.[119] Humans are the only reservoir of *Salmonella typhi*, the bacterium that causes typhoid fever. The infection is acquired by ingestion of contaminated food or water. Case fatality rates range from 1.3% to 8.4% and are highest in patients over 80 years of age. One to 3% of patients become chronic carriers.[120] Children less than 5 years of age may be more likely to have a mild illness than older children.[121]

Risk of contracting typhoid depends largely on travel destination and living circumstances during travel. Estimates of risk of contracting typhoid for short-stay travelers have ranged from 1 to 10 in 30,000 for trips to North Africa, India, and Senegal.[122] Another study showed the risk of disease to be decreased by immunization against typhoid prior to travel: incidence rates per visit ranged from 16 per 100,000 North American tourists, 92% of whom had received typhoid vaccine prior to travel, to 216 per 100,000 in Israeli tourists, 6% of whom had been immunized.[123]

The mainstay of prevention of typhoid fever is prevention of exposure. None of the currently available vac-

Table 22.2–9.   DOSAGE AND SCHEDULES FOR TYPHOID FEVER VACCINATION

VACCINATION	AGE	DOSE/MODE OF ADMINISTRATION	NUMBER OF DOSES	INTERVAL BETWEEN DOSES	BOOSTING INTERVAL
Oral live-attenuated Ty21a vaccine					
Primary series	≥6 yr	1 capsule*	4	48 hr	—
Booster	≥6 yr	1 capsule*	4	48 hr	Every 5 yr
Vi capsular polysaccharide vaccine					
Primary series	≥2 yr	0.50 mLA[†]	1	—	—
Booster	≥2 yr	0.50 mLA[†]	1	—	Every 2 yr
Heat-phenol-inactivated parenteral vaccine					
Primary series	6 mo–10 yr	0.25 mL[‡]	2	≥4 wk	—
	≥10 yr	0.50 mL[‡]	2	≥4 wk	—
Booster	6 mo–10 yr	0.25 mL[‡]	1	—	Every 3 yr
	≥10 yr	0.50 mL[‡]	1	—	Every 3 yr
	≥6 mo	0.10 mLA[§]	1	—	Every 3 yr

*Administer with cool liquid no warmer than 37°C (98.6°F).
[†] Intramuscularly.
[‡] Subcutaneously.
[§] Intradermally.

cines are fully effective, and immunity may be over-whelmed by ingestion of a large inoculum of bacteria.[124] Treatment of typhoid fever may be complicated by the emergence of multiresistant strains of *S. typhi*,[125] providing further impetus for prevention of the infection.

Three vaccines are available for prevention of typhoid; dosing schedules are presented in Table 22.2–9. Parenteral killed whole-cell typhoid vaccines have been available since 1896.[126] The parenteral heat-phenol-inactivated preparation is given in a series of two doses separated by 4 weeks, with booster doses at 3-year intervals. Vaccine trials performed by WHO in the 1960s in Yugoslavia, Guyana, and the U.S.S.R. revealed a vaccine efficacy of 51% to 77% for 2½ to 3 years after immunization.[126] Adverse reactions to this parenteral vaccine are frequent and include severe headache, moderate or severe local pain, swelling, or erythema. Thirteen to 24% of recipients may miss work or school following immunization.[127] The frequency of severe adverse reactions, plus the time required to provide the two-dose series, may have discouraged the use of this vaccine even in circumstances when it would otherwise be indicated. In some countries, whole-cell killed vaccine is no longer distributed because of these limitations and because of introduction of new products. It remains, however, the only vaccine available for protection of children under 2 years of age in some countries.

A newer parenteral vaccine containing the purified Vi antigen of *S. typhi* is available in some countries. It has been shown to have a protective efficacy of 60% to 72% in field trials conducted in Nepal and South Africa.[128,129] It is given as a single dose, and although local and rarely systemic adverse reactions may occur, they are less frequent than with killed whole-cell vaccine.[130] In some countries, the vaccine is indicated for children as young as 8 months old.

An oral live-attenuated vaccine made from an attenuated strain of *S. typhi*, Ty21a, is also available. The vaccine consists of a series of four enteric-coated capsules, taken one every other day. The capsules must be kept refrigerated and swallowed whole with a cool liquid, about 1 hour before a meal. Rare adverse reactions have included diarrhea, nausea, abdominal discomfort, vomiting, and rash. Although field trials of the vaccine in endemic areas, using a three-dose schedule, yielded protection rates of 43% to 96%,[130] the efficacy of the vaccine in travelers has not been studied systematically. Results of additional studies in Chile and Indonesia in children as young as 3 years of age suggest that a liquid preparation of oral Ty21a vaccine might provide greater protective efficacy than the enteric-coated preparation.[131,132] A recent study in Thailand demonstrated seroconversion rates of 83% to three doses of liquid vaccine preparation in 4- to 6-year-old schoolchildren and reported no adverse reactions to immunization.[133]

Vaccination against typhoid is currently recommended for travelers to countries where typhoid is a frequent risk (such as many countries in Africa, Asia, and Central and South America) and to those visiting other developing countries on nontourist itineraries where the risk of contaminated food and water is increased. Oral typhoid vaccine is recommended for most travelers who do not have specific contraindications. Parenteral whole-cell vaccine remains the only option available for infants. Development of protective antibody by this vaccine requires two doses of vaccine given 1 month apart. For individuals who do not have a month before departure to complete the primary series of parenteral whole-cell vaccine, three doses may be given at weekly intervals, but this schedule may not be as effective. The parenteral vaccine containing the Vi-antigen ideally should be given 10 days prior to departure. This vaccine would not provide protection against Vi-negative strains of *S. typhi*, but the pathogenicity of these strains is unclear.[134] A recent meta-analysis of efficacy of the three typhoid vaccines concluded that whole-cell vaccines are more effective but are associated more frequently with adverse events than either of the two newer preparations. Decisions about balancing added risk of adverse events and greater efficacy of whole-cell vaccines will be based primarily on careful consideration of the situation in which the vaccine is to be used.[135]

Oral typhoid vaccine should not be used in immunocompromised individuals including those infected with HIV. Antibacterial agents may interfere with immunogenicity of this vaccine, and, if possible, courses of these agents should be completed prior to taking vaccine. If this is not possible, doses of vaccine and antibacterial agents should be separated by as much time as possible. Concerns have been raised about the concurrent administration of the oral Ty21a vaccine with the antimalarial agent mefloquine, as mefloquine has been shown to inhibit the in vitro growth of typhoid strains, including Ty21a, at concentrations that might be expected after ingestion of a dose of vaccine. If all doses of vaccine cannot be taken before starting antimalarial drugs, ingestion of mefloquine and doses of oral typhoid vaccine should be separated by at least 24 hours. Simultaneous administration of yellow fever vaccine or immune globulin and oral typhoid vaccine does not seem to pose a problem. Currently, no data exist documenting interference with antibody response to oral polio vaccine by the oral typhoid vaccine. No experience has been reported about the use of typhoid vaccines in pregnant women, and immunization should be avoided if possible.

YELLOW FEVER VACCINE

A dramatic resurgence of yellow fever has occurred in the past decade, primarily in sub-Saharan Africa and tropical South America.[136] Outbreaks occurred in countries, such as Gabon, that had never had disease previously, and re-emergence of disease was noted in Senegal[137] and in Kenya, which had been yellow fever-free for nearly 50 years. Cases have also been reported from the West African countries of Nigeria, the Gambia, Mali, Burkina-Faso, Cameroon, Ghana, Sierra Leone, and Benin. In South America, the largest outbreak since the 1950s occurred in Peru in 1995, and cases were reported in Bolivia, Brazil, Colombia, Ecuador, and Peru from 1985 to 1994.[138] Urban yellow fever was confirmed in Santa Cruz, Bolivia, in 1997 and 1998.[139] Relaxation of eradication programs in the 1970s coupled with spread of the vector mosquito throughout South America has led to increasing concern about urbanization of yellow fever transmission.[140] Fatal cases of yellow fever have occurred in travelers.[141–143] Parts of the world where yellow fever is present are shown in Figure 25.1–3.

Yellow fever is a viral disease transmitted by mosquitoes. The case fatality rate may exceed 50%.[144] In South America, sporadic infections occur at the margins of or in riverine forests, whereas in West Africa, cases occur principally as endemic infections among children in the wet savanna. Large outbreaks occur at intervals in urban locations and villages in the dry savanna. Because areas reporting yellow fever change frequently, health providers are encouraged to consult national and local health departments for current information about local outbreaks. Travelers are at risk for contracting yellow fever and may be especially so in countries where yellow fever immunization is not required for entry but where disease transmission does occur.

International efforts to prevent the spread of yellow fever include mosquito control at airports and shipping ports and the requirement of documentation of immunization against yellow fever for travelers arriving from areas where disease is occurring. The WHO-approved yellow fever vaccines in current use are live vaccines made from the attenuated 17D strain of the virus and are prepared in chick embryos. Yellow fever vaccine is the only vaccine required by WHO for entry into some countries. Some endemic countries, however, such as Brazil and Senegal, do not require the vaccine for entry. Fatal cases in travelers have occurred in both countries.[141,142] A single 0.5-mL dose probably confers lifelong immunity, although immunization every 10 years is required to maintain validity of the International Certificate of Vaccination against Yellow Fever. Travelers to affected countries should receive a single dose of vaccine at least 10 days before departure. Vaccine is contraindicated in children under 4 months of age and should be used cautiously in children less than 1 year of age because of the risk of encephalitis following vaccination, which may occur in as many as 1% of infants less than 3 months of age.[145–147] Most countries will accept a medical waiver for individuals too young to be vaccinated or with a medical contraindication. The decision to immunize children less than 1 year of age must be based on individual circumstances. Children 9 months of age or older should be vaccinated routinely if traveling to or residing in areas where yellow fever is officially reported. Immunization may be deferred to 1 year of age if children will reside solely in urban areas where transmission has not been reported. Children between 4 and 9 months of age should be considered for vaccination if travel to areas with epidemic disease is anticipated and if protective measures against mosquitoes cannot be guaranteed. Infants less than 4 months of age should not be immunized.

Serologic response to yellow fever vaccine is not diminished by simultaneous administration of tetanus, diphtheria, pertussis, polio, BCG, hepatitis A, hepatitis B, or the Vi antigen capsular polysaccharide typhoid vaccines. Recent immunization with measles vaccine does not diminish response to yellow fever vaccine.[148] Immune globulin did not decrease the antibody response to yellow fever vaccine when given 0 to 7 days before immunization.[149] The antimalarial chloroquine has been shown not to affect adversely the antibody response to yellow fever vaccine.[150]

Reactions to yellow fever vaccine include mild side effects such as low-grade fever, myalgia, and headache in 2% to 5% of recipients within 5 to 10 days after immunization. Immediate hypersensitivity is extremely rare.

Individuals who are significantly immunocompromised should not be immunized due to the theoretical risk of encephalitis following immunization. Individuals with asymptomatic HIV infection may be offered vaccine if exposure to yellow fever cannot be avoided. Vaccine has been administered with good tolerance and efficacy to asymptomatic HIV-infected individuals.[151] Because yellow fever vaccine is produced in chick embryos, individuals who are hypersensitive to eggs should avoid the vaccine. Individuals with a questionable history of egg hypersensitivity who must receive vaccine may receive an intradermal test dose under close medical supervision.

Specific instructions for skin testing are available from the package insert.

Ideally, yellow fever immunization should be administered to nonpregnant women. A recent study documented fetal infection in 1 of 41 infants exposed to maternal vaccination; no abnormalities were identified in any of these infants.[152] The risk of contracting yellow fever, especially for women traveling to areas where there is active transmission, must be weighed against the theoretical risk of immunization. Measures to minimize exposure to insect bites, such as the use of long-sleeved clothing, permethrin-impregnated bednets, mosquito sprays, and repellents containing DEET, should be taken by those who will visit areas with endemic or epidemic yellow fever transmission.

COST EFFECTIVENESS OF TRAVEL IMMUNIZATIONS

Travel medicine experts have long observed the willingness of travelers to accept multiple vaccines for diseases for which they are at minimal risk. Although well-designed studies of cost effectiveness of travel immunizations are few, studies suggest that most travel-vaccine programs are not cost effective: the cost of immunizing all travelers exceeds the cost of treating illnesses in travelers who become ill in the absence of vaccination.[2,153]

Hepatitis A immunization has been studied most extensively with regard to cost-benefit of immunizing travelers. In one study, which also examined cost effectiveness of typhoid immunization, neither of the two vaccines was found to be cost effective; societal expenditures of over 67 million pounds was required to prevent a single death with either vaccine.[154] In contrast, a study from the Netherlands suggests that cost-effective choices are available with regard to hepatitis A immunization when frequency of travel, likelihood of prior immunity, and product used are taken into consideration.[155] Another study from the U.K. demonstrated that use of vaccine was more cost effective in travelers visiting high-risk areas more than five times in the next 10 years, and immune globulin use was more cost effective in travelers making fewer than five journeys in the next 10 years.[88] Cost effectiveness of pre-exposure rabies prophylaxis has been studied in Canada, with the conclusion that routine pre-exposure prophylaxis for most travelers is not indicated.[156]

Issues complicating performance of studies of cost effectiveness include difficulty estimating with accuracy the risk of vaccine-preventable diseases to travelers, difficulties in determining vaccine efficacy, especially for travelers who will have variable exposures in endemic areas, difficulties approximating costs associated with disease, and lack of sufficient experience with some newer vaccines to allow accurate estimation of incidence of vaccine-associated adverse events. Finally, some practitioners may be reluctant to omit any vaccine, no matter the risk of disease, for fear of liability. Until these issues are studied in greater detail, each travel medicine provider must continue to individualize recommendations for travel vaccination, taking into account the potential for adverse reactions to immunization and the patient's risk for the disease.

REFERENCES

1. Reid D, Keystone JS. Health risks abroad: general considerations. In: Dupont HL, Steffen R, eds. Textbook of travel medicine and health: Hamilton, ON: BC Decker, 1997:3–9.
2. Wiedermann G. Is vaccination worthwhile before travel? In: Steffen R, Lobel HO, Haworth J, Bradley DJ, eds. Travel medicine. Berlin: Springer-Verlag, 1989:208–215.
3. World Health Organization. International travel and health vaccination requirements and health advice. Geneva: WHO, 1994.
4. Centers for Disease Control and Prevention. Health information for international travel 1999–2000. Atlanta: Department of Health and Human Services, 1999.
5. Department of Health. Immunization against infectious disease. London: HMSO, 1992.
6. Société de Médecine des Voyages (Paris). Médecine des voyages: guide d'information et de conseils pratiques, format utile ed 4th edition, 1998.
7. King GE, Hadler SC. Simultaneous administration of childhood vaccines: an important public health policy that is safe and efficacious. Pediatr Infect Dis J 1994;13:394–407.
8. Centers for Disease Control and Prevention. General recommendations on immunization: recommendations of the Advisory Committee on Immunization Practices (ACIP). MMWR Morb Mortal Wkly Rep 1994;43(RR1):15–18.
9. Kaplan JE, Nelson DB, Schonberger LB, et al. The effect of immune globulin on the response to trivalent oral poliovirus and yellow fever vaccinations. Bull World Health Organ 1984;62:585–590.
10. American Academy of Pediatrics, Committee on Infectious Diseases. Recommended timing of routine measles immunization for children who have recently received immune globulin preparations. Pediatrics 1994;93:682–685.
11. Tsai TF, Bolin RA, Lazuick JS, Miller KD. Chloroquine does not adversely affect the antibody response to yellow fever vaccine. J Infect Dis 1986;154:726–727.
12. Centers for Disease Control and Prevention. Recommendations of the Advisory Committee on Immunization Practices (ACIP): use of vaccines and immune globulins in persons with altered immunocompetence. MMWR Morb Mortal Wkly Rep 1993;42(RR4):1–18.
13. Mileno MD, Bia FJ. The compromised traveler. Infect Dis Clin North Am 1998;12:369–412.
14. Brena AE, Cooper ER, Cabral HJ, Pelton SI. Antibody response to measles and rubella vaccine by children with HIV infection. J AIDS 1993;6:1125–1129.
15. Peters VB, Sood SK. Immunity to Haemophilus influenzae after reimmunization with oligosaccharide CRM197 conjugate vaccine in children with human immunodeficiency virus infection. Pediatr Infect Dis J 1997;16:711–713.
16. American Academy of Pediatrics Committee on Infectious Diseases. Recommended childhood immunization schedule—United States, January–December 2000. Pediatrics 2000;105:148–151.
17. Centers for Disease Control and Prevention. Immunization of adolescents: recommendations of the Advisory Committee on Immunization Practices, the American Academy of Pediatrics, the American Academy of Family Physicians, and the American Medical Association. MMWR Morb Mortal Wkly Rep 1996;45(RR-13):1–16.
18. Gardner P, Schaffner W. Immunization of adults. N Engl J Med 1993;328:1252–1258.
19. Fedson DS. Adult immunization: summary of the National Vaccine Advisory Committee Report. JAMA 1994;272:1133–1137.
20. Diphtheria acquired by US citizens in the Russian Federation and Ukraine—1994. MMWR Morb Mortal Wkly Rep 1995;44:237–244.

21. Lumio J, Jahkosa M, Vuento R, et al. Diphtheria after visit to Russia. Lancet 1993;342:53–54.

22. Diphtheria outbreak—Srarburi Province, Thailand, 1994. MMWR Morb Mortal Wkly Rep 1996;45:271–273.

23. Crossley K, Irvine P, Warren JB, et al. Tetanus and diphtheria immunity in urban Minnesota adults. JAMA 1979;242: 2298–3000.

24. Koblin BA, Townsend TR. Immunity to diphtheria and tetanus in inner-city women of child-bearing age. Am J Public Health 1989;79:1297–1298.

25. Christensson B, Bottiger M. Serological immunity to diphtheria in Sweden in 1978 and 1984. Scand J Infect Dis 1986; 18:227–233.

26. Ivanoff B, Robertson SE. Pertussis: a worldwide problem. Dev Biol Stand 1997;89:3–13.

27. Gangarosa EJ, Galazka AM, Wolfe CE, et al. Impact of the anti-vaccine movements on pertussis control: the untold story. Lancet 1998;351:356–361.

28. Centers for Disease Control and Prevention. Pertussis vaccination: use of acellular pertussis vaccines among infants and young children: recommendations of the Advisory Committee on Immunization Practices (ACIP). MMWR Morb Mortal Wkly Rep 1997;46(RR-7):1–25.

29. Certification of poliomyelitis eradication— the Americas, 1994. MMWR Morb Mortal Wkly Rep 1994;43:720–722.

30. Steffen R, Rickenbach M, Willhelm U, et al. Health problems after travel to developing countries. J Infect Dis 1987;156: 84–91.

31. Centers for Disease Control and Prevention. Recommendations of the Advisory Committee on Immunization Practices: revised recommendations for routine poliomyelitis vaccination. MMWR Morb Mortal Wkly Rep 1999;48(27):590.

32. Lange WR, Frame JD. High incidence of viral hepatitis among American missionaries in Africa. Am J Trop Med Hyg 1990; 43:527–533.

33. Steffen R. Risks of hepatitis B for travelers. Vaccine 1990;8: 31–32.

34. Grotto I, Mandel Y, Ephros M, et al. Major adverse reactions to yeast-derived hepatitis B vaccines—a review. Vaccine 1998; 16:329–334.

35. Chen RT. Safety of vaccines. In: Plotkin SA, Orenstein WA, eds. Vaccines. Philadelphia: WB Saunders, 1999:1144–1163.

36. Centers for Disease Control and Prevention. Prevention of varicella: recommendations of the Advisory Committee on Immunization Practices (ACIP). MMWR Morb Mortal Wkly Rep 1996;45(RR-11):1–36.

37. Fine PEM, Rodrigues LC. Mycobacterial diseases. Lancet 1990;335:1016–1020.

38. Snider DE, Rieder HL, Combs D, et al. Tuberculosis in children. Pediatr Infect Dis J 1988;7:271–278.

39. Colditz GA, Brewer TF, Berkey CS, et al. Efficacy of BCG vaccine in the prevention of tuberculosis: meta-analysis of the published literature. JAMA 1994;271:698–702.

40. Ponnighaus JM, Fine PEM, Sterne JAC, et al. Efficacy of BCG vaccine against leprosy and tuberculosis in Malawi. Lancet 1992;339:636–639.

41. Centers for Disease Control and Prevention. The role of BCG vaccines in the prevention and control of tuberculosis in the US: a joint statement by the Advisory Committee for Elimination of Tuberculosis and the ACIP. MMWR Morb Mortal Wkly Rep 1996;45(RR-4):1–18.

42. Crowley RG. Implication of the Vietnam War for tuberculosis in the United States. Arch Environ Health 1970;21:479–480.

43. Lobato MN, Hopewell PC. *Mycobacterium tuberculosis* infection after travel to or contact with visitors from countries with a high prevalence of tuberculosis. Am J Respir Crit Care Med 1998;158:1871–1875.

44. Driver CR, Valway SE, Morgan WM, et al. Transmission of *Mycobacterium tuberculosis* associated with air travel. JAMA 1994;272:1031–1035.

45. Kenyon TA, Valway SE, Ihle WW, et al. Transmission of multidrug-resistant *Mycobacterium tuberculosis* during a long airplane flight. N Engl J Med 1996;334:933–938.

46. Centers for Disease Control and Prevention. Prevention and control of influenza: recommendations of the Advisory Committee on Immunization Practices (ACIP). MMWR Morb Mortal Wkly Rep 1997;46(RR9):1–25.

47. Pneumococcal and influenza vaccination levels among adults aged ≥ 65 years— United States, 1995. MMWR Morb Mortal Wkly Rep 1997;46:913–919. (Erratum, MMWR 1997;46: 974).

48. Hall CB. Influenza: a shot or not? Pediatrics 1987;79:564–566.

49. Influenza A—Florida and Tennessee, July–August 1998, and virologic surveillance of influenza, May–August 1998. MMWR Morb Mortal Wkly Rep 1998;47:756–759.

50. Centers for Disease Control and Prevention. Outbreak of influenza A infection among travelers — Alaska and the Yukon Territory, May–June 1999. MMWR Morb Mortal Wkly Rep 1999;48:545–555.

51. Update: Outbreak of influenza A infection — Alaska and the Yukon Territory, July–August 1998. MMWR Morb Mortal Wkly Rep 1998;47:685–688.

52. Centers for Disease Control and Prevention. Prevention and control of influenza: recommendations of the Advisory Committee on Immunization Practices (ACIP). MMWR Morb Mortal Wkly Rep 1999;48(RR-4):8.

53. Palanche AM. Influenza vaccine: a reappraisal of their use. Drugs 1997;54:841–856.

54. Belshe RB, Mendelman PM, Treanor J, et al. The efficacy of live attenuated, cold-adapted, trivalent, intranasal influenza-virus vaccine in children. N Engl J Med 1998;338:1406–1412.

55. Centers for Disease Control and Prevention. Prevention of pneumococcal disease: recommendations of the Advisory Committee on Immunization Practices (ACIP). MMWR Morb Mortal Wkly Rep 1997;46(RR-8):1–24.

56. Shapiro ED, Berg AT, Austrian R, et al. The protective efficacy of polyvalent pneumococcal polysaccharide vaccine. N Engl J Med 1991;325:1453–1460.

57. Black S, Shinefield H, Greman B, et al. Efficacy, safety and immunogenicity of heptavalent pneumococcal conjugate vaccine in children. Pediatr Infect Dis J 2000;19:187–195.

58. Cholera Working Group, International Centre for Diarrhoeal Diseases Research, Bangladesh. Large epidemic of cholera-like disease in Bangladesh caused by *Vibrio cholerae* synonym Bengal. Lancet 1993;342:387–390.

59. Swerdlow DL, Ries AA. *Vibrio cholerae* non-O139—the eighth pandemic? Lancet 1993;3242:382–383.

60. Chongsa-nguan M, Chaicumpa W, Moolasard P, et al. *Vibrio cholerae* O139 Bengal in Bangkok. Lancet 1993;342:430–431.

61. Centers for Disease Control and Prevention. Imported cholera associated with a newly described toxigenic *Vibrio cholerae* O139 strain California, 1993. MMWR Morb Mortal Wkly Rep 1993;42:501–503.

62. Sack RB, Albert MI, Siddique AK. Emergence of *Vibrio cholerae* O139. Curr Clin Top Infect Dis 1996;16:172–193.

63. Wittlinger F, Steffen R, Watanage H, Handszuh H. Risk of cholera among Western and Japanese travelers. J Travel Med 1995;2:154–158.

64. Sanchez JL, Taylor DN. Cholera. Lancet 1997;349:1826–1830.

65. Mahon BE, Mintz ED, Greene DK, et al. Reported cholera in the United States, 1992–1994: a reflection of global changes in cholera epidemiology. JAMA 1996;276:307–312.

66. Steffen R, Dupont HL. Travel medicine: what's that? J Travel Med 1994;1:1–3.

67. Centers for Disease Control. Cholera vaccine: recommendations of the Immunization Practices Advisory Committee. MMWR Morb Mortal Wkly Rep 1988;37:617–624.

68. Snyder JD, Blake PA. Is cholera a problem for US travelers? JAMA 1982;247:2268–2269.

69. Weber JT, Levine WC, Hopkins DP, Tauxe RV. Cholera in the United States, 1965–1991; risks at home and abroad. Arch Intern Med 1994;154:551–556.

70. Swerdlow DL, Ries AA. Cholera in the Americas; guideline for the clinician. JAMA 1992;1495–1499.

71. Kollaritsch H, Que JU, Wiedermann G, et al. Safety and immunogenicity of live oral cholera and typhoid vaccines administered alone or in combination with antimalarial drugs, oral polio vaccine or yellow fever vaccine. J Infect Dis 1997; 175:871–875.

72. Cryz SJ, Que JU, Levine MM, et al. Safety and immunogenicity of a live oral bivalent typhoid fever (*Salmonella typhi* 21a)-cholera (*Vibrio cholerae* CVD103- HgR) vaccine in healthy adults. Infect Immun 1995;63:1336–1339.

73. Christenson B. Epidemiological aspects of acute viral hepatitis A in Swedish travelers to endemic areas. Scand J Infect Dis 1985;17:5–10.

74. Lange WR, Frame JD. High incidence of viral hepatitis among American missionaries in Africa. Am J Trop Med Hyg 1990; 43:527–533.

75. Steffen R, Kane MA, Shapiro CN, et al. Epidemiology and prevention of hepatitis A in travelers. JAMA 1994;272:885–889.

76. Hadler SC. Global impact of hepatitis A virus infection changing patterns. In: Hollinger FB, Lemon SM, Margolis H, eds. Viral hepatitis and liver disease: Proceedings of the 1990 International Symposium on Viral Hepatitis and Liver Disease: contemporary issues and future prospects. Baltimore: Williams & Wilkins, 1991:14–20.

77. Barnett ED, Holmes AH, Phillips SL, et al. Immunity to hepatitis A in travelers born and raised in hepatitis A endemic areas [abstract 280]. In: Proceedings of the Fifth International Conference on Travel Medicine. Geneva: International Society of Travel Medicine, 1997:207.

78. Hepatitis A: a vaccine at last. Lancet 1992;339:1198–1199.

79. Nalin DR. VAQTA, hepatitis A vaccine, purified inactivated. Drugs of the Future 1995;20:24–29.

80. Shouval D, Ashur Y, Adler R, et al. Single and booster dose responses to an inactivated hepatitis A virus vaccine: comparison with immune serum globulin prophylaxis. Vaccine 1993;11(Suppl 1):9–14.

81. Ellerbeck EF, Lewis JA, Nalin D, et al. Safety profile and immunogenicity of an inactivated vaccine derived from an attenuated strain of hepatitis A. Vaccine 1992;10:668–672.

82. Werzberger A, Mensch B, Kuter B, et al. A controlled trial of a formalin-inactivated hepatitis A vaccine in healthy children. N Engl J Med 1992;327:488–490.

83. Block SL, Hedrick JA, Tyler RD, et al. Safety, tolerability and immunogenicity of a formalin-inactivated hepatitis A vaccine (VAQTA) in rural Kentucky children. Pediatr Infect Dis J 1993;12:976–980.

84. Innis BL, Snitbhan R, Kunasol P, et al. Protection against hepatitis A by an inactivated vaccine. JAMA 1994;271:1328–1334.

85. Victor J, Knudsen JD, Nielsen LP, et al. Hepatitis A vaccine. A new convenient single-dose schedule with booster when long-term immunization is warranted. Vaccine 1994;12:1327–1329.

86. Clemens R, Sarary A, Hepburn A, et al. Clinical experience with an inactivated hepatitis A vaccine. J Infect Dis 1995; 171(Suppl 1):S44–49.

87. Centers for Disease Control and Prevention. Prevention of hepatitis A through active or passive immunization: recommendations of the Advisory Committee on Immunization Practices (ACIP). MMWR Morb Mortal Wkly Rep 1999; 48(RR-12):19.

88. Fenn P, McGuire A, Gary A. An economic evaluation of vaccination against hepatitis A for frequent travelers. J Infect 1998;36:17–22.

89. Bienzle U, Bock HL, Kruppenbacher JP, et al. Immunogenicity of an inactivated hepatitis A vaccine administered according to two different schedules and the interference of other "travellers" vaccines with the immune response. Vaccine 1996;14:501–505.

90. Bodsworth NJ, Neilsen GA, Donovan B. The effect of immunization with inactivated hepatitis A vaccine on the clinical course of HIV-1 infection: 1-year follow-up. AIDS 1997;11:747–749.

91. Bryan JP, Nelson M. Testing for antibody to hepatitis A to decrease the cost of hepatitis A prophylaxis with immune globulin or hepatitis A vaccines. Arch Intern Med 1994;154:663–668.

92. Monath TP. Japanese encephalitis—plague of the Orient. N Engl J Med 1988;319:641–643.

93. Umenai T, Krzysko R, Bektimirov TA, Assaad FA. Japanese encephalitis: current worldwide status. Bull World Health Organ 1985;63:625–631.

94. Trillin C. American chronicles: Zei-di-man. The New Yorker 1985;Oct 7:61–94.

95. Macdonald WBG, Tink AR, Ouvrier RA, et al. Japanese encephalitis after a two-week holiday in Bali. Med J Aust 1989;150:334–339.

96. Wittesjo B, Eitrem R, Niklasson B, et al. Japanese encephalitis after a 10-day holiday in Bali. Lancet 1995;345:856.

97. Falstead SB. Arboviruses of the Pacific and Southeast Asia. In: Feigin RD, Cherry JD, eds. Textbook of pediatric infectious diseases. 3rd Ed. Philadelphia: WB Saunders, 1992:1468–1475.

98. Centers for Disease Control and Prevention. Inactivated Japanese encephalitis virus vaccine. Recommendations of the advisory committee on immunization practices (ACIP). MMWR Morb Mortal Wkly Rep 1993;42(RR1):1–15.

99. McKinney WP, Barnas GP. Japanese encephalitis vaccine: an orphan product in need of adoption [letter]. N Engl J Med 1988;318:255–256.

100. Hoke CH, Nisalak A, Sangawhipa N, et al. Protection against Japanese encephalitis by inactivated vaccines. N Engl J Med 1988;319:608–614.

101. Poland JD, Cropp CB, Craven RB, Monath TP. Evaluation of the potency and safety of inactivated Japanese encephalitis vaccine in US inhabitants. J Infect Dis 1990;161:878–882.

102. Yamada A, Imanishi J, Juang RF, et al. Trial of inactivated Japanese encephalitis vaccine in children with underlying diseases. Vaccine 1986;4:32–34.

103. Koch S, Steffen R. Meningococcal disease in travelers: vaccination recommendations. J Travel Med 1994;1:4–7.

104. Moore PS, Harrison L, Telzak EE, et al. Group A meningococcal carriage in travelers returning from Saudi Arabia. JAMA 1988;260:2686–2689.

105. Serogroup W-135 meningococcal disease among travelers returning from Saudi Arabia—United States, 2000. MMWR Morb Mortal Wkly Rep 2000;47:345–346.

106. Twumasi PA, Kumah S, Leach, et al. A trial of a group A plus group C meningococcal polysaccharide-protein conjugate vaccine in African infants. J Infect Dis 1995;171:632–638.

107. De Moraes JC, Perkins BA, Camargo MCC, et al. Protective efficacy of a serogroup B meningococcal vaccine in Sao Paulo, Brazil. Lancet 1992;340:1074–1078.

108. Bjune G, Hoiby EA, Gronnesby JK, et al. Effect of outer membrane vesicle vaccine against group B meningococcal disease in Norway. Lancet 1991;338:1093–1096.

109. Fishbein DB, Robinson LE. Rabies. N Engl J Med 1993;329: 1632–1638.

110. Phanuphak P, Ubolyam S, Sirivichayakul S. Should travelers in rabies endemic areas receive pre-exposure rabies immunization? Ann Med Intern (Paris) 1994;145:409–411.

111. Sperizh RO, Morris JH, Lawhashwasdik. Rabies study SEATO. Medical Residence Laboratory, Annual Report, 1996.

112. Centers for Disease Control. Human rabies prevention—United States, 1999: recommendations of the Immunization Practices Advisory Committee (ACIP). MMWR Morb Mortal Wkly Rep 1999;48(RR-13):1–21.

113. Wilde H. Preexposure rabies vaccination. J Travel Med 1994; 1:51–54.

114. Pappaioanou M, Fishbein DB, Dreesen DW, et al. Antibody response to preexposure human diploid-cell rabies vaccine given concurrently with chloroquine. N Engl J Med 1986;314: 280–284.

115. Varner MW, McGuinness GA, Galask RP. Rabies vaccination in pregnancy. Am J Obstet Gynecol 1982;143:717–718.

116. Grandstrom M. Tick-borne zoonoses in Europe. Clin Microbiol Infect 1997;22:156–163.

117. McNeil JG, Lednar WM, Stansfield SK, et al. Central European tickborne encephalitis: assessment of risk for persons in the armed services and vacationers. J Infect Dis 1985;152: 650–651.

118. Le TP, Hoffman SL. Typhoid fever. In: Guerrant RL, Walker DH, Weller PF, eds. Tropical infectious diseases: principles, pathogenesis, and practice. 1st Ed. Philadelphia: Churchill Livingstone, 1999:277–295.

119. Ryan CA, Gargrett-Bean NT, Blake PA. *Salmonella typhi* infection in the United States, 1975–1984: increasing role of foreign travel. Rev Infect Dis 1989;11:1–8.

120. Rao N. Protecting travelers from typhoid fever. Infect Cont Hosp Epidemiol 1991;12:168–172.

121. Mahle WT, Levine MM. *Salmonella typhi* infection in children younger than five years of age. Pediatr Infect Dis J 1993; 12:627–631.

122. Typhoid in the United States and the risk to the international traveler. J Infect Dis 1983;148:599–602.

123. Schwartz E, Shlim DR, Eaton M, et al. The effect of oral and parenteral typhoid vaccination on the rate of infection with *Salmonella typhi* and *Salmonella paratyphi* among foreigners in Nepal. Arch Intern Med 1990;150:349–351.

124. Woodruff BA, Pavia AT, Blake PA. A new look at typhoid vaccination: information for the practicing physician. JAMA 1991;265:756–759.

125. Mandal BK. Modern treatment of typhoid fever. J Infect 1991;22:1–4.

126. Levine MM, Ferreccio C, Black RE, et al. Progress in vaccines against typhoid fever. Rev Infect Dis 1989;11(Suppl 3): S552–S567.

127. Centers for Disease Control and Prevention. Typhoid immunization. Recommendations of the immunization practices advisory committee. MMWR Morb Mortal Wkly Rep 1974;43:1–7.

128. Acharya IL, Lowe CU, Thapa R, et al. Prevention of typhoid fever in Nepal with the Vi capsular polysaccharide of *Salmonella typhi*. N Engl J Med 1987;317:1101–1104.

129. Klugman KP, Gilbertson IT, Koornhof HJ, et al. Protective activity of Vi capsular polysaccharide vaccine against typhoid fever. Lancet 1987;1165–1169.

130. Typhoid vaccination: weighing the options. Lancet 1992;340: 341–342.

131. Simanjuntak CH, Paleologo FP, Punjabi NH, et al. Oral immunization against typhoid fever in Indonesia with Ty21a vaccine. Lancet 1991;338:1055–1059.

132. Levine MM, Ferreccio C, Cryz S, Ortiz E. Comparison of enteric-coated capsules and liquid formulation of Ty21a vaccine in randomized controlled field trial. Lancet 1990;336: 891–894.

133. Olanratmanee T, Levine M, Losonsky G, et al. Safety and immunogenicity of *Salmonella typhi* Ty21a liquid formulation vaccine in 4- to 6-year old Thai children. J Infect Dis 1992; 166:451–452.

134. Arya SC. Typhoid Vi vaccine and infection by Vi-negative strains of *S. typhi*. J Travel Med 1997;4:207.

135. Engels EA, Falagas ME, Lau J, Bennish ML. Typhoid fever vaccines: a meta-analysis of studies on efficacy and toxicity. BMJ 1998;316:110–116.

136. Robertson SE, Hull BP, Tomori O, et al. Yellow fever: a decade of reemergence. JAMA 1996;276:1157–1162.

137. Thonnon J, Fontenille D, Tall A, et al. Re-emergence of yellow fever in Senegal in 1995. Am J Trop Med 1998;59:108–114.

138. Vasconcelos PFC, Rodrigues SG, Degallier N, et al. An epidemic of sylvatic yellow fever in the southeast region of Maranhao State, Brazil, 1993–1994: epidemiologic and entomologic findings. Am J Trop Med Hyg 1997;57:132–137.

139. Van der Stuykft P, Gianella A, Pirard M, et al. Urbanization of yellow fever in Santa Cruz, Bolivia. Lancet 1999;353: 1558–1562.

140. Monath TP. Facing up to re-emergence of urban yellow fever. Lancet 1999;353:1541.

141. McFarland JM, Baddour LM, Nelson JE, et al. Imported yellow fever in a United States citizen. Clin Infect Dis 1997;25: 1143–1147.

142. Salaun JJ, Germain M, Robert V, et al. La fievre jaune au Senegal de 1976 a 1980. Medecine Tropicale 1981;41:45–51.

143. Teichmann D, Grobusch MP, Wesselmann H, et al. A haemorrhagic fever, from the Côte d'Ivoire. Lancet 1999;354:1608.

144. McKee KT, Monath TP. Arboviruses of Africa. In: Feigin RD, Cherry JD, eds. Textbook of pediatric infectious diseases. Philadelphia: WB Saunders, 1992:1444–1446.

145. World Health Organization. Prevention and control of yellow fever in Africa. Geneva: WHO, 1986:55–65.

146. Thomson WO. Encephalitis in infants following vaccination with 17D yellow fever virus: report of a further case. BMJ 1955;2:182–183.

147. Stuart G. Reactions following vaccination against yellow fever. In: Smithburn JC, ed. Yellow fever vaccination. Geneva: World Health Organization, 1956:143–189.

148. Stefano I, Sato HK, Pannuti CS, et al. Recent immunization against measles does not interfere with the sero-response to yellow fever vaccine. Vaccine 1999;17:1042–1046.

149. Kaplan JE, Nelson DB, Schonberger LB, et al. The effect of immune globulin on the response to trivalent oral poliovirus and yellow fever vaccinations. Bull World Health Organ 1984;62:585–590.

150. Tsai TF, Bolin RA, Lazuick JS, Miller KE. Chloroquine does not adversely affect the antibody response to yellow fever vaccine [letter]. J Infect Dis 1986;154:726–727.

151. Goujon M, Tohr M, Feullie V, et al. Good tolerance and efficacy of yellow fever vaccine among subject carriers of human immunodeficiency virus [abstract 32]. In: Proceedings of the Fourth International Conference on Travel Medicine, 1995:63.

152. Tsai TF, Paul R, Lynberg MC, Letson GW. Congenital yellow fever virus infection after immunization in pregnancy. J Infect Dis 1993;168:1520–1523.

153. Beutels P, Van Damme P, Piper-Jenks N, Hilton E. Economic evaluation in travel medicine. In: Dupont HL, Steffen R, eds. Textbook of travel medicine and health. Hamilton, ON: BC Decker 1997:276–286.

154. Behrens RH, Roberts JA. Is travel prophylaxis worthwhile? Economic appraisal of prophylactic measures against malaria, hepatitis A, and typhoid in travelers. BMF 1994;309:918–922.

155. Van Doorslaer E, Tormans G, Van Damme P. Cost-effectiveness analysis of vaccination against hepatitis A in travelers. J Med Virol 1994;44:463–469.

156. LeGuerrier P, Pilon PA, Deshaies D, Allard R. Pre-exposure rabies prophylaxis for the international traveler: a decision analysis. Vaccine 1996;14:167–176.

22.3 ENTERIC VACCINES: PRESENT AND FUTURE

MYRON M. LEVINE AND ANN-MARI SVENNERHOLM

PRIORITIZATION OF VACCINES TO PREVENT ENTERIC INFECTIONS

Approximately one-third of all travelers to less-developed countries who stay for at least 1 week experience diarrheal illness caused mainly by bacterial pathogens and less often by viruses and protozoa. Hepatitis and typhoid fever are other enteric infections that pose risks for the traveler. New or improved vaccines against the following enteric infections are considered desirable to prevent disease among travelers: hepatitis A, enterotoxigenic *Escherichia coli* (ETEC), shigellosis, typhoid fever, cholera, giardiasis, and rotavirus (for pediatric travelers); vaccines against *Entamoeba histolytica*, *Campylobacter jejuni,* and caliciviruses such as the Norwalk gastroenteritis virus would also be welcome, whereas a need has not been clearly established for a vaccine against hepatitis E. Some of these enteric pathogens generally cause relatively mild clinical illness but occur at such a high incidence that suitable vaccines are needed (e.g., most episodes of ETEC diarrhea). Others among the above-listed enteric infections occur less frequently, yet vaccines are desirable because severe or fatal illness can rapidly ensue when a traveler is stricken (e.g., shigellosis, cholera, typhoid fever).

VACCINES AGAINST HEPATITIS A

RATIONALE

In less-developed regions of the world, infection by hepatitis A virus occurs almost universally in early childhood when clinical illness with this virus typically manifests as a mild, short-lived, nonicteric syndrome. In contrast, in the well-sanitated, hygienic environments of industrialized countries, most of the population reaches adulthood without having had contact with hepatitis A virus. If hepatitis A infection is acquired by nonimmune adults when they travel, a debilitating, clinical illness manifested by jaundice and extending for many weeks is likely to occur. For this reason, it is desirable to immunize travelers with vaccines against hepatitis A.

CURRENT VACCINES

Several parenteral vaccines that became available in the early 1990s (Table 22.3–1) consisting of formalin-inactivated whole hepatitis A virus, which are reviewed in the chapter on hepatitis, have had an extraordinary impact on providing travelers with active, long-lived protection from hepatitis A. However, the first generation of these vaccines, which require multiple spaced doses to elicit long-lived antibodies and immunologic memory, is relatively expensive to manufacture because the yield of virus in tissue culture is low. For this reason, research is continuing to develop vaccines that would be less expensive and might require the administration of fewer doses.

FUTURE VACCINES

Two broad strategies are being followed to develop improved hepatitis A vaccines (see Table 22.3–1). The first consists of formulating small amounts of inactivated virus in specialized antigen delivery systems in order to enhance immunogenicity. In this manner, it may be possible to immunize with a single dose of vaccine containing smaller amounts of hepatitis A antigen, thereby diminishing the cost of manufacture of vaccine. One such virosome vaccine against hepatitis A has recently become available and is already licensed in a number of countries.[1]

A second strategy being pursued independently by investigators in the U.S.A. and China is to develop attenuated strains of hepatitis A that will lead to subclinical infection followed by long-lived immunity.[2] If an appropriate level of attenuation can be attained with a replicating virus, it may be possible to immunize with a single dose of virus in relatively low titer; such a vaccine has the potential to be economical. Several candidate live strains tested in the U.S.A. were either insufficiently attenuated or hyperattenuated. An attenuated strain developed in China is undergoing large-scale clinical trials.

A combination parenteral hepatitis A/typhoid fever vaccine that consists of 1,440 units of inactivated hepatitis A virus and 25 µg of purified Vi capsular polysaccharide of *Salmonella typhi* was recently licensed in Europe.[3]

VACCINES AGAINST TYPHOID FEVER

RATIONALE

The risk of travelers acquiring typhoid fever varies widely throughout the less-developed world but is remarkably high in certain areas (e.g., Peru and the Indian subcontinent). The recent appearance throughout South and Southeast Asia and the Middle East of *S. typhi* exhibiting concomitant resistance to amoxicillin, trimethoprim/sulfamethoxazole, and chloramphenicol has emphasized the need for practical, highly effective vaccines. It is often forgotten that prior to 1950, when the efficacy of chloramphenicol in treating typhoid fever became widely recognized, the case fatality of typhoid fever worldwide was 10% to 20%. Thus, even today, a misdiagnosed, inappropriately treated case of multiply resistant typhoid fever can lead to fatality. The rising prevalence of these resistant *S. typhi* strains has increased the importance of having improved typhoid vaccines to offer to travelers.

Table 22.3–1.   CURRENTLY LICENSED ENTERIC VACCINES OR THOSE IN CURRENT CLINICAL TRIALS

TYPE OF VACCINE	ROUTE OF IMMUNIZATION	NUMBER OF DOSES	TRADE NAME (MANUFACTURER) OF LICENSED PRODUCT	SPONSOR OF EXPERIMENTAL VACCINE
Hepatitis				
Licensed vaccines				
Inactivated whole virus	Parenteral	2-3	Havrix (SKB); Vaqta (Merck)	
Inactivated virus in virosomes	Parenteral	1	Epaxal (SSVI)	
Experimental vaccines				
Attenuated	Parenteral	1	—	
Typhoid				
Licensed vaccines				
Live attenuated				
Ty21a	Oral	3–4	Vivotif, Typhoral (SSVI)	
Nonliving				
Vi polysaccharide	Parenteral	1	Typhim Vi (PMC)	
Experimental vaccines				
Live				
CVD 908-*htr*A	Oral	1		PT
Ty800	Oral	1		Avant
X4076	Oral	1		Megan
Nonliving				
Vi-protein conjugates	Parenteral	1	PMC	
Cholera				
Licensed				
Nonliving				
rBS-WC (01)	Oral	2	Dukoral, Colorvac	SBL Vaccin
Live				
CVD 103-HgR	Oral	1	Orochol, Mutacol	SSVI
Experimental				
Nonliving				
BS-WC O1/O139	Oral	2		SBL Vaccin
Live				
CVD 111 (O1, El Tor)	Oral	1		SSVI
CVD 112 (O139)	Oral	1		SSVI
Peru-15 (O1)	Oral	1		Avant
Bengal (O139)	Oral	1		Avant
Shigella				
Experimental				
Live attenuated *Shigella*				
icsA, iuc mutants	Oral	1–2		
guaBA, sen, set, virG mutants	Oral	1–2		Chiron
Nonliving				
Proteosomes	Oral	2		Intellivax
O Ps-protein conjugates	Parenteral	2		
ETEC				
Nonliving				
rBS-CFA ETEC	Oral	2		SBL Vaccin
Live				
Attenuated *E. coli*	Oral	1–2		Medeva
CFAs expresed in attenuated				
Shigella live vectors	Oral	1–2		

SKB = SmithKline Beecham, SSVI = Swiss Serum and Vaccine Institute, PMC = Pasteur Mérieux Connaught, PT = Peptide Therapeutics, SBL = Swedish Bacteriological Laboratory. This table lists most but not all experimental enteric vaccines in clinical trials.

CURRENTLY AVAILABLE VACCINES

The efficacy of typhoid vaccines has usually been evaluated in field trials in typhoid-endemic areas where older children and adults often have considerable prior contact with *S. typhi*. The efficacy of these vaccines in immunologically naive travelers may be lower. It is generally believed that a reasonable estimate of the level of efficacy that typhoid vaccines can confer upon travelers can be derived by considering their efficacy in young children in endemic areas.

Inactivated Whole-Cell Parenteral Vaccines

Parenteral vaccines consisting of heat-inactivated, phenol-preserved *S. typhi* bacteria have been in use for a century. In large-scale, randomized, placebo-controlled, double-blind field trials carried out in the 1960s, these vaccines were shown to confer a moderate (51%–67% efficacy) level of protection against typhoid fever. However, these whole-cell vaccines cause severe systemic adverse reactions at such a high frequency (25% develop fever, sometimes high; 15% remain absent from school or work) that they are considered unsuitable for routine use among travelers.[4]

Ty21a, Live Oral Typhoid Vaccine

Ty21a, an attenuated strain of *S. typhi* that is safe and protective as a live oral vaccine, was developed in the early 1970s by chemical mutagenesis of a pathogenic *S. typhi* strain. Ty21a has proven to be remarkably well tolerated in placebo-controlled clinical trials. Controlled field trials of Ty21a emphasize that the formulation of the vaccine and the number of doses administered markedly influence the level of protection that can be achieved.[4] In the first field trial of Ty21a in Alexandria, Egypt, 6- to 7-year-old schoolchildren received three doses of vaccine (suspended in a diluent) on Monday, Wednesday, and Friday of 1 week; to neutralize gastric acid, the children chewed a 1.0-g tablet of $NaHCO_3$ before ingesting the vaccine or placebo. During 3 years of surveillance, 96% protective efficacy against confirmed typhoid fever was observed.

The most widely available commercial formulation of Ty21a consists of lyophilized vaccine in enteric-coated, acid-resistant capsules. In a randomized, placebo-controlled field trial in schoolchildren in Santiago, Chile, three doses of this enteric-coated formulation given within 1 week (every other day schedule) provided 67% efficacy during the first 3 years of follow-up and 62% protection over 7 years of follow-up.[5] Based on these data, most countries use a three-dose schedule of enteric-coated Ty21a. However, in a large comparative trial, four doses of Ty21a in enteric-coated capsules given within 8 days (one dose every other day for four doses) were significantly more protective than two or three doses[4,6]; based on these data, the enteric-coated formulation of Ty21a was licensed in the U.S.A. and Canada with a recommended four-dose regimen.

To determine whether Ty21a administered as a liquid suspension (somewhat similar to that used in Alexandria) is superior to vaccine in enteric-coated capsules, two field trials were initiated in Chile and Indonesia. In both trials, the liquid formulation was superior.[4,7,8] In Chile, where the liquid formulation was administered on an every other day schedule, the vaccine conferred 78% protection over 5 years of follow-up.[5] The liquid formulation of Ty21a is becoming licensed in an increasing number of countries. In summary, orally administered, well-tolerated Ty21a offers a moderate level of protection against typhoid fever if one can ensure that the required three to four doses (every other day schedule) are taken. The salient characteristics of Ty21a vaccine (Vivotif®, manufactured by Swiss Serum and Vaccine Institute) are summarized in Table 22.3–2.

Purified Vi Polysaccharide Parenteral Vaccine

Vi antigen, a capsular polysaccharide found on the surface of *S. typhi*, is a recognized virulence property. When highly purified Vi antigen is administered parenterally, it is well tolerated. Purified Vi used as a parenteral polysaccharide vaccine was evaluated in randomized, placebo-controlled, double-blind field trials in Nepal (children and adults) and South Africa (school-aged children) where a well-tolerated single dose of 25 µg conferred circa 65% protection against typhoid fever for at least 17 to 21 months.[9,10] In South Africa, the vaccine conferred 55% protection over 3 years of follow-up.[11] Thus, the Vi vaccine provides a moderate level of protection with just a single dose.[4,11] The characteristics of purified Vi vaccine are summarized in Table 22.3–2. Originally, there was only a single manufacturer of Vi vaccine (TyphiViM®, Pasteur Mérieux Serums & Vaccins); however, presently, Vi vaccine is available from several sources. Vi polysaccharide elicits serum IgG antibodies in the majority of toddlers 12 to 18 months of age, but the titers fall rapidly and the protective effect of Vi in children < 18 months of age is not known. Purified polysaccharide vaccines derived from other bacteria (e.g., *Haemophilus influenzae* type b and *Streptococcus pneumoniae*) are poorly immunogenic and protective in infants.

VI POLYSACCHARIDE-CARRIER PROTEIN CONJUGATE VACCINES

Booster doses of purified Vi do not raise antibody titers over those elicited by a single dose of vaccine, that is, immunologic memory is not induced. To increase the immunogenicity of Vi by conferring T cell-dependent properties upon the antigen, including the induction of immunologic memory, Vi polysaccharide has been conjugated to carrier proteins, such as tetanus toxoid (see Table 22.3–1).[12] In children, booster doses of Vi conjugate vaccine clearly increase the titers of Vi antibody over those elicited by a priming dose of conjugate. A Vi conjugate vaccine developed by S. Szu, J. Robbins, and coinvestigators at the National Institute of Child Health and Human Development, Bethesda, MD, is being evaluated in a large-scale, randomized, controlled Phase 3 efficacy trial in Vietnam.[13]

NEW ATTENUATED *S. TYPHI* STRAINS AS LIVE ORAL VACCINES

New strains of *S. typhi* with precise attenuating mutations have been engineered that appear to immunize successfully following administration of just a single oral dose (see Table 22.3–1).[14–17] Four *S. typhi* strains, CVD 908, CVD 908-*htrA*, Ty800, and X4073, have completed phase 1 clinical trials in which they were shown to be well tolerated and immunogenic following ingestion of a single oral dose. Strain CVD 908-*htrA* has completed phase 2 trials with a lyophilized formulation that documented the clinical acceptability and strong immunogenicity of the candidate vaccine in eliciting serum antibodies, mucosal IgA, and cell-mediated immune responses (including cytotoxic T lymphocytes). It is expected that CVD 908-

Table 22.3–2. COMPARISON OF THE SALIENT CHARACTERISTICS OF TWO
FORMULATIONS OF LIVE ORAL VACCINE TY21A AND PARENTERAL VI
POLYSACCHARIDE VACCINE

	TY21A ENTERIC-COATED CAPSULES	TY21A LIQUID FORMULATION	VI POLYSACCHARIDE
Type of vaccine	Live	Live	Subunit
Route of administration	Oral	Oral	Parenteral
Immunization schedule	3 or 4 doses (every other day)	3 doses (every other day)	1 dose
Well tolerated	Yes	Yes	Yes
3-year efficacy	35%–67%	55%–77%	55%*
Duration of efficacy and level	7 yr, 62%	5 yr, 78%	3 yr, 55%
Evidence of a herd immunity effect	Yes	Yes	?
Interferes with use of serum Vi antibody as a screening test to detect chronic typhoid carriers	No	No	Yes

*Published data from the South African field trial demonstrated 64% vaccine efficacy over 21 months of follow-up.[10]

htrA will be evaluated in a phase 3 field trial of efficacy beginning in 2000.

VACCINES AGAINST CHOLERA

RATIONALE

Prior to 1991, the occurrence of cholera among travelers was uncommon. However, since the extension of cholera to Latin America, travel-related cases of cholera have greatly increased, particularly in the Western Hemisphere. Two recent studies suggest that the incidence of travelers' cholera is surprisingly high if appropriate bacteriologic methods are used to culture *Vibrio cholerae* and if denominators can be determined with reasonable precision.[18,19] Diminished gastric acidity and O blood group constitute important host risk factors for developing severe diarrhea during cholera infection. In the elderly patient with cardiovascular dysfunction, particularly those on digitalis and diuretics, even moderate cholera diarrhea can cause electrolyte imbalance leading to dangerous cardiac arrythmias or to cardiac dysfunction secondary to diarrheal dehydration and hypovolemia.

Data on the efficacy of cholera vaccines come from two sources: field trials in endemic areas (where adults and older children have had considerable prior antigenic contact with cholera antigens) and experimental challenge studies in immunologically naive adult volunteers. It has been argued that, with respect to the protection of immunologically naive travelers from industrialized countries who visit less-developed countries where cholera is endemic or epidemic, data from experimental challenge studies in immunologically naive volunteers may offer the best estimate of expected vaccine efficacy. Results of field trials of efficacy that have included young children (2–5 years of age) in endemic areas also provide useful data to estimate the efficacy of vaccines for travelers, although even young children typically manifest elevated

levels of antitoxin and higher baseline vibriocidal levels than travelers.

CURRENTLY AVAILABLE VACCINES

Killed Whole-Cell Parenteral Vaccines The fairly reactogenic inactivated whole-cell parenteral cholera vaccine that has been available for 90 years confers moderate (35%–70% vaccine efficacy) protection for a few months on adults and older children in endemic areas but provides little protection to children less than 5 years of age. The World Health Organization and other advisory agencies do not recommend the use of the parenteral killed whole-cell vaccine. Since *V. cholerae* O1 does not invade the intestinal mucosa and specific secretory IgA (SIgA) antibodies are deemed to be important, modern approaches have focused on oral vaccines to stimulate more efficiently SIgA antibodies locally in the intestine (see Table 22.3–1).

Nonliving Oral Vaccines Based on the detailed knowledge of the pathogenic and immune mechanisms in cholera, an oral inactivated cholera vaccine was developed during the early 1980s. This vaccine consists of a combination of killed vibrios representing the different serotypes (Inaba and Ogawa) and biotypes (classical and El Tor) of *V. cholerae* O1 and a toxoid, that is, the purified B subunits (BS) of cholera toxin.[20] In extensive clinical trials in Sweden, the United States, Bangladesh, and Peru, the BS-whole-cell (WC) vaccine was shown to be well tolerated and immunogenic in eliciting serum as well as intestinal antibodies.[21–23] The protective effect of three spaced doses of a pilot formulation of the BS-WC vaccine (that contained a fivefold greater amount of B subunit than subsequent formulations) was initially assessed in a small clinical trial in adult American volunteers; whereas overall efficacy against challenge with *V. cholerae* O1 El Tor was 64%, the BS-WC vaccine conferred complete

(100%) protection against moderate to severe cholera.[24] In a large field trial in Bangladesh during 1985 to 1988, another early formulation of the vaccine provided a high level of short-term protection, that is, 85% during the initial 6 months and 50% protection during 3 years.[25] Through its BS component, the vaccine also provided highly significant, although short-lasting, protection (67% for a 3-month period) against diarrhea caused by *E. coli* producing either LT alone or LT together with ST.[21,26] Similar protective effects have been induced by two doses of the BS-WC vaccine against *E. coli* LT diarrhea in Finnish travelers to Morocco (circa 60% protective efficacy)[27] and in U.S. citizens going to Mexico (~50% protection).[28]

In order to facilitate production of the oral BS-WC vaccine, BS produced by recombinant DNA technology (rBS) was used in the formulation of the vaccine that is currently commercialized so that the vaccine could be produced at lower cost and on a large scale (see Table 22.3–1).[29] Two doses of the rBS-WC vaccine given 2 weeks apart conferred on young adult Peruvian soldiers (710 vaccinees, 714 placebo controls) a high degree of short-term protection (86% protective efficacy) against epidemic cholera in the course of exposure to a common source vehicle of transmission.[30] In contrast, in a large placebo-controlled field trial of efficacy in Lima, Peru, that included children as well as adults, two doses of the rBS-WC vaccine did not confer significant protection during a 12-month period of follow-up (0% efficacy) against either hospitalized cases (detected by passive surveillance) or field cases (detected by active surveillance).[31] However, following the administration of a third dose of vaccine 1 year later, significant (61%) protection was conferred over the next year of observation, including against both hospitalized cases (82% efficacy) and against field cases (49% efficacy).[26,32]

The oral rBS-WC vaccine is produced by SBL Vaccin AB, Stockholm, Sweden, and marketed under the names Dukoral® or Colorvac®, and is licensed in six Latin American countries and in Sweden and Norway for use in travelers. The vaccine should be given in a glass of water together with an alkaline buffer in two doses 1 to 2 weeks apart; a booster dose is recommended after 1 or 2 years.

CVD 103-HgR Live Oral Cholera Vaccine   Single-dose recombinant live oral cholera vaccine CVD 103-HgR was engineered by deleting from wild-type *V. cholerae* O1 94% of the gene encoding the A subunit of cholera toxin and by inserting into the hemolysin A locus a gene encoding resistance to mercury ions. In a number of European and Asian countries, CVD 103-HgR is a licensed vaccine available to travelers under the trade name Orochol®; in North America (Canada), it is available under the name Mutacol® (see Table 22.3–1).[33,34]

A large body of evidence from randomized, placebo-controlled clinical trials in many countries established the safety and immunogenicity of this vaccine in subjects as young as 3 months and as old as 65 years of age. CVD 103-HgR was licensed for use in travelers based on evidence of efficacy generated in experimental cholera challenge studies in adult volunteers in North America. It was shown that a single dose of CVD 103-HgR confers on adult volunteers significant protection against experimental challenge with pathogenic *V. cholerae* O1 of either biotype or serotype.[33–36] Notably, almost complete protection (>95%) is conferred against moderate and severe diarrhea caused by either El Tor or classic biotype. In these experimental challenge studies, protection (against wild-type *V. cholerae* O1 of either El Tor or classical biotype) is evident as early as 8 days after vaccination and lasts for at least 6 months (the shortest and longest intervals tested).[36] The single-dose efficacy and rapid onset of protection make CVD 103-HgR an attractive vaccine for immunization of travelers.

A large-scale, randomized, placebo-controlled, double-blind field trial involving 67,508 pediatric and adult subjects was carried out in Jakarta, Indonesia, to evaluate the efficacy of a single dose of CVD 103-HgR in preventing cholera under natural challenge conditions in an endemic area. Unfortunately, so few cases of cholera (only six) occurred in the first 6 months of observation that efficacy could not be assessed during the period when the level of protection might be expected to be maximal and during the period of follow-up that was comparable to the experimental challenge studies in volunteers.[37] Under any circumstances, the vaccine did not confer significant long-term protection in this venue during a 4-year period of follow-up (13.5% vaccine efficacy overall).[37]

FUTURE CHOLERA VACCINES

Attenuated El Tor Vaccines   CVD 111 and Peru 15 are attenuated El Tor vaccine candidates that have been well tolerated, immunogenic, and protective (in small experimental challenge studies) when tested in preliminary phase 1 and 2 clinical trials involving small numbers of adult volunteers. A bivalent CVD 103-HgR/CVD 111 vaccine has been well tolerated and immunogenic in phase 2 trials.[38]

New Antigenic Strain of *Vibrio cholerae*   In late 1992, a new antigenic strain of *V. cholerae* emerged (serogroup O139) capable of causing epidemic cholera of notable severity. Immunity against *V. cholerae* O1, such as that conferred by natural infection or oral O1 vaccines, did not cross-protect against O139 cholera. Initially, there were well-founded fears that *V. cholerae* O139 might be responsible for an eighth pandemic of cholera. Fortunately, these concerns have not been realized, and O139 has not spread from South Asia to Indonesia, Africa, or Latin America. Moreover, since 1996, in the countries of South Asia, the incidence of O139 disease has greatly diminished, and *V. cholerae* O1 has clearly resumed its position as the predominant agent causing cholera. Nevertheless, the world vaccine community responded promptly to the O139 threat by developing candidate O139 vaccines.

An inactivated O139 plus O1/BS combination vaccine has been developed and shown to be well tolerated and immunogenic in early clinical trials in Sweden where the vaccine stimulated significant intestinal SIgA responses against *V. cholerae* O1 and O139 antigens in the majority of vaccinated subjects.[22,39]

Accelerated vaccine development programs have resulted in the engineering of two recombinant O139 strains for use as live oral vaccines (CVD 112 and Bengal 3). In preliminary studies, single-dose regimens of these candidates have been well tolerated, immunogenic, and highly protective against experimental challenge with *V. cholerae* O139 in volunteer studies.[40,41] However, due to the decrease in the relative importance of O139 as a cause of cholera, its very limited spread to other countries in Asia, and its lack of spread to Africa and Latin America, since 1997 efforts to develop a licensed vaccine for protection against *V. cholerae* O139 have been much less intensive.

SHIGELLA VACCINES

RATIONALE

Shigella infections can result in rather severe clinical illness (including full-blown bacillary dysentery) in which complications are not uncommon. Morever, antibiotic-resistant strains of *Shigella* are highly prevalent, rendering treatment difficult. Last, in several large surveys, *Shigella* infections were found to be second only to ETEC in frequency among travelers with diarrheal illness. A considerable body of evidence shows that an initial clinical *Shigella* infection induces approximately 70% to 80% protection against shigellosis on subsequent exposure to the same serotype of *Shigella*. For these reasons, there is interest in developing vaccines to prevent *Shigella* disease. Although no licensed *Shigella* vaccines are presently available, since 1995 considerable progress has been made, and several vaccine candidates are in clinical trials.

EARLY *SHIGELLA* VACCINES

In the 1960s and early 1970s, live attenuated strains of *Shigella*, including streptomycin-dependent mutants of several *Shigella* serotypes and the T$_{32}$ colonial mutant of *S. flexneri* 2a, were shown to be safe and protective when administered as live oral vaccines. Nevertheless, those pioneering vaccines exhibited a number of shortcomings and did not become licensed products for use in travelers.

MODERN VACCINE CANDIDATES DEVELOPED BY THE APPLICATION OF BIOTECHNOLOGY

Shigella are highly host adapted human pathogens that exhibit a complex pathogenesis involving an impressive array of bacterial virulence properties. Until recently, it has proven difficult to develop attenuated strains for use as live oral vaccines that manifest the proper balance of low reactogenicity but high immunogenicity. Nevertheless, recently, progress is being made and clinical trials are under way with several live oral *Shigella* vaccine candidates.

Attenuated *Shigella* Strains Harboring aro, guaBA, virG, and iut Mutations   *S. flexneri* candi-dates have been developed in Sweden, France, and the U.S.A. Some strains (e.g., with mutations in aro or guaBA) are impaired in their capacity to proliferate in vivo after invasion.[42–44] Further attenuation can be achieved by introducing deletions in virG (also called icsA) so that the *Shigella* vaccine strains are diminished in their ability to spread from enterocyte to enterocyte.[43–45] Similarly, the introduction of deletion mutations in iuc inhibits the ability of the *Shigella* strains to scavenge iron.[45] In general, such live vaccine candidates have proven to be well tolerated at low dosage levels that elicit modest to moderate immune responses but exhibit reactogenicity, including diarrhea and fever, when administered at high dosage levels; immune responses are stronger at the higher, more reactogenic dosage levels.[42,46,47] Administration of two or three doses of vaccine containing lower, well-tolerated numbers of vaccine organisms succeeds in eliciting acceptable immune responses. Yet further attenuation of *Shigella* vaccine candidates has been achieved by inactivating the genes that encode *Shigella* enterotoxin 2 (found on the invasiveness plasmid of all *Shigella* serotypes) and *Shigella* enterotoxin 1 (located on a pathogenicity island within the chromosome of *S. flexneri* 2a).[48,49]

One group of investigators is constructing a pentavalent *Shigella* vaccine that includes serotypes *S. dysenteriae* 1, *S. flexneri* 2a, *S. flexneri* 3a, *S. flexneri* 6, and *S. sonnei*.[50] Another team is preparing a trivalent vaccine with serotypes *S. dysenteriae* 1, *S. flexneri* 2a, and *S. sonnei*.[47] Individual component vaccine strains are in clinical trials.[47,51]

Proteosomes as a Nonliving Mucosal *Shigella* Vaccine   Proteosomes are derived from the highly hydrophobic outer membrane proteins of group B meningococcus. When mixed with the LPS of *Shigella*, meningococcal proteosomes noncovalently associate with the *Shigella* LPS to form membranous vesicles that are highly immunogenic in animals when administered as either oral or intranasal vaccines.[52] In phase 1 clinical trials, *S. flexneri* 2a proteosomes were well tolerated and quite immunogenic.

MODERN PARENTERAL VACCINES

O-Polysaccharide-Carrier Protein Conjugate Vaccines   Candidate parenteral *Shigella* vaccines that consist of the O repeat polysaccharide (derived from lipopolysaccharide) conjugated to carrier proteins such as tetanus toxoid have been tested for efficacy (see Table 22.3–1).[53] It has been hypothesized that the reason that parenteral killed whole-cell *Shigella* vaccines developed many decades ago were not effective is that they likely stimulated IgM (i.e., putatively nonprotective) O antibodies, whereas the conjugate vaccines elicit IgG (i.e., putatively protective) O antibodies.[54] In a preliminary controlled field trial involving young adult Israeli soldiers, a *S. sonnei* conjugate vaccine conferred approximately 70% serotype-specific protection for at least 3 months (the limit of the surveillance).[53]

VACCINES AGAINST ETEC

RATIONALE

ETEC, the most common cause of travelers' diarrhea (accounting for 20%–50% of cases), usually results in a short-lived, mild to moderately discomforting illness in which physical activity, ability to function, and mobility are compromised. The high incidence of ETEC diarrhea among travelers to less-developed, tropical regions of the world makes ETEC an important target for immuno-prophylaxis. Although no licensed ETEC vaccines are currently available, one candidate vaccine is in Phase 3 trials and another is in early clinical trials, so there is great expectation that within the next few years ETEC vaccines will indeed become a tool for preventing disease in travelers.

PATHOGENESIS OF ETEC AND EVIDENCE OF INFECTION-DERIVED ANTICOLONIZATION IMMUNITY

Two critical virulence properties that contribute to the pathogenesis of ETEC diarrhea are (1) the attachment of ETEC bacteria to the mucosa of the proximal small intestine by means of fimbrial colonization factors and (2) the elaboration of heat-labile (LT) or heat-stable (ST) enterotoxins leading to intestinal secretion. ETEC comprise many different O:H serotypes, multiple antigenic types of fimbrial colonization factors, and three different toxin phenotypes (LT only, ST only, or LT-ST).[55–57] To confer broad-spectrum protection, vaccines must immunize against this heterogeneous array of ETEC pathogens. Fortunately, epidemiologic evidence and results of experimental challenge studies in volunteers clearly demonstrate that strain-specific immunity follows ETEC infection; furthermore, the cumulative experience of multiple infections with antigenically diverse ETEC strains leads to broad-spectrum protection against ETEC diarrhea. In less-developed countries, infants and young children often experience up to three separate clinical ETEC infections per year during the first 3 years of life, after which the incidence of ETEC diarrhea drastically falls. The lower incidence in indigenous adults is due to acquired immunity rather than to other age-related host factors, since adults from industrialized countries who visit regions where pediatric ETEC diarrhea is endemic suffer high attack rates of ETEC travelers' diarrhea. In agreement with this thesis, travelers from industrialized countries who remain in less-developed countries for at least a year (and who therefore typically suffer multiple episodes of ETEC diarrhea) thereafter exhibit significantly lower incidence rates of ETEC diarrhea than newly arrived travelers.

The same antigenic types (O:H serotypes) and fimbrial colonization factors are observed among strains that cause endemic pediatric diarrhea as among those that cause travelers' diarrhea (Table 22.3–3). Protective immunity to ETEC appears to be mediated by SIgA antibodies directed against fimbriae, other surface antigens, and LT; heat-stable toxin ST, which is a small peptide, does not elicit neutralizing antibodies following natural infection. A few prospective epidemiologic field studies provide evidence that acquired immunity is largely directed against fimbrial colonization factors of ETEC.

ANTIGENIC DIVERSITY OF FIMBRIAL CFAS AMONG ETEC

To provide broad-spectrum protection, a vaccine must contain fimbrial antigens representative of the most prevalent ETEC pathogens. The most common fimbrial colonization factors (CFs) of human ETEC are colonization factor antigen I (CFA/I) and the different subcomponents of the CFA/II and the CFA/IV families of antigens.[55,56] CFA/I is a single antigenic moiety, whereas coli surface antigens 1 (CS1), CS2, and CS3 constitute the CFA/II family of antigens. All CFA/II strains express CS3, either alone or in conjunction with CS1 or CS2. CS4, CS5, and CS6 comprise the CFA/IV family of antigens and all CFA/IV strains express CS6, either alone or in conjunction with CS4 or CS5. Other fimbrial CFs such as CS7, CS12, CS14, and CS17 are much less frequent. Expression of particular fimbrial CFs by ETEC strains is closely correlated with the O:H serotype and toxin phenotype.[55,56]

Analysis of ETEC isolates from diverse geographic areas shows that CFA/I and CS1-6 are found on the majority of isolates (see Table 22.3–3). Approximately 90% of isolates that elaborate both LT and ST enterotoxins express these CFs, whereas they are found on circa 60% of ST-only strains.[55] Generally, only a small proportion of LT-only strains bear these CFs.[58] Thus, if a multivalent ETEC vaccine contained just CFA/I and CS1-6, it could theoretically provide protection against approximately 50% to 80% ETEC strains in most geographic areas (see Table 22.3–3). If an LT toxoid such as the nontoxic B subunit component of LT (LTB) or a mutant LT was included, and if such a vaccine was well tolerated and efficacious, the multivalent vaccine might provide relatively broad protection against circa 80% to 90% of ETEC strains worldwide. Inclusion of the less frequent fimbrial antigens (e.g., CS7, CS12, CS14, and CS17) in the multivalent vaccine (that would also include an LT antigen) might expand the potential spectrum of coverage to greater than 90% of ETEC strains.[56,59]

A number of distinct strategies are being taken to deliver fimbrial and toxin antigens of ETEC to the human immune system to elicit protective immune responses and functional immunologic memory (see Table 22.3–1). Several promising approaches for development of future ETEC vaccines for humans are summarized below.

INACTIVATED ETEC VACCINES

Purified CF fimbriae have drawbacks as oral immunogens for humans since they are expensive to prepare and sensitive to proteolytic degradation in the gut.[56,59] A more practical way is to construct vaccines that contain these fimbrial antigens in an immunogenic form on the surface of ETEC bacteria. Early "proof of principle" studies that confirmed the feasibility of this strategy were carried out

Table 22.3–3. PREVALENCE OF MAJOR FIMBRIAL COLONIZATION FACTOR ANTIGENS AMONG ENTEROTOXIGENIC *ESCHERICHIA COLI* STRAINS ISOLATED FROM ADULTS WITH TRAVELERS' DIARRHEA AND FROM CHILDREN WITH DIARRHEA IN LESS-DEVELOPED COUNTRIES

REPORT	GEOGRAPHIC SOURCE	TOXIN PROFILE	NUMBER OF ISOLATES	% OF ISOLATES EXPRESSING FIMBRIAL ANTIGENS			
				CFA/I	CFA/II	CFA/IV	CFA/I, II OR IV
Travelers' diarrhea							
Levine et al. 1983	Morocco, Honduras Kenya, Zaire	All	36	11	14	NT*	≥ 25–
		LT/ST	10	30	40	"	≥ 70
		ST	12	8	0	"	—
		LT	14	0	0	"	—
Wolf et al. 1993	Saudi Arabia, Egypt	All	189	12	34	31	77
		LT/ST	84	16	64	5	85
		ST	73	12	8	44	64
		LT	32	0	6	22	28
Pediatric diarrhea							
Qadri et al.[58]	Bangladesh	All	662	13	12	17	42
		LT/ST	162	23	23	13	59
		ST	327	15	12	28	55
		LT	168	0	0	0	0
Binsztein et al. 1991	Argentina	All	109	23	12	17	52
		LT/ST	15	0	80	0	80
		ST	71	35	1	27	63
		LT	23	0	0	0	0
Levine et al. 1993	Chile	All	93	12	27	5	44
		LT/ST	19	0	100	0	100
		ST	28	39	0	18	57
		LT	46	0	13	0	13
Travelers and pediatric							
Wolf[57]	18 locations	All	798	25	19	24	68
		LT/ST	231	24	575	86	
		ST	371	40	245	87	
		LT	196	0	85	13	

Adapted from Levine et al.[56]

by Evans et al., who used ETEC inactivated with colicin E1, which did not damage the fimbrial protein antigens.[60] Oral immunization with such colicin E1-inactivated ETEC induced intestinal IgA antibody response against the homologous CFA (and against LT) and protected volunteers against experimental challenge with wild-type ETEC. However, further development of the colicin-inactivated vaccine was not pursued. An alternative approach that was attempted in the late 1980s was to develop an oral ETEC vaccine consisting of cholera BS in combination with formalin-killed ETEC strains expressing prevalent CFs in immunogenic form on the bacterial surface. The rationale for including cholera BS was that this component had previously been shown to confer significant protection for several months against LT-producing ETEC.[26,27]

The initial prototype vaccine was subsequently replaced by an oral ETEC vaccine containing recombinant cholera B subunit (rBS) in combination with five different formalin-inactivated *E. coli* strains expressing CFA/I and the different subcomponents of CFA/II and CFA/IV, that is, CS1-CS6. Inactivation by mild formalin treatment has been shown to result in complete killing of the bacteria without significant losses in antigenicity of the different CFs (which retain antigenicity even after incubation in human gastrointestinal secretions containing acid and proteolytic enzymes). Phase 1 and 2 trials of this rBS-CF ETEC vaccine in Swedish, Bangladeshi, American, and Egyptian volunteers showed that the vaccine is well tolerated and gives rise to intestinal immune responses against all of the different CFs of the vaccine in most of the volunteers.[59,61,62] Analogous safety/immunogenicity clinical trials were carried out with this inactivated ETEC vaccine in Egyptian preschool children and infants, in whom it was similarly shown to be well tolerated and immunogenic.[63] Studies on the protective efficacy of the rBS-CFA ETEC vaccine are under-way in European and American travelers going to countries with a high risk of ETEC diarrhea (e.g., Kenya, Mexico, and Guatemala). A field trial of the efficacy of this vaccine is also in progress in children 6 to 18 months of age in Egypt.

In a placebo-controlled study, the ETEC vaccine was shown to provide 79% protection against ETEC diarrhea in European travelers going to 20 different countries in Africa, Asia, and Latin America. However, the protection was not statistically significant due to the small numbers of cases.[64]

MUTANT LT

LT not only induces antitoxic antibodies but serves as a powerful mucosal adjuvant that can augment the immune responses to coadministered antigens. Several investigators have introduced mutations in the LT molecule that greatly diminish its biologic toxicity (i.e., ability to elicit secretion) yet retain its adjuvanticity.[65,66] These mutant LT molecules can be coadministered with inactivated fimbriated ETEC or can be coexpressed from live ETEC vaccines that also express CFs.

In the 1980s and early 1990s, various attempts were made to produce immunogenic, yet nontoxic, ST antigens. However, these attempts met with little success, and this strategy has since been abandoned.[59]

LIVE ORAL VACCINES

Attenuated *E. coli* as Live Oral Vaccines Against ETEC   The potential of live ETEC vaccines was demonstrated when Levine et al. administered a prototype live vaccine strain expressing CS1 and CS3 fimbriae but lacking genes that encode LT and ST.[56] A single dose elicited impressive SIgA antifimbrial antibodies in the intestine and conferred 75% protection against experimental challenge with wild-type ETEC elaborating CS1 and CS3 fimbriae as well as LT and ST. Thus, one strategy involves assembling a collection of attenuated *E. coli* strains expressing the major fimbrial CFs and an LT antigen such as B subunit or mutant LT.

Attenuated *Salmonella* or *Shigella* Live Vectors Expressing ETEC Antigens   Because of their prolonged residence within the gut-associated lymphoid tissue, attenuated *Salmonella* make extremely attractive "live vectors" to express foreign genes encoding protective antigens of other bacterial enteropathogens and to deliver those antigens to the human immune system. As mentioned above, a new generation of attenuated *S. typhi* strains has appeared that are both well tolerated and highly immunogenic after administration of just a single oral dose. Such strains, such as CVD 908 and CVD 908-*htrA*, serve as suitable live vectors for expressing ETEC antigens. The genes necessary for expression of various CFs, including CFA/I and CS3, have been introduced into CVD 908 and CVD 908-*htrA* on stable plasmids and a high level of coexpression of these fimbriae has been demonstrated.[67]

Considerable success has been achieved recently in engineering strains of *Shigella* that are attenuated compared with their wild-type parent and in using these strains as live vectors to express ETEC antigens. Enlarging upon this strategy, a live *Shigella*-based multivalent *Shigella*/ETEC hybrid vaccine is being constructed wherein the important fimbrial CFs (see Table 22.3–1) are expressed along with mutant LT in attenuated *Shigella*.[68] The final multivalent live vector vaccine is expected to consist of a mixture of five attenuated *Shigella* strains (representing five different *Shigella* serotypes), each expressing two different CFs and mutant LT.

VACCINE AGAINST *CAMPYLOBACTER JEJUNI*

There is debate over the relative importance of *C. jejuni* as a cause of travelers' diarrhea, with some authorities attributing it to be an important pathogen, whereas others consider it to be of little consequence. U.S. investigators have begun Phase 1 clinical trials with a prototype vaccine consisting of inactivated *C. jejuni* bacteria combined with minute (subclinical) doses of *E. coli* LT as an adjuvant.[69]

VACCINES AGAINST *GIARDIA LAMBLIA* AND *ENTAMOEBA HISTOLYTICA*

RATIONALE

Giardia infections can cause an extended clinical illness with upper gastrointestinal symptoms, diarrhea, steatorrhea, malabsorption of nutrients, weight loss, and even megaloblastic anemia. For certain types of travelers, such as campers and those going to recognized high-risk areas (e.g., St. Petersburg), a vaccine against *Giardia* would be desirable. Basic research to develop a *Giardia* vaccine has been limited, and no candidate vaccines are approaching clinical trials.

Although symptomatic *E. histolytica* infections are generally uncommon, some individuals do develop amebic dysentery or amebic cysts in the liver consequent to travel in high-risk areas such as Natal Province, South Africa, and parts of India and Latin America. A vaccine against *E. histolytica* disease would be useful for certain travelers to high risk-areas. Several putative protective antigens of *E. histolytica* have been identified and have been shown to be protective in animal models. One promising approach is immunization with attenuated *S. typhi* or *Shigella* live vectors expressing these putative protective antigens.[70] Such candidate vaccines are expected to enter Phase 1 clinical trials in the near future.

VACCINES AGAINST ROTAVIRUS AND CALICIVIRUSES

Rotavirus is the single most important cause of dehydrating diarrhea among infants worldwide. Whereas severe clinical consequences of symptomatic rotavirus infection are limited when infants are in industrialized countries, because of access to health care, when they travel to developing countries rotavirus poses a serious risk for infant travelers, particularly if they do not have easy access to medical care. A tetravalent reassortant rotavirus vaccine was licensed by the Food and Drug Administration in August 1998 based on data demonstrating its safety and efficacy. In four randomized, placebo-controlled, double-blind field trials, a three-dose regimen (usually given at 2, 4, and 6 months of age) of the tetravalent rotavirus vaccine conferred circa 50% protection against all rotavirus diarrhea and approximately 85% protection against severe rotavirus diarrhea.[71,72] The American Academy of Pediatrics and the Advisory Committee on Immunization Practices recommended routine infant immunization with this vaccine in the U.S.A., and by June 1999, more than 1.8 million doses had been administered. Routine vaccination of American. infants was suspended in July 1999 because of reports of intussusception associated with the first dose of vaccine. In October 1999, following detailed epidemiologic investigations that established a clear-cut causal association between the administration of the tetravalent rotavirus vaccine and intussusception in some infants, the Advisory Committee on Immunization Practices concluded that the tetravalent rotavirus vaccine should no longer be given to infants in the U.S.A.[73]

Norwalk virus and other caliciviruses are important causes of viral gastroenteritis in both industrialized and developing countries, and all age groups are affected. The clinical illness may present either as mainly acute repetitive vomiting or as diarrheal illness. Although these agents do not typically cause dehydration and the illness is self-limited, the symptoms, particularly when accompanied by repetitive vomiting, are discomforting.

Some significant strides have been made in the use of virus-like particles composed of the nucleocapsid protein of Norwalk virus as a mucosal vaccine. In preliminary clinical trials, two different formulations of this antigen have been well tolerated and immunogenic. It is likely that further clinical development of candidate Norwalk virus vaccines will continue.[74]

REFERENCES

1. Loutan L, Bovier P, Althaus B, Gluck R. Inactivated virosome hepatitis A vaccine. Lancet 1994;343:322–324.
2. Lemon SM, Thomas DL. Vaccines to prevent viral hepatitis. N Engl J Med 1997;336:196–204.
3. Van Hoecke C, Lebacq E, Beran J, et al. Concomitant vaccination against hepatitis A and typhoid fever. J Travel Med 1998;5:116–120.
4. Levine MM, Taylor DN, Ferreccio C. Typhoid vaccines come of age. Pediatr Infect Dis J 1989;8:374–381.
5. Levine MM, Ferreccio C, Abrego P, et al. Duration of efficacy of Ty21a, attenuated *Salmonella typhi* live oral vaccine. Vaccine 1999;17(Suppl 2):S22–S27.
6. Ferreccio C, Levine MM, Rodriguez H, Contreras R. Comparative efficacy of two, three, or four doses of Ty21a live oral typhoid vaccine in enteric-coated capsules: a field trial in an endemic area. J Infect Dis 1989;159:766–769.
7. Levine MM, Ferreccio C, Cryz S, Ortiz E. Comparison of enteric-coated capsules and liquid formulation of Ty21a typhoid vaccine in randomised controlled field trial. Lancet 1990;336:891–894.
8. Simanjuntak C, Paleologo F, Punjabi N, et al. Oral immunisation against typhoid fever in Indonesia with Ty21a vaccine. Lancet 1991;338:1055–1059.
9. Acharya VI, Lowe CU, Thapa R, et al. Prevention of typhoid fever in Nepal with the Vi capsular polysaccharide of *Salmonella typhi*. A preliminary report. N Engl J Med 1987;317:1101–1104.
10. Klugman K, Gilbertson IT, Kornhoff HJ, et al. Protective activity of Vi polysaccharide vaccine against typhoid fever. Lancet 1987;2:1165–1169.
11. Klugman KP, Koornhof HJ, Robbins JB, Le Cam NN. Immunogenicity, efficacy and serological correlate of protection of *Salmonella typhi* Vi capsular polysaccharide vaccine three years after immunization. Vaccine 1996;14:435–438.
12. Szu SC, Taylor DN, Trofa AC, et al. Laboratory and preliminary clinical characterization of Vi capsular polysaccharide-protein conjugate vaccines. Infect Immun 1994;62:4440–4444.
13. Kossaczka Z, Lin FY, Ho VA, et al. Safety and immunogenicity of Vi conjugate vaccines for typhoid fever in adults, teenagers, and 2- to 4-year-old children in Vietnam. Infect Immun 1999;67:5806–5810.
14. Tacket CO, Hone DM, Losonsky GA, et al. Clinical acceptability and immunogenicity of CVD 908 *Salmonella typhi* vaccine strain. Vaccine 1992;10:443–446.
15. Tacket CO, Sztein MB, Losonsky GA, et al. Safety and immune response in humans of live oral *Salmonella typhi* vaccine strains deleted in htrA and aroC, aroD. Infect Immun 1997;65:452–456.
16. Tacket CO, Kelly SM, Schodel F, et al. Safety and immunogenicity in humans of an attenuated *Salmonella typhi* vaccine vector strain expressing plasmid-encoded hepatitis B antigens stabilized by the ASD balanced lethal system. Infect Immun 1997;65:3381–3385.
17. Hohmann EL, Oletta CA, Killeen KP, Miller SI. phoP/phoQ-deleted *Salmonella typhi* (Ty800) is a safe and immunogenic single-dose typhoid fever vaccine in volunteers. J Infect Dis 1996;173:1408–1414.
18. Taylor DN, Rizzo J, Meza R, et al. Cholera among Americans living in Peru. Clin Infect Dis 1996;22:1108–1109.
19. Wittlinger F, Steffen R, Watanabe H, Handszuh H. Risk of cholera among Western and Japanese travelers. J Travel Med 1995;2:154–158.
20. Holmgren J, Svennerholm AM, Lonnroth I, et al. Development of improved cholera vaccine based on subunit toxoid. Nature 1977;269:602–604.
21. Svennerholm A-M, Holmgren J. Oral B subunit whole cell vaccines against cholera and enterotoxigenic *Escherichia coli* diarrhea. In: Ala'Aldeen DA, ed. Molecular and clinical aspects of bacterial vaccine development. Chichester, UK: John Wiley & Sons, 1995:205–232.
22. Holmgren J, Jertborn M, Svennerholm A-M. Oral B subunit killed whole-cell cholera vaccine. In: Levine MM, Woodrow GC, Kaper JB, Cobon GS, eds. New generation vaccines. New York: Marcel Dekker, 1997:459–468.
23. Holmgren J, Osek J, Svennerholm A-M. Protective oral cholera vaccine based on a combination of cholera toxin B subunit and inactivated cholera vibrios. In: Wachsmuth IK, Blake P, Olsvik O, eds. *Vibrio cholerae* and cholera. American Society for Microbiology Publications, 1994:415–424.
24. Black RE, Levine MM, Clements ML, et al. Protective efficacy in humans of killed whole-vibrio oral cholera vaccine with and without the B subunit of cholera toxin. Infect Immun 1987;55:1116–1120.
25. Clemens JD, Sack DA, Harris JR, et al. Field trial of cholera vaccines in Bangladesh: results from three year follow-up. Lancet 1990;335:270–273.
26. Clemens JD, Sack DA, Harris JR, et al. Cross-protection by B subunit-whole cell cholera vaccine against diarrhea associated with heat-labile toxin-producing enterotoxigenic *Escherichia coli*: results of a large-scale field trial. J Infect Dis 1988;158:372–377.
27. Peltola H, Siitonen A, Kyrönseppä H, et al. Prevention of travellers' diarrhoea by oral B-subunit/whole-cell cholera vaccine. Lancet 1991;338:1285–1289.
28. Scerpella EG, Sanchez JL, Mathewson III, et al. Safety, immunogenicity, and protective efficacy of the whole-cell/recombinant B subunit (WC/rBS) oral cholera vaccine against travelers' diarrhea. J Travel Med 1995;2:22–27.

29. Sanchez J, Holmgren J. Recombinant system for overexpression of cholera toxin B subunit in *Vibrio cholerae* as a basis for vaccine development. Proc Natl Acad Sci U S A 1989;86: 481–485.

30. Sanchez JL, Vasquez B, Begue RE, et al. Protective efficacy of oral whole-cell/recombinant-B-subunit cholera vaccine in Peruvian military recruits. Lancet 1994;344:1273–1276.

31. Taylor DN, Cardenas V, Sanchez JL, et al. Two-year efficacy trial of the oral, inactivated whole-cell plus recombinant B subunit (WC/rCTB) cholera vaccine in Peru [abstract]. 1997; 33:57–62.

32. Taylor DN, Cardenas V, Sanchez JL, et al. Two year study of the protective efficacy of the oral whole cell plus recombinant B subunit (WC/rBS) cholera vaccine in Peru. J Infect Dis 2000 (in press).

33. Levine MM, Kaper JB. Live oral cholera vaccine: from principle to product. Bull Inst Pasteur 1995;93:243–253.

34. Levine MM, Tacket CO. Live oral vaccines against cholera. In: Ala'Aldeen DAA, Hormaeche CE, eds. Molecular and clinical aspects of bacterial vaccine development. Chichester, UK: John Wiley & Sons, 1995:233–258.

35. Tacket CO, Cohen MB, Wasserman SS, et al. Randomized, double-blind, placebo-controlled, multicentered trial of the efficacy of a single dose of live oral cholera vaccine CVD 103-HgR in preventing cholera following challenge with *Vibrio cholerae* O1 El Tor Inaba three months after vaccination. Infect Immun 1999;67:6341–6345.

36. Tacket CO, Losonsky G, Nataro JP, et al. Onset and duration of protective immunity in challenged volunteers after vaccination with live oral cholera vaccine CVD 103-HgR. J Infect Dis 1992;166:837–841.

37. Richie E, Punjabi NH, Sidharta Y, et al. Efficacy trial of single-dose live oral cholera vaccine CVD 103-HgR in North Jakarta, Indonesia, a cholera-endemic area. Vaccine 2000 (in press).

38. Taylor DN, Tacket CO, Losonsky G, et al. Evaluation of a bivalent (CVD 103-HgR/CVD 111) live oral cholera vaccine in adult volunteers from the United States and Peru. Infect Immun 1997;65:3852–3856.

39. Jertborn M, Svennerholm AM, Holmgren J. Intestinal and systemic immune responses in humans after oral immunization with a bivalent B subunit-O1/O139 whole cell cholera vaccine. Vaccine 1996;14:1459–1465.

40. Tacket CO, Losonsky G, Nataro JP, et al. Initial clinical studies of CVD 112 *Vibrio cholerae* O139 live oral vaccine: safety and efficacy against experimental challenge. J Infect Dis 1995;172:883–886.

41. Coster TS, Killeen KP, Waldor MK, et al. Safety, immunogenicity, and efficacy of live attenuated *Vibrio cholerae* O139 vaccine prototype. Lancet 1995;345:949–952.

42. Karnell A, Li A, Zhao CR, et al. Safety and immunogenicity study of the auxotrophic *Shigella flexneri* 2a vaccine SFL1070 with a deleted aroD gene in adult Swedish volunteers. Vaccine 1995;13:88–89.

43. Noriega FR, Wang JY, Losonsky G, et al. Construction and characterization of attenuated (aroA) virG *Shigella flexneri* 2a strain CVD 1203, a prototype live oral vaccine. Infect Immun 1995;65:5168–5172.

44. Noriega FR, Losonsky G, Lauderbaugh C, et al. Engineered (guaB-A) virG *Shigella flexneri* 2a strain CVD 1205: construction, safety, immunogenicity and potential efficacy as a mucosal vaccine. Infect Immun 1996;64:3055–3061.

45. Barzu S, Fontaine A, Sansonetti P, Phalipon A. Induction of a local anti-IpaC antibody response in mice by use of a *Shigella flexneri* 2a vaccine candidate: implications for use of IpaC as a protein carrier. Infect Immun 1996;64:1190–1196.

46. Kotloff KL, Noriega F, Losonsky GA, et al. Safety, immunogenicity, and transmissibility in humans of CVD 1203, a live oral *Shigella flexneri* 2a vaccine candidate attenuated by deletions in aroA and virG. Infect Immun 1996;64:4542–4548.

47. Coster TS, Hoge CW, VanDeVerg LL, et al. Vaccination against shigellosis with attenuated *Shigella flexneri* 2a strain SC602. Infect Immun 1999;67:3437–3443.

48. Nataro JP, Seriwatana J, Fasano A, et al. Identification and cloning of a novel plasmid-encoded enterotoxin of enteroinvasive *Escherichia coli* and *Shigella* strains. Infect Immun 1995;63:4721–4728.

49. Fasano A, Noriega FR, Maneval DR Jr, et al. *Shigella* enterotoxin 1: an enterotoxin of *Shigella flexneri* 2a active in rabbit small intestine in vivo and in vitro. J Clin Invest 1995;95: 2853–2861.

50. Noriega FR, Liao FM, Maneval DR, et al. Strategy for cross-protection among *Shigella flexneri* serotypes. Infect Immun 1999;67:782–788.

51. Kotloff KL, Noriega FN, Samandari T, et al. *Shigella flexneri* 2a strain CVD 1207 with specific deletions in virG, sen, set, and guaBA is highly attenuated in humans. Infect Immun 2000 (in press).

52. Orr N, Robin G, Cohen D, et al. Immunogenicity and efficacy of oral or intranasal *Shigella flexneri* 2a and *Shigella sonnei* proteosome-lipopolysaccharide vaccines in animal models. Infect Immun 1993;61:2390–2395.

53. Cohen D, Ashkenazi S, Green MS, et al. Double-blind vaccine-controlled randomised efficacy trial of an investigational *Shigella sonnei* conjugate vaccine in young adults. Lancet 1997;349:155–159.

54. Robbins JB, Schneerson R, Szu SC. Perspective: hypothesis: serum IgG antibody is sufficient to confer protection against infectious diseases by inactivating the inoculum. J Infect Dis 1995;171:1387–1398.

55. Gaastra W, Svennerholm AM. Colonization factors of human enterotoxigenic *Escherichia coli* (ETEC). Trends Microbiol 1996;4:444–452.

56. Levine MM, Giron JA, Noriega F. Fimbrial vaccines. In: Klemm P, ed. Fimbriae: adhesion, biogenics, genetics and vaccines. Boca Raton, FL: CRC Press, 1994.

57. Wolf MK. Occurrence, distribution, and associations of O and H serogroups, colonization factor antigens, and toxins of enterotoxigenic *Escherichia coli*. Clin Microbiol Rev 1997;10: 569–584.

58. Qadri F, Das SK, Faruque ASG, et al. Prevalence of toxin types and colonization factors in enterotoxigenic *Escherichia coli* isolated during a 2-year period from diarrheal patients in Bangladesh. Infect Immun 2000 (in press).

59. Svennerholm A-M, Ahren C, Jertborn M. Oral inactivated vaccine against enterotoxigenic *Escherichia coli*. In: Levine MM, Woodrow GC, Kaper JB, Cobon GS, eds. New generation vaccines. New York: Marcel Dekker, 1997:865–874.

60. Evans DG, Evans DJ Jr, Opekun A, Graham DY. Non-replicating whole cell vaccine protective against enterotoxigenic *Escherichia coli* (ETEC) diarrhea: stimulation of anti-CFA (CFA/I) and anti-enterotoxin (anti-LT) intestinal IgA and protection against challenge with ETEC belonging to heterologous serotypes. FEMS Microbiol Lett 1988;47:117–125.

61. Ahren C, Jertborn M, Svennerholm AM. Intestinal immune responses to an inactivated oral enterotoxigenic *Escherichia coli* vaccine and associated immunoglobulin A responses in blood. Infect Immun 1998;66:3311–3316.

62. Savarino SJ, Brown FM, Hall E, et al. Safety and immunogenicity of an oral, killed enterotoxigenic *Escherichia coli*-cholera toxin B subunit vaccine in Egyptian adults. J Infect Dis 1998;177:796–799.

63. Savarino SJ, Hall ER, Bassily S, et al. Oral, inactivated, whole cell enterotoxigenic *Escherichia coli* plus cholera toxin B subunit vaccine: results of the initial evaluation in children. PRIDE Study Group. J Infect Dis 1999;179:107–114.

64. Wiedermann G, Kollaritsch H, Kundi M, et al. Double-blind, randomized, placebo controlled pilot study evaluating efficacy and reactogenicity of an oral ETEC B-subunit inactivated whole cell vaccine against travelers diarrhea (preliminary report). J Travel Med 2000;7:27–29.

65. Douce G, Turcotte C, Cropley I, et al. Mutants of *Escherichia coli* heat-labile toxin lacking ADP-ribosyltransferase activity act as nontoxic, mucosal adjuvants. Proc Natl Acad Sci U S A 1995;92:1644–1648.

66. Dickinson BL, Clements JD. Dissociation of *Escherichia coli* heat-labile enterotoxin adjuvanticity from ADP-ribosyltransferase activity. Infect Immun 1995;63:1617–1623.

67. Giron JA, Xu J-G, Gonzalez CR, et al. Simultaneous constitutive expression of CFA/I and CS3 colonization factors of enterotoxigenic *Escherichia coli* by aroC, aroD *Salmonella typhi* vaccine strain CVD 908. Vaccine 1995;10:939–946.

68. Noriega FR, Losonsky G, Wang JY, et al. Further characterization of (aroA) virG *Shigella flexneri* 2a strain CVD 1203 as a mucosal *Shigella* vaccine and as a live vector vaccine for delivering antigens of enterotoxigenic *Escherichia coli*. Infect Immun 1996;64:23–27.

69. Scott DA, Baqar S, Burr DH, et al. Vaccines against *Campylobacter jejuni*. In: Levine MM, Woodrow GC, Kaper JB, Cobon GS, eds. New generation vaccines. New York: Marcel Dekker, 1997:885–896.

70. Zhang T, Stanley SL Jr. Oral immunization with an attenuated vaccine strain of *Salmonella typhimurium* expressing the serine-rich *Entamoeba histolytica* protein induces an antiamebic immune response and protects gerbils from amebic liver abscess. Infect Immun 1996;64:1526–1531.

71. Rennels MB, Wasserman SS, Glass RI, Keane VA. Comparison of immunogenicity and efficacy of rhesus rotavirus reassortant vaccines in breastfed and nonbreastfed children. US Rotavirus Vaccine Efficacy Group. Pediatrics 1995;96:1132–1136.

72. Vesikari T. Rotavirus vaccines against diarrhoeal disease. Lancet 1997;350:1538–1541.

73. Centers for Disease Control and Prevention. Withdrawal of rotavirus vaccine recommendation. MMWR Morb Mortal Wkly Rep 1999;48:1007.

74. Ball JM, Graham DY, Opekun AR, et al. Recombinant Norwalk virus-like particles given orally to volunteers: phase I study. Gastroenterology 1999;117:40–48.

22.4 FUTURE NONENTERIC NONMALARIAL VACCINES FOR TRAVELERS

TARÁZ SAMANDARÍ AND ROBERT EDELMAN

INTRODUCTION

Travelers to tropical and subtropical countries are often exposed to infectious agents that are unique to those environments. The greatest causes of morbidity and mortality are enteric microorganisms and malaria. However, a number of other important diseases include those dealt with in this chapter: group B meningococcus, dengue, leishmaniasis, tuberculosis, and HIV. At the end of the twentieth century, we are witnessing the geographic spread of some of these diseases or the threat of multidrug-resistant strains. In some areas of the world, the twin specter of HIV and tuberculosis is emerging. Concomitant with the expansion of global markets, we are witnessing an increase in travel to these areas and increased risk of exposure to these pathogens. The development of vaccines against these diseases is critical, and the status of these vaccines is described below. The results of clinical trials are narrated, whereas the status of candidate vaccines in preclinical trials is summarized in a table.

MENINGOCOCCUS GROUP B

Infection due to the gram-negative bacterium *Neisseria meningitidis* is a worldwide problem that occurs sporadically or as widespread epidemics. The organism is transmitted from person to person through inhalation of aerosolized droplets of infected nasopharyngeal secretions. The clinical manifestations may vary from transient bacteremia to fulminant disease, causing death in a matter of hours. Major outbreaks of meningococcal disease are regularly reported from Africa, China, and South America. Group B meningococcal meningitis causes 50% to 80% of sporadic cases of meningococcal meningitis in industrialized nations, and its incidence has risen recently in countries such as Cuba, Brazil, Colombia, Chile, and Argentina. Although chemoprophylaxis with rifampin (or ciprofloxacin or ofloxacin in adults) should be administered to close contacts of patients, their use in travelers is not warranted. A vaccine is available against four serogroups of meningococci (A, C, W-135,

Y); however, an effective group B vaccine has proved elusive thus far.

The existing vaccines for groups A, C, W-135, and Y meningococcus are all purified capsular polysaccharides. It is thought that the human immune response is poor toward group B meningococcus (GBM) capsular polysaccharide because it has the same structure as glycoproteins of certain human tissues, a phenomenon sometimes referred to as molecular mimicry. For this reason, candidate vaccines for GBM are based upon its outer membrane proteins (OMP) or the conjugation of the GBM capsular polysaccharide with other proteins.

The three vaccine candidates most intensely studied are composed of partially purified OMPs. One of these candidate vaccines was developed in Cuba. Early efficacy trials of this vaccine for prevention of GBM disease was estimated to be 83% (95% confidence interval [CI], 42%, 95%). However, this vaccine had no, or only modest, efficacy among children less than 4 years of age who are at the highest risk of meningococcal disease.[1,2] The other vaccine candidate developed in Norway had efficacies estimated to be 57% (lower 5% CI, 27%).[3] An international committee spearheaded by the Centers for Disease Control (CDC) compared the immunogenicity of the two vaccines in 408 15 to 20 year olds in Iceland.[4] At 12 months, the serum bactericidal antibody (SBA) and ELISA antibody levels were no different in the recipients of the Cuban vaccine than in controls. The Norwegian vaccine induced SBA in 47% of volunteers and ELISA antibodies in 34%. Although the protective efficacy of these vaccines against GBM disease was not evaluated in this study, the presence of SBA was important because SBA antibodies to meningococcus C correlated with protection against meningococcus C during the development of group C meningococcal vaccines. The third OMP candidate vaccine was tested in Chile by Walter Reed Army Institute of Research (WRAIR); 40,811 volunteers were given two doses of vaccine by jet injector. Although the protective efficacy was 70% for 5 to 21 year olds, there was no protection in 1 to 4 year olds.[5]

A number of other GBM vaccine candidates have undergone phase 1 trials that measured safety and immunogenicity in small groups of healthy adults but not protective efficacy. Investigators in Norway used GBM outer membrane vesicles, combined them with a purified GBM outer membrane protein called 5C, and induced high levels of bactericidal IgG.[6] The combination of GBM outer membrane protein vesicles with serogroup C *N. meningitidis* polysaccharide was highly immunogenic without the customary aluminum hydroxide adjuvant needed for other vaccine candidates.[7] GBM outer membrane vesicles administered in nose drops conferred nasal mucosal IgA in all volunteers tested, with almost half developing modest serum IgG.[8] Finally, Dutch investigators gave a synthetic peptide based on the amino acid sequence of an outer membrane protein (Por A) to volunteers who produced bactericidal antibodies against GBM.[9] Through clinical trials, careful choices of optimal adjuvants will have to be made for these newer experimental vaccines in order to demonstrate their protective efficacy. Finally, it is reasonable to hope for a single vaccine that will immunize the traveler against all five major meningococcal serotypes.

DENGUE FEVER

Four serologically distinct flaviviruses, dengue 1–4, are the causative agents of dengue fever and are transmitted by the mosquito *Aedes aegypti*. The disease typically causes sudden onset of fever, rash, headache, retro-orbital pain, arthralgia, and severe myalgia. A second dengue infection caused by a serotype different than the serotype causing the first infection may lead to hemorrhagic fever with shock (DHF/DSS). It is rare for Western travelers to suffer from DHF/DSS because they have not been naturally sensitized by prior exposure to dengue. In the past 20 years, dengue has spread in the Caribbean, South America, and Asia. In the early 1990s, U.S. military personnel were affected by dengue in Somalia.[10] Eighteen Israeli travelers to Thailand had to be evacuated due to severe dengue illness.[11] In the tropics, 1.5 billion people are at risk, and travelers to these areas are increasingly being infected during the daylight biting hours of the *Aedes* vector. Antiviral chemotherapeutic and chemoprophylactic agents are not available for dengue.

Protection against infection with dengue virus has been attributed to the presence of neutralizing antibodies to virion surface proteins, particularly the envelope protein. It is thought that if a vaccine confers immunity to all four serotypes at once, it is unlikely that DHF/DSS could result. Because there is limited cross-protection between the four serotypes, it is important to have all four represented in a candidate vaccine.

Clinical studies of attenuated dengue vaccines have been conducted for over 50 years. Most vaccine candidates have failed due to excessive reactogenicity or to overattenuation and poor immunogenicity. Commonly, viruses are attenuated by passaging them in in vitro cultures. The progressive decline in reactogenicity with increasing serial passage in primary dog kidney (PDK) cells of a dengue-1 vaccine candidate was demonstrated in volunteers.[12] Ten flavivirus nonimmune North American volunteers tolerated a dengue-2 strain passaged 53 times in PDK cell culture, and all 10 developed antibody and T-cell proliferative responses that lasted 2 years.[13] The Vaccine Center at Mahidol University in Thailand is now conducting phase II trials of its PDK-attenuated dengue serotypes 1-4 candidate vaccines combined into a tetravalent vaccine.[14]

Examples of novel candidate vaccines in preclinical trials are listed in Table 22.4–1. Some of these new vaccines may undergo clinical trials in the next 1 to 2 years.

LEISHMANIASIS

The intracellular protozoan *Leishmania* is transmitted in the tropics and subtropics by a sandfly bite. The insect transmits the flagellated promastigote, which enters the mammalian macrophage. The protozoan then transforms into the amastigote, which multiplies and infects other macrophages. Cutaneous leishmaniasis is manifested initially by papules, which then progress to nodules and then to slowly healing and often disfiguring ulcers. Visceral leishmaniasis may present as an acute, subacute, or chronic infection. In its manifestation as *kala-azar*, patients present with profound cachexia, fever, splenomegaly, and hepatomegaly. In areas where HIV is coendemic with leishmaniasis, the visceral form of the disease is becoming an important and an intractable opportunistic infection. The CDC reported 59 cases of American cutaneous leishmaniasis among civilian U.S. travelers between 1985 and 1990.[15] Preventive measures are limited to avoidance of outdoor activities from dusk to dawn and the use of screens and bednets. First-line therapy is pentavalent antimonial compounds. In areas where there is increasing resistance to antimony, amphotericin B or pentamidine is used as an alternative drug. These drugs are rather toxic. A *Leishmania* vaccine would be important for travelers to Central and South American jungles, such as researchers and military personnel.

A number of investigators are developing leishmanial vaccine candidates that consist of a mixture of killed *Leishmania* promastigotes and live Bacille Calmette-Guérin (BCG). BCG is attenuated *Mycobacterium bovis* used to prevent tuberculosis throughout the world as part of childhood immunization. It has been known for some time that BCG can partially or fully protect mice against leishmanial infections. In a phase II study conducted in Venezuela, 208 healthy volunteers from a *Leishmania*-endemic region were chosen because they were skin test negative for both leishmanial antigen and purified protein derivative of tuberculin (PPD).[16] They were administered a combined BCG-killed-promastigote vaccine in three doses. Over 85% of vaccinees had an immune response to *Leishmania*, not much better than individuals immunized with leishmanial antigens alone. A confounding issue was that significant numbers of control volunteers who received no vaccine had skin-test conversions to PPD and/or leishmanial antigens. It is suspected that this occurred due to the natural transmission of mycobacterial species, leishmanial species, and quite possibly to the antigens in the leishmanial skin-test preparation itself. An efficacy trial is now under way in Venezuela. Investigators in Iran performed a randomized, double-blind, efficacy trial in 3,637 leishmanin skin-test negative school-aged children using a vaccine consisting of killed *L. major* mixed with BCG . The vaccine afforded 55% protective efficacy in boys (who were at greater risk for becoming infected than girls) after a 2-year trial (95% CI: 19%, 75%). The vaccine was safe.[17] Brazilian investigators developed a subunit vaccine consisting of protein N antigen of a single strain of *L. amazonensis*.[18] In a phase I trial, they determined that the vaccine had minimal reactogenicity and induced 100% of vaccinees to develop positive Montenegro skin tests. However, 66% of controls also seroconverted, which confounds interpretation of vaccine immunogenicity results.

Because different species of *Leishmania* cause cutaneous and visceral leishmaniasis, and because the species in the Americas and the Old World vary, to be most useful, a *Leishmania* vaccine should confer cross-species protective immunity.

Table 22.4-1.   EXAMPLES OF SOME VACCINE CANDIDATES IN PRECLINICAL TRIALS*

DISEASE	VACCINE CHARACTERISTIC†	MODEL	REFERENCE
Dengue	Inactivated whole virus	Monkey	26
	Subunit protein	Mouse	27
	DNA	Mouse	28
	"Infectious" cDNA clones	Mouse	29
	Vaccinia virus vector	Mouse	30
Leishmania	Live attenuated	Mouse	31
	Killed parasite plus BCG	Monkey	32
	Subunit glycoprotein	Mouse	33
	Peptide or subunit	Mouse	34
	DNA	Mouse	35
	Live *Salmonella* vector	Mouse	36
Tuberculosis	Auxotrophic BCG	Mouse	37
	Lipopeptide	Mouse	38
	DNA	Mouse	39
Gonococcus	Live attenuated	Guinea pig	40
	Peptide	Rabbit	41
	Anti-idiotype	Mouse and rabbit	42
	Subunit	Rabbit	43

*All candidates demonstrated some degree of immunogenicity and/or protective efficacy in animal models.
†Vaccines were administered alone or formulated with one or more experimental adjuvants.

TUBERCULOSIS

Globally, tuberculosis causes more death than any infectious organism, some 30 million deaths each year. TB, transmitted by aerosolized droplets from infected individuals, is primarily manifested as pulmonary disease. A recent report of the transmission of multidrug-resistant TB from an index case during a long airplane flight highlights the ease of its spread.[19] Nevertheless, TB transmission on board airplanes is rarely documented. Individuals infected with HIV are particularly susceptible, and the HIV epidemic has fueled an increase in the incidence of TB. The specter of virulent, multidrug-resistant TB strains emphasizes the urgency of developing an effective vaccine.

The BCG anti-TB vaccine developed near the turn of the century is administered to 100 million infants each year. Although BCG appears to have significant efficacy against miliary TB and TB meningitis in children (46%–100% protective efficacies), its efficacy against adult pulmonary TB is less clear (0%–80%). Furthermore, BCG induces a positive PPD skin test, which makes the diagnosis of *M. tuberculosis* difficult in a BCG-vaccinated person. Because BCG is a live attenuated organism, it may cause serious disease in HIV-positive individuals and is contraindicated for immunocompromised individuals. The CDC does not recommend BCG as a vaccine for travelers.

No TB vaccine candidate has yet reached clinical trial. Numerous preclinical trials have been performed on candidate vaccines, some of which are listed in Table 22.4–1. Unfortunately, lack of a suitable animal model for human disease and the slow growth of the organism in vitro have hindered vaccine development.

GONORRHEA

The pilus of *N. gonorrhea* is important because it attaches the organism to mucosal tissue. Investigators at the WRAIR purified a gonococcal pilus vaccine and administered it intramuscularly to 3,250 individuals. Although a significant number of individuals developed antibody against the protein, it failed to protect men from gonococcal urethritis.[20] Examples of vaccine candidates at the preclinical phase are listed in Table 22.4–1. Sexually active travelers such as those in the military and tourists would be candidates for an effective gonococcal vaccine.

HIV

The development of an effective HIV vaccine remains a daunting task. The obstacles include a lack of markers for protective immunity to HIV; extreme sequence variability of the virus, even within the same individual; rapid and persistent replication of the virus; integration into the host genome and latency within certain cell types; and a lack of satisfactory animal models. However, recent advances in our understanding of the interaction of the virus with the immune system have revealed new possibilities.[21–23] In attempting to emulate the success of the recombinant hepatitis B vaccine, early efforts at constructing an HIV vaccine were focused on eliciting an antibody response to the viral surface glycoprotein. These efforts overlooked HIV's extreme genetic variability and were made before the discovery that the vast majority of infecting strains in primary HIV are selective for macrophages and not laboratory-derived T cells. Furthermore, effective HIV vaccines must elicit not only systemic immunity but mucosal immunity as well to prevent infection via mucosal surfaces.

The prevailing notion is that a vaccine must elicit cytotoxic T lymphocyte (CTL) activity against HIV. A nonreplicating recombinant canary pox virus vector carrying several HIV genes succeeded in eliciting both humoral and cellular immunity in human volunteers—even across clades. DNA vaccines hold great promise by showing protective efficacy in animal models. In a more recent development, human trials involving HIV-positive symptom-free volunteers, DNA vaccines elicited both antibody and CTL responses.[24,25] A natural mutant of HIV has been discovered that is defective in the Nef protein and appears to delay and possibly prevent the onset of AIDS in persons infected with this mutant. On this basis, a live attenuated virus with a *nef* deletion and/or with the deletion of another virulence gene may provide an effective vaccine. Another hopeful development is that a protective vaccine against another lentivirus (lentiviruses are the subfamily of retroviruses of which HIV is a member) has been made in the cat model, the feline immunodeficiency virus.

In summary, the goal of an HIV vaccine for travelers remains to elicit both antibody and CTL responses against multiple genetic variants of HIV existing in different parts of the world. Although there are those who doubt that an effective HIV vaccine can be developed, there remains hope that if a vaccine cannot prevent infection, it may at least prevent progression to AIDS.

CONCLUSION

Many new vaccines will become available in the coming years, and a travel medicine specialist will have to decide which vaccine is appropriate for the traveler and the destination. For instance, if the traveler is a health care worker and plans to practice at her/his destination, TB and HIV vaccination would be appropriate. If a traveler plans to visit Latin America, the Middle East, or Asia, a meningococcal B vaccine may give additional security to existing A and C vaccines. One approach to determining the traveler's needs is to distinguish whether he/she will be a long-term resident or short-term visitor. Long-term residents would include missionaries, Peace Corps volunteers, business persons, diplomatic staff, or military personnel. Vaccines against meningococcus, dengue, leishmaniasis, and gonococcus would be appropriate for short-term visitors, whereas the addition of HIV and TB vaccines would be appropriate for long-term residents of developing nations. The education of the traveler in behavior modification remains a cornerstone of prevention because no vaccine can guarantee protection.

REFERENCES

1. Noronha CP, Struchiner CJ, Halloran ME. Assessment of the direct effectiveness of BC meningococcal vaccine in Rio de Janeiro, Brazil: a case-control study. Int J Epidemiol 1995;24:1050–1057.

2. de Moraes JC, Perkins BA, Camargo MC, et al. Protective efficacy of a serogroup B meningococcal vaccine in Sao Paulo, Brazil. Lancet 1992;340:1074–1078 [published erratum appears in Lancet 1992;340:1554].

3. Bjune G, Hoiby EA, Gronnesby JK, et al. Effect of outer membrane vesicle vaccine against group B meningococcal disease in Norway. Lancet 1991;338:1093–1096.

4. Perkins BA, Jonsdottir K, Briem H, et al. Immunogenicity of two efficacious outer membrane protein-based serogroup B meningococcal vaccines among young adults in Iceland. J Infect Dis 1998;177:683–691.

5. Boslego J, Garcia J, Cruz C, et al. Efficacy, safety, and immunogenicity of a meningococcal group B (15:P1.3) outer membrane protein vaccine in Iquique, Chile. Chilean National Committee for Meningococcal Disease. Vaccine 1995;13:821–829.

6. Rosenqvist E, Hoiby EA, Wedege E, et al. The 5C protein of Neisseria meningitidis is highly immunogenic in humans and induces bactericidal antibodies. J Infect Dis 1993;167:1065–1073.

7. Rosenqvist E, Hoiby EA, Bjune G, et al. Effect of aluminium hydroxide and meningococcal serogroup C capsular polysaccharide on the immunogenicity and reactogenicity of a group B Neisseria meningitidis outer membrane vesicle vaccine. Dev Biol Stand 1998;92:323–333.

8. Haneberg B, Dalseg R, Oftung F, et al. Towards a nasal vaccine against meningococcal disease, and prospects for its use as a mucosal adjuvant. Dev Biol Stand 1998;92:127–133.

9. Rouppe van der Voort EM, Kuipers B, Brugghe HF, et al. Epitope specificity of murine and human bactericidal antibodies against PorA P1.7,16 induced with experimental meningococcal group B vaccines. FEMS Immunol Med Microbiol 1997;17:139–148.

10. Sharp TW, Wallace MR, Hayes CG, et al. Dengue fever in U.S. troops during Operation Restore Hope, Somalia, 1992–1993. Am J Trop Med Hyg 1995;53:89–94.

11. Schwartz E, Mendelson E, Sidi Y. Dengue fever among travelers. Am J Med 1996;101:516–520.

12. Edelman R, Tacket CO, Wasserman SS, et al. A live attenuated dengue-1 vaccine candidate (45AZ5) passaged in primary dog kidney cell culture is attenuated and immunogenic for humans. J Infect Dis 1994;170:1448–1455.

13. Vaughn DW, Hoke CHJ, Yoksan S, et al. Testing of a dengue 2 live-attenuated vaccine (strain 16681 PDK 53) in ten American volunteers. Vaccine 1996;14:329–336.

14. Bhamarapravati N, Sutee Y. Live attenuated tetravalent dengue vaccine. In: Gubler DJ, Kuno G, eds. Dengue and dengue hemorrhagic fever. New York: CAB International, 1997:367–377.

15. Herwaldt BL, Stokes SL, Juranek DD. American cutaneous leishmaniasis in U.S. travelers. Ann Intern Med 1993;118:779–784 [published erratum appears in Ann Intern Med 1993;119:173].

16. Castes M, Blackwell J, Trujillo D, et al. Immune response in healthy volunteers vaccinated with killed leishmanial promastigotes plus BCG. I: skin-test reactivity, T-cell proliferation and interferon-gamma production. Vaccine 1994;12:1041–1051.

17. Sharifi I, Fekri AR, Aflatonian M-R, et al. Randomised vaccine trial of single dose of killed Leishmania major plus BCG against anthroponotic cutaneous leishmaniasis in Bam, Iran. Lancet 1998;351:1540–1543.

18. Marzochi KB, Marzochi MA, Silva AF, et al. Phase 1 study of an inactivated vaccine against American tegumentary leishmaniasis in normal volunteers in Brazil. Mem Inst Oswaldo Cruz 1998;93:205–212.

19. Kenyon TA, Valway SE, Ihle WW, et al. Transmission of multidrug-resistant Mycobacterium tuberculosis during a long airplane flight. N Engl J Med 1996;334:933–938.

20. Boslego JW, Tramont EC, Chung RC, et al. Efficacy trial of a parenteral gonococcal pilus vaccine in men. Vaccine 1991;9:154–162.

21. Hilleman MR. A simplified vaccinologists' vaccinology and the pursuit of a vaccine against AIDS. Vaccine 1998;16:778–793.

22. Bangham CR, Phillips RE. What is required of an HIV vaccine? Lancet 1997;350:1617–1621.

23. Heilman CA, Baltimore D. HIV vaccines—where are we going? Nat Med 1998;4:532–534.

24. MacGregor RR, Boyer JD, Ugen KE, et al. First human trial of a DNA-based vaccine for treatment of human immunodeficiency virus type 1 infection: safety and host response. J Infect Dis 1998;178:92–100.

25. Calarota S, Bratt G, Nordlund S, et al. Cellular cytotoxic response induced by DNA vaccination in HIV-1-infected patients. Lancet 1998;351:1320–1325.

26. Putnak R, Barvir DA, Burrous JM, et al. Development of a purified, inactivated, dengue-2 virus vaccine prototype in Vero cells: immunogenicity and protection in mice and rhesus monkeys. J Infect Dis 1996;174:1176–1184.

27. Simmons M, Nelson WM, Wu SJ, et al. Evaluation of the protective efficacy of a recombinant dengue envelope B domain fusion protein against dengue 2 virus infection in mice. Am J Trop Med Hyg 1998;58:655–662.

28. Porter KR, Kochel TJ, Wu SJ, et al. Protective efficacy of a dengue 2 DNA vaccine in mice and the effect of CpG immunostimulatory motifs on antibody responses. Arch Virol 1998;143:997–1003.

29. Trent DW, Kinney RM, Huang CYH. Recombinant dengue virus vaccines. In: Gubler DJ, Kuno G, eds. Dengue and dengue hemorrhagic fever. New York: CAB International, 1997:379–403.

30. Fonseca BA, Pincus S, Shope RE, et al. Recombinant vaccinia viruses co-expressing dengue-1 glycoproteins prM and E induce neutralizing antibodies in mice. Vaccine 1994;12:279–285 [published erratum appears in Vaccine 1994;12:480].

31. Titus RG, Gueiros-Filho FJ, de Freitas LA, et al. Development of a safe live Leishmania vaccine line by gene replacement. Proc Natl Acad Sci U S A 1995;92:10267–10271.

32. Dube A, Sharma P, Srivastava JK, et al. Vaccination of langur monkeys (Presbytis entellus) against Leishmania donovani with autoclaved L. major plus BCG. Parasitology 1998;116:219–221.

33. Soong L, Duboise SM, Kima P, et al. Leishmania pifanoi amastigote antigens protect mice against cutaneous leishmaniasis. Infect Immun 1995;63:3559–3566.

34. Frankenburg S, Axelrod O, Kutner S, et al. Effective immunization of mice against cutaneous leishmaniasis using an intrinsically adjuvanted synthetic lipopeptide vaccine. Vaccine 1996;14:923–929.

35. Sjolander A, Baldwin TM, Curtis JM, et al. Induction of a Th1 immune response and simultaneous lack of activation of a Th2 response are required for generation of immunity to leishmaniasis. J Immunol 1998;160:3949–3957.

36. Gonzalez CR, Noriega FR, Huerta S, et al. Immunogenicity of a *Salmonella typhi* CVD 908 candidate vaccine strain expressing the major surface protein gp63 of *Leishmania mexicana mexicana*. Vaccine 1998;16:1043–1052.

37. Guleria I, Teitelbaum R, McAdam RA, et al. Auxotrophic vaccines for tuberculosis. Nat Med 1996;2:334–337.

38. da Fonseca DP, Joosten D, van der Zee R, et al. Identification of new cytotoxic T-cell epitopes on the 38-kilodalton lipoglycoprotein of *Mycobacterium tuberculosis* by using lipopeptides. Infect Immun 1998;66:3190–3197.

39. Tascon RE, Colston MJ, Ragno S, et al. Vaccination against tuberculosis by DNA injection. Nat Med 1996;2:888–892.

40. Chamberlain LM, Strugnell R, Dougan G, et al. *Neisseria gonorrhoeae* strain MS11 harbouring a mutation in gene aroA is attenuated and immunogenic. Microb Pathog 1993;15:51–63.

41. Heckels JE, Virji M, Tinsley CR. Vaccination against gonorrhoea: the potential protective effect of immunization with a synthetic peptide containing a conserved epitope of gonococcal outer membrane protein IB. Vaccine 1990;8:225–230.

42. Gulati S, McQuillen DP, Sharon J, et al. Experimental immunization with a monoclonal anti-idiotope antibody that mimics the *Neisseria gonorrhoeae* lipooligosaccharide epitope 2C7. J Infect Dis 1996;174:1238–1248.

43. Wetzler LM, Blake MS, Barry K, et al. Gonococcal porin vaccine evaluation: comparison of Por proteosomes, liposomes, and blebs isolated from rmp deletion mutants. J Infect Dis 1992;166:551–555.

Chapter 23

RESPIRATORY TRACT INFECTIONS

FLOYD W. DENNY JR. AND INGEGERD KALLINGS

Acute respiratory tract infections are the most common illnesses of the human host, but there is surprisingly little information in the medical literature regarding their incidence or etiology in travelers. Respiratory infections are not mentioned in most reports of illnesses in travelers, or if mentioned are not reported in detail. Notable exceptions are legionellosis and influenza. Information is available on the incidence and etiology of respiratory tract infections in nontravelers in developing and developed countries. These data, and those available from studies in travelers, will be used to construct a picture of respiratory infections in travelers.

GEOGRAPHIC CONSIDERATIONS

Data are not available to construct an accurate geographic picture of acute respiratory infections in travelers. Fortunately, data are available regarding the etiology and incidence of respiratory infections in many countries in the world, both developing and developed. The same microbial agents appear to cause infections of the respiratory tract all over the world. Furthermore, the incidence of respiratory infections is remarkably similar in developing and developed nations. However, there is an enormous difference in the morbidity and mortality from respiratory infections between advantaged and disadvantaged populations; severe or fatal infection may be several hundred times more frequent in poor nations. Factors such as malnutrition, indoor pollution, crowding, co-1infections with other agents that lead to suppression of host defenses, and certain vitamin or trace element deficiencies may play a role in this difference. Some travelers will have decreased host defenses, and some travel circumstances may increase the risk for certain infections. However, it seems reasonable to assume that most travelers will have respiratory infections due to the same agents and in at least the same numbers that they would have while not traveling.

INCIDENCE RATES

A limited number of published reports address the occurrence of respiratory infections in travelers, usually as a proportion of a population group, or more commonly the proportion of an ill group, with respiratory symptoms. The great majority of these illnesses are said to be of the upper respiratory tract and to be mild. Table 23–1 outlines the data from 13 such reports since 1972.[1–13] In two of these reports, acute respiratory infections were the most frequent type of illness.[8,12] In most of the others, respiratory infections were second only to diarrhea as causes of illnesses. Kendrick estimated the incidence of respiratory infections in travelers to be 3.7 per 1,000 travel days for those traveling only to Latin America, 3.5 for those traveling only to Oceania, and 3.1 for those traveling only to the Caribbean.[3] Steffen et al. estimated the rate of acute respiratory tract infections with fever to be 1,261 per 100,000 travelers for a stay of 1 month in a developing country.[10,11] These are exceedingly low figures (0.15 to 1.35 per person-year) when compared with figures from studies in the United States of infections of families in the home (Table 23–2), where it was shown that the incidence of respiratory infections in American families is related inversely to age: 6 to 8 per year in small children and 3 to 5 per year in older children and adults.[14] Selwyn reported studies in children in nine developing countries varying from 4.78 to 8.74 per child per year, with one exception in Thailand of 14.3 per child per year.[15] These rates were always inversely related to the age of the child. Thus, the incidence of respiratory infections appears to be relatively similar in developing and developed countries; however, the mortality rate due to respiratory infections is much increased in children in developing countries.

The reasons for the reported differences in respiratory infections in travelers and nontravelers are puzzling. It seems likely that most respiratory infections in travelers are mild, not incapacitating, and not reported. This has been a well-recognized problem in determining the incidence of respiratory infections by many investigators over many years and in many settings.

ETIOLOGIC AGENTS AND CAUSATIVE FACTORS

Outbreaks due to *Legionella pneumophila* and to influenza viruses in travelers have been well documented and will be covered in some detail below, as will infections due to *Mycobacterium tuberculosis* and *Corynebacterium diphtheriae*. Because few data are available on the etiology of respiratory infections in travelers, and because the etiology of respiratory tract infections in all countries studied has been the same, it seems reasonable to assume that travelers in foreign countries are infected with agents similar to those at home.

Table 23–1. REPORTED OCCURRENCE OF RESPIRATORY INFECTIONS IN TRAVELERS

AUTHOR	STUDY POPULATION DESCRIPTION	NO.	OCCURRENCE OF RESPIRATORY INFECTIONS	COMPARISON TO OTHER ILLNESSES	REFERENCE NUMBER
Caumes	French travelers to Nepal	12,437	17.55% of 838 ill travelers	Second to diarrhea (29.65%)	1
Hilton	U.S. travelers from immunization clinic	214	"Rare"; 4 of 10 travelers to China*	Diarrhea first	2
Kendrick	U.S. travelers	5,644	6.7%	Second to gastroenteritis (14.6%)	3
MacLean	Visit to clinic on return from tropics	587	12%	Second to malaria (32%)	4
Peltola	Visitors to Spain or Spanish Islands, North Africa, or Thailand	2,665	10% of 879 ill travelers	Diarrhea (18%) Sunburn (10%)	5
Reid	Package tourists and other travelers	2,211	16% of 951 ill travelers	Second to diarrhea (80%)	6
Sabate	Visitors to Tanzania: Children 0–14 yr Adolescents	335 158	16% 0	Parasites (22.45%) Digestive system (21.8%)	7
Smith	U.S. college student travelers: Developing countries Western Europe	453	39% 42%	Second to diarrhea (62%) More frequent than diarrhea	8
Steffen	Travelers from the tropics	10,500	12%	Third behind diarrhea (34%) and constipation (14%)	9
	Swiss travelers to:	7,886	15%		
	Developing countries		171 (2.2%)	Second only to gastro- intestinal problems	10, 11
	Greek or Canary Island		23 (1.0%)	Third behind gastrointestinal problems and dermatoses	
Christenson	Swedish passengers to southern Europe and northern Africa	418	88% of 335 ill passengers	Diarrhea and vomiting 33%	12
Cossar	Travelers returning to Scotland	13,816	4%	Gastrointestinal 28%	13

* In a personal communication with the authors in January 1995, Dr. T. Gherardin of the Australian Embassy in Beijing reported: "In the winter months, lower respiratory tract infections are certainly a leading cause of admission in foreigners' wards throughout Beijing and Shanghai. I am unable to provide you with actual admission/diagnostic data."

UPPER RESPIRATORY INFECTIONS

Table 23–3 lists the usual viral and bacterial agents that are isolated from patients with acute upper respiratory infections. Figure 23–1 shows a practical and useful classification of upper respiratory tract infections. Most acute upper respiratory infections, at any age, are not accompanied by the complications listed in Figure 23–1; the vast majority in older children and adults are uncomplicated. Uncomplicated infections are conveniently and practically separated into those due to the group A streptococcus and those that have nonstreptococcal etiologies. Only a small proportion of upper respiratory infections are caused by group A streptococci; most are caused by viruses. It is important to recognize group A streptococcal infections because they can be followed by acute rheumatic fever, which can be prevented with proper antibiotic treatment. Early treatment also ameliorates the

symptoms and shortens the clinical course of the infection. Classic streptococcal pharyngitis has an abrupt

Table 23–2. INCIDENCE OF COMMON RESPIRATORY DISEASES IN FAMILIES LIVING IN THE U.S.A., BY AGE

AGE (YEARS)	ILLNESSES PER PERSON YEAR
Under 1	6.7
1–4	7.93
5–9	6.28
10–14	5.15
15–16	4.7
Fathers	3.5
Mothers	4.8

From Dingle et al.[14]

Table 23–3. VIRUSES AND BACTERIA AS CAUSES OF ACUTE UPPER RESPIRATORY INFECTIONS

VIRUSES	BACTERIA
Adenoviruses	*Arcanobacterium haemolyticus*
Coronaviruses	*Chlamydia pneumoniae*
Enteroviruses	*Mycoplasma pneumoniae*
Epstein-Barr virus	*Streptococcus*, group A
Herpes simplex virus	*Streptococcus*, groups C and G
Influenza viruses	
Parainfluenza viruses	
Respiratory syncytial virus	
Rhinoviruses	

onset, pain on swallowing, tender and enlarged anterior cervical lymph nodes, and large, inflamed tonsils with patchy exudates. Only one-third to one half of infected patients have these classic findings; the remainder are asymptomatic or have atypical or milder symptoms. Detection of group A streptococcal antigen by a rapid strep test or the isolation of the organism on a sheep blood agar plate is the only dependable method of making an accurate diagnosis.

Arcanobacterium haemolyticus and *Chlamydia pneumoniae* are newly recognized, less frequent, bacterial upper respiratory pathogens. *A. haemolyticus* is of interest because it causes infections in older children and young adults that clinically resemble streptococcal pharyngitis, including a scarlet fever-like rash.[16,17] *C. pneumoniae* resembles *Mycoplasma pneumoniae*. It can cause pharyngitis, which is usually accompanied by tracheobronchitis and/or pneumonia—so-called atypical or walking pneumonia. Groups C and G streptococci can cause pharyngitis, which resembles group A disease, but

are more likely to occur in adolescents and young adults. Neither organism causes rheumatic fever. Group C infections have been associated infrequently with glomerulonephritis. Nonstreptococcal bacteria are infrequent causes of upper respiratory tract infections, are self-limited in their course, and, in general, cause few problems if left untreated. The causes of complications are most frequently secondary bacterial infections. *Streptococcus pneumoniae, Haemophilus influenzae,* and *Moraxella catarrhalis* are the most common infecting agents, but group A streptococcus and *Staphylococcus aureus* can also cause complications. Complications are more frequent in small children, and otitis media is the most frequent complication.

LOWER RESPIRATORY INFECTIONS

Acute infections of the lower respiratory tract are more difficult clinical problems; rapid, inexpensive, and effective methods for recognizing the etiologic agents are not available in most clinical settings. The viruses and bacteria that are common causes of acute lower respiratory infection are listed in Table 23–4; viruses cause most infections, especially in children. In small children, the listed viruses are frequently associated with a specific syndrome (croup, tracheobronchitis, bronchiolitis, pneumonia), are isolated in rather predictable seasons, and occur more frequently in children of certain ages in the United States. *M. pneumoniae* infections are infrequent in preschool children and are characterized by tracheobronchitis and pneumonia in older children and adults.

The big clinical problem in children and in adults is the etiology of pneumonia. It seems certain that most pneumonia cases are also caused by viruses, but bacteria play a more prominent role than in infections higher in the respiratory tract. *M. pneumoniae* and *C. pneumoniae* are well-recognized causes of pneumonia and have symptoms and signs that frequently suggest a diagnosis: gradual onset, cough progressing from dry to productive, chest film worse than symptoms, and a normal peripheral white blood cell count.

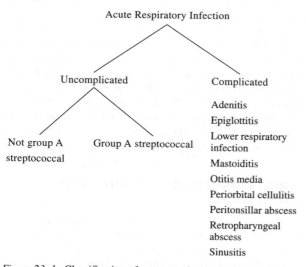

Figure 23–1. Classification of upper respiratory tract infections.

Table 23–4. VIRUSES AND BACTERIA AS CAUSES OF ACUTE LOWER RESPIRATORY INFECTIONS

VIRUSES	BACTERIA
Adenoviruses	*Chlamydia pneumoniae*
Enteroviruses	*Chlamydia trachomatis*
Influenza viruses	*Haemophilus influenzae*
Parainfluenza viruses	*Legionella pneumophila*
Respiratory syncytial virus	*Mycobacterium tuberculosis*
	Mycoplasma pneumoniae
	Streptococcus pneumoniae

S. pneumoniae and *H. influenzae* are well-recognized causes of pneumonia in patients over 2 years of age, *S. pneumoniae* being much more frequent than *H. influenzae*. The classic picture of pneumococcal pneumonia includes the abrupt onset of fever, cough, rapid respirations, and lobar consolidation on chest film. In the absence of a positive blood culture, a positive culture from a percutaneous needle aspirate from the infected lung, or a carefully obtained tracheal aspirate that is positive for pneumococci, the etiology remains in doubt. Diagnostic methods based on molecular technology are as yet not validated and adapted for broader clinical use.

Table 23–5 lists the microbial agents that can cause pneumonia under uncommon or special circumstances. Lower respiratory infections with these agents occur most frequently, but not exclusively in patients with depressed host defenses. These infecting agents should be considered in patients with depressed immunity and in normal hosts who do not respond readily to conventional therapy.

Factors that predispose the normal host to respiratory infections and the role of co-infections or superinfections are controversial. It has been shown rather convincingly that insults such as chilling are not important in predisposing patients to respiratory infections. Bacterial superinfections of patients with viral infections of the lower respiratory tract and co-infections with a virus and a bacterium are apparently uncommon in normal hosts. Patients with chronic tracheobronchial or pulmonary disease have infections with several bacteria that are infrequent causes of infections in normal hosts.

Table 23–5. AGENTS CAUSING RESPIRATORY INFECTIONS IN UNCOMMON OR SPECIAL CIRCUMSTANCES

VIRUSES	FUNGI
Cytomegalovirus	*Aspergillus* species
Epstein-Barr virus	*Blastomyces dermatitidis*
Herpes simplex virus	*Candida* species
Human immunodeficiency virus	*Coccidioides immitis*
Varicella-zoster virus	*Cryptococcus neoformans*
	Histoplasma capsulatum
	Malassezia furfur
	Zygomycetes

BACTERIA	PROTOZOA
Actinomyces species	Cryptosporidium
Anaerobes	*Pneumocystis carinii*
Atypical mycobacteria	*Strongyloides stercoralis*
Corynebacterium diphtheriae	*Toxoplasma gondii*
Enterobacteriaceae	
Group B streptococci	
Listeria monocytogenes	
Nocardia species	
Rickettsiae	
Staphylococcus aureus	

INFECTIONS FOR SPECIAL CONSIDERATION

Respiratory tract infections due to several microorganisms can pose special problems in travelers: influenza viruses, *Legionella pneumophila*, *M. tuberculosis*, *C. diphtheriae*, and *Coccidioides immitis*. Influenza viruses and *L. pneumophila* are important because they cause sharp outbreaks of infections if travelers take certain risks. *M. tuberculosis* is important because the traveler may have contact with infected natives, some of whom might have drug-resistant organisms. *C. diphtheriae* is included because many adults in developed countries have lost specific immunity and therefore are susceptible to infection. These four microorganisms are addressed in some detail because of their possible significance. *C. immitis* will not be addressed, except to point out that travelers can be at risk when visiting certain endemic areas of the world, such as the southwestern United States and certain areas in Central and South America.[18,19]

LEGIONELLA INFECTIONS

BACKGROUND

Legionella bacteria are ubiquitous environmental microorganisms that cause disease in humans when a susceptible individual is exposed to a sufficient inoculum of virulent organisms. Legionellae constitute a large group of bacteria with 31 species and 19 subgroups currently recognized. Since the first report in 1977, legionellae have been found in every part of the world where searches have been made.[20] *L. pneumophila*, serogroup 1, is the most common cause of infections in humans. Legionnaires' disease is the term used for pneumonia caused by *L. pneumophila* serogroup 1, whereas clinical syndromes and infections caused by other legionella species are referred to as legionella infections, which is the term used for diseases caused by any legionella species.

Legionella infections occur as endemic, sporadic cases, as clusters, and as large common-source outbreaks. Around 2% of community-acquired pneumonias are caused by legionellae as shown by studies in different countries. However, only a fraction of these cases is generally recognized. Early studies showed the most typical legionella patient to be a 55-year-old, smoking man. Immunosuppressed individuals are considerably more susceptible to legionellae, and several nosocomial clusters and outbreaks have been described. It is a rather uncommon disease in children.[21–23]

TRAVEL-ASSOCIATED LEGIONELLA INFECTIONS

An outbreak of legionella infections among travelers was recognized in 1978 among Scottish tourists on a package tour to Spain.[24] A number of outbreaks among travelers, comprising over 200 patients, have been reported in the literature since then (Table 23–6).[22,25–34] In an initiative by

Table 23–6. CLUSTERS OF LEGIONELLA INFECTIONS AMONG TOURISTS REPORTED IN THE INTERNATIONAL LITERATURE

YEAR OF OUTBREAK	COUNTRY/RESORT*	NUMBER OF CASES	NATIONALITY	REFERENCE NUMBER
1973–80	Spain, Benidorm	42+	Scottish, British	25
1973–87	Italy, several hotels and places	117	Tourists of different nationalities	32
1979	England, Corby	5	British	26
1979–82	U.S.A., Virgin Islands	24	American	27
1980–82	Italy, Lido di Savio	23	Italian	28
1980–82	Portugal, Quarteira	6	British	29
1980–83	Portugal, Quarteira	14	British	22
1981	Italy, Lake Garda	4	Danish	30
1986–90	Italy	6	German, Austrian, Swiss, Italian	31
1994	Cruise ships	50	U.S.A.	33
1995	Cruise ships	3	Italian cruise line	34

*For each cluster, one hotel was implicated as the source of infection. Some hotels were associated with cases over a period of months to several years despite control measures and temporary elimination of legionella bacteria in their domestic water system.

the European Working Group on Legionella Infections for an early warning system of travel-associated legionella infections, 485 cases were reported from 1987 to June 1993. Sixty-nine hotels in 56 cities or resorts in 18 countries were associated with clusters of more than one case. In 19 clusters, more than one nationality was represented by the patients. It was noted that cases associated with a certain hotel could occur over a period of several years, that is, the hotel in question was continuously contaminated with bacterial strains of low virulence, or there was an intermittent shedding of bacteria (Table 23–7). Among the 272 cases for which the outcome was known, the case fatality rate was 21%, which is higher than the overall case fatality rate of 5% to 15% in legionella infections. In England, Wales, and Sweden, 15% to 30% of all community-acquired legionella infections are related to travel, domestic or international.[23]

Early recognition of clusters and outbreaks with a common source is important in order to initiate control measures. Therefore, travel-associated legionella infections have been included in a European Community initiative. As soon as a legionella case has been diagnosed in a patient who has been traveling within the likely incubation period of 2 weeks, the case is reported together with geographic location and buildings suspected as sources of transmission.

A major problem in detecting occurrence of legionella infection in travelers is the incubation period. Passengers characteristically have left the region and returned home when symptoms develop. There are numerous reasons why there is an increased rate of legionella infection and pneumonia on cruises: passengers are often elderly or infirm, ports of call often include hotter tropical areas, and it is difficult to maintain safe water systems.[35,36] The most common diagnosis for passengers and crew seeking medical care from clinic staff on board ships is respiratory tract infection, found in 29% of clinic visits in one study.[37]

Table 23–7. TRAVEL-ASSOCIATED LEGIONNAIRES' DISEASE. DATABASE 1987–JUNE 1993*

No. of cases reported	485; single cases and clusters of >2 cases
No. of countries visited worldwide	41; 20 European countries, 21 countries
No. of clusters and cases involved	56; comprising 167 cases
No. of hotels associated with clusters	69; in 56 cities or resorts in 18 countries
No. of hotels associated with cases over a period of >12 months	20

*Reported at the 8th meeting, European Working Group on Legionella Infections, Vienna, Austria, May 10–12, 1993.

TRANSMISSION

The mode of transmission of legionella bacteria is evidently air borne. No other transmission route, including the spread of bacteria from person to person, has as yet been proven. The entrance of bacteria into the domestic water systems via the water plant is the most common mechanism of transmission.[38] Within a building, the bacteria may find a niche with suitable conditions for multiplication. Legionellae grow in water at a temperature of 25° to 42°C; growth is supported by biofilms found in a cooling tower or directly in waterpipe fittings and showers. From this amplification site, the bacteria are transmitted to humans via an aerosol, generated by a showerhead, a whirlpool, an ordinary faucet, or by the mist from a cooling tower.

Legionnaires' disease has been documented increasingly among passengers of cruise ships. Jernigan et al.[33] reported an outbreak affecting 50 cruise ship passengers that went unrecognized for 3 months. Exposure to whirlpool spas on board the ship was implicated in the disease transmission. In another study,[34] the water supply system was implicated in transmission of legionella infection on board ships.

CLINICAL COURSE

The major clinical symptom caused by legionellae is lobar pneumonia, clinically indistinguishable from a pneumonia caused by other organisms. The onset, after an incubation period of 2 to 10 days, is usually abrupt with high fever, chills, myalgia, and severe headache, often accompanied by confusion and hallucinations. Gastrointestinal symptoms are frequently present. Initially, respiratory symptoms may be absent, and half of the patients do not develop a cough. Many patients show no infiltrates on roentgenographs on admission to hospital. Gradually, a patchy, alveolar infiltrate increases to a lobar consolidation, bilateral in severe cases. Mortality is high, over 20%, if appropriate antibiotic treatment is delayed. Subclinical infections occur as well as pneumonia with a less severe course. Some legionella species may cause a self-limiting, influenza-like illness called Pontiac fever.

DIAGNOSIS

Clinical and epidemiologic suspicion of legionella infection must be confirmed by laboratory analysis, most commonly antibody detection, isolation of the organism, or antigen detection in urine. Reagents based on monoclonal antibodies have been used to detect bacteria by immunofluorescence microscopy directly on human secretions. Tests based on molecular technology for the detection of antigen or DNA components have been developed but are as yet not fully evaluated. Travel-associated legionella infection represents a challenge since sensitive diagnostic testing reagents are not widely available to diagnose cases occurring in travelers.

THERAPY

Erythromycin treatment has the best documented clinical effect, in combination with rifampin for severe cases with complications. Successful treatment with co-trimoxazole has been reported; reports of treatment with fluoroquinolones are controversial. Treatment may need to be continued for 3 weeks to avoid a relapse. Legionella bacteria are susceptible in vitro to many other antibiotics. However, due to the intracellular growth of the organisms, the clinical effect of antibiotic treatment does not always correspond with in vitro susceptibility. Most legionella species produce a beta-lactamase causing resistance of penicillins, ampicillin, and some other beta-lactam antibiotics.

PREVENTION

It is not possible to advise the individual traveler on how to avoid legionella infections. Prevention must be accomplished through control of bacterial amplification and of transmission. In order to initiate epidemiologic investigations to identify sources, it is important that cases are recognized and reported. Molecular techniques are being applied for matching patients' isolates with those from the environment. Control measures that have been proven effective are hyperchlorination in combination with flushing of the water system with hot water and thereafter maintaining an elevated hot water temperature. The construction of the water system should be reviewed and possible amplification sites eliminated. Unsuitable materials in tubings and fittings may need to be replaced. Cooling towers should be cleaned, decontaminated, and continuously subject to good maintenance practice.[38] Legionella infection should be preventable. Guidelines exist for maintaining safe water systems and spas in international tourist locations.[35]

There are currently four prototype vaccines of different designs that have been tested in animal models. Although people with an increased risk for legionella infections are easily defined, epidemiologic data on the accurate incidence of these infections are lacking, making it difficult to define a target group for immunization.

INFLUENZA VIRUS INFECTIONS

BACKGROUND

Influenza is an acute, usually self-limited, respiratory infection caused by influenza type A or B viruses that occur in outbreaks almost every winter or early spring. It is the most important of the viral respiratory infections because of its tendency to infect humans of all ages, to occur in epidemics involving a large proportion of the population, and to produce high morbidity and mortality in young children and the elderly.

TRAVEL-ASSOCIATED INFLUENZA INFECTIONS

Influenza appears to be unique among respiratory virus infections in travelers because it is the only one that has been described in detail, including the clinical, epidemiologic, and etiologic aspects. Several outbreaks in populations aboard ships or airplanes or in tour groups have been reported.[39–45] All of these outbreaks have been due to type A virus and are noted for involvement of a high proportion of the populations at risk and the short and explosive nature of their occurrence.

TRANSMISSION

There is some debate regarding the mode of spread of influenza viruses from host to host. The primary mode of spread is probably by close contact, either by direct contact or large droplets, as with other respiratory viruses. There is experimental evidence that the virus can be spread by the air-borne route, involving small or aerosolized droplets. The explosive nature of outbreaks in groups aboard ships, in airplanes, or in barracks is compatible with this mode of spread.

CLINICAL COURSE

The classic case of influenza has the sudden onset of fever, headache, cough, chills, and myalgia, but many cases are milder and cannot be differentiated from infections with other respiratory agents. The hallmark of influenza is the cough, resulting from involvement of the trachea and bronchi. Illness lasts from 3 to 5 days, with the cough lingering for several more days.

Most cases are relatively mild and uncomplicated, but influenza is noted for the severity of infections in infants and the elderly. Complications such as pneumonia, caused by the virus itself or a superinfection with a bacterium (*S. pneumoniae, H. influenzae, S. aureus*, or group A streptococcus), do occur, as do the complications of sinusitis and otitis media. Patients with chronic disease, especially cardiac conditions or chronic lung disease, are especially vulnerable to influenza infections.

DIAGNOSIS

Influenza outbreaks can usually be recognized by their epidemiologic and clinical characteristics. The classic clinical findings, described above, and the appearance of a large number of patients within a short period of time during the winter or early spring are very suggestive of influenza infections. These outbreaks can be confirmed tentatively by the use of one of the commercially available rapid diagnostic tests or more definitely by the isolation of the virus from respiratory secretions or by the appearance of specific antibodies in a convalescent-phase area.

TREATMENT

Treatment of most cases of influenza is entirely supportive; antivirals are not indicated.

Four antiviral agents are approved for treating severe influenza. Amantadine and rimantadine are approved for treating influenza A, whereas the neuramidase inhibitor drugs zanamivir and oseltamivir are approved to treat both influzena A and B. Ribavirin is effective against both types A and B viruses in the laboratory, but it is not approved for treatment of influenza at this time.

Adequate fluid intake, inhaled moisture, mild antitussives, and analgesics can be used to give patients relief of severe symptoms. Aspirin should not be used in children because of the association with Reye's syndrome.

PREVENTION

Two preventive measures are available: vaccine and chemoprophylaxis. It is recommended that patients at high risk for influenza infections—those with chronic cardiac or pulmonary conditions—and the elderly (65 years and older) receive yearly immunization with a vaccine containing the recommended virus strains. For those patients who are not immunized, amantadine or rimantadine is recommended as a prophylactic agent. The agent should be started as soon as the risk to influenza is recognized and continued until after the risk is past. Neither zanamivir nor oseltamivir is approved for prophylactic use.

Avoidance of contact with an infected patient should be practiced as much as possible.

M. TUBERCULOSIS INFECTIONS

BACKGROUND

Since the middle of the century, tuberculosis has decreased dramatically in industrialized countries, expressed both as actual numbers and as incidence rates. Globally, however, tuberculosis has increased to at least 40 million people with active disease, and the number of attributable deaths is calculated to be 3 million every year. Most infected people are found in tropical and subtropical areas such as East Asia, Oceania, and parts of Africa. Even in countries where tuberculosis was believed to be under control, there has been an upsurge during recent years due to the high prevalence of tuberculosis among AIDS patients and treatment difficulties caused by multiresistant *M. tuberculosis*.[46] Tuberculosis affects mainly young children, the elderly, and immunodeficient persons. Lung disease is the most common manifestation, but young children are at special risk to develop meningitis with a high case fatality rate or severe sequelae. Although treatment will usually effectively control disease, infection is lifelong and may recur later in life if the patient becomes immunocompromised.

TRANSMISSION

Transmission is air borne from person to person; the source is mainly patients with active lung disease who have not been treated. The risk of transmission is considered to be generally low and to occur mainly in families and people living in close contact. The infected person transmits infection only during active disease.

TUBERCULOSIS IN TRAVELERS

The risk of acquiring tuberculosis during travel is not very great, and there are not many reports of such cases, but it is known to have occurred. A recent publication reported the transmission of *M. tuberculosis* from an infected crew member to other crew members of an aircraft and concluded that transmission of *M. tuberculosis* to passengers cannot be excluded.[47] Transmission of *M. tuberculosis* was documented aboard a commercial aircraft from a highly infectious passenger during air travel.[48] Risk factors were long flight segments and close proximity of contacts to the index case. Transmission of tuberculosis has also been documented on commercial trains.[49,50] The spread of multiresistant mycobacteria has made consequences of even sporadic tuberculosis cases more alarming, and the disease must not be overlooked, especially when examining immunocompromised patients who might have been infected in a foreign country with *M. tuberculosis* a long time in the past.[51]

TREATMENT AND PREVENTION

Antituberculosis treatment according to general recommendation is usually effective if the patient is compliant. Epidemiologic data regarding the probable place of acquisition and antibiotic susceptibility must be considered when initiating therapy. Children of immigrants should be bacille Calmette Guérin vaccinated when visiting their parents' native country, if not sooner, and so should aid workers and vagabonds. The elderly and people with cancer, HIV/AIDS, or chronic diseases may not be vaccinated because of their immunocompromised state and the risk of side effects. The risk of being infected versus the risk with vaccination should be assessed individually and the traveler informed about the risks.

DIPHTHERIA

Immunization programs with diphtheria toxoid virtually eliminated diphtheria from most industrialized countries by the mid-1970s, despite the fact that up to 30% (age dependent) of the population lacked protective immunity. This deficient protection, in addition to the disease remaining endemic in developing areas, made possible the importation of cases and subsequent outbreaks in the United States.[52] In recent years, a major resurgence of diphtheria has been observed in Europe, mainly in the former Russian Federation and Ukraine; 19,046 cases occurred in 1993, a sixfold increase in 3 years. In 1992 to 1993, cases were identified in several Eastern European countries, including Poland, Finland, Germany, and Norway, that were epidemiologically linked to Belarus, Kazakhstan, Russia, and the Ukraine.[53]

A clinical suspicion of diphtheria should be raised when a patient presents with pseudomembranous pharyngitis, which would be strengthened by the presence of enlarged anterior cervical lymphnodes or bullneck (for further clinical description, see a textbook of infectious diseases). The diagnosis is confirmed in the laboratory by isolation of a toxigenic strain of *C. diphtheriae*. Early recognition, appropriate treatment, and epidemiologic control measures are required to prevent secondary cases.

PREVENTION

Four doses of diphtheria toxoid before 2 years of age have an efficacy of greater than 98% in young children. A booster should be given to school-aged children every 10 years, to persons traveling to known high-risk areas, and to refugees and immigrants arriving from such areas if they cannot provide documentation of sufficient immunization.

TRANSMISSION

The transmission of respiratory pathogens takes place mainly by human-to-human spread; animal sources play little or no role. Most respiratory infections are transmitted by close contact with an acutely infected host, either by direct contact or large droplets. An exception to this is the influenza virus, which probably can also be spread by small droplets; there are several examples of multiple infections following exposure on airplanes or ships as discussed above. Fomites do not appear to be important in most respiratory infections. The spread of *L. pneumophila* appears to be rather unique, as mentioned earlier.

Other respiratory infections may be spread during travel including measles,[54] rubella,[36] and coccidioidomycosis.[55]

SPECIAL POPULATIONS AT RISK

Populations at risk to more frequent or more severe respiratory infections include infants and small children, the elderly, and people with chronic diseases. Children in the first few years of life have more total respiratory infections, and a higher proportion of these will involve the lower respiratory tract than in later years. The elderly are also more prone to severe respiratory infections. Patients with chronic diseases, especially chronic pulmonary and cardiac conditions, are at risk for severe respiratory infections.

THERAPY AND PREVENTION

THERAPY

It is convenient to separate therapy of patients with respiratory infections into those with upper respiratory tract involvement and those with involvement of the lower tract. Figure 23–1 outlines a rational approach to patients with acute upper respiratory infections. Patients with any of the complications mentioned are likely to have a secondary bacterial infection, which warrants appropriate antimicrobials. For patients with uncomplicated upper respiratory infections, it is important to identify those due to the group A streptococcus by performing a rapid strep test or a culture on sheep blood agar in order to initiate appropriate antibiotic treatment. At the present time, penicillin for 10 days is the treatment of choice. Patients with nonstreptococcal infections, with the few exceptions outlined earlier, do not need an antibiotic and should be managed with supportive care only.

Complications of upper respiratory infections are caused most frequently by *S. pneumoniae*, *H. influenzae*, or *M. catarrhalis*, but group A streptococcus and *S. aureus* can be causative agents. Group A streptococcus remains exquisitively sensitive to pencillin G, which remains the treatment of choice. The other bacteria are more troublesome to treat because of evolving resistance to commonly used antimicrobials. In the management of these patients, the health care provider should be guided by the status of drug resistance locally.

Patients with lower respiratory tract involvement present a more complex clinical situation. Those with laryngitis, croup, tracheobronchitis, or bronchiolitis most probably have a viral infection. *M. pneumoniae* and *C. pneumoniae* are probably the only two bacteria that commonly infect these parts of the respiratory tract in normal hosts. Mycoplasma and chlamydia infections are effectively treated with erythromycin or a tetracycline if the patient is over 7 years old. All other patients can be managed with only supportive care.

Type b *H. influenzae* epiglottitis is a recognized entity in children and can resemble severe croup. Bacterial tracheitis, a clinical syndrome that resembles epiglottitis, has been rarely recognized and is caused by *H. influenzae*, *S. aureus*, *S. pneumoniae*, and group A streptococcus. These two clinical entities are medical emergencies and require antimicrobial therapy and measures to provide a patent airway.

Patients with pneumonia are more difficult to handle. Although most cases are due to viruses, it is difficult to separate those who require specific treatment. At present, patients with apparent pneumococcal infections and those severely ill with pneumonia due to an unknown etiology should receive appropriate antibiotic treatment until the causative microorganism is identified. As mentioned above, patients with mycoplasma or chlamydia infections can be treated with erythromycin or a tetracycline. Patients with complications such as pleural empyema or lung abscess require special treatment, almost always in hospital.

Antivirals effective against respiratory pathogens are limited. Ribavirin has been demonstrated to be effective against Rous saroma virus (RSV) in severely ill infants but probably has no role in patients either with milder infections or those managed out of the hospital. Ribavirin is also effective in the laboratory against the influenza and parainfluenza viruses, but its clinical effectiveness has not been demonstrated. Amantadine and rimantadine may be effective in treating infections with influenza virus type A but not type B, and should probably be used in severely ill patients. Neither drug has a role in treating mildly ill patients. Experience with zanamivir and oseltamivir has not been sufficient to allow a firm recommendation regarding their use in severely ill patients.

PREVENTION

Vaccines are available for the prevention of pneumococcal *H. influenzae* type b, influenza virus infections, and diphtheria. The presently available pneumococcal vaccine is recommended in the United States for children over 2 years of age who are at special risk for severe respiratory infections (cystic fibrosis, bronchopulmonary dysplasia, heart disease) and for all people 65 years or older. It is not effective in young children. A conjugated pneumococcal vaccine has been developed; it is effective in children of all ages and will be commercially available soon. All children should receive *H. influenzae* type b vaccine, beginning at 2 months of age. Influenza virus vaccine is recommended for all patients at high risk for respiratory infections, the elderly, and all others who are in vulnerable or critical positions such as health care givers or emergency personnel. All children should be immunized against diphtheria. A special toxoid is available for immunizing adults; it should be repeated every 10 years.

Amantadine and rimantadine are effective in preventing influenza A virus infections and should be used in people at high risk who have not received influenza vaccine. The drug should be started when it is clear that influenza is in the community and continued until the danger of infection is past.

Other methods of prevention, except avoidance of contact with infected individuals, are of no use. Ultraviolet light and antiseptics are ineffective.

SUPPORTIVE AND SELF-THERAPY

The use of analgesics, an adequate fluid intake, and inhaled moisture are available to make patients with respiratory infections more comfortable and are probably the most important. Nose drops, if used judicially, and antitussives that do not overly suppress the cough are also helpful.

FUTURE CONSIDERATIONS

Because most respiratory infections are self-limited and of short duration, it seems most likely that their control will be better accomplished by preventive measures, usually vaccines, rather than by treatment with antimicrobials. Antimicrobials will continue to play a role, most probably in severe infections due to viruses and bacteria. The effective vaccines that are now available are discussed above. A pneumococcal vaccine that is effective in young children is highly desirable and is in the final stages of development. Such a vaccine is now available for *H. influenzae* type b but not against other types and nontypable strains. An effective vaccine against group A streptococcus is probably many years away. Efforts are under way to develop vaccines against several of the respiratory viruses, especially RSV, but none are available commercially at this time. The presently available influenza vaccine, although usually quite effective, is not an ideal immunizing agent. It must be given annually, and choosing the correct virus strains for inclusion in the vaccine is not always successful. An improved vaccine is desirable. As mentioned above, amantadine, rimantadine, and other recently licensed anti-influenza drugs can be used prophylactically to prevent influenza virus type A infections, but no other antivirals effective against other respiratory viruses are available. Immunoglobulin preparations containing high titers of specific antibodies are being studied as prophylaxis against several respiratory viruses but are not available for routine use at this time.

SUMMARY AND ADVICE FOR TRAVELERS

1. A precise picture of the role of respiratory infections in travelers cannot be drawn at this time because of a paucity of information in the literature.
2. Most reported studies list respiratory infections second to diarrheal diseases as causes of illness in trav-

elers, but few data are available regarding microbiologic etiology of these infections. Comprehensive data on the incidence of these infections are also lacking.

3. Studies are available that show that acute respiratory infections have the same etiology and incidence in countries all over the world, including developing nations. The severity of these infections is much greater in developing countries, presumably because many people in these countries have decreased host defenses.

4. Most acute upper respiratory infections are due to viruses and are mild, and antibiotics are not indicated. Supportive measures such as nose drops, analgesics, antitussives, and adequate fluids may give some relief.

5. Group A streptococci are the most frequent causes of bacterial upper respiratory infections. They are important because adequate treatment will shorten the course of illness and prevent the occurrence of rheumatic fever. Patients with streptococcal pharyngitis should be under the care of an appropriate health care giver.

6. Acute infections of the larynx, trachea, bronchi, and bronchiole are usually due to viruses. *M. pneumoniae* and *C. pneumoniae* are the only bacteria that commonly infect these sites.

7. Most cases of pneumonia are also due to viruses, but bacteria play a larger role in infections higher in the respiratory tract. *M. pneumoniae, C. pneumoniae, L. pneumophila, S. pneumoniae, H. influenzae,* and *M. tuberculosis* are recognized causes of lower respiratory infections that require antimicrobial treatment. When an etiologic agent is not clear initially, antibiotics are frequently indicated until adequate studies have been done to indicate that they are not needed. Antibiotics given under these circumstances should be chosen with due consideration to the epidemiology of antibiotic susceptibility in the specific area visited (particularly with *S. pneumoniae, H. influenzae,* and *M. tuberculosis*).

8. People at high risk for respiratory infections—small children, the elderly, patients with chronic cardiac and pulmonary diseases—require careful attention while traveling.

9. Every effort should be made to prevent respiratory tract infections in travelers:

    a. Avoid close contact with ill people as much as possible.

    b. All children should receive routine childhood immunizations, including a conjugated *H. influenzae* type b vaccine.

    c. All adults should have been properly immunized against diphtheria within the past 10 years.

    d. All patients at high risk for respiratory infection should receive pneumococcal and influenza vaccines.

    e. High-risk patients with pulmonary and cardiac diseases who have not received influenza vaccine should receive prophylactic amantadine or rimantadine before and during travel to a country experiencing influenza infections.

REFERENCES

1. Caumes E, Brucker G, Brousse G, et al. Travel-associated illness in 838 French tourists in Nepal in 1984. Travel Med Int 1991;8:72–76.

2. Hilton E, Edwards B, Singer C. Reported illness and compliance in UN travelers attending an immunization facility. Arch Intern Med 1989;149:178–179.

3. Kendrick MA. Study of illness among Americans returning from international travel; July 11–August 24, 1971 (preliminary data). J Infect Dis 1972;126:684–685.

4. MacLean JD, Lalande RG. Fever in the tropics. In: Travel medical advisor. The physician's update on international health. Atlanta: American Health Consultants, 1992: 27.1–27.13.

5. Peltola H, Kyrönseppa H, Hösla P. Trip to the south—a health hazard morbidity of Finnish travelers. Scand J Infect Dis 1983;15:375–381.

6. Reid D, Dewar RD, Fallon R, et al. Infection and travel: the experience of package tourists and other travelers. J Infect 1980;2:365–370.

7. Sabate F. Health risks of children and adolescents in short-term travel or temporary residence in developing countries. In: Steffen R, Lobel HO, Haworth J, Bradley DJ, eds. Travel medicine: proceedings of the First Conference on International Travel Medicine. Berlin: Springer-Verlag, 1989:484–485.

8. Smith RP, Smith D, Bern K, et al. Health risks of international travel among United States college students. In: Steffen R, Lobel HO, Haworth J, Bradley DJ, eds. Travel medicine: proceedings of the First Conference on International Travel Medicine. Berlin: Springer-Verlag, 1989:67–70.

9. Steffen R, van der Linde F, Meyr HE. Erkrankungsrisiken bei 10,500 tropen und 1,300 Nordamerike-touristen. Schweiz Med Wochenschr 1978;108:1485–1495.

10. Steffen R. Health risks for short-term travelers. In: Steffen R, Lobel HO, Haworth J, Bradley DJ, eds. Travel medicine: proceedings of the First Conference on International Travel Medicine. Berlin: Springer-Verlag, 1989:27–36.

11. Steffen R, Rickenbach M, Wilhelm V, et al. Health problems after travel to developing countries. J Infect Dis 1987;156: 84–91.

12. Christenson B, Lidin-Janson G, Kallings I. Outbreak of respiratory illness on board a ship cruising to ports in southern Europe and northern Africa. J Infect 1987;14:247–254.

13. Cossar JH, Reid D, Fallon RJ, et al. A cumulative review of studies on travelers, their experience of illness, and the implications of these findings. J Infect 1990;21:27–42.

14. Dingle JH, Badger GF, Jordan WS Jr. Illness in the home. A study of 25,000 illnesses in a group of Cleveland families. Cleveland: The Press of Western Reserve University, 1964.

15. Selwyn BJ. The epidemiology of acute respiratory tract infection in young children: comparison of findings from several developing countries. Rev Infect Dis 1990;12:S870–S888.

16. Miller RA, Brancato F, Holmes KK. *Corynebacterium haemolyticum* as a cause of pharyngitis and scarlatinoform rash in young adults. Ann Intern Med 1986;105:867–872.

17. Karpathios T, Drakonaki S, Zervoudaki A, et al. *Acranobacterium haemolyticum* in children with presumed streptococcal pharyngotonsillitis or scarlet fever. J Pediatr 1992;121: 735–737.

18. Wiebe BM, Stenderup J, Grode GW, Jacobsen GK. Pulmonary coccidioidomycosis. Ugeskr Laeger 1993;155:1722–1723.

19. Bronnimann DA, Galgiani JN. Coccidioidomycosis. Eur J Clin Microbiol Infect Dis 1989;8:466–473.

20. McDade JE, Shepard CC, Fraser DW, et al. Legionnaires' disease: isolation of a bacterium and demonstration of its role in other respiratory disease. N Engl J Med 1977;297:1197–1203.

21. Rodgers FG, Pasculle AW. Legionella. In: Balows A, Hausler WJ Jr, Herrmann KL, Shadomy HJ, eds. Manual of clinical microbiology. 5th Ed. Washington, DC: American Society for Microbiology, 1991:442–453.

22. Bartlett CLR, Macrae AD, Macfarlane JT. Legionella infections. London: Edward Arnold, 1986.

23. Epidemiology, prevention and control of legionellosis: memorandum from a WHO meeting. Bull World Health Organ 1990;68:155–164.

24. Grist NR, Reid D, Najera R. Legionnaires' disease and the traveller. Ann Intern Med 1979;90:563–564.

25. Bartllett CLR, Swann RA, Casal J. Recurrent legionnaires' disease from a hotel water system. In: Thornsberry C, Balows A, Freeley CJ, Jakubowski W, eds. Legionella: proceedings of the 2nd International Symposium. Washington, DC: American Society for Microbiology, 1984:237–239.

26. Tobin JO, Bartlett CLR, Waitkins SA, et al. Legionnaires' disease: further evidence to implicate water storage and distribution systems as sources. BMJ 1981;282:573.

27. Schlech WF III, Gorman GW, Payne MC, Broome CV. Legionnaires' diseases in the Carribbean. An outbreak associated with a resort hotel. Arch Intern Med 1985;145:2076–2079.

28. Rosmini F, Castellani-Pastoris M, Mazzotti MF, et al. Febrile illness in successive cohorts of tourists at a hotel on the Italian Adriatic Coast: evidence for a persistent focus of legionella infection. Am J Epidemiol 1984;119:124–134.

29. Bartlett CLR, Bibby LF. Epidemic legionellosis in England and Wales 1979–1982. Zentralbl Bakteriol 1983;255:664–670.

30. Jorgensen KA, Korsager B, Johannsen G, et al. Legionnaires' disease imported to Denmark from Italy. Scand J Infect Dis 1981;13:133–136.

31. Castellani-Pastoris M, Benedetti P, Greco D, et al. Six cases of travel-associated legionnaires' disease in Ischia involving four countries. Infection 1992;20:73–77.

32. Passi C, Maddaluno R, Castellani-Pastoris M. Incidence of *Legionella pneumophila* infections in tourists: Italy. Public Health 1990;104:183–188.

33. Jernigan DB, Hofmann J, Cetron MS, et al. Outbreak of legionnaires' disease among cruise ship passengers exposed to a contaminated whirlpool spa. Lancet 1996;347:494–499.

34. Castellani-Pastoris M, LoMonaco R, Goldoni P, et al. Legionnaires' disease on a cruise ship linked to the water supply system: clinical and public health implications. Clin Infect Dis 1999;28:33–38.

35. Edelstein PH, Cetron MS. Sea, wind, and pneumonia. Clin Infect Dis 1999;28:39–41.

36. Minooee A, Rickman LS. Infectious diseases on cruise ships. Clin Infect Dis 1999;29:737–744.

37. Peake DE, Gray CL, Ludwig MR, Hill CD. Descriptive epidemiology of injury and illness among cruise ship passengers. Ann Emerg Med 1999;33:67–72.

38. Bhopal RS, Wagstaff R. Prospects for the elimination of legionnaires' disease [editorial]. J Infect 1993;26:239–243.

39. Klontz KC, Hynes NA, Gunn RA, et al. An outbreak of influenza A/Taiwan/1/86 (H1 N1) infections at a naval base and its association with airplane travel. Am J Epidemiol 1989;129:341–348.

40. Moser MR, Bender TR, Margolis HS, et al. An outbreak of influenza aboard a commercial airliner. Am J Epidemiol 1979;110:1–6.

41. Centers for Disease Control and Prevention. Acute respiratory illness among cruise-ship passengers—Asia. MMWR Morb Mortal Wkly Rep 1988;37:63–66.

42. Centers for Disease Control and Prevention. Outbreak of influenza-like illness in a tour group—Alaska. MMWR Morb Mortal Wkly Rep 1987;42:697–698, 704.

43. Ksiazek TG, Olson JG, Irving GS, et al. An influenza outbreak due to A/USSR/77-like (H1 N1) virus aboard a US Navy ship. Am J Epidemiol 1980;112:487–494.

44. Olson JG, Ksiazek TG, Irving GS, Rendin RW. An explosive outbreak of influenza caused by A/USSR/77-like virus on a United States naval ship. Mil Med 1979;144:743–745.

45. Miller J, Tam T, Afif C, et al. Influenza A outbreak on a cruise ship. Can Commun Dis Rep 1998;24:9–11.

46. Bloch AB, Cauthen GM, Onorato IM, et al. Nationwide survey of drug-resistant tuberculosis in the United States. JAMA 1994;271:665–671.

47. Driver CR, Valway SE, Morgan WM, et al. Transmission of *Mycobacterium tuberculosis* associated with air travel. JAMA 1994;272:1031–1035.

48. Kenyon TA, Valway SE, Ihle WW, et al. Transmission of multidrug-resistant *Mycobacterium tuberculosis* during a long airplane flight. N Engl J Med 1996;334:933–938.

49. Moore M, Valway SE, Ihle W, Onorato IM. A train passenger wth plumonary tuberculosis: evidence of limited transmission during travel. Clin Infect Dis 1999;28:52–56.

50. Witt MD. Trains, travel, and the tubercle. Clin Infect Dis 1999;28:57–58.

51. Bellin E. Failure of tuberculosis control. A prescription for change [editorial]. JAMA 1994;271:708–709.

52. Farizo KM, Strebel PM, Chen RT, et al. Fatal respiratory disease due to *Corynebacterium diphtheriae*: case report and review of guidelines for management, investigation and control. Clin Infect Dis 1993;16:59–68.

53. Plan of action for the prevention and control of diphtheria in the European Region (1994–1995). WHO Document ICP/EPI 038, Copenhagen, 1994.

54. Amler RW, Bloch AB, Orenstern WA, et al. Imported measles in the United States. JAMA 1982;248:2129–2133.

55. Cairns L, Blythe D, Kao A, et al. Outbreak of coccidioidomycosis in Washington state residents returning from Mexico. Clin Infect Dis 2000;30:61–64.

Chapter 24

SEXUALLY TRANSMITTED INFECTIONS

PER-ANDERS MÅRDH AND SUBHASH K. HIRA

INTRODUCTION AND OVERVIEW

Sexually transmitted infections (STIs) are a major public health problem. An estimated 200 million people contract an STI annually. Approximately 80% of these cases occur in developing countries. Medical professionals agree that traveling provides individuals with a greater opportunity to acquire an STI. The common view that STIs occurs mainly in sailors, soldiers, and prostitutes (so-called "core transmitters") has been proven wrong. In studies with diagnostic testing for all known STI agents in a general population and with a complete patient history taken, one-third of the subjects have had an STI or are currently a carrier of an STI agent, including bacteria, fungi, parasites, and viruses (Table 24–1).[1]

During travel, an STI can be acquired from contact with fellow travelers of the same group or other travelers who may be encountered. Often, tourists from another country may be the source of infection for local inhabitants as well as visitors.[2] Sex-for-pay is another route of acquiring an STI. Prostitutes may be citizens of the country that the traveler is visiting. However, migratory (mobile, international) prostitution has become an increasing phenomenon in many parts of the world.[3,4] Sexual services by such prostitutes are offered to tourists in recreational resorts and hotels.[5,6] Thus, a complex pattern exists for transmission of STIs to and among travelers.

IMPORTED CASE?

Some STIs are easily recognized as imported diseases, as occurrence is rare in the patient's country of residence. For example, chancroid, donovanosis, and, to a certain extent, HIV-2 infections are diseases of mainly tropic and subtropic origin. In contrast, some STIs, such as genital ulcers, present a similar epidemiologic situation in tropic areas as well as arctic regions.

Due to the long incubation period of many STIs (Table 24–2), an infection that presents clinically during a trip abroad or after the traveler has returned home may very well have been originally acquired at home, perhaps long before the traveler left. In the case of an STI with a short incubation period (e.g. gonorrhea), the infection may have been acquired immediately after returning home. When seeking medical treatment, a sexually active individual may be uncertain of when the infection was acquired and mistakenly believe that the infection was acquired during the trip.

FACTORS INFLUENCING THE SPREAD OF STIs BETWEEN DIFFERENT AREAS

In order to understand in detail the impact of traveling on the epidemiology of STIs, a large number of factors have to be analyzed (see Table 24–1). Obviously, the number of travelers moving from one spot to another and the epidemiologic situation on these locations are of importance, but also the number of infected travelers and the percentage of the latter who are contagious when arriving. The possible mixing pattern between travelers and locals and the sexual risk behavior of the latter has an impact on the spread of an infection once transferred to a new location. Sexual preference and mode of sexual performances by infected travelers, as highlighted by HIV infected, influence the transfer rate of STI agents. Even the number of sexual encounters during a short period of time can influence the transfer rate, as exemplified by gonorrhea. The immune status of the locals — induced either by natural infections or by vaccination, that is, against hepatitis B — and the use of various types of contraceptives can all influence the transfer rate of sexually transmitted agents. The access to health care units and their quality, as well as the availability of antibiotic drugs and suppressive antiviral therapy, are other factors that can have such an influence. Finally, the economy of locals who have acquired an STI from a traveler can also influence dissemination of such infections in the local population. That is, their economy may determine whether they will be able to seek health care or to pay for etiologic tests and curative drugs.

MICROBIAL MARKERS OF "IMPORTED STRAINS"

Few markers exist on sexually transmitted agents that may disclose their geographic origin, at least when dealing with markers that are easily detectable and that can be widely tested on a routine basis. Existing markers that are tested for are often of limited value (e.g., antibiotic susceptibility pattern and penicillinase-production in *Neisseria gonorrhoeae* [PPNG strains]).[7] However, determination of nucleic acid sequences in certain microbes have proved useful in epidemiologic investigations of international "routes" for transmission of STIs; for example, HIV-1 subtype C, which is dominant in Central Africa, is now widespread in India. HIV also may rapidly change its genetic identity.

In some countries, the majority of isolated PPNG strains of *N. gonorrhoeae* have traditionally been acquired

Table 24–1.   FACTORS THAT MIGHT INFLUENCE THE GEOGRAPHIC EPIDEMIOLOGY OF SEXUALLY TRANSMITTED INFECTIONS TRANSFERRED BY TRAVELERS

Number of infected persons traveling to and returning from a given destination per unit of time

Number of persons contagious when arriving

STI epidemiology at destination

Number of sexual contacts by traveler at destination (and when arriving home) and number of those partners being contagious

Sexual risk taking of consorts at destinations

Gender of traveler and of the new sexual contacts

Character of sexual performance(s) at contacts

Prostitution at destination and health promotion programs of prostitutes in the area

Private economy of travelers and locals, e.g., influencing health-seeking behavior, contraceptive use, etc.

Quality of local health care, e.g., knowledge among health providers, access to etiologic test services and to curative drugs

Immune status of locals, including vaccination programs (e.g., to hepatitis B) in locals

Access to contraceptives over the counter and traditions of prescribing contraceptives

Legal regulations of STIs and partner notification activities

Screening programs of STIs in population at destination

---

during trips abroad, mainly by contacts with prostitutes. For example, such strains are acquired by Europeans in Southeast Asia, Africa, and South America and spread domestically in Europe by travelers returning home. A similar situation is seen in American males traveling to the Caribbean and South America. The mean age of the infected males is usually higher than that of domestic cases of gonorrhea. One explanation is that older males usually have the economic resources required for travel to more remote areas. PPNG strains isolated from women in these men's home countries are often recovered from contacts with older male travelers. The age of these women is usually lower than that of their male consort.

SEX TOURISM VERSUS SEXUAL CONTACTS DURING TRAVEL

Often the focus on sexual activities by travelers has been on sex tourism, that is, tourists who make their trip with the intention to visit an area where sex is for sale.[2,3,8,9] Sex tourism has traditionally been concentrated in certain defined places. Sex tourists may acquire STIs that are exclusively seen in travelers who have also visited "local" prostitutes in remote areas. Most developing countries have a high rate of genital ulcer disease (GUD). For example, Mumbai (formerly known as Bombay) has reported GUD among 66% of STI clinic attendees. By comparison, GUD was reported in 40% of STI patients in Lusaka,

Zambia. In some countries, a high prevalence of hepatitis B[10] and C are found in such patients. Therefore, it is helpful to know the pattern of STIs existing at common tourist destinations.

The pedophilic sex tourist has attracted much attention during recent years as several organizations are trying to stop this form of child abuse, which is seen in the Far East, South America, and the Indian subcontinent. Some countries (e.g., Sweden) have laws that allow local prosecution of pedophiles to be based on foreign police reports documenting the purchase of sex from children in the foreign country.

TOURISTHOOD

The vast majority of STIs in travelers are seen in the "average" tourist, not the sex tourist. STIs are acquired during regular vacations, where "sun, sand, and sex" is a more or less expected ingredient for some of the regular holiday travelers. Increased risk taking in a foreign country is a part of the phenomenon of "touristhood."[11] The normal limits or restrictions on behavior are more likely to be ignored by the traveler at a foreign milieu. That is, the individual tends to be less inhibited abroad and might become engaged in, for example, sexual encounters that would be considered unacceptable at home by the individual or by society. This is just one reason why pre-travel STI counseling (see below) is especially important. It is notable that women often persist in their sexual risk-taking pattern, if any, from home when they travel abroad.[12]

SEXUAL CONTACTS ABROAD

Up to one-quarter of female charter tourists and inter-rail travelers from northern Europe have experienced one casual sexual contact abroad with a previously unknown partner.[2,12–19] This was a one-time experience, apart from in 2.1% of this one-quarter of the travelers who had more than one such sexual experience. In a group of young men from the same region, the same extent of sexual contacts abroad with female partners was observed. Various studies have shown that 5% of European travelers visiting developing countries have had casual sexual contacts abroad. In the mid-1980s, half of these contacts were unprotected intercourse; however, condom use appears to be increasing. Young male sex tourists are more likely to use condoms than men aged over 40 years. Likewise, unprotected sex is more common in younger than in older females.

For certain groups of female travelers, local males in the destination country are an important source for STIs. During the tourist season, some of these males seduce female tourists even on a more or less regular basis. As one group of tourists departs, the local males who prey on female tourists are waiting for new arrivals. During the off-season, when there are no tourists, sexual encounters are established by these men with local or migratory prostitutes. As a result, a link between nonpaying sexual contacts from female tourists and prostitutes exists in these areas. Male tourists, coming from high-income countries

Table 24–2.   STI AGENTS, INCUBATION PERIODS, MANIFESTATIONS

ORGANISM	INCUBATION PERIOD	CONDITION/DISEASE
Chlamydia trachomatis Serotypes D-K	5–21 d	Genital chlamydia infection: urethritis/cervicitis, endometritis, salpingitis, periappendicitis, perihepatitis, conjunctivitis, epididymitis, Reiter's syndrome, and neonatal pneumonia
Serotypes Ll-L3	0.5–4 wk	Lymphogranuloma venereum: bubo, fistula, lymphedema
Neisseria gonorrhoeae	3–10–(20) d	Gonorrhea: urethritis/cervicitis, endometritis, salpingitis, epididymitis, perihepatitis, septicemia, arthritis, pustules, conjunctivitis
Haemophilus ducreyi	4–14 d	Chancroid (ulcus molle): genital ulcer, inguinal lymphnodes (buboes), fistulas (seen in 50% of cases)
Calymmatobacterium inguinale	6 wk–1 yr	Donovanosis: subcutaneous nodules followed by granulating ulcer. Extragenital spread may occur.
Treponema pallidum	1.5–10 wk	Syphilis: painless genital ulcer (primary stage), rash (2nd stage); late in the course (3rd stage) a large variety of symptoms and signs from most organs may occur

Human papillomavirus (HPV),
  e.g., types 6, 11
  e.g., types 16, 18,
  and some types in the
  30-, 40-, and 50-ties series
	1 mo–1.5 yr	Genital warts (condyloma acuminata)
		Papillomatosis or flat condylomas (seen only by coloposcopy): ulcer, pain (strong statistical correlation to cervical cancer, particularly for types 16/18)

Herpes simplex virus, types 2 and 1	4–10 d	Painful ulcer, keratitis, encephalitis
Hepatitis B	(2)–3–6 mo	Acute hepatitis: jaundice, itching, tiredness
Hepatitis C	2 wk–2 mo	Acute hepatitis: jaundice, itching, tiredness Chronic hepatitis: associated with cancer of the liver
Hepatitis D	0.5–2.5 mo (unknown, but estimated to)	Acute hepatitis: jaundice, itching, tiredness
HIV 1	2 wk–10 yr	AIDS and its prestages
HIV 2	2 wk–10 yr	AIDS and its prestages
Trichomonas vaginalis	0.5–3 wk	Trichomoniasis: vaginal and urethral discharge, acute pain, irritation
Shigella, Salmonella, Entamoeba histolytica, Giardia lamblia	Different incubation times (days to weeks)	Gastroenteritis: diarrhea, septicemia, abscess formation, melena, weight loss
Sarcoptes scabiei	2–7 wk	Scabies: itching, excoriations
Phthirus pubis	1–2 wk	Pubic lice, "Papillon d'amour": itching

and areas where prostitution is not openly permitted, may for the first time meet young, attractive prostitutes offering sex for money. For male tourists, such migratory prostitutes may represent a novel temptation in their life.

THE PREVALENCE OF STIs IN MOST COUNTRIES IS GENERALLY POORLY DEFINED

Reliable figures for the prevalence of STIs are lacking for the majority of countries. Where such figures are available, they usually only exist for certain groups and almost never for all STI agents.

When data exist, they are usually only available for *N. gonorrhoeae* (gonorrhea), *Treponema pallidum* (syphilis), *Haemophilus dycreyi* (chancroid), *Chlamydia trachomatis,* serotypes L1-L3 (lymphogranuloma venereum), granuloma inquinale[20–22] and HIV (including AIDS). Data are, however, generally lacking for infections by *C. trachomatis,* serotypes D-K (representing the

vast majority of genital chlamydia infections), *Trichomonas vaginalis* (trichomoniasis), HPV (flat condylomas and genital warts caused by human papillomavirus), HSV (herpes), and hepatitis B, C, and D. Many of the latter diseases are more common than some of the ones that are tracked by health authorities.

In nearly all countries, STI prevalences are estimates based on data collected on selected groups, usually STI clinic patients. More rarely, such data come from sentinenel data. This latter type of data are generally more valuable for estimates of the prevalence of STIs on a national level than unreliable data submitted by various "nonspecified" clinics.

Prevalence figures for a given STI agent differ very much with age. The average sexual debut age is one of the most important nominators for the age-distribution pattern of STIs. The peak prevalence for most STIs in Western societies is seen in older teenagers and young adults, whereas in other areas for the same agent, prevalence may peak in early middle age. The prevalence of an STI within a given country may also differ greatly between ethnic groups and between rural and urban areas. As a result, the number of STI infections per 100,000 inhabitants in a country may have a restricted value when used for travel medicine counseling. However, travelers should still be made aware that STI rates are high. For example, STIs per 1,000 adults are 32 for Zambia and 60 for Papua New Guinea.

CHANGE IN SYPHILIS EPIDEMIOLOGY IN EAST EUROPE

Since the mid-1990s, there has been a remarkable increase in the number of reported cases of syphilis in East Europe (e.g., in Russia, in the three Baltic states, and in the Ukraine, Belrus, Moldavia, Kyrgystan, and Kazakktan).[22] In some of these countries, the increase in the prevalence has been as striking as 50- to 60-fold, that is, of only diagnosed and monitored cases. There may be some over-diagnosis due to unspecific test methods and difficulties in differentiating current active syphilis cases from healed infections. However, the dark number of nonlaboratory-confirmed syphilis cases and/or never reported cases is likely to outnumber the former cases several-fold. The increase in congenital syphilis cases in this region indicates, however, that the syphilis epidemic situation is real and is shown to embrace all socioeconomic classes. The increased reported prevalence has been blamed on promiscuity and flourishing prostitution (see also below), but also cease of sanctions again affected, for example, by obligatory long-term hospitalization and obligatory treatment in hospitals as well as monetary requests to the diseased by health providers in order not to report cases they have diagnosed. Also, recommendations allowing anonymous testing may have contributed.

Studies of the background and the education level of the mothers of the infants with congenital syphilis in Latvia showed that luetic infections have disseminated to all socioeconomic strata of the population.

As many of the East European sex workers will become mobile or so-called international prostitutes,[3] the epidemiology of syphilis in their home countries (like the high prevalence of other infections spread by sexual contacts in these women) is of concern also for other countries. With its currently open borders, this European region has become a frequent goal for both business and leisure trips, including that of sex tourists.

One encouraging tendency in the epidemiology of STIs in East Europe is the decrease in the prevalence of gonorrhea in non-hard-core groups, which still is a problem in hard-core groups (e.g., in prostitutes), as well as the levelling off of the increase in new syphilis cases.

CONTACT WITH PROSTITUTES INVOLVES A HIGH RISK

Syphilis was, for example, found in approximately 7% of Romanian migratory prostitutes working in Istanbul[23] and in 8.7% in a series of consecutively investigated commercial sex workers in the capital of Latvia,[24] who had all attended for a health check-up. Many of the prostitutes

may still have been within the incubation period of this disease. In Southwest Asia and in Africa, the percentage of prostitutes with active syphilis is also high. Twenty percent of prostitutes in Nepal and several cities in India have positive serologic tests for syphilis. Syphilis is also increasing in many industrialized countries. One reason may be increased drug use; for example, in the United States, young people using crack and offering sex-for-money to fund their drug habit were a common source of syphilis.

In the Scandinavian countries, up to 50% to 75% of all diagnosed syphilis cases have in recent years been contracted by males traveling abroad where they had used prostitutes or had homosexual contacts with non-prostitutes.

Prostitutes play an important role in the spread of chancroid in areas where this infection also occurs in the local population, including eastern and southern Africa, Southeast Asia, and some Pacific islands. The genital lesions in chancroid are highly infectious. The infection is, however, comparatively rare in tourists, and, when seen, it is usually found in travelers who have had sex with prostitutes.

The majority of adult males in Northwest Europe who develop hepatitis B and have returned home from abroad usually have had a sexual contact during their trip.

Lymphogranuloma venereum (LGV), another cause of genital ulcer, has been endemic in East and West Africa. At the present time, however, prevalence appears to be declining. LGV also occurs in India, the Far East, the Caribbean, and South America. LGV should be considered in the differential diagnosis of presumed syphilis and chancroid, as well as in other cases with GUD. The disease may be acquired by travelers who have had sexual contacts with individuals of the local populations in these areas, including prostitutes. Normally, however, LGV is rare in tourists.

A rapid increase in the prevalence of HIV has been seen among prostitutes in Southeast Asian brothels, especially in Thailand, where it increased from a low percentage to a situation where now more than half of the "sex workers" are infected with HIV. After seroconversion, young girls may be sent home to their villages, often in North Thailand, by the brothel owners. Also in East Europe, there has been a rapid increase in HIV-infected prostitutes. In a study in Kaleningrad, as many as 80% were found to be HIV positive.

Prevalence figures for certain STI agents and groups of individuals affected in certain areas change rapidly. The great mobility of groups of persons involved in spreading STIs further limits the usefulness of any existing prevalence data. The best data are frequently updated and the study population clearly defined.

MIGRATORY PROSTITUTION

In many countries, migratory prostitutes offer their services to travelers.[2,3] This is a business that, by its nature, is difficult for authorities to control. Cooperation on the part of different regional authorities may be nonexistent or weak and, as a result, totally ineffective against migratory prostitution. In Eastern Europe, a legal vacuum was created after the collapse of the communist leadership. Prior to the fall of communism, prostitution was a phenomenon that was not officially allowed to exist; therefore, laws were never enacted to control prostitution. However, prostitution did exist during the communist period, and women who worked as prostitutes had official permission to work in hotels reserved for foreign tourists. Now prostitutes in Eastern Europe offer their services at all types of facilities, including bars, cars, streets, parks, and illegal brothels.

One type of migratory prostitution that is growing and increasingly offered to travelers occurs along highways. Prostitutes either work in cars belonging to the customer or in vehicles provided by the prostitution ring. Services can be offered in caravans parked alongside the roads or in local establishments like motels. This type of prostitution has meant a rapid spread of HIV and other STI agents by travelers both inter- and intracontinentally (i.e., between countries and even between continents). At particular risk are truck drivers. In Africa, they have contributed to the rapid intracontinental spread of beta-lactamase-producing gonococci and of HIV. Major routes of diseases include travel from the Near East to Europe, from Western to Eastern Europe, within the Mediterranean basin, and among the Caribbean islands, and from there to North America and through the United States.

HIV TRANSMISSION PATTERNS IN DIFFERENT PARTS OF THE WORLD

Transmission of HIV has different predominating patterns, depending on the particular region of the world. In North America and Europe, the AIDS epidemic was initially dominated by homosexual men and persons who had received infected blood products, usually male hemophiliacs. Also affected were drug addicts and, in the case of addicted females who resorted to prostitution to pay for their drugs, their male clients. The present trend in some of these areas has been an increase in the percentage of heterosexual persons infected by HIV and a leveling off or a decrease in newly detected cases of HIV-positive homosexual men, as well as in the number of such men still living. That is, there have been less men entering the pool of known HIV-infected male homosexuals than those dying. In these societies, a smaller proportion of the HIV-infected persons have been females, some of whom have been female travelers to developing areas: European women going to West Africa have paid, either with cash or gifts, for sex with males of the local population.

Another pattern for spread of HIV has been seen in sub-Saharan Africa, Latin America, and in the Caribbean where the transmission has mainly been through heterosexual contacts. HIV infections may still, but less commonly, be transmitted by transfusion with nontested blood. As a consequence of the high prevalence of HIV infections in young women in these areas, perinatal infections with the HIV virus are also common.

In Southeast Asia and in some Moslem countries, prostitution has played a relatively more important role for the spread of HIV than in many non-Moslem countries. In the former countries, male customers may spread the infection to their families. The spread of the HIV infection has been very rapid during recent years in Southeast Africa. Now India has followed the pattern prevailing in sub-Saharan Africa with a predominance of heterosexual spread of HIV (i.e., a spread not dependent on prostitution). The possible influence of GUD and male circumcision on the transfer rate of HIV has been considered.[25–40]

AIDS may serve as an example of the importance of traveling for the spread of many STIs. The HIV epidemic has become pandemic as a consequence of migration, tourism, traveling for getting work (guest workers), and for educational purposes, and through persons having "mobility" as a profession (truck drivers, air company personnel, seamen, tourist industry field workers, as well as mobile, international prostitutes).

Although the origin of AIDS is a matter of dispute, some routes of importance for the initial intercontinental spread of the disease have been recognized. Major routes of the HIV virus have been by travelers for spread from Africa to Haiti, by homosexual male tourists from the United States to Haiti and by those traveling from the United States to Europe, and by European men returning home. Africans migrating as students, guest workers, or prostitutes have carried the HIV-1 and HIV-2 viruses to Europe. Heterosexual and homosexual "sex tourists" and business people have allowed HIV to "travel" to Asia from the United States, Europe, and Africa. HIV-2, which may be less pathogenic than HIV-1, is not as widespread as HIV-1. It occurs mostly in West Africa. HIV-2 has spread from there by mobile prostitutes and by their clients who have visited this region and have returned to Europe and other places.

STI VIRUS INFECTIONS OTHER THAN HIV

The role of inter- and intracontinental traveling or migration in the spread of viruses causing genital lesions, like herpes simplex (HSV) and human papillomaviruses (HPV), has been poorly studied. However, there are reasons to believe that migration has facilitated the global spread of these infectious agents.

ACQUISITION OF STIs BY NONSEXUAL CONTACTS DURING TRAVEL

The acquisition of STIs during travel may occur by routes that are rare or uncommon in the traveler's home country. For example, blood-borne infections, such as hepatitis B and HIV, can be transmitted by intravenous needle sticks for diagnostic and therapeutic reasons, when nondisposable needles are reused. There may be an increased risk for blood-borne STIs in travelers in need of regular injections of medical drugs if the travelers did not bring their own supply of sterile needles or if their supply runs out (thereby being forced to rely on local health care suppliers). Also, infected lancets (for fingertip sticks) used for diagnosing malaria may be one mode of transmission of such STIs, apart from the well-known mode of transmission of nontested blood. Surgery, as well as minor surgery like dental visits, can also result in transmission if nonsterile instruments are used.

It should also be remembered that some STI agents may be transmitted vertically in some populations and thus exclusively acquired by sexual transmission. For example, this is the case with the hepatitis B virus in some developing countries, including Eastern Europe and the Middle East, where the infection is endemic.

At risk for acquiring blood-borne viral infections (hepatitis B and C virus, HIV-1, and HIV-2) are injured travelers who require blood transfusions. This may also be true, even if blood is not given, when nonsterile operating instruments are used. Also, travelers in this category from whom blood is collected for diagnostic or therapeutic purposes, using nondisposable needles, are at risk (see also under HIV/AIDS).

CANDIDIASIS—INCREASED PREVALENCE IN TRAVELERS TO THE TROPICS

Candidiasis is a problem not only for immunocompromised persons but also for females prone to develop recurrent vaginitis by *Candida albicans*. When they travel to warm, humid (tropic and subtropic) areas, many of them experience increased problems. Women prone to candida vaginitis should carry therapeutic drugs that may be used in case infection develops. Tablets (e.g., Diflucan®) are usually preferable to vaginal applications, which may melt in a warm climate, creating problems of a cosmetic character. Although *C. albicans* is not regarded as an STI agent in its proper sense, balanitis may occur in partners of female travelers with genital candidiasis. Thus, *C. albicans* can be transmitted by sexual intercourse, with a higher frequency of infections being seen in couples traveling to warm and humid areas.

WHERE DO TRAVELERS WITH AN STI SEEK CARE?

Persons who have acquired an STI during travel may seek treatment at a variety of clinics according to the symptoms they may have developed (for example, at an ophthalmologic clinic with conjunctivitis or uveitis; at a surgical clinic with proctitis, periappendicitis, peritonitis, or perihepatitis; at a gynecologic department with genital discharge or symptoms of pelvic inflammatory disease [PID]; at an infectious disease unit with hepatitis; at a dermatologic clinic with skin manifestations; at a rheumatologic clinic with signs of arthritis; and at an STI venereal disease clinic or in a primary health care unit with urethritis symptoms or GUD). The symptoms and signs can easily be misunderstood as being related to a large number of non-STI conditions, particularly when the STI has caused extragenital manifestations. In patients returning home with gastrointestinal infections such as shigellosis, salmonellosis, amebiasis, and some other intestinal parasitic infections including giardiasis, the possibility of sexual transmission should be considered, particularly in homosexual men ("gay bowel syndrome"). In travel clinic practice, it should also be remembered that chronic inflammatory bowel disease may flare up and progress during or just after returning home from a journey abroad, particularly from developing areas.

HIV infections may first be detected when a person develops a sore throat (which turns out to be thrush), or with long-standing diarrhea caused by cyclospora or with respiratory symptoms due to an infection by *Pneumocystis carinii* or other mycobacterial species.

The risk of acquiring HIV is likely to be higher in travelers who already have an STI, which often results in an increased number of CD4+ lymphocytes and other cells with HIV receptors transudated into their genital secretion. Treatment of STIs before traveling may therefore, at least marginally, decrease the risk of getting infected by HIV when having coitus with an HIV carrier who is in an infectious stage (which can be right after having been infected and later in the prestages of AIDS).

COUNSELING TRAVELERS IN STI-RELATED MATTERS, INCLUDING CONTRACEPTIVE USE

The knowledge of what constitutes high sexual risk may differ from one country to another. Thus, estimations of the risk of acquiring a given STI based on the epidemic situation in a person's own home country may be misleading when counseling travelers for STI risks and also for estimations of the possibility that a traveler might have contracted an STI during a given trip.

Prophylactic measures for reducing the risk of contracting STIs should be integrated into counseling for travelers and should be routine and as "natural" as vaccinations and information regarding avoidance of, for example, intestinal infections. Advice about bringing condoms (also by females) as a preventive measure for travelers is often forgotten. Counseling before leaving home, perhaps in conjunction with required vaccinations, could involve instructions regarding appropriate use of a condom (which can be highly motivated in non- or infrequent users, remembering that some STIs may run a deadly course). Furthermore, one should inform travelers, both males and females, that in many countries, condoms may not be readily available, or if available, the quality may be poor (Table 24–3). Even if brought from home, condoms may remain forgotten in the hotel room while a sexual contact takes place elsewhere. The proper use of a condom requires "collaboration" between the partners, which may be more difficult in a situation where the partners may not know each other very well or not at all, particularly if there is a language barrier or alcohol intoxication.

Advice to travelers should include a discussion on contraceptives. It should be pointed out that contraceptives may not even be available due to religious and/or political reasons or simply due to poor distribution systems. In contrast to the traveler's domestic situation they may only be available by a prescription that may be difficult to arrange and/or may require a pelvic examination that a woman may not feel comfortable with when performed by an unknown gynecologist while traveling. It may also be mentioned that, like medical drugs, contraceptives should not be stored in checked-in luggage, which may disappear.

Attempts to encourage use of condoms has been a dominating message of many campaigns. Apart from

Table 24–3. FACTORS RELATED TO CONTRACEPTIVES THAT MAY INFLUENCE THE EPIDEMIOLOGY OF SEXUALLY TRANSMITTED INFECTIONS AND THEIR COMPLICATIONS AND SEQUELAE

Available at all in the country or at destination?

Price? Can be afforded and if so by whom in society?

Access over the counter and/or require a prescription?

Type(s) that can be purchased?

Available to tourists without great efforts? Condoms sold at hotels or even offered free in hotel rooms?

Quality of contraceptive, e.g., of condoms? Storage conditions used are okay?

Knowledge of how to best use contraceptives as STI protection?

Barrier contraceptives used by hard-core groups, including prostitutes?

Do prostitutes, by trading for a higher fee from clients, offer unprotected intercourse?

Condoms distributed free of charge to those who cannot afford to buy them, e.g., to teenagers at youth clinics?

Traditions in the society to use different types of contraceptives, e.g., hormonal and barrier contraceptives. Are spermicides and condoms with spermicides used?

spreading the message by mass media, condoms have been given to young backpack travelers of both genders when they purchase inter-rail tickets.[13] "Condomerias" and other activities to promote condom use at Mediterranean seaside resorts among charter tourists have been made, as a part of some Northern European countries' AIDS campaigns. In some, although still few countries, condoms have been made available in hotel receptions and free of charge even in the bathroom of hotel rooms.

The quality of contraceptives bought in certain areas may not be sufficient, like condoms that may easily break after being stored incorrectly, particularly in extreme climates, or that have been sold after the expiry date.

Although massive attempts have been made to increase condom use during casual sex, particularly with a previously unknown partner with whom the traveler established contact during a trip abroad, they have not been very encouraging. This is disappointing, because as many as 85% of a group of women with such an experience did not use a condom during casual sexual contacts abroad.

Barrier contraceptives are, however, believed to play a role in protection against the spread of infections transmitted by sexual contacts. Hormonal contraceptives may also positively influence the course of such infections in the female by hindering the spread of chlamydial infection to the upper genital tract and thereby cause development of pelvic inflammatory disease (PID).[41] The pill may also mask a PID[42,43] by decreasing the inflammatory response. However, hormonal contraceptives decrease the frequency of involuntary childlessness as a sequeale of

tubal adhesions and extrauterine pregnancies (which, untreated, are connected to a high mortality rate) in women infected with chlamydia.

Pill intake in a woman with diarrhea may not protect her from conceiving due to poor uptake of the drug. The rate by which this may occur is, however, poorly defined.

THE HIV-INFECTED OR OTHERWISE IMMUNOCOMPROMISED TRAVELER

The HIV-infected person, like others with immunodeficiency, has an increased risk of acquiring infectious diseases when traveling by being exposed to infectious agents not normally present in their home environment. Traveling may also lead to stress that can increase the risk of illness. HIV-infected persons with a decreasing number of CD4+ and CD8+ lymphocytes are exposed to an increased risk of acquiring infections by, for example, mycobacteria. The risk of meeting people with tuberculosis may be particularly high when traveling to underdeveloped areas. Persons with immunodeficiency, including persons with AIDS or its prestages, may be better off by taking prophylactic therapy like antibiotics for potential respiratory and gastrointestinal infections.[29]

When planning trips for HIV-infected and other immunocompromised individuals, one should remember that certain areas are known for being a source of geophilic fungal agents. Such travel destinations should, if possible, be avoided by this category of travelers.

TREATMENT OF STIs

Standard therapy for STIs is summarized in Table 24–4. In the table, alternative therapies are not listed for all correlations for those allergic or unable to tolerate the standard regimens for other reasons. It should also be noted that double or multiple concomitant STIs are common.[44] Therapy may be unsuccessful if drug selection for returning travelers is based on experience with "domestic" strains, as the antibiotic susceptibility pattern may be quite different in imported and domestic strains.[45,46] Likewise, the susceptibility pattern of infectious agents isolated in travelers seeking treatment abroad may involve the same risk of therapeutic failure if the susceptibility pattern is not known.

Lack of response to antibiotic therapy of some STIs may be due not only to the presence of resistant organisms but also to the fact that bogus or inferior drugs may be sold in some countries, such as drugs wrongly produced or stored under improper conditions. The risk of impaired drug absorption in those travelers with severe diarrhea and gastroenteritis may result in suboptimal antibiotic concentrations. Therapy-resistant cases of syphilis and genital chlamydial infection have been claimed to occur in some Eastern European countries, but never proved to be due to antibiotic-resistant strains (e.g., to penicillin and tetracycline, respectively). The novel possibility of instituting suppressive therapy in HIV-infected persons is discussed below.

Table 24–4.   TREATMENT REGIMENS FOR SOME STIs (IN NONPREGNANT PATIENTS)

Chlamydia trachomatis

Adults

Doxycycline, 100 mg twice daily for (7)–10–14 days, azithromycin 1 g orally as a single dose, or alternative therapy
Erythromycin, 500 mg orally twice daily for (7)–10–14 days or 250 mg 4 times daily or
Tetracycline hydrochloride, 500 mg 4 times daily for (7)–10–14 days

Children

Erythromycin syrup 50 mg/kg/day divided into 2 doses for 10–14 days (in case of pneumonia for 21 days)

Neisseria gonorrhoeae (uncomplicated genital infection)

Cefixime, 400 mg orally in a single dose
Ceftriaxone, 125 mg IM as a single dose
Alternative therapy:
Doxycycline, 200 mg twice daily for 7–(14) days or
Spectinomycin, 2 g IM as a single dose or
Azithromycin, 1 g orally in a single dose
For those allergic to penicillin:
Erythromycin, 500 mg orally 4 times daily for 7 days

Haemophilus ducreyi

Ceftriaxone, 250 mg IM as a single dose
Alternative therapy:
Erythromycin, 500 mg 4 times daily for 7 days or
Ciprofloxin, 200 mg IM as a single dose or
Trimethoprim/sulfamethoxazole (160/800 mg), orally 4 times daily for
7 days (less effective therapy than the other alternatives)

Treponema pallidum

Adults

Benzathine penicillin G, 2.4 million units IM as a single dose (in syphilis cases of less than 1 year of duration)
Benzathine penicillin G, 2.4 million units repeated 3 times 1 week apart (in syphilis cases of more than 1 year of duration)

Children

Aqueous crystalline penicillin G 200,000 units 1 g/day for 10–14 days. Infants are given 100,000–150,000 units (50,000 units
every 8–12 hours)

Trichomonas vaginalis

Metronidazole, 2 g orally as a single dose or
Metronidazole, 200 mg orally 3 times daily for 7–(14) days or
Tinidazole, 2 g orally in a single dose

Candida albicans

Clotrimazole, 1% cream 5 g intravaginally for 7–14 days
Clotrimazole, 100 mg vaginal tablet for 7 days
Tioconazole, 100 mg vaginal tablet daily for 7 days or
Fluconazole, 150 mg orally once daily for 5 days. Start with a 400-mg dose first day.

Flora change as in bacterial vaginosis

Metronidazole, 400 mg orally twice daily for 7 days or
Metronidazole, 2 g orally in a single dose, repeated after 48 hours
Clindamycin, vaginal cream (2%), one application (2 g) each night for 7 days

Herpes virus (in cases with normal immune defense)

Acute

Acyclovir, 200 mg orally 5 times daily for 5–10 days

Severe recurrent episodes

Acyclovir, 400 mg orally 5 times daily for several months

CHECK-UP OF RETURNING TRAVELERS

Post-travel check-up is an important field for travel medicine.[47,48] The varying incubation periods of different STIs require that patient examinations should be conducted several weeks or months after returning home (e.g., for serologic tests for syphilis and HIV infections). Since multiple infections with sexually transmitted agents are common, individuals who develop symptoms and signs of genital infection, such as genital discharge, may consult

and be treated soon after returning home, that is, for an STI with a short incubation period. Unless return visits are scheduled some time later, it may not be possible to establish if the person also had contracted any STIs with a long incubation period. As many STIs are asymptomatic, anyone who suspects that they may have acquired an STI should be encouraged to have a check-up.

The possibility that the HIV-infected may acquire opportunistic infections during travel should be remembered at post-travel check-ups.[49]

ETHICAL AND ECONOMIC PROBLEMS BY THE NOVEL HIV AND HEPATITIS THERAPIES

The novel possibility of prophylactically instituting combination drug therapy to prevent an HIV infection from developing in an exposed traveler has become a potential upcoming ethical and economic problem for the travel medicine physician, society, and the potentially infected. Thus, the possibility of hindering such an infection in persons who consult and claim that they might have acquired the infection, for example, by having had intercourse with high-risk persons, like prostitutes, in an area endemic for HIV, may be one such situation.[50] They may be informed about this possibility and may even require such therapy. If the person will be denied it and later develops AIDS, the health provider may encounter moral and legal dilemmas. Which will be the selection criteria for prescribing such therapy during indicated circumstances? Institution of suppressive therapy in those who have developed HIV/AIDS is already now an ethical problem in economically underprivileged areas, due to the extremely high costs for the therapy, especially as it must be given lifelong.

A situation similar to that discussed above for HIV is upcoming also for hepatitis B and C, where the use of long-term therapy with nucleoside analogues and interferon-alfa, apart from hypergammaglobulin and in case of hepatitis B vaccine, can prevent cirrhosis and thereby likely also liver cancer. The therapy is also very costly, not only for the drugs but also for delivering the drugs, which requires close contact with health care units and patients.

FUTURE CONSIDERATIONS

The spread of STIs by international travelers is likely to remain an important public health problem. The first reason for this is that there are so far no vaccines on the market for STIs (except for hepatitis B). Second, etiologic diagnosis of STIs is not widely made. If available, it is made only for the more common STI agents. Third, screening for STIs is seldom undertaken, in spite of the fact that many STI infections are asymptomatic. Finally, routinely notifying partners is not done or, in the case of travelers, partners may be impossible to identify.

In areas where condoms are not used, where diagnostic tests for STIs are not available, and where therapeutic agents are too expensive for many or even most infected individuals, conditions are created that allow STI epidemics to flourish. At the present time, Eastern Europe may serve as an example. In other geographic areas, public health measures such as screening activities, partner notification, free consultation, free testing, and free treatment, have resulted in a dramatic reduction of the prevalence of some of the treatable STIs (e.g., gonorrhea, genital chlamydial infections, and trichomoniasis). Such a trend has been seen in Scandinavian countries, where the prevalence of the two infections first mentioned in Sweden has dropped from 10% to 20% to a few percentages in patients presenting with signs of urethritis/cervicitis at gynecologic emergency rooms and venereal disease clin-

ics within the last decades. The figures for trichomoniasis in such persons dropped in fact to nearly undetectable levels during the same time.

Preventive health measures for travelers based on epidemiologic data should be evidence based.[51,52] To establish preventive programs for STIs,[53] including screening activities (particularly as the majority of such infections are asymptomatic), is essential, as it might decrease the transfer rate of HIV in STI agent carriers.[54] Health care of commercial sex workers constitutes a core group in STI health prevention.[55]

REFERENCES

1. Holmes KK, Mårdh P-A, Sparling F, et al., eds. Sexual transmitted diseases. New York: McGraw-Hill, 1990.
2. Hellberg D, Mårdh P-A. Casual travel sex, sex tourism and international prostitution. J Travel Med 1997;15:142–149.
3. Mårdh P-A, Gene M. Migratory prostitution with emphasis on Europe. J Travel Med 1995;2:28–32.
4. Tchudiomirova K, Domeika M, Mårdh P-A. Demographic data on prostitiutes from Bulgaria—an important recruitment area for national (migratory) prostitutes. Int J STD AIDS 1997;8:187–191.
5. Ford N, Inman M. Safer sex in tourist resorts. World Health Forum 1992;13:77–80.
6. Ford K, Nyoman Wirawan D, Fajans P, et al. AIDS knowledge, risk behavior, and factors related to condom use among commercial sex workers and male tourist clients in Bali, Indonesia. AIDS 1995;9:751–759.
7. Laar van de MJW, Dujnhoven YTHP van, Dessens M, et al. Surveillance of antibiotic resistence in *Neisseria gonorrhoeae* in the Netherlands 1977–95. Genitourin Med 1997;73:510–507.
8. Kleiber D, Wilke M. AIDS, Sex and Tourismus. Ergebnis einer Befragung deutscher Urlauber und Sextouristen. Schriftenreihe des Bundesministeriums für Gesundheit 33. Baden-Baden: Nomos Verlag, 1995.
9. Mulhall BP, Hu M, Thompson M, et al. Planned sexual behaviour of young Australian visitors to Thailand. Med J Aust 1993;158:530–535.
10. Kura M, Hira SK, Kohl MA, et al. High occurrence of HBV among STD clinic attenders in Mumbai, India. Int J STD AIDS 1998;9:101–103.
11. Hanefors M. "Touristhood" in the periphery of culture. In: Mårdh P-A, ed. Travel medicine. Uppsala: Scandinavian Association for Travel and Health, 1994:57–60.
12. Arvidson M, Hellberg D, Mårdh P-A. Sexually transmitted diseases in Swedish women with experience of casual sex with men of foreign nationalities within Sweden. Acta Obstet Gynecol Scand 1995;74:794–798.
13. Worm A-M, Lillelund H. Condoms and sexual behaviour of young tourists in Copenhagen. Aid Care 1989;1:3–6.
14. Daniels G, Kell P, Nelson, et al. Sexual behaviour amongst travellers: a study of genitourinary medicine clinic attenders. Int J STD AIDS 1992;3:437–438.
15. Tveit K-S, Nilsen A, Nyfors A. Causal sexual experience abroad in patients attending an STD clinic and at high risk for HIV infection. Genitourin Med 1994;70:12–14.
16. Stricker M, Steffen R, Hornung R, et al. Flüchtige sexuelle Kontakte von Schweizer Touristen in den Tropen. MMWR Morb Mortal Wkly Rep 1990;132:175–177.
17. Arvidson M, Hellberg D, Mårdh P-A. Sexual risk behaviour and history of sexually transmitted diseases during different

types of journeys. Acta Gynecol Obstet Scand 1996;75: 490–494.

18. DeSchryver A, Meheus A. International travel and sexually transmitted diseases. World Health Stat Q 1989;42:90–99.

19. Mulhall BP. Sexually transmitted diseases and travel. BMJ 1993;49:394–411.

20. World Health Organization. An overview of selected curable sexually transmitted diseases. WHO/GPA/STD 95.1 Geneva: WHO, 1995.

21. Jamkhedkar P, Hira SK, Shroff HJ, Langewar D. Clinicoepidemiologic features of granuloma inguinale in the era of AIDS. Sex Transm Dis 1998;25:196–200.

22. World Health Organization. Statistics on sexually transmitted diseases in the former Soviet Union. Copenhagen: WHO Europe, 1996.

23. Gene M, Agacfidan A, Gerikalmaz Ö, et al. A descriptive study on Rumanian women prostituting in Istanbul. Medical Dergi 1995;104:45–48.

24. Kurova T, Shoubnikova M, Makceva A, et al. Prostitution in Riga, Latvia—a socio-medical matter of concern. Acta Obstet Gynecol Scand 1998;77:83–86.

25. Pais P. HIV and India: looking into the abyss. Trop Med Int Health 1996;1:295–304.

26. Hira SK, Kamanga J, Macuacua R, et al. Genital ulcers and male circumcision as risk factors for acquiring HIV-1 in Zambia. J Infect Dis 1990;161:584–585.

27. Feachem RG, Phillips-Howard PA. Risk to UK heterosexuals of contracting AIDS abroad. Lancet 1988;2:394–395.

28. Behrens RH, Porter JDH. HIV infection and travel. BMJ 1990;301:1217.

29. Ellis CJ. HIV infection and travel. BMJ 1990;301:984–985.

30. Mitchell S, Band B, Bradbeer C, Barlow D. Imported heterosexual HIV infection in London. Lancet 1991;2:1614–1615.

31. Noone A, Gill ON, Clarke SE, et al. Travel, heterosexual intercourse and HIV-1 infection. Commun Dis Rep CDR Rev 1991; 1:39–43.

32. Wilson ME, Fordham von Rey, Fineberg HV. Infections in HIV-infected travelers: risk prevention. Ann Intern Med 1991; 114:582–592.

33. Allard R, Lambert G. Knowledge and belief of international traveller about the transmission and prevention of HIV infection. Can Med Assoc J 1992;146:353–359.

34. Gillies P, Slack R, Stoddart N, et al. HIV-related risk behaviour in UK holidaymakers. AIDS 1992;6:339–340.

35. Hake S, Malin A, Araru T, et al. HIV infection among heterosexual travellers attending the Hospital for Tropical Diseases, London. Genitourin Med 1992;68:309–311.

36. Hawkes S, Hart GJ, Johnson AM, et al. Risk behaviour and HIV prevalence in international travellers. AIDS 1994;8: 247–252.

37. Eng TR, O'Brien TR, Bernard KW, et al. HIV-1 and HIV-2 infections among U.S. Peace Corps volunteers returning from West Africa. J Travel Med 1995;2:174–177.

38. Ligthelm RJ, Bauer AGC, Wismans PJ. Case studies of acute HIV-1 infections acquired while visiting subsaharan Africa. J Travel Med 1995;2:196–198.

39. Hira SK, Dore GJ, Sirisanthana T. Clinical spectrum of HIV/AIDS in the Asia-Pacific region. AIDS 1998;12S:S145–S154.

40. Mastro TD, Satten GA, Nopkesorn T, et al. Probability of female-to-male transmission of HIV-1 in Thailand. Lancet 1994;343:204–207.

41. Wölner-Hansen P. Oral contraceptive use modifies the manifestations of pelvic inflammatory disease. Br J Obstet Gynecol 1986;93:619–624.

42. Wölner-Hansen P, Svenson L, Mårdh P-A. Laparoscopic findings and contraceptives use in women with signs and symptoms suggestive of acute salpingitis. Obstet Gynecol 1989;66: 233–238.

43. Mårdh P-A, Hogg B. Are oral contraceptives masking symptom of chlamydia cervicitis and pelvic inflammatory disease? Eur J Contracept Reprod Health Care 1998;3:41–43.

44. Mårdh P-A, Tchudimirova M, Elshibly S, et al. Symptoms and signs in single and mixed genital infections in attendees of family planning clinics and youth clinics. Int J Obstet Gynaecol 1998;63:145–152.

45. Bryan J, Hira SK, Brady W, et al. Oral ciprofloxacin versus ceftriaxone for the treatment of urethritis from resistant *Neisseria gonorrhoeae* in Zambia. Antimicrob Agents Chemother 1990;34:819–822.

46. Hira SK, Attili VR, Kamanga J, et al. Efficacy of gentamicin and kanamycin in the treatment of uncomplicated gonococcal urethritis in Zambia. Sex Transm Dis 1985;12:52–54.

47. Yung AP, Tilman AR. Travel medicine. 2. Upon return. Med J Aust 1994;160:206–212.

48. Churchill DR, Chiodini PL, McAdam KPWJ. Screening the returned traveller. BMJ 1993;49:465–474.

49. Lanjewar DN, Rodriques C, Saple DG, et al. Cryptosporidium, isospora, and strongyloides with AIDS. Nat Med J India 1996; 9:17–19.

50. Mårdh P-A. Travelling abroad—its impact on women's health, including that of prostitutes. Sex tourism, migratory prostitution and travel sex. In: Hawkins DF, Stray-Pederseon B, eds. Infections in obstetrics and gynaecology. J Obstet Gynecol 1994;14:76–77.

51. Steffens R. Travel medicine—prevention based on epidemiological data. Trans R Soc Trop Med 1991;85:156–162.

52. HIV. In: Loesch R, ed. Schützimpfungen und Reisemedicin. Balingen: Spitta Verlag 1998; Section 5, Chapter 4:1–27.

53. Hotz J, Lösch R, Demling L. Infektionen bei Fernreise. Prophylaxe und Therapie. Heidelberg, Leipzig: Johann Ambrosius Barth Verlag, 1995.

54. Mårdh P-A, Creatsas G, Guachino S. Wishful thinking on how to promote women's gynecological and reproductive health? Eur J Contracept Reprod Health Care 1998;3:1–6.

55. Mårdh PA, Shoubmikova M, Fenc M, et al. Health care of female commercial sex workers. Eur J Contracept Reprod Health Care 1999;4:165–180.

Chapter 25

VIRAL TROPICAL INFECTIONS

25.1 ARBOVIRUSES AND ZOONOTIC VIRUSES

THEODORE F. TSAI AND BO NIKLASSON

More than 150 arthropod-borne viruses (arboviruses) or zoonotic viruses, spread from animals without the agency of an arthropod vector, are known to cause human disease.[1-5] Although the majority of these infections are self-limited febrile illnesses whose principal consequence may be to inconvenience a journey, others result in potentially life-threatening neurologic or systemic illnesses or cause syndromes with subacute or chronic sequelae. In all instances, the epidemiologic context of travel and exposures is critical in both pretravel preparation and in post-travel counseling. In diagnosing and treating ill returned travelers, physicians should consider the geographic distribution, modes of transmission, and incubation period of infections with respect to the patients' itinerary, as well as their clinical manifestations. Practitioners should take special note of clinical manifestations that may have a delayed onset or subacute or chronic course. The most important of the zoonotic infections are the viral hemorrhagic fevers, which are potentially fatal. Rapid recognition and diagnosis of these infections are critical to initiate appropriate, potentially life-saving, antiviral therapy and to prevent secondary spread to health care workers and family members.

PRETRAVEL COUNSELING

Risks from the perspectives of time, place, and person in both broad and specific terms, such as the season and time of day in which activities are planned; the risk by country or region and the specific locales or geoecologic zones of the itinerary, and host factors such as age, pregnancy, or other intrinsic conditions of the traveler in addition to occupational and recreational activities on the itinerary should be considered. Most vector-borne infections cannot be prevented except by avoidance or adaptations to reduce exposure by using repellents, dressing in protective clothing, and other behaviors to reduce contact with vectors or rodents. Vaccines for yellow fever (YF) and Japanese encephalitis (JE) are commercially available in the United States and for tick-borne encephalitis (TBE) in Europe. Some countries require proof of vaccination for persons entering from a YF endemic area.[6-9]

AVOIDANCE

TIME

Most vector-borne diseases are transmitted seasonally or in association with monsoon rains or other weather phenomena. Travelers with some flexibility may choose to schedule their journeys accordingly. Travel during the dry season reduces risk of acquiring mosquito-borne infections in most locations. In Africa, YF is transmitted in savanna habitats during the late rainy and early dry season and in the tropical forests of South America, principally from January to March. Tick activity also may be seasonal; for example, the peak transmission season for Colorado tick fever (CTF) is April to May; fewer ticks will be encountered during late summer outdoor activity.[10] Rodent-borne infections due to hantaviruses and arenaviruses are also seasonal and can exhibit long cyclic patterns of incidence with the fluctuation of rodent populations (e.g., 300-fold changes in small rodent abundance are observed in 3- to 4-year cycles in some areas of Scandinavia).[11,12] Transmission patterns are highly variable from one location to another, even within a single country, and may also vary from year to year. Current information on transmission patterns often can be obtained from the sources cited below.

Host-seeking activity of specific mosquito vectors vary during the day. *Culex* mosquito vectors of JE and western equine encephalitis (WEE) are most active in the crepuscular period around sunset and evening.[13] *Aedes aegypti* and sylvatic *Hemagogus* vectors of yellow fever are diurnal (i.e., active during specific daylight periods). Principal vectors of Ross River virus, *C. annulirostris* in inland areas and *A. vigilax* near coastal saltmarshes, are crepuscular and diurnal, respectively.[14] With such vector activity patterns in mind, travelers can alter their outdoor activities or take special precautions accordingly.

PLACE

Although most travelers are unlikely to modify their itinerary significantly to avoid areas where specific diseases are endemic, it may be appropriate to avoid certain locales where epidemics are reported. Current reports of disease outbreaks can be obtained electronically on PROMED (promed@usa.healthnet.org), at the International Society of Travel Medicine site (http://www.istm.org/), or through various commercial travel medicine sources (e.g., http://www.tripprep.com/index.html). The World Health Organization (WHO) and its *Weekly Epidemiological Record* (http://www.who.ch/Welcome.html) and the Centers for Disease Control (CDC) homepage and *Morbidity and Mortality Weekly Report* (http://www.cdc.gov/) should be consulted to confirm reports from other sources.

Avoiding an endemic or epidemic location is the most sure approach to preventing infection; however, sources of information may be incomplete or inaccurate, and the precision of this advice usually is limited. Table 25.1–1 lists selected epidemiologic and clinical features of certain medically important arboviral and zoonotic viral infections. Transmission of specific diseases varies by location and microhabitat associated with the viral enzootic cycle. For example, in central and western Europe, TBE is transmitted in highly focal and relatively stable foci where vector *Ixodes ricinus* ticks are prevalent in sheltered forest-pasture ecotones (Figure 25.1–1). Similarly, foci of rodent-borne hemorrhagic fever with renal syndrome in Eurasia are highly focal, depending on rodent density and infection rates.[11] JE is transmitted throughout Asia, principally in rural areas, where pigs are abundant and rice fields provide breeding habitat for larval stages of vector *C. tritaeniorhynchus*[13] (Figure

25.1–2). YF also is transmitted in rural areas: mainly in forests in the Western Hemisphere and in Africa on savannas during the rainy season[15,16] (Figure 25.1–3). Dengue, chikungunya, and, potentially, YF are transmitted in the tropical urban environment in interhuman cycles vectored by *A. aegypti* mosquitoes, a species well adapted to human domiciles throughout the tropical zone[16–18] (Figure 25.1–4). Similarly, Oropouche and sandfly fevers are transmitted by peridomestic midges or sandflies.[19,20] Urban outbreaks of dengue, chikungunya, and Oropouche have produced tens of thousands of epidemic cases.

The rodent-borne, viral, hemorrhagic fevers are transmitted mainly in rural areas; close direct contact with rodents (e.g., by entering or sleeping in infested dwellings or temporary shelters) usually precedes acquisition of infection.[21,22] If the natural reservoirs of these infections cannot be avoided, potential risk in accordance with individual disease transmission patterns should be evaluated and patients advised of common sense behaviors to reduce exposure (e.g., avoiding unpasteurized milk products as a precaution against acquiring TBE and avoiding direct contact with slaughtered animals or their fluids and tissues because of risks of louping ill, Crimean-Congo hemorrhagic fever [CCHF], Rift Valley fever [RVF], and other diseases of livestock).[23–25] Preventive approaches against mosquito and tickbites and rodent exposure are described below. Details of transmission cycles for other viruses are available in a number of references.[1–5]

PERSON

Many arboviral infections are associated with high ratios of asymptomatic to symptomatic cases. For JE and other flaviviral encephalitides, several hundred subclinical infections occur for each symptomatic case; however, susceptibility increases with advanced age, resulting in a 10-fold higher risk in the elderly (aged >60 years), and a secondary increase in risk is seen in infants.[8,26] Although other risk factors are perhaps too modest to constitute a contraindication to exposure, some individuals may choose to modify their behaviors based on these and other factors. For example, chikungunya is more severe and more likely to result in chronic arthritis in older adults, as is dengue fever, which, in children, cannot be differentiated easily from other common febrile illness. Females appear to be at higher risk for developing symptomatic Ross river polyarthritis, and Caucasians may be at higher risk for developing dengue hemorrhagic fever (DHF).[27–29]

Pregnancy carries special risks for arenaviral hemorrhagic fevers, both for the woman, who may have a more severe course of illness, and for the fetus, which may be miscarried.[30] In addition, Junin and Machupo viruses are believed to be teratogenic, and lymphocytic choriomeningitis virus has been implicated as a cause of congenital hydrocephalus and chorioretinitis. First-trimester JE infections have led to fetal infection and spontaneous abortion, evidently without exacerbation of encephalitis in the expectant woman.[31] Hemorrhagic manifestations complicating pregnancy have been reported in dengue fever, and late-third infections occurring immediately prior to birth have been transmitted vertically,

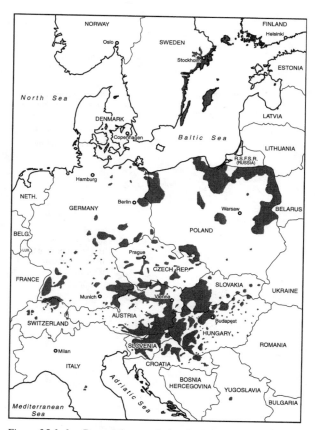

Figure 25.1–1. Reported transmission foci of tick-borne encephalitis (central European encephalitis) (source: WHO).

Table 25.1–1.   ARBOVIRAL AND ZOONOTIC VIRAL INFECTIONS BY GEOGRAPHIC AREA, MODE OF TRANSMISSION, AND CLINICAL SYNDROME

LOCATION AND VIRUS	FEBRILE ILLNESS			MENINGO-ENCEPHALITIS	HEMORRHAGIC FEVER	OTHER
	NON-DESCRIPT	WITH RASH	WITH ARTHRITIS			
North America						
Mosquito-borne						
Cache Valley	O					
California encephalitis				O		
Dengue 1–4		●				Hepatitis
EEE				O		
Everglades (VEE type II)				O		
Jamestown Canyon				O		Respiratory symptoms
Keystone				O		
LaCrosse				●		
St. Louis encephalitis				●		
Snowshoe hare				O		
Tensaw				O		
Trivittatus				O		Respiratory symptoms
Venezuelan equine encephalitis (sylvatic substypes ID, JE)				O		Pneumanitis
Western equine encephalitis				●		Perinatal illness after third-trimester infection
West Nile	●			●		Hepatitis, myocarditis; axonal neuropathy
Sandfly-borne						
Vesicular stomatits (New Jersey and Indiana)	O			O		Respiratory illness
Tick-borne						
Colorado tick fever	●			O	O	
Powassan				O		
Salmon River	O					
Zoonoses						
Lymphocytic choriomeningitis	O			O	O	Pneumonia, parotitis, orchitis, arthritis
Modoc				O		
Sin Nombre, Black Creek Canal, Bayou, New York						Noncardiogenic pulmonary edema; myositis, nephrosis
Rio Bravo	O			O		Pneumonia, orchitis
Seoul						Interstitial nephritis
Central and South America						
Mosquito-borne						
Bussuquara	O					
Cache valley	O					
Catu	O					
Cotia	O					
Dengue 1–4		●		O	●	Hepatitis; perinatal illness after congenital third-trimester infection
EEE				O		
Fort Sherman	O					
Group C viruses (Apeu, Caraparu, Itaqui, Madrid, Marituba, Murutucu, Nepuyo, Oriboca, Ossa, Restan)	O					
Guama	O					
Guaroa	O			?		Hepatitis
Ilheus	O			O		
Mayaro		●	●			
Mucambo (VEE type III)	O			O		
Piry	O					

continued

Table 25.1–1.   Continued

						Comments
Rocio				●		
StLE	○			○		
Tonate (VEE subtype III)	○			○		
Tacaiuma	○					Two cases with concurrent malaria fatal
Tucunduba				○		
VEE (epizootic subtypes IABC)	●			●		Abortion, CNS malformation after first-trimester infection
Western equine encephalitis				●		
Wyeomyia	○					
Xingu	○					
Yellow fever	●				●	Hepatitis? / Hepatitis
Sandfly-borne						
Alenquer	○					
Candiru	○					
Chagres	○					
Changuinola	○					
Morumbi	○					
Oropouche	●	○		○		
Punta Toro	○					
Serra Norte	○					
Vesicular stomatitis (New Jersey and Indiana)	○			○		
Vesicular stomatitis (Alagoas)				○		
Zoonoses						
Andes, Laguna Negra						Noncardiogenic pulmonary edema
Guanarito					●	
Junin					●	
Machupo					●	Fatal congenital infection
Rio Bravo	○			○		Fatal congenital infection
Sabia					○	Pneumonia, orchitis
Europe						
Mosquito-borne						
Batai	○			○		
Calovo	○					
Inkoo	○			○		
Sindbis (Ockelbo)	●	●	●			Respiratory illness
Snowshoe hare				○		
Tahyna	●			○		Respiratory illness
West Nile	○	○	○	●		Hepatitis, pancreatitis
Sandfly-borne						
Sandfly fever (Naples)	●					
Sandfly fever (Sicilian)	●					
Toscana	●			●		
Tickborne						
Bhanja	○			○		
Central European encephalitis	●			●		Hepatitis, thrombocytopenia
Crimean-Congo hemorrhagic fever					●	
Dhori	○			○		
Kemerovo				○		
Lipovnik				○		
Louping ill				○		
Thogoto	○			○		Hepatitis, optic neuritis
Zoonoses						
Erve				○		Thunderclap headache

Table 25.1–1.   Continued

	1	2	3	4	5	Remarks
Lymphocytic choriomeningitis	●			●	O	Pneumonia, arthritis, orchitis, parotitis, congenital CNS malformation
Belgrade-Dobrava	O				O	Interstitial nephritis, pantropic
Puumala	●			O	O	Interstitial nephritis, myocarditis; ocular disease
Seoul	O				O	Interstital nephritis, pantropic
Asia						
Mosquito-borne						
Batai	O			O		
Beijing				●		
Chandipura	O			O		
Chikungunya		●	●	O	O	
Dengue 1–4	●	●		O	●	Hepatitis common; perinatal illness after congenital third-trimester infection
Gansu				●		
Japanese encephalitis				●		Abortion after congenital first- and second-trimester infection
Kunjin		O	O	O		
Semliki Forest (MeTri)				O		
Sindbis	●	●	●		O	
Snowshoe hare				O		
Tahyna	●			O		Respiratory illness
West Nile	●	●	●	O		Hepatitis
Yunnan	O					
Zika		●				
Sandfly-borne						
Chandipura	O			O		
Sandfly fever (Naples)	●					
Sandfly fever (Sicilian)	●					
Tick-borne						
Alma-Arasan	O					
Banna				O		
Crimean-Congo hemorrhagic fever					●	
Dhori	O			O		
Ganjam	O					
Issyk-kul	O					
Karshi	O					
Kemerovo				O		
Kyasanur Forest				●	●	Pneumonitis, retinitis
Langat				O		
Negishi				O		
Omsk hemorrhagic fever				●	●	Pneumonia
Powassan				O		
Russian spring-summer encephalitis				●		
Syr-Darya valley		O				
Tamdy	O					
Wanowrie				O	O	
Zoonoses						
Nipah				●		Pneumonia
Hantaan					●	Pantropic interstitial nephritis
Lymphocytic choriomeningitis	O			O		Pneumonia, arthtritis, orchitis, parotitis; congenital CNS malformation

continued

Table 25.1–1.   Continued

Seoul					●	Pantropic, interstitial nephritis
Transmission cycle unknown						
Ebola (Reston)?						Asymptomatic infection
Africa						
Mosquito-borne						
Babanki	●	●	●			
Bangui		○				
Banzi	○					
Bhanja	○			○		
Bunyamwera		●		○		
Bwamba		●		○		
Chikungunya		●	●	○	○	
Dengue 1–4	●	●		○	●	Hepatitis; perinatal illness after congenital third-trimester infection
Germiston		○		○		
Igbo Ora	○					
Ilesha		●		○	○	
Koutango		○				
Lebombo	○					
Ngari				○		
Nyando	○					
O'nyong-nyong		●	●			
Orungo	●					
Pongola			○			
Rift Valley fever	●			●	●	Hepatitis, retinitis
Semliki Forest				●		
Shokwe	○					
Shuni	○					
Sindbis		●	●		○	
Spondweni		○				
Tahyna	●			○		Respiratory illness
Tataguine		●				
Usutu		○				
Wesselsbron	○					Hepatitis
West Nile	●	●	●	●		Hepatitis, pancreatitis
Yellow fever	●				●	Hepatitis
Zika		○				
Sandfly-borne						
Chandipura	○			○		
Sandfly fever (Naples)	●					
Sandfly fever (Sicilian)	●					
Tick-borne						
Abadina	○					
Bhanja	○			○		
Crimean-Congo hemorrhagic fever					●	
Dhori	○			○		
Dugbe	○			○		
Nairobi sheep disease	○					
Quaranfil	○			○		
Thogoto	○					Hepatitis, optic neuritis
Zoonoses						
Dakar bat	○					
Duvenhage				○		
Lassa					●	Pantropic
Lymphocytic choriomeningitis	○			○	○	Pneumonia, arthritis, orchitis, parotitis
Mokola				○		

continued

Table 25.1–1.   *Continued*

Monkeypox		●				
Tanapox		O				
Transmission cycle unknown						
Ebola (Zaire, Sudan, Ivory Coast)		●			●	Pantropic, abortion
Kasokero	O					
LeDantec				O		
Marburg		O			O	Pantropic
Australia and Oceania						
Mosquito-borne						
Barmah Forest			●	O		Glomerulonephritis
Dengue 1–4	●	●				Hepatitis; perinatal illness after third-trimester infection
Edge Hill			O			
GanGan			O			
Japanese encephalitis				O		
Kokobera			O			
Kunjin			O	O		
Murray Valley				●		
Ross River		●	●	O		Glomerulonephritis
Sepik	O					
Sindbis	O	O	O			
Trubanaman	O					
Zoonoses						
Ballina				O		
Hendra				O		Fatal pneumonia

O = rare, sporadic; ● = frequent, epidemic. Only arboviruses causing illness after natural infection are listed; viruses causing illness after laboratory exposure only are excluded.

producing perinatal illness, including hemorrhagic manifestations in the neonate.[32,33] Perinatal WEE also has been reported.[34] Anecdotal cases of eastern equine encephalitis (EEE) and St. Louis encephalitis (StLE) during pregnancy did not have more severe outcomes than expected, and the infections were not vertically transmitted. Asymp-

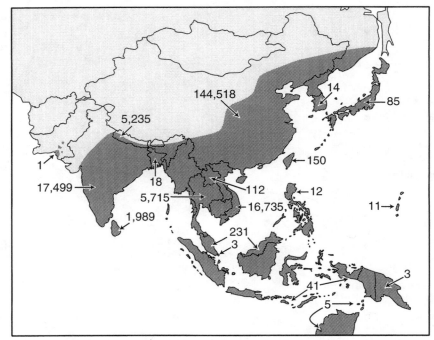

Figure 25.1–2.   Geographic distribution of Japanese encephalitis in Asia and the western Pacific and cases reported to WHO, 1986–1996.

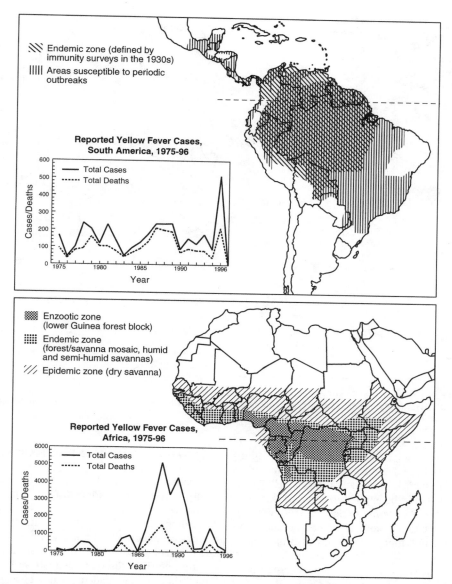

Figure 25.1–3.   Yellow fever (YF) transmission foci by phytogeographic zone and cases reported to WHO, 1975–1996. A resurgence of YF in Africa in the last decade has been followed in recent years by increased sylvatic transmission in South America. (Robertson SE, Hull BP, Bele O, et al. Yellow fever: a decade of reemergence. JAMA 1996;276:1157–1162).

tomatic congenital infection has been reported after Ross River viral infection and after YF immunization.[35–38] Spontaneous abortion has been reported following CTF in pregnancy; however, laboratory confirmation of a causal association was not shown.

GENERAL APPROACHES TO PREVENTION

MOSQUITO-BORNE INFECTIONS

Travelers may be unprepared for the presence of arthropod vectors around dwellings and indoors, even in good hotels with screens or air conditioning. Although hotels often supply mosquito bednets, travelers to tropical locations should consider bringing their own with string to hang it. Aerosol insecticidal space sprays can be used to kill indoor mosquitoes. Mosquito coils, typically containing pyrethrins, are effective and can be obtained locally; however, caution should be taken that they do not contain DDT or other potentially toxic ingredients. Travelers should be advised when outdoors to cover up by wearing long-sleeved shirts, long pants, and a hat when possible. Diethyltoluamide (DEET) is the most effective repellent, but dimethylphthalate ethylhexanediol and N butyl, N' acetyl 3 ethylamino propionate (35/35) also have activity, especially against anopheline mosquitoes.[39] Clothing should be sprayed with repellants containing DEET or permethrin, which is also insecticidal/acaricidal. Clothing, boots, and camping gear including sleeping bags, tents, and flies should be sprayed with permethrin to repel

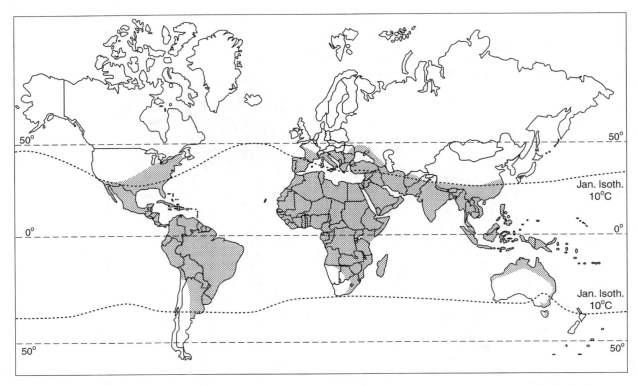

Figure 25.1–4.   Approximate distribution of *Aedes aegypti* mosquitoes and 10° isotherms representing area of potential distribution. (Modified from World Health Organization. Technical guide for diagnosis, treatment, surveillance, prevention and control of dengue haemorrhagic fever. 2nd Ed. Geneva: WHO, 1997.)

and kill insects and ticks. Local reductions in mosquito-biting activity have been demonstrated when all members of a party wore permethrin-treated clothing.[40] DEET-containing repellents should be applied to exposed skin only to minimize local and systemic toxicities. High concentrations applied to intertriginous areas can produce skin ulcerations, and acute allergic reactions also have been reported. Ingestion is associated with systemic and especially neurologic toxicities that have been potentially fatal.[41] In anecdotal cases, combined inhalation and mucous membrane exposure (spray used in a closed automobile) has led to acute encephalopathy and seizures, and, in others, encephalopathy has occurred after dermal exposure. The majority of cases have been reported in children; however, some cases also have been observed in adults. Although repeated use has been notable in some cases, in others, a single application of repellent was temporally associated with acute onset of seizures or encephalopathy. Risk factors have not been studied, and the pathophysiology of the neurologic toxicity has not been elucidated. Chronic dermal application also has been associated with psychological disturbances in adults (e.g., irritability, insomnia, anxiety). To reduce potential toxicity, and because higher concentrations provide a diminishing return of repellency, products containing less than 33% DEET should be recommended (<10% in children). Microencapsulated DEET provides a longer period of activity after application and minimizes absorption (e.g., 3M Ultrathon).[42] Other precautions to reduce potential repellent toxicity are listed in Table 25.1–2.

SANDFLY-BORNE INFECTIONS

Because of their small size, sandflies can penetrate ordinary screens and bednets. They typically feed during windless evenings and at night. They are common in the peridomestic environment and are frequently found in crevices and cracks of houses. Space and residual sprays to control malaria vectors are effective against phlebotomine flies. Spraying bednets and clothing with permethrin is recommended. Natural citronella products may be more effective than synthetic repellents in repelling sandflies.[43]

TICK-BORNE INFECTIONS

When entering habitats where ticks may be prevalent, travelers should be advised to wear light-colored clothing to facilitate finding and removing ticks. Clothing and gear should be inspected frequently and the entire body, including the scalp, at least once before retiring. Often, ticks will not have attached, and for nonviral infections such as Lyme disease and others, removal within 48 hours of tick attachment may prevent infection. Open sandals should be avoided, and because ticks climb upward, socks should be overlapped onto pantlegs and shirts tucked into pants. Repellents as described above should be used. Ticks on gear and clothing occasionally have been transported home where infections such as TBE and CTF have occurred in nontraveling family members.

Table 25.1–2. PRECAUTIONS TO MINIMIZE POTENTIAL ADVERSE REACTIONS FROM REPELLENTS

Apply repellent sparingly only to exposed skin or clothing.

Avoid applying high-concentration products (>35% DEET) to the skin, particularly of children.

Do not inhale or ingest repellents or get them into the eyes.

Wear long-sleeved shirts and long pants when possible; apply repellents (e.g., permethrin) to clothing to reduce skin exposure to DEET.

Avoid applying repellents to children's hands to reduce mucosal and oral contact.

Pregnant and nursing women should minimize use of repellents.

Never use repellents on wounds or irritated skin.

Use repellent sparingly; one application will last several hours. Saturation does not increase efficacy.

Wash repellent-treated skin after coming indoors.

If a suspected reaction to insect repellents occurs, wash treated skin and call a physician. Bring the repellent container to a physician.

RODENT-BORNE INFECTIONS

Close contact with infected rodent excretions generally is required for transmission of zoonoses due to hantaviruses and arenaviruses. Usually, these exposures occur while occupying infested dwellings and sometimes after simply entering an infrequently used infested shed or barn. The intensity of rodent infestation and the proximity of human-rodent contact are important determinants of risk. Poor house construction and heavy infestations, marked by rodent activity and droppings on counters, cabinets, and elsewhere indoors, possibly contaminating food, and close contact by sleeping on the floor increase risk.[11,12,21,22,44–48] Other cases occur occupationally, while working in fields where rodents gather during the harvest. Exposure may occur after infectious material is aerosolized by threshing or by direct contact.

A minority of travelers will face such conditions, among them backpackers or others residing with local people or in temporary camps for extended periods. Rodents may be attracted to tents, especially in cold weather and when food is scarce. Storing food in tight containers outside tents, disposing waste appropriately, and sleeping in cots above the ground are advised when tent camping for an extended period.

VACCINES

YELLOW FEVER VACCINE

YF vaccine, made from the attenuated 17D strain grown in chick embryos, is administered subcutaneously as a single 0.5-mL dose. Primary vaccination confers long-lived immunity, possibly lasting decades; however, international health requirements specify a current vaccination within 10 years. Vaccination is associated with a low rate of systemic and local side effects, except in infants, in whom the vaccine is contraindicated. Vaccination has pro-

duced encephalitis in 21 reported cases, 16 in infants less than 7 months old. The vaccine is recommended for infants younger than 9 months only during epidemics and is contraindicated in infants younger than 4 months. A recent review of Vaccine Adverse Events Reporting System (VAERS) reports suggests that the elderly also may be at increased risk for vaccine-associated severe multisystemic illness, including central nervous system (CNS) infection. Four such cases, including three fatalities temporally associated with vaccination, recently were reported in vaccinees >65 years. The observation appears to reflect an age-related pattern of risk seen in other flaviviral infections, rather than a general susceptibility of the elderly to severe vaccine-related adverse events (M. Cetron, personal communication, 1999). Allergic reactions, which have been reported in 1 in 116,000 vaccinees, probably occur principally in egg-allergic persons, although some cases might also involve allergy to gelatin, which is a vaccine component.[49] In such cases, immunization often has been successful when progressive vaccine dilutions were given intradermally and subcutaneously; however, proof of immunization should be confirmed by serologic testing. In anecdotal cases, vaccination of a diabetic patient was followed by ketoacidosis and in a patient with multiple sclerosis by a disease exacerbation.

Immunization of healthy HIV-infected persons with CD4 cell counts >200/mm has been well tolerated and followed by a good immune response without changes in CD4 cell counts or p25 antigenemia. However, in one study, asymptomatic HIV-infected children responded poorly to vaccination with a 17% seroconversion rate compared to 74% in controls.[50] Systematic studies of the vaccine's safety in other immunosuppressed conditions are unavailable, but, on theoretical grounds, immunocompromised persons should not receive the vaccine. Although the liver is a target organ for wild-type YF virus, in one study, experimental vaccination did not produce an elevation of liver enzymes.[51] However, the above cases in elderly vaccinees suggest the potential for rare multisystem infection including hepatic, renal, and cardiac and bone marrow involvement mimicking wild-type YF. Further studies are under way to characterize the frequency of such reactions and their pathogenesis. Often, a discussion of the traveler's itinerary and activities will reveal a low risk of exposure and little compelling need for vaccination, in which case a waiver letter should be provided in lieu of the international vaccination certificate (proof of YF vaccination is required for entry from YF endemic areas to certain countries). When travel to an endemic or epidemic area cannot be avoided, the theoretical risks of vaccination and risks of exposure and illness should be weighed to determine an appropriate course of action.

Pregnant travelers should be counseled in a similar fashion. Risks of vaccine-associated adverse events in pregnancy are uncertain, although, in one case, vertical infection after vaccination in the first trimester was documented serologically.[36–38] That neonate appeared normal; however, another study suggested an increased rate of abortions in pregnant vaccinees.[36] Immune suppression during pregnancy also may interfere with the formation of antibodies in the expectant woman.[37]

Concurrent vaccination with measles, hepatitis A or B meningococcal polysaccharide, or oral typhoid and cholera vaccines has not interfered with immune response to the individual antigens; simultaneous vaccination with parenteral typhoid vaccine is associated with an increased antibody response to YF vaccine.[8] Vaccination with outdated YF vaccine has not led to poor responses; nevertheless, revaccination with unexpired product is recommended. YF vaccines are produced locally in various countries and may be used if they meet WHO standards.

For most travelers, risk for acquiring YF is low; however, increasing numbers of itineraries now include an "adventure" component with attendant risks of sylvatic exposure, and several fatal cases have been reported recently in unimmunized individuals.[52,53] These wholly preventable cases were due, in one case, to the vaccine's restricted accessibility to a designated center, which inconvenienced the traveler, and in another (not yet reported) to the traveler's own disregard of the risk of exposure and refusal to be immunized.

JAPANESE ENCEPHALITIS VACCINE

The inactivated mouse-brain–derived vaccine produced by Biken (Osaka, Japan) and distributed in North America and Europe by Aventis Pasteur Inc. as JEVax has a 91% efficacy.[8,54] Three subcutaneous doses given within 2 or 4 weeks (days 0, 7, and 14 or 0, 7, and 28) provide protective neutralizing antibody levels in virtually all recipients, lasting for at least 2 to 3 years.[55] Local and mild systemic side effects are common (10% to 30% of vaccinees), but more serious hypersensitivity reactions consisting of generalized urticaria and angioedema occur in 0.5% of vaccinees.[8,56–58] Some cases have needed oral or parenteral steroids. In rare cases, reactions have led to respiratory obstruction and collapse, but no deaths have been directly attributed to such reactions. Because the onset of reactions may be delayed for 48 to 72 hours after vaccination, the last vaccine dose should be administered at least 1 week before departure. Acute disseminated encephalomyelitis has been temporally associated with vaccination in several anecdotal cases, but no causal association has been proved.[59] Risk for acquiring JE is low for most travelers. Only 11 cases have been reported in Americans since 1981, 7 in military personnel or their dependents. In seven studies, JE attack rates among western military personnel in Asia have ranged from 0.05 to 2.1 in 10,000 per week with a median of 0.9 (see below).[8] The low risk for acquiring the disease can be appreciated by considering that, typically, infection rates among vector mosquitoes are in the range of 5 in 1,000 and, after infection, only 1 in 500 cases is symptomatic (see above). Thus, risk for acquiring infection and especially for developing symptomatic infection is low. Because of the low incidence of disease and potential for vaccine side effects, routine vaccination of travelers to Asia is not recommended. Vaccination is advised only for expatriates living in endemic areas (persons residing through a transmission season or longer) and for travelers with an extended itinerary (arbitrarily, >30 days) or with extensive outdoor exposure in rural areas of an endemic area during the transmission season (camping, bicycle tours, outdoor occupational activities). Table 25.1–3 should be used to guide the decision, but there may be considerable local variation in viral activity geographically and seasonally. Available information should be interpreted with caution because of the uncertainties of local surveillance and reporting and secular changes in transmission patterns.

In studies of children, simultaneous administration with DTP, oral polio, and or measles vaccines did not interfere with immune responses to the individual vaccines and was not associated with increased side effects.[60] Other JE vaccines produced locally in China and other countries may not meet U.S. Food and Drug Administration standards, and, in general, they are not recommended.

OTHER VACCINES

Inactivated, cell-culture–derived vaccines against TBE virus are produced commercially in Austria and Germany and by a national institute in Russia. The commercial vaccines are available in most European countries but are not licensed in the United States. Estimates of efficacy have been drawn from national surveillance of case rates in populations given two doses in a month followed by a third dose 6 to 12 months later. Recently, three doses given over a month have been shown to be immunogenic.[61,62] Hemophiliacs with or without HIV infection have reduced immune responses to vaccination, with lower antibody titers and reduced cellular immune responses.[63] Cross-protection against related far eastern strains of TBE virus has been shown in immunized mice but not in humans.

Anecdotal TBE and Lyme disease cases, transmitted by the same tick vector in Europe, have been reported in returned travelers. However, spirochetal infection rates in *Ixodes ricinus* ticks are 10-fold higher than TBE viral infection rates; hence, comparative risks for the diseases may differ. A U.S. Army study of soldiers in Central Europe estimated the risk of acquiring symptomatic TBE as only 1 in 38,000 person-months of exposure.[64] An even lower risk for acquiring TBE probably holds for most travelers, and vaccination rarely is indicated. Expatriates can obtain the vaccine locally.

Passive immunization with TBE immune globulin is an alternative to protect travelers with a short and defined period of exposure. Immune globulin derived from vaccinees is available commercially in many European countries. For short-term protection, a traveler could arrange to receive intramuscular immune globulin in transit (e.g., at an airport clinic) or at a local clinic on arrival. The protective efficacy of passive pre-exposure immunization is uncertain. Although the immune globulin is also marketed for passive immunization within 96 hours after tickbite, postexposure prophylaxis after this interval may increase illness severity and is contraindicated. Safety and efficacy of postexposure prophylaxis at any interval have been questioned.[65]

An inactivated Hantaan virus vaccine for hemorrhagic fever with renal syndrome produced in Korea has uncertain immunogenicity and efficacy and cannot be recommended. Locally produced experimental vaccines for Argentine hemorrhagic fever and Kyasanur Forest disease are not available to travelers.

Table 25.1–3.   RISK OF JAPANESE ENCEPHALITIS BY COUNTRY, REGION, AND SEASON

COUNTRY	AFFECTED AREAS/JURISDICTIONS	TRANSMISSION SEASON	COMMENTS
Bangladesh	Few data, probably widespread	Possibly July–December as in northern India	Outbreak reported from Tangail district, Dacca division; sporadic cases in Rajshahi division
Bhutan	No data	No data; presumed to be similar to Nepal	Not applicable
Brunei	Pressumed to be sporadic—endemic as in Malaysia	Presumed year-round transmission	
Cambodia	Endemic—hyperendemic countrywide	Presumed to be May–October	Highly prevalent in rural areas near Phnom Penh; some JE cases confirmed in epidemics of uncertain etiology, Oct.–Dec. 1993–1998
Democratic Republic of Korea	Presumed countrywide chiefly in rural areas <800 m	July–October	Epidemics reported in the 1970s; few recent data
India	Reported cases from all states except Arunachal, Dadra, Daman, Diu, Gujarat, Himachal, Jammu, Kashmir, Lakshadweep, Meghalaya, Nagar Haveli, Orissa, Punjab, Rajasthan and Sikkim	*South India:* May–October in Goa October–January in Tamil Nadu August–December in Karnataka; second peak (April–June in Mandya district) *Andrha Pradesh:* September–December *North India:* July–December	Outbreaks in West Bengal, Bihar, Karnataka, Tamil Nadu, Andrha Pradesh, Assam, Uttar Pradesh, Maharashtra Manipure, Kerala, and Goa Urban cases reported (e.g., Lucknow)
Indonesia	Kalimantan, Bali, Nusa Tenggara, Sulawesi, Mollucas, and West Irian Java, Lombok	Probably year-round risk; varies by island; peak risks associated with rainfall, rice cultivation, and presence of pigs. Peak periods of risk, November–March; June–July in some years	Hyperendemic on Bali. Sporadic cases recognized elsewhere. Vaccine not recommended if travel is to only urban areas.
Japan*	Rare sporadic cases on all islands, except Hokkaido	June–September except Ryukyu islands (Okinawa) April–October	Vaccine not routinely recommended for travel to Tokyo and other major cities. Enzootic transmission without human cases observed on Hokkaido.
Laos	Presumed to be endemic—hyperendemic country wide	Presumed to be May–October	No data available
Malaysia	Sporadic—endemic in all states of Peninsula, Sarawak, and probably Sabah	November–January peak on peninsula	Most cases from Penang, Perak, Salangor, Johore, and Sarawak; differentiate cases from Nipah encephalitis
Myanmar	Presumed to be endemic—hyperendemic countrywide	Presumed to be May–October	Repeated outbreaks in Shan State in Chiang Mai Valley
Nepal	Hyperendemic in southern lowlands (Terai). Sporadic cases in Kathmandu Valley.	July–December	Vaccine not routinely recommended for travelers visiting high-altitude areas only
Papua New Guinea	Sporadic cases reported from D'entrecasteaux islands, Gulf, Milne Bay, South Highland, West Sepik, Western provinces	Unknown	Vaccine not routinely recommended
People's Republic of China	Cases in all provinces except Xizang (Tibet), Xinjiang, Qinghai. Hyperendemic in southern China; endemic—periodically epidemic in temperate areas. Rare cases in Hong Kong. New territories	*Northern China:* May–September *Southern China:* April–October (Guangshi, Yunnan, Gwangdong, and Southern Fujian, Szechuan, Guizhou, Hunan, Jiangsi provinces)	Vaccine not routinely recommended for travelers to urban areas only, including Hong Kong
Pakistan	May be transmitted in central deltas	Presumed to be June–January	Cases reported near Karachi. Endemic areas overlap those for West Nile virus.
Philippines	Presumed to be endemic on all islands	Uncertain, speculations based on locations and agroecosystems: *West Luzon, Mindoro, Negro Palowan:* April–November; *Elsewhere:* year-round—greatest risk April–January	Outbreaks described in Nueva Ecija, Luzon, and in Manila
Republic of Korea	Rare sporadic cases	July–October	Last major outbreaks in 1982–1983
Russia	Far eastern maritime areas south of Khabarousk	Peak period July–September	Sporadic transmission; differentiate cases from RSSE
Singapore	Rare cases; last indigenous cases in 1992	Year-round transmission no longer detected	Vaccine not routinely recommended
Sri Lanka	Endemic in all but mountainous areas; periodically epidemic in northern and central provinces	October–January; secondary peak of enzootic transmission May–June	Recent outbreaks in central (Anuradhapura) and northwestern provinces
Taiwan*	Endemic, sporadic cases; islandwide	April–October, June peak	Cases reported in and around Taipei
Thailand	Hyperendemic in north; sporadic—endemic in south	May–October	Annual outbreaks in Chiang Mai Valley; sporadic cases in Bangkok suburbs

continued

Table 25.1–3. Continued

Vietnam	Endemic hyperendemic in all provinces	May–October	Highest rates in and near Hanoi
Western Pacific and Australia	Discrete epidemics reported on Guam, Saipan (Northern Mariana Islands). Sporadic cases in the Torres Strait and Cape York, Australia	Uncertain, possibly September–January in the Pacific; February–April in northern Australia	Enzootic cycle may not be sustainable; epidemics may follow introductions of the virus. Single Australian mainland case reported in 1998.

*Local JE incidence rates may not accurately reflect risks to nonimmune vistitors because of high immunization rates in local populations. Humans are incidental to the transmission cycle. High levels of viral transmission may occur in the absence of human disease. Assessments are based on publications, surveillance reports, and personal correspondence. Extrapolations have been made from available data. Transmission patterns may change.

POST-TRAVEL COUNSELING

CLINICAL DIAGNOSIS

The differential diagnosis should take into account epidemiologic factors such as the transmission season, geographic distribution of diseases in relation to the itinerary, activities during travel, and, especially, the incubation period of clinically compatible illnesses in relation to the travel schedule (Table 25.1–4). It is beyond the scope of this chapter to review clinical features of each infection and the reader is referred to other sources.

To provide an approach to a differential diagnosis, diseases are listed in Table 25.1–1 by geographic distribution, clinical presentation (divided into general syndromes of nonspecific febrile illnesses, with or without rash; acute polyarthropathy; CNS infection; and hemorrhagic fever), mode of transmission, and disease frequency. After the patient's clinical illness is placed among the listed clinical syndromes, potential infections in the pertinent geographic regions can be narrowed further if a history of vector or animal exposure is given. Patients often give helpful clues about vector exposure. For tick-borne infections, a history of tickbite is typically given in 20% to 30% of cases, and tick exposure is reported in about three-quarters of cases. Sandflies make an impression because of their annoyance and small size. The rough gauge of disease frequency gives an indication of the likelihood of a given infection, but it should be interpreted with caution because reports of cases may be an artifact of their recognition through special investigations or sporadic availability of laboratory diagnosis.

ACUTE FEBRILE ILLNESS

A vast number of arboviruses have been described to cause a nonspecific and self-limited syndrome of fever and malaise, often with myalgias and headache. Clinical subtleties touted to be characteristic of some well-studied diseases (such as the 3-day duration of incapacity associated with sandfly fever—also called "three day fever") probably presume a higher degree of specificity than is warranted, and, in general, individual illnesses cannot be differentiated on a clinical basis. The most common acute febrile arboviral infection diagnosed in returned travelers is dengue fever, an *A. aegypti*-borne infection transmitted throughout the tropics, mainly in villages and urban areas (see Figure 25.1–4). In one study of returned febrile travelers, 5% of cases were due to dengue, but, in individual outbreaks among tourists or relief workers, attack rates of up to 50% have been observed. Attack rates of 1 in 1,000 per month have been reported among American servicemen.[66,67]

Four viral serotypes, dengue 1 to 4, produce a clinically identical illness of fever, malaise, chills, severe frontal headache, muscle and back pain leading to prostration, and abdominal tenderness 4 to 7 days after an infectious mosquito bite. The infection's severity varies with age, such that 80% of infections in children are asymptomatic, and the illness, which can include upper respiratory symptoms, cannot be easily differentiated from other common infections. The defervescence of fever 3 to 4 days after onset often is accompanied by the eruption of an indistinct macular rash, sparing the palms and soles. A recrudescence of illness frequently produces a saddleback pattern of fever. Illness may be complicated by minor bleeding from the gums, nares, and vagina, although, in rare cases, severe bleeding from preexisting peptic ulcers, hemoptysis, and even splenic rupture have been reported. Anicteric hepatitis with 10-fold elevations in transaminases have been reported in 10% of cases. Treatment is symptomatic, but medications prolonging bleeding time should be avoided.

Toscana and other sandfly fevers also have been reported frequently among returned travelers and military personnel stationed in the Mediterranean[68-72] (see Figure 25.1–5). Serologic evidence of Toscana viral infection has been reported in 1.5% of German tourists returning from that area and as high as 50% among Swedish tourists to Cyprus. The sandfly-borne infection is transmitted throughout the littoral and is the most common cause of childhood viral CNS infection in areas of Italy.

Other highly prevalent infections producing a nonspecific febrile illness syndrome are indicated in Table 25.1–1. Therapy is symptomatic.

ACUTE POLYARTHROPATHY

Several mosquito-borne alphaviruses—Sindbis, chikungunya, o'nyong nyong (ONN), Ross River, Barmah Forest, and Mayaro—cause a syndrome of acute symmetric polyarthropathy, often with rash and fever.[73-75] Infections in travelers have been reported with each of the viruses, although Ross River and chikungunya fevers have been reported more frequently, probably because those infections may be acquired in urban or suburban areas as well

Table 25.1–4. SALIENT EPIDEMIOLOGIC FEATURES OF SELECTED ARBOVIRAL INFECTIONS, VIRAL HEMORRHAGIC FEVERS, AND HANTAVIRUS PULMONARY SYNDROME

VIRAL FAMILY	DISEASE, VIRUS	GEOGRAPHIC DISTRIBUTION	ECOLOGY AND TRANSMISSION	INCUBATION PERIOD (DAYS)
Arenaviridae				
	Argentine hemorrhagic fever* (AHF), Junin	Argentina—Buenos Aires, Cordoba and Santa Fe Provinces	Rural; occupational disease of agricultural workers Rodent-borne	7–14
	Bolivian hemorrhagic fever* (BHF), Machupo	Bolivia—Beni Province	Rural peridomestic Rodent-borne	7–14
	Venezuelan hemorrhagic fever (VHF), Guanarito	Venezuela—Portuguesa and Baraquenas States	Rural peridomestic Rodent-borne	7–14
	Unnamed Sabía viral infection, Sabía	Brazil	Unknown	8
	Lassa fever,* Lassa	West and Central Africa	Rural peridomestic Rodent-borne	5–16
Bunyaviridae				
	Hantavirus pulmonary syndrome (HPS), Sin Nombre, Black Creek Canal, Bayou, others	United States, Canada, Argentina, Brazil, Paraguay	Rural peridomestic recreational and occupational infections Rodent-borne	7–21
	Hemorrhagic fever with renal syndrome (HFRS), Hantaan, Seoul, Dobrava, Puumala	Asia (Hantaan, Seoul); Europe (Puumula, Dobrava); Seoul virus infections worldwide	Rural campestral and sylvatic urban peridomestic Rodent-borne	4–42
	Rift Valley fever (RVF), Rift Valley fever	Africa	Rural Mosquito-borne, mechanically transmitted by other insects and directly from blood, tissues of infected livestock	3–5
	Crimean-Congo hemorrhagic fever* (CCHF), CCHF	Asia, Africa, Europe	Rural-sylvatic Tick-borne, directly from blood, tissues of infected livestock	2–7
	Toscana encephalitis, Toscana	Mediterranean littoral	Rural villages—peridomestic *Phlebotomus perniciosus* sandflies	
Filoviridae				
	Marburg hemorrhagic fever, *Marburg	Africa (imported to Europe in monkeys)	Rural Natural reservoir and primary transmission unknown	3–16
	Ebola hemorrhagic fever, *Ebola-Sudan, Ebola-Zaire, Ebola Ivory Coast	Africa	Rural Natural reservoir and primary transmission unknown	3–21
Flaviviridae				
	Dengue hemorrhagic fever (DHF), dengue types 1–4	Tropics, worldwide	Urban, peridomestic *Acdes aegypti*	2–7
	Yellow fever	South America, Africa	Forests and savanna, urban peridomestic Mosquito-borne	3–6
	Omsk hemorrhagic fever (OHF), OHF	Western Siberia	Sylvan Tick-borne, direct contact, water-borne	3–8
	Kyasanur Forest disease (KFD), KFD	India, Karnataka State ? Saudi Arabia	Human modified forests Tick-borne	3–8
	Japanese encephalitis (JE), JE	Asia	Rural Mosquito-borne	4–14
	Tick-borne encephalitis (central European/Russian spring-summer encephalitis), Absettarov, others	Scandinavia, western, central, and eastern Europe; eastern Russia, China, Korea, Japan	Sylvatic Tick-borne, directly from raw milk, butchering infected livestock	3–7
	West Nile (WN) fever, WN	Africa, Europe, Middle East, South Asia, U.S.	Rural Mosquito-borne, urban peridomestic	1–6
Togaviridae				
	Chikungunya (CHIK), CHIK	Africa, Asia	Rural, urban-peridomestic Mosquito-borne	2–10
	Ross River (RR) fever, RR	Australia, Oceania	Rural, suburban? Urban Mosquito-borne	3–21
	Sindbis (SIN) fever, SIN	Africa, Europe, Asia, Australia	Rural, sylvatic Mosquito-borne	? 2–7

*Documented nosocomial transmission.

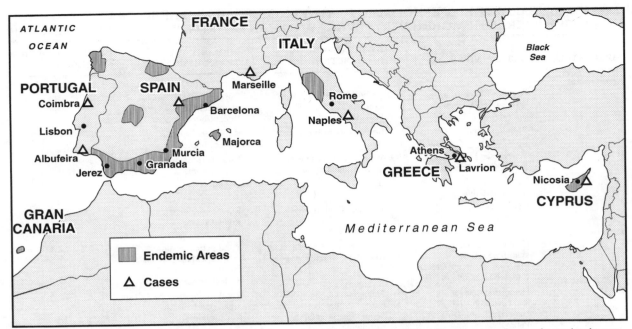

Figure 25.1–5. Areas with serologic evidence of Toscana viral transmission and reported locations of exposure for travel-associated cases.

as in sylvatic locations. Ross River virus, the most common arboviral infection in Australia, is transmitted principally on the eastern coast during the austral rainy season but sporadic infections may occur in the winter. Person-to-person transmitted outbreaks have appeared in the western Pacific, and such anthroponotic transmission in Australia has not been excluded. Chikungunya is considered to be endemic in Africa and Asia, but the pattern of transmission in Asia is one of periodic epidemic transmission followed by long intervals when the virus disappears. Transmission through its anthroponotic cycle by *A. aegypti*, often concurrently with dengue virus, has led to fearsome outbreaks, principally in Asian cities and less frequently documented in Africa. Enzootic transmission is maintained in a forest cycle. The rarity of ONN virus emergence in Africa, only twice in the last 50 years, represents an extreme of this periodicity. When outbreaks have arisen, however, they have been of a singular scale: an estimated 2 million cases were estimated in the initially recognized outbreak in 1959. Chikungunya and ONN viruses are closely related and cause similar syndromes of excruciating symmetric polyarthropathy, frequently leading patients to hobble and to minimize or limit all physical movement. Lymphadenopathy, especially in ONN fever, may be prominent, and a rash often appears several days after onset. Mayaro fever, transmitted in forested areas of Central and South America, produces a similar illness.

The polyarthropathies are self-limited without chronic sequelae except in anecdotal cases; however, resolution has taken up to a year in one-third of patients. The simultaneous occurrence of rash and polyarthritis frequently leads to misdiagnosis as rubella or parvoviral infection. Other etiologies in the differential diagnosis include rheumatoid arthritis, serum sickness, disseminated gonococcal infection, acute rheumatic fever, and symmetric polyarthropathies associated with infections with *Mycoplasma pneumoniae*, Epstein-Barr virus, enteroviruses, hepatitis A and B, and other viruses. Treatment with nonsteroidal anti-inflammatory compounds is sufficient in most cases.

CENTRAL NERVOUS SYSTEM INFECTION

Among the numerous arboviruses that produce a syndrome of CNS infection, three have been conspicuous as causes of neurologic infection in returned travelers and/or expatriates: JE, Toscana encephalitis, and TBE (see Figures 25.1–1, 2, 5).[8,70,76] The risk of JE to travelers and expatriates, which was recognized as early as 1933, is noteworthy for the number of reported cases and because cases in visitors to Beijing, China, in 1933 and, more recently, in an Australian child visiting Bali, Indonesia, were the first laboratory-confirmed cases to be recognized in those countries.[77,78] Sporadic and epidemic cases in western soldiers and their dependents stationed in Asia were reported in World War II and the Korean and Vietnam wars, and that risk stimulated development of a formalin-fixed mouse-brain–derived vaccine that was a prototype of the current commercial JE vaccine.[79] Since the Vietnam war, cases in military personnel and their dependents have comprised the majority of cases reported in the literature or informally to the authors, although no formal reporting mechanism exists and the number of unreported cases in private citizens is likely to be higher than has been notified.[8,57,80–84] Clinically, after an incubation period of 4 to 14 days, the illness begins with fever, vomiting, headache, and early disturbances in consciousness, evolving to profound coma in the majority of patients. Various motor disturbances, including bulbar and motor paralysis, cerebellar signs, and abnormal movements, may be present and convulsions may occur. A moderate cerebrospinal fluid (CSF) pleocytosis with elevated protein is found. Brain imaging studies have disclosed abnormalities in various structures, especially in the thalami, which may appear hemorrhagic. The diagnosis should be suspected in unvaccinated travelers to Asia during the transmission season—especially those with exposure to a rural area—who present with acute neurologic infection. Nipah encephalitis, caused by a novel zoonotic paramyxovirus spread from pigs and possibly from bats, which are the suspected vertebrate reservoir, is the principal alternative diagnosis to consider because it also occurs in rural areas of Asia, apparently with the same seasonality and in conjunction with pig husbandry. Therapy is supportive and consists of monitoring and treating elevated intracranial pressure, respiratory failure, and secondary infections, especially pneumonia. Even with good supportive care, 10% to 25% of cases may be fatal.

Infection with Toscana virus, which commonly produces aseptic meningitis or, less frequently, encephalitis, has been reported in numerous cases among travelers to the Mediterranean region. The illness is self-limited, with a favorable outcome in most cases.[68–72]

TBE has been reported in only one travel-acquired case; however, cases of Lyme disease, which is transmitted by the same tick vector (*I. ricinus*), also have been reported in travelers to areas of Europe where TBE is endemic.[85,86] Infection and illness in travelers are rare (see above), and, clinically, disease severity is age dependent. Infections in children are either asymptomatic or result principally in aseptic meningitis. The majority of all cases end abortively after a nonspecific grippe and only 5% to 30% develop a second phase of neurologic symptoms 2 to 8 days later (range 1 to 20 days), manifesting as encephalitis, bulbar or spinal paralysis, or a combination of those syndromes. A fatal outcome is reported in only 1% of all cases, but most severe and fatal cases are in elderly patients. Treatment is supportive. TBE immune globulin is licensed in various European countries for postexposure prophylaxis within 96 hours after a tick-bite; however, its administration after and, occasionally, even within this interval has been reported to exacerbate the illness.[65,87] Russian spring-summer encephalitis (RSSE), caused by a related *I. persulcatus*-transmitted virus, occurs in northeastern China, Russia, Korea, and Japan and differs clinically in its monophasic pattern and higher fatality rate of 20%.

In addition to the usual differential diagnosis of CNS infection, in returned travelers, special consideration should be given to bacterial meningitis (which may have been partially treated); listeria encephalitis (principally in the elderly and immunocompromised); typhoid fever; tuberculous meningitis; fungal meningitis; cerebral malaria; amebic meningoencephalitis; *Angiostrongylus*, Gnathostomal, and other eosinophilic meningitis; dengue encephalopathy; and HIV, herpes, and other viral encephalitis.

HEMORRHAGIC FEVER

Of all of the exotic viral infections potentially acquired during travel, the viral hemorrhagic fevers are of greatest concern because of their high fatality rate and, for some

infections, their capacity to be transmitted from person to person among family members, among health care workers, and, potentially, to the public. Since 1970, 12 cases have been imported to North America or European countries. The recognition and management of these infections are discussed below, but in addition to these principally rodent- and tick-borne viruses, mosquito-borne dengue and YF viruses can produce clinically similar illnesses that, fortunately, carry no risk for person-to-person spread. Cases in international travelers have been reported for YF and dengue, Lassa, Marburg, and Ebola hemorrhagic fevers. Early symptoms and signs of the viral hemorrhagic fevers are nonspecific, consisting of severe myalgias, asthenia, pharyngitis, dizziness, tachycardia, and postural hypotension. A high index of suspicion is indicated for ill patients who have returned with that history, especially if those symptoms are accompanied by epistaxis or minor mucosal or gastrointestinal bleeding.

Dengue hemorrhagic fever/dengue shock syndrome (DHF/DSS) is an immunopathologic disease arising from the phenomenon that immunity after infection with one dengue serotype is limited, so that second and third infections may occur due to other viral serotypes. The defervescence of fever after some secondary and tertiary infections may be followed by generalized hemorrhages and shock, the consequence of an immunopathologic response of cytokine release, complement activation, and endothelial cell dysfunction, leading to extravasation of fluid into tissues and pleural and peritoneal cavities.[88,89] Clinical signs of hypotension develop rapidly and shock may ensue, leading to death in 25% of untreated cases. Concurrently, petechial and purpuric bleeding into the skin and internal hemorrhages, hematemesis, and bleeding from venipuncture sites result from a combination of endothelial cell failure, platelet dysfunction, thrombocytopenia due to acute bone marrow suppression, and mild disseminated intravascular coagulation. If the patient is supported by careful monitoring and fluid support until the syndrome reverses spontaneously within 48 hours, the prognosis is good. However, adult respiratory distress syndrome and excessive fluid administration frequently complicate therapy. Radiographic or ultrasound detection of pleural fluid collections, thrombocytopenia, and rising hematocrit or serum proteins have been used as early indications of shock and to guide therapy, although when these abnormalities are detected, the onset of fluid extravasation usually has begun. Circulating cytokines have been studied as earlier prognostic indicators and as targets of intervention. In an individual case, the clinical syndrome in its early stages may be confused clinically with the more serious viral hemorrhagic fevers; however, the disease typically occurs in epidemics of numerous cases associated with ordinary dengue fever. Anecdotal cases have been reported in returned travelers, some in patients with a primary dengue viral infection. Infection is not transmitted from person to person; however, universal precautions should be sufficient to limit the hypothetical possibility of parenteral transmission from a viremic patient.

YF is transmitted only in South America and Africa, where cases are acquired principally from sylvatic or intermediate transmission cycles, mainly in forests or on rural savannas. However, epidemic transmission in the form of urban (*A. aegypti*-borne) YF is an extant threat with the increased ease of intracountry travel in countries at risk. Despite the recent occurrence of sizeable sylvatic outbreaks in Bolivia and in northern and western Brazil, cases imported to major cities, fortunately, have not led to epidemic spread. (Urban transmission reported from Santa Cruz de la Sierra, Bolivia, was discounted upon Pan American Health Organization [PAHO] tracing of cases; O. Oliva, personal communication, 1999.) Although recent cases in international travelers were acquired in sylvatic settings, the possibility of YF should be considered in all unimmunized travelers returning from any location within the endemic region. The majority of infections lead to no symptoms or to a self-limited severe flu-like illness with fever, myalgias, headache, and vomiting. Few physical signs characterize this early stage of infection except conjunctivitis, a slowed pulse, and a furrowed tongue. Recovery after several days is followed after a variable interval by a resumption of fever, severe vomiting (often of coffee ground material), jaundice, and proteinuria. From 25% to 50% of patients entering this phase of intoxication die, frequently with additional complications of spontaneous hemorrhages, shock, myocarditis and arrhythmias, encephalopathy, and secondary bacterial infection. Acute lobular hepatic necrosis, on average affecting half of the liver lobules, resolves without fibrosis and is no worse in hepatitis B antigen carriers. The hemorrhagic diathesis is complex, involving possibly disseminated intravascular coagulation, thrombocytopenia, platelet and capillary dysfunction, and depletion of vitamin K-dependent clotting factors. Supportive therapy with fluids and pressors may be life saving.

The arenaviral hemorrhagic fevers—Lassa fever, an endemic infection in rural West Africa, and Argentine, Bolivian, Venezuelan, and Brazilian hemorrhagic fevers, endemic and periodically hyperendemic infections in South American—are rodent-borne zoonoses (presumed for Brazilian hemorrhagic fever) transmitted to humans from infectious rodent secretions and excretions that are inhaled, ingested, or inoculated into skin abrasions.[12,47,48,90–93] Nosocomial outbreaks appear to have spread by a combination of air-borne parenteral and direct contact with infected fluids or excretions. The viruses are transmitted in geographically delimited areas of their respective countries or regions from persistently infected rodents when they enter human residences or, in the case of Argentine hemorrhagic fever, in fields disturbed by fall harvest activities. Cases are unlikely to occur in travelers except possibly in medical workers, backpackers, or those with similar activities. The illnesses overlap in their early nonspecific presentation with fever, headache, myalgias, and dysethesias and in their common features of hepatitis, mucosal hemorrhages, proteinuria, hypotension, effusions, and shock due to a capillary leak syndrome in patients with severe cases. The illnesses are fatal in approximately 20% of severe cases. Lassa fever may be complicated by encephalitis or encephalopathy and Argentine hemorrhagic fever by the delayed occurrence of a neurologic syndrome dominated by cerebellar disturbances. In recovered Lassa fever patients, deafness due to eighth nerve damage is a sequela in nearly one-third of cases. Vertically transmitted infection leading to spontaneous abortion has complicated the course of Lassa fever and Argentine and Bolivian hemorrhagic fevers acquired during pregnancy.

Although Marburg virus and the four subtypes of Ebola virus (Zaire, Sudan, Cote d'Ivoire, and Reston) are highly infectious when spread from infected monkey to person, or from person to person through nosocomial contacts, the natural reservoirs of the filoviruses are unknown, and the circumstances of infection in primary cases have remained elusive.[94] Until an outbreak in the Democratic Republic of the Congo occurred in 1999, cases in a traveler to Zimbabwe and two acquired in the same area of western Kenya were the sole reported naturally acquired Marburg fever cases; others were in laboratory workers or occurred through secondary spread.[95] The geographic distribution of the Ebola viruses is reflected in the subtype names, except for the Reston strain, which was traced from the source of infected monkeys to the Philippines. The virulence of the Ebola subtypes ranges widely, from a 90% case-fatality rate in cases infected with the Zaire strain, 50% with the Sudan strain, to only subclinical infection in the four persons who acquired a Reston virus infection. After an incubation period of 5 to 10 days, fever, myalgias, and headache begin abruptly, frequently accompanied by gastrointestinal and chest symptoms and pharyngitis. Conjunctivitis, lymphadenopathy, and jaundice also may be present. Spontaneous hemorrhages at injection sites develop with the progression of illness, and, unique among the hemorrhagic fevers, a prominent central maculopapular rash appears and later desquamates. Multiorgan failure resulting in anuria, hepatitis, disseminated intravascular coagulation, and CNS depression leads to death. Complications include orchitis, myelitis, relapsing hepatitis, and uveitis, which may be delayed in its onset and resolution.

Hemorrhagic fever with renal syndrome (HFRS) is caused by several hantaviruses endemic in Europe and Asia and carried by different species of wild rodents.[21,22,96–99] The dominant symptoms are fever, headache, severe abdominal pain, and renal dysfunction. Dobrava virus infection, endemic in central and eastern Europe, and Korean hemorrhagic fever (caused by Hantaan virus), endemic in Asia (Asian part of Russia, China, and Korea), are often complicated by shock and hemorrhagic manifestation with an overall mortality of 5% to 15%. Nephropathia epidemica caused by Puumala virus is a milder form of HFRS with a lower frequency of shock and clinical hemorrhage and a mortality of less than 1%, but not infrequently is complicated by ocular involvement, including uveitis. Large epidemics of HFRS often have occurred among military troops, and in the ongoing Balkan conflict both clinical forms of HFRS (Puumala and Dobrava virus infections) have circulated simultaneously. The incubation period typically is 2 weeks. After the onset of a flu-like illness, which may be accompanied by physical findings of conjunctival suffusion, facial flushing, and petechial hemorrhages, a phase of extreme vascular instability and increased hemorrhages ensues, with periods of sudden shock or hypertension. Leukocytosis and thrombocytopenia may be pronounced. Oliguria and frequently complete anuria follow reflecting interstitial nephritis and medullary tubular necrosis. A sudden reversal of urinary output with polyuria signals recovery. CNS hemorrhages, pulmonary edema, and secondary bacterial infections frequently complicate the illness and often are the proximal cause of death. Subtle tubular dysfunction resulting in an inability to concentrate the urine and electrolyte abnormalities may persist, and, in other cases, previous infection has been associated with hypertension. Balancing the maintenance of perfusion in the face of vascular instability and renal failure is a challenge to fluid and electrolyte management.

When administered early in the course of illness, ribavirin, a nucleoside analogue, has been shown to be clinically efficacious in Lassa fever and hemorrhagic fever with renal syndrome and may be effective in CCHF.[100-102] Oral ribavirin prophylaxis has been advocated for persons with exposure to Lassa and CCHF viruses. Early passive immunization with human convalescent plasma (within 8 days of onset) reduces mortality in Argentine hemorrhagic fever by 10-fold. No antiviral drug is yet available for filoviral infections with Marburg or Ebola viruses; however, an intensive search for different therapies including antiviral drugs is under way, and clinicians are advised to consult with CDC or WHO about compassionate use therapies if faced with a patient with suspected or confirmed VHF.

The viruses causing HFRS are not transmitted from person to person, nor have laboratory workers handling patient specimens been at risk. In contrast, secondary transmission of VHF to health care personnel, family members, and, in some cases, other hospitalized patients has been reported in Ebola, Marburg, Crimean-Congo, Lassa, and Machupo hemorrhagic fevers, with rates of 5% to 25% in filoviral outbreaks. Nosocomial transmission to other patients and to health care providers has involved close contact with patients, their blood, and body fluids, with the possibilities of direct percutaneous, mucosal, or respiratory infection.[103,104] In some cases, occult reuse of contaminated needles or syringes may have been involved. Surgical teams have been infected with CCHF virus following surgical exploration of patients with acute abdominal pain.[105,106] Secondary transmission to family members, especially in cases of Ebola hemorrhagic fever, has occurred principally while caring for acutely ill patients or their corpses in funeral rituals and by the same possibilities of transmission mechanisms mentioned previously.

Although among all body fluids, transmission risk and level (viral titer) and duration of infectiousness are best established for infected blood, virus also has been isolated variously from urine, feces, throat swabs, CSF, pleural fluid, and breastmilk in certain VHFs. During the incubation period and in early stages of the illness, risk of secondary transmission is believed to be low, except by direct contact with infected blood. With viral dissemination and progression of the illness, tissues and other fluids also may be sources of infection. Anecdotal cases in which other modes of infection seemed unlikely suggest

the possibility of air-borne spread from Lassa, Machupo, Junin, and Ebola fever patients. In addition, observational and experimental studies of monkeys indicate a possibility for air-borne Ebola virus transmission from animal to animal. Because the early clinical presentation of various VHFs is similar to other common infections, the initial approach must be based on an epidemiologic and a clinical assessment. The cardinal point is to ascertain a potential exposure within the 3 weeks before onset of symptoms by having visited an area where VHF recently had occurred, by direct contact with a suspected or confirmed VHF case, or by exposure in a laboratory that handles potentially infected clinical specimens or the viruses themselves. Treatable and common infections in the differential diagnosis, such as bacterial or parasitic infections (e.g., malaria, leptospirosis, rickettsial infections), must always be excluded expeditiously, regardless of the strength of suspicion of VHF.

Whenever possible, suspected patients should be referred to a hospital with good isolation facilities early in the illness to avoid the need for later transfer when the patient may be critically ill. The reported case-fatality rates for many hemorrhagic fevers are high (range 20% to 80%), but, in general, these figures have been recorded under primitive health care conditions with limited accessibility to intensive or even routine care. It is expected that intensive care would reduce mortality significantly. However, invasive monitoring and intensive supportive care, although likely to improve patient outcome, may introduce a new magnitude of exposure to health workers. Hospital transmission has occurred even under primitive conditions when little supportive treatment had been given. The complex physiologic derangements in critically ill VHF patients require supportive care that is technically difficult to provide in combination with biocontainment procedures.

Various countries have taken different approaches to this problem. Germany and the United Kingdom, for example, have central isolation facilities designed for care of VHF patients using plastic-film bed isolators (Figure 25.1–6). Sweden has taken another approach with a mobile support team that can be transported to local hospitals with a suspected or confirmed patient. The team

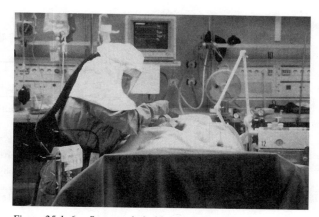

Figure 25.1–6.   Suspected viral hemorrhagic fever patient attended in hospital bed-isolator (courtesy of B. Niklasson).

brings protective equipment (respirators, protective clothing, and disinfectants) and serves as biocontainment advisors to local clinical and laboratory staff.

The recommended approach during the early stage of infection (before onset of hemorrhagic manifestations) is to use universal precautions with full face protection to prevent conjunctival and other mucous membrane infection. Direct contact with blood is believed to be the major mode of transmission during this stage. Risk of acquiring illness from an air-borne exposure is ill defined but, in most cases, appears to be low; risk apparently varies with individual hemorrhagic fever viruses and is greatest from patients with advanced disease. HEPA filter masks are suggested to block respiratory droplets and to minimize aerosol exposure in patients with prominent cough and respiratory symptoms. After the onset of hemorrhagic manifestations, additional nursing precautions are necessary. The number of health care staff at risk of exposure should be minimized, and those with patient contact should wear outfits that can resist massive contamination with blood or other potentially infectious fluids to prevent risk of direct physical contact. Full face protection is necessary, including a face mask with HEPA filter or a powered, air-purifying, protective respirator. Procedures for decontamination or destruction of excreta, linens, specimens, equipment, and other items exiting the room must be established. Procedures should be implemented to appropriately decontaminate, transport, and track clinical specimens. All laboratories handling patient specimens must be advised on decontamination procedures to minimize aerosols in specimen preparation and testing and on appropriate specimen storage and disposal. Patient contacts should be identified and placed under surveillance. Oral ribavirin prophylaxis may be indicated in some cases. Clinicians are advised to inquire about national contingency plans for case and contact management. With increasing awareness of VHF and its consequences, the number of false alarms is likely to increase. A suspected case of VHF in the absence of a contingency plan may create concern and even panic among nursing and laboratory staff. In two recent case reports, one in the U.S.A. and another in Europe, clinical laboratories have refused to analyze specimens from critically ill patients because VHF was listed in the differential diagnosis.

DELAYED CLINICAL MANIFESTATIONS

Most arboviral infections are preceded by short incubation periods and are self-limited without subacute or chronic manifestations; however, delayed or subacute manifestations of certain diseases may be the presenting feature in returned travelers (Table 25.1–5). After remission from the initial febrile illness, 30% of TBE cases develop a second clinical phase with neurologic symptoms.[26,76] One case imported to the United States and others to various European countries have been reported.[85] Neurologic symptoms develop monotonically in RSSE and Powassan encephalitis, but recovery may be complicated by subacute progression of limb and girdle weakness and atrophy.[107,108] RVF frequently is biphasic with a recrudescence of symptoms several days after remission. The second phase may be complicated by meningoencephalitis and, rarely, hemorrhagic manifestations.[109,110] Days or weeks after recovery from the acute febrile illness, diminished visual acuity and blurred vision develop in a small percentage of cases.[111] Retinitis, retinal vasculitis, and vascular occlusion have been described leading to exudates and scarring, sometimes in a macular or perimacular distribution. Permanent visual impairment or loss may result. Ocular symptoms have been the presenting complaints of RVF in several returned travelers. Ocular disorders, although self-limited, may follow a subacute course after Puumula viral infection. Symptoms may also recrudesce in Kyasanur Forest disease with the appearance of neurologic signs in some cases.[112] Chikungunya, Ross River, Sindbis, Mayaro, and Barmah Forest fevers cause acute polyarthritis that resolves within weeks or months in most cases but that persists for years in some individuals, especially in the elderly.[73–75,113] Symptoms are limited to morning stiffness and gelling in most cases. In rare instances, erosive changes have developed. A lengthy convalescence with asthenia and easy fatiguability is common after dengue, Ross River, Colorado tick, and Oropouche fevers. Chronic fatigue may be the presenting complaint of these infections after a mild, undifferentiated, febrile illness.

Clinical relapses several months after recovery from the acute illness have been reported in anecdotal JE cases.[114] Viremia was detected in symptomatic and

Table 25.1–5. DELAYED OR SUBACUTE CLINICAL MANIFESTATIONS OF ARBOVIRAL INFECTIONS

DISEASE	DELAYED OR SUBACUTE MANIFESTATION	INTERVAL AFTER INITIAL DEFERVESCENCE
Tick-borne encephalitis, louping ill	Meningitis, encephalitis, polyneuritis	1–20 d
Russian spring-summer encephalitis	Chronic progressive encephalitis	Months to years
Kyasanur Forest disease	Meningoencephalitis	9–21 d
Omsk hemorrhagic fever	Meningismus, hemorrhages	3–18 d
Rift Valley fever	Retinitis, optic atrophy, uveitis, meningoencephalitis	~1–3 wk
Alphaviral polyarthropathy	Polyarthralgias, polyarthritis	Relapses for 1 yr in 33%, 2–3 yr in 15% (chikungunya)

asymptomatic recovered patients months after resolution of the initial illness. Laboratory evidence of subacute CNS infection has been found in more than 40% of JE cases, and latent CNS abnormalities such as persistent electroencephalogram changes have been reported in JE and also in TBE.[115] Sensorineural deafness is a sequela in 30% of recovered Lassa fever patients and could potentially present as an isolated finding in a returned expatriate who had had an unrecognized Lassa fever case.[116] Persistent renal tubular dysfunction and hypertension have been reported in patients with hantaviral infection (nephropathia epidemica and hemorrhagic fever with renal syndrome).[117]

Sexual transmission of Junin and Marburg viruses has been reported—in the former case, 1 to 3 weeks after onset of illness in the primary case. In recovered cases of Marburg and Ebola infection, a longer interval of infectiousness was demonstrated; these respective viruses were isolated from semen 83 and 61 to 74 days after onset. In addition, Marburg virus was isolated from the anterior chamber of the eye 80 days after onset in one case. There is no direct evidence for persistent shedding and transmission of the viruses, but these anecdotal observations suggest means by which chains of transmission could be maintained in the absence of acute infection.

LABORATORY DIAGNOSIS

Arboviral infections rarely are persistent or latent; hence, direct detection of virus, viral antigen, or genomic sequences in blood or tissues of an acutely ill patient is specific evidence of recent infection. Virus can frequently be recovered from acute phase blood specimens in dengue, yellow fever, chikungunya, ONN, Ross River fever, Mayaro fever, sandfly fever, Venezuelan equine encephalitis, Kyasanur Forest disease, RVF, and arenaviral hemorrhagic fevers.[118,119] However, in most cases, the procedures should be carried out in specialized laboratories, and results may be unavailable in a timely interval. Neurotropic arboviruses rarely can be isolated from acute CSF, but attempts using cell lines available in routine virology laboratories sometimes are successful, and isolation attempts can be made providing that sufficient volume is preserved for serologic procedures on the sample. IgM capture ELISAs, whether applied to CSF or acute phase serum samples, are, in general, the serologic procedure of choice, yielding a high level of sensitivity and good to moderate specificity. Viral-specific IgM usually develops by 7 to 10 days after onset of illness but, in specific infections, may remain elevated for an extended interval (e.g., specific IgM declines by 60 to 90 days in dengue fever but may persist for a year in Sindbis fever, St. Louis and West Nile encephalitis, and for several years in YF). Other serologic procedures, such as hemagglutination inhibition (HI) and complement fixation (CF), may have value in diagnosing past infections. The neutralization test, usually the most specific serologic procedure, is of value in differentiating cross-reactions to closely related antigens, a situation that frequently arises because immunity in persons who previously resided in or traveled to tropical locations and immunization against YF, JE,

and/or TBE can interfere with the interpretation of serologic tests.

Viral-specific IgM in CSF, however, reflecting intrathecal synthesis, is considered diagnostic of recent CNS infection. A laboratory diagnosis can be confirmed by demonstrating fourfold changes between acute and convalescent serum samples by various serologic procedures, including ELISA, immunofluorescence, HI, CF, or neutralization (in increasing order of specificity). Under certain circumstances, an elevated antibody titer in a single serum specimen in a clinically compatible case is also interpreted as presumptive evidence of recent infection.

Acute specimens from hemorrhagic fever patients also should be evaluated by direct detection methods to make a timely diagnosis and because antibodies may appear late in the evolution of arenaviral infections. Negative serologic results from such cases are potentially misleading and falsely reassuring. Examples of available direct detection assays include polymerase chain reaction (PCR) of blood and tissues, direct electron microscopic examination of blood for filoviruses, and immunohistochemical and electron microscopic examination of tissues and skin (for filoviruses) for evidence of viral antigen and virions. Clinical evaluations of PCR in diagnosis of arboviral CNS infections are limited; in preliminary observations, PCR assays of CSF have been insensitive, although greater success has been reported in bunyaviral infections (e.g., Toscana and California serogroup viruses). The hemorrhagic fever viruses and many arboviruses are laboratory biohazards that should be confined to biosafety level 3 or 4 containment. Consultation should be sought from one of the following reference laboratories: Special Pathogens Branch, CDC, Atlanta (404-639-1511 [days], 639-2888 [evenings]); U.S. Army Medical Research Institute for Infectious Diseases (USAMRIID), Ft. Detrick, MD (301-619-2833); National Institute for Virology, Special Pathogens, Republic of South Africa (27-11-882-99-10; fax: 27-11-882-05-96); and the Centre for Applied Microbiology and Research, Porton Down, United Kingdom (44-1098-612224; fax: 44-1980-612731). The European Network for Diagnosis of Imported Viral Diseases (see homepage) publishes an updated list of European laboratories performing diagnostics on hemorrhagic fever viruses. Advice also can be sought from the WHO Division of Emerging and Other Communicable Diseases (41-22-791-21-11; fax: 41-22-791-0746).

REFERENCES

1. Monath TP, ed. The arboviruses: epidemiology and ecology, Vol I–V. Boca Raton, FL: CRC Press, 1983.
2. Karabatsos N. International catalogue of arboviruses and certain other viruses of vertebrates. 3rd Ed. San Antonio, TX: American Society of Tropical Medicine and Hygiene, 1985.
3. Richman DR, Whitley R, Hayden F, eds. Clinical virology. New York: Churchill Livingston, 1996.
4. Feigin RD, Cherry JD, eds. Textbook of pediatric infectious diseases. 4th Ed. Philadelphia: WB Saunders, 1998.
5. Schwarz TF, Siegel G, eds. Imported virus infections. Arch Virol 1996;(Suppl 11):3–202.

6. World Health Organization. International travel and health—vaccination requirements and health advice, 1999. Geneva: WHO, 1999.

7. Centers for Disease Control. Health information for international travel, 1999–2000. Atlanta: U.S. Department of Health and Human Services, CDC, 1999.

8. Plotkin SA, Orenstein WA, eds. Vaccines. 3rd Ed. Philadelphia: WB Saunders, 1999.

9. Jong EC. Travel immunizations. Med Clin North Am 1999;83:903–922.

10. Goodpasture HC, Poland JD, Francy DB, et al. Colorado tick fever: clinical, epidemiological and laboratory aspects of 228 cases in Colorado in 1973–1974. Ann Intern Med 1978; 88:303–310.

11. Niklasson B, Hornfeldt B, Lindkvist A, et al. Temporal dynamics of Puumala virus antibody prevalence in voles and of nephropathia epidemica incidence in humans. Am J Trop Med Hyg 1995;53:134–140.

12. Maiztegui JL. Clinical and epidemiological patterns of Argentine hemorrhagic fever. Bull World Health Organ 1975; 52:567–576.

13. Rojanasuphot S, Tsai TF, eds. Regional workshop on control of strategies for Japanese encephalitis. Southeast Asian J Trop Med Public Health 1995;26(Suppl):3.

14. Mackenzie JS, Lindsay MD, Coelen RJ, et al. Arboviruses causing human disease in the Australian zoogeographic region. Arch Virol 1994;136:447.

15. Monath TP. Yellow fever: Victor, Victoria? Conquerer, conquest? Epidemics and research in the last 40 years and prospects for the future. Am J Trop Med Hyg 1991;45:1–43.

16. Monath TP. Yellow fever and dengue—the interactions of virus, vector and host in the re-emergence of epidemic disease. Semin Virol 1994;5:133–145.

17. Halstead SB. The XXth century dengue pandemic: need for surveillance and research. World Health Stat Q 1992; 45:292–298.

18. Gubler DJ. Dengue and dengue hemorrhagic fever. Clin Microbiol Rev 1998;11:480–496.

19. Watts DM, Phillips I, Callahan JD, et al. Oropouche virus transmission in the Amazon River basin of Peru. Am J Trop Med Hyg 1997;56:148–152.

20. Schwarz TF, Gilch S, Jager G. Aseptic meningitis by sandfly fever virus, serotype Toscana. Clin Infect Dis 1995;21; 669–671.

21. Mertz GJ, Hjelle BL, Bryan RT. Hantavirus infection. Adv Intern Med 1997;42:369–421.

22. Peters CJ, Mills JN, Spiropoulou C, et al. Hantaviruses. In: Guerrant RL, Walker DH, Weller PF, eds. Tropical infectious diseases: principles and practice. New York: WB Saunders, 1999:1189–1212.

23. Davidson MM, Williams H, MacLoed JA. Louping ill in man: a forgotten disease. J Infect 1991;23:241–249.

24. Gresikova M, Sekeyova M, Stupalova S, et al. Sheep milk-borne epidemic of tick-borne encephalitis in Slovakia. Intervirology 1975;5:57–60.

25. Fisher-Hoch SP, McCormick JB, Swanepoel R, et al. Risk of human infections with Crimean-Congo hemorrhagic fever virus in a South Africa rural community. Am J Trop Med Hyg 1992;47:337.

26. Tsai TF. Flaviviruses. In: Mandell GL, Bennett JE, Dolin R, eds. Principles and practice of infectious diseases. Philadelphia: Churchill Livingstone, 2000:1714–1736.

27. Brighton SW, Prozesky OW, de la Harpe, et al. Chikungunya virus infection. A retrospective study of 107 cases. S Afr Med J 1983;63:313.

28. Fraser JRE. Epidemic polyarthritis and Ross River disease. Clin Rheum Dis 1986;12:369.

29. Bravo JR, Guzman MG, Kouri GP. Why dengue hemorrhagic fever in Cuba? I. Individual risk factors for dengue hemorrhagic fever/dengue shock syndrome. Trans R Soc Trop Med Hyg 1987;81:816–820.

30. Price ME, Fisher-Hoch SP, Craven RB, McCormick JB. A prospective study of maternal and fetal outcome in acute Lassa fever infection during pregnancy. BMJ 1988; 297:584–587.

31. Chatuverdi VC, Mathur A, Chandra A, et al. Transplacental infection with Japanese encephalitis virus. J Infect Dis 1980;141:712–715.

32. Poli L, Chungue E, Soulignac O, et al. Dengue materno-foetale: a propos de J cas observes pendant l'epidemie de Tahiti (1989). Bull Soc Pathol Exot 1991;84:513–521.

33. Thaithumyanon P, Thisyakorn V, Deerojinawong J, Ennis B. Dengue infection complicated by severe hemorrhage and vertical transmission in a parturient woman. Clin Infect Dis 1994;18:243–249.

34. Copps SC, Giddings LE. Transplacental transmission of western equine encephalitis. Pediatrics 1959;24:31.

35. Aaskov JG, Nair K, Lawrence GW, et al. Evidence for transplacental transmission of Ross River virus in humans. Med J Aust 1981;2:20.

36. Tsai TF, Paul R, Lynberg MC, Letson GW. Congenital yellow fever virus infection after immunization in pregnancy. J Infect Dis 1993;168:1520–1523.

37. Nasidi A, Monath TP, Vandenberg J, et al. Yellow fever vaccination and pregnancy: a four year prospective study. Trans R Soc Trop Med Hyg 1993;87:337–339.

38. Nishioka S, Nunes-Araujo FRF, Pires WP, et al. Yellow fever vaccination during pregnancy and spontaneous abortion: a case-control study. Trop Med Int Health 1998;3:29–33.

39. Fradin MS. Mosquitoes and mosquito repellents: a clinician's guide. Ann Intern Med 1998;128:931–940.

40. Schreck CE, Kline DL. Personal protection afforded by controlled release typical repellents and permethrin treated clothing against natural populations of Aedes taeniorhynchus. J Am Mosq Control Assoc 1989;5:75–80.

41. Tenenbein M. Severe toxic reactions and death following the ingestion of diethyltolamide-containing insect repellents. JAMA 1987;258:1509–1571.

42. Gupta RK, Rutledge LC. Laboratory evaluation of controlled release repellent formulations on human volunteers under three climatic regimens. J Am Mosq Control Assoc 1989; 5:52–55.

43. Wirtz RA, Rowton ED, Hallam JA, et al. Laboratory testing of repellents against the sandfly Phlebotomus papatasi (Diptera: Psychodidae). J Med Entomol 1986;1:64–67.

44. Ruo SL, Li YL, Tong Z, et al. Retrospective and prospective studies of hemorrhagic fever with renal syndrome in rural China. J Infect Dis 1994;170:527–534.

45. Tsai TF. Hemorrhagic fever with renal syndrome: mode of transmission to humans. Lab Animal Sci 1987;37:428–430.

46. Khan AS, Ksiazek TG, Peters CJ. Hantavirus pulmonary syndrome. Lancet 1996;347:739–741.

47. Mills JN, Ellis BA, McKee KT, et al. A longitudinal study of Junin virus activity in the rodent reservoir of Argentine hemorrhagic fever. Am J Trop Med Hyg 1992;47:749–763.

48. Vainrub B, Salas R. Latin America hemorrhagic fevers. Infect Dis Clin North Am 1994;8:47–59.

49. Kelso JM, Mootrey GT, Tsai TF. Anaphylaxis from yellow fever vaccine. J Allergy Clin Immunol 1999;103:698–701.

50. Sibailly TS, Wiktor SZ, Tsai TF. Poor antibody response to yellow fever vaccination in children infected with human immunodeficiency virus type 1. Pediatr Infect Dis J 1997; 16:1177–1179.

51. Freestone DS, Ferris RD, Weinberg AL, Kelly A. Stabilized 17D strains of yellow fever vaccine: dose response studies, clinical reactions, and effects on hepatic function. J Biol Stand 1977;5:181–186.

52. McFarland JM, Baddour LM, Nelson JE, et al. Imported yellow fever in a United States citizen. Clin Infect Dis 1997;25:1143–1147.

53. Barros ML, Boecken G. Jungle yellow fever in the central Amazon. Lancet 1996;348:969–970.

54. Hoke CH, Nisalak A, Sangawhipa N, et al. Protection against Japanese encephalitis by inactivated vaccines. N Engl J Med 1989;319:609–614.

55. Gamble JM, deFraites R, Hoke C, et al. Japanese encephalitis vaccine: persistence of antibody up to 3 years after a three dose primary series. J Infect Dis 1995;171:1074.

56. Centers for Disease Control. Inactivated Japanese encephalitis virus vaccine: statement of the ACIP. MMWR Morb Mortal Wkly Rep 1993;42(RR1):1–15.

57. Berg SW, Mitchell BS, Hanson RK, et al. Systemic reactions in US Marine Corps personnel receiving Japanese encephalitis vaccine. Clin Infect Dis 1997;24:265–266.

58. Plesner AM, Ronne T. Allergic mucocutaneous reactions to Japanese encephalitis vaccine. Vaccine 1997;15:1239–1243.

59. Plesner AM, Soborg PA, Herning M. Neurological complications and Japanese encephalitis vaccine. Lancet 1996;348:202–203.

60. Rojanasuphot S, Nachiangmai P, Srijaggrawalong A, Nimmannitya S. Implementation of simultaneous Japanese encephalitis vaccine in the Expanded Program of Immunization of infants. Mosq-Borne Dis Bull 1992;9:86–92.

61. Girgsdies OE, Rosenkranz G. Tick-borne encephalitis: development of a paediatric vaccine. A controlled randomized, double-blind and multicentre study. Vaccine 1996;14:1421–1428.

62. Stephenson JR, Lee JM, Easterbrook LM. Rapid vaccination protocols for commercial vaccines against tick-borne encephalitis. Vaccine 1995;13:743–746.

63. Wolf HM, Pum M, Jager R, et al. Cellular and humoral immune responses in haemophiliacs after vaccination against tickborne encephalitis. Br J Haematol 1992;82:374–383.

64. McNeil JG, Lednar WM, Stansfield SK, et al. Central European tick-borne encephalitis: assessment of risk for persons in the Armed Forces and vacationers. J Infect Dis 1985;152:650–651.

65. Valduega JM, Weber JR, Harms L, Bock A. Severe tickborne encephalitis after tickbite and passive immunization. J Neurol Neurosurg Psychiatr 1996;60:593–594.

66. Eisenhut M, Schwarz TF, Hegenscheid B. Seroprevalence of dengue, chikungunya and Sindbis virus infections in German aid workers. Infection 1999;27:82–85.

67. Gambel JM, Drabick JJ, Swalko MA, et al. Dengue among United Nations mission in Haiti personnel, 1955: implications for preventive medicine. Mil Med 1999;164:300–302.

68. Schwarz TF, Jager G, Gilch S, Pauli C. Serosurvey and laboratory diagnosis of imported sandfly fever virus, serotype Toscana, infection in Germany. Epidemiol Infect 1995;114:501–510.

69. Eitrem R, Niklasson B, Weiland O. Sandfly fever among Swedish tourists. Scand J Infect Dis 1991;23:451–457.

70. Braito A, Corbisiero R, Corradini S, et al. Toscana virus infections of the central nervous system in children: a report of 14 cases. J Pediatr 1998;132:144–148.

71. Schwarz TF, Gilch S, Jager G. Travel-related Toscana virus infection. Lancet 1993;342:803–804.

72. Mendoza-Montero J, Gamez-Rueda M-I, Navarro-Mari J-M, et al. Infections due to sandfly fever virus serotype Toscana in Spain. Clin Infect Dis 1998;27:434–436.

73. Tesh RB, Watts DM, Russel KL, et al. Mayaro virus disease: an emerging mosquito-borne zoonosis in tropical South America. Clin Infect Dis 1999;28:67–73.

74. Kiwanuka N, Saners EJ, Rwaguma EB, et al. O'nyong-nyong fever in south-central Uganda, 1996–7: clinical features and validation of a clinical case definition for surveillance purposes. Clin Infect Dis 1999;29:1243–1250.

75. Flexman JP, Smith DW, Mackenzie JSA. Comparison of the diseases caused by Ross River virus and Barmah Forest virus. Med J Aust 1998;169:159–163.

76. Gunther G, Haglund M, Lindquist L, et al. Tick-borne encephalitis in Sweden in relation to a septic meningo-encephalitis of other etiology: a prospective study of clinical course and outcome. J Neurol 1997;244:230–238.

77. Kuttner AG, T'sun T. Encephalitis in north China. Results obtained with neutralization tests. J Clin Invest 1936;15:525–530.

78. MacDonald WBG, Tink AR, Ouvrier RA, et al. Japanese encephalitis after a two-week holiday in Bali. Med J Aust 1989;150:334–336.

79. Sabin AB. Epidemic encephalitis in military personnel. Isolation of Japanese B virus on Okinawa in 1945, serologic diagnosis, clinical manifestations, epidemiologic aspects, and use of mouse brain vaccine. JAMA 1947;133:281–293.

80. Ognibene AJ. Japanese B encephalitis. In: Ognibene AJ, Barrett O, eds. Internal medicine in Vietnam: general medicine and infectious diseases. Washington, DC: U.S. Army Office of Surgeon General and Center for Military History, 1982.

81. Sabin AB, Schlesinger RW, Ginder DR, Matumoto M. Japanese B encephalitis in American Soldiers in Korea. Am J Hyg 1947;46:356–375.

82. Long AP, Hullinghorst RL, Gauld RL. Japanese B encephalitis, Korea 1950. Army Medical Science Graduate School Medical Science Publication No. 4;2:317–329. Recent advances in medicine and surgery. Washington, DC: Walter Reed Army Medical Center, 1954.

83. Halstead SB, Grosz CR. Subclinical Japanese encephalitis. I. Infection of Americans with limited residence in Korea. Am J Hyg 1962;75:190–201.

84. Benenson MW, Top FH, Gresso W, et al. The virulence of Japanese B encephalitis virus in Thailand. Am J Trop Med Hyg 1975;24:974–980.

85. Cruse RP, Rothner AD, Erenberg G, et al. Central European tickborne encephalitis: an Ohio case with history of foreign travel. Am J Dis Child 1979;133:1070–1071.

86. Cimperman J, Marapsin V, Lotric-Furlan S. Concomitant infection with tick-borne encephalitis virus and *Borrelia burgdorferi* sensu lato in patients with acute meningitis or meningoencephalitis. Infection 1998;26:160–164.

87. Arras C, Fescharek R, Gregersen JP. Do specific hyperimmunoglobulins aggravate clinical course of tick-borne encephalitis? Lancet 1996;347:1331.

88. Vaughn DW, Green S, Kalayanarooj S, et al. Dengue viremia titer, antibody response pattern, and virus serotype correlate with disease severity. J Infect Dis 2000;181:2–9.

89. Rothman AL, Ennis FA. Immunopathogenesis of dengue hemorrhagic fever. Virology 1999;257:1–6.

90. McCormick JB, King IJ, Webb PA, et al. A case-control study of the clinical diagnosis and course of Lassa fever. J Infect Dis 1987;155:445–455.

91. Monson MH, Cole AK, Frame JD, et al. Pediatric Lassa fever: a review of 33 Liberian cases. Am J Trop Med Hyg 1987;36:408.

92. Barry M, Russi M, Armstron L, et al. Treatment of a laboratory-acquired Sabia virus infection. N Engl J Med 1995;333:294–296.

93. Fulhorst DB, Bowen MD, Ksiazek TG, et al. Isolation and characterization of Whitewater Arroyo virus, a novel North American arenavirus. Virology 1996;224:114–120.

94. Peters CJ, LeDuc JW, eds. Ebola: the virus and the disease. J Infect Dis 1999;Suppl 1:S1–S288.

95. Anonymous. Marburg fever, Democratic Republic of the Congo. Wkly Epidemiol Rec 1999;74:145,157–158.

96. Peters CJ, Simpson G, Levy H. Spectrum of hantavirus infection: hemorrhagic fever with renal syndrome and hantavirus pulmonary syndrome. Annu Rev Med 1999;50:531–545.

97. Settergren B, Ahlm C, Alexeyev O, et al. Pathogenetic and clinical aspects of the renal involvement in hemorrhagic fever with renal syndrome. Ren Fail 1997;19:1–14.

98. Linderholm M, Sandstrom T, Rinnstrom O, et al. Impaired pulmonary function in patients with hemorrhagic fever with renal syndrome. Clin Infect Dis 1997;25:1084–1089.

99. Kontkånen M, Puustjarvi T, Kauppi P, Lahdevirta J. Ocular characteristics in nephropathia epidemica or Puumala virus infection. Acta Ophthalmol Scand 1996;74:621–625.

100. McCormick JB, King IJ, Webb PA, et al. Lassa fever: effective therapy with ribavirin. N Engl J Med 1986;314:20–26.

101. Huggins JN, Hsiang CM, Cosgriff TM, et al. Prospective, double blind, concurrent, placebo-controlled clinical trials of intravenous ribavirin therapy of hemorrhagic fever with renal syndrome. J Infect Dis 1991;169:1119–1127.

102. Fisher-Hoch SP, Khan JA, Rehman S, et al. Crimean-Congo hemorrhagic fever treated with oral ribavirin. Lancet 1995;346:372–475.

103. Peters CJ, Jahrling PB, Khan AS. Patients infected with high-hazard viruses: scientific basis for infection control. Arch Virol Suppl 1996;11:141–168.

104. Centers for Disease Control. Update—management of patients with suspected hemorrhagic fever—United States. MMWR Morb Mortal Wkly Rep 1995;44:475–479.

105. Schwarz TF, Nsanze H, Ameen AM. Clinical features of Crimean-Congo haemorrhagic fever in the United Arab Emirates. Infection 1997;25:364–367.

106. Van Eeden PJ, Joubert JR, van de Wal BW, et al. A nosocomial outbreak of Crimean-Congo hemorrhagic fever at the Tygerberg hospital I. Clinical features. S Afr Med J 1985;68:711.

107. Ogawa M, Okubo H, Tsuji Y, et al. Chronic progressive encephalitis ocurring 13 years after Russian spring-summer encephalitis. J Neurol Sci 1973;19:363–373.

108. Anonymous. Leg weakness associated with Powassan virus infection—Ontario. Can Dis Wkly Rep 1989;15:123–124.

109. Riou O, Phillipe B, Jouan A, et al. Les formes neurologiques et neurosensorielles de la fievre de la Vallee du Rift en Mauritanie. Bull Soc Exot Pathol 1989;82:605–610.

110. Siam AL, Meegan JM, Gharbawi RF. Rift Valley fever ocular manifestations during the 1977 epidemic in Egypt. Br J Ophthalmol 1980;64:366–374.

111. Mahdy MS. A case report of Rift Valley fever with retinopathy. Can Dis Wkly Rep 1979;5:189–192.

112. Webb HE, Rao RL. Kyasanur Forest disease: a general clinical study in which some cases with neurological complications were observed. Trans R Soc Trop Med Hyg 1981;55:284–298.

113. Niklasson B, Espmark A, Lundstrom J. Occurrence of arthralgia and specific IgM antibodies three to four years after Ockelbo disease. J Infect Dis 1988;157:832.

114. Ravi V, Desai AS, Shenoy PK, et al. Persistence of Japanese encephalitis virus in the human nervous system. J Med Virol 1993;40:326.

115. Lehtinen L, Halonen JP. EEG findings in tick-borne encephalitis. J Neurol Neurosurg Psychiatry 1984;47:500–504.

116. Cummins D, McCormick JB, Bennett D, et al. Acute sensorineural deafness in Lassa fever. JAMA 1990;264:2093–2096.

117. Lahdevirta J, Collan Y, Jokinen EJ, et al. Renal sequelae to nephropathia epidemica. Acta Pathol Microbiol Scand 1978;86:265–271.

118. Tsui TF. Arboviruses. In: Murray PR, Baron EJ, Pfaller MA, et al., eds. Manual of clinical microbiology. 7th Ed. Washington, DC: American Society of Microbiology Press, 1999:1107–1124.

119. Jahrling PB. Filoviruses and arenaviruses. In: Murray PR, Baron EJ, Pfaller MA, et al., eds. Manual of clinical microbiology. 7th Ed. Washington, DC: American Society of Microbiology Press, 1999:1125–1136.

25.2 OTHER IMPORTANT VIRAL INFECTIONS

CHRISTOPH F.R. HATZ, USA THISYAKORN, CHULE THISYAKORN, AND HENRY WILDE

Various infections play an important role in travel medicine. A few of the more important viral infections will be considered in this chapter.

VIRAL HEPATITIS

Infectious hepatitis is common among travelers to less developed countries and is caused by a variety of organisms. The vast majority are of viral origin.[1,2] These include the hepatotrophic viruses causing hepatitis A (HAV), B (HBV), C (HCV), D (HDV, "Delta"), E (HEV), members of the herpes virus group (herpes simplex, varicella zoster, Epstein-Barr, and cytomegaloviruses), coxsackie, adeno, echo, paramyxo, measles, rubella, dengue, yellow fever, and other agents. The association of some viruses with liver disease such as HGV (GBV-C) and TTV is doubtful. Hepatitis can also be a manifestation of infection with *Leptospira, Mycobacteria, Rickettsia,* and hantaviruses and in bacteremia. The clinical picture of amebic liver abscess is distinct and only rarely confused with viral hepatitis. The acute illness of hepatitis A-E is similar in all. Prodromal symptoms include fever, headache, and fatigue followed by anorexia, nausea, vomiting, right upper quadrant discomfort, pain, or tenderness. Dark urine, light-colored stools, and jaundice may appear shortly after prodromes but subclinical forms are also common. Jaundice can be prolonged and hepatic failure leading to coma and death may occur. All forms are found worldwide, although HAV and HEV are more common in countries with poor sanitation.

HEPATITIS A

HAV is responsible for roughly 50% of acute hepatitis cases in the U.S. and for about 60% of hepatitis in returning travelers to Western Europe. Transmission of this RNA picornavirus is by fecally contaminated water or food. There is only one serotype, and mutants capable of resisting monoclonal antibody-mediated neutralization do not occur in nature.[3] Outbreaks can often be traced to poor kitchen hygiene. Raw or undercooked shellfish cultivated in sewage-contaminated water and vegetables grown in soil fertilized with human excreta are risk factors. HAV has been transmitted by unsterile needles among drug addicts. The incubation period is between 3 to 5 weeks. All age groups are susceptible. In many developing countries, almost all of the adult population have antibodies to HAV. This is not true in the developed countries of Europe, North America (except for the Arctic), Japan, and Australia. Populations born after 1945 are found to have an HAV-antibody prevalence of less than 20% in some industrialized countries[4]; however, the pattern may vary substantially. Travelers from these regions are thus at risk of HAV when visiting less developed countries (including those in the former communist block region). Although the risk of infection is higher in the more adventurous, it is occasionally also seen in travelers returning from luxury tours.[4] The average disability from HAV infections is 1 month in young adults and longer in older patients.[5] The overall mortality is low but is higher in alcoholics, subjects with preexisting liver disease, and the aged.[6] HAV does not cause persistent infection or chronic liver disease. Subclinical infections are common, particularly in children, and may be associated with a rheumatoid-like arthritic syndrome. Diagnosis is by detection of IgM antibodies in the acute and early convalescent phase. Prevention is by good personal hygienic practices and avoidance of ingestion of high-risk water and food and by HAV vaccine or immune globulin.[4,7] Several vaccines containing formalin-inactivated and lyophilized, alum- and nonalum-adsorbed virus grown in cell culture and one influenza-virosome–complexed vaccine are now available. Combined hepatitis A and B vaccines are also available. Treatment for hepatitis A is symptomatic and supportive.

HEPATITIS B

This DNA hepadnavirus is transmitted via blood and body fluids. It is common among subjects who engage in high-risk sexual behavior, who are also at risk of HIV infection. HBV is worldwide in prevalence but more common in poor regions (tropics to Arctic), where carrier rates may reach 20% of the population. Animal vectors such as mos-

quitoes, leeches, and bedbugs are unlikely but not impossible vectors. Transmission from a carrier mother to her infant is common, and the newborn has a 90% chance of developing chronic liver disease and late hepatocellular cancer. The virus is more resistant to inactivation and more readily transmitted than HIV. The incubation period varies between 50 and 160 days. Cautious short-term travelers who avoid unsterilized needles, uncertain blood products, tattoo parlors, careless dentists, and hazardous sexual practices are not at low risk,[8,9] whereas the prevalence of seropositivity appears to increase with the length of stay, especially in long-term male residents in tropical countries. Among a group of 105 men living in Southeast Asia, the seroprevalence was 0% in those who had been living there for up to 1 year, rising to 47% in those in the fifth year.[10] Small wounds may occasionally lead to transmission, as illustrated by continuously increasing seroprevalence in children living in high-endemicity countries. The incidence of chronic hepatitis B is, however, only 5% to 10% among adults who developed clinical HBV. Anecdotal reports describe travelers with chronic HBV liver disease who took chloroquine for malaria prophylaxis and then experienced flare-ups of liver disease when the drug was discontinued.[11] Inactivated plasma-derived hepatitis B vaccines are still being manufactured in some developing countries.[12] An association between hepatitis B vaccine and multiple sclerosis has not been proven scientifically. A small number of individuals do not respond to vaccination with any of the plasma-derived or recombinant products. Whereas some slow responders will start to develop antibodies after repeated (up to 12) doses of vaccine, others will not respond at all to revaccination with any product. Their inability to produce HBV antibodies is genetically determined. In persons likely to be exposed to HBV, it is prudent to determine antibody titers approximately 1 month after completion of the vaccine series so that the subject can be told of his or her antibody status. Both active and passive immunization with HBV immune globulin are indicated in newborns if the mother is a known carrier. Treatment of acute HBV disease is supportive and symptomatic. Antiviral drugs have been used with promising results.[13] Chronic active HBV liver disease may respond to alpha-interferon therapy, and such patients need to be followed with periodic alpha fetoprotein determinations and ultrasonography since they have a high incidence of late hepatocellular cancer.

HEPATITIS C

This RNA flavigroup virus is spread via blood and body fluids, sexually, and perinatally.[14] The incubation period is 6 to 8 weeks. The infection can be mild and even subclinical but severe life-threatening disease also occurs. Twenty percent to 30% of patients develop chronic disease resulting in cirrhosis after 20 to 30 years. Hepatocellular carcinoma has a yearly incidence of approximately 3%. Current readily available diagnostic tests are antibody based and do not detect all infected cases and carriers. HCV-RNA is detectable in serum, but the cost of such tests is high. Transmission occurs among drug users and patients who receive organ transplants. HCV is now the major cause of transfusion-induced hepatitis world-wide. The development of an effective vaccine is hindered by extensive genetic and possibly antigenic diversity among different strains of HCV.[15] The preventive efficacy of immune globulins has not been established. The same precautions recommended for HBV apply to HCV. Treatment of the acute disease is symptomatic and supportive. Alpha-interferon suppresses chronic HCV liver disease, but the beneficial response is often only transient. Combinations of interferon with antiviral drugs (amantadine, ribavirin) are promising but carry a high prevalence of adverse reactions.

HEPATITIS D

This is caused by a defective RNA virus that can only replicate in the presence of HBV. It has a spotty worldwide distribution, is transmitted by blood and body fluids, and may cause life-threatening flare-ups of liver disease in subjects with chronic HBV. Known areas with high prevalence of HDV are parts of the Mediterranean region and South America.

HEPATITIS E

This calcivirus-like agent causes water-borne outbreaks in South Asia, parts of Africa, and Latin America. It is also encountered in immigrants to industrialized countries.[16,17] Long-term expatriates were found to have a prevalence of up to 10% in certain endemic countries.[18] The epidemiology and clinical picture of HEV, except for a higher number of cholestatic cases in HEV, is virtually identical to that of HAV. The incubation period ranges from 2 to 9 weeks. It appears to affect mainly young adults. Less than 5% of household contacts develop HEV infection, whereas the figure for HAV is 15%, indicating a lower person-to-person transmission or a dependence on a higher viral load ingested.[19] HEV differs from HAV mostly in that it is pernicious in the pregnant, where the mortality may reach 20%. Antibody-based diagnostic kits and more sophisticated research laboratory procedures can diagnose HEV but are not generally available where this disease is endemic. Diagnosis is thus on the basis of the travel history, clinical picture, and exclusion of HBV and HBC by common tests. Precautions for the traveler are the same as for HAV. There is no vaccine, and immune globulins are not likely to be effective as they are manufactured from donors from regions with a low prevalence of HEV.

HEPATITIS F AND G

Hepatitis F (French) virus was isolated from a French patient with sporadic non-A, non-B hepatitis.[20] Clinically and epidemiologically, it appears to be close to HAV and HEV. The geographic distribution is unknown. No commercial test system is available. More information is needed to classify HFV as a distinct hepatitis virus. Hepatitis G virus (identical with GBV-C) belongs to the flavivirus group and is distantly related to HCV.[21] HGV has been documented in the Americas, Europe, and Aus-

tralia. It may have a prevalence of 1% to 2% in the general population and up to 32% among frequently transfused children. Diagnosis is based on detection of HGV-RNA (RT-PCR). HGV-RNA is frequently associated with HBV and HCV infections. No serologic tests to detect antigen or antibodies exist. The role of HGV in acute and chronic non–A-E liver disease is not yet understood. Patients with hepatitis of unknown origin are not routinely investigated for HGV-RNA.

DENGUE AND DENGUE HEMORRHAGIC FEVER

Dengue hemorrhagic fever (DHF) is an acute febrile illness of children. It is characterized by fever, a hemorrhagic diathesis, and a tendency to develop a potentially fatal shock syndrome. The disease is a major public health problem in South and Southeast Asia, the Western Pacific regions, and Central and South America. It is among the 10 leading causes of hospitalization and death in children in many infected countries.

The etiologic agents include all four dengue serotypes that belong to the genus flavivirus in the family *Flaviviridae*. Infection with a particular dengue serotype confers long-lasting homotypic immunity. Heterotypic immunity lasts for a few months, after which patients are susceptible to infection with another serotype. The principal vector is the mosquito *Aedes aegypti*, which breeds largely indoors in clean water and artificial water containers. It feeds on man in the daytime.

Extensive epidemiologic studies in Southeast Asia have shown that DHF occurs when two or more dengue serotypes are simultaneously endemic or sequentially epidemic and where ecologic conditions favor efficient virus transmission by the vector. Serologic studies demonstrate that there is an association between DHF and a secondary type antibody response in most cases. These epidemiologic and serologic observations clearly link DHF to individuals who have had a previous dengue infection or have acquired maternal dengue antibody. The manifestations of dengue fever, which have been known for more than a century in Asia, are largely age dependent. The disease is mild in children and more severe in adults. Infants and children with dengue fever have symptoms ranging from an undifferentiated fever to a mild febrile illness, sometimes associated with a rash. Older children and adults frequently suffer a more severe form with the triad of high fever, pain in various parts of the body, and a maculopapular rash. The infection is only rarely fatal.

In comparison, DHF is considered a distinct disease because of its unusual hemorrhagic manifestations and the associated dengue shock syndrome. DHF mostly affects children under the age of 14 years and causes significant mortality.[22] Evidence from every country in which DHF has been recorded indicates a strong association between good nutritional status and an increased risk of developing dengue shock syndrome. DHF and dengue shock syndrome is rarely seen in the critically malnourished child.[23]

The critical pathophysiologic abnormality of DHF is an acute increase in vascular permeability without an inflammatory response, ultimately resulting in hypovolemic shock. Supporting evidence of plasma leakage includes serous effusions found at autopsy, pleural effusions and ascites on chest and abdominal x-rays (Figure 25.2–1), and hemoconcentration and hypoproteinemia. The exact mechanism responsible for the increased permeability is not known. Activation of the complement system with profound depression of C3 and C5 levels in serum and the formation of immune complexes are constantly found. The peak in complement activation and the presence of C3a and C5a anaphylatoxins coincide with the onset of shock and plasma leakage. The levels of C3a correlate closely with disease severity. Platelets, in the acute phase of DHF, contain on their surface fragments of C3. Their amount also correlates with disease severity.[24]

It has been proposed that the immunologic response plays a central role in disease pathogenesis, but the immunopathogenesis of DHF is still debated. Some investigators have suggested that DHF is a form of systemic Arthus reaction in which viral antigen and antidengue IgG complexes interact with the complement system to generate anaphylatoxins.[25] Others attribute shock to both immune complexes and IgE-mediated reactions.[26]

A phenomenon known as "immune enhancement" of virus infection has also been associated with the pathogenesis of DHF. The most significant evidence for this is the demonstration that dengue virus shows enhanced replication in human and simian peripheral blood leukocytes (most likely monocytes) in the presence of subneutralizing concentrations of specific antibody.[27,28] Halstead[29,30] proposed that an immune elimination response, probably mediated by T lymphocytes, activates these dengue-infected monocytes to release a variety of factors that produce hemorrhage and shock. These include vascular permeability factor, complement activating factors, and thromboplastin. However, DHF has been diagnosed in patients with primary dengue infection. Carefully designed epidemiologic studies are needed to further evaluate the possible interaction of immune enhancement with risk factors such as viral virulence, other environmental or infectious agents, genetic susceptibility, or unknown host factors.

Another hypothesis proposes the involvement of a delayed hypersensitivity reaction in the pathogenesis of DHF. It has also been shown that cytotoxic T lymphocytes are activated. It is possible that these dengue virus-specific T cells contribute to the pathogenesis of DHF/dengue shock syndrome by producing interferon-gamma and lysis of dengue virus-infected cells during secondary infections.[31] Further investigation needs to be carried out to fully understand the pathogenesis of the disease.

The incubation period of DHF is 4 to 6 days (range 3 to 10 days). Clinical and laboratory criteria for the diagnosis of DHF are as follows:

Clinical Criteria

- Fever—acute in onset, high, continuous, lasting for 2 to 7 days.
- Hemorrhagic manifestations, including a positive tourniquet test and any of the following: petechiae, purpura, ecchymosis, epistaxis, bleeding gums, hematemesis, and/or melena.
- Hepatomegaly, observed at some stage of the illness in 90% to 96% of Thai children and 60% of Thai adults.
- Shock—a rapid, weak pulse with a narrow pulse pressure and hypotension with cold, clammy skin and restlessness.

Laboratory Criteria

- Thrombocytopenia (platelet < 100,000/cu mm).
- Hemoconcentration (hematocrit increased by > 20%).

A diagnosis based on these criteria can be confirmed in the laboratory in 90% of patients. The presence of the first two or three clinical criteria with thrombocytopenia and hemoconcentration is sufficient to establish the diagnosis of DHF. This diagnosis is highly likely when shock occurs with high hematocrit levels (except in patients with severe bleeding).

Other common laboratory findings are hypoproteinemia, hyponatremia, and mildly elevated concentrations of liver enzymes and blood urea nitrogen levels. Metabolic acidosis may be found in patients with prolonged shock. The white blood cell count is variable, ranging from leukopenia to mild leukocytosis. An increase in the proportion of lymphocytes, with the presence of atypical forms, is common.[32] Hematologic findings include vascu-

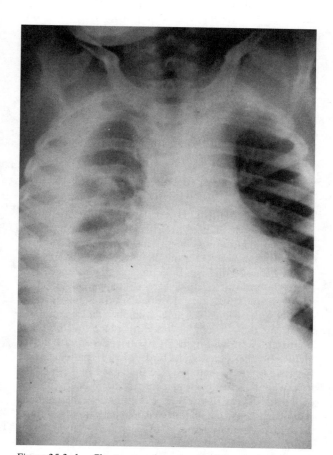

Figure 25.2–1.   Chest x-ray of a patient with dengue hemorrhagic fever showing right pleural effusion.

lopathy, increased capillary fragility (a positive tourniquet test), and coagulopathy (prolonged partial thromboplastin time and prothrombin time and platelet abnormalities). Assays of clotting factors show variable patterns of reduced levels of factors I, II, V, VII, VIII, IX, X, and XII. Thrombocytopenia is the most constant finding. The occurrence of disseminated intravascular coagulation, leading to uncontrolled and fatal hemorrhage, occurs only in patients with severe and prolonged shock.[33]

The specific diagnosis of dengue can be confirmed by serologic tests or by isolation of the virus from blood specimens. Virus isolation is easier during the early febrile phase. The enzyme-linked immunosorbent assay (ELISA) for dengue antibodies offers an improvement over the previous hemagglutination inhibition assay.[34]

There have been increasing reports of dengue with unusual cerebral, renal, and hepatic manifestations. Patients with these manifestations have tended to be in the younger age group and have a significantly higher mortality rate than those with the more common form of the infection.[35]

Treatment is essentially symptomatic and supportive. In most cases, early and effective replacement of lost plasma with plasma, plasma expander, and/or fluid and electrolyte solutions results in a favorable outcome. High doses of steroids do not help to reduce mortality in severe dengue shock syndrome.

Prognosis depends on early recognition of infection and careful monitoring. Serial determinations of platelet and hematocrit levels are essential for the early recognition and prevention of shock. Blood transfusion, preferably using fresh whole blood, is indicated for patients with significant clinical bleeding, mostly from the gastrointestinal tract. Fresh frozen plasma and/or platelet concentrates may be needed in some cases when consumptive coagulopathy causes massive bleeding. Persistent shock, despite adequate fluid administration, and a decline in the hematocrit level suggest significant clinical bleeding, which requires prompt intervention. Disseminated intravascular coagulation is usually associated with severe shock and may play an important role in the development of massive bleeding and irreversible shock. The coagulogram should be studied in all cases of shock to document the onset and severity of disseminated intravascular coagulation, which determines the outcome. Blood grouping and matching should be carried out as a routine precaution for every patient in shock. In general, there is no need for fluid therapy beyond 48 hours after the cessation of shock. Reabsorption of extravasated plasma takes place, manifested by a further drop in the hematocrit level after intravenous administration of fluid has been discontinued. Hypervolemia, pulmonary edema, or heart failure can result if more fluid is given. It is extremely important that a drop in the hematocrit level at this stage is not taken as a sign of internal hemorrhage. A strong pulse and blood pressure, with a wide pulse pressure and diuresis, are good prognostic signs in this phase. They rule out the likelihood of gastrointestinal hemorrhage, mostly found during the stage of shock. Prevention of DHF depends on control of the mosquito vector. Dengue vaccines that are under investigation include live attenuated tetravalent and recombinant dengue virus candidates.[36,37]

EPSTEIN-BARR VIRUS INFECTION

The Epstein-Barr virus (EBV) belongs to the herpes family and causes a variety of diseases.[38–40] They include the primary infection or "mononucleosis syndrome," mostly in developed countries, and nasopharyngeal carcinoma in Asia, Pacific Islands, and circumpolar region. Nasopharyngeal cancer is one of the most common malignancies of men in some of these regions,[41,42] Burkitt's lymphoma in Africa, and a variety of hematologic malignancies worldwide. It is also related to hairy-cell leukoplakia, progressive lymphoproliferative syndrome, and B cell lymphomas in patients with HIV.[43–45] There is a rare familial disorder that represents a genetic inability to cope with EBV infection resulting in fatal polyclonal lymphoproliferation when exposed to the virus.[46] Chronic fatigue syndrome had been linked to EBV infection, but no proof for this has ever come forth.[47] Children in the poor world acquire the virus when they are very young, and the infection is usually not detected. The virus then becomes a lifelong resident and incorporates into the cell genomes of the host, eventually generating oncogenes and leading to malignancies later in life. Genetic and external cofactors also play a role in the etiology of nasopharyngeal cancer and Burkitt's lymphoma.[48] It is not known why EBV infection after the teen years does not increase one's risk of these malignancies.

EBV disease is of no great importance to the travelers, virtually all of whom acquire the virus during their teens back home, but physicians in developed countries should be aware of it when they care for immigrants from Africa or Asia. Several candidate vaccines for EBV are now under study, and a variety of sensitive serologic tests are useful for diagnosis and follow-up of patients.

JAPANESE ENCEPHALITIS

Japanese encephalitis (JE) is a flaviviral infection of the central nervous system. The virus (JEV) is transmitted to man through mosquito bites. JE has long been endemic in South and Southeast Asia and the Western Pacific regions. It is a zoonotic disease, infecting man as an incidental host. The ratio of overt disease to inapparent infection varies from 1:300 to 1:1,000. Culicine mosquitoes, notably *Culex tritaeniorhynchus*, are the main vector. Rice fields are their principal breeding place and pigs are important amplifying hosts. Other vertebrate hosts include bovines, horses, and birds. Most JE patients come from areas where there are rice fields and pigs. In countries where JE has been present for many years, annual peaks of cycles have been irregular. In hot tropical regions, there is no apparent seasonal pattern. In contrast, there is a seasonal incidence of JE in northern moderate regions, and outbreaks have been associated with rainfall or irrigation and floods. The following factors are involved in the changing epidemiology of JE in many countries:

1. Changes in agriculture such as adoption of paddy (rice) cultivation, use of pesticides, and establishment of large, unscreened pig farms.
2. Changes in socioeconomic status involving a shift to rice cultivation from dry land crops and the promotion of pig breeding as food source.
3. Climate, including changes in temperature and rainfall.
4. Vaccination of humans and pigs.
5. A possible role of additional amplifying hosts other than pigs (e.g., horses, cattle, and buffaloes).
6. The wide variety of mosquito species in Southeast Asia and their vector efficiency.

The age-specific rate is highest in children 5 to 9 years old. The male to female ratio is 1.5:1. The case-fatality rate in symptomatic patients with encephalitis is in the range of 10% to 30%.[22,49] The incubation period following mosquito bites varies from 5 to 15 days. The course of the disease is divided into three stages:

- *Prodromal stage.* Acute onset of high fever is common. Other features at this stage are malaise, headache, nausea, and vomiting. The duration of the prodromal stage is usually between 1 and 6 days.
- *Acute encephalitic stage.* The main features are continuous fever, signs of meningeal irritation, alteration of consciousness, convulsions, spasticity, pyramidal tract signs, flaccid paralysis with diminished deep tendon reflexes, and focal neurologic deficits (e.g., hemiplegia and cranial palsies). The first two stages usually last no more than 2 weeks.
- *Late stage and sequele.* At this stage, fever subsides, and neurologic signs become stationary or tend to improve. Permanent sequelae of intellectual impairment, emotional instability, motor neuron lesions, and aphasia are common (Figure 25.2–2). Blood counts show a moderate to high leukocytosis and neutrophilia

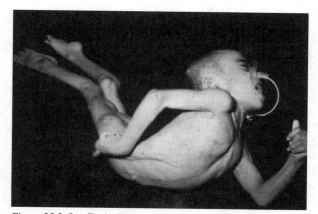

Figure 25.2–2. Tonic fits in a 4-year-old Thai boy with Japanese encephalitis: opisthotonos with head retracted, extended legs, and arms flexed at the elbow.

in the majority of cases. The cerebrospinal fluid is usually clear, colorless, and has a pleocytosis with cell counts ranging between 10 and 1,000 per cu mm. Most cases show a predominance of lymphocytes. Cerebrospinal proteins may be elevated but the sugar is usually normal.[50] No distinction can be made between JE and encephalitis caused by other agents on clinical grounds or by routine cerebrospinal fluid examination. Confirmation of JE is by demonstration of anti-JE IgM in the cerebrospinal fluid. Eighty percent of cases at the time of admission will show a positive test for specific IgM in the cerebrospinal fluid.[51]

Only symptomatic and supportive treatment is available. There is no benefit in terms of mortality and days to return of alert state from using high-dose dexamethasone.[52] Interferon-alpha has been shown to inhibit the replication of the JE virus in vitro and a clinical trial of interferon-alpha on JE patients in Thailand showed encouraging results.[53] Risk factors present on hospital admission and associated with a fatal outcome are infectious virus in cerebrospinal fluid, low levels of JEV-specific IgG and IgM in cerebrospinal fluid and serum, and a severely depressed sensorium.[54] Immunocytochemical studies of viral antigen and inflammatory cells in fatal cases showed that viral antigen was localized in neurons. The greatest involvement was in the thalamus and brain stem. Quantitation of the perivascular inflammatory response showed a preponderance of T cells, but only 7% to 30% of these cells were T suppressor/cytotoxic cells. Inflammatory cells invading the parenchyma were predominantly macrophages with small numbers of T cells. B cells remained localized to perivascular cuffs. Viral antigen disappeared in patients who survived 6 days or more.[55]

Control measures include reduction of vectors, protection of animal reservoirs by screening of pigstalls, prevention of mosquito bites, and vaccination of animals and man. For primary immunization, two doses of inactivated JE vaccine should be administered at an interval of 7 to 14 days. The primary immunization should be completed at least 1 month before the epidemic season or travel to an endemic region. A third injection should be given a few months after primary vaccination (before 1 year) in order to develop full protection by a booster effect. This may be all that is necessary for individuals living in endemic areas. They will likely have "natural boosters" from mosquito bites. Those in a nonendemic zone who travel frequently may need further periodic boosters.[56]

Although there is a high ratio of inapparent infection, clinical encephalitis, when present, is usually severe and results in a high mortality rate. Long-term disability, in the form of residual neuropsychiatric sequelae, occurs in 30% of survivors.[57] In endemic areas, children are the principal victims of JE, presumably because they have not yet developed protective levels of antibodies from inapparent infections. Virtually 100% of nonimmune piglets exposed to mosquitoes in all regions of Thailand seroconvert to JE within 2 weeks. Human seroprevalence studies indicate nearly universal exposure by adulthood. In areas where children are protected by immunization, a secondary increase in the incidence of JE has been observed in the elderly.[58] This observation suggests an increased JE risk with age because of waning immunity. JE acquired in the first or second trimester of pregnancy carries a high potential for intrauterine infection and fetal death.[59]

Travelers of all ages from nonendemic areas are nonimmune and as vulnerable as children to JE infection. In 1969, at least 10,000 Americans were infected in Vietnam and 57 encephalitic cases were reported.[60] Since then, cases have occurred in expatriates in Thailand, Burma, India, Sri Lanka, Cambodia, Vietnam, Indonesia, Singapore, Philippines, Okinawa, China, Manchuria, and Far Eastern Siberia.[61] This reflects the fact that viral transmission occurs across a broad part of Asia. JE may well be the most common form of encephalitis in the world today. Indeed, it is apparent that JE is expanding its range. It is now endemic in most of the Indian subcontinent and may "jump" to other parts of the world where suitable *Culex* mosquito vectors and pigs or other amplifying hosts are abundant.

Asia is popular with tourists, including backpackers, who often visit rural regions. Nonetheless, rice paddies and pig farms are also found near cities and cases of JE are seen in city dwellers. Although the risk of acquiring JE among the majority of travelers is low, the risk for any individual is variable and depends on factors such as the season, location and duration of travel, efforts at protection from mosquito bites, and the activities of the travelers. Travel during the transmission season and exposure in rural areas, especially for extended periods of time, are the principal factors contributing to risk. However, cases have occurred in the absence of obvious risk factors. One such example occurred in an Australian traveler who made only a few excursions into rural areas while on a 2-week vacation in Bali.[62] Another one involved an embassy secretary in Beijing, China, who rarely traveled outside the city.

The Biken JE vaccine (Research Foundation for Microbial Diseases, Osaka, Japan) is an inactivated preparation of Nakayama-NIH virus grown in suckling mice. It has been licensed in Japan since 1954[63] and was made available in the United States after 1983 through travel clinics in collaboration with the U.S. Centers for Disease Control (CDC).[64] Millions of Japanese, Thai, Chinese, and Korean children have been vaccinated with only minor adverse reactions. The immunologic or other mechanisms underlying the rare adverse events have not been defined. Some resemble delayed-type hypersensitivity reactions, perhaps to an antigenic component of the vaccine to which adults have previously been sensitized. An additional question is whether the reactogenicity of JE vaccine was associated only with certain lots or whether a uniform pattern of reactogenicity has gone undetected. Adverse reactions in expatriates from JE vaccine have been comprehensively reviewed by the CDC.[61] The Thai Red Cross Immunization Clinic in Bangkok has administered over 2,000 doses of JE vaccine from the Biken Institute without a single severe adverse event.

The recommended dose schedule for adults from nonendemic countries consists of three injections (days 0, 7, and 28); a slightly less efficacious regimen can also be employed (days 0, 7, and 14).The present JE vaccine is not an ideal product, and rare adverse reactions have been seen such as redness at injection sites (usually with the second or third dose), fever, and headache. The rare adverse side effects of JE vaccine were emphasized in a report from the American Institute of Medicine, which, at the request of the U.S. Congress, reviewed adverse reactions of pertussis and rubella vaccines.[65] Individuals anticipating long-term stays in JE endemic regions, or who plan to travel extensively in rural areas, should obtain JE vaccine prior to departure. They should, however, be informed of the small risk of adverse reactions. Individuals who had previous mouse brain JE vaccine series or any other mouse brain-derived vaccines (suckling mouse brain rabies vaccine, the old French yellow fever vaccine, or experimental Hantaan virus vaccines) should probably not be given the present mouse brain JE vaccine. It should also be used with caution in atopic individuals and is contraindicated in those allergic to the preservative thimerosol. No specific information is available on the safety of JE vaccine in pregnancy, and vaccination may pose a theoretical risk to the fetus.[65] There is an obvious need for a tissue culture or recombinant JE vaccine. It has been shown that the JE envelope glycoprotein E produces neutralizing antibodies and is apparently protective in a mouse system. Several studies have been done to express protein E or fragments by recombinant DNA techniques. Mice were effectively immunized with these products, and the development of a recombinant vaccine for human use may be expected.[66] Primary baby hamster kidney cell JE vaccine is being manufactured and widely used by the Wuhan Institute for Biological Products in China. Unfortunately, we are not aware of any studies of its safety, efficacy, and adverse reaction rates published in international peer-reviewed journals, and it has not been licensed or marketed abroad. A JE vaccine manufactured on microspheres and *vero* cells is now undergoing human trials.

The Biken JE vaccine was fully licensed by American authorities in December 1992 "in order to meet the needs of increasing numbers of U.S. residents traveling to Asia and to accommodate the needs of the U.S. military." Travelers to endemic areas should also reduce their risk of exposure by the appropriate use of bednets, insect repellents, and protective clothing.

An epidemic of encephalitis that killed over 100 persons in Malaysia and Singapore in 1999 and resulted in the culling of over 1,000,000 pigs was not due to JE virus. It was shown to have been caused by a new paramyxovirus related to the Australian hendravirus. It has now been named nipavirus. The natural host is still unknown; pigs were responsible for the recent epidemic. This virus is not mosquito borne and transmission to man is by direct contact with flesh, blood, and excretions of pigs.

MEASLES

Measles virus is an RNA virus of one antigenic type. It is classified as a morbillivirus of the paramyxovirus family. Measles is transmitted by droplets spread by coughing and sneezing. The incubation period is 8 to 12 days. The characteristics of the infection and its potential complications are well known. Most cases used to occur in children, but the introduction of attenuated viral vaccines against measles in the 1960s resulted in a dramatic reduction in the incidence of the disease in countries with high vaccine coverage. However, there also was a higher average age of cases in incompletely vaccinated communities. Measles outbreaks are still being reported from developed countries and from the developing world. Imported infections have resulted in case clusters. Measles is a concern in travel medicine.

Imported measles played an important role in the United States where between 1980 and 1985 approximately 100 international measles importations were recorded each year, accounting for 0.7% to 6.9% of the annual number of total reported measles cases.[67] Approximately 20% of these resulted in secondary spread. As many as 43% of reported cases were epidemiologically linked to an imported case. The importation rate per million travelers varied between less than 1 to 3 when the traveler came from Europe or Mexico to greater than 30 in travelers from India or the Philippines. The number of reported measles cases in the United States in 1995 was a historic low. However, there was a resurgence of measles during 1989–1991, when the incidence was highest among unvaccinated preschool-age children. A report in 1995 documents important epidemiologic trends, including a shift in age distribution and the continued occurrence of importations.[68]

Travelers to countries with a poorly implemented Expanded Program on Immunization (EPI) should ensure that they are immune to measles. For young children traveling to areas where measles is endemic or epidemic, the age for initial measles vaccination may need to be lowered. Children 12 to 15 months old should be given their first dose of measles-mumps-rubella (MMR) vaccine before departure. Infants 6 to 11 months old should receive a dose of monovalent measles or MMR vaccine before departure. They should be revaccinated with MMR vaccine (at least 4 weeks after the initial measles vaccination) at 12 to 15 months and again at 4 to 6 years. Children 12 months of age or older, who have received one dose and are traveling to areas where measles is endemic or epidemic, should receive their second dose before departure, provided that the interval between dosages is 4 weeks or more. Postexposure prophylaxis with immune globulin can be given to prevent or modify measles in a susceptible person within 6 days of exposure. Vaccine, if given within 72 hours of measles exposure, can provide protection.[69]

The authors have seen several cases of "atypical measles" in expatriates and tourists who had received an old inactivated vaccine. This vaccine resulted in inadequate or incomplete antibody titers and caused susceptibility to infection with wild virus. Atypical measles can present with unusual manifestations such as hemorrhagic rashes, pulmonary infiltrates, and a severe multisystem illness difficult to diagnose. These patients are not infectious to others and are characterized by extremely high antibody titers early in the disease course. Travelers to developing countries, who have had inactivated measles vaccine, should therefore receive one dose of the live vaccine. They should be aware that moderately severe local injection site and febrile reactions are common in this group.[70]

POLIOMYELITIS

Polioviruses are enteroviruses and consist of the antigenic types 1, 2, and 3. Humans are the only known reservoir of poliovirus. Transmission is by fecal-oral route. Clinical disease occurs in decreasing order of frequency as follows: inapparent infection (> 95%), nonspecific febrile illness, aseptic meningitis, and paralytic disease involving lower motor neurons (1% to 2%). Diagnosis can be made by isolation of virus from blood or CSF or by serologic means. Viral isolates serve to distinguish wild virus from vaccine strain illness.[71]

A survey reviewing poliomyelitis infections in industrialized countries between 1975 to 1984 revealed that 8.7% were imported from abroad.[72] Among 175 cases, 96 (55%) were diagnosed in foreign workers or their family, 47 (27%) in nationals traveling on holiday or business, 11 (6%) in immigrants, and 21 (12%) either in contacts without a travel history or in unclassified groups. Among the 47 travelers, 11 were below 10 years of age, whereas 16 were over 40 years old. Six of the patients had received a complete series of poliomyelitis vaccine, but the last dose was given at least 16 years prior to paralysis. The risk of paralytic poliomyelitis in international travel was estimated to be 0.3 per million, whereas the risk of infection was 7 to 336 per million. As shown in Figure 25.2–3, poliomyelitis in 1993 continued to occur in Eastern Europe, the Netherlands, and large parts of Africa and Asia. Travelers to such destinations need to be protected until global eradication of poliomyelitis will be achieved.[73–75]

RABIES

Rabies is caused by a neurotropic virus that can infect all mammals. It is present in North America as a zoonosis in

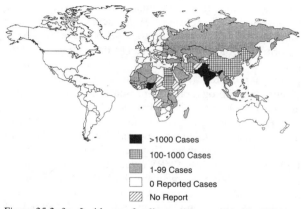

Figure 25.2–3. Incidence of poliomyelitis—worldwide, 1993. From MMWR Morb Mortal Wkly Rep 1994;43:501.

raccoons, foxes, and skunks, in wolves and dogs in the Arctic, and in dogs, coyotes, and cats along the Mexican border. Insectivorous, fruit-eating, and vampire bats harbor the agent in parts of the Americas, Europe, Africa, Asia, and Australia. Rabies has been virtually eradicated in Western Europe since oral vaccines for foxes became available. New Zealand, Japan, Hawaii, England, Ireland, Norway, and some islands in the Pacific and Atlantic are rabies free.[76] However, rabies remains a major public health problem in most parts of Asia, South and Central America, Africa, and some Pacific Islands where unvaccinated dogs roam freely. There are over 60,000 annual human deaths from rabies worldwide.[76] India alone accounts for at least 30,000[77]; the number for Africa, where wild animals are also involved, is not known. Rabies causes more annual human deaths than meningococcal meningitis, dengue fever, Japanese encephalitis, polio, and yellow fever.[78] Well over 1 million people receive postexposure rabies vaccination every year.[76] Rabies deaths among travelers returning to Europe, America, and Australia from endemic regions have been reported.[79] Hatz et al.[80] studied the incidence of animal bites among Swiss and German expatriates living in the tropics and found that these could be as high as 18.2 per 1,000 person-years. Phanuphak et al.[81] reported an airport survey of 1,882 travelers to Thailand, the majority from Europe, who spent an average of 17 days in the Kingdom. Only 1.6% had pre-exposure rabies vaccination and 1.3% had experienced a possible rabies exposure (bite, scratch, or lick from a mammal). Thus, any traveler who ventures past the luxury hotel environment in a rabies-endemic region may be at risk.[80,81]

Tissue and avian culture rabies vaccines are safe and effective but only when postexposure treatment with vaccine and immune globulin is carried out promptly following vigorous wound cleansing.[82] Modern rabies vaccines and immune globulins are expensive, and this is a major reason why locally made sheep and suckling mouse brain vaccines are still being used. These crude neural-tissue–derived vaccines are not only dangerous but often poorly immunogenic.[83] Human and equine rabies immune globulins are needed to provide protective antibodies during the first critical week after infection.[79,82,84] However, they are often not available in regions where they are needed the most.[83] Incubation periods can be very short, and more than half of the human victims in Thailand die within 6 weeks of exposure.[83] Well-documented unusually long incubation periods, up to 7 years, have also been reported.[85] Prolonged anxiety can be difficult to deal with if there is later doubt about the quality of postexposure treatment rendered. It is beyond the scope of this essay to discuss the virology, clinical presentations, and the hitherto near futile treatment of human rabies.[86]

The following rabies vaccines are widely used and are interchangeable: human diploid cell vaccine (HDCV) made in France, Germany, Canada, and Switzerland; purified vero cell vaccine (PVRV) made in France and India; purified duck embryo vaccine (PDEV) made in Switzerland (soon also in India); and purified chick embryo vaccine (PCEC) made in Germany, India, and Japan. All of these are approved by national drug regulatory authorities,

are of high potency and safety, and are administered using one of the following WHO-accepted schedules[82,87]:

1. The "gold standard" intramuscular regimen (also known as the Essen schedule). It is administered as one full ampoule on days 0, 3, 7, 14, and 28. This is the only U.S. Food and Drug Administration-approved method.[82]

2. The reduced-dose Thai Red Cross intradermal schedule. It is given intradermally at two sites on days 0, 3, and 7 and at one site on days 28 and 90. It uses 0.1-mL vaccine solution intradermally for each injection when the diluent provided with the vaccine is 0.5 mL and 0.2 mL if the diluent is 1.0 mL. This regimen is approximately 75% less expensive than when the same vaccine is used in full dose intramuscularly. It is now used widely in many developing countries where it has been shown to be as immunogenic and effective as the Essen schedule.[87,88]

3. The Oxford schedule consists of 0.1 mL of tissue culture vaccine (HDCV, PVRV, PDEV, or PCEC) given intradermally at eight different sites on day 0, at four sites on day 7, and at one site on days 28 and 90.[87] It has the disadvantage, like the "2-1-1" schedule, that the patient is not seen on day 3 when most bite-wound infections become apparent.

4. The 2-1-1 intramuscular regimen, also known as the Zagreb schedule, is given as one dose at two sites on day 0 and at one site on days 7 and 21. This method saves one ampoule of vaccine and two clinic visits. Suppression of the antibody titer by rabies immune globulin has been reported with this method, but this is probably clinically not significant.[87,89,90]

Rabies vaccines are given into deltoid or lateral thigh muscle. As much human rabies immune globulin (HRIG) or purified equine rabies immune globulin (ERIG) as possible is infiltrated into and around the wounds and the rest is given by deep intramuscular injection at a different site than the vaccine.[82,87] HRIG is given at 20 IU/kg and ERIG at 40 IU/kg.[85] Adverse reactions to current tissue culture vaccines are uncommon and mild. Rare serum sickness-like reactions have been reported in subjects who received booster doses of HDCV.[91] They have not been a problem in our experience with PCEC, PDEV, PVRV, and the Swiss-made albumin-free HDCV. Our institution therefore uses PVRV, PCEC, or PDEV as boosters in subjects whose occupational exposure mandates a continuous high antibody titer and repeat boosters. Local injection-site reactions, including mild regional lymphadenopathy, are more common when one is using the intradermal routes.[84,88] There are no contraindications to postexposure rabies vaccination, and it is safe during pregnancy.[92] HRIG is virtually free of side effects. Modern purified and pepsin digested ERIG is safe and cost effective when compared to HRIG. It is often the only immune globulin available in many countries.[93] Some developing countries in Asia, Africa, and South America still manufacture crude unpurified ERIG, which has a high adverse reaction rate. A skin test using 0.2 mL of a 1:100 dilution of ERIG is usually performed but does not predict serum sickness, which is seen in 1% to 3% of recipients given purified ERIG.[94] Anaphylaxis from modern ERIG preparations has been extremely rare. We have seen only one case among over 80,000 patients treated with purified and pepsin digested ERIG manufactured either by Pasteur (Paris), Berna (Switzerland), or the Thai Red Cross.[94] Serum sickness usually appears 1 week after injection and is treated with antihistamines and analgesics without any change in the postexposure vaccine regimen.[93]

If there are extensive and multiple wounds, where the calculated dose of immune globulin (by weight) is inadequate in volume to infiltrate all wounds, the HRIG or ERIG must be diluted in normal saline to create an adequate volume.[95] Wound infection is no contraindication for immune globulin infiltration as long as appropriate antibiotics are also administered.[96] Rabies immune globulin is normally given with the first dose of vaccine but can be given up to 7 days later if delay is unavoidable.[97] Corticosteroids, chloroquine, and mefloquine should be avoided since they may interfere with the immune response to vaccine.[82] Travelers may return after having been started on a postexposure regimen using a tissue or avian culture vaccine that is not available at home. One should then continue the schedule using one of the available WHO-approved vaccines (HDCV, PVRV, PCEC, PDEV). If a vaccine of dubious origin, one known to be of marginal potency (hamster kidney cell vaccines from China or CIS — former USSR) or suckling mouse brain or Semple vaccine had been used, the patient should be started on a full course of HDCV, PVRV, PCEC, or PDEV. Serum for rabies antibody testing should also be collected on the first visit. Patients presenting with delay after a rabies exposure are treated with immune globulin and vaccine as if the exposure occurred that day.[82] Management of dog and cat bites in a canine rabies endemic region may differ from that used in developed countries. Some of the reasons for this are:

1. The probability of a biting dog or cat being rabid is much greater.
2. Animals that are not usually considered a rabies risk in Europe or America may be rabid since there is "spillover" from canine and feline rabies to other mammals. Monkeys, bandicoots, and other large rats that live in close proximity to dogs and humans have been found rabies positive.[98,99] There has been one documented recent human rabies death from the bite of a rat in Central Thailand (Dr. Thavatchai Kamoltham, Ministry of Public Health, personal communication).
3. Vaccine failures in dogs are common. For example, 3% to 6% of rabies-positive dogs in Thailand had a vaccine history.[84,100] This is one reason why an attacking dog should not be observed in this environment without first starting treatment. If possible, have the animal killed and a fluorescent antibody test on brain performed in a reliable laboratory. Alternately, it is best to start full treatment with immune globulin and vaccine and discontinue it if the animal is found well after 10 days of observation.[82,84]
4. The biting animal does not need to act overtly rabid at the time of the attack.[101]
5. Any transdermal bite at any site or mucous membrane exposure in a canine rabies endemic region must be considered a potential exposure. It requires immediate vigorous wound cleansing, immune globulin (with wound injection), and vaccine treatment.[82,84]

Rabid vampire bats present an enormous economic problem for cattle ranchers as well as a risk to humans in Central and South America.[102] Bats are now the major cause of human rabies in North America and have also caused casualties among humans and domestic animals in northern and eastern Europe.[103] Rabies is known to be present among bats in Thailand[104] and has been reported from Omsk, Siberia (Ivan Kuzmin, personal communication) and from "rabies-free" Australia.[105] Both insect and fruit-eating bats are involved. Management of bat exposures present special problems as they are often not recognized, and it is not always known how transmission has taken place.[106,107] Current recommendations are that bat-cave explorers and handlers of bats should all receive pre-exposure vaccination. Subjects bitten by bats or those with close contact with a bat, particularly one that behaves unusually, are also potentially exposed. Subjects infected with HIV are at increased risk of rabies. They are known to develop a poor or no antibody response to rabies vaccination that correlates with low CD4 counts and a high viral load.[107,108] There are no scientifically proven guidelines that help manage a possible rabies exposure in such an individual. Exceptionally good wound care and infiltration with immune globulin and doubling the dose of vaccine is currently being recommended.[82,107,108]

Travelers to canine rabies endemic regions should consider having pre-exposure vaccination. This consists of one full intramuscular dose of any of the tissue or avian culture vaccines on days 0, 7, and 28.[108,109] The reduced-dose (less costly) intradermal regimen, using 0.1 mL of the vaccine on the same schedule, can also be used. However, it yields lower antibody titers with shorter endurance unless annual boosters are given.[110,111] If a person who had a prior pre-exposure or postexposure series has been rabies exposed, only two intramuscular or intradermal boosters on days 0 and 3 are given. There is no need to administer immune globulin to such a patient. Having received a full-dose intramuscular pre-exposure or intramuscular or intradermal postexposure series, using tissue culture vaccines, the patient maintains immune memory for at least 10 years.[112] Advantages of having pre-exposure vaccination when extensive travel or residence in a rabies endemic region is planned are:

1. There is no need for HRIG or ERIG if the subject is later exposed. Both may not be available or of unknown quality in many developing countries.
2. One eliminates the risk entailed in receiving a vaccine of uncertain quality or a dangerous nerve-tissue–derived product.

Persons moving to rabies-free countries with a valued pet face special problems. Most such destinations used to require quarantine for up to 6 months for any mammal.

This can be traumatic and costly. New studies by Blancou and Aubert in France have shown that a vaccinated dog, which has a high neutralizing rabies antibody titer, is not incubating rabies and is protected.[113] Efforts to change animal import regulations are now leading to revision of outdated quarantine rules.

REFERENCES

1. Shapiro CN. Transmission of hepatitis viruses. Ann Intern Med 1994;120:82–84.
2. Teo CG. The virology and serology of hepatitis: an overview. Commun Dis Rep CDR Rev 1992;2:109–114.
3. Lemon SM, Thomas DL. Vaccines to prevent viral hepatitis. N Engl J Med 1997;336:196–204.
4. Steffen R, Kane MA, Shapiro CN, et al. Epidemiology and prevention of hepatitis A in travelers. JAMA 1994;272:885–889.
5. Gutersohn T, Steffen R, Van Damme P, et al. Risk of hepatitis A infection in aircrews. Aviat Space Environ Med 1966;67:153–156.
6. Forbes A, Williams R. Increasing age — an important adverse prognostic factor in hepatitis A virus infection. J R Coll Physicians Lond 1988;22:237–239.
7. Jilg W, Deinhardt F, Hilleman MR. Hepatitis A vaccine. In: Plotkin, Mortimer, eds. Vaccines. 2nd Ed. WB Saunders, 1994:583–595.
8. Larouze B, Gaudebout C, Mercier G, et al. Infection with hepatitis A and B viruses in French volunteers working in tropical Africa. Am J Epidemiol 1987;126:31–37.
9. Steffen R. Risk of hepatitis B in travellers. Vaccine 1990;8(Suppl):S31–S32.
10. Dawson DG, Spivey GH, Korelitz JJ, Schmidt RT. Hepatitis B: risk to expatriates in South East Asia. BMJ 1987;294:547.
11. Helbling B, Reichen J. Reaktivierung einer Hepatitis B nach Absetzen von Chloroquin. Schweiz Med Wochenschr 1994;124:759–762.
12. Krugman S, Stevens CE. Hepatitis B vaccine. In: Plotkin, Mortimer, eds. Vaccines. 2nd Ed. WB Saunders, 1994:583–595.
13. Omata M. Treatment of chronic hepatitis B infection [editorial]. N Engl J Med 1998;339:114–115.
14. Choo QL, Weiner AJ, Overby LR, et al. Hepatitis C virus — the major causative agent of viral non-A, non-B hepatitis. Br Med Bull 1990;46:423–441.
15. Bukh J, Miller RH, Purcell RH. Genetic heterogeneity of hepatitis C virus: quasispecies and genotypes. Semin Liver Dis 1995;15:41–63.
16. Krawczynski K. Hepatitis E. Hepatology 1993;17:932–941.
17. Coursaget P, Depril N, Buisson Y, et al. Hepatitis type E in a French population: detection of anti-HEV by a synthetic peptide-based enzyme-linked immunosorbent assay. Res Virol 1994;145:51–57.
18. Jaenisch T, Preiser W, Berger A, et al. Emerging viral pathogens in long-term expatriates (I): hepatitis E virus. Trop Med Int Health 1997;2:885–891.
19. Skidmore SJ. Tropical aspects of viral hepatitis: hepatitis E. Trans R Soc Trop Med Hyg 1997;91:125–126.
20. Deka N, Sharma MD, Mukerjee R. Isolation of a novel agent from stool samples that is associated with sporadic non-A, non-B hepatitis. J Virol 1994;68:7810–7815.
21. Miyakawa Y, Mayumi M. Hepatitis G virus — a true hepatitis virus or an accidental tourist? N Engl J Med 1997;336:795–796.
22. Thisyakorn U, Thisyakorn C. Diseases caused by arboviruses-dengue haemorrhagic fever and Japanese B encephalitis. Med J Aust 1994;160:22–26.
23. Thisyakorn U, Nimmannitya S. Nutritional status of children with dengue hemorrhagic fever. Clin Infect Dis 1993;16:295–297.
24. Malasit P. Complement and dengue hemorrhagic fever/shock syndrome. Southeast Asian J Trop Med Public Health 1987;18:316–320.
25. Russel PK, Brandt WR. Immunopathologic processes and viral antigens associated with sequential dengue virus infection. Perspect Virol 1973;7:263–277.
26. Pavri KM, Prasad SR. T suppressor cells: role in dengue hemorrhagic fever and dengue shock syndrome. Rev Infect Dis 1980;2:142–146.
27. Halstead SB, O'Rourke EJ. Dengue virus and mononuclear phagocytes. I. Infection enhancement by non-neutralizing antibody. J Exp Med 1977;146:201–217.
28. Halstead SB, O'Rourke EJ, Allison AC. Dengue viruses and mononuclear phagocytes. II. Identity of blood and tissue leukocytes supporting in vitro infection. J Exp Med 1977;146:218–229.
29. Halstead SB. Immunological parameters of togavirus disease syndrome. In: Schlesinger RW, ed. The togaviruses. New York: Academic Press, 1980:107–173.
30. Halstead SB. The pathogenesis of dengue: molecular epidemiology in infectious disease. Am J Epidemiol 1981;114:632–648.
31. Ichiro K, Innis BL, Nimmannitya S, et al. Human immune responses to dengue viruses. Southeast Asian J Trop Med Public Health 1990;21:658–662.
32. Thisyakorn U, Nimmannitya S, Ningsanond V, Soogarun S. Atypical lymphocyte in dengue hemorrhagic fever: its value in diagnosis. Southeast Asian J Trop Med Public Health 1984;15:32–36.
33. Mitrakul C, Thisyakorn U. Hemostatic studies in dengue hemorrhagic fever. In: Suvatte V, Tuchinda M, eds. Proceedings of the 1st International Congress of Tropical Pediatrics, 1989 Nov 8–12, Bangkok, Thailand. Bangkok: Ruen Kaew Press, 1989:215–217.
34. Innis BL, Nisalak A, Nimmannitya S, et al. An enzyme-linked immunosorbent assay to characterize dengue infections where dengue and Japanese encephalitis co-circulate. Am J Trop Med Hyg 1989;40:418–427.
35. Thisyakorn U, Thisyakorn C. Dengue hemorrhagic fever: unusual manifestation and problems in management. JAMA SEA 1994;10:102–103.
36. Bhamarapravati N, Yoksan S. Live attenuated tetravalent dengue vaccine. In: Gubler DJ, Kuno G, eds. Dengue and dengue hemorrhagic fever. Oxon: CAB International, 1997:367–377.
37. Trent DW, Kinney RM, Huang CYH. Recombinant dengue virus vaccines. In: Gubler DJ, Kuno G, eds. Dengue and dengue hemorrhagic fever. Oxon: CAB International, 1997:379–403.
38. Ablashi DV, Huang AT, Pagano JS, et al. Epstein-Barr virus and human disease. Clifton, NJ: Humana Press, 1990.
39. Dan R, Chang S. A prospective study of primary Epstein-Barr virus infection among university students in Hong Kong. Am J Trop Med Hyg 1990;42:380–385.
40. Committee in Infectious Diseases, American Academy of Pediatrics. Epstein-Barr virus infections. In: Report of the Committee on Infectious Diseases. 24th Ed. Elk Grove Village: American Academy of Pediatrics, 1997:199–201.
41. Lanier A, Bender T, Talbot M, et al. Nasopharyngeal carcinoma in Alaskan Eskimos, Indians and Aleuts. Cancer 1980;46:2100–2106.

42. Li Lung M, Chang RS, Huang ML, et al. Epstein-Barr virus genotypes associated with nasopharyngeal carcinoma in Southern China. Virology 1990;177:44–53.

43. Henle W, Henle G, Lennette T. The Epstein-Barr virus. Sci Am 1979;241:48–57.

44. Evans AS, Mueller NE. Viruses and cancer. Casual association. Ann Epidemiol 1990;1:71–92.

45. Epstein-Barr virus and AIDS-associated lymphomas [editorial]. Lancet 1991;2:979–980.

46. Miller G. The switch between latency and replication of Epstein-Barr virus. J Infect Dis 1990;161:833–844.

47. Landay AL, Jessop C, Lennette ET, Levy JA. Chronic fatigue syndrome: clinical condition associated with immune activity. Lancet 1991;2:707–711.

48. Sham JST, Wei WI, Yong-Sheng Z, et al. Detection of subclinical nasopharyngeal carcinoma by fiberoptic endoscopy and multiple biopsy. Lancet 1990;1:371–374.

49. Thisyakorn U, Thisyakorn C. Studies on flaviviruses in Thailand. In: Miyai K, Kanno T, Ishikawa E, eds. Progress in clinical biochemistry: proceedings of the 5th Asian-Pacific Congress of Clinical Biochemistry, Sep 29–Oct 4, 1991, Kobe, Japan. Amsterdam: Excerpta Medica, 1992: 985–987.

50. Thisyakorn U, Nimmannitya S. Japanese encephalitis in Thai children, Bangkok, Thailand. Southeast Asian J Trop Med Public Health 1985;16:93–97.

51. Burke DS, Nisalak A, Ussery MA. Antibody capture immunoassay detection of Japanese encephalitis virus immunoglobulin M and G antibodies in cerebrospinal fluid. J Clin Microbiol 1982;16:1034–1042.

52. Hoke CH, Vaughn DW, Nisalak A, et al. The effect of high-dose dexamethasone on the outcome of acute encephalitis due to Japanese encephalitis virus. J Infect Dis 1992;165:631–637.

53. Harinasuta C, Nimmannitya S, Thisyakorn U, Hiranyachote U. A clinical trial of interferon-alpha on Japanese encephalitis in Thailand. Southeast Asian J Trop Med Public Health 1989;20:656–657.

54. Burke DS, Lorsomrudee W, Leake CJ, et al. Fatal outcome in Japanese encephalitis. Am J Trop Med Hyg 1985;34: 1203–1210.

55. Johnson RT, Burke DS, Elwell M, et al. Japanese encephalitis: immunocytochemical studies of viral antigen and inflammatory cells in fatal cases. Ann Neurol 1985;18:567–573.

56. Hoke CH, Nisalak A, Sangawhipa N, et al. Protection against Japanese encephalitis by inactivated vaccines. N Engl J Med 1988;319:608–614.

57. Burke DS, Leake CJ. Japanese B encephalitis. In: Monath TP, ed. The arboviruses: epidemiology and ecology. Boca Raton, FL: CRC Press, 1988:3:63–92.

58. Kitaoka M. Shift of age distribution of cases of Japanese encephalitis in Japan during the period 1950–1967. In: Hammon McD, Kitaoka M, Downs WG, eds. Immunization for Japanese encephalitis. Amsterdam: Excerpta Medica, 1972:285–291.

59. Chatavedi UC, Mathur A, Chandra A, et al. Transplacental infection with Japanese encephalitis virus. J Infect Dis 1980;141:712–725.

60. Ketel WB, Ognibene AJ. Japanese B encephalitis in Vietnam. Am J Med Sci 1971;261:271–279.

61. Centers for Disease Control. Inactivated Japanese encephalitis vaccine. Recommendations of the advisory committee on immunization practices. MMWR Morb Mortal Wkly Rep 1993;42:1–15.

62. MacDonald WBG, Tink AR, Ouvrier RA, et al. Japanese encephalitis after a two-week holiday in Bali. Med J Aust 1989;150:334–336.

63. Oya A. Japanese encephalitis vaccine. Acta Pediatr Jpn 1988;30:175–184.

64. Marcus LC. Liability for vaccine-related injuries. N Engl J Med 1988;318:191.

65. Thisyakorn U, Thisyakorn C, Wilde H. Japanese encephalitis and international travel. J Travel Med 1994;2:37–40.

66. Brandt WE. World Health Organization. Development of dengue and Japanese encephalitis vaccines. J Infect Dis 1990;162:577–582.

67. Markowitz LE, Tomasi A, Hawkins CE, et al. International measles importations United States, 1980–85. Int J Epidemiol 1988;17:187–192.

68. Centers for Disease Control. Measles—United States, 1995. MMWR Morb Mortal Wkly Rep 1996;45:306–307.

69. Committee on Infectious Diseases, American Academy of Pediatrics. Measles. In: Report of the Committee on Infectious Diseases. 24th Ed. Elk Grove Village: American Academy of Pediatrics, 1997:344–357.

70. Hatz C, Wilde H, Thisyakorn C, et al. Other important viral infections in travelers. In: DuPont HL, Steffen R, eds. Textbook of travel medicine and health. Hamilton, ON: BC Decker, 1997:215–222.

71. Committee on Infectious Diseases, American Academy of Pediatrics. Poliovirus infections. In: Report of the Committee on Infectious Diseases. 24th Ed. Elk Grove Village: American Academy of Pediatrics, 1997:424–433.

72. Kubli D, Steffen R, Schar M. Importation of poliomyelitis to industrialized nations between 1975 and 1984: evaluation and conclusions for vaccination recommendations. BMJ 1987; 295:169–171.

73. Gardner P, Schaffner W. Immunization of adults. N Engl J Med 1993;328:1252–1258.

74. Canada Communicable Disease Report. Community surveillance for wild poliovirus in Ontario, 1993. Can Med Assoc J 1995;152:1997–2000.

75. Wright PF, Kim-Farley RJ, de Quadros CA. Strategies for the global eradication of poliomyelitis by the year 2000. N Engl J Med 1991;325:1774–1779.

76. World Health Organization. World survey of rabies no. 32. Geneva: WHO, 1996.

77. Sehgal S, Bhattacharya D, Bhardwaj M. Ten year longitudinal study of efficacy and safety of purified chick embryo cell vaccine for pre and postexposure prophylaxis of rabies in Indian population. J Commun Dis 1995;27:36–43.

78. World Health Organization. The world health report. Life in the 21st Century. Geneva: WHO, 1998.

79. Fishbein DB, Robinson DVM. Rabies. N Engl J Med 1993;329:1632–1638.

80. Hatz CF, Bidaux JM, Eichenberger K, et al. Circumstances and management of 72 animal bites among long-term residents in the tropics. Vaccine 1995;13:811–815.

81. Phanuphak P, Ubolyam S, Sirivichayakul S. Should a traveler in rabies endemic areas receive preexposure rabies immunization? Ann Med Intern 1994;145:409–411.

82. World Health Organization. WHO expert committee on rabies. WHO technical report series 824. Geneva: WHO, 1992.

83. Parviz S, Luby S, Wilde H. Postexposure treatment of rabies in Pakistan. Clin Infect Dis 1998;27:751–756.

84. Wilde H, Chutivongse S, Tepsumethanon W, et al. Rabies in Thailand. Rev Infect Dis 1991;13:644–652.

85. Smith JS, Fishbein DB, Rupprecht CE, et al. Unexplained rabies in three immigrants in the United States; a virological investigation. N Engl J Med 1991;324:205–211.

86. Hemachudha T, Mitrabhakdi E. Rabies. In: Davis LE, ed. Infectious diseases of the nervous system. Oxford: Butterworth, Heinemann, 2000.

87. World Health Organization. Recommendations on rabies post-exposure treatment and the correct technique of intradermal immunization against rabies. WHO/EMC/Zoo 96.6. Geneva: WHO, 1996.

88. Chutivongse S, Wilde H, Supich C, et al. Postexposure prophylaxis for rabies with antiserum and intradermal vaccination. Lancet 1990;335:896–898.

89. Chutivongse S, Wilde H, Fishbein DB, et al. One-year study of the 2-1-1 intramuscular postexposure rabies vaccine regimen in severely exposed Thai patients using rabies immune globulin and Vero cell rabies vaccine. Vaccine 1991;9: 573–576.

90. Wilde H, Tipkong P, Khawplod P. Economic issues in postexposure rabies treatment. J Travel Med 1999;6:238–242.

91. Langs J, Simanjuntak S, Soerjosembodo C, et al. Suppressant effect of human or equine rabies immunoglobulins on the immunogenicity of post-exposure rabies vaccination under the 2-1-1 regimen: a field trial in Indonesia. Bull WHO 1998; 76:491–495.

92. Fishbein DB, Yenne KM, Dreesen DW, et al. Risk factor for systemic hypersensitivity reactions after booster vaccinations with human diploid cell rabies vaccine: a nationwide prospective study. Vaccine 1993;11:1390–1394.

93. Chutivongse S, Wilde H, Benjavogkulchai M, et al. Postexposure rabies vaccination during pregnancy; experience with 202 cases and their infants. Clin Infect Dis 1994;20: 818–820.

94. Wilde H, Chomchey P, Punyaratabandu P, et al. Purified equine rabies immune globulin; a safe and affordable alternative to human rabies immune globulin. Bull WHO 1989; 67:731–736.

95. Tantawichien T, Benjavongkulchai M, Wilde H, et al. Value of skin testing for predicting reactions to equine rabies immune globulin. Clin Infect Dis 1995;21:550–562.

96. Wilde H, Sirikawin S, Sabcharoen A, et al. Failure of postexposure treatment of rabies in children. Clin Infect Dis 1996; 22:228–232.

97. Wilde H, Bhanganada K, Chutivongse S, et al. Is injection of contaminated animal bite wounds with rabies immune globulin a safe practice? Trans R Soc Trop Med Hyg 1992;86: 86–88.

98. Khawplod P, Wilde H, Chomchey P, et al. What is an acceptable delay in rabies immune globulin administration when vaccine alone has been given previously? Vaccine 1996;14: 389–391.

99. Smith PC, Lawhaswasdi K, Vick WE, Stanton JS. Enzootic rabies in rodents in Thailand. Nature 1968;217:954–955.

100. Wimalaratne O. Is it necessary to give rabies postexposure treatment after rodent (rats, mice, squirrels and bandicoots) bites? Ceylon Med J 1997;42:144.

101. Sage G, Khawplod P, Wilde H, et al. Immune response to rabies vaccine in Alaskan dogs; failure to achieve a consistently protective antibody response. Trans R Soc Trop Med Hyg 1993;87:593–595.

102. Sivasontiwat D, Lumbertdacha B, Polsuwan C, et al. Rabies: is provocation of a biting dog relevant for risk assessment? Trans R Soc Trop Med Hyg 1992;86:443.

103. Schneider MC, Santos-Burgoa C, Aron J, et al. Potential force of infection of human rabies transmitted by vampire bats in the Amazonian region of Brazil. Am J Trop Med Hyg 1996; 55:680–684.

104. Noah DL, Drenzek CL, Smith JS, et al. Epidemiology of human rabies in the United States 1980–1996. Ann Intern Med 1998;128:922–930.

105. Smith PC, Lawhaswadi K, Vick WE, Stanton JS. Isolation of rabies virus from fruit bats in Thailand. Nature 1967;216:384.

106. Torvaldsen S, Watson T. Rabies prophylaxis in Western Australia; the impact of Australian bat lyssavirus. Commun Dis Intell 1998;22:149–152.

107. Debbie JG, Trimarchi CV. Prophylaxis for suspected exposure to bat rabies. Lancet 1997;350:1790–1791.

108. Jaijaroensup W, Khawplod P, Tantawichien T, et al. Rabies postexposure vaccination in patients with human immunodeficiency virus infection. Clin Infect Dis 1999;28:913–914.

109. Thisyakorn U, Ruxrungtham K, Khawplod P, et al. Safety and immunogenicity of preexposure rabies immunization in HIV1-infected children. Clin Infect Dis 2000;30:218.

110. Bernard KW, Fishbein DB. Preexposure rabies prophylaxis for travelers; are the benefits worth the cost? Vaccine 1991;11:833–836.

111. Wilde H. Preexposure rabies vaccination. J Travel Med 1994;1:51–54.

112. Kositprapa C, Limsuwun K, Wilde H, et al. Immune response to simulated postexposure rabies booster vaccination in volunteers who received preexposure vaccination. Clin Infect Dis 1997;25:614–616.

113. Bernard KW, Fishbein DB, Miller KD, et al. Preexposure rabies immunization with human diploid cell vaccine; decreased antibody responses in persons immunized in developing countries. Am J Trop Med Hyg 1985;34:633–647.

Chapter 26

BACTERIAL INFECTIONS

GIAMPIERO CAROSI, ALBERTO MATTEELLI, AND HENRY WILDE

INTRODUCTION

Bacterial infections continue to cause considerable morbidity and mortality despite the availability of effective therapeutic and preventive measures. The geographic distribution of a few bacterial infections is limited to the tropical belt, and primary cases of the disease are not observed outside the respective endemic areas. However, most bacterial infections, although widespread worldwide, are more prevalent in the Southern Hemisphere. Both environmental and socioeconomic factors (i.e., poorer hygiene and living conditions, lower coverage of childhood immunization campaigns, wider spreading of zoonotic infections) may account for these differences.

The most frequent bacterial infections acquired in the tropics are probably infected wounds, caused by common streptococcal and staphylococcal bacteria. Bacteria are also responsible for the majority of cases of travelers' diarrhea, sexually transmitted diseases, and cases of community-acquired meningitis and respiratory tract infections. These conditions are dealt with in other chapters of this book. Here we review bacterial infections of specific tropical interest and a few cosmopolitan bacterial infections that frequently affect travelers.

The awareness of the importance of some of these conditions has increased considerably in recent years. The number of cases of active disease and late consequence of Buruli ulcer has increased, bringing this disease high on the agenda of national governments and international organizations. During the 1990s, human plague and epidemic typhus have re-emerged from the past and caused large epidemics, resulting in travel and trade disruption with severe economic repercussions. New bacterial pathogens continue to emerge as a cause of significant mortality and morbidity: new insight is now available on several species of the genus *Bartonella* (strictly related to the agent of Carrión's disease) and on the members of the new genus, *Ehrlichia*. Finally, a renewed interest in anthrax has emerged for the potential use of its lethal toxin in biologic warfare and the associated risks of unpredictable recurrences in the future from soil reservoirs.

BURULI ULCER

ETIOLOGY, TRANSMISSION, AND PATHOGENESIS

Mycobacterium ulcerans, a slow-growing photochromogen *Mycobacterium* belonging to Group II of the Runyon classification, is the etiologic agent of Buruli ulcer, an emerging cutaneous disease of specific tropical interest, first reported in 1948 from Australia. *M. ulcerans* is thought to be present in the soil,[1] vegetation, and water.[2] It is thought to penetrate the dermis through thorn pricks or other injuries. Case-to-case transmission is unusual.

The pathogen multiplies in the dermis, developing a necrotizing panniculitis; extension to bone or dissemination through the blood stream is rare. Unlike other mycobacteria, *M. ulcerans* produces a necrotizing toxin that suppresses the immune system. In the dermis necrosis of fat and fibrous tissues and vasculitis are the prominent pathologic features. Infiltration with macrophages similar to a typical tuberculin-like granuloma is present. The inflammatory reaction is responsible for the development of the chronic, ulcerated lesions, which may heal spontaneously or may progress until large areas of skin are destroyed. Spontaneous healing often occurs due to a specific host immune reaction.

GEOGRAPHIC DISTRIBUTION AND SPECIAL POPULATIONS AT RISK

Buruli ulcer affects immunocompetent hosts and is the third most common mycobacterial infection after tuberculosis and leprosy.[3] It occurs in isolated foci of Africa, Asia, Latin America, and the Western Pacific.[4] In the African continent, it was first extensively described from Uganda (the name is derived from a Ugandan region) and Zaire, but it is now common in West Africa along the Gulf of Guinea (Benin, Ghana, Cameroon, Gabon, Nigeria, Liberia, and Ivory Coast). In some villages of Ghana, up to one-quarter of the entire population may be affected.

The disease is mainly reported in children and women who live in rural tropical villages close to rivers and wetlands. There is no evidence of an increased risk of infection in subjects living in the same household with patients. Although long-term travelers may occasionally be affected, short-term travelers have a very limited risk of infection.

CASE MANAGEMENT

In Buruli ulcer, the lesion is localized to the limbs and less frequently to the thorax or abdomen.[5] It starts as a painless swelling of the skin and develops into a nodule and then an ulcer in a few weeks or months. Ulcers are usually single and painless, may reach 20 cm in diameter, and have characteristic deep, undermined edges with possible tunnel formation (Figure 26–1). Subcutaneous tissues are necrotic. Local lymphadenopathy is present when bacterial superinfection occurs. The duration of the ulcer ranges from a few months to years. Scars and tendon retractions due to spontaneous or surgical healing represent a major problem in Buruli ulcers.

Buruli ulcer should be considered in the diagnosis of tropical ulcers and should be differentiated from many other diseases: ecthyma (staphylococcal or streptococcal infection), cutaneous leishmaniasis, tropical phagedenic ulcer, yaws, and fungal infections. Diagnostic investigation starts with direct microscopic examination of a swab of the base of the ulcer, which demonstrates acid-fast bacilli; differentiation from other mycobacteria is not possible morphologically. Biopsy and histologic examination may reveal typical granulomata. Culture isolation of the pathogen is difficult and slow. Identification by polymerase chain reaction (PCR) has recently been described.[6]

The treatment of Buruli ulcer is difficult.[7] Many antibiotics are active against *M. ulcerans* in vitro but have little effect in vivo. No antibiotic combination has demonstrated clinical effectiveness to date. Surgical excision and repeated skin grafting are the treatment of choice, but scars and tendon retractions cause restricted movements of the limbs and other permanent disabilities. Current control approaches therefore focus on early recognition and excision of nodules. Education is essential to motivate individuals to seek treatment at an early stage of the disease. The World Health Organization (WHO) has established the Global Buruli Ulcer Initiative to raise awareness of the importance of the diseases and to coordinate control efforts.

PREVENTION

Bacille Calmette-Guérin (BCG) vaccination was reported to provide some short-term protection and to decrease the duration of the ulcer. In general, however, there are no specific measures to prevent Buruli ulcer and other atypical mycobacteria infections due to the widespread distribution of the agents and an incomplete understanding of specific risk behaviors.

LEPROSY

ETIOLOGY, TRANSMISSION, AND PATHOGENESIS

Leprosy is one of the most feared human diseases, which has affected deeply the history of medicine and is still of interest at the beginning of the third millennium. *M. leprae*, the causative organism of leprosy, is an acid-fast bacillus that shares several antigenic properties with other mycobacteria. Its classification in the genus *Mycobacterium* is based on antigenic characterization and recently confirmed by genetic analysis. *M. leprae* has never been isolated by culture; it only replicates in the footpad of the normal mouse and produces systemic infection in the early-thymectomized mouse and in the nine-handed armadillo. It has a remarkably slow rate of growth in the animal model (the generation time has been calculated as 12 days), which is consistent with the extremely long incubation period of the disease in humans.

Man is the only source and reservoir of infection. Person-to-person transmission occurs through inhalation

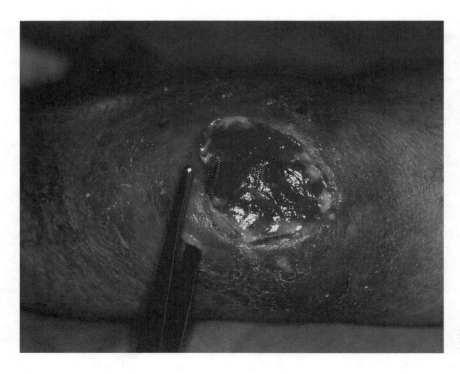

Figure 26–1. Cutaneous lesion in Buruli ulcer disease. To view this figure in color, refer to CD-ROM.

or skin-to-skin contact. The relative importance of these two methods has not been clearly established. However, it is thought that most cases are caused by inhalation of mycobacteria discharged from the nasal mucosa of infected patients.

M. leprae is a pathogen with poor pathogenicity. Serologic studies in populations of endemic areas show a high rate of infection, but development of the disease occurs in a very small proportion of infected subjects. In addition, self-healing of early lesions is common. *M. leprae* is an intracellular pathogen that penetrates through the intact mucosa or skin and invades Schwann cells of the peripheral nervous system and subsequently interferes with neural cell functions, causing significant damage to peripheral nerves and leaving patients with disabilities and deformities.[8] The bacterium may be phagocytized by macrophages, where it survives apparently in an inactive stage; infected macrophages develop into epithelioid cells, merge to form multinucleated giant cells, and determine the formation of typical granulomas.

Resistance to disease is probably multifactorial, including genetic determinants of susceptibility and environmental factors such as crowding, diet, and the intensity and duration of exposure to the organism. Most, if not all, of the pathogenicity of *M. leprae* is thought to be determined by the host immune response. The immune system may completely overwhelm the infection so that no sign of disease occurs. Alternatively, a few bacilli may survive and develop new granulomas that will appear in the tuberculoid clinical form of leprosy. In the case of a deficient immune response, bacteria can spread freely through the skin and into peripheral nerves and diffuse to multiple sites via the bloodstream, giving the lepromatous form of the disease. In these cases, the lack of cellular immune response is not a passive process but is the result of a local prevalence of CD8+ lymphocytes conferring a suppressive action over CD4+ lymphocyte helper action.

GEOGRAPHIC DISTRIBUTION AND SPECIAL POPULATIONS AT RISK

Leprosy is prevalent only in regions situated in the intertropical belt, and highest detection rates are observed in some Pacific Islands, Southeastern Africa, West Africa, and Southeast Asia.[9] Throughout the world, the leprosy prevalence rate was reduced by 85% since 1985, mainly as a consequence of the implementation of multidrug chemotherapy.[10] In 1997, 113 countries notified to WHO a total number of 642,167, which represents an increase of 16% in leprosy detection rate compared to the previous year.[11] The top three leprosy-endemic countries, Brazil, India, and Indonesia, report 85% of the global leprosy case detection.

Since prolonged and intimate contact with infectious cases is required for transmission of the disease, travelers are not considered at risk for leprosy. Sporadic reports of leprosy in tourists visiting the tropics do not affect the general validity of this statement.

CASE MANAGEMENT

Leprosy is a disease with a wide clinical spectrum. A five-group classification system based on bacteriology, immunology, and histology has been devised that shows remarkable correlation with clinical features.[12] Indeterminate leprosy corresponds to the first appearance of disease and may develop toward spontaneous healing, lepromatous leprosy, or tuberculoid leprosy. It is characterized by isolated or occasionally multiple skin lesions. These lesions are hypopigmented macules with sharp margins, hypoesthesia on the margins, and sometimes hyperesthesia in the interior. On biopsy, granulomas may be seen, but bacilli are rare. Bacilli are not recovered from the nasal mucosa and the Mitsuda skin reaction is negative. In progressive disease, lepromatous or tuberculoid leprosy develops within a few months. These forms represent the poles of a unique entity. All of the intermediate situations are possible, and one form may turn into the other as a consequence of therapy or precipitating conditions like pregnancy, which change the immune response to infection. Tuberculoid leprosy is determined by an active immune response. Neuropathy is represented by peripheral polyneuritis, which is characteristically superficial and hypertrophic (nerves may be palpated as thick and firm cords). Nerve pain and paraesthesia are followed by anesthesia when the distal segments of peripheral nerves are replaced by fibrous tissue. Sensory nerve loss is responsible for traumatic injuries with progressive mutilation of the extremities. Late manifestations of neuropathy are paralysis, amyotrophy, and tendon retraction. Skin lesions consist of scanty infiltrated macules with relevated borders. Histologically, epithelioid granulomas are prevalent with very few or absent bacilli. The Mitsuda reaction is strongly positive. Lepromatous leprosy is determined by a decrease of the specific immune response to the organism. Skin manifestations predominate with numerous symmetric papular lesions that develop into nodules and frequently ulcerate. Sensation is preserved or slightly decreased. The nodules contain a large number of bacilli in the absence of granulomas. Bacilli are found in nasal mucosa and the Mitsuda reaction is frequently absent. Neurologic signs are similar to those of the tuberculoid form but occur later and progress more slowly.

Leprosy is a chronic disease that should first be suspected on clinical grounds. The association of skin lesions and peripheral nerve palsies is evocative, especially in subjects with possible exposure to the pathogen. Diagnosis and clinical classification of the disease is based on the presence of acid-fast bacilli in epithelial biopsies, the presence of granulomas on pathologic section, and the Mitsuda reaction. A species-specific antigen, designated by Gly-1, has been recently identified and may become important for serodiagnosis in the future.

As in the case of tuberculosis, leprosy treatment is based on regimens containing two or more drugs for prolonged periods of time. Rifampin and, to a lesser extent, clofazimine are the drugs with the highest bactericidal action against *M. leprae*. They have recently joined dapsone, the major drug for treatment of leprosy since the late 1940s. Treatment schedules depend on the clinical form of disease. Multibacillary cases are usually treated with three drugs for at least 2 years or until smears are negative. Paucibacillary cases usually need a rifampin-dapsone combination for a 6- to 36-month period. Beyond chemotherapy for the mycobacterial infection, leprosy still raises great concern for the estimated 2 to 3 million patients who have residual deformities as a result of past leprosy and who need specific rehabilitation programs.

PREVENTION

There is consistent evidence that improved socioeconomic conditions contribute to the reduction of leprosy in the community irrespective of the intensity of leprosy control activities. Only patients with multibacillary lepromatous leprosy who do not receive specific treatment are likely to transmit the disease by direct human contact. Transmission by indirect contact by bacilliferous patients cannot be ruled out but is uncommon. For this reason, the isolation of patients is ineffective, expensive, and not recommended. Infection control measures are based on early detection and effective treatment of cases. The efficacy of multidrug therapy in curing patients, preventing relapses, and minimizing side effects has prompted WHO to endorse a goal of global elimination of leprosy as a public health problem by the year 2000.

ENDEMIC TREPONEMATOSIS

ETIOLOGY, TRANSMISSION, AND PATHOGENESIS

The term nonvenereal treponematosis designates a group of three diseases: yaws, pinta, and bejel (or endemic syphilis), potentially disabling and disfiguring infections caused by closely related spirochetes belonging to the genus *Treponema*, *Treponema pertenue*, *Treponema carateum*, and *Treponema pallidum*, respectively. Although the etiologic agents of bejel and syphilis are designated with the same species name, they are thought to be biologically different. All treponema, however, are believed to have evolved from a common ancestor spirochete and are very closely related to the agent of venereal syphilis from which they are morphologically indistinguishable.

The major characteristic of nonvenereal treponematoses is that they are not transmitted by sexual intercourse. They are acquired during childhood by skin-to-skin contact with infected individuals with primary lesions. Humans are the only known reservoir of the infections.

Spirochetes enter the body through the skin and replicate actively at the site of initial inoculation, producing a primary lesion. Such lesions, which possess peculiar characteristics for each of the treponematosis, contain large numbers of bacteria and are highly infectious. At a secondary stage, spirochetes invade the bloodstream and disseminate to the target organs. After several years, 10% to 20% of untreated patients develop late complications typical of the tertiary phase. There are many similarities between the pathogenicity of syphilis and nonvenereal

treponematosis, probably due to a hypersensitivity immune reaction to spirochetal antigens. Granulomatous lesions developing in deep organs lead to fibrosis, tissue destruction, and necrosis. These lesions contain very few spirochetes and carry a small risk of infection. The histologic features are similar to that of syphilitic gummas.

GEOGRAPHIC DISTRIBUTION AND SPECIAL POPULATIONS AT RISK

In the 1950s, there were an estimated 50 million cases of nonvenereal treponematosis worldwide. With a WHO-UNICEF-assisted global control program, the burden of endemic treponematosis was drastically reduced by the mid 1960s; however, none were eradicated and endemic foci remained, giving the chance of resurgence of the disease in patchy areas. The geographic distribution of nonvenereal treponematosis in the early 1990s is shown in Figure 26–2. Bejel is confined to Africa and pinta to South and Central America, where most cases are detected in isolated indian tribes of Mexico and the Amazon basin. Yaws is widespread in the tropics. Central and West Africa are the regions most affected by the resurgence of the disease and residual foci persist in Chad, Ethiopia, and Sudan. Asia, the Pacific rim, Pakistan, the Solomon Islands, and Indonesia continue reporting cases of yaws.

Nonvenereal treponematoses are presently confined to poor populations with low standards of hygiene. Cases are located in remote areas where access to health care is difficult or nonexistent.[13] Children 5 to 15 years of age are most often affected.

CASE MANAGEMENT

The incubation period is 3 to 5 weeks. The primary lesion in yaws is a small, raised, nonindurated papule that grows and ulcerates superficially. It is not painful unless secondary bacterial infections occur. In bejel, the primary lesion at the site of inoculation is rarely seen. In the case of pinta, the initial lesion is an erythematous papule that does not ulcerate, increases in size, and assumes psoriasis-like features. The secondary stage is characterized by the septicemic dissemination of spirochetes to the skin and mucosa and the development of multiple lesions far from the inoculation site.[14] Any region can be affected, but moist areas are the most common site of disseminated lesions. Papillomata and maculopapular lesions are observed in yaws and bejel. These lesions resolve spontaneously in a few months. Yaws and bejel, but not pinta, are characterized by osseous involvement. Early lesions include periostitis of the long bones (tibia), giving nocturnal pain and polydactylitis of the small joints of the hand and foot. Both yaws and bejel develop late, characteristic, skeletal abnormalities like the saber tibia. In all treponematosis, systemic constitutional symptoms are not present during either the primary or the secondary stage. In the tertiary stage, several years later, gummas develop in the bones, joints, and facial cartilages causing severe destruction and deformity. Secondary lesions in pinta initially resemble the primary one. They do not disappear

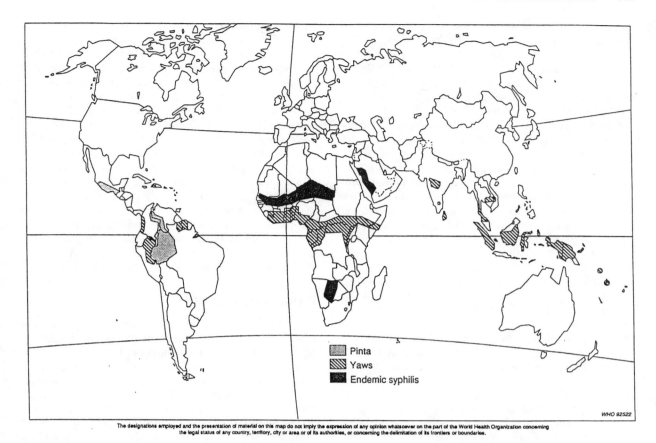

Figure 26–2. Map distribution of endemic treponematosis.

and represent the only late sign of the disease, evolving into large dischromic areas of atrophic skin.

Treponemes cannot be grown in culture, but direct identification from primary and secondary skin lesions is usually possible. The method of choice is the dark-field examination of the exudate, which shows actively motile spirochetes. During latent or tertiary stages, positive serologic tests are the only diagnostic clue. The same nontreponemic (VDRL, RPR) and treponemic (TPHA, FTA-ABS) tests used for syphilis are helpful for serologic diagnosis. Cross-reactivity (but not cross-protection) between all treponematosis is thought to be complete, raising important problems of test interpretation, at least in the sexually active populations from endemic areas who may be exposed to several treponemes.

Treatment is based on long-acting parenteral penicillin G. Single doses of 0.6 to 1.2 million units are considered universally effective in eradicating the infection, although reduced susceptibility to penicillin of *T. pertenue* has recently been reported from Papua New Guinea.[15] In penicillin-allergic patients, tetracyclines and erythromycin given for a 10-day course may be used.

PREVENTION

At the community level, case finding, contact tracing, and treatment of cases and contacts are the latest strategies for control of endemic treponematoses, following the previ-

ously successful mass treatment campaign of the 1950s and 1960s. At the individual level, prevention is based on avoidance of close personal contact with subjects who have primary or secondary lesions. Since affected populations are poor inhabitants in isolated communities, nonvenereal treponematoses do not represent a significant hazard to travelers.

RELAPSING FEVER

ETIOLOGY, TRANSMISSION, AND PATHOGENESIS

The agents of relapsing fever are spirochetes of the genus *Borrelia*. They measure 5 to 40 μm in length and 0.5 μm in diameter and display active corkscrew-like motility due to the presence of flagella. Like other spirochetes (*Treponema* and *Leptospira*), *Borreliae* are best seen in wet preparations by dark-field or phase-contrast microscopy; however, they can also be seen in fixed preparations using aniline dyes. Relapsing fever diseases may be grouped according to the vector species responsible for transmission, being either lice or ticks. *B. recurrentis* is the only species of the louse-borne relapsing fever (LBRF), transmitted by the human body louse (*Pediculus humanus*). There is no known animal reservoir of *B. recurrentis*. Tick-borne relapsing fever (TBRF) presents as an endemic or sporadic disease due to several other species of *Borrelia* with different geographic distribution: *B. duttoni* in tropical Africa, *B. hispanica* in the Mediterranean, *B. persica* in Middle-East Asia, *B. hermsi* in North America, and *B. venezuelensis* in Central South America are among the most diffused ones. In TBRF, the vector is a soft tick of the genus *Ornithodoros* and the reservoir of infection are wild rodents; an exception is represented by *B. duttoni* in tropical Africa, for which humans appear to be the only natural reservoir.

The cycle of borrelia spirochetes differs in LBRF and TBRF. In the first case, the cycle of infection is simply from person to person via the louse. Lice acquire the infection by biting a spirochetemic human: spirochetes survive in the louse for its entire lifespan, distributed in the hemolymph but not in the salivary glands. Transmission occurs when an infected louse is crushed on the skin; spirochetes are released and penetrate through a bite site or the intact skin. In the case of ticks, on the contrary, the bacteria are present in the saliva and are transmitted while the vector assumes its blood meal. The bacteria are maintained in the tick for its entire life up to 15 years; transovarian transmission to the offspring of the tick has also been demonstrated, so that ticks that had never come in contact with infected animals may be infested.

The periodic cycling of acute and afebrile episodes that names the disease is associated with dramatic changes in the abundance of spirochetes circulating in the blood; each new cycle is due to spirochetes showing critical changes in serotype and major immunogenic lipoprotein of the bacterial outer surface.[16] Borrelia spirochetes are confined predominantly to the plasma space of their mammalian hosts. They have no recognized endo- or exotoxins, do not elicit acute inflammation, and do not produce abscesses. The pathogenic mechanism is represented by the activation of plasma proteins and stimulation of cytokine production. Interleukin-1, produced by mononuclear phagocytes, is responsible for fever. Hypotension and disseminated intravascular coagulation are seen in severe cases and during the Jarisch-Herxheimer reaction (JHR). Such reaction, during which patients are at greatest risk of dying, is due to the massive liberation of tumor necrosis factor provoked by bacterial lysis.[17] Immunity develops after few relapses but is short-lasting and is strictly species-specific. It is represented mainly by antiborrelial antibodies that can agglutinate, opsonize, or kill the spirochetes. The spleen and other organs of the reticuloendothelial system play an important role in clearance of opsonized bacteria.

GEOGRAPHIC DISTRIBUTION AND SPECIAL POPULATIONS AT RISK

LBRF is virtually cosmopolitan and presents as epidemic outbreaks. After the last large epidemic during World War II, the number of notified cases decreased significantly in recent years, but LBRF is still observed in Ethiopia and Sudan where it determines an estimate of more than 10,000 cases per year. LBRF is a condition linked to poverty, overcrowding, poor hygiene, and housing. Epidemics are reported among troops involved in war campaigns in Africa and in refugee camps. Health personnel in the camps may be at increased risk of the disease.

TBRF is widespread worldwide, presenting as endemic disease with focal outbreaks. Cases are reported from most of Africa, central Asia, the Mediterranean, and South, Central, and North America. Only Oceania is thought to be free from relapsing fever. Tropical Africa is particularly affected: in the region of Dodoma, Tanzania, more than 60,000 cases are reported per annum[18]; in Rwanda, up to 6% of all consultations at a health center were due to TBRF[19]; and during an outbreak in Zaire, more than half of the acute fever cases were due to TBRF.[20] In TBRF, humans represent an occasional host: those at risk of infection are campers in rural areas who can come in contact with wild rodents and their ticks. The exception is TBRF due to *B. duttoni*, as exposure is in this case linked to housing conditions: in Tanzania, up to 90% of village houses may be infested by ticks.[18]

CASE MANAGEMENT

The clinical presentation of different forms of relapsing fever is similar. The severity of the disease is usually higher in LBRF. The incubation period varies from 4 to 18 days. Fever is the most important clinical sign of the acute phase with an abrupt onset accompanied by shaking chills, headache, and fatigue. Most symptoms of a flu-like illness, such as myalgia, arthralgia, dry cough, and abdominal pain, are also present. Fever and the other symptoms last for a period of 1 to 17 days (with a mean of 3); in most patients, they are continuous during the day. The fatality rate of untreated cases may be as high as 30% during LBRF. Complications consist of hypotension, disseminated intravascular coagulation, liver failure, neurologic impairment, lethargy, and polyneuritis. Neurologic involvement (primarily demonstrated by meningismus and facial palsy) is present in up to one-quarter of patients with relapsing fever, a proportion that is similar to that observed during the course of Lyme disease.[21] Thrombocytopenia is common in TBRF but major bleeding complications are rare in this condition.[22] The first access is followed by a period of 7 to 9 days during which fever is absent. Eventually, relapses occur, few in the case of LBRF, up to 18 in the case of TBRF. Symptoms are similar to those of the first attack but are milder and complications are uncommon.

The diagnosis of relapsing fever depends on the demonstration of spirochetes in the blood of patients. Routine blood smears for malaria hemoscopy are suitable; otherwise, spirochetes may be seen in wet mounts at dark-field microscopy or at fluorescence microscopy (Figure 26–3). Culture of spirochetes and detection of bacterial DNA by PCR are primarily a research tool. Serologic tests do not play a diagnostic role in relapsing fever; moreover, significant cross-reactivity between *B. burgdorferi*, an agent of Lyme disease, and other borreliosis have been described, leading to possible misdiagnoses.[23]

Tetracycline and doxycycline are the treatment of choice for all relapsing fevers. Administered as a single dose of 500 mg and 100 mg, respectively, they terminate

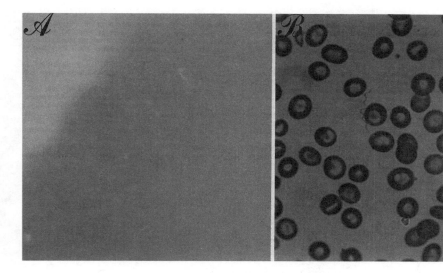

Figure 26–3. Spirochetes (*Borrelia* spp) seen in peripheral blood at fluorescence microscopy (*A*) and at Giemsa stain (*B*). To view these figures in color, refer to CD-ROM.

the acute attack, but relapse rates may be as high as 40%; therefore, multiple doses for 3 to 4 days are recommended.[21] Whenever tetracycline is contraindicated (pregnancy, children under 8 years of age), erythromycin, chloramphenicol, and ampicillin, all as single-dose treatment, may be used. Treatment is effective in clearing spirochetemia and prevent relapses. JHR, characterized by abrupt onset of temperature >40°C, rigors, tachycardia, and hypotension, is a very frequent complication of treatment.[22] JHR is observed shortly (frequently within 2 hours) after drug administration in nearly all patients with LBRF and half of those with TBRF.

PREVENTION

Personal hygiene measures are important to prevent lice infestation and subsequent LBRF. In the course of epidemics, especially in refugee camps and during military campaigns, intensive antivectorial measures are indicated. TBRF is prevented by personal protection measures, like avoidance of cabins inhabited by wild rodents and by applying topical tick repellants to the skin. The lack of natural reservoir for *B. duttoni* and the close association of *Ornithodoros* with humans in their dwellings make house residual spraying a possible method of TBRF control in tropical Africa.[18]

RICKETTSIAL DISEASES AND SCRUB TYPHUS

ETIOLOGY, TRANSMISSION, AND PATHOGENESIS

Rickettsial diseases are widely distributed throughout the world in endemic foci with sporadic and often seasonal outbreaks, occasionally re-emerging in epidemic form in human populations. Rickettsiae are small gram-negative bacteria characterized by obligate intracellular parasitism in both mammalian and arthropod hosts. Recently, a rearrangement of the phylogenetic tree of *Richettsia* has

been proposed, to show the similarities with the genera *Ehrlichia* and *Bartonella* (Figure 26–4).[24] The complete genome sequence of *Rickettsia prowazekii* has recently been reported and a fascinating hypothesis of the role of this parasite in the origin of mitochondria has been postulated.[25]

Rickettsiae differ considerably in terms of arthropod vectors, geographic distribution, and clinical diseases (Table 26–1).[26] The etiologic agents of the typhus fever group, comprising epidemic typhus, murine typhus, and scrub typhus, are described below.

Epidemic typhus is caused by *R. prowazekii* and transmitted by body lice. The cycle of infection is basically from person to person via the louse. Since lice die of *R. prowazekii*, humans represent the only reservoir: infection is lifelong, the parasite sequesters in its human host despite strong and long-lasting immunity, and patients with recrudescent typhus (Brill-Zinsser disease) are the occasional origin of new infections in the vector.[27] The role of animal reservoirs such as flying squirrels in North America is still debated. Infection occurs when a louse drops infected feces onto the skin while feeding, and the parasite penetrates through abrasions of the skin or mucosa. Murine typhus is caused by *R. typhi*, formerly named *R. mooseri*. The reservoir of the infection is the domestic rat and the vector is a rodent flea, usually *Xenopsylla cheopis*. Humans are occasional hosts of this agent. *Orientia tsutsugamushi* is the causative agent of scrub typhus. The transmission cycle includes the mite (primary host), which acquires the infection from domestic and sylvatic rodents (secondary host) to which they attach as parasites. Humans become accidental secondary hosts when they are parasitized by the larval stage of an infected mite.

The pathogenetic mechanisms of rickettsiae are similar: the parasites multiply at the initial site of inoculation, are released into the circulation at the end of the incubation period, and disseminate throughout the vascular system. Endothelial cells of small blood vessels are the usual site of rickettsial involvement. This causes endothelial cell degeneration and swelling, thrombus formation, and

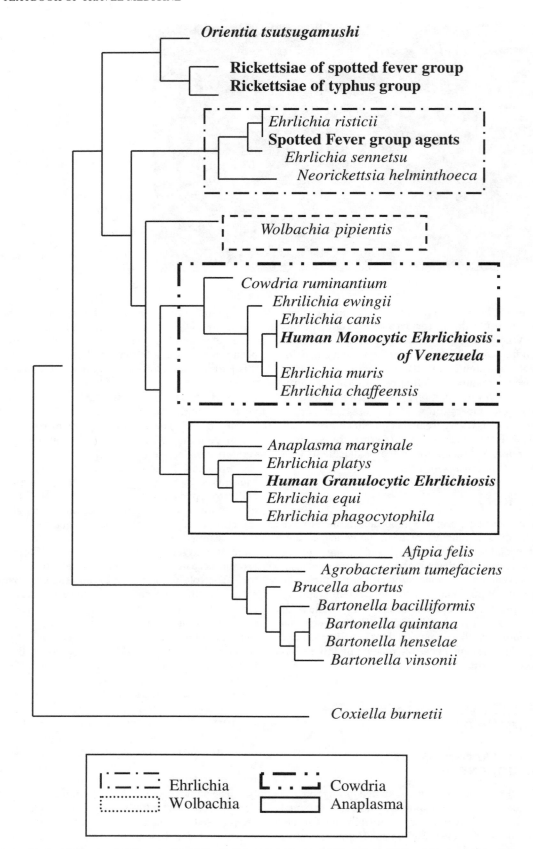

Figure 26–4. Phylogenetic tree of *Rickettsia*, *Ehrlichia*, and *Bartonella* based on the analysis of the *16S RNA* gene. From Brouqui P, Raoult D. Ehrlichia. Ehrlichiosis. In: Encyclopédic médical chirurgie maladies infectieuses. Paris: Elsevier, 1999;1–10.

Table 26–1.   VECTOR, GEOGRAPHIC DISTRIBUTION, AND CLINICAL DISEASE OF RICKETTSIAE AND EHRLICHIAE

RICKETTSIA SPECIES	DISEASE	VECTOR HOST	DISTRIBUTION
R. prowazekii	Epidemic typhus	Human body lice (humans)	Worldwide
R. typhi	Murine typhus	Fleas (rodents)	Worldwide
Ehrlichiosis			
E. chaffeensis	Human monocytic ehrlichiosis	Ticks (humans, deer)	U.S.A., Europe
E. species	Human granulocytic ehrlichiosis	Ticks (humans, deer, rodents)	U.S.A., Europe
Others			
O. tsutsugamushi	Scrub typhus	Mites (rodents)	Asia, Australia
C. burnetii	Q fever	Ticks (mammals)	Worldwide

Rickettsiae of the spotted fever group are not listed here.
Adapted with permission from Azad and Beard.[26]

partial or complete vessel occlusion. The inflammatory component is represented by a mononuclear leukocyte infiltration of the adventitia. Vasoconstriction, plasma leakage, and hemoconcentration are also observed and are caused by a specific toxin released by the organism. Focal parenchymatous abnormalities are caused by minute cellular infarcts that occur in all tissues but are most conspicuous in the brain, lung, and kidney. The skin rash of rickettsial diseases is caused by angiitis. Cell-mediated immunity is thought to be important for inhibition and eradication of rickettsiae in tissues. However, it is also suggested that delayed hypersensitivity reactions may contribute to the vasculitis.

GEOGRAPHIC DISTRIBUTION AND SPECIAL POPULATIONS AT RISK

Epidemic typhus fever has been reported during the 1990s from the cold environments of Africa (the highlands of Ethiopia, Rwanda, Burundi, Uganda, Nigeria, and Algeria) and South America (Bolivia, Ecuador, and Peru).[28] A gigantic outbreak of epidemic typhus occurred in Burundi from 1995 to 1997,[29] confirming that the parasite is transmitted under epidemic conditions whenever breakdown of social, economic, or political systems occur. Poverty, overcrowding, poor hygienic conditions, and housing are the usual predisposing conditions that provoke widespread body-louse infestation. Travelers are at increased risk for the disease following even transient exposure to body lice during typhus epidemics, as suggested by the report of a fatal case in a health care worker during the outbreak in Burundi.[30]

In contrast to epidemic typhus, human cases of murine typhus occur sporadically worldwide, although nowadays the number of reported cases is very low. Conditions facilitating contacts between humans and infected rodents and their fleas are usually encountered in port cities with high densities of human and rodent populations. Murine typhus is reported occasionally in travelers with imported fever,[31] but most infections are likely to remain unrecognized due to the unspecific clinical presentation.

Scrub typhus became well known during the Vietnam war, when it was diagnosed in 10% of febrile American soldiers. The disease is endemic in Southeast Asia and is known to occur in Australia, the Pacific Region, and Japan. Suspected cases have been reported from Africa,[32] but the presence of the parasite has not been conclusively documented in this continent so far. Scrub typhus is acquired by humans who come in contact in the mite's habitat, such as rain forests, river banks, seashores, and agricultural fields. Travelers are readily affected by the infection, but most cases go unrecognized.[33]

CASE MANAGEMENT

Human rickettsiosis are potentially severe diseases that constitute a significant, but often unrecognized, cause of acute febrile illness. The clinical presentation of the typhus group of rickettsiosis is similar, although epidemic and scrub typhus are more severe and life-threatening diseases. The incubation period is from 3 to 20 days. A primary lesion with local lymphadenitis may be noted in scrub typhus. Prodromata are represented by malaise and headache, which precedes the abrupt onset of high fever, chills, prostration, myalgia, and arthralgia. Severe frontal headache is very common. Fever remains high for as many as 7 to 14 days, then becomes remittent with defervescence occurring by slow lysis. A distinctive rash may appear by the fourth day of fever, but it occurs in not more than 50% of the patients with either epidemic[29] or murine typhus.[31] When present, the rash begins on the trunk and the axillae and later involves the arms and legs, sparing the periphery. The lesions are flat, delicate, pink macules from 2 to 6 mm in diameter. Disturbances of the central nervous system are typical and more pronounced in severe cases. They include irritability, restlessness, inability to sleep, and mental confusion, which may progress to coma. In untreated cases during the second week of illness, vascular abnormalities develop, causing a weakened pulse rate, hypotension, and cyanosis. Renal failure may be heralded by oliguria, albuminuria, and azotemia. Petechial skin lesions appear and gangrene of extremities may occur as a consequence of vasculitis. Disseminated intravascular coagulation (DIC) may complicate severe cases, leading to thrombocytopenia, reduced prothrombin time, and fibrinogenolysis.

Important epidemiologic clues to suspect typhus include a history of louse infestation in a known endemic area, flea bites in a rat-infested population, or exposure to mites in a rural tropical setting. Isolation requires inoculation in laboratory animals and subculturing onto hen eggs or tissue culture systems. In practice, the diagnosis is made on a clinical basis with confirmatory serologic tests. The Weil-Felix test, an agglutination reaction that detects antibodies to Proteus OX-19 (positive in cases of epidemic and murine typhus) and Proteus Ox-K (positive in cases of scrub typhus), has low sensitivity. A fourfold rise in titers between sera collected in the acute and convalescent phases is confirmatory. An indirect fluorescent antibody technique for diagnosis of epidemic typhus and scrub typhus is available in reference centers. A commercial dot-blot ELISA dipstick test compares favorably with the IFAT test for the diagnosis of scrub typhus.[34]

Antibiotic treatment significantly shortens the duration of fever, prevents the development of vascular complications, and significantly lowers mortality of epidemic typhus.[29] A single dose of 200-mg doxycycline is highly effective. Doxycycline-resistant and chloramphenicol-resistant strains of *O. tsutsugamushi* have been reported from Thailand[35]; the clinical significance of this report is still unclear. The management of severely ill patients requires support circulation, renal and cerebral functions, and correction of DIC.

PREVENTION

The most important preventive intervention for epidemic typhus consists in the strengthening of personal hygiene measures to prevent lice infestation. In the course of epidemics, especially in refugee camps and during military campaigns, intensive antivectorial measures (lindane powder) are recommended. A vaccine for epidemic typhus, consisting of inactivated *R. prowazekii*, is available but has no clear-cut indication for travelers.

Murine typhus is prevented by personal protection measures, such as rodent-proof accommodations or topical application of a flea repellent.

Scrub typhus is prevented by avoidance of bites by wearing protective and insecticide-impregnated clothes or by the application of topical repellent.

EHRLICHIOSIS

ETIOLOGY, TRANSMISSION, AND PATHOGENESIS

Ehrlichiae are intracellular organisms closely related to the Richettsiae (see Table 26–1) that may infect a variety of mammalian hosts. The emergence of two new human ehrlichial infections has recently been reported: human monocytic ehrlichiosis (HME) is caused by *E. chaffeen-*

sis,[36] whereas human granulocytic ehrlichiosis (HGE) is caused by a still unclassified *Ehrlichia* species closely related to the animal pathogens *E. phagocytophila* and *E. equi*.[37]

Both diseases are a tick-borne zoonosis: HGE transmission occurs through the bites of *Ixodes* ticks, the same arthropod vectors of *Borrelia burgdorferi*.[38] White-tailed deers and small mammals may serve as primary reservoir. Perinatal transmission has been described, although the route of infection (intrauterine, intrapartum, or through breastfeeding) has not been determined.[39] HME is transmitted by the tick *Amblyomma americanum*, a vector that is not found outside the American continent; in Europe, the tick *Ixodes persulcatus* has been proposed as a putative vector for *E. chaffeensis*.

E. chaffeensis infects mononuclear phagocytes, whereas the agent of HGE replicates within granulocytes circulating in peripheral blood but the agent has been recovered from body fluids and tissues. Ehrlichiae penetrate into the cell by phagocitosis, multiply into the phagosome, and are actively responsible for inhibition of phagolisosomial fusion. A life cycle similar to that of *Chlamydia* is recognized: an elementary body is the resistant, biologically inactive form responsible for infection, which turns into a reticular body, the intracellular, biologically active form. Ehrlichiae have no endotoxic factors. Tissues of the reticuloendothelial system infected by HME may reveal granulomas with no caseous necrosis. Immune mechanisms in the human host seems to involve a T cell response; high antibody titers are found during active disease, showing that humoral response has no protective activity. Ehrlichial infections have a potential for immune suppression and inflammatory cell disfunctions, demonstrated in animal models, which may determine the activation of underlying viral infections.

GEOGRAPHIC DISTRIBUTION AND SPECIAL POPULATIONS AT RISK

HGE is becoming an emerging public health problem in the United States and Europe. Incidence rates of clinical disease in Wisconsin have been estimated to range between 1 and 16 cases per 100,000, with picks in some counties as high as 60.[40] In Europe, infection has been reported from Slovenia, Switzerland, Italy, United Kingdom, Norway, and Sweden, in the same areas where Lyme borreliosis and tick-borne encephalitis are reported. HME is basically confined to the American continent.

Risk factors for the acquisition of HGE and HME are probably similar to those recognized for Lyme borreliosis. People exposed to tick bites through outdoor activities or employment are at increased risk for infection. The most important risk factor is residence or temporary stay in areas where the population density of ticks is high. Infection has a seasonal distribution with picks during the summer months. Preliminary observations suggest that children are less affected than adults, although it is unclear whether this is due to reduced exposure, reduced risk of infection, or reduced risk of progression to disease.

CASE MANAGEMENT

HGE is an acute, febrile, nonspecific illness that may be severe enough to cause hospitalization and death, particularly in the elderly.[40] Clinical severity seems to be milder in European compared to American cases. Seroepidemiologic studies indicate that the infection is quite common, and most infected subjects develop subclinical or mild infection.[40] The incubation period seems to range between 1 and 4 weeks. When symptoms are present, the typical presentation is that of an indifferentiated febrile illness with headache, malaise, myalgias, and arthralgias. The clinical examination is usually unremarkable. Laboratory findings include leukopenia, thrombocytopenia, and elevated transaminase levels. Severe and fatal complications have been described, including pancarditis, seizures, brachial plexopathy, and demyelinating polineuropathy. The clinical presentation of HME is similar to that reported for HGE.

Several diagnostic techniques have been described. Direct examination of buffy-coat smears stained with Wright's stain can be examined for intragranulocytic morulae, although the sensitivity of this test is questionable. Ehrlichial DNA can be demonstrated by a PCR assay on whole blood samples.[41] The pathogen can be grown in HL-60 cell cultures from blood samples, detecting the growing bacteria by either Wright's microscopy or PCR.[42] Diagnosis can also be based on serologic criteria, using sequential indirect-immunofluorescence assays. Cross-reactivity with antibodies to *B. burgdorferi* is possible.

Antibiotic treatment is recommended for febrile cases: doxycycline 100 mg twice daily for 7 days has been proven effective. Rifampin may be considered for pregnant women and children, although evidence of efficacy is based on few case reports.[43] Interestingly, antibiotics that are frequently prescribed after tick bites, including ampicillin, amoxicillin, and ceftriaxone, are not effective in vitro.

PREVENTION

Personal efforts to avoid tick bites are the mainstay of prevention of ehrlichiosis, especially for temporary residents of tick-infested areas. Routine antibiotic prophylaxis with doxycycline after tick bites has no demonstrable utility. No vaccine for either HME or HGE is currently available.

CARRIÓN'S DISEASE AND OTHER *BARTONELLA* INFECTIONS

Bartonella species are considered emerging pathogens. Renewed interest is prompted by the recent description of new clinical manifestations caused by old and new *Bartonella* species that are pathogenic for humans (see Table 26–1). Of the five *Bartonella* species considered potential human pathogens, *B. bacilliformis,* the causative agent of Carrión's disease, was the only known species of the genus till 1993. Later, *B. quintana* was recognized as the causative agent of trench fever and for indifferentiated fever with or without endocarditis among homeless people (called urban trench fever).[44] *B. henselae* is responsible for the cat scratch disease[45]; both *B. quintana* and *B. henselae* determine bacillary angiomatosis/peliosis.[46] Bartonellae are transmitted under several conditions.[47] *B. bacilliformis* and *B. quintana* are insect-borne disease, transmitted, respectively, by the sandfly *Lutzomia* and the body louse *Pediculus*; *B. henselae*'s primary reservoir is the cat, and the bacteria are transmitted as a result of cat scratches and bites. Infections due to *B. quintana* and *B. henselae* have a worldwide distribution. Carrión's disease is restricted to the tropical belt and is described in more details below.

CARRIÓN'S DISEASE

Etiology, Transmission, and Pathogenesis *Bartonella bacilliformis* is an intracellular, flagellated, coccoid gram-negative bacterium that penetrates and replicates in erythrocytes and endothelial cells.

Carrión's disease is a vector-borne disease transmitted by phlebotomine sandflies of the *Lutzomyia* genus, which also transmit leishmaniasis. The habitat of the vector has a geographic distribution very similar to that of the disease, suggesting that vector availability may be the major determinant of the limited local endemicity of Carrión's disease. Only female sandflies seek a blood meal. They have night-biting behavior, weak flight, and a dispersal area limited to a few hundred meters from their breeding sites. Humans are the only recognized reservoir of *B. bacilliformis*, and 10% to 15% of asymptomatic persons in endemic areas have been reported as chronic carriers due to positive blood cultures. It is estimated that in hyperendemic zones, people receive 20 to 50 sandfly bites per night and that 0.5% to 3% of wild vectors are infected.

B. bacilliformis actively adheres, penetrates, and ruptures the erythrocytes during the septicemic phase of Oroya fever. It also has a specific tropism for endothelial cells, which is related to the capacity to determine proliferation of these cells, typical of verruga peruana.

Geographic Distribution and Special Populations at Risk Endemic areas are limited to certain valleys of Peru, Ecuador, and Colombia from latitude 54N to 13S on both slopes of the Andes between 1,000 and 3,000 meters above sea level.[48] Natural resistance to infection has not been reported. Populations resident in endemic areas are at significant risk for the disease. Carrión's disease has sporadically been described in short-term travelers to endemic areas.[49]

Case Management *B. bacilliformis* is responsible for cases of acute, severe, febrile illness with hemolytic anemia (Oroya fever) and for a dermatologic disease characterized by cutaneous papules and nodules (verruga peruana). Oroya fever should be included in the differential diagnosis of patients who have visited endemic areas and present with fever, progressive hemolytic anemia, and generalized lymphadenopathy.

Diagnosis of Oroya fever is based on a high degree of clinical suspicion. A Giemsa-stained peripheral blood film, the same used to diagnose malaria, may reveal endo-erythrocytic blue or reddish violet rods and rounded forms. Massive bacteremia with close to 100% parasitism is common. Conclusive diagnosis is made by isolation of the organism by blood culture, although *Bartonella* is a fastidious agent, growing on media enriched by hemin, at 28°C in a CO_2-enriched atmosphere, after not less than 2 to 3 weeks. Bartonellae may be detected by the use of a PCR technique, although this does not apply to the management of individual cases.

The fatality rate of untreated Oroya fever is as high as 40% to 80%. Treatment must be started early since the prognosis of untreated cases is poor. Chloramphenicol is the drug of choice; 500 mg four times a day for 14 days is the usual adult dose. Tetracyclines and erythromycin are effective on other human diseases caused by *Bartonella*. No clinical experience is available with gentamicin, although this is the only antibiotic with bactericidal activity in vitro. Concurrent infections resulting from the temporary immunodeficiency caused by the disease are often encountered with Oroya fever. Diagnosis and treatment of associated disease caused by *Salmonella* (up to 40% of cases), *Brucella*, *Plasmodia*, *Mycobacteria*, and *Entamoeba* are important components of case management.

Verrucous lesions (verruga peruana) present months after an apparent or inapparent septicemic phase. They usually present as diffuse, rapidly disseminating muco-cutaneous papules and nodules. Some develop into vegetating, painless, purple nodules a few centimeters in diameter (Figure 26–5). The disease is recognized on the basis of the clinical picture, the patient's history, and the histopathologic findings (proliferation of epithelioid cells of angioblastic nature). Verrucous lesions are benign and treatment is not essential.

Prevention   No vaccine is currently available for any *Bartonella* disease. Prevention of Carrión's disease is based on individual protection using measures to prevent man/vector nocturnal contacts similar to those used to prevent malaria. Use of proper clothing and insect repellent, screening of premises, and bednets are encouraged. Because sandflies are smaller than mosquitoes, ordinary screens and netting of 14 to 18 meshes per inch are inadequate, and those of 25 to 30 meshes per inch should be used.

MELIOIDOSIS

ETIOLOGY, TRANSMISSION, AND PATHOGENESIS

Burkholderia pseudomallei (Pseudomonas pseudomallei) is an aerobic gram-negative bipolar staining bacillus that is free living in earth and water in many tropical and subtropical countries.

The disease is properly termed a zoonosis since many mammals (rats, cows, horses, pigs, and others) may be

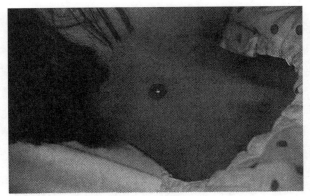

Figure 26–5.   Verruga peruana of the neck.

affected. The role of the animal reservoir and its importance as a cause of human disease are not known. The organism is a pathogen for domestic and wild animals that, like humans, acquire the infection by inhalation, by ingestion, or from contaminated injuries. Human-to-human transmission is extremely rare.[50-52] The bacillus is able to actively penetrate the skin, even in the absence of macroscopic lesions, and to survive inside the cells of the reticuloendothelial system. *B. pseudomallei* is responsible for abscess formation; it also produces a heat-stable endotoxin and a thermolabile exotoxin that are thought to contribute to the lethality of the disease in humans.

The majority of infected persons remain asymptomatic, and the organism may remain quiescent for decades, similar to tuberculosis. It may later recrudesce and present as acute and overwhelming, subacute, or chronic disease. This is more likely if the patient develops diabetes, renal disease, or alcoholism or is immunocompromised. However, this disease is not a common opportunistic infection in Thai patients with AIDS.

GEOGRAPHIC DISTRIBUTION AND SPECIAL POPULATIONS AT RISK

Melioidosis was first reported from Burma in 1912 and remained poorly known in the western world until the Vietnam war, where it was recognized as an environmental hazard for soldiers. The main endemic regions for melioidosis are Southeast Asia and Northern Australia, but isolated cases have been reported in animals and man from Africa and even the Americas.[53,54] A serologic survey of 1,000 children in Northeast Thailand showed an increasing seroconversion rate ranging from 12% at <6 months to a plateau of 80% at 4 years of age.[55]

Reactivation melioidosis has been reported among tourists, immigrants, and Vietnam veterans decades after leaving endemic regions. Patients who develop melioidosis outside endemic regions often undergo prolonged and expensive diagnostic studies and inappropriate treatment before a correct diagnosis is made. A recent study of expatriates living in northern Thailand and Laos revealed a high prevalence of seropositivity depending on length of stay and rural travel.[56] However, seropositivity among expatriate residents of Bangkok was found to be very rare (ongoing study, unpublished, by N. Riesland et al.). A cluster of melioidosis cases was recently reported from Western Australia and carried a high mortality rate.[53,54] Delay in diagnosis and in rendering appropriate treatment was thought to have contributed to this. Awareness of this disease and considering it in the differential diagnosis of febrile illness in a subject who is or has lived in an endemic region are vital.

CASE MANAGEMENT

The most common clinical manifestations of melioidosis among rural Thais are localized infection with regional lymphadenitis and abscess formation; granulomatous or necrotizing lesions of skin, muscles, and internal organs (spleen, liver, kidney); acute airspace or blood-borne pneumonias; chronic granulomatous or fibrosing lung disease mimicking tuberculosis; obscure fever; and overwhelming rapidly fatal sepsis. Unusual manifestations such as pericarditis, meningitis, osteomyelitis, and pyomyositis have also been reported.[50,53,57–60]

Any fever of undetermined origin, acute or chronic lung disease (particularly if it involves upper lobes), or integumental or organ abscess (particularly of liver and spleen) should suggest melioidosis in such a subject. The suspected diagnosis can be confirmed by aspiration, gram stain (gram-negative bipolar stained safety-pin appearance), and culture of a lesion. Culture is not difficult since the bacterium grows after 24 to 48 hours on ordinary bacteriologic media (EMB or MacConkey media) and by serology (IHA or ELISA). A presumptive diagnosis of melioidosis may be supported by positive serology. However, IHA titers above 1:80 are suggestive of active infection but can also be seen in asymptomatic subjects in endemic regions.[61–63]

Current therapy recommendations are ceftazidime or imipenem plus trimethoprim-sulfamethoxazole, doxycycline, or amoxicillin-clavulanic acid.[64–66] Parenteral therapy is continued for 2 to 6 weeks, depending on the severity and clinical response. This must be followed by maintenance therapy for 3 to 6 months to prevent relapse. The most commonly used drugs for maintenance are either trimethoprim-sulfamethoxazole, doxycycline, or amoxycillin clavulanic acid. Large abscesses require aspiration and/or surgical debridement. Recurrences are not uncommon and usually are associated with inadequate or not long enough treatment.[50]

Clinically manifest melioidosis cases are uncommon among tourists and expatriates residing in Southeast Asia. They are, however, not unknown. Subjects who have lived in this region and later develop an obscure acute or chronic febrile illness should inform their physicians that they have resided in a melioidosis-endemic region.

PREVENTION

A vaccine against melioidosis is not available, and the authors know of no current efforts to make one. There is no known role for chemoprophylaxis. High-risk behavior, such as bathing or walking in rice paddies and still water, should be discouraged.

PLAGUE

ETIOLOGY, TRANSMISSION, AND PATHOGENESIS

Plague is a zoonotic infection caused by *Yersinia pestis*, a gram-negative, nonmotile bacillus belonging to the Enterobacteriaceae family.[67] Several species of domestic and sylvatic rodents represent the natural hosts of the infection, but many other animals, including dogs and cats, may be infected. *Y. pestis* is transmitted from one host to another by vectors of the flea genera either specific to rodents (*Xenopsylla cheopis*) or, more rarely, to humans (*Pulex irritants*). The dynamics of plague transmission are explained by the existence of an enzootic reservoir, usually small-animal species that do not develop severe disease, and by an epizootic reservoir, where the disease propagates cyclically in epidemic forms. At least three epidemiologic settings of plague are recognized. In the sylvatic form, the infection is transmitted from and to sylvatic animals by specific vectors and humans are rarely involved. One exception is when children play with dead animals killed by plague. In the rural form, the infection extends to village rodents and may accidentally be carried to humans by domestic rodent fleas. The urban form develops and propagates in epidemic forms transmitted among humans by human fleas. In addition to vectorial transmission, plague may be acquired by inhalation from coughing patients. This causes the pulmonary form of the disease. After inoculation by a flea bite, *Y. pestis* diffuses through the lymphatic vessels, reaches the regional lymph nodes, and causes a pyogenic reaction. Systemic signs are mediated by a potent lipopolysaccharide endotoxin.

GEOGRAPHIC DISTRIBUTION AND SPECIAL POPULATIONS AT RISK

Plague spreads by worldwide epidemics. The present epidemic started at the end of the last century in China and has extended to the rest of Asia, Europe, Africa, and North and South America (Figure 26–6). Plague is now considered a re-emerging disease because of the increase in the worldwide number of reported cases, the occurrence of epidemics (such as the one in India in 1994), and the gradual expansion in areas of low endemicity (such as in the United States). The total number of plague cases reported to WHO in 1996 by 10 countries was 3,017, with a slight increase over the previous year and a considerable increase over the average figure per year of the previous 10 years.[68] Over 85% of the cases of 1996 were reported from Africa, where more than 85% of the cases occurred in just two countries, Madagascar and United Republic of Tanzania.[68] The major worldwide plague epidemic occurred in India, where a total of 5,150 suspected pneumonic or bubonic cases occurred from August to October 1994, causing travel and trade disruption and resulting in severe economic repercussions.[69] Plague notifications are slightly increasing in the southern states of the United States, where 390 cases have been reported from 1947 to 1996, with 60 (15.4%) deaths.[70]

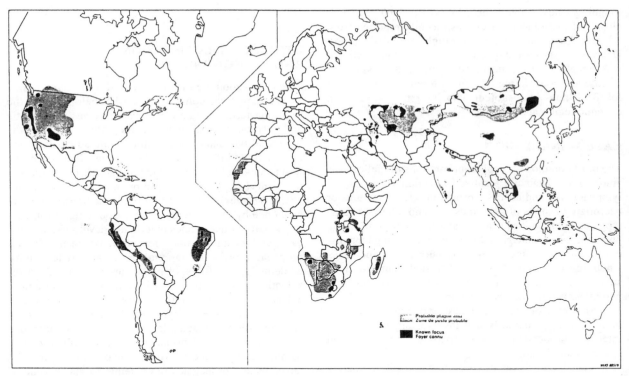

Figure 26–6.   Map distribution of plague (from WHO).

Children are most often affected possibly because of their propensity to come in contact with rodents. There are seasonal peaks in transmission, coincident with the moderately hot and humid seasons (e.g., the monsoon period in India and Tanzania). Under these conditions, the reservoir animals get closer to human houses, the vectors find optimal conditions for replication, and the bacteria are in optimal temperature conditions.

Travelers are rarely affected by plague while visiting endemic areas; for example, no visitors were affected during the 1994 epidemic in India.[71] Campers or visitors staying in rodent-infested lodges are exposed to the highest risk of infection.

CASE MANAGEMENT

In humans, *Y. pestis* causes an acute, regional lymphadenitis that may be complicated by pneumonia, septicemia, and endotoxic shock. Three clinical forms are recognized: bubonic, septicemic, and pneumonic. In bubonic plague, axillary, cervical, and groin lymph nodes are the most commonly affected. Plague buboes may be single or a group of confluent nodes, swelling from 1 to 10 cm in length. They are extremely painful so that movements of the involved area are avoided. The overlying skin is reddish and warm. Buboes are initially firm, but they eventually become fluctuant and, in favorable cases, open spontaneously to the skin during the convalescent phase. The disease has a sudden onset 2 to 6 days after infection, characterized by high fever, chills, headache, and weakness. This occurs usually before lymph nodes assume char-

acteristic features. Prostration may be prominent with signs of cerebral involvement ranging from agitation to lethargy. Complement activation and disseminated intravascular coagulation cause tissue damage and general failure of the vascular system. Intermittent bacteremia occurs and is responsible for secondary foci. Pneumonia may follow septicemic events or may be a primary event in the case of air-borne transmission.

Plague should be suspected in febrile patients who have been exposed to rodents or other mammals in the known endemic areas of the world. The presence of buboes in this setting is highly suspicious. The bacterium may be isolated on standard bacteriologic media from culture samples of blood and bubo aspirate. In the bubo aspirate, the gram stain easily reveals gram-negative coccobacilli with polymorphonuclear leukocytes. Rapid diagnostic tests are more useful than culture in guiding case management in individual patients: a direct immunofluorescence test for the presumptive identification of *Y. pestis* F1 antigen should be applied to blood films, lymph node aspirates, or culture isolates.[72] Serologic tests to detect antibodies to the F1 antigen by passive hemoagglutination assay or enzyme-linked immunosorbent assay methods are available. A fourfold increase in titer (or a single titer of 1:16 or more) may provide presumptive evidence of plague in culture-negative cases.[73]

Untreated plague has a fatality rate of over 50%. Antibiotic treatment effectively reduces mortality of plague and should be started on the basis of clinical suspicion. Streptomycin 30 mg per kg per day intramuscularly in two divided doses for 10 days is the drug of choice. Whenever streptomycin is contraindicated due to allergy, tetracyclines or chloramphenicol should be administered. Classically, *Y. pestis* isolates are uniformly susceptible to antibiotics. One clinical isolate from Madagascar with high-level, plasmid-mediated resistance to multiple antibiotics including all of the drugs recommended for plague therapy and prophylaxis has recently been reported.[74]

PREVENTION

A formalin-killed whole-cell vaccine is licensed and available for subjects at specific risk for plague, but its efficacy is questionable.[75] Those who may have contact with rodents in endemic areas and laboratory personnel handling live *Y. pestis* cultures are candidates for vaccination. Personal hygiene (avoidance of lice by using insect repellants) and safe behaviors (avoidance of contacts with rodents) represent the most important preventive measures for travelers. Plague is an internationally quarantinable disease. Pulmonary infections present a particular risk for human epidemics due to the contagiousness of the organism. Doxycycline (100 mg twice daily for 7 days) prophylaxis of family members of index cases is indicated within the standard 7-day maximum plague incubation period.

TRACHOMA

ETIOLOGY, TRANSMISSION, AND PATHOGENESIS

Trachoma is a communicable, chronic keratoconjunctivitis due to *Chlamydia trachomatis* serotypes A, B, Ba, and C. Overcrowding, poor personal and communal hygiene, and poor access to water (which prevents face washing) facilitate the spread of the infection and enhance the severity of the disease. Bacterial superinfections of the cornea are important causes of late scarring lesions. *C. trachomatis* is a strict intracellular pathogen that infects the epithelial cells and develops small reactive follicles in the subepithelial strata of the conjunctiva. Histologic studies reveal an infiltrate with T lymphocytes, plasma cells, and macrophages. The necrosis of follicle germinal centers is responsible for the scarring process. The determinants of disease and disease severity after chlamydial infection are still largely unknown. Although repeated infections have frequently been considered to determine most of trachoma morbidity, persistent *C. trachomatis* infection (with high bacterial burden for prolonged periods) has been suggested to directly contribute to disease severity.[76]

GEOGRAPHIC DISTRIBUTION AND SPECIAL POPULATIONS AT RISK

With improvement of living standards, the incidence of trachoma has decreased in the last 30 years in many areas worldwide. However, at least 100 million children still suffer from active trachoma with inflammation and 30 million adults, mostly women, have trichiasis. Trachoma is the major cause of preventable blindness in poor communities located in hot, dry, and dusty environments. Most recent estimates reported a prevalence of about 6 million blind people due to trachoma.[77] The disease is typically found in large areas of North and sub-Saharan Africa, the Middle East, parts of India and central and south Asia, Indonesia, and Northern Australia. There are also foci in Central and South America. The disease mainly affects young children and the women who look after them[78] in poor communities in the tropical belt. Environment and culture may predict the frequency and severity of the disease. Poor drainage systems, the habit of cooking on an open fire in the living quarters, and inadequate water supply are usually associated with a higher incidence of trachoma. The prevalence of trachoma is lower in children with clean faces, and a face-washing program significantly reduces trachoma incidence.[79] Short-term travelers are not usually at risk for the disease. However, trachoma may affect children and adult immigrants from endemic areas.

CASE MANAGEMENT

Trachoma consists of a wide range of ocular pathology. WHO has recently proposed a simplified grading scheme for clinical classification of trachomatous lesions.[80] It includes two inflammatory (T-follicular and T-intense follicular) and three cicatricial grades (TS—presence of scars, TT—one eyelash rubs on the eyeball, and TO—presence of corneal opacity). Inflammatory lesions are characterized by large yellow or white spots of 1 mm in the upper tarsus and limbus. At advanced stages of cicatricial trachoma, entropion (inward curvature of the eyelid) and trichiasis (eyelash turned inward) occur. Xerosis (loss of lacrimal glands and ducts) is also frequently present. Trichiasis and xerosis are responsible for secondary corneal injury, bacterial infection, and scarring. The inflammatory reaction may extend from the upper bulbar conjunctiva toward the cornea, determining a vascularization process known as "pannus," which determines, over a period of months to years, corneal opacity.

Cases of trachoma are recognized on clinical grounds. Direct identification of the bacterium on Giemsa-stained smears or isolation of *Chlamydia* in cell culture is usually not necessary. Individual management of patients with trachoma is medical in the inflammatory stages and surgical in the cicatricial stages. Classical medical treatment consists of topical tetracycline eye ointment 1% three times daily for 3 to 6 weeks. Azithromycin at a single dose or by repeated doses (weekly for 3 weeks or monthly for 6 months) is as effective as tetracycline ointment[81] and represents a useful alternative for trachoma control programs. The efficacy of chemotherapy should be assessed from 3 to 6 months after the end of treatment since trachomatous hyperplasia takes a long time to disappear. Trachoma and chlamydial infection rapidly reappear in a large proportion of those treated. Surgical treatment consists of repair of entropion, trichiasis, and stricture of the lacrimal duct to prevent future visual loss.

PREVENTION

No effective vaccine against *C. trachomatis* is currently available. At an individual level, the priority is to prevent blindness by recognizing and treating the inflammatory stages of the disease. At the community level, improvement of global socioeconomic conditions seems to be the most important factor toward the eradication of trachoma. Dramatic falls in disease occurrence may be seen as a consequence of improvements of sanitation, water supply, education, and access to health care in absence of specific disease control programs.[82]

ANTHRAX

ETIOLOGY, TRANSMISSION, AND PATHOGENESIS

A renewed interest in anthrax has recently emerged, originated by the potential use of its lethal toxin in biologic warfare.[83] Anthrax is a zoonotic disease due to *Bacillus anthracis*, a gram-positive, capsulated, spore-forming bacillus. Spores are responsible for resistance in the environment and transmission of the organism.[84]

In animals, transmission occurs primarily through fecal-oral modalities. Humans usually acquire the infection accidentally either from animal secretion, carcasses, products (skins, hair, wool), or from a contaminated environment (soil). Cutaneous anthrax is the most prevalent clinical form, but pulmonary and gastrointestinal disease are also sporadically reported. In cutaneous anthrax, spores penetrate the subcutaneous tissues through existing wounds or are carried by foreign bodies. Spores may also be inhaled, producing primary pulmonary and mediastinal disease, or ingested, producing primary gastrointestinal disease.

The pathogen is able to spread locally through the lymphatics and can spread to tissues following bacteremia. The virulence of the vegetative form of *B. anthracis* is due to the capsular material. However, most of the pathologic effects of anthrax are due to an exotoxin, which is responsible for local tissue necrosis and, after hematogenous dissemination, generalized toxemia. Anthrax spores are produced in a dry form for bacteriologic warfare.

GEOGRAPHIC DISTRIBUTION AND SPECIAL POPULATIONS AT RISK

Epidemiologically, anthrax is classified as either industrial or agriculturally acquired. The first situation occurs in industrialized countries where small epidemics are due to importation of contaminated animal material for industry. The reported number of cases of industrial anthrax is at present low and still decreasing. A few cases have been described in travelers who import souvenirs.[85] Agricultural anthrax is more common in developing countries where the risk is still significant in parts of Asia, Africa, Eastern Europe, and South and Central America as a result of contaminated soil.[86]

CASE MANAGEMENT

Anthrax can occur in three forms: cutaneous, inhalation, and gastrointestinal. In cutaneous anthrax, the primary lesion develops 1 to 10 days after infection. It is usually situated on exposed skin (arms, legs, face) and consists of a small, painless papule over the site of inoculation. After several days, the papule develops into a vesicle with a surrounding erythematous and edematous base that is characteristically painless.[87] The extension of edema depends on the site of infection (loose subcutaneous tissue is the most affected) and correlates with the severity of disease due to the effects of the toxin. A few days later, the vesicle becomes hemorrhagic, ulcerates, and reveals a necrotic area (a painless, nonsuppurative black eschar). Cutaneous anthrax heals spontaneously in about 80% of the cases. However, severe cases are not uncommon. They are characterized by extensive edema and induration at the inoculation site, followed by hematogenous spread leading to sepsis, meningitis, and subsequent death in 20% of the cases in the preantibiotic era.

Inhalation anthrax results in an extremely severe mediastinitis due to the penetration of the pathogen from the pulmonary alveoli and its spread to hilar lymph nodes. The incubation period is shorter, 2 to 5 days, and the presenting symptoms are nonspecific, with mild fever, malaise, and a nonproductive cough. After a period of a few days in which the patient's condition apparently improves, a second phase begins with high fever, respiratory distress, cyanosis, and subcutaneous edema of the neck and thorax. Crepitant rales are evident on auscultation. The chest film reveals mediastinal widening and frequently a pleural effusion. Inhalation anthrax is almost always fatal with a very short time between the onset of the second phase, mediastinal signs, and death.

Gastrointestinal anthrax, at present a very rare disease, is due to ingestion of spores. The primary lesion is located on the mucosal surface at any site between the oropharynx and large intestine. An extremely severe disease follows, with a short incubation period (2–5 days) and clinical manifestations consisting of fever, anorexia, nausea, and vomiting. Ascites is often present. The disease progresses to a toxic shock state leading to death within a week from the onset of symptoms.

Cutaneous anthrax should be suspected in exposed professionals presenting with skin lesions.[86] The differential diagnosis includes staphylococcal skin infections, contagious pustular dermatitis, tularemia, and plague. Culture for *B. anthracis* should be performed from the vesicular fluid on ordinary media. Identification may be confirmed by direct fluorescent antibody staining or by bacteriophage testing. Direct examination of the vesicular fluid may reveal gram-positive bacilli with slightly rounded ends. Spores are not seen in fresh materials. Culture of the organism from sputum, vomit, or fecal material should be attempted in suspected cases of pulmonary or gastrointestinal anthrax, but results are often negative. A serologic ELISA test is available, although a significant increase in titer is usually obtained only in convalescent subjects who survive.

B. anthracis is sensitive to penicillin: 1.2 million units (or intravenously 18–24 million units daily in severe cases) for 7 to 10 days. In penicillin-allergic subjects, tetracyclines or erythromycin may be used. Penicillin resistance in *B. anthracis* has rarely been reported.[88] Ancillary treatment to sustain vascular volume, cardiac, pulmonary, and renal functions is essential in severe cases.

PREVENTION

In industrialized countries, human anthrax is a disease of blue-collar workers manipulating animal products. Good hygiene practices are effective in reducing the risk for acquiring the infection and in preventing the development of severe disease. These include appropriate clothing, control of sources of animal material, and prevention of wounds. In developing countries, local farmers and stock keepers are exposed. Prevention mainly focuses on control of the disease in animals. A human vaccine is available that is prepared by whole-cell, killed bacteria and is reported to be 93% effective against cutaneous anthrax. The vaccine is recommended for professionals having regular contact with potentially infected animals. The U.S. Department of Defense recently announced a program of systematic vaccination of all U.S. military personnel.

COSMOPOLITAN INFECTIONS

TUBERCULOSIS

Tuberculosis is a widespread infection caused by mycobacteria of the tuberculosis complex. *M. tuberculosis* is transmitted mainly as an air-borne infection by bacilliferous cases. *M. bovis* is found in cattle and is transmitted to humans via contaminated milk and dairy products. Whereas food-borne tuberculosis is presently an uncommon disease and transmission is limited to developing countries, air-borne tuberculosis is in a new epidemic phase throughout the world. WHO estimates that the yearly number of new tuberculosis cases will rise from 7.5 million in 1990 to 10.2 million by the year 2000. Similarly, the number of yearly deaths due to tuberculosis will rise from 2.5 to 3.5 million over the same years. The predicted increase in new cases is due mainly to population growth and changes in the age of populations in developing countries. The HIV pandemic and the failure of infection control programs are also expected to play an important role. Industrialized countries account for only 2% of the total morbidity and less than 1% of total mortality of tuberculosis. In this setting, tuberculosis is increasing among HIV-infected people, immigrants, and ethnic minorities. Only 5% of the people infected by *M. tuberculosis* progress to active tuberculosis in their lifetime. Infected subjects may develop the disease immediately after infection or after a latency period that may last several years. In most cases, tuberculosis presents as a subacute pulmonary disease, but extrapulmonary spread is not uncommon, especially in immunocompromised hosts. Almost every organ can be affected via blood dissemination. Important advances have been made in the recent past in the field of chemotherapy, and now short-course regimens with very effective drugs are available so that tuberculosis is a curable disease. There is concern about the emergence of multidrug-resistant strains of *M. tuberculosis*, as recently reported from the United States and other industrialized countries. Prevention of tuberculosis at a public health level is based on vaccination of children and on case finding and appropriate treatment of active tuberculosis cases. Vaccination (to be considered for noninfected subjects only) is effective in preventing the development of primary disease but does not prevent infection. This technique is used throughout the world, except in the United States, where it has been decided to perform skin testing to determine people at risk. The cure of sputum-positive subjects is considered the most effective tool to reduce morbidity and mortality and to prevent circulation of the mycobacteria in the environment. Although tuberculosis is a highly communicable disease, tight contacts in closed environments with bacilliferous subjects are usually necessary to ensure transmission. Although the risk for *M. tuberculosis* transmission on aircrafts is not greater than in other confined spaces, recent investigations indicate that exposure to persons with infectious pulmonary tuberculosis may result in infection of others traveling on the same aircraft. Short-term travelers from areas of low endemicity to high endemicity are not considered at increased risk of infection, and there is no evidence that travelers with past exposure are at greater risk of developing disease during short stays. Therefore, BCG vaccination and other preventive measures are not recommended in the setting of travel.

BRUCELLOSIS

Brucellosis is caused by several species of the genus *Brucella*. It primarily affects farm animals, causing severe veterinary diseases and economic loss. Most farm animal species are susceptible to the infection, including cattle, sheep, and goats. Humans acquire the infection by consuming contaminated milk and dairy products or by direct contact with animals with the illness. In spite of programs to eradicate brucellosis in animals, human *Brucella* infections are increasing worldwide. Although animal and human brucellosis are still reported from virtually all world countries, the prevalence of human infection varies. It is closely determined by the efficiency of policies concerning stock keeping and milk production and is therefore higher in developing countries in general. Brucellosis is mainly an occupational disease affecting farmers and veterinarians. Food-borne brucellosis is not a rare event in travelers to *Brucella*-endemic areas. Travelers with persisting fever after exclusion of malaria and failure to isolate an organism in cultures over 72 hours should raise suspicion of brucellosis. They should be questioned about consumption of raw milk and soft cheese, and serologic tests for *Brucella*, and prolongation of blood cultures for at least 3 weeks should be performed. Pasteurized milk is safe, as are products from pasteurized milk. In fresh milk, brucellae can survive for several days and in cheese they survive for several months. On an individual traveler level, avoidance of potentially contaminated food and beverages is effective in preventing brucellosis. Effective prevention, however, will be achieved only when well-known policies for elimination of the infection in animals will be effectively applied throughout the world.

LEPTOSPIROSIS

Leptospirosis is a zoonosis of worldwide dimensions affecting both wild and domestic animals, due to several serovars of a spirochetal bacteria, *Leptospira interrogans*. The infection in animals is mild and persists in the kidney. Rodents may shed bacteria in the urine throughout their lifetime. Domestic animals may also be infected, but they usually remain leptospiruric for a few months to a year. Rodents and domestic animals are the major reservoirs and the source for human infection. Transmission occurs by accidental contact with urine, contaminated water, and soil. In temperate areas, leptospirosis is either a professional disease of farmers/veterinarians or affects fishermen and hunters. In the tropics, the pathogen is widespread in moist soil and water, and the infection is more common in the general population. The bacteria penetrate through the skin or mucosa and cause a systemic infection, the severity of which may range from asymptomatic to fulminant. Severe cases are characterized by liver and renal failure with mortality, in untreated cases as high as 30%. Some leptospira serovars are responsible for lymphocytic meningitis. Prevention of leptospirosis is difficult, especially in tropical areas where the disease is not limited to high-risk groups. Livestock and other domestic animals may be vaccinated, but the vaccine should contain antigens specific for the serovars that are prevalent in the area. Prevention of rodent-human contacts is also important. A human vaccine and the use of tetracycline chemoprophylaxis (200 mg/week) are available but are indicated for well-defined, high-risk populations only.

REFERENCES

1. Portaels F. Epidemiology of mycobacterial diseases. Clin Dermatol 1995;13:207–222.
2. Roberts B, Hirst R. Immunomagnetic separation and PCR for detection of *Mycobacterium ulcerans*. J Clin Microbiol 1997;35:2709–2711.
3. Meyers WM, Tignokpa N, Priuli GB, Portaels F. *Mycobacterium ulcerans* infection (Buruli ulcer): first reported patients in Togo. Br J Dermatol 1996;134:1116–1121.
4. Portaels F. Epidemiologie des ulceres à *Mycobacterium ulcerans*. Ann Soc Belge Med Trop 1989;69:91–103.
5. van der Werf TS, van der Graaf WTA, Groothuis DG, Knell AJ. *Mycobacterium ulcerans* infection in Ashanti region, Ghana. Trans R Soc Trop Med Hyg 1989;83:410–413.
6. Bar W, Rush-Gerdes S, Marquez de Bar G, et al. *Mycobacterium ulcerans* infection in a child from Angola: diagnosis by direct detection ad culture. Trop Med Int Health 1998; 3:189–196.
7. Aguiar J, Stenou C. Les ulceres de Buruli en zone rurale au Benin: prise en charge de 635 cas. Med Trop (MARS) 1997; 57:83–90.
8. Rambukkana A, Yamada H, Zanazzi G, et al. Role of α-dystroglican as a Shwann cell receptor for *Mycobacterium leprae*. Science 1998;282:2076–2079.
9. World Health Organization. Global leprosy distribution in 1998. Wkly Epidemiol Rec 1998;73:188–190.
10. Noorden SK. Epidemiology and control of leprosy — a review of progress over the last 30 years. Trans R Soc Trop Med Hyg 1993;Suppl 7:515–517.
11. World Health Organization. Trend in leprosy detection. Wkly Epidemiol Rec 1998;73:169–175.
12. Ridley DS. Jopling WH. Classification of leprosy according to immunity: a five group system. Int J Lepr Other Mycobact Dis l966;34:255–273.
13. Meheus A, Antal GM. The endemic treponematoses: not yet eradicated. World Health Stat Q l992;45:228–237.
14. Perine PL, Hopkins DR, Niemel PLA, et al. Handbook of endemic treponematoses: yaws, endemic syphilis and pinta. Geneva: World Health Organization, 1984.
15. Backhouse JL, Hudson BJ, Hamilton PA, Nesteroff SI. Failure of penicilline treatment of yaws on Karkar island, Papua New Guinea. Am J Trop Med Hyg 1998;59:388–392.
16. Schwan TG, Hinnebusch BJ. Bloodstream versus tick-associated variants of a relapsing fever bacterium. Science 1998; 280:1938–1940.
17. Vidal V, Scragg IG, Catler SJ, et al. Variable major lipoprotein is a principal TNF-inducing factor of louse-borne relapsing fever. Nat Med 1998;4:1416–1420.
18. Talbert A, Nyange A, Molteni F. Spraying tick-infested houses with lambda-cyhalothrin reduces the incidence of tick-borne relapsing fever in children under five years old. Trans R Soc Trop Med Hyg 1998;92:251–253.
19. Goubeau PF. Relapsing fevers. A review. Ann Soc Belge Med Trop 1984;64:347–355.
20. Tissot Dupont H, La Scola B, William R, Raoult D. A focus of tick-borne relapsing fever in Southern Zaire. Clin Infect Dis 1997;25:139–144.
21. Cadavid D, Barbour AG. Neuroborreliosis during relapsing fever: review of the clinical manifestations, pathology, and treatment of infections in humans and experimental animals. Clin Infect Dis 1998;26:151–164.
22. Dworkin MS, Anderson DE Jr, Schwan TG, et al. Tick-borne relapsing fever in the northwestern United States and southwestern Canada. Clin Infect Dis 1998;26:122–131.
23. Rath PM, Rogler G, Schonberg A, et al. Relapsing fever and its serologic discrimination from Lyme borreliosis. Infection 1992;20:283–286.
24. Brouqui P, Raoult D. Ehrlichia. Ehrlichiosis. In: Encyclopédie medical chirurgie maladies infectieuses. Paris: Elsevier, 1998:1–10.
25. Andersson SGE, Zomorodipour A, Andersson JO, et al. The genome sequence of *Rickettsia prowazekii* and the origin of mitochondria. Nature 1998;396:133–140.
26. Azad FA, Beard CB. Rickettsial pathogens and their arthropod vectors. Emerg Infect Dis 1998;4:179–186.
27. Perine PL, Chandler BP, Krause DK, et al. A clinico-epidemiological study of epidemic typhus in Africa. Clin Infect Dis 1992;14:1149–1158.
28. World Health Organization. Global surveillance of rickettsial diseases: memorandum from a WHO meeting. Bull World Health Organ 1993;71:293–296.

29. Raoult D, Ndihojubwayo JB, Tissot-Dupont H, et al. Outbreak of epidemic typhus associated with trench fever in Burundi. Lancet 1998;352:353–358.

30. Zanetti G, Francioli P, Tagan D, et al. Imported epidemic typhus. Lancet 1998;352:1709.

31. Parola P, Vogelaers D, Roure C, et al. Murine typhus in travelers returning from Indonesia. Emerg Infect Dis 1998; 4:677–680.

32. Ghorbani RP, Ghorbani AJ, Jain MK, Walker DH. A case of scrub typhus probably acquired in Africa. Clin Infect Dis 1997;25:1473–1474.

33. Thiebaut MM, Bricaire F, Raoult D. Scrub typhus after a trip to Vietnam. N Engl J Med 1997; 336:1613–1614.

34. Pradutkanchana J, Silpapojakul K, Paxton H, et al. Comparative evaluation of four serodiagnostic tests for scrub typhus in Thailand. Trans R Soc Trop Med Hyg 1997;91:425–428.

35. Watt G, Chouriyagune C, Ruangweerayud R, et al. Scrub typhus infections poorly responsive to antibiotics in Northern Thailand. Lancet 1996;348:86–89.

36. Anderson BE, Dawson JE, Jones DC, Wilson KH. Ehrlichia chaffeensis, a new species associated with human ehrlichiosis. J Clin Microbiol 1991;29:2838–2842.

37. Chen SM, Dumler JS, Bakken JS, Walker DH. Identification of a granulocytic Ehrlichia species as the etiologic agent of human disease. J Clin Microbiol 1994;32:589–595.

38. Schwartz I, Fish D, Daniels TJ. Prevalence of the richettsial agent of human granulocytic ehrlichiosis in ticks from a hyperendemic focus of Lyme disease. N Engl J Med 1997; 337:49–50.

39. Horowitz HW, Kilchevsky E, Haber S, et al. Perinatal transmission of the agent of human granulocytic ehrlichiosis. N Engl J Med 1998;339:375–378.

40. Bakken JS, Krueth J, Wilson-Nordskog C, et al. Clinical and laboratory characteristics of human granulocytic ehrlichiosis. JAMA 1996;275:199–205.

41. Sumner JW, Nicholson WL, Massung RF. PCR amplification and comparison of nucleotid sequences from the groESL heat shock operon of Ehrlichia species. J Clin Microbiol 1997;35:2087–2092.

42. Goodman JL, Nelson C, Vitale B, et al. Direct cultivation of the causative agent of human granulocytic ehrlichiosis. N Engl J Med 1996;334:209–215.

43. Buitrago MI, Ijdo JW, Rinaudo P, et al. Human granulocytic ehrlichiosis during pregnancy treated successfully with rifampin. Clin Infect Dis 1998;27:213–215.

44. Brouqui P, Lascola B, Roux V, Raoult D. Chronic Bartonella quintana bacteriemia in homeless patients. N Engl J Med 1999;340:184–189.

45. Wong MT, Dolan MJ, Lattuada CP, et al. Neuroretinitis, aseptic meningitis, and lymphoadenitis associated with Bartonella (Rochalimea) henselae infection in immunocompetent patients and patients infected with human immunodeficiency virus type 1. Clin Infect Dis 1995;21:352–360.

46. Koelher JE, Sanchez MA, Garrido CS, et al. Molecular epidemiology of Bartonella infections in patients with bacillary angiomatosis-peliosis. N Engl J Med 1997;337:1876–1883.

47. Maurin M, Raoult D. Bartonella infections: diagnostic and management issues. Curr Opin Infect Dis 1998;11:189–193.

48. Amano Y, Rumbea J, Knobloch J, et al. Bartonellosis in Ecuador: serosurvey and current status of cutaneous verrucous disease. Am J Trop Med Hyg 1997;57:174–179.

49. Matteelli A, Castelli F, Spinetti A, et al. Verruga peruana in an Italian traveler from Peru. Am J Trop Med Hyg 1994;50:143–144.

50. Punyagupta S. Melioidosis: review of 689 cases and presentation of a new clinical ciassification. In: Punyagupta S, ed. Melioidosis. Bangkok: Bangkok Medical Publishers, 1989.

51. Thummakul T, Wilde H, Tantawichien T. Melioidosis, an environmental and occupational hazard in Thailand. Mil Med 1999;164:658–662.

52. Chaowagul W, White NJ, Dance DAB, et al. Melioidosis: a major cause of community-acquired septicemia in northeastern Thailand. J Infect Dis 1989;159:890–899.

53. Woods ML, Bart W, Howard DM, et al. Neurological melioidosis: seven cases from the northern territory of Australia. Clin Infect Dis 1992;15:163–169.

54. Ashdown LR, Guard RV. The prevalence of melioidosis in northern Queensland. Am J Trop Med Hyg 1984;33: 474–478.

55. Kanaphum P, Thirawattanasuk N, Suputtamongkol Y, et al. Serology and carriage of Pseudomonas pseudomallei: a prospective study in 1,000 hospitalized children in northern Thailand. J Infect Dis 1993;167:230–233.

56. Thummakul T, Wilde H, Tantawichian T. Melioidosis, an environmental and occupational hazard in Thailand. Mil Med 1999; 164:658–662.

57. Osetraas GR, Hardman JM, Bass JW, et al. Neonatal melioidosis. Am J Dis Child 1971;122:446.

58. Osterberg LG, Chau PY, Raffin TA. Pulmonary melioidosis. Chest 1995;108:1420–1424.

59. Vatcharapreechasakul T, Supputamongkol Y, Dance DAB, et al. Pseudomonas pseudomallei liver abscess: a clinical, laboratory and ultrasound study. Clin Infect Dis 1992;14:412–417.

60. Kosuwon W, Saengnipanthkul S, Mahaisavariya B, et al. Musculoskeletal melioidosis. J Bone Joint Surg 1993;75-A: 1811–1815.

61. Dharakul T, Anuntagool SS, Chaowagul N, et al. Diagnostic value of an antibody enzyme-linked immunosorbent assay using affinity-purified antigen in an area endemic for melioidosis. Am J Trop Med Hyg 1997;56:418–423.

62. Appassakij H, Silpojakul KR, Wansit R, et al. Diagnostic value of indirect hemagglutination test for melioidosis in an endemic area. Am J Trop Med Hyg 1990;42:248–253.

63. Wuthiekanun V, Dance D, Chaowagul W, et al. Blood culture techniques for the diagnosis of meliodosis. Eur J Clin Microbiol Infect Dis 1990;9:654–658.

64. Suputtamongkol Y, Rajchanuwong W, Chaowagul DAB, et al. Ceftazidime vs amoxicillin in the treatment of severe melioidosis. Clin Infect Dis 1994;19:846–853.

65. Suputtamongkol Y, Dance DAB, Chaowagul W, et al. Amoxycillin-clavulanic acid treatment of melioidosis. Trans R Soc Trop Med Hyg 1991;85:672–675.

66. Chaowagul W, Supputamongkul Y, Smith MD, et al. Oral fluoroquinolone for maintenance treatment of melioidosis. Trans R Soc Trop Med Hyg 1997;91:599–601.

67. Perry RD, Fetherston RD. Yersinia pestis — etiologic agent of plague. Clin Microbiol Rev 1997;10:35–66.

68. World Health Organization. Human plague in 1996. Wkly Epidemiol Rec 1998;47:366–369.

69. Campbell GL, Hughes JM. Plague in India: a new warning from a old nemesis. Ann Intern Med 1995;122:151–153.

70. Centers from Diseases Control and Prevention. Fatal human plague—Arizona and Colorado, 1996. JAMA 1997; 278:230–232.

71. Centers for Diseases Control and Prevention. Detection of notifiable diseases through surveillance for imported plague—New York, September/October 1994. MMWR Morb Mortal Wkly Rep 1994;43:805–807.

72. Chanteau S, Rabarijaona L, O'Brien T, et al. F1 antigenaemia in bubonic plague patients, a marker of gravity and efficacy of therapy. Trans R Soc Trop Med Hyg 1998;92:572–573.

73. William JE, Gentry MK, Braden CA, et al. Use of enzyme linked immunosorbent assay to measure antigenaemia during acute plague. Bull World Health Organ 1984;62:463–466.

74. Galimand M, Guiyoule A, Gerbaud G, et al. Multidrug resistance in *Yersinia pestis* mediated by a transferable plasmid. N Engl J Med 1997;337:677–680.

75. Heath DG, Anderson GW Jr, Mauro JM, et al. Protection against experimental bubonic and pneumonic plague by a recombinant capsular F1-V antigen fusion protein vaccine. Vaccine 1998;11:1131–1137.

76. Bobo LD, Novak N, Munoz B, et al. Severe disease in children with trachoma is associated with persistent *Chlamydia trachomatis* infection. J Infect Dis 1997;176:1524–1530.

77. Thylefors B, Negril AD, Pararajasegaram R, Dadzie KY. Global data on blindness. Bull World Health Organ 1995;73:115–121.

78. Munoz B, Aron J, Turner V, West S. Incidence estimates of the late stages of trachoma among women in a hyperendemic area of central Tanzania. Trop Med Int Health 1997;2:1030–1038.

79. West S, Munoz B, Lynch M, et al. Impact of face washing on trachoma in Kongwa, Tanzania. Lancet 1995;345:155–158.

80. Thylefors B, Dawson CR, Jones BR, et al. A simplified system for the assessment of trachoma and its complications. Bull World Health Organ 1987;65:477–483.

81. Dawson CR, Schachter J, Sallam S, et al. A comparison of oral azithromycin with topical oxytetracycline/polymyxin for the treatment of trachoma in children. Clin Infect Dis 1997;24:363–368.

82. Dolin PJ, Faal H, Johnson GJ, et al. Reduction of trachoma in a sub-Saharan village in absence of a disease control programme. Lancet 1997;349:1511–1512.

83. Wise R. Bioterrorism: thinking the unthinkable. Lancet 1998;351:1378.

84. Van Ness GB. Ecology of anthrax. Science 1971;172:1303–1307.

85. Paulet R, Caussin C, Coudray JM, et al. Visceral form of human anthrax imported from Africa. Presse Med 1994;23:477–478.

86. Longfield R. Anthrax. In: Syrickland GT, ed. Hunter's tropical medicine. Philadelphia: WB Saunders, 1991:434–438.

87. Smego RA, Genrian B, Desmangels G. Cutaneous manifestations of anthrax in rural Haiti. Clin Infect Dis 1998;26:97–102.

88. Lalitha MK, Thomas MK. Penicillin resistance in *Bacillus anthracis*. Lancet 1997;349:1522.

Chapter 27

PARASITIC TROPICAL INFECTIONS

MARY ELIZABETH WILSON AND THOMAS LÖSCHER

INTRODUCTION AND OVERVIEW

The term parasite is used in many ways. This chapter will focus on infections caused by protozoa and helminths (worms) and will include arthropods and other ectoparasites that infest the skin and superficial tissues. Discussion will encompass those parasites found exclusively in tropical regions as well as many others that are widely distributed but may be especially common in tropical and developing countries.

Only a few of the infections discussed in this section require urgent intervention; many are subacute or chronic; some require only explanation and reassurance. One of the most important parasitic infections in the world, malaria, is discussed separately in Chapter 21. Parasitic infections that cause diarrhea are also discussed in Chapter 20. Separate chapters address the evaluation of patients with fever and eosinophilia.

Many protozoa and helminths have a focal geographic distribution. As a consequence, only a portion of the world's population may be regularly exposed to these infections, and many travelers and their physicians may be unaware of the existence of these parasites, their modes of transmission, and disease caused by them.

Short-term travelers to an area may be at little risk for parasitic infections that are highly endemic in the local population. Some of the reasons include the fact that travelers use accommodations and engage in activities that allow little contact with soil, vectors, animals, and highly risky foods; duration of stay is brief; repeated exposures may be necessary to cause disease with some parasites; and some infections are found in remote areas inaccessible to most travelers. Most parasites that infect short-term travelers are those that can be transmitted by a single arthropod bite or single water exposure and those that commonly contaminate food and drink.

Many helminths and some protozoa have the capacity for prolonged survival in the human host. As a consequence, symptoms may develop months or years after a person has left an endemic area. The clinical incubation period (interval between exposure and first symptoms of infection) can be more than a year for some infections. Some parasites may cause prominent symptoms during a stage of parasite development when infection is difficult to diagnose (e.g., pulmonary migration phase of ascaris, hookworm or strongyloides, or early schistosomiasis). Especially in helminth infections, the prepatent period (interval between exposure and beginning of the produc-

tion of sexual products; e.g., eggs or larvae) has to be taken into consideration (Table 27–1). Repeated investigations over a period of time may be necessary before a definite parasitologic diagnosis can be made.

Many parasitic infections occur primarily in persons who have had prolonged exposures in tropical or developing countries, have traveled to remote areas, or have engaged in unusual activities that have brought them in close contact with the local environment. Unlike bacteria, viruses, and protozoa, adult forms of most helminthic pathogens (e.g., schistosomes, filariae, ascaris) are unable to multiply in the human host. Eggs or immature forms produced by the adult parasites may contribute to the symptoms and pathologic changes in tissue. In many instances, clinical expression in the human host is determined by the burden of parasites; intense or repeated exposures may be needed to cause clinical disease. For some parasitic infections, such as filariasis, a heightened immune response characterizes infection in persons from nonendemic regions in contrast to residents from an area who may have been exposed since early childhood.[1] Tissue-invasive helminthic infections frequently are associated with eosinophilia (see Chapter 42.4, Table 42.4–4).

Intestinal protozoan infections (e.g., amebiasis, giardiasis) may be transmitted directly from person to person by the fecal-oral route, although indirect transmission through fecally contaminated food or water is much more common. Other protozoan infections generally are not transmissible from person to person through casual contact. Transmission can occur via blood transfusions (e.g., malaria, toxoplasmosis, Chagas' disease), from mother to fetus, and through shared needles (e.g., malaria), organ transplantation, and other unusual means. A few of the helminthic infections can be spread in a shared environment through the fecal-oral route (e.g., cysticercosis). In most instances, however, patients can be reassured that these infections are not casually transmissible; most pose no risk to household contacts, especially if good hygienic practices are followed.

Parasites commonly enter the human host through the skin or mucous membranes or via the gastrointestinal tract after ingestion of contaminated food or drink. The mode of transmission will be used as the organizing principle for the discussion of specific diseases because it allows a way of integrating information about risky activities and preventive strategies. An arthropod vector frequently is required to inoculate the parasite into the human host (or to facilitate its entry); essential stages of

Table 27–1.   PREPATENT PERIODS OF
IMPORTANT HELMINTH INFECTIONS

HELMINTH INFECTION	PREPATENT PERIOD
Nematode infections	
Enterobiasis	1–4 weeks
Ascariasis	2–3 months
Trichuriasis	2–3 months
Hookworm infection	3–8 weeks
Strongyloidiasis	2–4 weeks
Trichostrongyliasis	3–4 weeks
Capillariasis	2–3 weeks
Trichinelliasis	1 week (larvae in the blood)
Wuchereriasis	7–24 months
Brugiasis	3–12 months
Onchocerciasis	7–34 months
Loiasis	5 months to several years
Dracunculiasis	8 months to 2 years
Trematode infections	
Schistosomiasis	5–10 weeks
Paragonimiasis	8–10 weeks
Fascioliasis	2–4 months
Opisthorchiasis	3–6 weeks
Fasciolopsiasis	2–3 months
Cestode infections	
Taeniasis	2–4 months
Hymenolepiasis	2–4 weeks
Diphyllobothriasis	3–5 weeks
Diphylidiasis	2–3 weeks

parasite development may occur in the arthropod as well. Parasite forms found in water, soil, or sand may be able to penetrate skin if direct contact occurs. Ingestion of parasites (eggs, larvae, or other infective form) remains an important means of transmission via fecally contaminated food and drink or from fingers, in raw or undercooked flesh, fruits, and vegetables, and parasite-contaminated water. The routes of transmission (blood transfusion, transplacentally, tissue transplantation, etc.) noted above are rare and infrequently affect the traveler.

GEOGRAPHIC CONSIDERATIONS

The focal geographic distribution of many parasites reflects the need for certain climatic conditions, specific insect vectors (e.g., malaria, Chagas' disease), or appropriate intermediate hosts (e.g., right kind of snails for schistosomiasis). Often, the requirements for persistence and spread in an area involve a complex interplay of socioeconomic, cultural, dietary, climatic, environmental, and other factors. The geographic distribution of most diseases is not fixed and may expand or contract or even skip to new regions. Many examples exist of extension of parasitic infections into new regions at times of change, such as displacement of populations, social and economic

collapse, change in land use (e.g., clearing of forests, building of dams), and introduction of new animals into an area. The fluidity of distribution of many diseases can complicate the process of developing an informed differential diagnosis in a person who has had diverse geographic exposures.

Access to information about the geographic distribution of diseases is essential in the evaluation of patients who have traveled or lived in distant regions. Many sources are available,[2–8] including Web sites. All are limited by the inevitable lag period between occurrence of events and dissemination of data, by lack of resources and diagnostic expertise for many diseases in many areas of the world, and by incomplete reporting.

Maps displaying data currently available from the World Health Organization (WHO) about the distribution for several diseases are shown in Figures 27–1, 27–2, 27–5, 27–6, 27–8, 27–10, and 27–14, including WHO maps for cutaneous leishmaniasis, visceral leishmaniasis, filariasis, onchocerciasis, American trypanosomiasis, African trypanosomiasis, and schistosomiasis. These maps provide a useful starting point in deciding whether specific diseases should be considered.

CAUSATIVE AGENTS AND TRANSMISSION MECHANISMS

ENTRY THROUGH SKIN

Arthropod vectors transmit the parasites that cause malaria, filariasis, leishmaniasis, and trypanosomiasis (African and American). After inoculation locally, all of these parasites can spread systemically and cause disease that can result in serious sequelae or death. After malaria, leishmaniasis is the most common of these in travelers.

Leishmaniasis   Leishmaniasis is a protozoan infection transmitted by the bite of an infective female sandfly. The three major clinical syndromes, visceral, cutaneous, and mucosal, reflect the location of infected macrophages. Infection is typically subacute to chronic. Findings may first be recognized weeks to months or longer after exposure.

According to WHO, in 1996 leishmaniasis was present in 88 countries. Annual estimates of cases were 500,000 cases of visceral leishmaniasis (VL) and 1 to 1.5 million cases of cutaneous leishmaniasis (CL). More than half of the cases of VL in recent years have been in the Sudan and India.[9] Infection in travelers is uncommon. In the United States between 1990 and 1995, the Centers for Disease Control and Prevention (CDC) released sodium stibogluconate for treatment of 167 patients with leishmaniasis.[9] CL acquired in the Americas accounted for 70% of these, reflecting the travel patterns of U.S. citizens. An earlier analysis of American CL found that the risk estimates varied greatly by country from about 1 in 1,000 travelers to Suriname to fewer than one per million for travelers to Mexico. Among the 58 persons interviewed in detail, the median time spent abroad was 54 days (range 4 days to 3 years).[10]

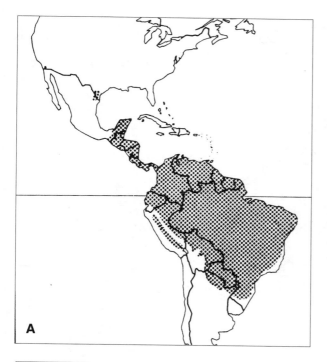

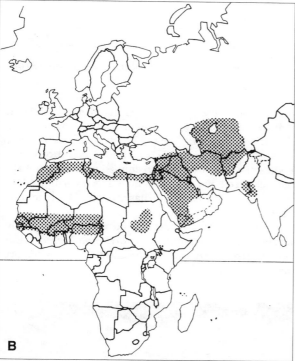

Figure 27–1. A, Distribution of cutaneous and mucocutaneous leishmaniasis in the New World. *B,* The distribution of Old World cutaneous leishmaniasis. From *Control of the leishmaniases: report of a WHO Expert Committee.* WHO Technical Report Series, No. 793, 1990:105, 108.

Depending on the species of leishmania and on host factors, infection may remain localized, manifesting as a cutaneous ulcer, or may spread hematogenously to involve viscera, causing fever and other systemic symptoms, or may infect mucocutaneous surfaces leading to

mucocutaneous leishmaniasis (MCL) with disfiguring, progressive destruction of tissues. The geographic distribution of CL, MCL, and VL is given in Figures 27–1 and 27–2.

CL typically begins with a papule that enlarges to a nodule with a central crust, which drops off to expose an ulcer that is painless, chronic, and may have a raised border and satellite lesions (Figure 27–3). Regional lymphadenopathy may be present. Because some New World leishmania that cause cutaneous ulcers can be complicated by late mucocutaneous disease, it is important to identify the infecting species if possible (Figure 27–4).

Symptoms of VL often begin insidiously and include fever, malaise, weight loss, and sweats. Disease is often subacute or chronic; symptoms may wax and wane. Diarrhea may be prominent. Splenomegaly, hepatomegaly, and lymphadenopathy are common findings on physical examination. The majority of patients have pancytopenia (anemia, leukopenia, thrombocytopenia) and elevated total serum-IgG levels. Symptoms may begin months or years after exposure in an endemic region. Persons infected with HIV are at increased risk for symptomatic infection, which may be difficult to diagnose. Mortality reaches 75% to 90% in untreated persons with symptomatic infection. The number of persons co-infected with HIV and leishmania has increased as HIV-infected persons have moved into rural areas and VL has spread into urban areas. In southern Europe, for example, 1.5% to 9% of AIDS patients have VL, which can reflect either recent acquisition or reactivation of latent infection.[11]

Diagnosis of CL and MCL can be made by finding amastigotes in tissue or on smears, although sensitivity of a single investigation is low (14% to 18%), especially in MCL. Biopsy specimens can also be cultured for *Leishmania* organisms using special media. In VL, bone marrow, lymph nodes, and other tissues can be examined for the characteristic amastigotes or cultured. Serology (e.g., indirect immunofluorescent antibody test [IFT], ELISA, immunoblot) usually is positive in VL and MCL; however, it may be negative in patients co-infected with HIV. Polymerase chain reaction (PCR) can detect leishmania DNA in all forms of leishmaniasis with high sensitivity. Species differentiation of the morphologically indistinguishable parasites is possible by zymodeme-typing, monoclonal antibodies, or PCR. The most commonly used treatment is with pentavalent antimonials (sodium stibogluconate or meglumine antimonate), but antimony resistance of VL is spreading in Sudan and India.[12]

Filarial Infections Filarial infections are transmitted to humans by the bite of an infective mosquito or fly. The larvae mature to adult worms whose progeny, the microfilariae, may contribute to the pathologic changes. Infections are usually chronic and characterized by eosinophilia, often high grade. Most filarial infections are uncommon or rare in short-term travelers. Filarial infections and their manifestations are described in Table 27–2. Figures 27–5 and 27–6 depict the geographic distributions for several of these infections.

Diagnosis typically relies on identification of microfilariae in blood or skin. Adult worms are rarely found

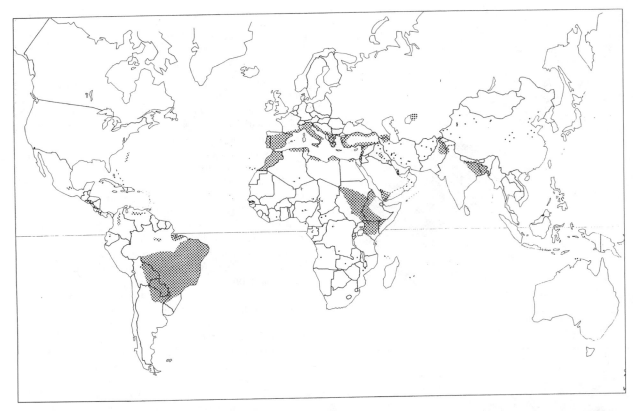

Figure 27–2. Distribution of Old World and New World visceral leishmaniasis. From *Control of the leishmaniases: report of a WHO Expert Committee.* WHO Technical Report Series, No. 793, 1990:97.

except in *Loa loa*, where they may be seen traversing the eye, in onchocerciasis in subcutaneous nodules, and in *Wuchereria bancrofti*, when they are found (often unexpectedly) in a surgically excised mass (e.g., scrotal mass). Figure 27–7 shows swelling of the hand caused by loiasis. Blood can be examined for microfilariae in suspected infections with *Brugia malayi, W. bancrofti, Loa loa,* and mansonelliasis. The timing of the blood specimens should correspond to the peak blood levels of microfilariae for that species. Use of special filters can increase the yield. Superficial skin snips are used to diagnose skin microfilariae. Currently available tests for the detection of antibodies may be useful for screening diagnosis in travelers but lack specificity. Recently, more specific antigen detection assays for lymphatic filariasis have become available.[13]

The mainstays of therapy have been diethylcarbamazine for *W. bancrofti, B. malayi, Loa loa,* and *Mansonella streptocerca,* and ivermectin for onchocerciasis and *M. ozzardi.*

Table 27–2. FILARIAL INFECTIONS

PATHOGEN	MAIN CLINICAL MANIFESTATIONS
Wuchereria bancrofti	Lymphangitis, recurrent, often with fever; hydroceles, late elephantiasis; pulmonary infiltrates
Brugia malayi	Similar to *W. bancrofti*
Brugia timori	Similar to *W. bancrofti*
Loa loa	Localized areas of angioedema that may be pale or red, itchy, painful; visible subconjunctival migration of adult worm
Mansonella ozzardi	Itching
Mansonella perstans	Itching, angioedema
Mansonella streptocerca	Itching, papular rash
Onchocerca volvulus	Itchy rash, recurrent fevers; lymphadenopathy; nodules, chronic infection associated with lichenification of skin, visual impairment (river blindness)

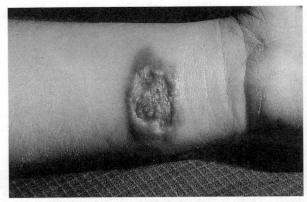

Figure 27–3. Cutaneous leishmaniasis ulcer in *Leishmania tropica* infection.

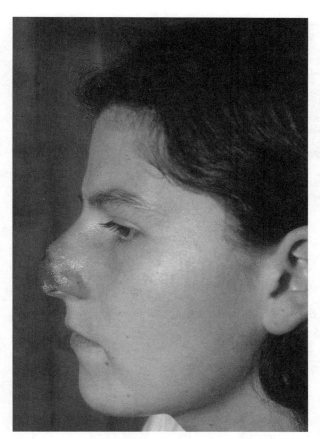

Figure 27–4.   Mucocutaneous leishmaniasis of the nose.

Trypanosomiasis *Trypanosoma cruzi*, a protozoan, is transmitted when parasites in feces of the reduviid bug enter the human host through mucous membranes, conjunctivae, or breaks in the skin. *T. cruzi* is widely distributed in many mammalian species in Mexico and Central and South America (Figure 27–8). The reduviid bug inhabits dwellings primarily in rural areas and seeks its blood meal at night (Figure 27–9). Although high rates of infection exist in some areas (more than 40% of the population infected in some countries), infections in short-term travelers are rare. Of 15 cases of acute American trypanosomiasis (Chagas' disease) reported to the CDC over a 20-year period, none occurred in returning tourists. Disease can be acute (fever, lymphadenopathy, hepatosplenomegaly, meningoencephalitis, myocarditis), subacute, or chronic. Sequelae of chronic infection involve primarily the heart (arrhythmias, congestive heart failure) and gastrointestinal tract (megacolon, megaesophagus).[14] Persons who are immunocompromised because of drugs or underlying diseases, such as HIV infection, can develop reactivation of latent infection. HIV-infected persons may develop *T. cruzi* brain abscesses, which resemble cerebral toxoplasmosis on imaging studies.[15] Blood collected by blood banks in endemic areas may contain parasites that can be transmitted by blood transfusion.

In parts of Africa (Figure 27–10), *T. brucei gambiense* and *T. brucei rhodesiense* cause African trypanosomiasis, also known as sleeping sickness because of the lethargy associated with central nervous system infection with the parasite. Infection is transmitted by the bite of an infective tsetse fly in rural areas. In the U.S., of the 15 patients with trypanosomiasis diagnosed and treated between 1967 and 1987, 73% had acquired infection during short-term travel (2–28 days) while participating on organized safaris. Infections were acquired in eight different countries in East Africa. In Germany, 11 imported cases have been reported since 1970. The usual interval between exposure and onset of fever is 1 to 3 weeks, although onset of symptoms may be delayed for months. A chancre at the site of the tsetse bite may begin 2 to 3 days after the bite and persist 2 to 4 weeks (Figure 27–11). Manifestations of infection include fever, headache, arthralgias, and generalized lymphadenopathy. A rash may wax and wane. Untreated infection can progress to involve the central nervous system. Diagnosis is made by identifying the parasite in blood, bone marrow, lymph node aspirate, or cerebrospinal fluid (CSF). Serology may be negative initially, especially in *T. brucei rhodesiense* infection. Treatment is available but toxic. Consultation with persons with expertise in treating the infection is recommended.

Besides the avoidance of known endemic areas of sleeping sickness, specific measures to prevent tsetse bites are limited. Wearing clothing that covers the arms and legs is advised, although tsetse flies can bite through most clothing except for heavy khaki. Repellents containing N,N-diethyl-3-methylbenzamide (DEET) apparently have some activity but cannot be relied on to prevent bites. During safaris in infested game parks, travelers can reduce risk by staying inside a vehicle with windows and outlets closed or screened. Tsetse flies bite during the day and seem to be attracted to dark colors and by moving vehicles.

DIRECT PENETRATION OF PARASITE THROUGH SKIN

Schistosomiasis Schistosomiasis, also known as snail fever or bilharziasis, is caused by trematodes (flukes). Snails are essential for some developmental stages of the parasite. Tiny, free-swimming cercariae (the infective larvae of the parasite) in fresh water penetrate human skin, undergo development, and migrate to venous plexes where mature worm pairs begin to produce eggs 1 to 3 months after the parasites entered the human host. The human response to eggs in tissues is characterized by granulomas and abundant eosinophils. The site of residence in the human host and the location of the main pathologic changes vary with the species of schistosome. Currently, WHO has listed 74 countries as endemic for schistosomiasis, although transmission is focal in many countries. Infection in travelers is usually acquired by bathing, swimming, boating, or rafting in cercaria-infested waters. The risk of infection is usually highest along the margins of lakes, slow moving streams, and irrigation ditches, although transmission has also occurred far from the shores of lakes, in swamps, dams, rivers, and flooded paddy fields. Swimming pools and even tap water can contain viable cercariae when there is an influx of water from contaminated sites and inadequate water

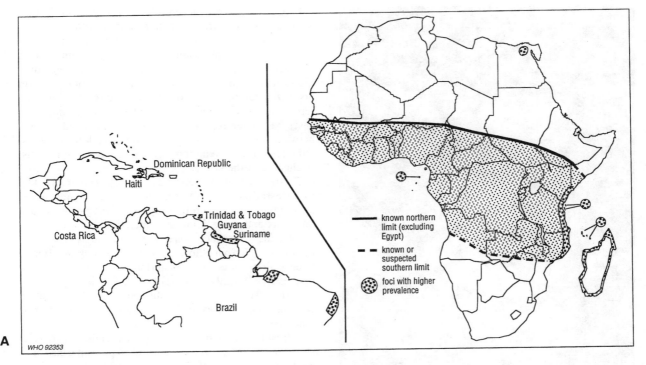

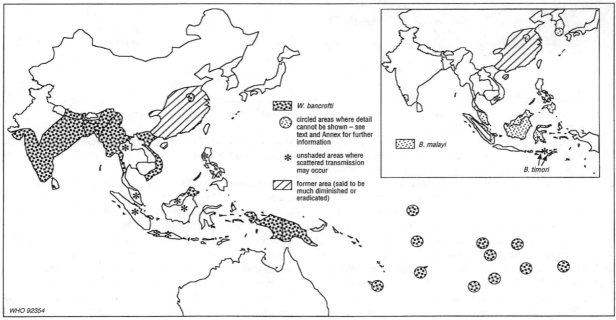

Figure 27–5.   A, Distribution of *Wuchereria bancrofti* in the African region and in the Americas. *B*, Distribution of filariasis in Southeast Asia and Western Pacific. From *Lymphatic filariasis: the disease and its control. Fifth report of the WHO Expert Committee on Filariasis.* WHO Technical Reports Series, No. 821, 1992.

treatment. Chlorinated pools that are properly maintained should be safe. Although seawater does not pose a risk, infection can be acquired near the mouths of rivers and in brackish waters.

Even persons with brief water exposure have become infected.[16] The cercariae penetrate skin over a period of 30 seconds to 10 minutes. An itchy, urticarial or maculopapular rash may follow contact with cercariae in water,

especially in persons previously sensitized (Figure 27–12). An acute illness (Katayama fever) characterized by fever, malaise, and eosinophilia can be seen during early infection quite often in travelers and expatriates[17] but is uncommon in the indigenous population. Other symptoms may include cough, diarrhea, hepatosplenomegaly, and sometimes urticaria. Neurologic findings can occur in early infection (e.g., transverse myelitis) and

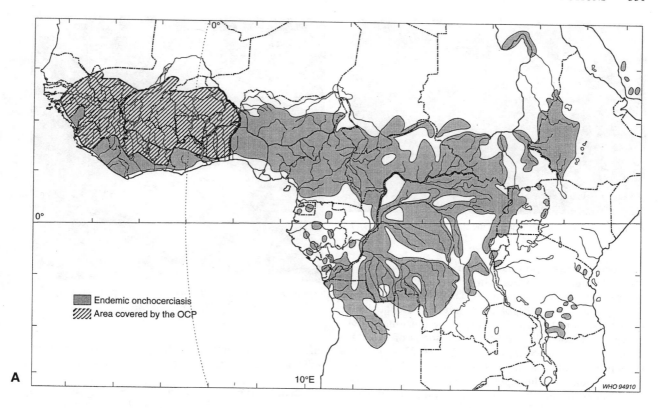

A

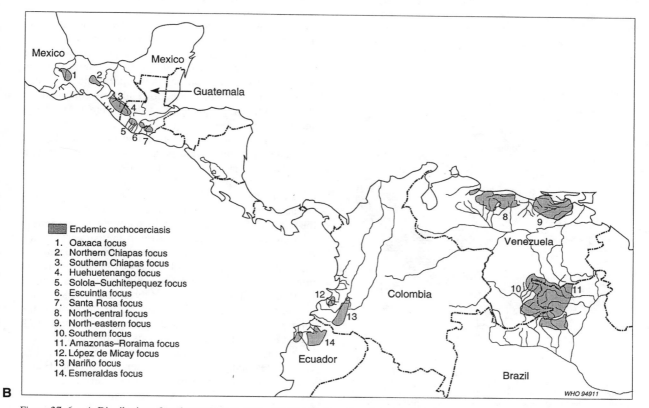

B

Figure 27–6. *A,* Distribution of onchocerciasis in Africa. *B,* Distribution of onchocerciasis in Latin America. From *Report of a WHO Expert Committee on Onchocerciasis Control.* WHO Technical Report Series, No. 852, 1995.

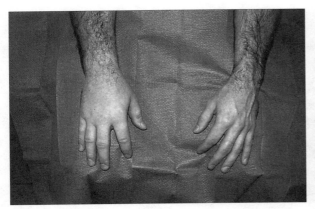

Figure 27–7.   Calabar swelling of the right hand in loiasis.

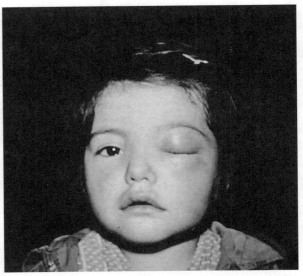

Figure 27–9.   Unilateral conjunctivitis at the portal of entry in *Trypanosoma cruzi* infection (Romaña's sign).

can also develop months to years after exposure to infested water and may occur in the absence of fever and other symptoms.[18] Eosinophilia is useful if present but is found in less than 50% of those infected. Hepatosplenomegaly, portal and pulmonary hypertension, bowel polyps, and strictures can be complications of *Schistosoma mansoni* and *S. japonicum* (Figure 27–13). Late complications of *S. haematobium* involve the urinary tract (e.g., hematuria, chyluria, renal stones, obstructive uropathy, bladder cancer). The geographic distribution of these parasites is shown in Figure 27–14.

Infection is diagnosed by identifying eggs in feces, urine, rectal biopsy, or other tissue. However, in acute schistosomiasis, fever and eosinophilia typically begin during the prepatent period, before eggs are produced. Sensitive and specific serologic tests are available, although they may be negative in the first week or so of symptomatic

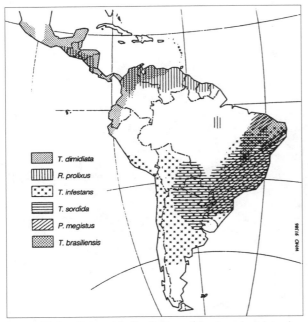

Figure 27–8.   Geographic distribution of the six major triatomine vectors of Chagas' disease (American trypanosomiasis). From *Control of Chagas disease. Report of a WHO Expert Committee.* WHO Technical Report Series, No. 811, 1991.

infection. Praziquantel is the drug of choice for treatment, although it has limited activity in early infection.

Hookworm Infection and Strongyloidiasis

Filariform larvae of two nematodes, strongyloides and hookworm (*Ancylostoma duodenale*, *Necator americanus*), gain entry into the human host by penetrating skin. The larvae have a pulmonary migration phase before the parasites reach maturity and settle in the gut. Hookworm infections are usually associated with mild or no symptoms, unless infection is heavy, a condition seen almost exclusively in persons who have been repeatedly exposed in developing countries. Then, severe hookworm anemia can develop. Eosinophilia may be present in hookworm infection and more commonly in strongyloidiasis. Diagnosis is made by detection of eggs and larvae in feces. Strongyloidiasis can be difficult to detect and coproculture may be necessary. Serology is available for strongyloidiasis (ELISA). Treatment is with albendazole, ivermectin, or thiabendazole.[19]

Strongyloidiasis has unique characteristics that make it a formidable clinical challenge.[20] Because rhabditiform larvae can mature directly to invasive filariform larvae in the human host, infection can be maintained indefinitely without the need for re-exposure to the parasite. Filariform larvae have the capacity to invade skin and can disseminate to all organs and tissues in persons who are immunocompromised. An itchy skin rash may develop at the time of initial penetration of the skin. Episodic, itchy, urticarial, or serpiginous lesions occur throughout the time of infection, often on the buttocks or in the groin area. Movement in the skin lesions, up to 5 to 10 cm per hour, may be observed (larva currens) (Figure 27–15). Gastrointestinal symptoms are often nonspecific. Heavy infection causes malabsorption. In the hyperinfection syndrome, often complicated by bacteremia, larvae may be found in sputum, CSF, and throughout the body. Persons on steroids and with other conditions that compromise the

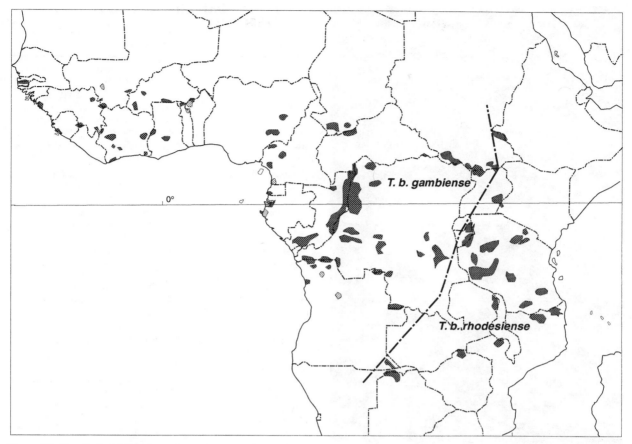

Figure 27–10. Foci of African trypanosomiasis. From *Epidemiology and control of African trypanosomiasis. Report of a WHO Expert Committee.* WHO Technical Report Series, No. 739, 1986.

immune system are more likely to develop disseminated infection. To completely eradicate infection, repeated or extended treatment courses may prove necessary, especially in hyperinfective strongyloidiasis.

Larval nematodes that are unable to penetrate deeper than the epidermis cause the clinical syndrome of cutaneous larva migrans, also known as creeping eruption (Figure 27–16). The third-stage larvae of dog and cat hookworms (*Ancylostoma caninum* and *Ancylostoma*

braziliense) most commonly cause this eruption. The infective larvae that contaminate moist sandy soil penetrate the skin, typically causing a linear or serpiginous, pruritic track. Diagnosis is made clinically. Patients are treated with albendazole or ivermectin orally or topical thiabendazole.

Parasitic infections causing fever may require urgent intervention. Some of the associated findings and causes are described in Table 27–3.

INGESTION

A long list of parasitic infections can be acquired by ingestion (Table 27–4). Among the most important in travelers are giardiasis and amebiasis. Infections causing diarrhea are also discussed in the Chapter 20 Travelers' Diarrhea.

Amebiasis   Amebiasis is caused by *Entamoeba histolytica*, a protozoan parasite that frequently lives as a commensal within the large intestine. Geno- and phenotypic analysis has proved that there are two morphologically indistinguishable species, *E. histolytica* and *E. dispar*.[21] Only *E. histolytica* (sensu strictu) is pathogenic and able to invade the colonic wall and to cause amebic dysentery, liver abscesses, and, more rarely,

Figure 27–11. Trypanosome chancre of the leg in *Trypanosoma brucei rhodesiense* infection.

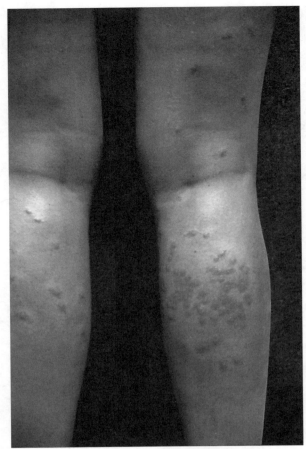

Figure 27–12.   Cercarial dermatitis in schistosomiasis.

other extraintestinal manifestations, whereas *E. dispar* is nonpathogenic. The two species can be differentiated genetically (DNA probes, PCR), by distinct isoenzyme patterns (zymodemes), and immunologically (monoclonal antibodies).

Infection is acquired by ingestion of cysts, which most commonly are excreted by asymptomatic cyst

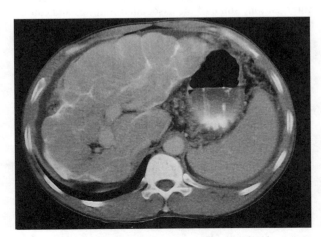

Figure 27–13.   Abdominal computed tomography showing hepatic schistosomiasis (inactive) in a Filipino man who also had mesenteric tuberculosis.

Table 27–3.   **PARASITIC INFECTIONS CAUSING FEVER**

INFECTION	COMMENTS
Amebiasis	Liver abscess. Hepatic findings may be minimal or absent. Chest x-ray may suggest pulmonary process
Clonorchiasis	Epigastric and right upper quadrant discomfort; alkaline phosphatase usually elevated; eosinophilia
Fascioliasis	Right-sided abdominal pain, diarrhea; tender liver; eosinophilia
Filariasis, lymphatic	Local soft-tissue findings (or pulmonary infiltrates) may accompany fever
Gnathostomiasis	Early fever; intermittent, migratory swellings in skin and subcutaneous tissues
Leishmaniasis, visceral	Hepatosplenomegaly; weight loss; diarrhea and cough may be prominent; anemia, leukopenia, and thrombocytopenia are common
Malaria	Fever and chills; splenomegaly; thrombocytopenia common in falciparum malaria
Opisthorchiasis	Epigastric and right upper quadrant discomfort; eosinophilia
Schistosomiasis	Gastrointestinal and respiratory symptoms may accompany fever; neurologic deficits
Trichinosis	Severe myalgias, facial swelling
Toxoplasmosis	Fever, lymphadenopathy, lymphocytosis
Trypanosomiasis, African	Episodic fevers, headache, myalgias, lymphadenopathy, central nervous system changes
Trypanosomiasis, American (Chagas')	Acute: hepatosplenomegaly, lymphadenopathy, chagoma (25%)
Visceral larva migrans (toxocariasis)	Cough, wheezing, myalgias, tender enlarged liver, eosinophilia

Some flukes and other worms (e.g., ascaris) precipitate fever when they enter bile ducts and obstruct bile flow.

passers. Transmission occurs most often through fecally contaminated water but also through contaminated food and through direct fecal-oral transmission from person to person.

The worldwide prevalence of *Entamoeba* infection is approximately 10%. However, a smaller percentage of persons (10% or less) are infected with *E. histolytica* and at risk of developing invasive disease. Infection rates in travelers vary from 0% to 4% and are highly dependent on the area visited, hygienic practices, and intensity and duration of exposure.[22] Infections with *E. histolytica* are acquired almost exclusively in warm climates, do not cause disease in all persons, and may persist asymptomatically for long periods.

The incubation period is days to years. The course of amebic dysentery may be acute, chronic, or intermittent. In travelers, common findings are a few diarrheal stools per day streaked with mucus and blood. Fever and severe constitutional symptoms are usually absent, although

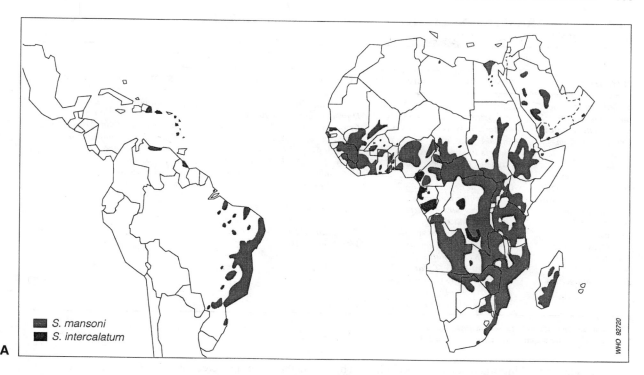

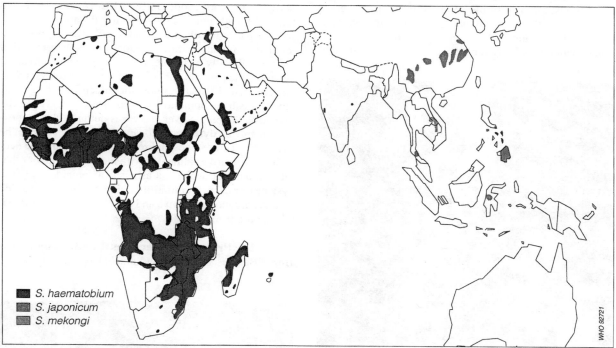

Figure 27–14.   *A*, Distribution of schistosomiasis (*S. mansoni* and *S. intercalatum*). *B*, Distribution of schistosomiasis *(S. haematobium, S. japonicum,* and *S. mekongi).* From *The control of schistosomiasis. Second report of the WHO Expert Committee.* WHO Technical Report Series, No. 830, 1993.

infection can be severe, causing frequent bloody diarrhea, fever, vomiting, dehydration, tenesmus, generalized abdominal tenderness, and prostration. Complications include hemorrhage, perforation, and peritonitis. Fulminant disease is more common in malnourished people, during pregnancy and puerperium, and in patients taking steroids or other immunosuppressive drugs. Amebic liver abscesses may develop in persons without a history of dysentery, sometimes after a latency period of months or even years (Figure 27–17). The main symptoms are fever, upper abdominal pain, and tenderness and enlargement of the liver. Complications are rupture into the peritoneum, the pleural space or the pericardium, peritonitis, and secondary bacterial infection.

Table 27–4.   PARASITIC INFECTIONS ACQUIRED BY INGESTION OF CONTAMINATED SOIL, FOOD, OR WATER

| PROTOZOA | HELMINTHS | | |
	NEMATODES (ROUNDWORMS)	TREMATODES (FLUKES)	CESTODES (TAPEWORMS)
Acanthamoeba spp*	*Ancylostoma duodenale* [†]	*Clonorchis sinensis*	*Diphyllobothrium latum, D. pacificum*
Balantidium coli	*Angiostrongylus cantonensis*	*Dicrocoelium dendriticum*	*Dipylidium caninum*
Blastocystis hominis	*Angiostrongylus costaricensis*	*Echinostoma* spp (*E. ilocanum*)	*Echinococcus granulosus, E. vogeli*
Cryptosporidium spp (*C. parvum*)	*Anisakis simplex*	*Fasciola hepatica, F. gigantica*	*Echinococccus multilocularis*
Cyclospora (*C. cayetanensis*)	*Ascaris lumbricoides*	*Fasciolopsis buski*	*Hymenolepis nana, H. diminuta*
Dientamoeba fragilis	*Baylisascaris procyonis*	*Gastrodiscoides hominis*	*Multiceps* spp
Entamoeba histolytica	*Capillaria philippinensis*	*Heterophyes* spp (*H. heterophyes*)	*Spirometra* spp
Giardia intestinalis	*Capillaria hepatica*	*Metagonimus yokogawai*	*Taenia saginata*
Isospora belli	*Dracunculus medinensis*	*Metorchis conjunctus*	*Taenia solium*
Microsporidia (several genera)	*Enterobius vermicularis*	*Nanophyetus salmincola*	
Naegleria fowleri *	*Gnathostoma spinigerum*	*Opisthorchis viverrini, O. felineus*	
Sarcocystis spp	*Oesophagostomum* spp	*Paragonimus* sp (*P. westermani*)	
Toxoplasma gondii	*Pseudoterranova decipiens*	*Watsonius watsoni*	
	Ternidens diminutus		
	Toxocara canis, T. cati		
	Trichinella spp (*T. spiralis*)		
	Trichostrongylus sp		
	Trichuris trichiura		

*Via mucosal membranes (i.e., nasopharynx, conjunctiva).
[†]Most infections are acquired by penetration of the skin.

The diagnosis of intestinal amebiasis is confirmed by the demonstration of trophozoites or cysts in the feces. Morphologically, *E. histolytica* cannot be differentiated from *E. dispar*, unless hematophagous trophozoites are found, which are highly suggestive of *E. histolytica*. New methods for the detection of *E. histolytica* and *E. dispar* antigens in stool (coproantigen-ELISAs) have shown high, although not absolute, sensitivity and specificity when used for the diagnosis and differentiation of *E. histolytica*.[23] As long as methods for species determination are not generally available, it seems prudent to treat all symptomatic patients, including those with nondysenteric amebiasis, and also asymptomatic infections when serology is positive. Immunodiagnosis is most useful in the diagnosis of amebic liver abscesses but may also be positive in amebic dysentery. However, serologic tests can be negative at early stages and repeated testing may be necessary. Standard treatment is with metronidazole or other nitroimidazoles, which act as tissue amebicides. To cure cyst passers, intraluminal amebicides, like diloxanide furoate, are more effective and may be given in combination with nitroimidazoles.

Other Protozoan Infections Acquired by Ingestion   Besides giardiasis and amebiasis, other intestinal

Figure 27–15.   Larva currens in strongyloidiasis.

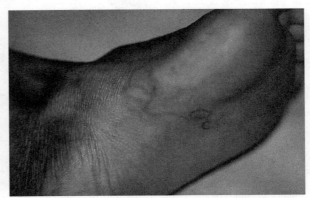

Figure 27–16.   Cutaneous larva migrans (creeping eruption).

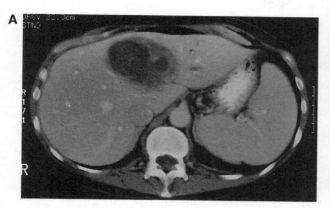
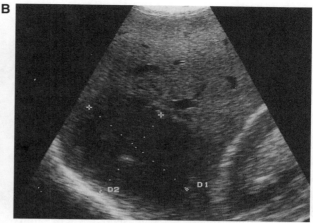

Figure 27–17.   Amebic liver abscesses in two different patients shown by *A,* computed tomography and by *B,* ultrasound.

protozoa may cause disease in travelers (Table 27–5). Many may be found in asymptomatic persons. Some (e.g., cryptosporidiosis, isosporiasis, microsporidiosis) cause chronic and debilitating disease in HIV-infected and other immunocompromised patients.

Ascariasis and Trichuriasis   The eggs of the roundworm *Ascaris lumbricoides* and the whipworm *Trichuris trichiura* are not infective at the time they are excreted in the feces by an infected individual. It takes 10 to 30 days in the environment for development of infective larvae. Infection is acquired by ingestion of embryonated eggs with contaminated food, water, or soil. Like hookworms and strongyloides, ascaris larvae have a pulmonary migration phase before they mature and reach the small intestine. Trichuris larvae migrate down the intestinal wall to reach the mucosa of the colon. Ascariasis and trichuriasis are the most frequent helminth infections in travelers and expatriates returning from the tropics. Infection rates may reach 1% in adults and about 2% in children. Both parasites can be found in the same individual.

In some patients, transient pulmonary symptoms and significant eosinophilia are present during the migration phase of ascaris. In travelers, the number of adult ascaris and trichuris usually is low and intestinal infection remains asymptomatic. Sometimes, an adult ascaris, measuring 10 to 30 cm, is passed per rectum or orally. Both ascaris and trichuris eggs are easy to detect in feces. However, there is a prepatent period of 2 to 3 months between the time of ingestion of the infective larvae and the beginning of egg production by the adult worms. For treat-

Table 27-5.   INTESTINAL PROTOZOAN INFECTIONS IN TRAVELERS

INFECTION	PARASITE	DISEASE	COMMENTS
Amebiasis	*Entamoeba histolytica*	Amebic dysentery, liver abscess	See text
Balantidiasis	*Balantidium coli*	Diarrhea, dysentery, liver abscess	Infection may be asymptomatic
Blastocystosis	*Blastocystis hominis*	Uncertain pathogenicity, diarrhea	Infections are usually asymptomatic
Cryptosporidiosis	*Cryptosporidium parvum*	Acute self-limited enteritis in the immunocompetent	Chronic enteritis and extra-intestinal manifestations in immunocompromised patients
Cyclosporiasis	*Cyclospora cayetanensis*	Acute self-limited enteritis	Prolonged or chronic course in some cases
Dientamoebiasis	*Diaentamoeba fragilis*	Diarrhea, abdominal cramps, flatulence	Most infections are asymptomatic
Giardiasis	*Giardia intestinalis*	Acute or chronic nondysenteric enteritis	See chapter on travelers' diarrhea
Isosporiasis	*Isospora belli*	Acute or protracted nondysenteric enteritis	Chronic enteritis and malabsorption in immunocompromised patients
Microsporidiosis	*Enterocytozoon bieneusi* and other species	Disease is rare in the immunocompetent	Chronic enteritis and extraintestinal manifestations in immunocompromised patients
Sarcocystosis	*Sarcocystis hominis* and other species	Acute self-limited enteritis	

ment, drugs of choice are benzimidazoles, like mebendazole or albendazole, which are effective against most intestinal nematode infections.

Enterobiasis *Enterobius vermicularis* has a worldwide distribution and occurs most frequently in children. The pinworms inhabit the large bowel, and the adult female deposits its eggs in the perianal area at night. Transmission is by ingestion of eggs through fecal-oral contamination directly from person to person or via contaminated food, toys, or fomites, or by swallowing eggs from the air or with dust. Eggs are infective shortly after being deposited, and autoinfection may be common, especially in young children. The risk of infection in travelers is generally low, unless there is a close contact, for example, from staying in a household where family members are infected. The most important symptom is perianal pruritus. Women may develop vulvovaginitis. Diagnosis is made by recovery of eggs from perianal swabs (scotch tape test) and by detection of adult worms in feces or on perianal skin. Various antihelminthics, like pyrantel pamoate, pyrvinium, and benzimidazoles, are effective.

Flukes The trematode parasites can be grouped according to the organ site they tend to inhabit (e.g., liver, lung, or intestinal flukes). Snails play an essential role in their development. The cercariae encyst as metacercariae in aquatic animals like fish and crabs, or on vegetation, which are sometimes eaten by humans.[24]

Infections with the oriental liver flukes *Clonorchis sinensis* and *Opisthorchis viverrini* are common in Southeast Asia. The cat liver fluke *O. felineus* is endemic also in Siberia and parts of Eastern Europe. Human infection results from consumption of raw freshwater fish, used in local dishes in endemic areas. There are only few reports of infections in tourists, although the prevalence in immigrants and refugees from endemic areas may reach 50%. Most infections are asymptomatic. Complications of heavy infections are cholangitis, biliary obstruction, and liver abscesses. Diagnosis rests on finding the small characteristic eggs in feces. The drug of choice for treatment is praziquantel.

The large liver fluke *Fasciola hepatica* occurs worldwide, primarily as a zoonosis. Occasional infections in travelers are usually acquired by eating raw watercress or other aquatic plants. Depending on the number of metacercariae ingested, fever, abdominal pain, hepatomegaly, eosinophilic leukocytosis, and abnormal liver function tests may develop.[25] Ectopic migration to other organs (e.g., lung, heart), biliary obstruction, and liver abscesses are possible complications. Diagnosis is made by the identification of the eggs in feces and more readily in bile. Serology is positive in most cases. Praziquantel is not effective. Emetine, bithionol, and albendazole have been tried with variable success. Triclabendazole, an investigational drug in humans, seems to be highly effective.

Infections with the lung flukes of the genus *Paragonimus* (e.g., *P. westermani*) occur as a zoonosis in many parts of the world. However, human infection is common only in East Asia, due to local eating habits. Infective metacercariae are ingested with raw or undercooked freshwater crabs and crayfish. Infections in travelers are rare, although cases in immigrants and refugees have been reported more frequently. Chronic cough and rusty sputum are the main symptoms. Radiographic findings can mimic tuberculosis. Complications may result from ectopic migration of flukes (e.g., to the brain or abdominal organs). Eosinophilia and specific antibodies are usually present. Eggs may be seen in sputum or feces. Therapy is with praziquantel.

Infections with a variety of intestinal flukes (e.g., *Fasciolopsis buski*, *Heterophyes* spp, *Echinostoma* spp) are common in Asia and some other parts of the world. Human infection occurs through the ingestion of metacercariae, which, depending on the species, are encysted in fish, in snails, or on vegetables. The occasional infections in travelers usually are light and asymptomatic. Diagnosis relies on the detection of eggs in feces and treatment is with praziquantel.

Tapeworm Infections The beef tapeworm, *Taenia saginata*, and the pork tapeworm, *Taenia solium*, are the most common intestinal cestodes affecting humans. Most carriers are asymptomatic and become aware of infection only when tapeworm segments (proglottides) are passed with feces. The eggs of *T. solium* passed within proglottides or free in the feces are infective to humans and can cause cysticercosis, with the human serving as the intermediate host for the larval stage of *T. solium*. When larval cysts (cysticerci) develop in the central nervous system, serious manifestations of neurocysticercosis (e.g., seizures, cerebral hypertension) may evolve after a period of a few months to many years.

Adult taenia infection is acquired by eating raw or undercooked beef (*T. saginata*) or pork (*T. solium*) containing cysticerci. Canine meat, which is eaten in parts of Southeast Asia, can be another source of infection with *T. solium*. Cysticercosis results from ingestion of *T. solium* eggs with fecally contaminated food or water or by direct fecal-oral transmission from person to person. Whereas *T. saginata* occurs worldwide, *T. solium* has a more focal distribution in areas with low hygienic standards and where pork is eaten raw or undercooked. The most important endemic regions are Latin America (e.g., Mexico), Africa (e.g., South Africa), India, China, Southeast Asia (e.g., northern Thailand), and Irian Jaya. Taeniasis does occur in travelers, mainly caused by *T. saginata*. Cysticercosis has rarely been observed in travelers and is more commonly seen in immigrants from endemic areas.[26]

Diagnosis of taeniasis is by identification of proglottides or eggs in feces. Taenia eggs are morphologically indistinguishable and species differentiation should be done with proglottides. Treatment is with praziquantel or niclosamide.

The diagnosis of neurocysticercosis relies on imaging techniques (CT, MRI) (Figure 27–18) and serology (ELISA, Western blot). Many patients can be successfully treated with albendazole or praziquantel, but neurosurgery may still prove necessary in patients with treatment failures and complications.

Other intestinal tapeworm infections that may occur in travelers are caused by fish tapeworms of the genus

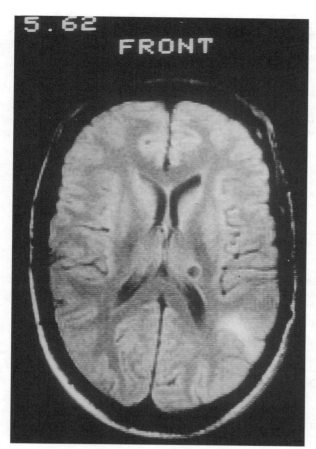

Figure 27–18.   Parenchymal brain cyst in *Taenia solium* cysticerosis shown by magnetic resonance imaging.

Diphyllobothrium and by the dwarf tapeworm *Hymenolepis nana.* Diphyllobothriasis is acquired by eating raw freshwater or sea fish in endemic areas (coastal and riverine regions of Russia, Northern Europe, Canada, Alaska, and the Pacific coast of South America). Infection may also result from imported fish. In 1980, salmon imported from Alaska caused a multistate outbreak in the U.S.[27]

Hymenolepiasis is common in warm climates. Both adults and larval stadia (cysticercoids) are present in the intestines. Eggs are infective when passed with the feces and may hatch in the intestinal tract, causing endogenous autoinfection. Infection is acquired through direct fecal-oral transmission from person to person but also through fecally contaminated food and water. Heavy infections, which occur predominantly in children, may cause abdominal cramps and diarrhea. Diagnosis of both diphyllobothriasis and hymenolepiasis is by finding the characteristic eggs in stools. The drug of choice is praziquantel.

Echinococcosis is a serious larval cestode infection in humans. Cystic hydatid disease (CHD) is caused by *Echinococcus granulosus.* The adult worms parasitize the intestines of dogs and other canids that excrete proglottides and eggs with feces. Human infection results from ingestion of eggs with contaminated food or water or from direct contact with infected animals (muzzle, fur). The slowly growing cysts in liver, lungs, and other organs usually cause clinical manifestations of a space-occupying lesion only after years, depending on the size and local-

ization of larval cysts. *E. granulosus* is enzootic worldwide and circulates between canids and ungulates as intermediate hosts. Human infection is common where hygienic practices are inadequate and feeding of infected ruminant viscera to dogs is common. Infections in travelers are rare. CHD may be seen more frequently in immigrants from highly endemic areas.

Alveolar hydatid disease (AHD) is caused by *Echinococcus multilocularis,* which is endemic in some parts of Central Europe, Russia, China, Canada, and Alaska. Final hosts are foxes and sometimes also dogs and cats. AHD in humans primarily affects the liver, which is infiltrated by the tumor-like larval tissue. Clinical manifestations, which include hepatomegaly and jaundice and mimic malignancy, usually evolve only after many years. AHD is a rare disease and is seen almost exclusively in people living in endemic areas.

Diagnosis of CHD and AHD is made by imaging techniques and serology. Sensitive and specific tests are available (ELISA, Western blot, Em2-ELISA). First-line treatment still is by surgery. However, a considerable percentage of patients are inoperable at the time of diagnosis, especially in AHD. Recent advances that have complemented surgical approaches include biliary stenting, percutaneous inactivation of *E. granulosis* hydatid cysts with ethanol (the PAIR procedure = puncture-aspiration-injection-reaspiration), and chemotherapy for inoperable and nonresectable infections.[28] Such patients may benefit from treatment with albendazole or mebendazole.

Trichinosis   *Trichinella* is enzootic in Africa, America, and Eurasia. Human infections with *T. spiralis* and rarely other *Trichinella* species result from eating raw or undercooked meat containing larvae. The main source is pork, but infection may also result from meat of wild boar, bears, game, and other carnivorous or omnivorous animals. Several outbreaks have been traced to horse meat.[29] Light infections (< 10 larvae/g) are usually asymptomatic. The incubation period varies from a few days to several weeks. Clinical manifestations include diarrhea, myalgia, fever, periorbital edema, splinter hemorrhages, and skin rash. Encephalitis and myocarditis may be dangerous complications. Diagnosis is made by serology and by detection of larvae in blood or muscle biopsy or in the incriminated meat product. Treatment is with benzimidazoles and steroids. Occasional infections in travelers have been reported.[30] Often, several persons are infected at the same time, belonging to a family or a group of travelers.

ECTOPARASITES

Infestations with arthropod ectoparasites (Table 27–6) more commonly seen in travelers are scabies (Figure 27–19), myiasis (Figure 27–20), tungiasis (Figure 27–21), pediculosis, and phthiriasis. In addition to the usually localized manifestations caused by these ectoparasites, many arthropods are vectors for the transmission of a variety diseases (e.g., Chagas' disease, arbovirosis, rickettsiosis, borreliosis, plague). Venomous arthropods are discussed in Chapter 30 Envenoming and Poisoning Caused by Animals.

Table 27–7 lists several types of skin lesions and describes the parasitic causes of each.

Table 27–6.   ECTOPARASITES IN TRAVELERS

INFECTION PARASITE	GEOGRAPHIC DISTRIBUTION	TRANSMISSION	MANIFESTATIONS
Scabies *Sarcoptes scabiei*	Worldwide	Close contact with infected persons	Pruritic skin eruptions (mite burrows)
Trombiculosis *Trombicula* spp	Worldwide	Contact with infested animals or vegetation	Itchy dermatitis
Myiasis			
Furuncular myiasis			
Dermatobia hominis (human bot fly)	Latin America	Ova are transported via mosquitoes	Furuncular swellings, secondary bacterial infection
Cordylobia anthropophaga (tumbu fly)	Africa	Ova are deposited on ground or clothes	Furuncular swelling, secondary bacterial infection
Creeping myiasis			
Hypoderma spp (cattle bot fly) *Gasterophilus* spp (horse bot fly)	Worldwide Worldwide	Penetration of larvae from ova deposited on skin	Cutaneous/subcutaneous larva migrans, furuncular swelling, rarely central nervous system invasion
Ophthalmic/nasopharyngeal myiasis *Oestrus ovis* and other species	Worldwide	Larviposition during flight onto eyes/nose	Conjunctivitis, rhinitis, rarely invasion of the eye
Wound myiasis *Callitroga, Cochliomyia, Chrysomyia, Wohlfahrtia,* and other species	Worldwide	Larviposition onto wounds	Extensive local destruction, secondary bacterial infection
Tungiasis *Tunga penetrans* (sand flea, chigoe fleas)	Tropical Africa, Latin America	Female flea penetrates skin at the foot	Itchy pea-sized swelling, secondary bacterial infection
Pulicosis *Pulex irritans,* animal-infesting fleas	Worldwide	Infestation of human dwellings (or animals)	Pruritic papules, often in clusters
Phthiriasis *Phthirus pubis* (pubic lice)	Worldwide	Close (mainly sexual) contact with infected persons	Pruritic dermatitis of pubic area; regional lymphadenitis; lice can also attach to eyelashes
Pediculosis *Pediculus humanus corporis* (body lice) *Pediculus humanus capitis* (head lice)	Worldwide	Close contact with infected persons or with infested clothes	Pruritic, eczematous dermatitis of body/scalp

SPECIAL POPULATIONS AT RISK

Three main factors influence risk of infection during travel: duration of stay, activities and lifestyle, and host factors, such as age and immunity. In general, likelihood of infection rises with increasing length of time spent in an area endemic for a parasitic infection. For example, a study of expatriates and visitors to Malawi found that the risk of schistosome infection, as indicated by serologic studies, increased with length of stay in Malawi. Persons who had resided there for 1 year or less had a seroprevalence of 11% as compared with 48% in those who had lived in Malawi 4 years or longer.[31] Travel to remote areas of developing countries, intimate contact with the resident population, and adoption of local eating habits all increase the risk for acquiring parasitic infections. Risks are usually higher in backpackers and expatriates working in remote areas, such as Peace Corps volunteers, missionaries, construction workers, hunters, and scientists. When infection occurs, the course of disease may be more severe in the very young and the aged, during pregnancy (e.g., malaria, toxoplasmosis, amebiasis), and when underlying diseases are present (e.g., cardiovascular, diabetes, immunosuppression).

PREVENTION

Individual protection from infection and disease may be feasible through vaccination, chemoprophylaxis, and avoidance of exposure. At the moment, there is not a single vaccine available against a human parasitic infection or disease, although several are under development.

In travelers, chemoprophylaxis plays a major role only in preventing malaria (see Chapter 21). Chemoprophylaxis to prevent lymphatic filariasis and onchocerciasis with diethylcarbamazine (medicated salt) and ivermectin has been successfully applied in mass campaigns for indigenous populations in highly endemic areas. This is not recommended routinely for travelers because the risk of acquiring filariasis is low.

Table 27–7.   COMMON SKIN FINDINGS IN PARASITIC INFECTIONS AND ARTHROPOD INFESTATIONS*

Maculopapular eruption
  Cercarial (schistosomal) dermatitis
  Hookworm
  Onchocerciasis
  Strongyloidiasis
  Ectoparasites (scabies, lice, myiasis)

Ulcer
  Amebiasis, cutaneous (painful, rapidly growing)
  Leishmaniasis, cutaneous and mucocutaneous

Nodules and cysts
  Cysticercosis   Myiasis
  Dracunculiasis   Onchocerciasis
  Echinococcosis   Paragonimiasis
  Filariasis (mass in scrotum) Scabies
  Gnathostomiasis   Sparganosis
  Leishmaniasis   Tungiasis
  Loiasis

Migratory swellings or serpiginous lesions
  Cutaneous larva migrans
  Gnathostomiasis
  Loiasis
  Strongyloidiasis
  Visceral larva migrans

*For more details of skin lesions, see Chapter 42.5.

Interventions that prevent exposure are the most important ways to minimize the risk of most parasitic infections. Travelers should adhere to the following rules that are simple to state but difficult to carry out consistently, especially during a long stay:

1. Avoid direct skin contact with fresh water (in schistosomiasis-endemic regions), soil, and sand. Walking barefooted and other skin contact with soils that may be contaminated with human and animal feces carries the risk of infection with helminth larvae (e.g., hookworm infection, strongyloidiasis, cutaneous larva migrans), tungiasis, and myiasis.
2. Avoid biting arthropods. Available means to protect against arthropod bites include bednets, window screens, appropriate clothing, repellents applied to skin and clothing, and insecticides (see Chapter 21.2).

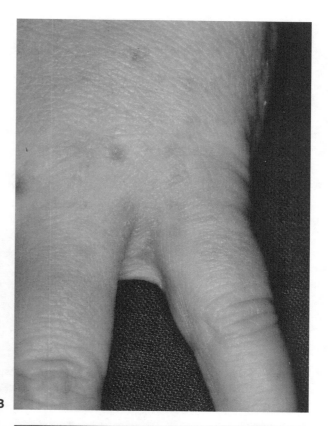

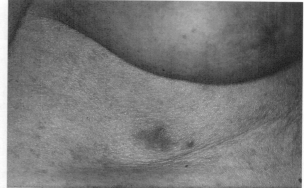

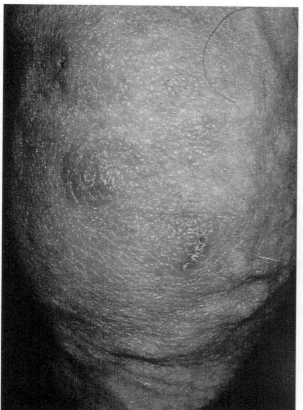

Figure 27–19.   Mite burrows in scabies in three body sites: penis (*A*), interdigital (*B*), and breast (*C*).

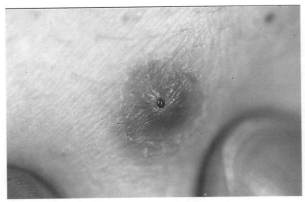
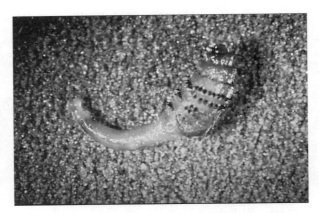

Figure 27–20.   Myiasis due to *Dermatobia hominis*: *A*, subcutaneous nodule with typical respiratory aperature; *B*, extracted second-stage instar.

Exposure also can be reduced by avoiding outdoor activities at peak biting times for arthropods and by avoiding colors (in clothing) and aromas (e.g., perfumes, aftershave lotions) that attract insects.

3.   Avoid raw and undercooked foods; drink only boiled water (stored in clean container) or other safe beverages. This will reduce infection with parasites transmitted by ingestion (see Table 27–4). Travelers should be instructed to avoid foods sold by street vendors and from buffets and other places where food is held at ambient temperatures for prolonged periods. Even if food has been safely prepared, it can become contaminated through improper storage or handling. It is often easier to give travelers information about foods and beverages that are safe rather than trying to list all relevant prohibitions. Travelers should be reminded that it is best to consume dishes immediately after preparation and while still steaming hot. Some of the helminth larvae transmitted by raw or undercooked meat or fish (e.g., liver and lung flukes, intestinal flukes, trichinosis, anisakiasis, taeniasis) may be killed by extended freezing. However, for travelers, it is usually impossible to learn if these preventive measures have been properly applied. Therefore, dishes with raw or undercooked meat or fish that are popular in Southeast Asia, for example, although local delicacies, should be avoided.

SELF-THERAPY

Malaria is the only parasitic disease for which self-therapy by the traveler may be applied in special emergency situations (see Chapter 21). Most parasitic diseases are difficult to diagnose clinically and require sophisticated laboratory techniques for definite diagnosis (exceptions: dracunculiasis, cutaneous larva migrans, myiasis). Drugs used for treating many parasitic infections are unfamiliar to most travelers and can have serious toxicity (Table 27–8). Fortunately, most parasitic infections do not require urgent treatment (exceptions: malaria, amebic liver abscess, African trypanosomiasis, and neurologic involvement with schistosomiasis). In some developing areas with limited or no laboratory facilities, empiric therapy with a broad anithelminthic drug may be given to persons with a history of passing worms. In a remote area lacking laboratory facilities, it could be reasonable to give presumptive treatment with metronidazole (or tinidazole) for suspected amebiasis to a person with dysentery not responding to antibiotics. These are not infections for which travelers should carry medications for self-treatment. Generally, there is enough time to seek evaluation and medical advice.

FUTURE CONSIDERATIONS

The expanding knowledge of the molecular basis of parasitic diseases and host-parasite interactions gives reason for optimism. It should be possible to generate more effective tools, such as vaccines, diagnostic tests, and better treatment, to combat these diseases that afflict the majority of people in the world. To successfully control these diseases, developing countries need the cooperation and support of industrialized countries for scientific collaboration and resources to improve the socioeconomic conditions that contribute to persistence of parasitic infections.

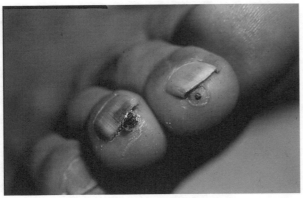

Figure 27–21.   Tungiasis of the toes of the right foot.

Table 27–8.   LIST OF DRUGS AND DOSAGES

PARASITIC DISEASE/INFECTION	DRUG(S) OF CHOICE	DOSAGE FOR ADULTS	ALTERNATIVE OR ADDITIONAL DRUGS
Amebiasis			
Dysentery/extraintestinal	Metronidazole, tinidazole	500 mg tid, 7–10 d	Dehydroemetine, chloroquine
Cyst passers	Diloxanide furoate	500 mg tid, 10 d	Nitroimidazoles, paromomycin
Ascariasis	Mebendazole	100 mg bid, 3 d	Albendazole, pyrantel pamoate
Clonorchiasis/opistorchiasis	Praziquantel	25 mg/kg tid, 1 d	
Cutaneous larva migrans	Topical: tiabendazole	10%–15% ointment tid	
	Oral: albendazole	400 mg qd, 3 d	Ivermectin
Cysticercosis	Albendazole	7 mg/kg bid, 7–14 d	Praziquantel
Diphyllobothriasis	Praziquantel	5–10 mg/kg single dose	Niclosamide
Echinococcosis			
Cystic hydatid disease	Albendazole	7 mg/kg bid, 3–6 m	Mebendazole
Alveolar hydatid disease	Mebendazole	15–20 mg/kg tid, ≥ 2 yr	Albendazole
Enterobiasis	Pyrantel pamoate	5-mg base/kg single dose	Mebendazole, albendazole, pyrvinium
Fascioliasis	Triclabendazole*	10-mg/kg single dose*	Bithionol
Filarial infections			
Lymphatic filariasis	Diethylcarbamazine	2 mg/kg† tid, 2–3 w	Albendazole, ivermectin
Loiasis	Diethylcarbamazine	2 mg/kg† tid, 3–4 w	Ivermectin, mebendazole,
Onchocerciasis	Ivermectin	150–200-μg/kg single dose	Diethylcarbamazine, suramin
Hookworm infection	Mebendazole	100 mg bid, 3 d	Albendazole, pyrantel pamoate
Hymenolepiasis	Praziquantel	25-mg/kg single dose	Niclosamide
Leishmaniasis			
Visceral and mucocutaneous	Sodium stibogluconate or meglumine antimonate	10 mg Sb/kg bid, 30 d	Pentamidine, aminosidine, amphotericin B
Paragonimiasis	Praziquantel	25 mg/kg tid, 3 d	
Schistosomiasis	Praziquantel	20 mg/kg tid, 1 d	Oxamniquine, metrifonate
Strongyloidiasis	Ivermectin	200 μg/kg/d, 1–2 d	Albendazole, tiabendazole
Taeniasis	Praziquantel	10-mg/kg single dose	Niclosamide
Trichinosis	Albendazole	5–7 mg/kg bid, 1–2 w	Tiabendazole, mebendazole
Trichuriasis	Mebendazole	100–200 mg bid, 3 d	Albendazole
Trypanosomiasis			
American (Chagas' disease)	Nifurtimox	3-5 mg/kg tid, 2–4 m	Benzimidazole
African (sleeping sickness)			
without central nervous system involvement	Suramin	1-g single dose at day 0, 3, 7, 14, and 21‡	Pentamidine, eflornithine
with central nervous system involvement			
T. b. rhodesiense infection	Melarsoprol	Various regimens	Eflornithine
T. b. gambinense infection	Eflornithine	Various regimens	Melarsoprol

*Investigational drug.
†Initial test dose (25–50 mg), slowly increase to full dosage.
‡Initial test dose (possible idiosyncrasia).
The Medical Letter, readily available in the United States, provides regularly updated recommendations for treatment of parasitic infections. It also provides information on drugs available (in the U.S.A.) only from the manufacturer or through the CDC Drug Service, Centers for Disease Control and Prevention, Atlanta, GA, U.S.A. Most recent update was published January 2, 1998.

REFERENCES

1. Klion AD, Massoubougbodji A, Sadeler B-C, et al. Loiasis in endemic and non-endemic populations: immunologically mediated differences in clinical presentation. J Infect Dis 1991;163:1318–1325.

2. Centers for Disease Control and Prevention. Health information for international travel. Revised every 1–2 years. Avail-able through Superintendent of Documents, U.S. Government Printing Office, Washington, DC.

3. World Health Organization. International travel and health. Vaccination requirements and health advice. Updated annu-ally. Available through WHO Publication Center USA, 49 Sheridan Avenue, Albany, NY 12210.

4. Wilson ME. A world guide to infections: diseases, distribution, diagnosis. New York: Oxford University Press, 1991.

5. International Association for Medical Assistance to Travellers. Publishes regularly updated summaries that include material about several parasitic infections, e.g., schistosomiasis, American trypanosomiasis, malaria. Canada: 40 Regal Road, Guelph, ON N1K 1B5 (519-836-0102); U.S.: 417 Center Street, Lewiston, NY 14092 (716-754-4883).

6. ProMED (The Program for Monitoring Emerging Diseases) and ProMED-mail (continuous information via e-mail). http://www.promedmail.org.

7. Gideon (Global Infectious Disease and Epidemiology Network). http://www.cyinfo.com/index.html (kommerzieller Anbieter).

8. Berger SA. GIDEON: a computer program for diagnosis, simulation, and informatics in geogaphic medicine. J Travel Med 1998;7:383–386.

9. Herwaldt B. Verbal communication. Presented at the annual meeting of the American Society of Tropical Medicine and Hygiene, December 1997, Lake Buena Vista, FL.

10. Herwaldt B, Stokes SL, Juranek DD. American cutaneous leishmaniasis in U.S. travelers. Ann Intern Med 1993;118:779–784.

11. World Health Organization. Leishmania/HIV co-infection. Epidemiological analysis of 692 retrospective cases. Wkly Epidemiol Rec 1997;72:49–54.

12. Berman JD. Human leishmaniasis: clinical, diagnostic, and chemotherapeutic developments in the last 10 years. Clin Infect Dis 1997;24:684–703.

13. More SJ, Copeman DB. A highly specific and sensitive monoclonal antibody-based ELISA for the detection of circulating antigen in bancroftian filariasis. Trop Med Parasitol 1990;41:403–406.

14. Kirchhoff LV. American trypanosomiasis (Chagas' disease). Gastroenterol Clin North Am 1996;25:517–533.

15. Rocha A, DeMeneses ACO, Da Silva AM, et al. Pathology of patients with Chagas disease and acquired immunodeficiency syndrome. Am J Trop Med Hyg 1994;50:261–268.

16. Visser LG, Polderman AM, Stuiver PC. Outbreak of schistosomiasis among travelers returning from Mali, West Africa. Clin Infect Dis 1995;20:280–285.

17. Jelinek T, Nothdurft HD, Löscher T. Schistosomiasis in travelers and expatriates. J Travel Med 1996;3:160–165.

18. Centres for Disease Control. Schistosomiasis in U.S. Peace Corps volunteers—Malawi, 1992. MMWR Morb Mortal Wkly Rep 1993;42:565–570.

19. DeSilva N, Guyatt H, Bundy D. Anthelminthics. A comparative review of their clinical pharmacology. Drugs 1997;53:769–788.

20. Mahmoud AAF. Strongyloidiasis. Clin Infect Dis 1996;23:949–952.

21. Tannich H, Horstmann RD, Knobloch J, Arnold HH. Genomic DNA differences between pathogenic and nonpathogenic *Entamoeba histolytica*. Proc Natl Acad Sci U S A 1989;86:5118–5122.

22. Weinke T, Friedrich-Jänicke B, Hopp P, Janitschke K. Prevalence and clinical importance of *Entamoeba histolytica* in two high-risk groups: travelers returning from the tropics and male homosexuals. J Infect Dis 1990;161:1029–1031.

23. Jelinek T, Peyerl G, Löscher T, Nothdurft HD. Evaluation of an antigen-capture enzyme immunoassay for detection of *Entamoeba histolytica* in stool samples. Eur J Clin Microbiol Infect Dis 1996;15:752–755.

24. WHO Study Group on the Control of Foodborne Trematode Infections. Control of foodborne trematode infections: report of a WHO study group. Geneva: WHO, 1995.

25. Arjona R, Riancho JA, Aguado JM, et al. Fascioliasis in developed countries. A review of classic and aberrant forms of the disease. Medicine (Baltimore) 1995;74:13–23.

26. Sorvillo JF, Waterman SH, Richards FO, Schantz PM. Cysticercosis surveillance: locally acquired and travel-related infections and detection of intestinal tapeworm carriers in Los Angeles County. Am J Trop Med Hyg 1992;47:365–371.

27. Centers for Disease Control. Diphyllobothriasis associated with salmon—United States. MMWR Morb Mortal Wkly Rep 1981;30:331–338.

28. WHO Informal Working Group on Echinococcosis. Guidelines for treatment of cystic and alveolar echinococcosis in humans. Bull WHO 1996;74:231–242.

29. Ancelle T, Dupouy-Camet J, Desenclos JC, et al. A multifocal outbreak of trichinellosis linked to horse meat imported from North America to France in 1993. Am J Trop Med Hyg 1998;59:615–619.

30. McCauly JB, Michelson MK, Schantz PM. Trichinella infection in travelers. J Infect Dis 1991;161:1013–1016.

31. Cetron MS, Chitsulo L, Sullivan JJ, et al. Schistosomiasis in Lake Malawi. Lancet 1996;348:1274–1278.

Chapter 28

PSYCHIATRIC ILLNESS AND STRESS

ROBERT L. DUPONT, THOMAS H. VALK, AND JON HELTBERG

International travel is a geographic uprooting that often produces mental and physical stresses. For many people, international travel encourages the dream of getting away from limitations in their lives and finding new, even magical, opportunities, from the educational and the economic to the romantic and the recreational. Other people dread international travel as a loss of familiar places and people, as well as a time of frightening uncertainty. Travel can expose people to new dangers, from accidents to infectious diseases. Travel may exacerbate or even precipitate psychiatric illness, and frequent international travel has been associated with increased numbers of insurance claims for psychological illnesses.[1] The experience of overseas travel has recently been reviewed with a focus on the psychological danger signals.[2–4]

Primary care physicians dealing with international travelers can deliver valuable mental health services in two settings: (1) counseling prior to travel and (2) evaluation and treatment of mental disorders during or after travel. Proper evaluation of preexisting psychiatric difficulties prior to travel can lead to prevention of common psychiatric problems encountered overseas. Treatment of mental disorders during or subsequent to travel must take into account not only the major psychiatric syndromes and their presentations but also how treatment of these disorders may be affected by the travel itself. In this chapter, we focus on the mental health problems most likely to arise in international travel and make suggestions for how to deal with them.

To some extent, the duration and geographic scope of travel determine what issues need to be addressed in pretravel counseling. For those about to travel for relatively brief periods of time, such as the tourist or business traveler, the clinician's history taking should focus on preexisting psychiatric disorders that have been or are under treatment and that could lead to serious illness in the overseas environment should there be a recurrence. Since most countries do not have mental health services that are culturally compatible for all travelers, any illness characterized by psychotic episodes, significantly impaired judgment (including manic episodes or substance abuse), bizarre behavior, or any mental illness that would normally require hospitalization is cause for concern. The stability of the psychiatric illness under treatment should also be assessed. Travelers on medication should take adequate supplies with them, since even commonly used medications in some countries are not available in other countries. If the stability of a current mental illness is in doubt, consideration should be given to the postponement of travel or the purchase of international travelers' air ambulance insurance in case decompensation occurs, since evacuation can be both difficult and expensive.[5]

Pretravel counseling should review issues related to diet, exercise, sleep, sexuality, and the use of alcohol and other nonmedical drugs. Travel medicine physicians can help prevent problems by encouraging sound mental health practices in these fundamental behaviors, which are often disturbed during travel. In particular, discouragement by their physicians of excessive alcohol consumption and use of illicit drugs can be helpful to prospective travelers.[6] Healthy eating, adequate sleep, and regular exercise can make the difference between a successful and an unsuccessful trip. Also, for short-term travelers, straightforward recommendations from their physicians to avoid promiscuous sexual activity and to use a condom to reduce the risk of sexually transmitted diseases can be helpful.

The effect of travel in terms of diet, activity, and climatic changes on some psychiatric medications should be specifically addressed. For travelers taking monoamine oxidase (MAO)-inhibitor antidepressants, dietary restrictions should be reviewed carefully, especially in light of the fact that foods in foreign countries may not be easily recognizable as containing high concentrations of tyramine. Signs and symptoms of hypertensive crisis should be reviewed, and consideration should be given to restriction of travel to those countries with adequate emergency room facilities. Patients taking lithium, valproic acid, or carbamazepine should consider restricting travel to countries where serum levels of these mood-stabilizing medications can be obtained. Patients using lithium should be re-educated about the effects of change in sodium intake, activity levels, dramatic changes in ambient temperatures, and travelers' diarrhea on blood lithium levels, with due attention to signs and symptoms of lithium intoxication.

For families that intend to reside abroad, the list of issues to be covered includes but extends beyond those addressed for the tourist or business traveler. Stressors face families as a result of cultural and language differences, feelings of loss of the home and social network left behind, and the need to cope with new jobs, neighborhoods, social settings, and schools. Pretravel counseling should focus on the culture shock syndrome because all members of relocating families will experience it regardless of prior overseas travel and independent of the culture of the host countries.[7] As this predictable syndrome is usually limited to the first 6 to 12 months of overseas living, counseling ahead of time can relieve considerable distress and may prevent the need for later psychiatric intervention.

The culture shock syndrome is best understood as an adjustment disorder, usually with only limited dysfunction in terms of the ability to meet the demands of everyday living. Individuals should be counseled to expect fluctuations in mood, sleep patterns, energy level, sex drive, and appetite. Symptoms are age dependent, however, with preschool children more likely to experience regressive behaviors, such as the recurrence of bed-wetting in the previously adequately toilet-trained child. Other regressive behaviors in young children include clinging to parents and an increase in fears and nightmares. School-age children also may exhibit regressive behaviors such as declines in academic performance, behavioral problems at school, separation anxiety, increased friction with siblings, and an increase in "bad" behavior at home. Teenagers are more likely to have symptoms seen in adults, except that they may engage in acting out behaviors, especially involving the abuse of alcohol and other drugs as well as high-risk sexual activity. The fact that all members of a family go through adjustment difficulties at the same time makes for a heady brew. Despite this, however, advance preparation for the vicissitudes of the culture shock syndrome is often all that is necessary to prevent serious difficulties and to promote successful adjustment to the new environment.[8–11]

A variant of the culture shock syndrome is re-entry adjustment when families that have resided abroad move back to their country of origin. Surprisingly to some, such homeward moves can cause just as many, if not more, adjustment difficulties as the outbound move. The clinical characteristics are essentially the same. Advance preparation can help a great deal.[12–14]

As with the tourist traveler, careful attention must be paid to the management of any preexisting psychiatric disorders. Issues to address include the following:

1. Are culturally compatible mental health services available in the host country?
2. Are laboratory facilities available to monitor medication blood levels?
3. Are there adequate family or sponsoring agency resources if psychiatric evacuation becomes necessary?
4. Do children within the family require specialized schooling as a result of either emotional problems or learning disorders? Are there adequate schools in the host country, either within the country's own educational system or as international schools?
5. Is it likely that the culture shock syndrome, superimposed on preexisting psychiatric or marital problems, will jeopardize the stability of an individual or a family?

It is often helpful to provide a family that has experienced prior mental health problems with the names, addresses, and telephone numbers of specific mental health care providers in the host countries in case problems develop so that the search for help does not have to

begin in the midst of a crisis in the family. In particularly complex situations, specialists in mental health with experience in dealing with overseas populations should be consulted prior to departure. It may help to keep in contact with mental health professionals on whom family members have relied at home. Modern communications make this possible by telephone and the Internet. Some families should reconsider living abroad if preexisting difficulties are serious and/or the host country care is particularly tenuous.

The issues of child and spousal abuse occurring overseas present significant difficulties for the responsible physician. To some extent, the definition of what behaviors constitute abuse varies by culture and country, so that abuse as defined by home country laws and practice may not constitute behavior that a host country's legal or social system will address. Since many domestic abuse situations involve considerable denial on the part of both the abuser and the abused, the clinician may be left with little in the way of legal or social agency leverage with which to protect the suspected victim or bring the alleged abuser to evaluation and treatment. In such difficult situations, it may be useful for the institution sponsoring the family to handle the matter administratively in order to ensure culturally compatible evaluation. Repatriation may prove to be necessary.

EVALUATION AND TREATMENT OF PSYCHIATRIC DISORDERS IN TRAVEL MEDICINE

Once overseas, either as tourists or new residents, travelers suffer from the same psychiatric disorders as do people who stay home. For the most part, these disorders present in the same manner as do those occurring in the general population. Incidence and prevalence data for the tourist and the nonmilitary expatriate population are virtually nonexistent, although it is known that psychiatric disorders result in significant numbers of psychiatric evacuations in some populations.[15–17] The physician caring for travelers should be able to recognize the major psychiatric syndromes and should have practical strategies to handle each of them.[18]

MAJOR PSYCHIATRIC SYNDROMES

The major psychiatric syndromes are as follows:

- *Affective disorders*, including major depression and manic depression or bipolar disorder;
- *Anxiety disorders*, including panic disorder and agoraphobia, specific phobia, social phobia, generalized anxiety disorder, and obsessive-compulsive disorder;
- *Substance use disorder*, including alcohol and other drug abuse and dependence;
- *Psychotic disorders*, including schizophrenia.

Affective disorders show up as disorders of mood, most often as depression with loss of pleasure in things one would ordinarily enjoy (such as food, sex, hobbies, and other interests), and sadness, as well as loss of energy and hope for the future. Less commonly, affective disorders present as a manic episode with elevated mood and impulsivity. Both depression and mania are commonly associated with severe insomnia in addition to disturbances of eating and sexuality. Recent studies have suggested that mania is more commonly triggered by traveling from west to east, whereas depression is more common following air travel from east to west.[19,20]

Anxiety disorders are associated with extreme worry, often with panic, tension, and avoidance. Clinically significant anxiety may be triggered by stress in a travel setting but, like affective disorders, it is usually apparent before the onset of travel. The anxiety disorders are divided into five major categories: agoraphobia/panic disorder (the fear of being away from a safe person or a safe place and episodes of intense panic, often out of the blue); specific phobia (fear of a specific experience or situation, such as fear of flying, fear of heights, or claustrophobia); social phobia (fear of embarrassment, including either public speaking phobia or more general extreme shyness); obsessive-compulsive disorder (obsessions are unwanted intrusive and repugnant thoughts while compulsions are senseless rituals repeated to ward off anxiety, such as perpetual hand washing); and generalized anxiety disorder (waxing and waning anxiety without panic, phobic avoidance, or obsessions and compulsions).[21]

About 15% of adults in the United States experience fear of flying sufficiently severe to limit or stop air travel.[14,22] People with chronic phobic and panic disorders often do not travel at all. The stress of travel may precipitate an initial attack of what later proves to be panic disorder. Often, patients with panic disorder present in the setting of international travel as possible cardiac or neurologic emergencies because they fear that they are dying. A careful evaluation and diagnosis can be helpful, as can a respectful education of the patients that their anxiety symptoms are real and distressing but not medically dangerous.

Substance use disorder is associated with denial and/or dishonesty about use of alcohol and/or other drugs, as well as with continued use despite negative consequences of this use. Substance abusers are reluctant to give up their substance use. Use of alcohol and other drugs, like out-of-control sexual activity, may have been a major reason for the decision to travel, in the hope that the restrictions on potentially dangerous behaviors at home will be escaped abroad.

Psychotic disorders show up with bizarre behavior, sometimes with delusions (often paranoid) and hallucinations (often auditory and persecutory). One recent study found a higher rate of psychosis in French travelers to Asia than other destinations.[23]

All four major groups of mental disorders tend to have onsets between about ages 15 and 30 and to be lifelong, showing a fluctuating course over time. They range in severity from mild to debilitating. In evaluating the need and site for treatment for psychiatric disorders, the physician must consider the severity of the illness as well as its timing in relation to travel. Virtually all persons moving overseas will experience relatively mild symptoms within the first year of residence due to the culture shock syndrome and may be more likely to seek medical or psychiatric care during this period.[16] For those mental health problems that appear to exceed the level of a relatively mild adjustment disorder, however, treatment will depend on the mental health capabilities of the host country's health care system with due regard to cultural compatibility and the availability of appropriate medications and psychotherapy, as well as, in some instances, laboratory facilities.

If the mental illness is severe or if the host country's mental health care system cannot provide the necessary care, psychiatric evacuation to the home country may be the best course of action. Within the U.S. Foreign Service population, a medically prescreened group, substance abuse and affective disorders ranked as the two principal causes of such evacuations. Of those evacuated, nearly 58% were unable to return to their postings overseas.[15] Table 28–1 ranks the top causes of psychiatric evacuations in this population by broad DSM-III diagnostic categories.[24]

Temporary treatment aimed at stabilization of an acute disorder prior to travel home, especially those disorders with psychotic features, may be necessary. Creative use of an individual's family members to provide care may be an important option, especially if the use of host country hospitals is not appropriate. Often, a careful history will point the way to the most appropriate treatment because patients are likely to have suffered from the same disorders at earlier times in their lives, and they or their families will have useful thoughts based on what has helped them in the past.

Depression is likely to respond to antidepressant medications, but this response often does not occur until the medicine has been taken daily for several weeks. An active manic episode is less likely to be handled on an outpatient basis, but if the manic patient has been treated before and has a relatively mild case, it may be possible to handle it with acute use of an antipsychotic medication (e.g., haloperidol) while an antimanic medicine such as lithium carbonate is being instituted. In instances that require evacuation because local hospitalization is not feasible, the treating physician may need to rely on an antipsychotic medication until repatriation is accomplished since the response to lithium carbonate does not

Table 28–1. PSYCHIATRIC MEDICAL EVACUATIONS BY DIAGNOSTIC CATEGORY (NOT INCLUSIVE)

DIAGNOSTIC CATEGORY	PERCENTAGE OF MEDEVACS
Substance use disorder	28.0
Affective disorder	22.3
Adjustment disorder	19.4
Personality disorder	10.3
Somatiform disorder	4.0
Paranoid disorder	3.4

Adapted from Valk TH. Psychiatric medical evacuations within the Foreign Service. Foreign Service Med Bull 1987;268:9–11.

occur quickly and frequent serum lithium levels are necessary in the start-up period.

Phobias are avoidance behaviors that are the result of anxiety and panic. Phobias fit under the diagnoses of agoraphobia, specific phobias, or social phobia depending on the activity or situation that is avoided. Travel may trigger panic and heightened anxiety among patients suffering from anxiety disorders so that travel is commonly avoided by people with agoraphobia and other anxiety disorders. The anxiety disorders are the most prevalent of the major mental disorders, affecting an estimated 26.9 million Americans (14.6%) during their lifetimes.[25] The anxiety disorders produce the highest social costs of any group of mental disorders in the United States, estimated at $46.6 billion in 1990.[26] The anxiety disorders are underrepresented in travel medicine since they often lead to the avoidance of travel.

Travel medicine physicians can help people suffering from anxiety disorders manage their illnesses so as to permit travel for both work and recreation. Physicians can relieve the guilt of clinically anxious patients by characterizing these disorders as common, often crippling, biologic disorders for which effective treatments are available. All too often, anxiety disorders are hidden by patients and family members because of shame and a deeply entrenched hopelessness. Travel medicine physicians can provide a valuable service to these patients by encouraging them to find and use effective treatments that will permit travel, including air travel, to become an enjoyable experience. There are many excellent self-help books available for anxious patients, including books by Claire Weekes, R. Reid Wilson, Jerilyn Ross, and Robert DuPont.[27–30] Standard medical and psychiatric texts offer advice to physicians about the treatment of the anxiety disorders.[31–33]

Travel medicine physicians can provide understanding and support to patients suffering from anxiety disorders by referring them to specialized treatment and/or self-help books.[34,35] A simple principle of the behavioral treatment of phobias is to break the overwhelming anxiety-provoking experience down into smaller, more manageable steps and then to encourage patients to expose themselves to these small steps, gradually and repeatedly, as they "practice their phobias." This progressive, voluntary exposure is best done with the help of a family member, a friend, or a therapist since even small steps can be frightening to phobic people. Anxious patients need to learn that their sensitized nervous systems will not make them go crazy, lose control, or die, as they commonly fear.

Some airlines offer courses to help fearful flyers overcome their phobic fears of flying.[36,37] Patients can call the major airlines serving their communities to inquire about courses and/or therapists who can help them. Once they have overcome the phobic problem, many formerly fearful flyers are avid air travelers who fly with no residual symptoms of anxiety. Some phobic flyers are helped by visiting airports repeatedly and even sitting in parked airplanes so that they become familiar with the terminals and planes. A recent study explored the measurement of physiologic correlates of anxiety in flying, concluding that such measurement is possible, but that self-reported anxiety was a better discriminator between phobic and control flyers.[18]

Because many airline ground personnel are familiar with helping fearful flyers, they will gladly permit them to practice their phobias in this way if the patients identify themselves as fearful flyers. Sometimes it helps if the patients have a note from their physicians stating that they are being treated for this problem. Fearful flyers can board early when they fly along with other passengers "needing extra assistance." They can meet the flight crew and pilots, telling each of them that they are working to overcome their fear of flying. These strategies break down the shame and isolation that most phobic people feel and turn the otherwise alien flight crew into their allies in their efforts to overcome their phobic fears. Flying phobics may also find it helpful to use therapeutic audiotapes, which they can use first for practice and later on their flights.[38–40]

Anxiety disorders respond to a variety of treatments.[41] Many anxiety problems can be treated with daily doses of antidepressants even in the absence of depression. This approach is especially useful in the prevention of panic attacks and the treatment of obsessive-compulsive disorder, which can be treated with the serotonin reuptake inhibitors, such as clomipramine, sertraline, and fluoxetine. The benzodiazepines, such as alprazolam or diazepam, can be useful in the treatment of clinically significant anxiety because their beneficial effects are experienced within 30 minutes of taking the medicine. Flying phobics may benefit from the use of 2 to 5 mg of diazepam or 0.25 to 0.5 mg of alprazolam 1 hour before a flight. For many anxious patients, having access to an effective antianxiety medicine makes otherwise difficult situations manageable. The use of alcohol to reduce anxiety should be discouraged since such "self-medication" can produce disturbing intoxication and promote alcoholism. Cognitive-behavioral techniques often help phobic/anxious patients.[42,43] These techniques can sometimes be mastered by travel medicine physicians, but often patients need to be referred to a psychotherapist or psychiatrist who has mastered these treatments.

Substance use disorders can be handled successfully on an outpatient basis only if the patient is willing and able to stop use of alcohol and other intoxicating drugs. Commitments to "reduce" the dose or to eliminate one or another specific nonmedical drug while continuing to use others are certain to fail. If the patient can stop the use of alcohol and other nonmedical psychoactive drugs, then the disorder may be controlled, at least temporarily, in the context of travel. It is often useful to meet with family members or friends about substance use problems.

Referrals to addiction specialists and/or to 12-step programs such as Alcoholics Anonymous are often useful, although the availability of such programs varies widely by country and city. Alcoholics Anonymous meetings can now be found in many urban areas worldwide. Attendance at meetings can be of great value to addicted patients who are willing to attend meetings, especially if they have made use of 12-step fellowships prior to travel. Drug and alcohol tests are also useful in managing substance abusers over time to ensure that patients are remaining abstinent.

Psychotic disorders (including schizophrenia) sometimes can be handled with antipsychotic medicines on an outpatient basis if the patient is cooperative. On the other hand, when the patient's behavior is out of control, evacuation or hospitalization is usually the best course of action. In all mental disorders, an experienced travel medicine physician can handle the milder cases, but referral to a psychiatrist often is necessary for the more serious cases, especially if patients do not respond to initial treatment by the primary care physician. Because all of the mental disorders are characterized by stigma and shame, it is important that travel medicine physicians approach patients suffering from these illnesses with compassion, respect, and realistic hope for living a good life. When treated in this way, patients suffering from mental disorders can be among the travel medicine physician's most rewarding patients.

Standard medical and psychiatric texts provide useful information about the presentation, diagnosis, and treatment of the major mental disorders, all of which are seen in the context of travel. Since these conditions usually are chronic, the patients and their families, as well as physicians who have treated them previously and who can often be contacted by telephone, can provide help to the travel medicine physician, as can local psychiatrists for more difficult cases.

REFERENCES

1. Liese B, Mundt KA, Dell LD, et al. Medical insurance claims associated with international business travel. J Occup Environ Med 1997;54:499–503.
2. Gomez J. Why is it so popular? The psychology of travel. Travel Med Int 1993;26–29.
3. Sauteraud A. Occurrence and management of psychiatric pathology in travelers. Med Trop (Mars) 1997;57(4Bis):457–460.
4. Rayman RB. Passenger safety, health, and comfort: a review. Aviat Space Environ Med 1997;68:432–440.
5. Lavernhe JP, Ivanoff S. Medical assistance to travelers: a new concept in insurance—cooperation with an airline. Aviat Space Environ Med 1985;56:367–370.
6. Lange WR, McCune BA. Substance abuse and international travel. Adv Alcohol Subst Abuse 1989;8(2):37–51.
7. Steward L, Leggat PA. Culture shock and travelers. J Travel Med 1998;5:84–88.
8. Arnold CB. Culture shock and a Peace Corps field mental health program. Community Mental Health J 1967;3–1:53–60.
9. Locke SA, Feinsod FM. Psychological preparation for young adults traveling abroad. Adolescence 1982;17:815–819.
10. Rigamer EF. Stresses of families abroad. In: Steffen R, Lobel H, Haworth J, Bradley D, eds. Travel medicine. Berlin: Springer, 1989:409–413.
11. Valk TH. Adjusting to the overseas move. State Magazine 1993;369:6–7.
12. Werkman SL. Coming home: adjustment of Americans to the United States after living abroad. In: Coelho GV, Ahmed PI, eds. Uprooting and development: dilemmas of coping with modernization. New York: Plenum Press, 1980:233–247.
13. Westwood MJ, Lawrence WS, Paul D. Preparing for re-entry: a program for the sojourning student. Int J Adv Couns 1986;9:221–230.
14. Uehara A. The nature of American student reentry adjustment and perceptions of the sojourn experience. Int J Intercultural Rel 1986;10:415–438.
15. Heltberg J, Steffen R. Psychiatric and psychological problems in travellers. In: Mårdh P-A, ed. Proceedings of the First Scandinavian Symposium on Travel Medicine and Health, Uppsala, May 21–22, 1992; 1994.
16. Valk TH. Psychiatric medical evacuations within the Foreign Service. Foreign Service Med Bull, 1987;268:9–11.
17. Valk TH. Psychiatric practice in the Foreign Service. Foreign Service Med Bull 1990;280:6–11.
18. Kaplan HI, Sadock BJ, Grebb JA. Kaplan and Sadock's synopsis of psychiatry — behavioral sciences/clinical psychiatry. 7th Ed. Baltimore: Williams & Wilkins, 1994.
19. Wilhelm FH, Roth WT. Taking the laboratory to the skies: ambulatory assessment of self-report, autonomic, and respiratory responses in flying phobia. Psychophysiology 1998;35:596–606.
20. Young DM. Psychiatric morbidity in travelers to Honolulu, Hawaii. Compr Psychiatry 1995;36:224–228.
21. American Psychiatric Association. Diagnostic and statistical manual of mental disorders, fourth edition (DSM-IV). Washington, DC: American Psychiatric Association, 1994.
22. Cummings TW, White R. Freedom from fear of flying. New York: Pocket Books, 1987.
23. Sauteraud A, Hajjar M. Psychotic disorders. Higher incidence during travels in Asia. Presse Med 1992;21:805–810.
24. American Psychiatric Association. Diagnostic and statistical manual of mental disorders. 3rd Ed. Washington, DC: American Psychiatric Association, 1980.
25. National Institute of Mental Health. Epidemiologic Catchment Area (ECA) Program community surveys in five sites: St. Louis, MO; Baltimore, MD; New Haven, CT; Durham, NC; and Los Angeles, CA 1980–1985. Public use tapes.
26. DuPont RL, DuPont CM, Rice DP. The economic costs of anxiety disorders. In: Stein DF, Hollander E, eds. Textbook of anxiety disorders. Washington, DC: American Psychiatric Press, in press.
27. Weekes C. Hope and help for your nerves. New York: Hawthorne Books, 1969.
28. Wilson RR. Don't panic — taking control of anxiety attacks. New York: HarperPerennial, 1987.
29. Ross J. Triumph over fear — a book of help and hope for people with anxiety, panic attacks, and phobias. New York: Bantam Books, 1994.
30. DuPont RL, Spencer ED, DuPont CM. The anxiety cure — an eight-step program for getting well. New York: John Wiley and Sons, 1998.
31. The Merck manual of diagnosis and therapy. 16th Ed. Rahway, NJ: Merck Sharp & Dohme Research Laboratories, Merck & Co., Inc., 1992.
32. American Psychiatric Association. Treatments of psychiatric disorders: a task force report of the American Psychiatric Association. Vols. I–IV Washington, DC: American Psychiatric Association, 1989.
33. Kaplan HI, Sadock BJ, eds. Comprehensive textbook of psychiatry/IV. Baltimore: Williams & Wilkins, 1985.
34. Elkus B, Tieger ME. The fearful flyers resource guide. Cincinnati: Argonaut Entertainment, 1991. (To order by phone: 800-776-9800.)
35. Windsor N. How to fly — for adults: relaxed and happy from takeoff to touchdown. Burbank, CA: CorkScrew Press, 1993. (Distributed by Globe Pequot Press, Old Saybrook, CT. To order by phone: 800-243-0495.)
36. USAir's Fearful Flyers Program. For information: Box 100, Glenshaw, PA 15116, 412-366-8112. USAir book based on the program Fly Without Fear.

37. The American Airlines AAir Born program. For information: 800-451-5106.

38. Cummings TW. Audio cassettes, booklet, seminars. For information: Freedom from Fear of Flying, Inc., 2021 Country Club Prado, Coral Gables, FL 33134, 305-261-7042.

39. Pathway Systems. Self-help program on tape, informational booklet. For information: P.O. Box 269, Chapel Hill, NC 27514-0269, 800-394-2299.

40. Thairapy. Tape program. For information: 4500 Campus Dr., Suite 628F, Newport Beach, CA 92660, 714-756-1133.

41. DuPont RL. Choosing the right treatment for the patient with anxiety. Mod Med 1992;60:64–76.

42. Marks IM. Cure and care of neuroses — theory and practice of behavioral psychotherapy, New York: John Wiley & Sons, 1982.

43. Greist JH, Jefferson JW, Marks IM. Anxiety and its treatment: help is available. Washington, DC: American Psychiatric Press, 1986.

Chapter 29

TRAVEL-RELATED INJURIES (MOTOR VEHICLE CRASHES, FALLS, DROWNINGS): EPIDEMIOLOGY AND PREVENTION

STEPHEN W. HARGARTEN AND ROBERT D. GRENFELL

INTRODUCTION

Although the majority of travel-related morbidity is due to infectious diseases,[1-4] travel-related mortality and serious morbidity is primarily due to injuries.[5-12] Every year, thousands of international travelers die or become disabled from injuries.[6-8] Motor vehicle crashes, drownings, aircraft crashes, homicides, and burns account for the overwhelming majority of injury deaths.[6,9] Motor vehicle crashes, falls, and recreational injuries are common causes of nonfatal injuries.[13,14]

This chapter is devoted to an examination of the major travel-related injuries, their epidemiology, and prevention. The science of injury control and prevention will be introduced and discussed in this chapter. Specifically excluded from this chapter are marine hazards and other less common injury events. Emergency medical services and their impact on the care of the injured patient are discussed in other chapters of this text.

TRAVEL-RELATED INJURIES: SCOPE OF THE PROBLEM

Travel-related mortality has been a constant risk of travel since individuals and groups began to journey by foot, animals, ship, carriage, train, automobile, or airplane. Only recently, however, has there been a critical examination and description of the nature and scope of travel-related injuries.

Published studies describing travel-related deaths of Swiss, Scottish, Australian, and United States nationals indicates that injuries consistently account for 20% to 25% of all travel-related deaths.[6,7,8,11] For selected host countries, injuries to travelers are the number one cause of travel-related deaths.[10] These injury deaths are primarily motor vehicle crashes and drownings (Table 29-1). Other far less common causes of travel-related injury death include homicides, suicides, airplane crashes, and animal and marine bites.

Travel-related injury mortality rates have had limited examination. However, for U.S. citizens traveling abroad, there appears to be a higher injury death rate when compared to injury death rates of U.S. citizens at home.[5,6] U.S. Peace Corps volunteers had a significantly higher death rate for motorcycle crashes than did their age and sex control group in the United States.[5] In one country, the proportional mortality rates for drownings and aircraft crashes of U.S. citizen tourists were significantly increased.[10] In one analysis of deaths of international visitors to one state of Australia, it was found that in an 18-month period, there were 7 deaths due to injury, in comparison to 20 by medical causes (almost solely cardiovascular).[12]

Travel-related injury morbidity has had limited examination as well. A Swiss study demonstrated that injuries were the most common reason for air medical evacuations.[13] In a study of air-transported U.S. citizen tourists, injuries accounted for 44% of all air transports.[14] In this study, motor vehicle crashes were the most common injury cause (45%), followed by falls (21%) and sports injury (8%).

There is significant geographic variation between countries for nonfatal injuries. Motor vehicle crash injuries account for 15% to 65% of all travel-related injuries depending on which region or country of origin. For Mexico, 65% of injured tourists were motor vehicle related, compared to only 15% of the injuries from the Bahamas. Falls accounted for 13% to 32% of all nonfatal injuries transported.[14] The Bahamas had the greatest percentage of injuries due to falls (32%) and Mexico had the

Table 29–1. INJURY DEATHS OF U.S. CITIZENS FOR 1975 AND 1984

CAUSE OF DEATHS	NUMBER OF DEATHS	% OF TOTAL
Motor vehicle crash	163	26.8
Drowning	96	16.1
Airplane crash	43	7.2
Homicide	52	8.6
Poisoning*	39	6.5
Suicide	20	3.4
Burns	21	3.6
Electrocution	3	0.5
Others	164	27.4
Total	601	100.0

*The category of poisoning includes unintentional acute alcohol intoxication, drug overdose, and carbon dioxide intoxication.

least (13%). These variations in injury patterns reflect the variable exposure of travelers to injury risk and possibly age and gender differences in the groups of travelers to those countries. Tourists to Mexico tend to drive. There may be more elderly traveling to the Bahamas.

More recent analysis of U.S. citizen travel-related deaths revealed that homicide is emerging as a leading cause of injury death in selected countries such as Columbia and South Africa.[9]

Overall, injuries account for less than 2% of all travel-related morbidity.[1] Yet, compared to other causes of travel-related morbidity, travel-related injuries have higher case fatality rates and higher rates of hospitalization.[1]

PUBLIC HEALTH APPROACH TO TRAVEL-RELATED INJURIES

Increasingly, travel-related health problems are being addressed by using the classic methods of epidemiology.[2,7,15] Over the past 50 years, physicians, public health advocates, and researchers have been applying the science of epidemiology to the study of injuries and injury control. Only recently have travel-related injuries and their prevention been addressed in the context of injury prevention and public health.[15]

The control and prevention of travel-related injuries can be addressed by examining the host, agent/vehicle, and environmental components of the injury event. This paradigm has been applied to infectious disease prevention for decades. Dividing injuries into the classic public health model increases the scope and focus of prevention strategies, which can lead to a reduction in deaths and nonfatal injuries (Table 29–2).[15,24] For the remainder of the chapter, the epidemiology and prevention of selected travel-related injuries will be described.

TRAVEL-RELATED INJURIES: EPIDEMIOLOGY AND PREVENTION

MOTOR VEHICLE CRASHES

Epidemiology   Motor vehicle crash deaths are a constant travel risk that change significantly from country to country.[16,17,31,34,35] There is significant motor vehicle crash death rate variation between countries[31] (from 10 to 20 times), largely due to variations in roadways and their construction,[35] vehicle safety standards,[18] the presence or absence of standardized emergency medical services,[19] and driver abilities. In addition, roadways in many countries have additional challenges: animals obstructing the road, poor or variable lighting, animal-drawn carts with no lights or reflecting material, and pedestrians using the roads with motorized vehicles. Further compounding the risk of motor vehicle crashes is the individual's unfamiliarity with the destination's driving conditions, the influence of alcohol, and the effects of fatigue and jet lag.

Motor vehicle crashes are the leading cause of travel-related injury death. For U.S. travelers to Mexico, motor vehicle crashes are the leading cause of all travel-related injury deaths, accounting for 18% of all deaths.[10] In one study involving Peace Corps volunteers, motorcycle crashes were a major subset of the motor vehicle crash problem, accounting for 33% of all crash deaths.[5]

There are no specific studies that verify travel-related death rate variability between countries, yet in-country motor vehicle crash death rates vary considerably. There has been a significant increase in motor vehicle crash deaths in Eastern Europe during the years 1987–1993. An average increase of 60% has been experienced ranging from 24% (Hungary) to 190% (Ukraine).[31] Significantly high rates occur in other countries such as Guatemala, Peru, and other areas in Central and South America, as well as the Middle East.[16,17] From 1989 to 1993, Lithuania, Pakistan, Thailand, and Iceland had the highest percentage increase in motor vehicle crash injuries in the world.[31]

In an analysis of motor vehicle crashes involving international visitors to Australia, it was determined that approximately 32 deaths occur per year.[32] In one Australian state, over a 5-year period there were 39 deaths and 1,161 injuries from motor vehicle crashes involving international visitors. The estimated cost of these injuries in 1997 for this Australian state alone was almost $19 million AUS. The significance of this is heightened by the low overall in-country crash rate in Australia.[32]

As less developed countries become more industrialized, the trend of increased motor vehicle use predictably leads to more motor vehicle crashes and injuries.[20] These trends and variations impact on tourists who use motorized vehicles to explore their countries of destination.

Pedestrian deaths also vary considerably between countries. For Europe, there is a greater than fourfold difference in pedestrian deaths, with Portugal, the former Yugoslavia, and Greece having the highest rates (respectively 6.4, 5.9, and 4.6 per 100,000 population), and Luxembourg, Sweden, and the Netherlands having the lowest rates (respectively 2.2, 1.8, 1.5 per 100,000).[34]

Table 29–2.   MALARIA PREVENTION AND MOTORCYCLES, HEAD INJURY PREVENTION: EPIDEMIOLOGIC MODEL

HOST	AGENT	VEHICLE	INJURY EVENT	INJURY
Man	*Plasmodium falciparum*	Mosquito	Mosquito bite	Malaria
Man	Kinetic energy	Motorcycle	Motorcycle crash	Skull fracture

Prevention There is a great need for the establishment of international standards for safe motor vehicle design, roadways, and drivers' licensing. Safety evaluation and surveillance of all motorized vehicles should occur.[18] All countries should cooperate in the design, testing, and manufacture of safe vehicles. Safety equipment such as air bags, safety belts, and child restraints should be mandatory features for all motor vehicles yet are not routinely available when tourists seek to rent and drive motor vehicles.[25] Helmets should be available and used whenever motorbikes, motorcycles, and bicycles are used by tourists.

Emporiatric health care providers need to stress seat belt and helmet use advice and integrate it into their overall educational activities. Travelers need to inquire about the availability of seat belts, air bags, car seats, and helmets when renting cars, motorcycles, and bicycles. Travel agents need to request safe cars and helmet availability for their clients.

Creative injury prevention programs should be implemented. An example would be a travel charter group providing motorcycle and bicycle helmets when clients go to countries where these forms of transportation are likely to be used.

WATER-RELATED INJURY

Epidemiology Epidemiology studies describing the risk of travel-related drownings and near drownings are limited. Drownings are consistently a significant cause of travel-related deaths, accounting for 18% of all injury deaths in U.S. Peace Corps volunteers.[5] One study that examined U.S. tourists traveling to Mexico showed a significant increase in the proportional mortality ratio of drownings for all ages of travelers.[10] An Australian study of rescues and drownings identified that 10% of rescues and 10% of drownings involved international visitors. Considering that the beach population of international visitors is less than 0.9%, these rescues and drownings appear to be significantly more frequent among visitors than in-country beach users.[22]

One study examining beach-related injuries found that 18% of the incidents involved rescue from near drownings, whereas lacerations, sprains, and sunburn accounted for 60% of the beach-related injuries.[23]

Far less frequent, but with significantly greater morbidity, are injuries from outboard motor propellers.[30] Every year, scuba divers and other travelers who are water skiing, fishing, or boating are killed or seriously injured by outboard propellers.[36]

Prevention Prevention strategies for water-related injuries can be divided into swimming, boating, and beach-related events.

The use of flotation devices during water skiing and other activities of boating is crucial in preventing drownings. Resort areas where boats are rented and water skiing activities are promoted should have life jackets available.

Propeller guards should be used on all boats with outboard and inboard motors (Figure 29–1).

At-risk alcohol use (alcohol intake while swimming and boating) is unfortunately common among travelers and is a significant risk factor for drowning.[21] Concurrent use of alcohol during water-related activities should be actively minimized or discouraged.

Beach areas can be dangerous. Preventive strategies can focus on individual awareness (education, informational brochures placed in airplanes and hotels), hazard identification and control (clear and visible signs, barriers, safety equipment), and service provision (lifeguards).[23]

FALLS

Epidemiology Travel-related falls account for a small percentage of travel-related deaths but comprise approximately 8% of all tourist-related air medical evacuations and can result in permanent disability from spinal cord injury.[14]

Mountain climbing is a popular travel-related activity, unfortunately resulting in death and nonfatal injury. Reliable data describing these events are not uniformly available.

Prevention Tourists should be encouraged to wear good fitting, firm shoes while hiking and when walking on irregular or slippery surfaces.

Hotels and other structures should establish standards for balcony railings so that the height of the railing exceeds the midway height of most people.

SPECIAL ISSUES

Alcohol and travel often go hand in hand. Yet defining and reducing tourist at-risk alcohol use can be challenging. In one country, tourism was positively associated with elevated alcohol-related motor vehicle fatality rates.[26] Travel-related alcohol consumption is directly correlated with higher alcohol consumption rates and high crash rates and death.[27]

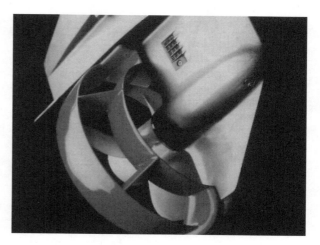

Figure 29–1. Propeller guard.

Violence (intentional injury) is increasingly becoming a health issue for travelers, especially in areas of political instability. Studies have demonstrated that homicide and assaultive injuries are significant causes of travel-related morbidity and mortality.[5,11] Avoiding nighttime travel and traveling in groups are two ways that tourists can reduce their risk of intentional injuries.

Special travel destinations involving wilderness areas and ecotours represent unique injury risk. Special populations with unique health conditions are increasingly traveling to challenging destinations with injury risk.[28]

Injury prevention advocacy is crucial for the travel medicine specialist. Emporiatric professionals need to address all aspects of travel-related risks. The traveler needs accurate and complete advice on injury prevention. Travel medicine specialists need to advocate for consistent safety standards for vehicles and roadways and uniform driver licensure procedures throughout all countries.[29]

INJURIES ARE NOT ACCIDENTS

Injury prevention is crucial for travel medicine.[7,15,24] Injuries are predictable events and amenable to prevention strategies using classic public health science similar to what has been done in the field of infectious diseases.[15,24] Prevention strategies need to address both the agent (mechanical energy, thermal energy, chemical energy, and radiation energy) and vehicles (cars, airplanes, guns, motorcycles, and bicycles).

The environment of the host country plays a crucial role in determining injury risk and should be an important focus of prevention strategies.

Personal behavior change has been the traditional approach for injury prevention but is only one component of comprehensive injury prevention strategies. It is important for emporiatric health professionals to craft educational strategies specific for travelers (Table 29–3).

Control of injury risk requires a multifaceted approach. Not only should the individual receive information on risk reduction, but a concerted effort is required to control hazards through safety equipment, barriers and signs, and other engineering solutions. There also needs to be a focus on the emergency medical services provided for injury management. Although many of these factors are out of the immediate control of the individual travel health practitioner, they are not out of the control of the profession. Health professional advocacy to tourist operators and local and national governments has been shown to institute positive change in the control of injury risk and death.[37]

REFERENCES

1. Steffen R, Rickenbach M, Wilhelm U, et al. Health problems after travel to developing countries. J Infect Dis 1987;156: 84–91.
2. Steffen R, Lobel HO. The epidemiologic basis for the practice of travel medicine. J Wilderness Med 1994;5:156–166.
3. Cossar JW, Reid D, Grist NR, et al. Illness associated with travel: a ten-year review. Travel Med Int 1985;3:1,13–18.
4. Kendrich MA. Study of illness among Americans returning from international travel. J Infect Dis 1972;126:684–687.
5. Hargarten S, Baker S. Fatalities in the Peace Corps. JAMA 1985;254:1326–1329.
6. Hargarten SW, Baker TD, Gupthill K. Overseas fatalities of United States citizen travelers: an analysis of deaths related to international travel. Ann Emerg Med 1991;20:622–626.
7. Steffen R. Travel medicine prevention based on epidemiologic data. Trans R Soc Trop Med Hyg 1991;85:156–162.
8. Paixao MLT DA, Dewar RD, Cossar JH, et al. What do Scots die of when abroad? Scot Med J 1991;36:114–116.
9. Holliman CJ, Messina J, Fresh L, et al. Injury death risk for U.S. travelers in other countries in 1996 [abstract]. Presented at the 6th Conference of the International Society of Travel Medicine, Montreal, June 1999.
10. Guptill KS, Hargarten SW, Baker TD. American travel deaths in Mexico: causes and prevention strategies. West J Med 1991; 154:169–171.
11. Prociv P. Deaths of Australian travelers overseas. Med J Aust 1995; 163(1):27–30.
12. Grenfell R, Ranson D, Hargarten S. Mortality of visitors to Victoria, Australia [abstract]. Presented at the International Society of Travel Medicine Conference, Geneva, March 1997.
13. Seiler O, Hofliger C. Aeromedical evacuation: 40 years experience of Swiss Air Rescue (RECA). Travel Med Int 1990;8: 3–7.
14. Hargarten S, Bouc G. Emergency air medical transport of U.S. citizen tourists: 1988–1990. Air Med J 1993; Oct:398–402.
15. Hargarten SW. Injury prevention: a crucial aspect of travel medicine. J Travel Med 1994;1:48–50.
16. Hargarten SW. International travel and motor vehicle crash deaths: the problem, risks, and prevention. Travel Med Int 1991;9:106–110.
17. Jacobs GD, Sayer I. Road accidents in developing countries. Accid Anal Prev 1983;15:337–353.
18. Egun G. Conditions of vehicles in Saudi Arabia. Accid Anal Prev 1987;19:343–358.
19. Gursu KG. Accident prevention and emergency services. In: Pasini W, ed. Tourist health. 1990:338–344.
20. Wintemute GJ. Is motor vehicle-related mortality a disease of development? Accid Anal Prev 1985;17:223–237.
21. Dietz PE, Baker SP. Drowning: epidemiology and prevention. Am J Public Health 1974;64:303–312.
22. Short AD, May A, Hogan CL. NSW beach safety program. A three-year study into the circumstances behind surf-based rescues. Report 91-1. Sydney: University of Sydney Coastal Studies Unit, 1991.
23. Grenfell RD, Ross KN. How dangerous is that visit to the beach? A pilot study of beach injuries. Aust Fam Physician 1992;21:1145–1148.

Table 29–3. INJURY PREVENTION STRATEGIES (AVOIDANCE VS. CONSTRUCTIVE BEHAVIORS)

AVOIDANCE BEHAVIORS	CONSTRUCTIVE BEHAVIORS
Avoid nighttime driving	Select safe rental cars Use helmets and seat belts Use designated drivers
Avoid traveling alone at night	Travel in groups at night
Avoid swimming and alcohol usage	Use life jackets
Avoid unscheduled aircraft	Use scheduled aircraft when possible

24. Gursu KG. Accidents and traveling. In: March PA, ed. Travel medicine. 1994:147–148.

25. Hargarten SW. Availability of safety devices in rental cars: an international survey. Travel Med Int 1992:109–110.

26. Colon I. The role of tourism in alcohol-related highway fatalities. Int J Addictions 1985;20:577–582.

27. Lowenfels AB, Wynn PS. One less for the road: international trends in alcohol consumption and vehicular fatalities. Ann Epidemiol 1992;2:249–256.

28. Welch TR. Climbing harness fit in kidney transplant recipients. Wilderness Environ Med 1999;10(1):2.

29. Association for Safe International Road Travel (ASIRT). www.asirt.org. May 27, 1999.

30. Hargarten SW, Karlson T, Vernick J. Motorboat propeller injuries in Wisconsin: enumeration and prevention. J Trauma 1994;37:187–190.

31. International Road Federation. World road statistics 1989–1993. Washington, DC: IRF, 1994.

32. Wilks J, Watson B. Road safety and international visitors in Australia: looking beyond the tip of the iceberg. Travel Med Int 1998;16:194–198.

33. Reid D, Cossar JH. Epidemiology of travel. Br Med Bull 1993;49:257–268.

34. Automobile Association of Great Britain and National Safety Council, 1986.

35. Swaddiwudhipong W, Nguntra P, Mahasa Kpan P. Epidemiologic characteristics of drivers, vehicles, pedestrians, and road environments in road traffic accidents in rural Thailand. Southeast Asian J Trop Med Public Health 1994;25(1):37–44.

36. Hargarten SW, Karlson T, Vernick JS, Aprahamian C. Motorboat propeller injuries in Wisconsin: enumeration and prevention. J Trauma Injury Infect Crit Care 1994;37:187–190.

37. Australian National Water Safety Plan. Sydney: Australian Water Safety Council, July 1998.

Chapter 30

ENVENOMING AND POISONING CAUSED BY ANIMALS

MAURO BODIO AND THOMAS JUNGHANSS

INTRODUCTION

Travelers increasingly explore the most remote places of the world. A horrifying diversity of venomous and poisonous animals far away from medical help is added to other more well-known risks.[1–3]

Thousands of animal species, taxonomically as different as Portuguese men o'war and Patagonian lance head vipers or yellow scorpions and red snappers, are known to cause accidents. Toxic liquids, combined with specialized teeth, stings, arrows, or nematocysts for injection, are used by various venomous animals to fulfill essential biologic needs as prey catching or self-defense. Many marine creatures lack such injection devices but possess toxins dispersed in their body tissues and are thus poisonous to eat.

Travelers, however, are not exposed to bites and stings to the same extent as the local population. For the latter, such accidents are associated closely with daily living and work. Being bitten by a snake or stung by a scorpion during a lifetime is almost inescapable. Protecting oneself against snake bites, for example, with footwear and clothing, is unrealistic for many reasons. Boots are unacceptable because of the heat or unaffordable for economic reasons.

There are no good data available that tell us much about the risks of being envenomed as a traveler in various regions of the world. From the daily experiences of travel clinics, it appears, however, that accidents in the marine environment head the list, in particular, stings by venomous fish and skin eruptions caused by jellyfish. Intoxication due to ingestion of poisonous fish also seems among the more frequent encounters that tourists make. In terms of pure numbers of incidents, bee, wasp, and ant stings are clearly the most important causes of accidents. Strictly speaking, the majority of those are allergies, however, rather than envenoming in the true sense.

DIVERSITY AND CLASSIFICATION OF VENOMOUS AND POISONOUS ANIMALS

Venomous and poisonous animals have evolved in a fascinating diversity over a wide range of the animal kingdom. They inhabit a large variety of aquatic or terrestrial ecologic niches worldwide. The diversity of venomous and poisonous animals is highest in tropical and subtropical regions.

Most clinicians feel overwhelmed by the taxonomic diversity of venomous and poisonous animals. It is therefore important to tailor taxonomic work-up of the culprit of an accident to the needs of clinical problem solving. In this respect, the ultimate necessity for identification is determined by the availability of a specific antidote (antivenom). We need to sort out this question in every patient before we confine ourselves solely to supportive treatment.

For this purpose, it is reasonable to divide the whole range of venomous and poisonous animals into animal groups in a first step (Figure 30–1). These groups are distinguishable from each other by a simple set of criteria. This should allow a rapid classification in an individual case of envenoming or poisoning. The group of venomous terrestrial snakes comprises a large number of dangerous species and the number of available specific antivenoms is equally high. It thus appears useful to further subdivide venomous terrestrial snakes into regional subgroups (see Figure 30–1).[1]

VENOMS, POISONS, AND THEIR CLINICAL EFFECTS

Most animal venoms are complex, species-specific mixtures of pharmacologically active substances that display a confusing range of clinical signs and symptoms. In contrast to venoms, poisons show little or no variability over wide taxonomic ranges (genera, families, orders, classes, or even phyla); hence, the clinical presentation is remarkably uniform.[4] This is explained by the fact that most poisonous animals do not produce their poisons by themselves but accumulate toxic microorganisms via the food chain.

The biologic function of animal venoms is related to prey catching, prey digestion, defense against predators, brood care, protection from microbial infestation, or various other interactions in an ecosystem. They frequently consist of compounds belonging to different chemical classes. Relating individual venom components to single and specific pharmacologic actions is rarely possible. Some, for example, phospholipase A, display a whole range of actions. Moreover, venom components with low toxicity may act synergistically with others and thus exert actions that cannot be observed in isolation.[5,6]

Criteria	Venomous / poisonous animals of medical importance									
	Poisoning (per oral)	Envenoming (parenteral)								
		Aquatic animals				Terrestrial animals				
		Area of contact	Sting / bite			Arthropods				Vertebrates
Animal groups	Poisonous animals	Cnidarians	Other aquatic animals	Venomous fish	Sea snakes	Scorpions	Spiders	Hymenopterans	Other terrestrial animals	Terrestrial venomous snakes / Regional groups

Figure 30–1.   Dividing venomous and poisonous animals into animal groups.

In human envenoming, there is still a long way to go until particular chemical compounds, pathophysiologic mechanisms, and clinical signs and symptoms can clearly be related to each other. For the time being, a practical classification of venoms and poisons needs to rely on observations of clinical effects that they cause.

The wide range of signs and symptoms that venoms and poisons produce in humans have been grouped into seven classes of venom/poison effects[1]: (1) autopharmacologic, (2) local, (3) hemostatic, (4) neurologic, (5) muscular, (6) cardiac, and (7) renal.

POISONOUS ANIMALS

Most animals that are poisonous to eat live in the marine environment. Although edible, in general, they may become poisonous during certain seasons. Fish (Figure 30–2) and shellfish are common causes of poisoning in tropical and subtropical regions. Mussels and clams, instead, may also cause poisoning in colder climates. The toxins involved originate mostly from protozoans or bacteria and accumulate via the food chain. Poisonings are covered in detail in Chapter 14.2 Seafood Infection and Intoxication.[1-5,7]

VENOMOUS ANIMALS

CNIDARIANS

Biology   Jellyfish, anemones, corals, and their relatives hunt and defend themselves with the help of nematocysts. Besides nematocysts with gluing or wrapping threads, a venomous type is widely used in this group. The species-specific venoms are packed into tubular cells that are connected to harpoons. On contact with trigger hairs, they rupture and penetrate the touching surface (Figure

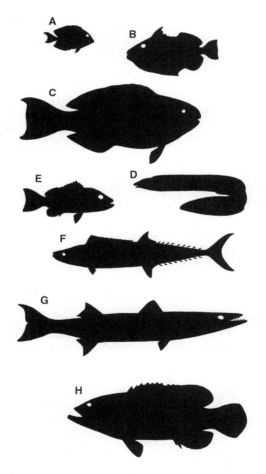

Figure 30–2.   Potentially ciguatoxic fish. Various forms of tropical reef fish may become poisonous to eat during some unpredictable seasons: *A, Acanthurus* sp (surgeonfish); *B, Ballistoides* sp (triggerfish); *C, Scarus* sp (parrotfish); *D, Muraena* sp (moray); *E, Lutjanus* sp (snapper); *F, Scomberomorus* sp (Spanish mackerel); *G, Sphyraena* sp (barracuda); *H, Cephalophis* sp (sea bass); and *I, Caranx* sp (jack).

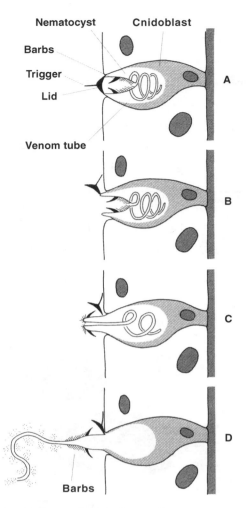

Figure 30–3. Discharge sequence of a nematocyst.

30–3). Up to millions of nematocysts cover the surface of big jellyfish.[1,8–10]

Prevention   Where dangerous jellyfish are suspected, one should never swim or dive unprotected. Stinger suits that are very much in use in Australia are fully protective.

Clinical Features and Epidemiology   Corals or anemones cause local burning or scratching. Most jellyfish species also cause only local envenoming of the skin. Some, however, may inflict systemic envenoming with neurologic or cardiac signs and symptoms besides massive local effects on the skin (Figure 30–4). Such accidents have been reported from the Pacific and Carribean shores (box jellyfish) and the Atlantic and Indopacific coastal waters (Portugese man o'war). *Chironex fleckeri* has caused 70 reported deaths in Australia alone. Death may occur within 3 minutes (!) after massive nettling. *Carukia barnesi*, a box jellyfish of the size of a thumb, frequently causes the Irukandji syndrome in tropical Australia, which is characterized by massive catecholamine release. Seabathers' eruption, which has been repeatedly

reported from Florida, is also worth mentioning since the clinical features might be very puzzling for those who have never come across this skin eruption. This skin rash is caused by *Linuche unguiculata* (sea lice). All cnidarians may cause hypersensitivity type I reactions after repeated exposure including anaphylactic shock. Less well known are allergic reactions of the delayed type that cause flare-up reactions and may produce clinical features that resemble rheumatic diseases.[1,10–14]

First Aid   Unfortunately, there is no universally effective and safe first-aid measure available. Interestingly, vinegar has been found to inactivate nematocysts of box jellyfish very effectively and is widely recommended and used in Australia. It is ineffective against Pacific Portuguese man o'war, however, and even activates nematocysts of the Atlantic variety of the same species. Because of the rapid cause of envenoming with death as early as minutes (box jellyfish) after the stinging, the application of antivenom through paramedical workers has been introduced. This is unique to Australia, however. If respiratory or cardiovascular failure ensues, ventilation and blood pressure must be maintained or restored. Ventilation and cardiac massage should be continued as long as possible since the toxins involved are heat labile, and very favorable results have been reported even after prolonged periods of resuscitation.[1,11]

Clinical Management   Local envenoming needs pain control and straightforward wound management including tetanus prophylaxis if the skin is broken.

In severe systemic envenoming, treatment is mostly symptomatic, aiming to maintain respiration and blood circulation. Specific antivenom is available only for box jellyfish envenoming. Only its effect on pain control and possibly skin damage is of proven value. Calcium antagonists (verapamil hydrochloride) have been suggested to counteract the action of box jellyfish venom. Their use, however, is still highly experimental and increasingly controversial.[1,11]

VENOMOUS FISH

Biology and Epidemiology   This group comprises all fish species that are fitted with venom gland-bearing fin rays for self-defense. The venom glands are mainly located on the dorsal fin but may also be present in the ventral and anal fins (scorpionfishes, lionfishes, stonefishes) (Figure 30–5) or in the pectoral fin (catfishes). Most catfishes are freshwater species living in rivers and lakes. Stingrays have one or more serrated stings on their whip-like tails, stings that may exceed 30 cm in length in large species (Figure 30–6). Freshwater stingrays (*Potamotrygon* spp) are only found in rivers and lakes of the South American continent. The weeverfishes of the Mediterranean and Eastern Atlantic coastal waters and toadfishes possess venomous stings on their gill covers in addition to those located in their dorsal fins.

In many species, the venom apparatus seems to have evolved along with a sedentary lifestyle in shallow waters for protection from enemies attacking from above.

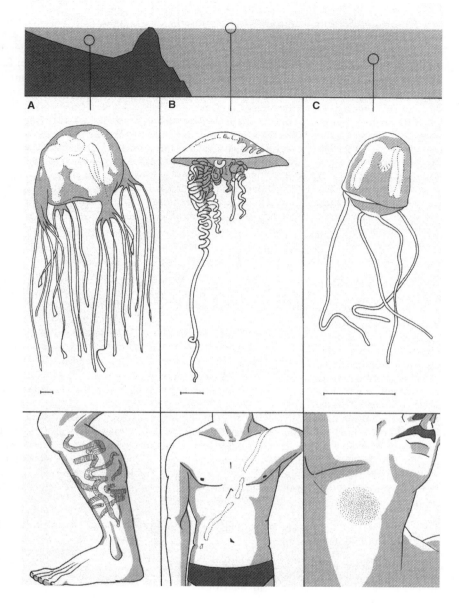

Figure 30–4. Ecologic, morphologic, and clinical features of dangerous jellyfish in the Indoaustralian region. *A, Chironex fleckeri* may reach a bell diameter of 20 cm and prefers shallow coastal waters. Tentacle prints show the typical ladder pattern. *B, Physalia* sp—in fact, not a single individual but a colony of symbiotic polyps—is floating on the water surface with the help of a gas-filled bladder. Whip-like tentacle prints. *C,* The Irukandji, a pelagic box jellyfish, has the size of a thumb. After heavy storms, it may also be found in the inward zone of a reef. The nematocysts of the bell produce a faint print on the skin.

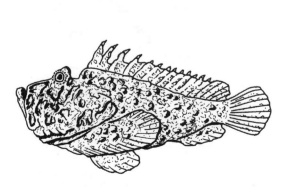

Figure 30–5. Stonefish (*Synanceia horrida*) with erected dorsal spines.

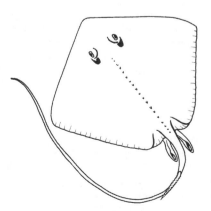

Figure 30–6. Stingray (*Dasyatis americana*).

Bathers are therefore mainly stung in the foot, ankle, or calf while wading. Divers who do not keep respectful distance to the slowly swimming lionfishes of tropical reef areas risk being stung in a sudden attack. Venomous fishes can also cause stings when handled inappropriately on fish markets or in the kitchen since venoms may still be active.[1,7,15]

Prevention Avoid wading in shallow waters. Flippers and bathing shoes can be penetrated by fish stings: they do not reliably protect. Diving masks are useful to identify potential dangers. Do not touch venomous animals even when they are dead.

Clinical Features As a rule, stings of venomous fish are extremely painful. Soft-tissue damage is twofold. There is mechanical injury caused by the sting itself and, additionally, tissue necrosis following deposition of venom, often deep in the wound. In rare instances, deeply penetrating stings can be complicated by injuries to large blood vessels and major nerves. Systemic venom effects are uncommon and are restricted to a few species.[1,10,16,17]

First Aid Injured persons should be brought ashore as quickly as possible to save them from drowning. Pain may be so excruciating that people often panic.

The debate around the effectiveness of immediate pain control has still not abated. Applying heat of about 45°C to the stung area continues to have its supporters, who argue that the heat-labile toxins can thus be inactivated. Others hold against this view that this method has never been formally evaluated and is potentially dangerous since it may cause further tissue damage.[1,10,16,17]

Clinical Management In most instances, pain control and straightforward wound management including tetanus prophylaxis will suffice. Where appropriate, nerve block with a local anesthetic is ideal. Revision of the wound might be necessary when nerve, large vessel, and organ damage is involved or when necrosis due to deep deposition of venom is suspected—similarly, when hard or soft tissue of the sting has remained in the wound. There is always a chance of bacterial infection, including deep abscess formation. Treatment is along the usual lines. The range of bacteria that might be implicated might differ, however, from what is usually expected due to the marine origin of the bacterial wound contamination.

An antivenom is available for stonefish envenoming. Its efficacy has never been formally evaluated; however, case series suggest pronounced pain relief.[1,10,16–18]

SEA SNAKES

Biology and Epidemiology The approximately 50 species of sea snakes form a specialized snake family that probably derived from elapid snakes. They secondarily conquered the marine environment as their habitat. Some species also enter river mouths. Two species, *Hydrophis semperi* and *Laticauda crockeri*, are freshwater species. They live in Lake Taal on Luzon, Phillippines,

and Lake Tenago, Solomon Islands, respectively. The pelagic sea snake (*Pelamis platurus*) is the only species found in the open ocean. It is drifted across the Indian and Pacific Oceans over large distances by currents and reaches the coasts of Eastern and Southern Africa and the Pacific coasts of central and northern South America. The habitat of all other species is restricted to coastal waters from the Persian Gulf to Japan and southward to Australia and New Zealand, where they hunt for bottom-dwelling fish or fish roe.

The most obvious morphologic feature that distinguishes sea snakes from terrestrial snakes is their paddle-like, laterally flattened tail (Figure 30–7). Their venom fangs in the front of the upper jaw are very tiny. In many species, they are far too small to penetrate human skin. Moreover, they are known to be good tempered and inoffensive when not handled inappropriately.

Accidents in bathers or divers are extremely rare. Sea snakes are mainly a hazard to professional fishermen in subtropical and tropical zones. They are bitten when removing sea snakes from their nets or when wading in shallow muddy waters. Epidemiologic studies exist from Penang in the northwest of Malaysia. The beaked sea snake (*Enhydrina schistosa*) and the annulated sea snake (*Hydrophis cyanocinctus*) have been identified as the main culprits.[1,19–22]

Clinical Features Extensive clinical experience with sea snake envenoming exists only with *Enhydrina schistosa* bites. The predominant feature is muscular paralysis, respiratory failure due to respiratory muscle involvement, and renal failure. All features can be fully explained by extensive myolysis, which is the main effect caused by the venom of *Enhydrina schistosa*. Local swelling is absent, and the bite marks are so tiny that they

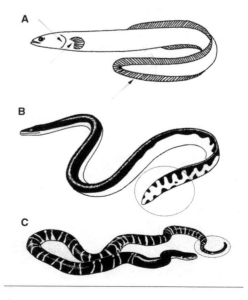

Figure 30–7. Pelagic sea snake *A*, Morphologically, sea snakes are easily distinguishable from eel-like fish since they lack fins and gills. *B*, *Pelamis platurus*. *C*, In contrast to terrestrial snakes, they possess a laterally compressed tail.

often cannot be detected. If the bites take place while wading, they can pass unnoticed until muscular pain and paresis ensue.

From the few case reports of *Astrotia stokesi* bites, it seems that they mainly cause neurotoxic signs and symptoms.[1,23]

Prevention   Wading in shallow muddy waters has to be avoided. Sea snakes should never be handled, even when they appear dead.

First Aid   Since local swelling is absent, crepe bandage should be a safe method to locally fix injected venom until medical help, including antivenom, is in place.[1,16]

Clinical Management   Antivenom is clearly indicated as soon as signs and symptoms of systemic envenoming become obvious. Dialysis might be necessary if renal failure precipitates. Patients with advanced envenoming regularly need artificial ventilation. Early muscle straining interferes with regeneration of skeletal muscles and should be avoided.[1,10,16,22]

SCORPIONS

Biology and Epidemiology   The order of scorpions comprises about 1,500 species. They represent an archaic group of arthropods that is related to the spiders and thus possess four pairs of legs. Morphologically characteristic are large pincers on the head pole and a tail consisting of five segments and bearing a venomous sting (telson) at its tip.

Most medically important species belong to the family *Buthidae*, which, as a rule of thumb, possesses more slender and smooth pincers than their less dangerous relatives.

Scorpions are present on all continents with the exception of Antarctica and may inflict painful stings when squeezed or handled. Systemic envenoming, however, is restricted to the medically important species in (1) Southwest U.S.A. (*Centruroides exilicauda* in Arizona, Western New Mexico, Southern California, and Southern Nevada), (2) Mexico (*Centruroides* sp) (Figure 30–8), (3) Brazil and Trinidad (*Tityus* sp, also *Bothriurus* sp in Brazil, although much less of a problem), (4) Northern Africa and the Near and Middle East (*Androctonus* sp, *Buthus occitanus*, *Leiurus quinquestriatus*, *Nebo hierochonticus*), (5) Southern Africa (*Parabuthus* sp), and (6) the Indian Subcontinent (*Mesobuthus tamulus*).

Residents are the main risk group, since these nocturnal arthropods live in or near houses. In urban areas of Mexico and India and in villages of the Sahara belt, dangerous species may reach high population densities. Very high incidences of envenoming are reported from Leon, a city in the Mexican State Guanajuato, where thousands of victims suffer from scorpion envenoming every year.[1,24–27]

Prevention   Always check shoes, clothing, luggage, and beds for scorpions, which might hide there.

Holes and cracks in walls are also hiding places and should be sealed. Walking barefoot is a risk.

Clinical Features   Local effects of envenoming are pain, erythema, and swelling. Bacterial infection may later complicate a scorpion sting.

Features of systemic envenoming can be readily explained by endogeneous acetylcholine and catecholamines, which are set free by scorpion venom. Two stages are observed: (1) cholinergic effects with vomiting, sweating, hypersalivation, priapism, bradycardia, and arterial hypotension and (2) adrenergic effects with arterial hypertension, tachycardia, and cardiac failure. Additionally, cranial nerves and neuromuscular junctions may be affected. Respiratory failure may follow due to failure of respiratory muscles and bronchial hypersecretion.[1,27]

First Aid   There is no clear evidence for the efficacy of routine first-aid measures like splinting of the affected limb and crepe bandage.[1]

Clinical Management   Local pain can be very well controlled by local anesthetics and regional anesthesia. Wound management and tetanus prophylaxis follow the usual lines.

Treatment of patients with systemic envenoming continues to be highly controversial. Experts from Israel have extensive experience in *Leiurus quinquestriatus* stings with symptomatic control of the effects of an overstimulated autonomic nervous system with hydralazine and/or nifedipine. They strongly discourage the use of antivenom. Similarly in favor of symptomatic treatment are clinicians in India (*Mesobuthus tamulus*) who use the α-blocker prazosin hydrochloride to control catecholamine effects.

Controversially, the Saudi Arabian (*Leiurus quinquestriatus*) and Mexican (*Centruroides* sp) experiences favor the use of antivenom. The use of drugs that control potentially lethal catecholamine effects such as hydralazine, prazosin hydrochloride, and calcium antagonists is undoubtedly a big step forward in the treatment

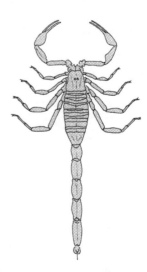

Figure 30–8.   Bark scorpion (*Centruroides* sp).

of scorpion envenoming. Immediate relief can be achieved and problems with antivenom use (availability, side effects) are avoided.[1,27–33]

SPIDERS

Biology and Epidemiology Most spider species —about 30,000 in all—possess venom glands connected to their mouth claws for prey catching and self-defense. Only a few, however, are medically important since in most species, the claws are either too small to penetrate human skin or the venoms are too weak to produce substantial envenoming.

Brown spiders (Figure 30–9), cosmopolitan in warm and tropical regions, and some species of other genera can cause necrotic lesions around the bite site. This is known as necrotic arachnidism. Some bird spiders ("tarantulas") possess urticating hairs on their abdomen that they rub off with their hind legs when disturbed. Otherwise, these fearsome large spiders do not cause serious envenoming (with the exception of *Atrax* sp and *Hadronyche* sp).

Systemic neurotoxic envenoming is regularly caused by (1) widow spiders (*Latrodectus* sp; cosmopolitan between 50°N and 45°S latitude) (Figure 30–10), (2) wandering spiders (*Phoneutria* sp; tropical and subtropical South America), and (3) funnel web spiders (*Atrax* sp and *Hadronyche* sp; South Eastern Australia).

Spider bites occur in or around houses since some of the dangerous species like *Latrodectus* spp or *Loxosceles* spp prefer habitats near human dwellings, but also during outdoor activities like camping, field work, or military exercises, when people may be bitten while squeezing spiders unintentionally. Bites may remain unnoticed until clinical signs and symptoms develop.[1,34–37]

Prevention Always check shoes, clothing, luggage, and beds for spiders that might hide there. Holes and cracks in walls are also hiding places and should be sealed. Walking barefoot is a risk.

Clinical Features Pain is not a constant feature of spider bites. Trivial local signs include erythema and swelling. Bacterial infection might be introduced through bites. In particular, *Loxosceles* bites have a record of local tissue necrosis. There are numerous reports on this problem from the Americas. Bird spiders may cause irritation of the skin and mucous membranes by tiny hairs that they can rub off.

Systemic envenoming in *Latrodectus*, *Phoneutria*, *Atrax*, and *Hadronyche* bites very much resembles that of scorpion stings. The clinical course is also predominantly triggered by catecholamine release.[1,18,38–44]

First Aid Again, few evidenced-based recommendations can be given apart from *Atrax* bites, for which experimental studies have shown beneficial results for crepe bandage. Crepe bandage and splinting appear to delay transport away from the bite site.

Clinical Management Local venom effects are either trivial and need routine wound management including tetanus prophylaxis or can cause severe problems due to tissue necrosis around the bite site. Treatment of necrosis is still controversial, but there are strong arguments for routine wound management alone.

Systemic envenoming appears to respond very well to antivenom treatment according to fairly well-documented case series from Australia and South Africa. In particular, the excruciating painful muscle spasms can be brought under control. Equally beneficial is funnel-web spider antivenom in *Atrax* and *Hadronyche* bites.[1,18,38–45]

HYMENOPTERANS (WITH A FOCUS ON BEES, WASPS, AND ANTS)

Biology and Epidemiology Hymenopterans form a large order that belongs to insects. They comprise the highly social bees (Figure 30–11), wasps, and ants (Figure 30–12). Their venom apparatus consists of a complex stinging apparatus connected to venom glands in the terminal part of the abdomen. During phylogenetic evolution, some bees (*Melliponinae*) and ants secondarily lost their stings.

Since honey bees and wasps are widely and numerously distributed from cold to tropical climates, most humans have experienced a sting at some stage. Single stings are only dangerous if they are located in the throat or in people with severe forms of allergy to the venom of this group. For toxic effects of the venom to become life

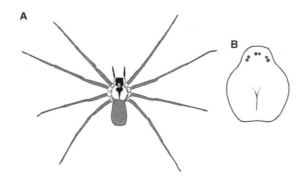

Figure 30–9. *A,* Brown spider (*Loxosceles reclusa*). Like the widow spiders, brown spiders grow up to only 1.5 or 2 cm. Note the characteristic violin-shaped drawing on the forebody. Six eyes in pairs (*B*).

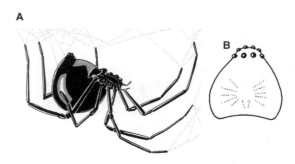

Figure 30–10. *A,* Black widow (*Latrodectus mactans*). *B,* The composition of the eight eyes on the head pole.

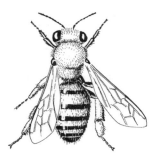

Figure 30–11.   The cosmopolitan honey bee (*Apis mellifera*).

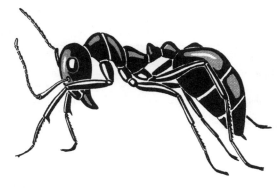

Figure 30–12.   The imported fire ant (*Solenopsis* sp).

threatening, hundreds or even thousands of stings are needed. These accidents account for less than 5% of all deaths due to hymenopteran stings.

In the first half of this century, the red and black imported fire ants (*Solenopsis* sp; see Figure 30–12) were accidentally introduced from South America into Mobile, Alabama. Spreading continued since then into other warm zones of the U.S., where they today cause the majority of all hymenopteran sting allergies.[1,46–51]

Prevention   People known to be allergic should get advice with respect to desensitization. Moving fast, perfumes, and certain colors may be alarming signs for bees and wasps. Walking barefoot is a risk.

Clinical Features   In most patients, allergic reactions to hymenopteran venom are restricted to the skin around the sting with pain, itching, erythema, and swelling. In sensitized persons, reactions to stings can be life threatening. The prevalence of honey bee and wasp venom allergies in the North American population is around 3.3% in adults and 0.8% in children. In moderate to severe allergic reactions, the whole range of hypersensitivity type I reactions can develop. In its most severe form, this can lead to anaphylactic shock and death. Larynx edema can develop after stings in the oral cavity, pharynx, or larynx.

Multiple stings induce toxic effects (venom dose!) in addition to allergic problems. Extensive swelling may lead to hypovolemia and hypovolemic shock. Toxic effects are extensive swelling with hypovolemia, hemolysis, neurologic disturbances, myolysis, and renal failure.[1,46,51–54]

First Aid   Effective first aid needs some knowledge and an emergency kit. Persons who are known to have moderate to severe reactions certainly need advice. First aid has to consider the severity of the reaction:

• Allergic reactions are restricted to the site of the sting: locally applied cold packs or ice will usually do.
• Sting in the oral cavity or pharynx/larynx: seek medical help immediately. If larynx edema develops, give adrenaline.
• In a patient with known allergy to hymenopteran venom with previous extended local reactions of > 10 cm in diameter and of > 24 hours duration, urticaria, and

angioedema: give antihistamine plus steroid immediately after the sting.
• In a patient with known allergy to hymenopteran venom with previous cardiovascular or respiratory reactions: give antihistamine plus steroid immediately after the sting, as well as adrenaline for self-injection as soon as systemic signs and symptoms ensue. Seek medical help immediately.

Stings should be carefully removed. Compression of the venom glands should be avoided in bee stings.[1,46,53]

Clinical Management   Clinical management is supportive. As in first-aid antihistamines, steroids and adrenaline are the mainstems of counteracting the allergic effects of the venom. Local wound management and tetanus prophylaxis should be appropriately applied.[1,46,53]

VENOMOUS TERRESTRIAL SNAKES

Snakes form the medically most important group among all venomous animals (Tables 30–1 and 30–2; Figures 30–13 to 30–17). It is estimated that 50,000 to 100,000 people die each year from snake bites alone and many more suffer from permanent disability. Rural areas of the tropics are particularly affected. The incidence of snake bites in the Savannah region of Nigeria, for example, is in the order of 600/100,000 inhabitants, with a mortality of above 12%. More than 10% of an estimated 6,050 snake bite victims die each year in Sri Lanka. Dangerous species are comparably numerous in Australia, less so also in the U.S. On average, 3,000 snake bite accidents are annually reported from Australia, of which 0 to 5 end fatally. In the U.S., less than 10 people die each year from snake bites.

Most accidents happen during field work in the tropics in workers lacking protective clothing and footwear. Travelers are extremely rarely affected. In Europe and the U.S., pet owners handling snakes are the main risk group. Differences in medical treatment between developing and industrial countries are enormous and explain differences of outcome after bites. High-technology medicine and the availability of antivenom is standard in Western countries but not so in developing countries.

Table 30–1. CHECKLIST OF MEDICALLY IMPORTANT VENOMOUS TERRESTRIAL SNAKES

	COMMON NAME	GENERAL DESCRIPTION
Colubrids		
Dispholidus	Boomslang	Arboreal in Savannah or bushland. Slender body up to 1.8 m. Inflates neck when disturbed. Bites only when handled.
Rhabdophis	Keelbacks	Mainly in forests but also in grasslands and rice fields. Up to 1.3 m. Reluctant to bite. Common pet snake.
Thelotornis	Vine snake	Arboreal mainly in rainforests. Slender body up to 1.8 m. Well camouflaged as a branch. Inflates neck when disturbed. Inoffensive.
Elapids		
Acanthophis	Death adders	Heavy bodied similar to viperid snakes. Does not try to flee when approached. From dry bushland to moist rainforests.
Bungarus	Kraits	Nocturnal. Slender snakes between 70 and 90 cm, up to 2 m. Very reluctant to bite during the day. Envenoming often in sleeping persons.
Dendroaspis	Mambas	Slender and very fast moving snakes up to 2 m or even 4 m. Arboreal. Black mamba mainly ground dwelling. Very dangerous when threatened.
Micrurus	Coral snakes	Mainly nocturnal. Often striking coloring with alternating red, black, and pale rings. Inoffensive. Some harmless colubrids show similar coloring (mimicry).
Naja	Cobras	Common snake in many different habitats. Slender or sturdy body up to 2 m. Typical warning posture with inflated neck and raised forebody.
Notechis	Tiger snakes	Sturdy body up to 1.5 m. Many have dark cross stripes. Usually does not flee when approached. Slightly inflates neck.
Ophiophagus	King cobra	Habitus and defense behavior similar to cobras (*Naja* sp) but up to 5-m body length! Mainly living in dense forest, never in densely populated areas. Only rarely cause of venomous snake bite.
Oxyuranus	Taipans	Slender and very fast moving snakes up to 2.5 m. Living in dry open habitats but also in forests and sugar cane plantations. May bite several times when threatened.
Pseudechis	Black snakes	Mainly diurnal in many different habitats. The mulga (*P. australis*) is the largest species of black snakes with a length of up to 3 m. Mulgas are easily provoked to bite.
Pseudonaja	Brown snakes	Slender and fast moving snakes. Mainly diurnal in many different habitats. Often in suburbs. Warns with open mouth and slightly raised forebody.
Viperids		
Bitis	Puffadder, gaboon viper, and others	Mainly heavy bodied species. *B. arietans*, the puffadder, is a very common species in savannahs and grasslands. Does not flee and puffs loudly when disturbed. Common cause of venomous snake bite.
Causus	Night adders	Nocturnal vipers of moderate size. Common cause of snake bite with local effects.
Cerastes	Horned and sand viper	Mainly nocturnal in sandy and stony deserts. Between 30 and 50 cm length. Produces a bright warning sound by rubbing its body loops continuously to each other.
Echis	Saw scaled viper	Dry areas, agricultural areas, and gardens. Small snakes with an average length of 35 cm. Population density may by extremely high. Bright warning sound produced by rubbing body loops to each other. May bite several times when threatened. One of the most dangerous snakes worldwide.
Vipera	European and Asian vipers	Larger Asian species up to 1.6 m. Usually in dry habitats, also in mountain regions. *V. russelli*, a very dangerous Asian species, often in plantations and rice fields.
Crotalids		
Agkistrodon	Moccasins and Asian pit viper	Dry habitats, forests. The North American *A. piscivorus* in swamps and near water. The Asian *A. blomhoffi* in humid forests and plantations, mainly rice fields.
Bothrops	Lance heads	Mainly nocturnal. Sturdy body up to 2 m. Mainly in humid forests, but also in plantations and near settlements. Easily provoked to bite, jerking forward.
Calloselasma	Malayan pit viper	Mainly nocturnal. In forests, open areas, and plantations. Sturdy body under 1 m. Most accidents in plantations.
Crotalus	Rattle snakes	Massive body with characteristic rattle at the tip of the tail. Large species up to 1.5 m. Mainly in dry areas from lowlands to mountainous regions. Produces bright warning sound with the rattle when threatened.
Deinagkistrodon	Chinese copperhead	In wooded mountain regions, mainly in rocky zones. Sturdy body with typical pointed protuberance at the tip of the snout. Since this snake is used regularly in Chinese medicine, snake catchers are often bitten.
Lachesis	Bushmaster	Nocturnal. Secretive snake from the rainforests. Never near civilization. Up to 3.5 m!
Trimeresurus	Asian lance head vipers	Most species are arboreal in forests, open areas, but also in parks of cities. Under 1 m. Medically most important species are uniformly green colored.

Table 30–2. GEOGRAPHIC DISTRIBUTION OF MEDICALLY IMPORTANT VENOMOUS TERRESTRIAL SNAKES

	NORTH AMERICA	MEXICO AND CENTRAL AMERICA	SOUTH AMERICA	EUROPE	NORTH AFRICA AND NEAR AND MIDDLE EAST	CENTRAL AND SOUTH AFRICA	FAR EAST	INDIA AND SOUTHEAST ASIA	AUSTRALIA
Colubrids									
Dispholidus						X			
Rhabdophis							X	X	
Thelotornis						X			
Elapids									
Acanthophis									X
Bungarus							X	X	
Dendroaspis						X			
Micrurus	X	X	X						
Naja					X	X	X	X	
Notechis									X
Ophiophagus						X	X		
Oxyuranus									X
Pseudechis									X
Pseudonaja									X
Viperids									
Bitis					X	X			
Causus					X	X			
Cerastes					X	X			
Echis					X	X		X	
Vipera				X	X		X	X	
Crotalids									
Agkistrodon	X	X		(X)	X		X	X	
Bothrops		X	X						
Calloselasma								X	
Crotalus	X	X	X						
Deinagkistrodon							X	X	
Lachesis		X	X						
Trimeresurus							X	X	

Venomous snakes bear venom fangs in the front of the upper jaw. There is a venom duct running inside these specialized fangs. In elapids and hyrophiids, the fangs are fixed and of small or moderate size. In vipers (viperids) and pit vipers (crotalids), the fangs are mostly large and mobile. Pit vipers possess a characteristic heat-sensitive pit organ between the eye and the nostril (see Figure 30–13). Many species of the large *Colubrid* family (*Colubridae*; around 2,000 species) possess toxic products in their salivary glands that mound at the base of the teeth in the hind part of the upper jaw.[1,55–64]

For short descriptions and common names of the medically important snake genera, see Table 30–1.

Prevention Boots and long, thick trousers are certainly helpful. Carrying a torch at night is essential. Hitting the ground hard when walking might help since snakes are sensitive to vibration. One should exert great care when lifting objects from the ground. Check where you step and what you touch. Bednets also protect from snakes that wander around at night.

Clinical Features Clinical signs and symptoms that are produced by the wide range of active components in snake venoms are manifold. To begin with, venom components that act around the bite site induce erythema, swelling, and necrosis. In bites of some species, the absence of swelling around the bite site a few hours after the bite clearly indicates that no venom has been injected by the offending snake. This is true for most viperids and crotalids but does not apply to a number of elapids. Venom components might cause anaphylactoid responses that resemble very closely true hypersensitivity reactions. Compromised blood clotting and impairment of respira-

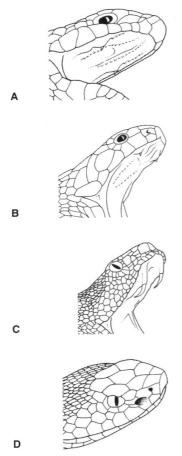

Figure 30–13.   Dentition in the different families of venomous snakes: A, colubrids (back fanged snakes); B, elapids and hydrophiids; C, viperids; D, crotalids (similar dentition as viperids; note pit organ, which distinguishes colubrids from viperids).

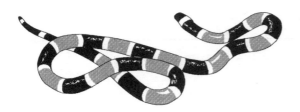

Figure 30–14.   Harlequin coral snake (*Micrurus fulvius*) from southern U.S.A. and Mexico.

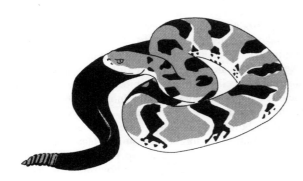

Figure 30–15.   Timber rattlesnake (*Crotalus horridus*).

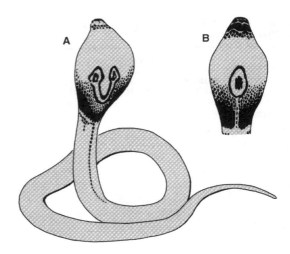

Figure 30–16.   Indian (A, *Naja naja*) and monocled cobra (B, *Naja kaouthia*) in warning position.

tory muscle function present the major clinical problems of systemic envenoming and are the predominant causes of death. For an overview of clinical impacts of snake venoms, see Table 30–3.[1,3,16,65–68]

First Aid   There is no universally applicable method that delays transport of venom from the bite site into systemic circulation effectively and without causing damage. Tourniquets cause severe tissue destruction depending on the pressure exerted. Devices that operate with cutting and suction to remove venom from the tissue are not only completely ineffective but are also harmful. In summary, of the many first-aid procedures that are on offer to inhibit venom action, few can be recommended. Calming the bitten patient and avoiding any further movements after an accident are of utmost importance. Transport of venom that depends on the muscle pump is thereby slowed down. Splinting bitten limbs and carrying patients are sensible methods from this point of view. Even more effective is the so-called crepe bandage, which works by fixing injected venom at the bite site by exerting gentle pressure (55 mm Hg) to the tissue with elastic bandages. The efficacy of the method has been experimentally estab-

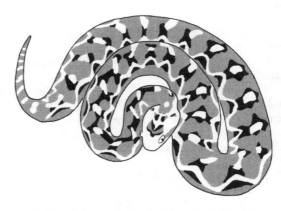

Figure 30–17.   Saw scaled viper (*Echis carinatus*) in defense posture.

Table 30–3.   VENOM EFFECTS CAUSED BY MEDICALLY IMPORTANT VENOMOUS TERRESTRIAL SNAKES

	AUTOPHARMACOLOGIC	LOCAL	HEMOSTATIC	NEUROLOGIC	MUSCULAR	CARDIAC	RENAL
Colubrids							
Dispholidus	X	(X)	X				
Rhabdophis		X	X				
Thelotornis		X	X				
Elapids							
Acanthophis	X			X			
Bungarus				X			
Dendroaspis				X			
Micrurus				X			
Naja		X	X[a]	X		?[b]	
Notechis	X		X	X	X		
Ophiophagus		X		X			
Oxyuranus	X		X	X	X		
Pseudechis	X	X	(X)		X		
Pseudonaja	X		X	(X)			X
Viperids							
Bitis	X	X	X			X	X
Causus	(X)	X	(X)		(X)		
Cerastes	(X)	X					
Echis	X	X	X				
Vipera	X	X	X[c]	X[d]	X[e]	X[f]	X[g]
Crotalids							
Agkistrodon	(X)	X	(X)	X[h]	?[i]		
Bothrops	X	X	X		?[j]		X
Calloselasma		X	X			?	
Crotalus	X[k]	X[k]	X	X[l]	X[m]		?[n]
Deinagkistrodon		X	X				
Lachesis		X	X				
Trimeresurus	X	X	X				

[a]Only reported from the African black necked spitting cobra (*Naja nigricollis*).
[b]May be present in Asian Cobras (*Naja naja* ssp).
[c]Not reported from European vipers.
[d]Only reported from the Russel's viper in Southern India and Sri Lanka and from some populations of European vipers.
[e]Only reported from the Russel's viper in Southern India and Sri Lanka.
[f]Only reported from European vipers.
[g]Only reported from the Asian Russel's viper (*Vipera russelli*).
[h]Only reported from *Agkistrodon blomhoffi* in the Far East.
[i]May be present in some species of the Far East.
[j]May be present in the South American *Bothrops moojeni*.
[k]Not reported from the South American rattlesnake (*Crotalus durissus* ssp).
[l]Only reported from the South American rattlesnake (*Crotalus durissus* ssp) and from specific populations of the North American *Crotalus scutulatus scutulatus*.
[m]Only reported from the South American rattlesnake (*Crotalus durissus* ssp) and from the North American *Crotalus horridus*.
[n]May be present in the South American rattlesnake (*Crotalus durissus* ssp).
Crosses in parentheses indicate that effect is less pronounced.

lished in Australia. There are queries, however, as to whether this method is safe when injected venom is locally cytotoxic and when swelling ensues, which builds up occlusive pressures under the bandage. In any case, medical help should be sought as quickly as possible after a snake bite.[1,3,16,64–67]

Clinical Management   The first step after a snake bite is to find out if specific antivenom is available and to

decide on its use. For this purpose, the culprit needs to be identified to the level that is determined by the range of antivenoms that are available for a given region. Polyspecific antivenoms need less precision, whereas monospecific antivenoms might require identification to subspecies level. Indications for antivenom use include signs and symptoms of systemic envenoming: (1) neurotoxicity, (2) spontaneous systemic bleeding, (3) incoaguable blood, (4) cardiovascular abnormalities, and (5) impaired consciousness. Local signs and symptoms of envenoming might present an indication for antivenom use if the species that inflicted the bite is known to cause local necrosis: (1) swelling involving more than half the bitten limb, (2) rapidly progressive swelling, and (3) bites on fingers and toes. In particular with respect to local envenoming, efficacy of antivenom is doubtful.

One has to be well aware that signs and symptoms of envenoming might be very much delayed. Observation of patients between 24 and 48 hours after a bite is therefore strongly recommended. If the decision is made to give antivenom, side effects have to be carefully observed and controlled. The range and severity of side effects depend very much on the quality of antivenoms. Quality ranges from crude antivenoms with a high rate of often severe side effects to very refined antivenoms with virtually no serious adverse effects at all. Pretesting for allergic reactions is unreliable. The value of premedication with adrenaline, instead, has recently been clearly established. Repeated doses of antivenom are often required because of prolonged absorption of venom from the bite site. In travel clinics, the question is often put forward if antivenoms should be carried along when traveling in remote areas where snake bites are a problem. As a rule, the answer is clearly "no," since the decision to give antivenom, its application, and the management of side effects need medical skills and appropriate equipment.

In addition to antivenom treatment, supportive medical care is regularly needed. Among the life-threatening effects of envenoming this applies particularly to the impairment of respiratory muscle function as in most elapid bites. Antivenom, as a rule, is not very effective to counteract these venom activities, and in severe neurotoxic envenoming, artificial ventilation is regularly needed. If successful, respiratory muscle function is restored completely. Prolonged and heavy bleeding is a difficult problem when unresponsive to antivenom treatment. Renal failure is also among the problems after snake bites requiring prolonged supportive treatment with dialysis. Needs for local tissue damage around the bite site range from straightforward wound management and tetanus prophylaxis to debridement for extensive necrosis. Compartment syndrome is rare and should be diagnosed only after careful compartmental pressure measurements.[1,3,16,64–67,69,70]

REFERENCES

1. Junghanss T, Bodio M. Notfallhandbuch Gifttiere. Diagnose—therapie—biologie. Stuttgart: Thieme Verlag, 1996.
2. Meier J, White J, eds. Handbook of clinical toxicology of animal venoms and poisons. Boca Raton, FL: CRC Press, 1995.
3. Warrell DA. Injuries, envenoming, poisoning, and allergic reactions caused by animals. In: Weatherall DJ, Ledingham JGG, Warrell DA, eds. Oxford textbook of medicine. 3rd Ed. Vol. 1. Oxford: Oxford University Press, 1996:1124–1151.
4. Mills AR, Passmore R. Pelagic paralysis. Lancet 1988; i:161–164.
5. Shier WT, Mebs D, eds. Toxins acting on ion channels and synapses. Handbook of toxinology. New York: Marcel Dekker, 1990.
6. Stocker K, ed. Medical use of snake venom proteins. Boca Raton, FL: CRC Press, 1990.
7. Halstead BW. Poisonous and venomous marine animals of the world. Princeton, NJ: Darwin Press, 1988.
8. Cleland JB, Southcott RV. Injuries to man from marine invertebrates in the Australian region. Canberra: Commonwealth of Australia, 1965.
9. Heeger T. Quallen—gefährliche Schönheiten. Stuttgart: Wissenschaftliche Verlagsanstalt, 1998.
10. Williamson J. The marine stinger book. 3rd Ed. Newstead: Surf Live-Saving Association of Australia, Queensland State Center Inc., 1985.
11. Williamson J, Burnett J. Clinical toxinology of marine coelenterate injuries. In: Meier J, White J, eds. Handbook of clinical toxicology of animal venoms and poisons. Boca Raton, FL: CRC Press, 1995:89–115.
12. Ohtaki N, Oka K, Sugimoto A, et al. Cutaneous reactions caused by experimental exposure to jellyfish, *Carybdea rastonii*. J Dermatol 1990;17:108–114.
13. Reed KM, Bronstein BR, Baden HP. Delayed and persistent cutaneous reactions to coelenterates. J Am Acad Dermatol 1984;10:462–466.
14. Auerbach PS, Hays JT. Erythema nodosum following a jellyfish sting. J Emerg Med 1987;5:487–491.
15. Helfman GS, Collette BB, Facy DE. The diversity of fishes. MA: Blackwell Science, 1997.
16. Sutherland SK. Australian animal toxins. Melbourne: Oxford University Press, 1983.
17. Edmonds C. Dangerous marine creatures. Frenchs Forest, New South Wales: Reed, 1989.
18. Sutherland SK. Antivenom use in Australia. Premedication, adverse reactions and the use of venom detection kits. Med J Aust 1992;157:734–739.
19. Dunson WA. The biology of sea snakes. Baltimore: University Park Press, 1975.
20. Gasperetti J. Snakes of Arabia. In: Büttiker W, Krupp F, eds. Fauna of Saudi Arabia, Vol. 9. Basel: Pro Entomologia, 1988: 169–450.
21. Reid HA, Lim KJ. Sea-snake bite. A survey of fishing villages in Northwest Malaya. BMJ 1957;2:1266–1272.
22. Reid HA. Epidemiology and clinical aspects of sea snake bites. In: Dunson WA, ed. The biology of sea snakes. Baltimore: University Park Press, 1975:417–462.
23. Audley I. A case of sea-snake envenomation. Med J Aust 1985; 143:532.
24. Polis GA. The biology of scorpions. Stanford: Stanford University Press, 1990.
25. Keegan HL. Scorpions of medical importance. Jackson, MS: University of Mississippi Press, 1980.
26. Stahnke HL. Biology of scorpions (*Scorpionida*). In: Nutting WB, ed. Mammalian diseases and arachnids. Vol 1. Boca Raton, FL: CRC Press, 1984:41–57.
27. Gueron M, Ilia R, Sofer S. The cardiovascular system after scorpion envenomation. A review. Clin Toxicol 1992;30: 245–248.
28. Dehesa-Davila M. Epidemiological characteristics of scorpion sting in Leon, Guanajuato, Mexico. Toxicon 1989;27:281–286.
29. Freire-Maia L, Campos JA, Amaral CFS. Approaches to the treatment of scorpion envenoming. Toxicon 1994;32:1009–1014.
30. Banner W. Scorpion envenomation. In: Auerbach PS, Geehr EC, eds. Management of wilderness and environmental emergencies. 2nd Ed. St. Louis: CV Mosby, 1989:303–316.
31. Gueron M, Margulis G, Ilia R, Sofer S. The management of scorpion envenomation 1993. Toxicon 1993;31:1071–1083.
32. Ismail M. Serotherapy of the scorpion envenoming syndrome is irrationally convicted without trial. Toxicon 1993;31: 1077–1083.

33. Bawaskar HS, Bawaskar PH. Severe envenoming by the Indian red scorpion *Mesobuthus tamulus*: the use of prazosin therapy. Q J Med 1996;84:701–704.

34. Bücherl W. Spiders. In: Bücherl W, Buckley EE, eds. Venomous animals and their venoms. Vol. 3. New York: Academic Press, 1971:197–277.

35. Preston-Mafham R, Preston-Mafham K. Spiders of the world. London: Blandford Press, 1984.

36. Levi HW, Levi LR, Zim HS. Spiders and their kin. New York: Golden Press, 1968.

37. White J, Cardoso JL, Fan HW. Clinical toxicology of spider bites. In: Meier J, White J, eds. Handbook of clinical toxicology of animal venoms and poisons. Boca Raton, FL: CRC Press, 1995:259–329.

38. Clark RF. Clinical presentation and treatment of black widow spider envenomation: a review of 163 cases. Ann Emerg Med 1992;21:782–787.

39. Müller GJ. Black and brown widow spider bites in South Africa, a series of 45 cases. S Afr Med J 1993;83:399–405.

40. Hartman LJ, Sutherland SK. Funnel-web spider (*Atrax robustus*) antivenom in the treatment of human envenomation. Med J Aust 1984;141:796–799.

41. Rees R, Campbell D, Rieger E, King LE. The diagnosis and treatment of brown recluse spider bites. Ann Emerg Med 1987;16:945–949.

42. Futrell JM. Loxoscelism. Am J Med Sci 1992;304:261–267.

43. King Jr LE, Rees RS. Dapsone treatment of a brown recluse bite. JAMA 1983;250:648.

44. Chang PCT, Kaz Soong H, Barnett JM. Corneal penetration by tarantula hairs. Br J Ophthalmol 1991;75:253–254.

45. Wille RC, Morrow JD. Case report: dapsone hypersensitivity syndrome associated with treatment of the bite of a brown recluse spider. Am J Med Sci 1988;296:270–271.

46. Mueller UR. Insect sting allergy: clinical picture, diagnosis and treatment. Stuttgart: George Fischer Verlag, 1990.

47. Akre RD, Reed HC. Biology and distribution of social *Hymenoptera*. In: Tu AT, ed. Handbook of natural toxins. Vol. 2. New York: Marcel Dekker, 1984:3–47.

48. O'Toole C, Raw A. Bees of the world. London: Blandford, 1991.

49. Gould JL, Gould CG. The honey bee. New York: Scientific American Library, 1988.

50. Spradbery JP. Wasps. An account of the biology and natural history of social and solitary wasps. Chichester: Packard, 1973.

51. DeShazo RD, Butcher BT, Banks WA. Reactions to the stings of the imported fire ant. N Engl J Med 1990;323:462–466.

52. Golden DBK, Marsh DG, Kagey-Sobotka A, et al. Epidemiology of insect venom sensitivity. JAMA 1989;262:240–244.

53. Müller U, Mosbech H, Blaauw P, et al. Emergency treatment of allergic reactions to *Hymenoptera* stings. Clin Exp Allergy 1991;21:281–288.

54. França FOS, Benvenuti LA, Fan HW, et al. Severe and fatal mass attacks by "killer" bees/Africanized honey bees—*Apis mellifera scutellata* in Brazil: clinicopathological studies with measurement of serum venom concentrations. Q J Med 1994; 87:269–282.

55. Warrell DA, Fenner PJ. Venomous bites and stings. Br Med Bull 1993;49:423–439.

56. Pugh RNH, Theakston RDG. A clinical study of viper bite poisoning. Ann Trop Med Parasitol 1987;81:135–149.

57. De Silva A. Snake bites and antivenom treatment in Sri Lanka. Snake 1980;12:134–137.

58. Sutherland SK. Epidemiology of snakebite in Australia. Snake 1980;12:138–139.

59. Minton SA. Snakebites in the USA. Snake 1980;12:141.

60. Coborn J. The atlas of the snakes of the world. Neptune, NJ: TFH, 1991.

61. Seigel RA, Collins JT, Novak SS, eds. Snakes: ecology and evolutionary biology. New York: Macmillan, 1987.

62. Bauchot R, ed. Schlangen. Augsburg: Weetbild Verlag, 1998.

63. Minton SA, Dowling HG, Russell FE. Poisonous snakes of the world. Washington, DC: U.S. Government Printing Office, 1965.

64. Meier J, Stocker KF. Biology and distribution of venomous snakes of medical importance and the composition of snake venoms. In: Meier J, White J, eds. Handbook of clinical toxicology of animal venoms and poisons. Boca Raton, FL: CRC Press, 1995:367–412.

65. Warrell DA. Clinical toxicology of snakebite in Africa and the Middle East/Arabian Peninsula. In: Meier J, White J, eds. Handbook of clinical toxicology of animal venoms and poisons. Boca Raton, FL: CRC Press, 1995:433–492.

66. Warrell DA. Clinical toxicology of snakebite in Asia. In: Meier J, White J, eds. Handbook of clinical toxicology of animal venoms and poisons. Boca Raton, FL: CRC Press, 1995:493–594.

67. White J. Clinical toxinology of snakebite in Australia and New Guinea. In: Meier J, White J, eds. Handbook of clinical toxicology of animal venoms and poisons. Boca Raton, FL: CRC Press, 1995:595–617.

68. Russell FE. Snake venom poisoning. Great Neck, NY: Scholium, 1983.

69. Malasit P, Warrell DA, Chanthavanich P, et al. Prediction, prevention, and mechanism of early (anaphylactic) antivenom reactions in victims of snake bites. BMJ 1986;292:17–20.

70. Premawardhena AP, de Silva CE, Fonseka MMD, et al. Low dose subcutaneous adrenaline to prevent acute adverse reactions to antivenom serum in people bitten by snakes: randomised, placebo-controlled trial. BMJ 1999;318:1041–1043.

Chapter 31

MEDICAL ASPECTS OF AIR TRAVEL

ALEXANDER GRAHAM DAWSON

INTRODUCTION

Modern aircraft technology features extraordinary sophistication and reliability. For example, engines on twin-engine widebody (more than one aisle) aircraft flying more than 120 minutes from land must demonstrate a rate of in-flight shutdown less than 1 in 50,000 hours, and engines today operate for 25,000 hours without removal from the wing for maintenance. This reliability has contributed to the exemplary safety of air transport so that, as the other chapters of this book testify, the destination is typically more hazardous than getting there!

However, there are limitations in aircraft technology—and human physiology—that persist in spite of the combined efforts of aircraft manufacturers, regulatory authorities, and airlines. These limitations during flight may particularly affect people with specific illnesses, injuries, and disability. Physicians advising travelers should be aware of the significant characteristics of the cabin environment and the possible options for minimizing or eliminating adverse consequences from air travel itself.[1] There are several texts with more specific and detailed information, and the medical care of professional aircrew is beyond the scope of this book.

In general, it is important to choose a reputable airline that is able to offer passengers the range of services that may be required for their specific medical problems. Many airlines have medical departments or contracted medical services that are available to assist passengers—and their travel medicine advisors.

This chapter will describe the aircraft cabin environment as it affects human physiology, review the assessment of fitness for flying for people with significant illness, and briefly note the medical aspects of emergencies.

MEDICAL ASPECTS OF THE CABIN ENVIRONMENT

Modern widebody subsonic aircraft operate at altitudes up to approximately 41,000 ft (12,500 meters), where the outside air pressure is less than 25% of sea level pressure and the outside air temperature may be approximately −60°C (−76°F). Ionizing radiation from cosmic and solar sources is significantly raised at these altitudes. The atmosphere has very low levels of industrial and biologic pollutants but is very dry (because it is so cold) and contains more ozone than normally present at sea level.[2] The atmosphere may also be turbulent—around mountains, in bad weather, and at higher cruise altitudes around the "jet-streams" of high-speed wind that are associated with clear air turbulence.

CABIN ENVIRONMENT

Cabin pressurization systems are essentially very sophisticated air-conditioning systems that modify the pressure and temperature of the external atmosphere and distribute the air in controlled flows from ceiling to floor-level exits.

Cabin pressurization systems vary with aircraft type: the maximum cabin (equivalent) altitude in widebody aircraft (aircraft with two passenger aisles) is typically less than 8,000 ft (comparable with ski-fields in many parts of the world), and the cabin altitude changes progressively as the aircraft climbs and descends (Figure 31–1).

Smaller aircraft (such as the Swearingen "Metroliner") may maintain sea level pressure in the cabin until their maximum pressure differential is reached (16,000 ft in the case of a Metroliner).

Unpressurized aircraft are limited by regulation to 10,000 to 13,000 ft unless oxygen is used.

Cabin Pressure and Barotrauma At 7,000 ft, cabin altitude gas trapped at sea level in a perfectly elastic body cavity would expand by about 25%, and any resulting injuries are termed barotrauma. Ears, sinuses, and the gastrointestinal tract normally contain air/gas that

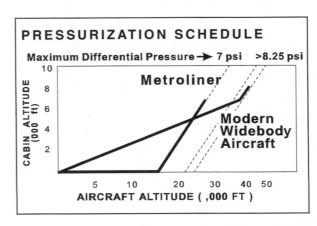

Figure 31–1. Graph demonstrating the pressurization schedule of the Metroliner vs. modern widebody aircraft (simplified).

can ventilate to the outside environment, but in some circumstances the air/gas may be trapped. Trapped gas may also be present in other locations (pneumothorax, gas gangrene, under poorly applied dental fillings, intraocular gas after retinal detachment surgery, etc.). There is no practical method to avoid this cabin pressure change during commercial widebody airline flights. Medical assessment should concentrate on determining the presence of gas and the therapeutic steps to ensure that gas is not trapped in a body cavity (see the section that follows on the assessment of fitness to fly).

Cabin Air Quality and Passenger Health The most common concerns are about disease transmission, low humidity, ozone levels, cigarette smoke, and disinsection (where this is required by governments).[3] Modern airliners recirculate 50% of their cabin air and typically exchange the air completely every 3 to 4 minutes. Air is recirculated from the cabin and not from galley or toilet areas (all of this air is ducted overboard). Ventilation rates are constrained by the requirement to avoid drafts in the passenger cabin, and carbon dioxide levels average 1,500 microliters/liter,[7] which is of no direct physiologic significance in the presence of low levels of other pollutants.

Recirculation may be switched off, for example, in an attempt to clear cigarette smoke or an air-borne allergen like peanut, but humidity levels may fall as a result.

Disease Transmission. Air from the atmosphere is compressed by the fan blades of turbine engines or by engine-driven compressors. Air from the cabin for recirculation passes through High Efficiency Particle (HEPA) filters that effectively retain bacterial size particles and aerosols. Specifications for modern filters vary but typically exceed 99.97% for 0.3 micron particles and 98% for the most penetrating particle size of 0.1 microns. Viruses (0.01–0.02 microns) and larger bacteria/mold (0.1–1.0 micron) particles are retained even more effectively.[4] Microbiologic surveys of airline cabin air demonstrate levels of colony-forming units and molds that are much less than for public areas on the ground.[5,7] Nevertheless, disease transmission has been documented for influenza[6] and tuberculosis[7] but is presumably directly person to person. It seems appropriate to recommend the same precautions for passengers with compromised immune function as would apply to cinemas and bus travel.

Low Humidity. The relative humidity in widebody aircraft falls to very low levels within 1 to 2 hours of reaching cruise altitudes—5% to 10% relative humidity in first class and up to 25% in economy[7] (passenger seating density is the relevant variable). This dryness has been very widely publicized. One study found that even experienced subjects find it difficult to discriminate between dry and normal air humidity in climatic chambers until 8 hours have elapsed; normal thirst mechanisms were easily able to cope with fluid loss associated with dry air, and whole-body dehydration was not shown to occur[8] (actually, subjects normally retain fluid). However, regardless of extra water consumption, water does evaporate from skin, eyes, and nasopharynx, and this may cause local symptoms. Dry skin is best treated with moisturizing

creams and dry eyes (most common in contact lens wearers who may be better using spectacles) can be treated with artificial tears solutions, but the nasopharynx is difficult to treat. Breathing through a moist towel or using water sprays may offer transient relief.

Ozone. Ozone (triatomic oxygen) is present in the atmosphere at the cruise altitudes used by airliners and at concentrations that would produce symptoms after long flights. Fortunately, some ozone may be converted to oxygen by the heat generated as the outside air is compressed before it enters the cabin, and many long-range airliners now have catalytic converters to further reduce the levels of ozone in the cabin. Ozone levels measured in airlines are approximately 0.01 microliters/liter,[7] and are typically less than those measured on the beach in Los Angeles.

Cigarette Smoke. This is clearly a health issue of concern to flight attendants, but nicotine and other markers of smoking in cabin air[7] are well within the limits for building standards.[9] The International Civil Aviation Organization has suggested that all civil aviation air transport should be nonsmoking from July 1996. Airlines are reluctant to ban smoking on flights between countries with high smoking rates (mainly in Asia), but, increasingly, flying is smoke-free by legislation or airline policy.

Disinsection. Some governments require aircraft disinsection for international arrivals, and a World Health Organization-approved "Standard Reference Aerosol" was commonly sprayed before or after flight. One sudden death on a British aircraft has been attributed to an anaphylactic reaction to this spray. Increasingly, airlines are using a residual surface disinsection of 2% permethrin (a stable synthetic pyrethroid).[10,11] The levels of permethrin in cabin air after residual disinsection are much too low to harm even insects, which must land on sprayed surfaces to be killed. No harm has ever been scientifically demonstrated to passengers from residual disinsection procedures, but people who consider themselves at risk should contact the airline and agriculture authorities for the countries they plan to visit.

Ionizing Radiation in the Cabin.[12] Radiation levels in flight vary with altitude and latitude but may be six times higher at cruise altitudes of 40,000 ft compared with sea level. The radiation arises from cosmic sources, with contributions from the sun that are most marked during solar flares. Radiation levels over the pole are higher than over the equator (Figure 31–2).

As a consequence, international aircrew in most countries are typically the occupational group most heavily exposed to ionizing radiation. The major radiation dose is of high energy with a significant neutron component; it is not therefore practicable to screen passengers or to reliably monitor levels with portable monitors. The International Commission on Radiation Protection (ICRP) has published recommendations for maximum exposures[13]: frequent flyers on business would need to fly at least 2,000 hours a year to exceed the ICRP 60 limits, but pregnant women should limit flying on subsonic aircraft to less than 200 hours during the pregnancy (depending on routes and altitudes, more flying may be appropriate).

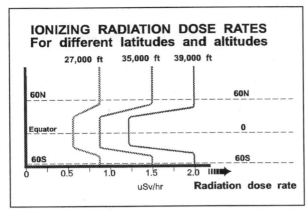

Figure 31–2. Ionizing radiation dose rates.

ASSESSMENT OF FITNESS TO FLY

There are very few absolute contraindications to air travel if the need to travel is sufficiently great, and the airline is willing! Many airlines will accept passengers who require intensive care in flight from a dedicated medical escort team (see Chapter 42.1 on aeromedical evacuation), but more frequently the problems relate to less serious conditions and unaccompanied passengers.

As with most aspects of medicine, the important foundation is a good history, and it is important to review a patient's experience during previous flying. This chapter contains selected information about routine preparations, chronic illness, and air travel.

Some basic guidelines about fitness for flying include:

1. Severe illness that would be significantly exacerbated by travel (e.g., decompression sickness or a significant pneumothorax) or that might prove fatal. Clearly, the treatment of the decompression sickness, or venting of trapped gas, would be important before flight at reduced cabin pressures.
2. Any infectious disease during the period of infectivity or where it would prove unacceptable to health authorities at the destination airport. This includes chicken pox and infectious diseases of childhood. No airline will knowingly accept an infectious passenger for travel, and this is a cause of huge disruption to travel plans.
3. Any disease or ailment that would cause serious offense to other travelers on commercial flights, such as infections or tumors with foul-smelling discharges. Smell is a difficult problem to counter on an airline with other passengers in close proximity. Equally, people with behavioral problems that may cause offense to other passengers need careful assessment before flight, and some may require sedation and/or escorting.

The important principle is that any patient to be carried by air should be properly prepared to cope with the constraints and adjustments necessary in flight and to ensure that medical control of illness is maintained at an appropriate level at all times during the journey.

Cabin crew are trained in cabin service and the best of them are wonderfully helpful, but as food handlers with no medical training, they cannot be expected to help people who require assistance with toileting, hygiene, or administering medications. In these circumstances, an escort may also be required.

FITNESS TO FLY FOR SPECIFIC MEDICAL CONDITIONS

HYPOXIA AND ISCHEMIC CONDITIONS

At a 7,000-ft cabin altitude, healthy people will experience an asymptomatic fall in hemoglobin saturation from a normal 98% at sea level to 92% to 94%.[14] However, due to the nature of the hemoglobin dissociation curve, people with even subclinical hypoxia (most commonly as a result of chronic obstructive airways disease) may develop symptoms at normal cabin altitudes.[15] Ischemic heart or cerebrovascular disease is rarely significantly affected by cabin altitudes in people with normal lung function, but oxygen is often suggested for 2 to 4 weeks after myocardial infarct or stroke. Profound anemia (less than 7 g/dL) and major sickle cell trait may also cause symptoms.

Assessment is based primarily on the history (especially of previous air travel), exercise tolerance, and blood gas measurements (pulse oximetry). For chronic stable lung disease, the ability to walk 100 meters on the flat without stopping, and/or an arterial oxygen pressure of more than 9 kPa (70 mm Hg), does not normally require supplementary oxygen for airline travel.

If necessary, a High Altitude Simulation Test using a hypoxic gas mixture with an oxygen partial pressure equivalent to that in the cabin (i.e., about 15% oxygen at sea level) should be considered.[16]

People with major sickle cell trait should also be carefully assessed before air travel.

If there is a medical indication, most airlines will provide continuous oxygen for passengers on payment of a fee. The travel agent should provide a "Medical Fitness for Air Travel" form for the passenger and doctor to complete (for IATA airlines, these are called MEDIF forms). Airlines do not generally allow the use of oxygen equipment in the cabin that does not have air-worthiness certification. Airline equipment may only allow predetermined fixed flow rates from portable cylinders, and the connectors (i.e., for nasal prongs) are not compatible with those used for domiciliary oxygen. Transit stops may also need specific arrangements, with a contingency plan in the event of a flight delay. Talk to the airline, and if they will not help, change airlines to one that will!

PREGNANCY

*   No later than 36/40 for international flights (check with the airline).

- No later than 38/40 for domestic flights (check with the airline).
- Airline policies vary and sometimes can be negotiated.

Note that most inadvertent in-flight deliveries are to women who are less than 36 weeks pregnant because premature labor is then likely to be precipitate!

Long-distance travel is contraindicated for pregnant mothers after 36/40, or even earlier if there is a history of premature delivery, for the following complex maternity cases:

- a grand multiparous patient,
- a parous patient with a history of precipitate labor,
- an elderly multiparous patient, and
- a patient with a complicated pregnancy.

Healthy mothers without symptoms of complicated pregnancy can usually be carried safely up to 38/40, depending on the sectors to be flown. However, it is important that women considering a return flight (i.e., an overseas holiday before the baby is born) appreciate the risk that an obstetric problem (e.g., threatened labour) at their destination may make the return flight inadvisable or expensive (because an escort may be required).

Women who are frequent flyers should be advised about radiation risks for pregnancy (see earlier).

Traveling in the first 2 weeks postpartum is not advisable, mainly because of travel-associated hazards to the neonate.

INFECTIOUS DISEASE

- any infectious disease during the infectious phase.

This applies to infections like chicken pox as well as serious illnesses like tuberculosis. In the event of persisting symptoms or obvious signs like jaundice or a rash, it is good advice to obtain a letter from a medical practitioner confirming for the airline that the passenger is not infectious.

RESPIRATORY DISEASE

- large untreated pneumothorax (the pneumothorax will expand and may cause symptoms),
- respiratory failure (increased hypoxia is possible), and
- recent chest surgery (especially if there is risk of pneumothorax).

In rare circumstances, it may be appropriate after specialist assessment to fly with a stable small pneumothorax, but typically the passenger will be well advised to have the pneumothorax treated. Some airlines will accept passengers with a Heimlich valve and a medical escort.

CARDIOVASCULAR DISEASE

- acute myocardial infarction (less than 10 days previously if uncomplicated, up to 40 days if complicated),

- congestive cardiac failure (uncontrolled),
- cardiac or cor pulmonale, and
- recent cerebrovascular accident.

A general rule for patients with cardiorespiratory illness is that if they can walk 100 meters to the aircraft with their hand luggage without assistance, they are fit for even an international flight.

GASTROINTESTINAL DISEASE

- recent intraperitoneal surgery and
- irreducible hernia.

Gas in the gastrointestinal tract will expand in flight, but it is rarely a problem.

NEUROLOGIC DISEASE

- recent bleeding or ischemia.

OPHTHALMOLOGY

- intraocular gas,
- perforating eye injury,
- retinal detachment.

Patients with intraocular gas should be advised by an ophthalmologist, but flying is not invariably contraindicated.[17]

PSYCHIATRIC DISEASE

- If unstable, unless escorted.

DECOMPRESSION ILLNESS

People who have recently been SCUBA diving or working in hyperbaric conditions (e.g., caisson work tunneling under pressure) may develop decompression illness in flight if they travel by air before excess body nitrogen is dissipated (see Chapter 14.1).

VENOUS STASIS AND THROMBOSIS RISK

There is extensive (if not conclusive) evidence that long-distance air travel is associated with a risk of venous thrombosis and thromboembolism,[18] and this has been called "the economy class syndrome."[19] Arterial thrombosis is also implicated. Smokers, obese people, women on oral contraceptives, people with previous DVT, and perhaps tall people may be at greater risk of venous thrombosis.[20] Lower leg swelling occurs as a result of prolonged sitting posture during ground simulations: it may not be pathologic, and calf exercise had no significant effect in one study.[21] No change in clotting parameters has been demonstrated during or after flight, but this was in a small sample of hematologists en route to a conference. A case-controlled study investigating preceding long-distance travel in patients with thromboembolism compared with a control group would be invaluable to establish an estimate of relative risk.

Meanwhile, it still seems wise to advise people to drink adequate water without excess alcohol, to exercise calf/thigh muscles in flight to promote venous return, to recommend graduated support stockings for people affected by ankle swelling, and to consider anticoagulation for people at high risk of venous thrombosis—especially those with previous thrombosis after flying! In the absence of specific trials in flight, the recommendations for prophylaxis after surgery or bed rest are most relevant[22]: aspirin has no proven benefit for prophylaxis of venous thombosis but may be reasonable for very low-risk patients (smokers, oral contraceptive users, tall people) on longer flights. Low molecular weight heparin subcutaneously provides about 24 hours protection and should be considered for moderate-risk patients, and full anticoagulation with warfarin (coumarin) may be indicated for some high-risk passengers (usually, these people will be anticoagulated anyway).

ENT DISORDERS

- recent middle ear surgery or infection (in case of ear barotrauma—unless grommets are patent, the ear drum is perforated, or the middle ear is filled with fluid),
- recent severe sinusitis (sinus barotrauma may be extremely painful in flight),
- fixed wiring of jaws (in case of vomiting from air sickness),
- recurrent ear or sinus barotrauma.

People who are not able to clear their middle ears (usually as a result of viral or allergic rhinitis) should not fly unless the aircraft cabin can be maintained at ground level pressure and the risk of emergency depressurization is acceptable.

The middle ear is the most common site of barotrauma, and this occurs as a result of eustachian tube dysfunction, most commonly as a result of upper respiratory tract infections or allergic rhinitis. The eustachian tube behaves functionally as a flap valve and this explains why "blocked ears" are almost exclusively a problem during aircraft descent.

Mechanisms for equalizing middle ear pressure include jaw movement (swallowing, yawning, etc.), the Valsalva maneuver (holding the nose closed and blowing into the nose to increase pressure in the nasal airway), Frenzel maneuver (Valsalva and swallowing simultaneously), and decongestant medication such as sprays, tablets, or inhalants.

If the middle ear pressure does not equalize, there is ongoing pain (from the periphery of the retracted eardrum), conductive hearing loss, and possibly vertigo. On the ground afterwards over the next few hours, the middle ear progressively develops a serous otitis. The fluid typically increases the lowered middle ear pressure and reduces pain, but there is still discomfort, a sensation of fluid movement when the individual shakes his/her head, and a risk of subsequent infection. On examination, the drum is retracted and inflamed, and often air bubbles or a fluid level can be seen behind the drum as the person tilts his/her head.

The appropriate treatment is conservative and includes decongestant medication, with antibiotics either prophylactically or as soon as increasing symptoms or signs suggest superimposed infection (the author's preference). The patient should be instructed in the Valsalva maneuver and should repeat it frequently once the eustachian tube is patent again to allow air to displace any persisting middle ear fluid down the eustachian tube. Typically, eustachian function will return to normal in 5 to 10 days (Table 31–1).

Other specialist treatment options from specialists include "pulitzerization" (insufflating air into the nasal airway with a special "pulitzer bag" while the patient swallows), eustachian tube canulation (may be difficult in acute barotrauma), or a tympanotomy. Grommets—either temporary or permanent types—may be useful for persistent eustachian dysfunction, or, alternatively, nasal surgery may be indicated.

Fortunately, the size of an eardrum perforation during descent in the aircraft is usually very small, presumably because as soon as the drum starts to perforate the air pressure equalizes, the ear drum reverts to a normal position, and the perforation will usually heal after 5 to 10 days on the ground.

Sinus Barotrauma   Sinus barotrauma is less common but may be much more painful. It can occur during climb or (more commonly) descent, and treatment in the cabin is by Valsalva maneuver (if the problem occurs during descent) or decongestant medication. If the person is not able to equalize sinus pressure once on the ground, then subsequent sinus infection is predictable enough to prescribe antibiotics routinely for 10 days.

Tomography, or computed tomography, of the sinuses is the most useful investigation when the problem is not obviously associated with allergic rhinitis or an upper respiratory tract infection. Endoscopic sinus surgery or conventional antrostomy may help persistent sufferers.

Table 31–1.   **TREATMENT FOR EAR OR SINUS BAROTRAUMA**

Medication: oral or nasal decongestants

Oral
    Pseudoephedrine tablets: 60 mg q8h

Nasal spray/drops
    Oxymetazoline nasal spray/drops: 0.05% or 0.25%
    Xylometazoline nasal spray/drops: 0.1% or 0.05%
    Eucalyptus/menthol inhalant capsules

Consider antibiotics (if infection develops or for prophylaxis, especially sinus barotrauma)

Treat for allergic rhinitis if present

Instruct in Valsalva/Frenzel maneuvers

Specialist referral for tympanotomy, grommets, or nasal surgery if persistent or recurrent

MEDICAL EMERGENCIES IN FLIGHT

Travel medicine physicians may be asked to assist with in-flight medical emergencies. Most emergencies for air travelers occur in airport terminals, but it is incomparably more difficult for anyone to respond to medical emergencies during the cramped and noisy environment in flight.

The most common medical problems are syncope, gastrointestinal, and angina/cardiac problems. These comprise over half of the conditions that a medical practitioner may be asked to assist. Many airlines also have access to ground-based medical advice using the aircraft communication systems, and these are a valuable source of second opinions! The aircraft crew should be trained in basic first aid and medical assistance, and the captain will advise about options for diversion.

Medical kits on airlines are not standardized internationally, and the Aerospace Medical Association has produced a recommendation.

Approximately 0.31 deaths per million airline passengers are reported to IATA, and over half are sudden cardiac death. Increasingly, international airlines are providing semiautomatic external defibrillators (AEDs) and training cabin crew in their use. Unfortunately, in-flight arrests are often unwitnessed and 80% do not have a shockable rhythm, but a third of those in ventricular fibrillation will survive long term. Some AEDs also provide basic ECG displays that are useful to diagnose dysrhythmias but not ischemia.

TURBULENCE AND IN-FLIGHT INJURY

Turbulence at lower altitudes during climb and descent is usually caused by bad weather, and the aircraft weather radar provides adequate warning to ensure that passengers are strapped in and trolleys secured. Fortunately, the majority of the cruise for modern airlines is in the stratosphere, and so above the weather. However, there are intense, localized areas of extreme turbulence in the stratosphere not associated with classic weather patterns—the so-called "clear-air turbulence" (CAT). The problem with CAT is that it is not detectable either visually or on weather radar, and so the aircraft hits severe turbulence with little or no warning. CAT is particularly dangerous because passengers may be standing in aisles or toilets, loose articles may be flung from open lockers, or the weight of articles in the overhead lockers may cause them to burst open. Food and drinks from trays or trolleys may themselves be a serious hazard. Serious injury and death may result from hitting severe CAT.

PASSENGER SAFETY IN AIRCRAFT ACCIDENTS

Cabin safety has substantially improved with better crew training, stronger 16 "G" passenger seats, safer materials with lower flammability and smoke emission, and better brace positions.

In 90% of potentially survivable accidents, there will be a major postcrash fire. This often starts 10 to 30 seconds after the aircraft has crashed and may take a little time to develop fully. About 15% of all airline fatalities are caused directly by aircraft fire, and another 10% are caused by smoke and fumes. If the aircraft cabin has remained intact at the end of the impact sequence, this will offer some degree of protection from external fire, and passengers may be able to escape through emergency exits on the other side of the cabin or at the other end of the aircraft and survive quite intense fires owing to the shielding of the aircraft fuselage.

Fire hardening does not protect entirely against smoke and fire generation but merely delays its onset, buying time of about 60 seconds or so—perhaps not long enough for evacuation to be completed. The use of smoke hoods can protect against the effect of the inhalation of toxic fumes but does not prevent these fumes from building up until they reach concentration where "flashover" is likely to occur. This is an explosive combustion of the fumes that have been given off from heated and burning plastic, as a sufficient density and temperature is reached that the gas mixture ignites spontaneously.

Table 31–2.   EMERGENCY MEDICAL KIT

MEDICATION	EQUIPMENT
1. Without Defibrillator / Monitor	
Epinephrine 1:1000	Stethoscope
Antihistamine injection	Sphygmomanometer
Dextrose 50% injection 50 mL	(electronic preferred)
Nitroglycerine tablet or spray	Airways, oropharyngeal
Major analgesic injection	(3 sizes)
Moderate analgesic PO	Syringes (1 mL, 3 mL, 10 mL)
Sedative/anticonvulsant	Needles (18, 20, 25)
injection	IV catheter (16, 18, 20)
Antiemetic injection	Antiseptic wipes
Bronchial dilator inhaler	Gloves (disposable)
Atropine injection	Needle disposal box
Adrenocortical steroid injection	Urinary catheter
Diuretic injection	IV administration set
Antispasmodic tablet	Tourniquet
Ergotamine/oxytocin	Sponge gauze (4 × 4)
Sodium chloride 0.9%	Tape adhesive
ASA PO	Surgical mask
	Flashlight and battery
	Glucostix set
	Emergency tracheal catheter
	(large gauge intracatheter)
	Cord clamp
	ACLS cards
	Bag-valve-mask
	List of contents
2. With Defibrillator / Monitor	
Same as list 1, adding:	Same as list 1
Lidocaine injection	
Bretylium injection 10 mL	
Sodium bicarbonate injection	
Diltiazem injection	

Evacuation procedures must be prearranged to include indicators that are obvious to a passenger escaping by crawling along the floor. Emergency lights at floor or seat level that can be easily followed to exits and the use of wider spacings between seats at the emergency-exit level can help a passenger locate an over-wing exit, even though it cannot be seen directly from the crawling position.

Passenger behavior in an emergency can affect survivability significantly. Passengers should know how to operate emergency exits and where at least two exits are located closest to them. Passengers should also be prepared to use any opportunities to make the best of their survival prospects; this may include climbing over seats to get to the exits first and knowing how to use survival equipment.

Airlines should offer counseling and other support to survivors in the event of an accident.

REFERENCES

1. AMA Commission on Emergency Medical Services. Medical aspects of transportation aboard commercial aircraft. JAMA 1982;247:1007–1011.
2. Ernsting J, King P, eds. Aviation medicine 2nd Ed. London: Butterworths, 1988.
3. Geomet Technologies Inc. Airliner cabin environment: contamination measurements, health risks and mitigation options. Washington, DC: U.S. Department of Transportation, 1989.
4. Needleman WM. New technologies for airliner cabin air contamination control. In: Proceedings of the International Seminar on Cabin Air Quality in Commercial Airliners.
5. Wick RL, Irvine LA. The microbiological composition of airliner cabin air. Aviat Space Environ Med 1995;66:220–224.
6. Moser MR, Bender TR, Margolis HS, et al. An outbreak of influenza aboard a commercial airliner. Am J Epidemiol 1979;110:1–5.
7. Centers for Disease Control. Exposure of passengers and flight crew to *Mycobacterium tuberculosis* on commercial aircraft 1992–1995. MMWR Morb Mortal Wkly Rep 1995;44:137–140.
8. Stroud MA, Belyavin AJ, Farmer EW, Sowood PJ. Physiological and psychological effects of 24 hour exposure to a low humidity environment. RAF Institute of Aviation Medicine Report no. 705, May 1992.
9. Crawford WA, Holcomb LC. Environmental tobacco smoke (ETS) in airliners—a health hazard evaluation. Aviat Space Environ Med 1991;62:580–586.
10. World Health Organization. Recommendations on the disinsecting of aircraft. Wkly Epidemiol Rec 1985;60(7):45–47.
11. World Health Organization. Recommendations on the disinsecting of aircraft. Wkly Epidemiol Rec 1985;60(45):345–346.
12. Radiation exposure of civil aircrew—proceedings of a workshop held at Luxembourg, June 25–27, 1991. Radiat Protect Dosim 1993;48:
13. International Commission on Radiological Prevention. 1990 recommendations of the International Commission on Radiological Protection. ICRP Publication 60. Oxford: Pergammon, 1991.
14. Cottrell JJ, Lebovitz BL, Fennell RG, Kohn GM. In flight arterial saturation: continuous monitoring by pulse oximetry. Aviat Space Environ Med 1995;66:126–130.
15. Gong H Jr. Air travel and oxygen therapy in cardiopulmonary disease. Chest 1992;101:1104–1113.
16. Gong H Jr, Tashkin DP, Lee EY, Simmons MS. Hypoxia altitude simulation test: evaluation of patients with chronic airway obstruction. Am Rev Respir Dis 1984;130:980–986.
17. Kokame GT, Ing MR. Intra-ocular gas and low altitude air flight. Retina 1994;14:356–358.
18. Sarvesvaran R. Sudden natural deaths associated with commercial air travel. Med Sci Law 1986;26:35–38.
19. Cruickshank JM, Gorlin R, Jannett B. Air travel and thrombotic episodes: the economy class syndrome. Lancet 1988;11:497–498.
20. Sahiar F, Mohler SR. Aeromedical grand rounds: economy class syndrome. Aviat Space Environ Med 1994;65:957–960.
21. Landgraf H, Vanselow B, Schulte-Huerman D, et al. Economy class syndrome: rheology, fluid balance, and lower leg oedema during a simulated 12 hour long distance flight. Aviat Space Environ Med 1994;65:930–935.
22. Silver D. An overview of venous thromboembolism prophylaxis. Am J Surg 1991;161:537–540.

31.1 MOTION SICKNESS

WILHELMUS J. OOSTERVELD AND JACK P. LANDOLT

INTRODUCTION AND OVERVIEW

Motion sickness is a disorder characterized primarily by pallor, cold sweating, nausea, and vomiting that occurs in individuals exposed to real or apparent unfamiliar motions. Other less dependable but frequent signs and symptoms of motion sickness could include drowsiness, yawning, increased salivation, headache, stomach awareness, belching, flatulence, general malaise, social indifference, and mental confusion. Furthermore, cardiovascular, respiratory, and other effects may result, as well as a variety of other sensations, emotions, and performance changes.

Signs and symptoms of motion sickness may range from mild discomfort to severe sickness, and the effect may range from lowered enthusiasm for work to complete incapacitation for any useful activity. The mildest form of motion sickness is the sopite syndrome, which is restricted to some gasping, some drowsiness, a decreased interest in the environment, and general inactivity. The most severe form can lead to dehydration through excessive vomiting, and, in extreme cases, such as in survival situations, the side effects can lead to a loss in morale and even to death. It should be noted that all of the signs and symptoms given above might not be the same or even present in different modes of real or apparent motion or in every individual.

Almost everyone who enjoys traveling has experienced motion sickness to some degree. Moreover, it is a significant problem in every major form of modern transportation: in ships and boats, in aircraft, in automobiles and buses, in trains, and even during camel and elephant rides. It will affect tourists in the 21st century who embark on space journeys. (An aeronautical company in the United States is currently booking commercial space flights that will commence in the year 2001!) It even impacts on individuals exposed to entertainment situations where the motion is only apparent, as is the case of total immersal in a virtual reality environment, when viewing cinerama films or in handling modern simulators employing moving visual scenes. It may be quite a challenge for future space and cruise ship designers and travelers to find ways to counteract the deleterious effects of both real and apparent motion if such entertainment devices are employed in these modes of transportation.

Motion sickness is a self-inflicted condition. It is a consequence of the enormous capacity of human beings to modify their environment and to increase the extent of their natural powers of locomotion. The human nervous system and, in particular, the spatial senses are those of a self-propelled animal designed to move at a footpace through an essentially two-dimensional terrestrial environment under normal gravity conditions. Motion sickness arises because of the disparity between the time scales of evolutionary progress and those of technological advancement. Evolution has taken place over millions of years and has adapted humankind extremely well to a particular way of life for a certain kind of environment. Technological advancement can be measured in decades; nevertheless, it has altered the natural circumstances so that many of the slowly acquired adaptations that have evolved have been rendered inappropriate: sometimes, these are even dangerous to present lifestyle changes. Motion sickness is the penalty for going beyond the design specifications of human locomotion and of doing something for which the human being is not specifically adapted to by the evolutionary process. It is a normal response to an abnormal motion environment, and it occurs from a wide variety of physical stimuli, most of them acceleratory.

Who suffers from motion sickness? The answer is rather simple: almost everyone. Of the normal population, 5% suffer considerably, 5% suffer minimally, and the rest suffer moderately. Motion sickness was mentioned by Homer, Galen, and Pliny. Julius Caesar, Cicero, Admiral Nelson, Charles Darwin, Winston Churchill, and Lawrence of Arabia are all reported to have been severely affected by motion sickness through sea travel, camel riding, or whatever means of transportation was available to them. Charles Darwin is reported to have "discovered" evolution after insisting on being let off the ship Beagle

to quell his sea sickness: this is further proof that illnesses have had a sometimes hidden influence on world events.

A consistent finding by many authors is that women are more susceptible than men. Women appear to have a higher susceptibility near menstruation and during pregnancy. Moreover, provocative motions may enhance the inappropriate vomiting in the morning sickness of pregnancy. Aerobic fitness training in both men and women increases their susceptibility to motion sickness.[1] Even race may be a factor; for example, the Chinese appear to be significantly more susceptible to unfamiliar motion stimuli than European-American individuals.[2]

Motion sickness is rare before the age of 2 years. It increases to a maximum by about the age of 12 years, then declines between 12 and 21 years, and declines still further before the age of 40 years. Beyond the age of 50 years, motion sickness is rare in civil aviation. Age does not confer immunity to highly provocative motions, but the declining incidence of motion sickness in advancing age may be related to a decreasing function of the organs of balance—the vestibular system—with increasing age.

The onset and severity of motion sickness depends on a number of factors: the intensity and frequency of the motion, the duration and direction of the motion, individual susceptibility to the motion, and the nature of the task being performed. Predisposing factors such as odors, fatigue, alcohol, a variety of drugs, and emotional state may enhance motion sickness. Sleep deprivation also renders many people more susceptible to this disorder.

Not only does humankind suffer from motion sickness, but many animals also have the problem: birds, fish, horses, pigs, cats, dogs, and even reptiles are susceptible to this disorder.

ETIOLOGIC THEORIES

Many different theories have attempted to explain the origin of motion sickness. The 19th century especially was a time of weird theories and bizarre remedies. The only aspect that the theories of that time had in common was that the root cause was motion. Which part of the body was primarily affected was the subject of many different theories, including a mechanical disturbance of the viscera, the "gut shift theory," irritation of the circulatory system, irritation of the gastric mucosa, and a battering of the liver causing an excessive discharge of bile into the small bowel. These were supposed to provoke nausea and vomiting.

A satisfactory theory of motion sickness has to explain a number of factors. First, it must consider the fact that not only motion alone but also visual stimuli alone can produce the disorder. Second, it must include the presence of a viable vestibular apparatus as individuals missing this sensory organ do not become motion sick. Third, the phenomenon of adaptation, that is, the ability to adjust to the real or apparent motion environment with cessation of motion sickness by most individuals within 3 to 4 days of provocative exposure, must be taken into account. Last, it must recognize the reality of mal de débarquement, the transient feeling of unsteadiness and queasiness occurring when individuals return to their normal environment following adaptation to a different real or apparent motion environment. (Mal de débarquement is a common feature following disembarkment from a ship following prolonged exposure to sea travel, in pilots after simulator training, and in astronauts returning to earth following lengthy stays in orbit.)

The neural mismatch theory is the most satisfactory construct that takes into account the essential features of the factors cited above that provoke the signs and symptoms of motion sickness.[3] This theory starts from the basic premise that situations that provoke motion sickness are all characterized by a condition of sensory information incongruence, in which the current motion information signaled by the vestibular receptors, the eyes, and the nonvestibular proprioceptors is at variance with the kinds of input that are expected by the central nervous system on the basis of past experience.

In an individual's normal environment, according to the neural mismatch construct, the relevant sensory information is congruent and compatible with expectations. As soon as there is an unfamiliar real or apparent motion such as air turbulence or rough seas, a "mismatch" signal occurs in the central nervous system that slowly diminishes over a period of 3 to 4 days until the individual has adapted to the new environment, and, consequently, the signs and symptoms of motion sickness will cease. Should the motion environment change, as in the case of a change in sea state during a cruise, or a return to the familiar as evidenced by mal de débarquement, a new set of mismatch signals are produced. In this case, the adaptation process will likely proceed more quickly than initially because of expectations derived from past experiences accumulated in memory stores.

Although the nonvestibular proprioceptors, that is, the receptors in the tendons, muscles, and joints, also contribute to motion sickness, it is the mismatches involving the eyes and vestibular apparatus that will most affect the traveling public. Accordingly, the focus of this chapter will be on the two categories of neural mismatch that are usually recognized as being most important. They are intersensory incongruence between visual and vestibular sensory information and intrasensory incongruence within the vestibular apparatus between the semicircular canals (angular movement detectors) and the otoliths (linear movement and gravity sensors).

Table 31.1–1 provides examples of common, unfamiliar, real and apparent motions that signal these two categories of mismatch.

The neural mismatch theory is a useful construct for visualizing the different circumstances under which motion sickness may occur. However, it fails to explain why incongruence in sensory information should lead to the signs and symptoms inherent in motion sickness. In this regard, Treisman has proposed that nausea and vomiting in response to motion are "accidental byproducts" of a system designed to rid the body of ingested toxins that has evolutionary survival advantage.[5] He has stated that the brainstem mechanisms of orientation and motion normally perform an additional function beside the maintenance of bodily equilibrium and the stability of gaze. This additional function is to detect and respond to certain poisons. In motion sickness, the theory goes, conflict in sensory inputs simulates poisoning in those brainstem neural mechanisms. Similar reactions to those of motion sickness are known from studies of smell and taste. A so-called bad odor or taste is able to provoke the motion sickness syndrome.

In line with Treisman's hypothesis is some current thinking, which argues that "... motion sickness can be seen as a poison response that occurs, inappropriately, in response to certain kinds of motion. The signs and symptoms form two groups, (1) stomach-emptying phenomena and (2) stress-response phenomena" that are triggered by

Table 31.1–1. EXAMPLES OF PROVOCATIVE REAL AND APPARENT MOTION STIMULI THAT CONTRIBUTE TO INCONGRUENT SENSORY INFORMATION LEADING TO MOTION SICKNESS SIGNS AND SYMPTOMS*

	SENSORY INCONGRUENCE	
TYPE OF INCONGRUENCE	VISUAL (A)—VESTIBULAR (B) MISMATCH	SEMICIRCULAR CANAL (A)—OTOLITH (B) MISMATCH
A and B together but uncorrelated	Wave watching at shipside	Head movements in abnormal acceleratory environments
	Reading handheld texts or displays in turbulent flight	
	Observing from side or rear window in moving vehicle	
	Employing immersive virtual reality devices in moving vehicle	
A without B	Watching cinerama films	Head movements in microgravity (space travel)
	Operating a fixed-base simulator having dynamic visual display	Lying down following ingestion of alcohol
B without A	Lacking external visual reference as below deck in boat	Low-frequency (<0.5 Hz) translational oscillation

*Modified from Benson.[4]

the vestibular system interacting with the autonomic nervous system.[6] The stress response of motion sickness involves the sympathetic part of the autonomic nervous system that results in pallor, cold sweating, and an increased blood flow in skeletal muscles and heart rate. The stomach-emptying phenomena involve increases in the parasympathetic activity of the autonomic nervous system such as nausea and the sensation of vomiting.

If the central vestibular mechanisms—the brainstem mechanisms of orientation and motion—do, in fact, respond to motion as well as facilitate the emetic response to poison, then it follows that removal of the peripheral vestibular apparatus should render such individuals immune to nausea and vomiting from both poison and motion. There is evidence that some vestibular brainstem mechanisms may respond to certain poisons. Surgical removal of the peripheral vestibular apparatus in dogs has impaired the emetic response to certain poisons injected intramuscularly.[7] Dogs, like humans, respond to inappropriate motion by vomiting; removal of the vestibular apparatus renders them immune to emesis during such motion. It should be noted, however, that the results in labyrinthectomized dogs were inconsistent: with three administered poisons, the emetic response was markedly lowered; however, with two other emetics, there was no effect at all or only a marginal one. This indicates that there are neural pathways that do not involve the vestibular system in evoking emesis during ingestion of toxins. These findings may also indicate that central brainstem mechanisms that coordinate information on orientation and motion from the vestibular system, eyes, and nonvestibular proprioceptors are colocated with the vomit control center in the brain stem that is responsible for all emesis. Therefore, one of the processes leading to emesis may be one that provides a graded response according to the degree of activation provided indirectly by toxins

through vestibular afferents on the vomit control center. The most likely prospect, however, is that the vomit control center coordinates the activities of numerous orientations, visual and autonomic nerve pathways, and mechanisms that converge to evoke the motor responses for emesis (Figure 31.1–1).

Some studies in animals suggest that the main vomit control center, and perhaps that of nausea, lies in the nucleus tractus solitarius (NTS), a brainstem region that receives its signals via a number of pathways.[8] The area postrema, which is also in the brain stem, detects neurotransmitters released by blood-borne toxins that cross the blood-brain barrier. The nearby NTS receives signals from the area postrema, the vagus nerve, which is stimulated by serotonin released by gut cells triggered by toxins, from cortical centers that provide information about "anticipatory" nausea and vomiting, and, possibly, through other neural pathways (see Figure 31.1–1).

Anticipatory nausea and vomiting is a conditioned response that occurs in individuals who associate an event with a previous bad experience. For example, it occurs in many cancer patients who associate the memory of receiving chemotherapy drugs with health care workers and hospital settings, and it occurs with individuals who associate a past illness with a particular type of food or other experience that is vigorously avoided. It also occurs in individuals susceptible to extremes in motion sickness (see below).

Much current research is focusing on the role of the vestibular system in regulating the autonomic nervous system.[9] Recent electrophysiologic and neuroanatomic studies in animals have demonstrated that vestibular input integrates with other signals at numerous stages (see Figure 31.1–1). In particular, the NTS communicates with the vestibular nuclei, the former of which receives nerve signals from gastrointestinal afferents via the vagus nerve

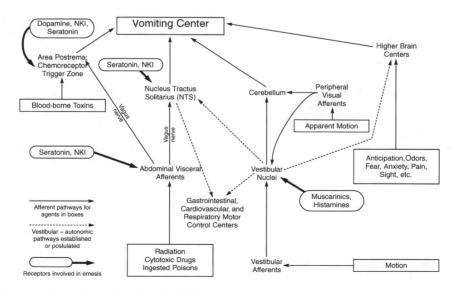

Figure 31.1–1 Nervous system pathways for vomiting and autonomic reflexes. Many authorities consider the NTS to be the vomiting center. Modified from Veyrat-Follet et al.[8] and Balaban and Porter.[9]

and is interconnected with the area postrema. This opens up the possibility that nausea and vomiting from motion sickness are elicited, in part, through nerve pathways in the NTS that mediate emesis induced by gastrointestinal inputs. Vestibular-autonomic influences also appear to have a role in maintaining or detecting disturbances in homeostasis of cardiovascular, respiratory, and muscle function. Higher cortical centers may also affect vestibular-autonomic influences. For example, motion sickness is not as severe in many experienced travelers who have learned postural counter measures than it is in inexperienced individuals. Similarly, unpleasant odors or anticipatory effects associated with bad motion environments may provoke nausea and vomiting.

Graybiel has proposed a link between the perceptual-motor adaptive processes and the onset of motion sickness.[10] There is some consensus about a linking threshold in a conceptual model of motion sickness. There is also evidence that the threshold linking perceptual-motor adjustments to the motion sickness syndrome is subject to conditioning. Some authors have reported on the occurrence of sea sickness at the sight of a ship or even after walking the gangway. Such reports are frequently heard as anecdotes about persons who have previously been sick at sea. There are also volunteer subjects who previously had severe motion sickness experiences in experimental rotation experiments assessing the effects of protective drugs who demonstrate similar patterns of behavior. These individuals become sick in anticipation of the consequences on seeing the rotation device and have to be removed from further participation in the experiments. In these cases, the sickness can be considered to be an ordinary conditioned response in which the primary and associated stimuli together give the same response as the associated stimulus alone.[11]

Notwithstanding that motion sickness may be a by-product of protective mechanisms against neurotoxins, it seems inconsistent with the consideration of motion sickness susceptibility as a product of a disturbed psychological function. The presence of psychological correlates, causal or otherwise, suggests that motion sickness is, at least in part, an enduring psychological trait. The reaction to motion stress is individualistic. High scores on neuroticism, anxiety, feminism, and introversion scales correlate well with a high motion sickness susceptibility. Air sickness, much more than sea sickness, may be a weakness associated with certain personality types (e.g., anxiety neuroses) who are more susceptible to the effects of psychological factors involved in flying. Anxiety disorders have recently been linked clinically to vestibular dysfunction.[12]

THERAPY

As long as man has suffered from motion sickness, methods of prevention and ways of treatment have been developed and many of these are still under examination. A wide variety of behaviors, potions, and drugs have been advocated for lessening the problems of motion sickness. Many recommendations appearing in the early scientific literature were based on personal experiences or anecdotes and are not supported by controlled studies. Today, many individuals traveling still adopt measures that have not been proven to be effective scientifically. Statistically significant benefits to travelers, from the consumption (or avoidance) of certain foods and drinks to the use of various commercial devices, have yet to be proven in many instances. For example, old prevention methods concern behavior activities such as the need for controlled respiration, as well as the intake of onions to avoid an abdominal vacuum. Other common practices encountered in previous centuries included the carrying of a horse chestnut in the left pocket or fixed on a necklace, the wearing of special wristlets, and an endless list of a variety of diets.

The use of a drug was first mentioned in 1869 in *The Lancet*, in which a combination of chloroform and tincture of belladonna was recommended in a letter to the editor. Moreover, between 1829 and 1900, *The Lancet* revealed that practically everything that could be carried, worn, or swallowed was prescribed for motion sickness at one time or another, including opium, cocaine, strychnine, creosote, quinine, nitrous oxide, amyl nitrite, hydrocyanic acid, nitroglycerine, warm salt water, and strong tea or coffee, as well as a variety of alcoholic beverages. Not only did these potions fail to alleviate motion sickness, but many of them were dangerous to one's health.

Usually, the best and safest nonpharmacologic treatment for motion sickness is the process of protective adaptation. For example, when at sea in rough conditions, most people adapt to its changeable motions in a few days. However, 5% of the population do not adapt to any form of motion. This raises the question as to whether there is a transfer of adaptation, that is, does adaptation to motion on a large ship transfer automatically to adaptation against motion sickness on board a smaller ship or other means of transportation? This is the case up to a certain level: when the motion patterns differ considerably, there is no transfer of adaptation as, for example, in a change of sea state or wind direction during sailing. Adaptation to motion sickness does not last a lifetime. When leaving a ship, adaptation usually fades away gradually. After being away from the provocative motion for 3 months or more, susceptibility will increase again, possibly considerably.[13]

Adaptation trainers are able to facilitate adaptation both to motion sickness in the microgravity of space and on earth. However, the fact that artificial adaptation training is time consuming and costly makes this method unattractive for the traveling public.[13,14]

There are other nonpharmacologic ways, consistent with the neural mismatch concept, that can lessen the impact, or delay the onset, of motion sickness. Low-frequency translational oscillations of 0.5 Hz or less are very nauseagenic. This suggests that faster or slower oscillatory motions are less likely to make individuals motion sick. Therefore, the chance of becoming sick from the rocking motion of a sailboat will be much greater than that of a cruise ship. Moreover, remaining close to the center of a ship or boat to lessen the rocking motion may further reduce nauseagenicity, as choosing a seat over the wings of an aircraft reduces the effects of turbulence. In land vehicles, such as cars and buses, reducing speed particularly on winding roads can lessen the rocking motion. Traveling on large ships and aircraft reduces the possibilities of encountering provocative motions and, consequently, decreases the incidence of motion sickness. Other strategies have been suggested to reduce sensory information mismatch such as restricting head motions in turbulent or rocking conditions by means of head supports,[15] avoiding reading during turbulence in aircraft or in land vehicles, visually fixating on a stable reference such as the horizon at sea, avoiding cabins on board ship without an outside view, etc. (see Table 31.1–1).

Recent controlled studies at Farnborough (RAF Institute of Aviation Medicine) have shown that vehicular motion direction, body axis, and posture are important considerations in inducing motion sickness during provocative low-frequency translational oscillations.[16] The results show that an upright seating position is more nauseagenic than a supine body posture, as is a motion through a body axis from the nose to the back of the head (X-axis) compared to one along the spine (Z-axis). The potential for nausea is greatest for X-axis stimulation when seated upright. This supports the age-old notion that lying down supine provides protection (e.g., on board ship). However, this does not take into consideration that closing the eyes when lying down on board ship below deck may further reduce sensory mismatch and, accordingly, lessen even more the nauseagenic potential of the motion environment. Travelers should be aware too that alcohol introduces a gravity effect on the semicircular canals causing dizziness while lying down. This, in combination with rocking vehicular motion, increases the chance of becoming motion sick.

Pharmacotherapy is the first choice in most cases where prevention or treatment of motion sickness is involved (Table 31.1–2).

Oral hyoscine (called scopolamine in the United States and Canada) is the single most effective prophylactic drug against motion sickness. It is a belladonna alkaloid with a long history as an antimuscarinic. Drowsiness, inattentiveness, dry mouth, and blurred vision are associated with the use of hyoscine. A very effective anti–motion-sickness preparation for short-term protection in severe motion environments is the combination (taken orally) of hyoscine (0.3–0.6 mg) and dextroamphetamine (5–10 mg), which does not have most of the side effects associated with hyoscine taken by itself.

The short duration of effect of oral hyoscine and hyoscine dextroamphetamine (4 hours) is a major impediment to extended protection in provocative motion environments. This has led to the development of the transdermal therapeutic patch (Transderm Scop®) that delivers hyoscine through the skin at consistent serum levels for protection up to 72 hours. The long onset time associated with these patches necessitates anticipating the need well in advance of application.

These patches are placed behind the ear in a hairless dry area. The amount of drug that penetrates through the skin differs considerably between individuals and can be excessive. It is advisable to prescribe these patches only when oral drugs have no effect. In children, patches are not advisable, and, in the elderly, they should be used with care because of the toxic psychotic effects that have been reported.[18] There are also indications that the hyoscine patch, although initially protecting against motion sickness, only delays the occurrence of protective adaptation.[19]

Included in the class of antihistamines are the drugs cyclizine, meclozine, dimenhydrinate, promethazine, and cinnarizine. Although less effective prophylactically than hyoscine, these drugs are safer, longer lasting, and, with the exception of drowsiness, have fewer side effects.[20] However, neither cinnarizine nor cyclizine is available in the United States.

Comparisons of cinnarizine to hyoscine have shown that cinnarizine is better tolerated, with less marked side effects.[21] Cinnarizine has been known for a very long time as a drug with strong anti–motion-sickness effects.[22–24] However, notwithstanding the fact that hyoscine is more effective in protecting against sea sickness, cinnarizine remains the drug of choice among seafarers in many countries including the United Kingdom because it is better tolerated.

Individuals with severe motion sickness can be relieved of their symptoms by intramuscular injections of promethazine or hyoscine.[4] Intramuscular promethazine is the method and drug of choice for astronauts to counteract space motion sickness. Concern that promethazine may delay or retard the acquisition of protective adaptation is unfounded.[25]

Dimenhydrinate is available both as a tablet and as a chewing gum. The active chewing movements may have a positive psychological effect, since the individual is actively involved in fighting the onset of motion sickness.

The anticonvulsant phenytoin has been shown to give very good protection during sea trials and in flights simulating weightlessness. At anticonvulsant blood levels (9–15 mg/mL), there are none of the usual side effects associated with the anti–motion-sickness drugs listed in Table 31.1–2 (other than ginger—see below). Phenytoin

Table 31.1–2 ANTI–MOTION-SICKNESS DRUGS*

DRUG	ROUTE	ADULT DOSE (MG)	ONSET	DURATION (HR)
Cinnarizine	Oral	15–30	4 hr	8
Cyclizine	Oral	50	2 hr	12
Dimenhydrinate	Oral	50–100	2 hr	8
Hyoscine	Oral	0.3–0.6	30 min	4
	Patch	1.5	6–8 hr	72
	Injection	0.2	15 min	4
Meclozine	Oral	25	2hr	8
Promethazine				
Theoclate	Oral	25	2hr	24
Hydrochloride	Oral	25	2 hr	18
	Injection	50	15 min	18
Phenytoin	Oral	300–1200	15 min	24
Ginger	Oral	500–2000	30 min	4

*Modified from Stott.[17]

is very inexpensive and can be administered prophylactically.[17,26]

One has to keep in mind that all anti–motion-sickness drugs have slight to moderate drowsiness as a side effect. Alcoholic beverages and medications that depress the central nervous system must be avoided when taking these drugs.

Most drugs listed in Table 31.1–2 influence the central nervous system. The mode of action likely involves the inhibition of sensory afferent activity via the vestibular nuclei that prevents emesis by the vomiting mechanisms. Consequently, it is not surprising that side effects such as drowsiness, gastrointestinal disturbances, visual troubles, etc. are prevalent when taking these drugs.

Ginger used as a prophylactic for motion sickness does not affect the central nervous system. Most investigators believe that the pharmacologically active components of ginger act on the digestive tract, providing a calming effect by relaxing the smooth muscles and improving circulation. No side effects have been reported following ingestion of ginger.[27] Several controlled studies have demonstrated the prophylactic effectiveness of ginger as a sea sickness antidote. In one particular study involving participants on a whale safari in high seas, 250 mg of ginger rhizome (root) was as effective as cinnarizine, hyoscine, dimenhydrinate, meclozine, and cyclizine.[28] Of those who took the ginger rhizome by mouth before departure, 78% did not experience sea sickness. Ginger preparations are also used to relieve a variety of other gastrointestinal disorders, including the vomiting of morning sickness during pregnancy. Because ginger preparations are extremely safe medicines, they should be considered seriously for pregnant women and children, unless contraindicated otherwise, if a drug is required for the prevention of motion sickness when traveling.

Much hope is being placed on new drugs that will completely ameliorate nausea and vomiting once and for all.[29,30] A set of drugs known as the neurokinin (NK1) receptor antagonists are promising as they seem to eliminate vomiting caused by motion sickness, radiation, or drugs used in chemotherapy in a variety of animals. These drugs are believed to work directly on the NTS, affecting the mechanisms producing motion sickness by blocking the neurokinin transmitter, Substance P, from triggering vomiting (see Figure 31.1–1). Clinical trials are currently under way by several drug companies to determine the efficacy of the NK1 antagonists in preventing both nausea and vomiting from all causes.

In the area of nonpharmacologic treatments, there are two experimental methods, acupressure and acustimulation, that rely on acupuncture to control motion sickness. Both methods stimulate the P6 (Neiguan) point on the wrist, which is known from Chinese medicine to be an important acupuncture site for the control of nausea and vomiting. Trials employing acupressure applied to the wrist of subjects by means of "Sea Bands," which were developed in the United Kingdom, were ineffective in decreasing motion sickness in laboratory experiments using reliable motion-sickness-provoking equipment.[31] In the other trial, subjects reported decreased symptoms of sea sickness in field trials when using an acustimulation "wrist-watch" (Relief Band®) that delivered mild electrical pulses to the P6 point.[32] This latter method may modulate the autonomic nervous system, which affects pathways that mitigate the response of nausea and vomiting and other motion sickness responses.

A few words on the clinical features of mal de débarquement are in order.[33,34] Whereas true sea sickness is dominated by nausea and vomiting, mal de débarquement is subtler in that it appears as a sensation of rocking, swaying, and unsteadiness.

Mal de débarquement is more prevalent in those susceptible to sea sickness and appears to be more often found in females. Normally, mal de débarquement is a transient feeling and does not require medical attention. When it is a persistent dysfunction in individuals, mal de débarquement may be alleviated through vestibular exercises such as walking. The drug amitriptyline hydrochloride (Elavil®) is helpful in assisting recovery in extreme cases.

The working mechanism of drugs preventing motion sickness is not known in most cases. The assumption that a drug can alter the susceptibility of a sense organ is difficult to accept. Nevertheless, the effect of some drugs in ameliorating motion sickness has been proven in many studies. As long as humans have a desire to travel, it must be accepted that motion sickness is a fact of life in modern traveling.

ACKNOWLEDGMENTS

We thank Mrs. N. Wisteard, DCIEM, for typing the manuscript, and Miss S. Bolsen, DCIEM, for preparing the illustration. Copyright is held by the Canadian Government, but permission to use this material has been provided by the authors and the Department of National Defence on behalf of the Crown.

REFERENCES

1. Cheung BSK, Money KE, Jacobs I. Motion sickness susceptibility and aerobic fitness: a longitudinal study. Aviat Space Environ Med 1990;61:201–204.
2. Stern RM, Hu S, LeBlanc R, Koch KL. Chinese hyper-susceptibility to vection-induced motion sickness. Aviat Space Environ Med 1993;64:827–830.
3. Reason JT, Brand JJ. Motion sickness. London: Academic Press, 1975.
4. Benson AJ. Motion sickness. In: Ernsting J, King P, eds. Aviation Medicine. 2nd Ed. London: Butterworths, 1988:318–338.
5. Treisman M. Motion sickness: an evolutionary hypothesis. Science 1977;197:493–495.
6. Money KE, Lackner JR, Cheung RSK. The autonomic nervous system and motion sickness. In: Yates BJ, Miller AD, eds. Vestibular autonomic regulation. Boca Raton, FL: CRC Press, 1996:147–173.
7. Money KE, Cheung BS. Another function of the inner ear: facilitation of the emetic response to poisons. Aviat Space Environ Med 1983;54:208–211.
8. Veyrat-Follet C, Farinotti R, Palmer JL. Physiology of chemotherapy-induced emesis and antiemetic therapy: pre-

dictive models for evaluation of new compounds. Drugs 1997;53:206–234.

9. Balaban CD, Porter JD. Neuroanatomic substrates for vestibulo-autonomic interactions. J Vestibul Res 1998;8:7–16.

10. Graybiel A. Structure elements in the concept of motion sickness. Aerospace Med 1969;40:351–367.

11. Money KE. Motion sickness. Physiol Rev 1970;50:1–39.

12. Furman JM, Jacob RG, Redfern MS. Clinical evidence that the vestibular system participates in autonomic control. J Vestibul Res 1998;8:27–34.

13. Oosterveld WJ, Graybiel A, Cramer DB. The influence of vision on susceptibility to acute motion sickness studied under quantifiable stimulus-response conditions. Aerospace Med 1972;43:1005–1007.

14. Harm DL, Parker DE. Preflight adaptation training for spatial orientation and space motion sickness. J Clin Pharmacol 1994;34:618–627.

15. Johnson WH, Taylor NBG. The importance of head movements in studies involving stimulation of the organ of Galance. Acta Otolaryngol (Stockh) 1961;53:211–218.

16. Golding JF, Markey HM, Stott JRR. The effects of motion direction, body axis, and posture on motion sickness induced by low frequency linear oscillation. Aviat Space Environ Med 1995;66:1046–1051.

17. Stott JRR. Management of acute and chronic motion sickness. In: Motion sickness: significance in aerospace operations and prophylaxis. AGARD-LS-175, NATO, France 1991:11-1–11-7.

18. Sennhauser FH, Schwarz HP. Toxic psychosis from transdermal scopolamine in a child. Lancet 1986;2:1033.

19. Van Marion WF, Bongaerts MCM, Christiaanse JC, et al. Influence of transdermal scopolamine on motion sickness during seven days' exposure to heavy seas. Clin Pharmocol Ther 1985;38:301–305.

20. Lucot JB. Pharmacology of motion sickness. J Vestibul Res 1998;8:61–66.

21. Pingree BJ, Pethybridge RJ. A comparison of the efficacy of cinnarizine with scopolamine in the treatment of seasickness. Aviat Space Environ Med 1994;65:597–605.

22. Oosterveld WJ. The combined effect of cinnarizine and domperidone on vestibular susceptibility. Aviat Space Environ Med 1987;58:218–223.

23. Shupack A, Doweck I, Gordon CR, Spitzer O. Cinnarizine in the prophylaxis of seasickness: laboratory vestibular evaluation and sea study. Clin Pharmacol Ther 1994;55:670–680.

24. Doweck I, Gordon CR, Spitzer O, et al. Effect of cinnarizine in the prevention of seasickness. Aviat Space Environ Med 1994;65:606–609.

25. Lackner JR, Graybiel A. Use of promethazine to hasten adaptation to provocative motion. J Clin Pharmacol 1994;34:644–651.

26. Knox GW, Woodward D, Chelen W, et al. Phenytoin for motion sickness: clinical evaluation. Laryngoscope 1994;104:935–939.

27. Langner E, Griefenberg S, Gruenwald J. Ginger: history and use. Adv Ther 1998;15:25–44.

28. Schmid R, Schick T, Steffen R, et al. Comparison of seven commonly used agents for prophylaxis of seasickness. J Travel Med 1994;1:203–206.

29. Andrew PLR, Naylor RJ, Joss RA. Neuropharmacology of emesis and its relevance to anti-emetic therapy: consensus and controversies. Support Care Cancer 1998;6:197–203.

30. Bountra C, Gale JD, Gardner CJ, et al. Towards understanding the aetiology and pathophysiology of the emetic reflex: novel approaches to antiemetic drugs. Oncology 1996;53(Suppl 1):102–109.

31. Bruce DG, Golding JF, Hockenhull N, Pethybridge RJ. Acupressure and motion sickness. Aviat Space Environ Med 1990;61:361–365.

32. Bertolucci LE, DiDario B. Efficacy of a portable acustimulation device in controlling seasickness. Aviat Space Environ Med 1995;66:1155–1158.

33. Gordon CR, Spitzer O, Doweck I, et al. Clinical features of mal de débarquement: adaptation and habituation of sea conditions. J Vestib Res 1995;5:363–369.

34. Murphy TP. Mal de débarquement syndrome: a forgotten entity? Otolaryngol Head Neck Surg 1993;109:10–13.

31.2 JET LAG

ANDREA SUHNER AND KEITH J. PETRIE

INTRODUCTION

Rapid transmeridian flights across several time zones lead to a mismatch between bodily systems and the external environment. This condition, commonly known as jet lag, is characterized by sleep disturbances, daytime fatigue, reduced performance, gastrointestinal problems, and generalized malaise, which can last up to a week following travel. Considering the millions of passengers who fly transmeridian routes each year, the prevalence of jet lag symptoms has not been well researched. Evidence suggests, however, that it affects the vast majority of aircrew and the traveling public.

SYMPTOMS

A study[1] of the effects of a 6-hour eastward time zone shift in soldiers found that the most common symptoms reported were fatigue, weakness, headache, sleepiness, and irritability. Some motivational decrements were also noted as well as reductions in physical performance capabilities. Most symptoms had disappeared by the fifth day following travel, apart from tiredness and irritability. A study in athletics[2] also showed that mood state, anaerobic power and capacity, and dynamic strength were affected by rapid transmeridian flight and that even highly trained athletes suffered from jet lag.

A study[3] on pilots' efficiency following transmeridian flight showed a significant performance decrement of 8.5% after an eastward flight over eight time zones. The most common symptoms reported by pilots flying transmeridian routes were sleepiness, low energy, mental slowness, concentration problems, and grouchiness or irritability.[4] The problem of jet lag in pilots is an important issue with clear safety implications, as there is a close association between fatigue and the likelihood of errors and accidents.[5] Sleep problems and jet lag are exacerbated when aircrews have to operate transmeridian flights in close succession.

Transmeridian travel generally causes sleep problems, both with difficulty getting off to sleep and sleep maintenance. Many travelers report feelings of sudden tiredness and hunger at unusual times as well as lightheadedness and irritability. The constant time zone changes inherent in the work of international aircrew can be a major source of occupational stress for this group of workers.

JET LAG: DESYNCHRONIZATION OF THE CIRCADIAN SYSTEM

Jet lag may be thought of as a combination of desynchronization of the circadian system and sleep loss due to travel disrupting the normal sleep routine. Sleep is often best on the first night following travel due to sleep deficit and physical exhaustion, but circadian dysruption often causes difficulty getting to sleep or inappropriate waking on subsequent nights. Many of the symptoms experienced following travel are a direct result of the dissociation between the environmental time cues, which have been phase-advanced or phase-delayed, and the internal body clock.

Jet lag occurs because the circadian system is unable to adapt to phase-shifts immediately. Without specific jet lag countermeasures, it normally takes 4 to 6 days after a transmeridian flight to re-establish a normal sleep pattern,[6–9] and daytime sleepiness is reported for up to 4 days post-travel.[7,9] The resynchronization of the endogenous circadian rhythms takes even longer: for temperature rhythm, the resynchronization time after an 8-hour time shift was 11 to 15 days, depending on the flight direction[10]; the melatonin rhythm had adjusted by the 11th day after a 7-hour shift,[11] whereas the adrenocorticotropic hormone and cortisol rhythms were still measurably affected after 3 weeks.[12]

The severity and duration of the jet lag symptoms are most strongly influenced by the number of time zones crossed and the direction of travel. Adaptation is easier after westbound compared to eastbound flights.[10] This phenomenon is explained by the fact that the endogenous circadian system naturally adopts a longer day (approx. 24.3 hours)[13] in isolation, and that it is, therefore, easier to lengthen the day required for adaptation after westward flights (phase-delay) than to shorten the day to advance circadian rhythms after eastward flights. Additionally, eastward flights are usually scheduled as night flights, resulting in more pronounced sleep loss and, consequently, greater fatigue post-travel. Moreover, the susceptibility to jet lag depends on various individual characteristics (summarized in Comperatore and Krueger[14]) such as age, rhythm stability, rhythm chronotype, and sleep habits.

PREVENTION AND TREATMENT OF JET LAG

To minimize the effects of jet lag, various pharmacologic and nonpharmacologic countermeasures (Table 31.2–1) have been proposed, although only a few have been scientifically validated. The three main treatment approaches are resynchronization of the body clock, promotion of sleep, and enhancement of alertness.

RESYNCHRONIZATION OF THE CIRCADIAN SYSTEM: LIGHT AND CHRONOBIOTICS

In mammals, the circadian rhythms (e.g., melatonin, core body temperature) are generated by the suprachiasmatic nucleus (SCN), the most important endogenous pacemaker. The human circadian period is longer than 24 hours in isolation but is normally entrained to the 24-hour solar day by external environmental synchronizers, so-called zeitgebers. In humans, the light/dark cycle is undoubtedly the most important zeitgeber. The pineal hormone melatonin, which is secreted only during the dark phase of the day, also plays an important role in regulating circadian rhythms in that it transduces the light-dark information and modulates the SCN by a pineal feedback. Melatonin is a chronobiotic, which is defined as a chemical substance capable of therapeutically re-entraining short-term dissociated or long-term desynchronized circadian rhythms or prophylactically preventing their disruption following environmental insult (for a review on the circadian system and chronobiotics see Dawson and Armstrong[15]).

The use of chronobiotics or other therapies that accelerate the adaptation process after a time zone transition is only appropriate when travelers plan to stay for an extended period at the new time zones. For short trips,

Table 31.2–1. OPTIONS TO ALLEVIATE JET LAG

Nonpharmacologic

Bright light therapy: either using portable light sources or by light seeking or avoiding at appropriate times of the day

Jet lag diet (Ehret and Scanlon[33])

Exercise

Strategic napping (especially for airline personnel)

Adaptation to social time cues (e.g., sleep-wake cycle, meal timing)

Pharmacologic

Melatonin 3- to 5-mg fast-release formulation (if the stay at the new destination is longer than 3 days)

Short-acting hypnotics (zolpidem 10 mg is recommended, but individual tolerability has to be checked)

---

and for aircrew constantly changing time zones, adaptation to the new environment is not desirable, and chronobiotics should be used only after arrival home.

MELATONIN

Due to its synchronizing effect on the internal body clock, melatonin would appear to be suitable for the alleviation of jet lag as it accelerates the adaptation process after a time zone transition. Orally administered melatonin has been shown to shift circadian rhythms according to a phase-response curve (PRC)[16]: melatonin delays circadian rhythms when administered in the morning and advances them when administered in the afternoon or early evening.

In addition, melatonin has an acute soporific effect, which is independent of the phase-shifting properties and has been shown by changes in the electoencephalogram after administration of pharmacologic doses of melatonin.[17] The mechanism by which exogenous melatonin increases sleepiness is still unknown. This soporific effect may either be mediated by a hypothermic effect or modulating receptors, thereby potentiating the effects of endogenous aminobutyric acid (GABA).[18]

Features of melatonin that enhance its use in alleviating jet lag include excellent tolerability, short half-life, and lack of residual effects. A negative feature is the large interindividual variation in bioavailability.[19]

Some have expressed concern about purity and quality control of melatonin. Indeed, quality analysis of 19 commercial melatonin products point to a deficit in pharmaceutic quality.[20] Whereas in the U.S.A., melatonin is sold over the counter as a "dietary supplement" without premarket approval by the Food and Drug Administration,

in other countries, melatonin would be considered as a drug and has not been approved by governmental agencies.

The efficacy of melatonin for the alleviation of jet lag has been tested in several placebo-controlled and uncontrolled studies with the majority,[7,9,21–26] demonstrating a superior overall recovery from jet lag. Critical for the successful treatment of jet lag is the correct dosage and timing of melatonin administration. A large jet lag field study[9] comparing various melatonin dosage forms showed that fast-release formulations of this hormone were more effective in reducing jet lag symptoms than a controlled-release formulation. Furthermore, the hypnotic properties such as sleep quality and sleep latency (Figure 31.2–1) were significantly better with a pharmacologic dose of 5-mg melatonin compared to a physiologic dose of 0.5 mg. Based on these results, 3 to 5 mg of melatonin are recommended at bedtime for approximately 4 days following eastbound and westbound flights. One could imagine that daytime melatonin intake before traveling would initiate adaptation to the local time at the destination. However, no melatonin administration prior to intercontinental flights is recommended, since ingestion of melatonin results in increased subjective sleepiness.[27] Other treatment regimes using melatonin for the alleviation of jet lag have been suggested.[28]

LIGHT THERAPY

Light is the most important zeitgeber. It entrains the endogenous clock (SCN) directly or indirectly by suppressing melatonin production. The PRC of light is opposite to that of melatonin and is related to the core body temperature minimum: bright light in the very early morning (slightly after the temperature minimum) causes a phase advance in body rhythms, whereas in the late

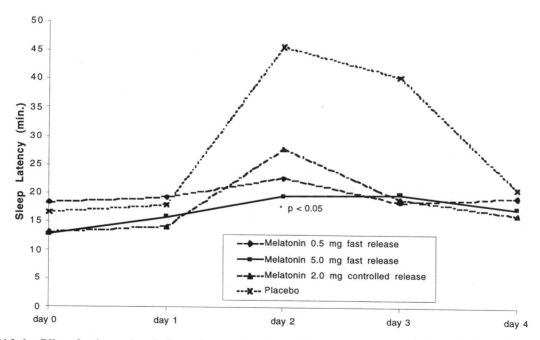

Figure 31.2–1.   Effect of various melatonin dosage forms and placebo on sleep latency on a baseline day (day 0) and 4 days postflight (days 1–4).

evening (slightly before the temperature minimum), it causes a phase delay in body rhythms.[29] Although light is very potent in phase shifting under laboratory conditions, after a real transmeridian flight, light therapy is not very feasible because portable light sources are generally cumbersome and natural light conditions can be unreliable. Only very few field studies on light treatment as a jet lag countermeasure have been performed and results are unsatisfactory.[30]

As a supplement to melatonin or any other jet lag treatment, on the first day, post-travel light seeking (daylight) or light avoiding (sunglasses, staying indoors) at correct times to promote adaptation to the new time zone should be considered. The strategy is easy for westward flights, since there is no need to deviate from natural light; however, after eastward flights of five to nine time zones, morning light should be avoided and light in the afternoon sought. For eastward flights crossing more than nine time zones, evening light should be avoided and light in the late morning and early afternoon should be sought because it is better to promote phase delays and phase advances.[28]

OTHER POSSIBLE ZEITGEBERS

Social influences, physical activity, and meal timing are other external time cues that may have an influence on the circadian system.

In rodents, exercise has been shown to be effective in phase shifting and synchronizing circadian rhythms.[31] Recent studies[32] in humans support the hypothesis that increased physical activity during the habitual rest period is capable of altering clock function. However, since little is known about the optimal amount and timing of exercise and the interactions between photic and nonphotic zeitgebers, no specific recommendations regarding exercise to promote adjustment of the body clock can be made.

Another treatment approach is the jet lag diet proposed by Ehret and Scanlon.[33] Its exact routine depends on the flight schedule and is based on the fact that carbohydrates induce sleep by facilitating serotonin synthesis and proteins promote alertness by stimulating the synthesis of catecholamines. The effectiveness of this diet remains controversial; however, it appears that the exact timing rather than the composition of meals is responsible for hastening resynchronization.

PROMOTION OF SLEEP: GENERAL SLEEP ADVICE AND HYPNOTICS

Because loss of sleep by itself due to traveling is in part responsible for the performance impairment after intercontinental flights, sleep hygiene is very important (see Final Recommendations). Short naps (<1 hour) may help to compensate for cumulative sleep deprivation. Studies by NASA have shown that the use of naps by aircrew does reduce cumulative sleep deficit when travel involves a large number of time zone changes over a short period.[34]

Short-acting benzodiazepines such as temazepam, triazolam, and midazolam have been promoted and used to minimize sleep loss after transmeridian flights.[35] Although these substances are found to be effective in reducing sleep problems, there are some concerns about safety. Residual effects of short-acting benzodiazepines have been reported.[36] Consequently, the use of these drugs should be carefully considered for those who must perform complex psychomotor or intellectual tasks the next day (e.g., pilots). Recently, a novel hypnotic agent, zolpidem, which is an imidazopyridine with selective binding on omega 1 GABA receptors, has been proposed for pilots and military personnel due to the absence of residual effects.[37] Another field study[38] comparing the efficacy and tolerability of melatonin and zolpidem for the alleviation of jet lag demonstrated that zolpidem is a suitable alternative for melatonin to alleviate sleep disorders associated with jet lag and that it was most effective to facilitate in-flight sleep. However, zolpidem showed a higher incidence of adverse events than melatonin; therefore, individual tolerability should be checked before prescribing zolpidem. Due to the risk of dependence, benzodiazepines should not be taken longer that three to four consecutive nights.

Whether benzodiazepines have only sleep-inducing effects or whether they also act as chronobiotics is unclear. The presence of GABA-type-a receptors in the SCN may suggest a direct action of benzodiazepines on the endogenous pacemaker. Phase-shifting effects of triazolam have been demonstrated in hamsters,[39] but to date there is no evidence that benzodiazepines are able to modify the human circadian system.[35]

PROMOTION OF ALERTNESS: ALERTNESS-ENHANCING DRUGS

To combat daytime sleepiness associated with jet lag or shift work, several pharmacologic countermeasures have been discussed.[40] A common practice to improve alertness during work and to delay sleep onset is the use of caffeine. Its use is usually uncontrolled in the form of cups of coffee, and there are still few data on its systematic application. Very potent and well-known psychostimulants are the amphetamines, which are unsuitable for use in normal work situations because of side effects and abuse potential. A very new alternative for amphetamines is modafinil, an α-receptor-agonist. Modafinil is as effective as amphetamines in enhancing alertness but causes no sleep impairment, and few side effects have been observed. Since this substance is not registered in most countries and only a few clinical studies have been conducted, it is premature to discuss a routine use of modafinil. Little is known about chronic use and tolerability of alertness-enhancing drugs, and further investigation is needed to optimize dosage regimens.

FINAL RECOMMENDATIONS

To reduce jet lag symptoms after transmeridian flights, it is recommended to take 3- to 5-mg melatonin (fast-release) at bedtime for approximately 4 days after eastbound and westbound flights. No daytime administration

Table 31.2–2. PHARMACOLOGIC TREATMENT OF JET LAG

Preflight	No medication
In-flight (night flights)	Zolpidem 10 mg (or other short-acting hypnotics)
Postflight (during 3–4 days at bedtime):	Melatonin 3–5 mg (fast-release formulation) or zolpidem 10 mg (for short trips)

of melatonin prior to intercontinental flights is recommended. On eastbound flights, which are usually scheduled as night flights, one dose of melatonin may be taken in the late afternoon to advance the body clock and to initiate adaptation to new environmental time cues. Since melatonin did not significantly improve in-flight sleep quality, a short-acting hypnotic such as zolpidem is considered first choice for facilitating sleep on night flights.

As an alternative to melatonin, especially for short trips, when adaptation to the new local time is not desirable, zolpidem 10 mg can be recommended if tolerated. Similar to melatonin administration, it should be taken at bedtime for 3 to 4 days after an intercontinental flight. The dosage regimens for the pharmacologic treatment of jet lag are summarized in Table 31.2–2.

From a theoretical point of view, a combination of a chronobiotic (melatonin) and a hypnotic (e.g., a benzodiazepine), which means the combination of two mechanisms of action, might be the most powerful treatment for jet lag. A jet lag field study[38] where a combination of melatonin 5 mg plus zolpidem 10 mg was tested concluded that this combination cannot be recommended due to poor tolerability. Morning sleepiness, confusion, and nausea were significantly increased in participants taking this combination compared to those taking melatonin or zolpidem alone.

In addition to pharmacologic treatments of jet lag, a few other measures may help to synchronize with local time. A good night's rest before the trip is necessary. During the flight, try to sleep at night, but when the day is much prolonged, a short nap should also be considered. Adopt local time and routines immediately upon arrival (meals, bedtime, etc.). Allow plenty of time to sleep and rest in the new location in order to compensate for reduced sleep quality and delay important work or touring activities for a couple of days to allow for adjustment.

REFERENCES

1. Wright JE, Vogel JA, Sampson JB, et al. Effects of travel across time zones (jet-lag) on exercise capacity and performance. Aviat Space Environ Med 1983;54:131–137.
2. Hill DW, Hill CM, Fields KL, Smith JC. Effects of jet-lag on factors related to sport performance. Can J Appl Phys 1993;18:91–103.
3. Klein KE, Brüner H, Holtmann H, et al. Circadian rhythm of pilots' efficiency and effects of multiple time zone travel. Aerospace Med 1970;41:125–132.
4. Petrie KJ, Dawson AG. Symptoms of fatigue and coping strategies in international pilots. Int J Aviat Psychol 1997; 7:251–258.
5. Dinges DF. An overview of sleepiness and accidents. J Sleep Res 1995;4(Suppl 2):4–14.
6. Nicholson AN, Spencer MB, Pascone PA, et al. Sleep after transmeridian flights. Lancet 1986;22:1205–1208.
7. Petrie K, V Conaglen JV, Thompson L, Chamberlain K. Effect of melatonin on jet lag after long haul flights. BMJ 1989;298:705–707.
8. Spencer MB, Rogers AS, Pascone PA. Effects on sleep of a large eastward time zone transition. J Sleep Res 1996;5(Suppl 1):219.
9. Suhner A, Schlagenhauf P, Johnson R, et al. Comparative study to determine the optimal melatonin dosage form for the alleviation of jet-lag. Chronobiol Int 1998;15:655–666.
10. Klein KE, Wegmann HM, Bonnie IH. Desynchronization of body temperature and performance circadian rhythm as a result of outgoing and homegoing transmeridian flights. Aerospace Med 1972;43:119–132.
11. Fèvre-Montagne M, Van Cauter E, Refetoff S, et al. Effects of jet-lag on hormonal patterns. II. Adaptation of melatonin circadian periodicity. J Clin Endocrinol Metab 1981;52:642–649.
12. Désir D, Van Cauter E, Fang VS, et al. Effects of jet-lag on hormonal patterns. I. Procedures, variations in total plasma proteins, and disruption of adrenocorticotropin-cortisol periodicity. J Clin Endocrinol Metab 1981;52:628–641.
13. Klermann EB, Dijk DJ, Kronauer RE, Czeisler CA. Simulations of light effects on the human circadian pacemaker: implications for assessment of intrinsic period. J Physiol 1996; 39:R271–R282.
14. Comperatore CA, Krueger GP. Circadian rhythm desynchrosis, jet lag, shift lag, and coping strategies. Occup Med 1990;5:323–341.
15. Dawson D, Armstrong SM. Chronobiotics—drugs that shift rhythms. Pharmacol Ther 1996;69:15–36.
16. Lewy AJ, Ahmed S, Jackson JM, Sack RL. Melatonin shifts human circadian rhythms according to a phase-response curve. Chronobiol Int 1992;9:380–392.
17. Waldhauser F, Saletu B, Trinchard-Lugan I. Sleep laboratory investigations on hypnotic properties of melatonin. Psychopharmacology 1990;100:222–226.
18. Cajochen C, Kräuchi K, Wirz-Justice A. The acute soporific action of daytime melatonin administration: effects on the EEG during wakefulness and subjective alertness. J Biol Rhythms 1997;12:636–643.
19. Di WL, Kadva A, Johnston A, Silmann R. Variable bioavailability of oral melatonin. N Engl J Med 1997;336:1028–1029.
20. Suhner A, Werner IA, Wilde AM, Schlagenhauf P. Over-the-counter melatonin — quality or quackery? Pharmazie 1999; 54:863–864.
21. Armstrong SM. Melatonin — the internal zeitgeber of mammals? Pineal Research Reviews 1989;7:157–202.
22. Arendt J, Aldhous M, English J, et al. Some effects of jet-lag and their alleviation by melatonin. Ergonomics 1987;30: 1379–1393.
23. Skene DJ, Aldhous M, Arendt J. Melatonin, jet lag and sleep-wake cycle. In: Horne J, ed. Sleep 88. Proceedings of the Ninth European Congress of Sleep Research; Jerusalem 1988. Stuttgart: Gustav Fischer Verlag, 1989:39–41.
24. Claustrat B, Brun J, David M, et al. Melatonin and jetlag: confirmatory result using a simplified protocol. Biol Psychiatry 1992;32:526–530.
25. Petrie K, Dawson AG, Thompson L, Brook R. A double blind trial of melatonin as a treatment for jet lag in international cabin crew. Biol Psychiatry 1993;33:526–530.

26. Arendt J, Deacon S. Treatment of circadian rhythm disorders—melatonin. Chronobiol Int 1997;14:185–204.

27. Suhner A, Schlagenhauf P, Tschopp A, et al. Impact of melatonin on driving performance. J Travel Med 1998;5:13:7–13.

28. Waterhouse J, Reilly T, Atkinson G. Jet-lag. Lancet 1997; 350:1611–1616.

29. Minors DS, Waterhouse JM, Witz-Justice A. A human phase-response curve to light. Neurosci Lett 1991;133:36–40.

30. Samel A, Wegmann HM. Bright light a countermeasure for jet-lag? Chronobiol Int 1997;14:173–183.

31. Reebs S, Mrosovsky N. Effects of induced wheel-running on the circadian activity rhythm of Syrian hamsters: entrainment and phase-response curve. J Biol Rhythms 1994;4:39–48.

32. Buxton MB, L`Hermite-Baleriaux M, Hirschfeld U, Van Cauter E. Acute and delayed effects of exercise on human melatonin secretion. J Biol Rhythms 1997;12:568–574.

33. Ehret CF, Scanlon LW. Overcoming jet-lag. New York: Berkley, 1983.

34. Rosekind MR, Gander P, Dinges DF. Alertness management in flight operations: strategic napping. SAE technical paper 912138. Warrendale, PA: Society of Automotive Engineers, 1991.

35. Donaldson E, Kennaway DJ. Effects of temazepam on sleep, performance, and rhythmic 6-sulphatoxymelatonin and cortisol excretion after transmeridian travel. Aviat Space Environ Med 1991;62:654–660.

36. Wehli L, Knüsel R, Schelldorfer K, Christeller S. Comparison of midazolam and triazolam for residual effects. Arzneimit-telforschung 1985;35:1700–1704.

37. Sicard BA, Trocherie S, Moreau J, et al. Evaluation of zolpidem on alertness and psychomotor abilities among aviation ground personnel and pilots. Aviat Space Environ Med 1993;64:371–375.

38. Suhner A, Schlagenhauf P, Höfer I, et al. Efficacy and tolerability of melatonin and zolpidem for the alleviation of jet-lag. In: Suhner A, ed. Melatonin and jet-lag. Dissertation No. 12823. Zurich: Swiss Federal University of Technology, 1998: 85–103.

39. Turek FW, Losee-Olsen S. A benzodiazepine used in the treatment of insomnia phase-shifts the mammalian circadian clock. Nature 1986;321:167–168

40. Akerstedt T, Ficca G. Alertness-enhancing drugs as a countermeasure to fatigue in irregular work hours. Chronobiol Int 1997;14:145–158.

Chapter 32

VERY SHORT-TERM TRAVEL

JOHN COTTRELL-DORMER AND ROSMARIE WYSS

Historically, travel to foreign countries took months or years; now, transport by aircraft enables access to trips of great distance and very short duration. "Very short-term" travel is defined by the editors of this text as a stay lasting 4 days or less. Little has been written about the special health issues for these travelers. Business travelers and air crews (pilots and cabin attendants) probably make up the majority of very short-term travelers; others include VIP travelers, pilgrims, some news journalists and television crews, sporting groups, and travelers making a stopover in a "high-risk" country (Table 32–1). This group of travelers includes a significant proportion for whom very short-term travel occurs frequently: these may be exposed briefly and recurrently to important and exotic avoidable health risks.

More than 400 million persons per year travel on international flights. Although clear estimates of the number of very short international trips (a duration of 4 days or less) are not available, it is reported that 10% to 25% of international travel is for trips of less than 1 week duration. In addition, air crews (pilots and cabin attendants) are often excluded from arrival and departure data: this group, however, represents approximately an additional 5% of total travel on international flights. The growth rate in total international travel has been around 7% annually for several years. Rapid economic growth and demand for industrialized technology are being experienced in many developing countries, particularly in South and East Asia, leading to rapid growth in very short-term business travel from industrialized countries to these areas.

Travel health epidemiology varies greatly with the origin and destination: the greatest risk of morbidity is when there is a cultural and climatic contrast between the country of origin and a tropical or Eastern European destination. Very short-term travelers often enjoy protected environments, sheltered from the larger "unhealthy environment of the surrounding countryside."[1] Their stays in developing countries are most commonly only overnight or a few days in good hotels. For VIP travel and very short business travel, the trip is likely to be of considerable strategic and financial importance; thus, when ill health might ruin the trip, avoidance of health impairment during brief trips is very desirable. Jet lag due to rapid extensive transmeridian travel can mar a very short trip, as can sunburn, security, accidental injury, and other environmental risks discussed in other chapters of this text. It is interesting to consider the example of international airlines using a wide range of strategies to minimize the possible impingement of health problems in aircrew and hence minimize costly interruptions to airline schedules and passengers' safety. For pilots, the critical need is for optimal psychomotor performance; for cabin attendants, safety protocols during possible emergency, hygienic food service, and high levels of customer service are required.

EPIDEMIOLOGY

Published data specifically related to travel of less than 1 week in duration are scarce, as are data about aircrew illness in international airlines. In a study[2] comparing medical claims by 4,738 World Bank business travelers to claims by 6,146 nontraveling colleagues, male travelers had 80% more claims than male nontravelers, there were more claims with greater numbers of trips, and psychological claims were most prominent: greater perceived workload and demands on the travelers' time were possible explanations. In long-haul airline crews, respiratory illness is the most common cause of lost work time, with gastrointestinal illness second and trauma third. Self-reported health problems in a Norwegian study[3] found that dry skin, lower back pain, colds, fatigue, and sleep disturbances were "often" noted by more than 30% of airline crew members; crews flying long distances were more likely to report health problems, and transmeridian air travel was associated with digestive disturbances. There are case reports of in-cabin transmission of both tuberculosis and influenza. However, air-borne transmission is thought to be by direct contact, not by recirculated and filtered air: the concentration of microorganisms in airline cabin air appears[4] to be much lower than on ordinary city locations. Unpublished data from various French airlines indicate that the risk of malaria infection during a 30-year career was only slightly lower than that seen in tourists,

Table 32–1. VERY SHORT-TERM TRAVELERS

Business travelers
VIPs, politicians, and entertainers
Sportsmen and sportswomen
Stopovers
Pilgrims
Pilots and aircraft cabin attendants

and that a substantial proportion of cockpit and cabin crew acquired malaria at least once, most commonly in tropical African destinations. In a study[5] of 2,268 tourists returning from Mombasa to Europe, 38% had experienced diarrhea in their first week. In a large study[6] of short-term international business travelers, the reported incidence of travelers' diarrhea was 5.8% for trips of 1 week or less, much less than rates for tourists, students, and first-time travelers; experienced travelers appeared much less susceptible to travelers' diarrhea; and no reduction in the incidence of travelers' diarrhea was observed using prophylactic antibiotics. In another study of international corporate travel,[7] where 90% traveled for less than 1 month, 51% used travel health kits and 35% suffered diarrhea, 25% upper respiratory infection, and 3% injuries.

Unpublished data from British Airways found no significant difference in hepatitis A seropositivity between an international crew and a control group of ground crew based in London; however, the airline's expatriate staff had an increased hepatitis A virus (HAV) seroprevalence. Among 3,322 Swiss international airline staff[8] who spent an average of 45 nights in developing countries from 1987 to 1991, 22 cases of hepatitis A infection were reported, finding in male cabin attendants a threefold higher rate of hepatitis A infections compared to the airline's pilots and female cabin attendants; no cases of infection were reported in 734 noninternational flying crew of whom 33% were already HAV seropositive. Other studies have revealed that homosexual and heterosexual males and business travelers are at a higher (up to 200-fold) risk of casual sex encounters and of acquiring sexually transmitted diseases while traveling.

CONTRAINDICATIONS

Some travelers should be discouraged by their medical advisors from making even very short trips or stopovers in high-risk countries. Unstable medical conditions, especially life threatening, provide a relative or absolute contraindication to travel generally. Some travelers' health might be adversely affected by the hypobaria or hypoxia of air travel (see Chapter 31); others might be subject to unacceptable risks even for a very short stay at some proposed destinations. Even brief travel to malaria areas is relatively contraindicated for immunosuppressed or splenectomy patients and pregnant women: these patients might be advised not to travel or to visit an alternative destination. Although Parkins et al.[9] raised the concern that a small proportion of infants might develop significant hypoxia in commercial passenger aircraft or at high altitude, there are insufficient data to regard airline carriage of full-term infants beyond 7 days old as contraindicated or hazardous.

PREVENTION

Each traveler needs individual preventive advice based on his or her medical and vaccination history and the destination and activities proposed. International airlines employ to varying extents a range of little known strategies to minimize crew health impairment (Table 32–2). The diverse strategies that have arisen illustrate that a surprisingly thorough approach is required in order to maximize the chance of healthy travel. The complexity, depth, and breadth of airline crew health logistics contrasts ironically with the carefree image of travel presented by these airlines to their consumers. Meanwhile, travel agents might not mention health issues to their potential customers unless prompted, and the content and extent of other sources of travel health advice, including from consulates and general practitioners, can be of poor quality, limited, conflicting, and confusing. However, some Internet sources now provide an acceptable standard of basic travel health advice for advisers and travelers.

The rate of health impairment[10] in travelers from western Europe to less affluent countries has remained constant, reinforcing the important benefit of providing a medical kit to enable self-treatment by the traveler to reduce the duration of incapacitation. Given the importance of very short-term trips to the traveler (and to his or her employer), the carriage of a basic medical kit should be encouraged even for these very short trips. Although studies of pretravel safe sex advice demonstrate little effect on the travelers' sexual behavior, it seems important to advise all travelers about travel sex issues, even for very short trips; likewise, general basic safety advice and travel insurance should be encouraged for all.

The 24-hour operations of international airlines mean that crew fatigue is a potential danger,[11] as it might adversely impinge on pilots' psychomotor performance. In an effort to combat the possibility of fatigue, international air navigation rules include limitations on maximum flying duty hours, minimum rest periods, maxi-

Table 32–2. AIRLINES' CREW HEALTH STRATEGIES

Training in
   Food hygiene
   Behavioral and environmental risks
   First aid
   Infectious diseases
Work schedules with generous rest periods
Food safety
   Crew education
   Different pilot meals
   Hotel kitchen audits
Vaccination
Malaria
   Education
   Exposure prophylaxis
   Chemoprophylaxis
   Standby self-treatment
Accommodation of crew
   Physical and food safety
Destination-specific briefings
Extensive central and local back-up

mum flying time over several days, and minimum off-duty rest periods. Persons not familiar with the airline industry are often surprised at the apparent generosity of rest days during and after transmeridian trips (in contrast to the relentless work demands on international corporate air travelers). Although aircrew rest periods cannot allow sufficient time for circadian resynchronization, crew are recommended to minimize sleep deficit by taking naps when possible and by remaining on home time if their schedule permits. Accommodation at crew hotels is selected to ensure that various safety standards are met in addition to adequate rest and safe food. At any destination where crew have rest days, international airlines will arrange for a 24-hour local medical service to be available. In some international airlines, recurrent training is given to both pilots and cabin attendants in tropical diseases including malaria, first aid, and hygienic food handling. International airline crews include a hierarchy of senior and more junior crew members (both among pilots and cabin crew) whose combined problem-solving experience is considerable. Twenty-four-hour home-base telephone and radio contact for assistance with medical or logistic problems is also routinely available for aircrews.

Extensive preparation—not just athletic—is deployed by sporting groups[12] traveling internationally, for sometimes very brief competition, in order to maximize the chance of victory. In addition to immunization, advice topics ought to include jet lag; food hygiene and perhaps travelers' diarrhea chemoprophylaxis; vector-borne diseases such as malaria, rabies, and dengue fever; climatic and cultural acclimatization including appropriate clothing, the need for sunscreens, and avoidance of dehydration in tropical destinations; and sexual risk advice.

TRAVELERS' DIARRHEA

Gastrointestinal illness occurs most commonly on the third day following arrival and so is an important cause of preventable morbidity in even very short trips. The potential hazard of contaminated food for passengers and crew—the latter eating both in flight and during rest periods in a less hygienic country—means that international airlines go to great lengths to maintain food safety. Those measures include menu selection and preparation to ensure that food is safe to eat even if not reheated in flight, different meals for each pilot, investigation of any food poisoning notification, and independent site and microbiologic analysis of food preparation techniques both at commercial in-flight food preparation kitchens and at airline crews' hotel kitchens.

Efforts to reduce diarrhea-related travel morbidity generally include education about food safety, chemoprophylaxis, and self-treatment (see Chapter 20.2 Prevention of Travelers' Diarrhea: Risk Avoidance and Chemoprophylaxis). Attempts by most travelers to maintain dietary restrictions are very short lived—typically for only 48 hours. Even experienced travelers find dietary restriction difficult, but experienced travelers tend to have diarrhea less frequently. Short-term chemoprophylaxis,

usually quinolones, can prevent at least 80% of travelers' diarrhea. For occasional very important trips of only a few days or less, the benefit of diarrhea chemoprophylaxis may outweigh concern about potential side effects including fluoroquinolone photosensitivity and tendonitis. Thus, fluoroquinolone chemoprophylaxis might be suggested for VIPs, politicians, sporting travelers, and other very short-term travelers who cannot afford such illness interfering with the brief course of their trip. In the absence of such chemoprophylaxis, self-treatment of diarrhea is the most effective means of limiting its resultant morbidity in very short-term travelers. Fluoroquinolones are the choice for antimicrobial drug and loperamide for antimotility agent and relief of crampy abdominal pain (see Chapter 20.3). Self-treatment for the very short-term traveler can begin following the passage of the first unformed stool. Both a fluoroquinolone and loperamide can be taken if the traveler has no fever or blood in the stool; otherwise, the antimicrobial drug alone should be taken for 3 days.

MALARIA

Cases of malaria infection are reported in the literature when the duration of exposure was minimal. Airport malaria is a well-reported event and refers to travelers who are infected without visiting a malaria area; the presumed transmission is from the bite of a mosquito transported by aircraft to a nonmalarious country. Runway malaria was first described in the literature in 1990 and refers to a traveler who has contracted malaria when the only apparent exposure has been while the aircraft landed transiently in a malarious zone. Some authors[13] have suggested that all transit passengers at international airports be warned of this rare possibility and raise the issue of malaria with their doctor if a febrile illness occurs. There are also reports[14] of "ship-board malaria" in merchant seamen whose exposure is thought to be of very short duration and who are at a high mortality risk when no effective malaria treatments are on board.

Armengaud[15] argues, perhaps controversially, that when the stay in a malaria area is less than 1 week, no chemoprophylaxis is needed as the disease will appear after returning home where diagnosis and therapy can be instituted if fever occurs and an informed physician consulted. Certain short-term travelers seem to prefer this approach: those who are familiar with the disease process and its treatment, those who eschew medication, and experienced travelers who make frequent very short trips to endemic areas. The Thai government has advised similarly on malaria prevention for short-term travelers to Thailand.[16] Most short-term travelers are on an organized tour, follow tour schedules with daytime excursions, and are essentially at no risk. Even for those increasing numbers of adventure travelers (elephant riding, trekking, remote rural camping) who may be significantly exposed to the disease, the Thai recommendation is to avoid mosquito bites without chemoprophylaxis: in the event of a febrile illness, the traveler is advised to attend a malaria treatment clinic, present in all endemic areas in Thailand, for rapid diagnosis and appropriate free treatment.

Malaria infection in international airline crews occurs infrequently. In these travelers, malaria exposure varies but is usually limited to only a few days or less. There is no consensus among commercial or military medical aviation advisors regarding chemoprophylactic regimens for aircrews transitting in malaria endemic areas. Malaria prevention needs to be tailored to each airline's requirements as appropriate to each crew member's current health status, destination, and the activities abroad; unpublished very low malaria chemoprophylaxis aircrew compliance rates are reported (e.g.,12% for Central, East, and West Africa). Although it would be desirable to cluster flight crew schedules with repeated rotations to the same area in order to minimize the number of crews going to high-risk areas, in practice, this is rarely feasible. Mefloquine prophylaxis is regarded as contraindicated for pilots due to concern about possible neuropsychiatric side effects. However, in a cockpit simulator study[17] of 23 trainee Swissair pilots, no significant performance deficit was noted using mefloquine at steady state; some airlines will consider a pilot's use of mefloquine for prophylaxis in high-risk areas when the pilot has tried and tolerated the medication during a nonflying period.

Some advisers advocate carriage of medication for emergency self-treatment when the minimum incubation period of malaria—6 days—exceeds the duration of the trip, but carriage of emergency self-treatment is infrequently suggested for very short-term travelers and is only sometimes employed by airline crews. Very recently, two new options have been added to the methods of minimizing malaria-related mortality and morbidity: first, Malarone™ (atovaquone and proguanil) provides another option for emergency self-treatment (and perhaps in the future might be used as a causal prophylactic); second, self-testing kits are available for highly accurate diagnosis or exclusion of *Plasmodium falciparum* infection. For recurrent very short-term travelers, regular prophylactic medication is unappealing given the intermittent long-term risk. Nonetheless, for brief exposures, malaria chemoprophylaxis should be considered (1) if there are recurrent very short trips over a relatively short period of time and (2) for high-risk areas (e.g., tropical Africa, Solomon Islands) when there is more than one night's stay. Few new prophylactic medications will be available in the near future, so the usefulness of currently available drugs needs to be prolonged by rational use: in Australia, doxycycline is very commonly prescribed for travel, especially very short term, to high-risk areas in the western Pacific Islands and Papua New Guinea at 100 mg per day from 2 days before until only 14 days after travel, a simple 3-week regimen that might gain more widespread use globally for similar types of brief intense malaria risk.[18] *P. falciparum*, of course, is responsible for one of the most common infectious diseases worldwide and can rapidly progress to coma and death. Table 32–3 summarizes the approach to malaria prevention when the risk is four nights or less. Whatever strategy is chosen—chemoprophylaxis, febrifuge, or standby self-treatment—very short-term travelers need advice on insect avoidance and careful instructions in case a febrile illness develops.

Table 32–3. MALARIA STRATEGIES IN VERY SHORT-TERM TRAVEL

Inform all about
  Destination-specific risks
  Insect avoidance
  Fever protocol
No medication
  Experienced travelers
  Minimal risk intensity or duration
Standby self-treatment
  Recurrent very short trips
Chemoprophylaxis
  Recurrent trips over a short period
  High-risk areas 1–5 nights' stay
  Consider 3-week course of doxycycline (100 mg/day)

Global warming, deforestation, and increasing urbanization are factors encouraging other vector-borne diseases worldwide. Dengue fever has undergone a resurgence, causing between 50 million and 100 million infections annually, predominantly in the world's tropical cities, especially in the Americas and Asia: very short-term travelers to such destinations need mosquito avoidance advice.

VACCINATIONS

All persons in industrialized countries should be up to date with vaccinations against polio, tetanus, and diphtheria and should prefer to be immune to measles, mumps, and rubella either through past infection or by appropriate vaccination; only 50% of those over 50 years of age in the U.S.A. and Australia are reported to have protective antitetanus titers. Influenza, hepatitis B, and *Haemophilus influenzae* vaccination may be appropriate for some persons regardless of travel. Influenza vaccine (and or amantadine) should be offered to those in at-risk groups in travelers to the tropics, given that influenza transmission occurs year round in the tropics; the brief incubation period of influenza viruses gives potential for symptoms interfering with even very short trips.

A valid yellow fever vaccination is mandatory for travel to some countries within the zone and required for entry into other countries outside the yellow fever zone. During the annual Muslim Hajj pilgrimage to Mecca, more than 1 million travelers from diverse parts of the globe converge to spend several weeks in Saudi Arabia; in addition, throughout the rest of the year, many tens of thousands of Umra pilgrims pay homage at Mecca for 1 or just a few days. The Saudi government requires vaccination against meningococcal disease for all pilgrims and prophylaxis against diphtheria and yellow fever for some.

Because hepatitis A is the most commonly occurring vaccine preventable disease in travelers, and as most reports come from short-term travelers from industrialized countries to developing countries staying at middle and upper level hotels, it follows that travelers for even very short duration to high-risk destinations should be made aware of hepatitis A prevention options. There is debate about the cost-benefit of the highly effective vaccine versus partially effective immunoglobulin related to an extent to the number and duration of trips (see Chapter 22). Immunoglobulin and or vaccine should be offered for single trips and vaccination advised for recurrent very short-term travel.

CONCLUSION

The effort and expense of long-distance travel means that short trips are only undertaken in important circumstances. Even minor health impairments can ruin such important trips (and/or mar health after travel). Very short-term travelers' health risks will vary with destination and activities, but the general focus should particularly be as outlined in Table 32–4. Pertinent and accurate health advice is hard to find but can be of significant advantage to the outcome of the important trips taken by very short-term travelers.

Table 32–4. **PRETRAVEL HEALTH FOCUS FOR VERY SHORT-TERM TRAVEL**

Destination and activity-specific risks

Travel insurance

Malaria

    Chemoprophylaxis or self-treatment

    Insect avoidance advice

Sexual risk advice

Travelers' diarrhea

    Chemoprophylaxis for some

        or

    Self-treatment with fluoroquinolone on first unformed stool

Vaccinations

    Hepatitis A

    Routine and mandatory vaccines

Basic medical kit

REFERENCES

1. Berger SA. Emporiatrics versus geographic medicine: interface or spectrum. J Travel Med 1995;2:153.
2. Liese B, Mundt KA, Dell LD, et al. Medical claims associated with international business travel. Occup Environ Med 1997;54:499–503.
3. Haugli L, Skogstad A, Hellesoy OH. Health sleep and mood perceptions reported by airline crews flying short and long hauls. Aviat Space Environ Med 1994;64:27–34.
4. Wick Jr RL, Irvine LA. The microbiological composition of airliner cabin air. Aviat Space Environ Med 1995;66:220–224.
5. Angst F, Steffen RL. Update on the epidemiology of traveler's diarrhea in east Africa. J Travel Med 1997;4:118–120.
6. Balassanian N. Traveler's diarrhea in international corporate business travelers. J Travel Med 1995;2:109.
7. Kemmerer T, Cetron M, Harper L, et al. Health problems of corporate travelers: risk factors and management. J Travel Med 1995;2:110.
8. Gutersohn T, Steffen R, van Damme P, et al. Hepatitis A infection in aircrews. Aviat Space Environ Med 1996;67:153–156.
9. Parkins KJ, Poets CF, O'Brien LM, et al. Effects of exposure to 15% oxygen on breathing patterns and oxygen saturation in infants. BMJ 1998;316:887–894.
10. Bruni M, Steffen R. Impact of travel-related health impairments. J Travel Med 1997;4:61–64.
11. Harding RM, Mills FJ. Aviation medicine. 2nd Ed. London: British Medical Association, 1988.
12. Young M, Flicker P, Maughan R, et al. The travelling athlete: issues relating to the Commonwealth Games, Malaysia 1998. Br J Sports Med 1998;32:77–81.
13. Connor MP, Green AD. Runway malaria in a British serviceman. J R Soc Med 1995;88:415–416.
14. Deseda CC, Lobel HO. Shipboard malaria, Puerto Rico. J Travel Med 1995;2:133.
15. Armengaud M. Arguments against chemoprophylaxis in areas at low risk for chloroquine–resistant plasmodium falciparum. J Travel Med 1995;2:4–5.
16. Thimasarn K, Jatapadma S, Vidjaykadga S, et al. Epidemiology of malaria in Thailand. J Travel Med 1995;2:59–65.
17. Schlagenhauf P, Lobel H, Steffen R, et al. Tolerance of mefloquine by Swissair trainee pilots. Am J Trop Med Hyg 1997;56:235–240.
18. Lobel HO, Kozarsky PE. Update on prevention of malaria for travelers. JAMA 1997;278:1767–1771.

Chapter 33

EXPATRIATES AND LONG-TERM TRAVELERS

DAVID R. SHLIM AND THOMAS H. VALK

INTRODUCTION

People who travel or move abroad for an extended period of time to areas of medical risk have concerns beyond those of the short-term traveler. Those people who take up residence abroad will have even more concerns: finding a house, hiring staff, moving their belongings, arranging schools for the children, finding something meaningful for the nonemployed spouse to do, and becoming familiar with the various methods of trying to avoid illness. In addition, moving abroad involves leaving family, friends, and jobs behind. Long-term adventure travelers often have concerns about the effects of protective measures (malaria prophylaxis) over a longer period and are concerned about the repeated use of antibiotics or other drugs to treat the inevitable illnesses that occur while traveling. Both groups often have concerns about appropriate medical screening upon returning home from a long tour.

A person who moves from his home country and takes up residence abroad is usually referred to as an expatriate in his or her adopted country. Expatriates can move to another country based on a wide variety of motivations and goals: embassy staff, missionaries, geologists looking for oil and other mineral resources, refugee relief workers, business people looking for new markets or production capabilities, photographers, journalists, film makers, spiritual seekers, anthropologists, military, and others. Destinations and environments vary from the capitals of Western Europe to sub-Saharan Africa, the islands of the Pacific, the rain forests of South America, the Himalayas, the Andes, and beyond. Families may or may not be involved in the move. Increasingly, older persons are choosing to retire abroad. Obviously, each of these groups requires an individual approach. However, if one becomes the medical consultant to an organization, then group standards may need to be developed to streamline the care of people both coming and going. Medical-legal issues arise if a person with a known disorder is placed in a setting where adequate care is not available, or, after the fact, as one tries to prove that the person was fit and healthy prior to being posted abroad and is not harboring any persistent problems from his/her posting.

Employers undertake a great expense to move a family abroad and get them settled. In one survey of major corporations, respondents indicated that the cost of an expatriate assignment ranged from $250,000 or less to over $500,000.[1] Given these costs, medical consultation may be a prudent investment prior to moving abroad,[2] and preexisting conditions such as asthma, diabetes, heart disease, hypertension, seizure disorders, and a variety of psychiatric disorders must be balanced with the stressor of the move itself and the receiving country's medical and mental health facilities to determine whether a particular posting is appropriate for an individual.[3,4]

PREDEPARTURE MEDICAL EVALUATIONS

The predeparture medical evaluation has become standard for most organizations sending someone abroad. Although the motivation should be to discover and document any problems that might impact the posting abroad, these examinations have taken on a medical-legal aspect. Organizations want to document that either the person is healthy enough to undertake the posting or is disqualified based on medical reasons. Preexisting conditions need to be documented so that the person cannot later claim that the posting caused medical harm. How thorough these examinations need to be should be based on an understanding of the health risks and health care facilities and providers in the destination country and any concerns that arise from the review of systems of the patient. Many adults do not undergo rigorous physical examinations regularly, so the pretravel examination is a chance to review the entire health picture and not just the travel-related risks. Long-term expatriates who spend the bulk of their adult life working abroad may "fall through the cracks" in terms of getting recommended health screenings such as sigmoidoscopy, prostate examinations, breast cancer screening, pap smears, and heart disease risk factor testing. These routine tests are often overlooked when the focus is on the more dramatic-sounding risks of malaria, dengue fever, typhoid, etc. It should not be assumed that this testing is available in most third-world destinations.

Predeparture evaluations should include a psychiatric component. Preexisting disorders that involve psychotic states, impaired judgment, bizarre behavior, or substance abuse can be very problematic in an overseas setting. The factors and disorders to be considered are covered elsewhere in this text in Chapter 28, Psychiatric Illness and Stress.

Likewise, dental care prior to travel is extremely useful, as dentistry abroad can be either unavailable or of extremely poor quality. Recommending a complete dental examination, along with fixing all existing problems prior to travel, is one of the most important recommendations that the travel health professional can make.

In addition, it is a good idea to get one's vision checked and glasses changed as needed. Many destinations do not have the ability to fit eyeglasses expertly. The patient should carry an extra pair of glasses and a copy of his/her prescription. Contact lens wearers should try to determine if the supplies they will need are available at their destination and, if not, to carry adequate supplies for the length of their trip.

Persons who take medication on a regular basis should take adequate supplies with them. Occasionally, the same medications are available abroad, and the cost is often a fraction of the cost at home. However, quality control in third-world-manufactured drugs is poor, and trial and error may be the only way to know if the new drug is effective. An independent study of the quality of selected antimalarials and antibiotics in Thailand and Nigera found that 36.5% of the samples were substandard.[5] If there are clinics that specialize in the care of expatriates in the given destination, the staff may be able to recommend which drugs they have found to be reliable. If the person has been stable on a particular brand for a long time, it makes sense not to change brands and then wait to see if symptoms are experienced. Drugs that should probably not be sought abroad are thyroid hormone replacement and coumadin.

Some doctors are reluctant to prescribe large quantities of drugs, and some patients are reluctant to carry them through customs. Carrying drugs in their original containers is not usually a problem for customs officials, who are more often looking for smuggled electronic gear, gold, and illicit drugs. Having pharmaceuticals mailed to a person living abroad is an option, but mail is often unreliable: both carelessness and theft account for nondelivery. Organizations usually have people traveling back and forth on a regular basis, and these people could act as couriers for other people stationed in the country.

SCREENING CONCERNS

For long-term travelers and expatriates heading to developing countries for an extended period of time, the rationale for extended pretrip testing has never been firmly established. Recommendations are based on conventional wisdom. However, it makes sense to have some baseline studies so that certain diseases can be ruled in or out at the end of the trip or posting. Tuberculosis (TB) is making a resurgence around the world, and multidrug-resistant strains are a growing concern. Patients with a negative purified protein derivative (PPD) skin test can be retested upon return to see if they have been exposed to the TB bacillus. Patients who are already PPD positive can have that documented in their chart so that they will not be alarmed that they may have acquired TB on their journey. Although the use of condoms to prevent HIV infection is reducing the number of other venereal infections, it can also be a good idea to test a patient's VDRL status prior to travel.

Whether international travelers should be screened for their HIV status remains controversial. However, the topic should be discussed, and counseling about safe sex and avoidance of unsafe needles should take place. Some countries require HIV testing for certain classes of people entering the country.[6] An unofficial list of these countries has been compiled by the U.S. State Department (available at http://travel.state.gov/HIVtestingreqs.html). If there is a chance that HIV testing will be required to obtain a visa to stay in the destination country, the test should be done at home before travel, where there are no concerns of unsafe needles and inaccurate testing and where counseling will be available for positive results. Persons who know that they are HIV positive should be evaluated individually by someone who is an expert in the issues of treating HIV infection. Travel abroad is not automatically prohibited, but the destination, length of stay, availability of and monitoring for HIV treatment, etc. require a very individualized approach.

CONCERNS OF EXPATRIATES LIVING IN DEVELOPING COUNTRIES

ENVIRONMENTAL CONCERNS

Living in developing countries is, in some ways, like going back in time to an ecologically naive era. There is little concern about the environment and almost no effective government regulation of health hazards.[7] Garbage disposal is haphazard, and toxic substances from batteries, motor vehicle oil, paints, and worse are strewn across the landscape.[8] In order to keep up crop production, pesticides are used widely and often applied just prior to harvesting.[9,10] Where industries are developing, there is no regulation of industrial wastes.[11] Expatriates and long-term travelers have become aware of these issues mainly in recent years, when the consequences of pollution have become inescapable in many third-world cities. Thus, to the usual concerns about enteric illness and infectious diseases are added the more imponderable worries about the effects of air pollution[12,13] and the possibility of gradual poisoning through water and food.

SETTING UP THE EXPATRIATE KITCHEN

In the absence of reliable testing facilities and the lack of governmental regulation, what steps can the expatriate take to help alleviate these concerns? Most expatriates boil their water prior to drinking, but this does not eliminate most toxins. The American Foreign Service supplies its workers with water distillers in some situations, which creates pure water. These machines are expensive, large, and impractical for most expatriate families. However, the combination of charcoal filtration with boiling should create reasonable protection. Charcoal filters should be used in conjunction with prefilters so that they do not rapidly fill up with silt. These devices can be purchased in one's home country and a local plumber can usually fit them to the destination house.[14,15] Sophisticated water filters are starting to become available overseas.

If expatriates want to find out if their water is contaminated with chemicals, lead, or pesticides, commercially available test kits can be obtained in their home country. Then, just prior to flying home, the containers can be filled with tap water and then mailed within their home country. There is usually too much delay in transporting the containers home to reliably test for coliforms, which are assumed to be present in any case in developing countries.

Fruits and vegetables can be soaked in an iodine solution to kill microorganisms, allowing expatriates to enjoy salads and raw vegetables. But this step will not eliminate pesticides or other pollutants. Therefore, all fruits and vegetables should be washed in water treated with a small amount of dish soap, then rinsed thoroughly with tap water, and finally soaked in water that has been treated with iodine. The concentration of iodine required is four to eight parts per million, which can be achieved with different products. There is evidence that *Cyclospora* and *Cryptosporidium* are not killed by iodine or chlorine, so this method may not prevent these infections in areas where these organisms are endemic. In areas with poor sanitation, flies may be a major source of fecal contamination and infection. Kitchens should be screened, and portable screens should be placed over food that has to sit out. Kitchen staff should be taught to wash their hands any time they have been out of the house and after they go to the toilet or change the children's diapers. Refrigeration is usually available in developing countries, but power outages are common, and stored food may deteriorate more rapidly after a long power cut.

RESPIRATORY CONCERNS

People who have asthma should try to get some idea about the asthma risk in their particular destination. Particulate counts alone do not give a clear idea of the risk. For example, the Kathmandu Valley in Nepal has proven to be a very provocative place for people with reactive airway disease. However, as soon as these people fly to Bangkok, Thailand, they begin to feel better immediately, even though Bangkok has what appears to be more vehicle pollution than Kathmandu. Adults and children with no prior history of asthma have had attacks in Kathmandu for the first time in their lives and never had trouble again after leaving that environment. Expatriates and long-term travelers who plan to bicycle or spend a lot of time in open vehicles in traffic may want to invest in a good-quality breathing mask to reduce the quantity of pollutants taken into the lungs.

LIVING WITH CHILDREN ABROAD

Parents are justifiably concerned about the health consequences to their children while living abroad. Small children (0–5 years) should have their usual childhood immunizations on schedule, as well as the travel-related immunizations appropriate to their destination and age. Parents should be counseled that diarrheal disease may occur more frequently abroad but that it also occurs in this age group in one's home country. Parents should bring with them a good-quality car seat and use it in their own vehicle, and whenever possible in other vehicles.

Schooling is the second most prominent concern. Many destinations have international schools of excellent quality. However, the ability and willingness of these schools to handle children with either learning or emotional disorders varies considerably. In such situations, placement overseas in many areas may be difficult or impossible, and parents should investigate their options carefully and well ahead of time. Home schooling is a major commitment on the part of the parents. Placing the child in local school is almost always too difficult for the child, and the education may not be adequate to return to the home school system without losing ground. Special counseling may be required prior to traveling abroad with teenage children, as leaving one's high school, set of friends, sports, and activities and starting over again somewhere else can be very traumatic for all involved.

Expatriate living may induce a closer relationship among siblings and family, particularly when accompanied by frequent overseas moves. Expatriates may have more generous vacation allowance and paid home leaves. The family gets used to traveling long distances together, and the children become more sophisticated in terms of their exposure to foreign cultures and their ability to move around the world. The downside of an entire childhood abroad can be the absence of an identifiable "home" culture. Such children, who live neither in their home culture nor in close contact with the host country culture, have been deemed to be "Third Culture Kids." They grow up in an "interstitial culture" composed of the adults and children of the expatriate community in which they live and go to school.[16] The move back to their "home" culture can be difficult, especially if it is superimposed on their first going away to college.

If parents plan to leave their children in the care of staff or friends while in a country that has an inadequate medical infrastructure, they should make sure that the caregiver has access to the children's passports and a recent letter authorizing them to travel with the children in the event of a medical emergency.

HOUSEHOLD STAFF

One of the positive sides of foreign postings in developing countries is the affordable availability of household staff. Parents suddenly discover a freedom that they could only dream of before: clothes are washed and pressed, meals are shopped for and prepared, dishes cleared and washed, houses cleaned, and, most importantly, children have continuous care. The parents are free to go and come without arranging further babysitters and day care. The availability of so much support may be one reason why many expatriates decide to start or expand their families while posted abroad. On the other hand, some families find that having staff is intrusive and requires more management skills than they possess or are willing to use.

New expatriates are often concerned about the potential for their household staff to pass illnesses onto themselves and their families. An effort is sometimes made to have them "screened" for communicable diseases. However, the ability for healthy people to infect others in a household is relatively limited. Expatriates should be reassured that household staff who appear healthy probably are and do not need chest x-rays, stool cultures, and blood tests as a condition of employment.

VEHICULAR SAFETY

An additional problem facing expatriates and long-term travelers in developing countries is vehicular safety. In most instances, one cannot have control over one's local transportation options. Taxis may not have seatbelts, buses may not have brakes, and drivers may have blood alcohol levels well above the legal limit. Most expatriates will acquire their own vehicles and learn to drive in the chaos that represents most third-world driving situations. It is important to counsel these people that although many aspects of driving safety are out of their control, they should maximize the things that are within their control. Seatbelts should always be worn when available, cars should be as well maintained as possible, and one must practice an extreme form of defensive driving—which basically means assuming that every other vehicle on the road is going to constantly violate the rules of common sense. Motorcyclists must always wear helmets, and small children should not be carried in backpacks on motorcycles.

PERSONAL HEALTH CONCERNS

Expatriates and long-term travelers are often people who have enjoyed good health throughout most of their lives. When they move overseas, they frequently experience illness and are emotionally unprepared for the experience. They often overestimate the severity of the illness or the frequency (e.g., expatriates may complain that they are having "constant diarrhea," but when you examine their history, they may have had two or three brief episodes in a month). Although short-term travelers can shrug off illness and look forward to regaining their health upon return, long-term travelers and expatriates must try to recover their health while living at constant risk of further illness.

Diarrhea is the most common of the illnesses acquired abroad. A prospective cohort study among expatriates in Nepal showed that they experienced an average of 3.2 episodes of diarrhea per person per year in the first 2 years of moving to Nepal.[17] This figure is comparable to the rate of diarrhea among third-world children. Some expatriates experience much more diarrhea than that. Bacterial pathogens are the most common cause of diarrhea,[18,19] and expatriates and long-term travelers can be taught how to recognize probable bacterial diarrheal infections and treat themselves with antibiotics. Bacterial diarrhea is almost always characterized by the abrupt onset of relatively uncomfortable diarrheal symptoms. In contrast, protozoal diarrhea usually has an insidious onset of a few loose stools per day, with fewer constitutional symptoms. When bacterial diarrhea is suspected, treatment with 1 or 2 days of a quinolone antibiotic can dramatically shorten the illness.[20]

Expatriates and long-term travelers should be counseled that immunity to diarrheal pathogens is acquired slowly. The risk of acquiring diarrhea remains constant for at least 1 year and then gradually declines over a number of years.[21] Of importance, however, is the fact that not only the frequency of diarrhea declines but the severity. Long-term expatriates rarely experience the combination of high fevers, severe abdominal pain, watery diarrhea, and vomiting that terrorizes shorter-term visitors to high-risk countries.

Are there long-term consequences to the intestines of individuals residing in high-risk developing countries? Rarely written about is the fact that many expatriates experience a relatively constant loosening of their stools during a long-term residence in a third-world country. This can be distressing to some individuals and may lead them to seek treatment repeatedly to find a cure. However, these patients can be reassured that if they feel well, have good energy, are not losing weight, and merely have one to two loose stools per day, this is not likely due to a treatable pathogen. The etiology of this chronic loosening of the stools is unknown: is it due to low-grade infection, the effects of repeated infection, or some environmental factors? In the majority of cases, the stools gradually firm up and return to normal after the person returns to his/her home country.

Many expatriates harbor concerns about intestinal worms and take treatment every 6 months or so to eliminate worms. Although intestinal worms are ubiquitous in most developing countries, the risk for foreigners to acquire worms has not been adequately assessed. At the CIWEC Clinic Travel Medicine Center in Kathmandu, helminth eggs were found in fewer than 5% of the 1,200 stool samples that were processed each year (unpublished data). In a study of Peace Corps volunteers in Nepal, a total of 18% of volunteers had a worm diagnosed during their 2-year stint. However, worms were almost never found in the first 6 months, and the average amount of time in the country before the diagnosis of worms was almost 20 months.[22] Despite the low incidence of and severity of worm infections, many expatriates and travelers are distressed by the thought of harboring worms. Both mebendazole and albendazole have high safety profiles, and concerned expatriates and travelers can be allowed to self-medicate if it helps them psychologically. They should be warned, however, that worms could appear in their stool after successful treatment. Self-treatment is probably not necessary more than once per year. The other reassuring information to point out is that the most common worms—ascaris, trichuris, and hookworm—do not have the capability of reproducing within the intestine. Eggs have to go outside the body to complete their life cycles. Therefore, foreigners almost never acquire more than a few adult worms.

PROLONGED USE OF ANTIMALARIALS

The safety of long-term continuous use of antimalarials (beyond 2 years) has not been well documented. This does not mean that they are not safe to use, but only that careful follow-up has not been carried out in this group.

Studies of U.S. Peace Corps volunteers in West Africa showed that mefloquine was safe and effective for up to 2 years.[23] There are anecdotal cases of continuous mefloquine prophylaxis of up to 8 years, with no apparent ill effects. The long-term safety of doxycycline has not been formally studied, but experience with various tetracyclines prescribed for the prevention of teenage acne has not revealed any adverse effects associated with prolonged treatment.

Several studies have looked at the safety of mefloquine taken while pregnant.[24–28] These studies found no adverse effects from mefloquine taken at any point during pregnancy. Since malaria can have severe consequences to the fetus and the mother during pregnancy, the risk of prophylaxis must be weighed against the risk of acquiring malaria while pregnant. For long-term travelers and expatriates, pregnancy raises some difficult issues: should the mother remain in a malaria risk area while pregnant, and if she chooses to stay, should she continue to take malaria prophylaxis while pregnant? A recent survey, reported as an abstract, found that of 276 missionary women who spent at least part of their pregnancy in a malaria risk area, 25 (9%) contracted malaria while pregnant. Eighty percent of the 276 women had received inadequate or no malaria prophylaxis. Outcomes of the pregnancies and infections were not given.[29]

Long-term travelers who are traveling for less than 2 years can be reasonably reassured about the safety of taking an antimalarial for that length of time. Travelers who become pregnant while taking mefloquine can be reassured that no birth defects have been associated with mefloquine use in hundreds of pregnancies. For expatriates with a longer-term commitment in areas of continuous risk, they will just have to weigh the necessity of their living there against the risk of malaria and the unknown risk of continual antimalarial use. For reassurance, expatriates can be informed that there are no published reports of adverse effects of antimalarials due to continuous use over a prolonged period of time when taken at the appropriate dosage level.

RABIES

Most of the countries in Asia, Africa, and South America harbor street dog populations that are endemic for rabies. The risk of rabies appears to be highest in the Indian subcontinent, including India, Bangladesh, Pakistan, and Nepal.[30] Street dogs can have contact with other animals, making almost any mammalian bite a risk for rabies. Expatriates should be counseled about avoiding contact with street animals and to make sure that their own household pets are vaccinated against rabies. A recent study from Nepal demonstrated that expatriates had a threefold higher risk of wounds requiring rabies postexposure prophylaxis (Pandey P, unpublished data). Reasons that expatriates might be at higher risk for rabies exposures include owning pets that become ill, children taking in street puppies, and visiting friends' homes where dogs are kept. Because expatriates may be at risk for rabies exposures, predeployment advice should include advice about the benefits of thorough wound washing in any possible rabies exposure. Rabies virus never enters the bloodstream but remains for a variable length of time at the wound site, where it can be physically removed by thorough washing.[31]

For expatriates in high-risk countries, pre-exposure rabies immunization would be a worthwhile investment.[32,33] Preimmunized individuals do not require human rabies immune globulin (HRIG) and only require two tissue culture vaccine boosters after a potential rabies exposure. HRIG is rarely available in any developing countries. Good-quality tissue culture rabies vaccines are now available in most places, so rabies immune prophylaxis after a bite could be handled without emergency travel.

It is usually recommended that all expatriate children should be preimmunized with rabies vaccine for the following reasons: (1) children's short stature makes them at risk for high-risk exposures around the face and neck and (2) children may not report an encounter with an animal due to lack of knowledge or fear of parental anger. Although unproven, parents can take some comfort in the knowledge that a recent pre-exposure rabies vaccine may create high enough antibody titers to protect against an unreported exposure. A case of rabies that occurred in a 10-year-old Australian boy 16 months after his return from a trip to India and Nepal is a sobering reminder of both the risk of rabies in these countries and the fact that a child may not report a possible exposure.[34]

PSYCHOLOGICAL PROBLEMS

An overseas assignment can create an enormous amount of stress as familiar supports are removed and adjustments are made to a new culture, job, and living situation. All family members can expect to experience the vicissitudes of "culture shock" within the first 6 to 12 months overseas. This predictable syndrome occurs virtually independent of the difference between the home culture and the host country culture and usually results in only mild dysfunction. In this setting, anyone with a significant psychiatric history can be at risk of exacerbation in this new environment, and preexisting marital or family problems can be expected to worsen. The travel medicine practitioner should firmly refute the notion that someone with psychological difficulties might do better by moving overseas. As always, the travel medicine practitioner must balance the nature and stability of the disorder against the potential exacerbating effects of the move itself and the availability of adequate, culturally compatible mental health care providers and facilities in the host country. Readers are referred to Chapter 28 Psychiatric Illness and Stress for further details on culture shock and psychiatric issues.

Alcohol abuse can be an increased risk of an overseas posting due to the increased stress, absence of counseling options, an expatriate community that may get together mainly to drink alcohol, and an absence of supervision when alcohol begins to become a problem. Other substance abuse disorders, in adults or teenagers, can be particularly troublesome, especially if they involve the use of illicit substances. In some countries, the penalties for use of illicit substances are severe and persons with such problems should be well into a stable sobriety before they risk assignment. There may also be a temptation to self-medicate, especially with tranquilizers or sedative-hypnotics that may be readily available without prescription in some countries. Such activity is to be discouraged as it risks addiction, dysfunction, and a delay in the necessary adaptation to the new overseas environment.

Overall, expatriates and long-term travelers may indulge in risky behavior including increased alcohol and drug use, starting or resuming cigarette smoking, riding motorcycles without helmets, driving without seatbelts, and indulging in casual sex without adequate protection. Part of the reason that this behavior may suddenly seem acceptable is a phenomenon that occurs when people move from a familiar environment to a totally new environment without familiar cultural restraints. The new environment may seem so foreign that one's behavior in this environment may be thought of as not having consequences in one's "normal" life. This kind of "magical thinking" may account for indulging in risky behavior that would not even be considered at home. Informing long-term travelers and expatriates that this type of thinking may ensue may help "inoculate" them against suddenly taking up self-destructive behavior in the new environment. This advice might have saved the life of a 28-year-old Swedish tourist at the Thai beach island of Ko Samui, who rented a motorcycle, drove it wearing only a T-shirt and shorts, and, being unused to driving on the left side of the road, swerved the wrong way to avoid an oncoming truck and was killed instantly.

Surprising to some, the repatriation phase, coming home after a tour overseas, involves many of the same signs and symptoms as does "culture shock." Indeed, many experienced expatriates consider this leg of their journey as difficult or even more trying as the outbound leg. Travel medicine practitioners can help in this setting by helping the returning family understand the nature of their distress, its normality, and its causes. These include that the family and each of its members have been changed by their extended contact with a foreign culture and may not find aspects of their home culture enjoyable or even tolerable anymore. There are frequently major financial changes as well as significant changes in the roles of the employee at work and of the spouse at work or at home.

Another shock, frequently discovered by those returning, is that their compatriots have no referent experience with which to relate to the expatriate's experiences and quickly tune out in conversations. Finally, what is regarded as "home" usually has changed in a number of unpredictable ways. For teenagers, the latest fads, fashions, and slang are strange and unfamiliar. For adults, neighborhoods, schools, and political and social concerns can all be new. The results are significant. Recent surveys indicate a high rate of executive turnover after repatriation, up to 25%.[35] In a survey of corporate managers, 82% were satisfied with their expatriate assignment, whereas only 35% were satisfied with the repatriation process.[36]

INSURANCE COVERAGE

Persons planning to live abroad for an extended period of time should review their medical and evacuation insurance options. For short-term travel, most health insurance policies will cover an illness or accident abroad and may even cover the costs associated with repatriation. However, these insurance companies may not be in a position to offer any assistance to the person who is abroad in obtaining medical care or arranging evacuation. In addition, they may have a provision that requires prior authorization for evacuation or hospitalization, even though the company may not maintain 24-hour phone answering services. For these reasons, long-term travelers should consider the benefits of an evacuation insurance policy.

Evacuation insurance usually does not cover the costs of medical treatment and hospitalization abroad. However, these companies can help arrange all aspects of finding medical treatment, getting to a hospital, or getting evacuated home. They maintain 24-hour contact desks and immediate access to medical consultants and can arrange air ambulance evacuation in appropriate cases. Since air-ambulance flights can cost between $50,000 to $100,000, this option is usually unaffordable for the uninsured traveler. Evacuation insurance is usually quite affordable, with rates under $300 per year. The combination of expert help in an emergency and the possibility of using expensive air evacuation options makes this insurance appealing to most long-term travelers or expatriates.

Health insurance for long-term expatriates is a tricky issue. Many U.S. health insurance carriers will not offer health insurance to persons who take up residence overseas. This leaves the person with the option of (1) maintaining U.S. health insurance and not informing the company of the move or (2) dropping U.S. coverage and obtaining a special expatriate health insurance package. The first option results in anxiety as to whether a claim will be honored or the insurance cancelled if the person is discovered to be living outside his/her home territory. The second option poses two problems: international health insurance companies usually limit the coverage that they provide within the United States, and serious medical problems that might develop while living overseas, such as diabetes, cancer, or ischemic heart disease, may be excluded from coverage when one returns to the U.S., or one may find oneself completely unable to obtain health insurance upon returning home. A healthy pregnant woman who returns to the U.S. may find that health insurance will be denied to both her and her immediate family until after the baby is born. Therefore, maintaining a U.S. policy should be a priority for most Americans. Some Americans who were initially told by a company that they could not be insured if they lived overseas were later granted health insurance by someone higher up in the company.

Most other countries have government-sponsored health care that is available to all residents of that country. Persons from countries with national health care need to determine whether they are covered while outside that country, and, if not, they will need to arrange for expatriate or travel health insurance.

"WESTERN-STYLE" HEALTH CARE FOR FOREIGNERS ABROAD

The term "Western-style" health care has come to mean personalized health care in a clean, sanitary environment with appropriate sterilization, record keeping, cold chain for vaccines, and appointments for consultations. The CIWEC Clinic Travel Medicine Center in Kathmandu, Nepal, was one of the first of these types of clinics. Western doctors created a "medical oasis" in an otherwise underserved area and were able to treat most illnesses and to supervise the care and evacuation of more serious conditions. The doctors at the clinic were able to develop relationships with local specialist physicians, steering their patients to the best care available. After a 3-year sponsorship period by a Canadian aid agency, the clinic was able to become self-supporting. In recent years, similar clinics have been created in destinations that have developing international business interests: Moscow, Beijing, Almaty. Even more recently, clinics have been established as an extension of medical evacuation companies.

The chances of success of these clinics depends on (1) an inadequate local medical structure, (2) a concentration of expatriates and tourists in a major city, and (3) permission from the local government to operate. When the clientele is mostly business people from large corporations, the clinic can charge what it needs to provide the service and cover salaries. When the clientele are mainly tourists, patients tend to be more cost conscious, and the clinic may not generate a lot of income. Local doctors inevitably pay attention to the success of these clinics, and "Western-style" clinics marketed to tourists may begin to appear, even though the local doctor may have no special expertise in travel-related problems.

A well-run destination travel clinic makes an ideal learning environment for persons interested in travel medicine. Travel medicine practitioners may want to spend time in one of these clinics in a high-risk destination in order to become more familiar with the risks of travel, the presentation of common illnesses, and the limitations of providing medical care abroad.

RETURN HEALTH ASSESSMENT

Just as in the predeparture physical assessment, the return examination can have a dual agenda: screening the patient for the patient's own benefit and the more legalistic concerns of proving that the person is free of health consequences from this particular posting. The tests that should be run will differ with the risks of the destination country. A repeat PPD, if negative, is adequate to rule out TB, and a chest x-ray would be redundant. Schistosomiasis serology might be appropriate for at-risk expatriates from parts of Africa. If appropriate, syphilis screening should be performed. In the absence of intestinal symptoms, the travel medicine literature differs as to whether stool screening is of any value in preventing a longer-term problem. If the person has any ongoing medical complaints, they should be investigated vigorously, but in the absence of any complaints, the likelihood of benefiting the patient with extensive examinations is minimal. Realistic standards, based on studies of the outcomes of expatriates returning home, will hopefully someday better define this problem.

REFERENCES

1. National Foreign Trade Council, SRI Selection Research International. International sourcing and selection practices: 1995 survey reports. September 1995.
2. Steffen R. Travel medicine—prevention based on epidemiological data. Trans R Soc Trop Med Hyg 1991;85:156–162.
3. Peppiatt R, Byass P. A survery of the health of British missionaries. Br J Gen Pract 1991;41:159–162.
4. Lange WR, Franenfield D, Contoreggi CS. Psychological concerns of overseas employees and families. Travel Med Int 1994;12:176–181.
5. Shakoor O, Taylor RB, Behrens RH. Assessment of the incidence of substandard drugs in developing countries. Trop Med Int Health 1997;2:839–845.
6. Centers for Disease Control and Prevention. Health information for international travel 1999–2000. Atlanta: Department of Health and Human Services, 1999.
7. Pinnock MA. Environmental health: catching up with the developed world. West Indian Med J 1998;47 (Suppl 4):25–27.
8. Hunter JM, Arbona SI. Paradise lost: an introduction to the geography of water pollution in Puerto Rico. Soc Sci Med 1995;40:1331–1355.
9. Kannan K, Tanabe S, Giesy JP, Tatsukawa R. Organochlorine pesticides and polychlorinated biphenyls in foodstuffs from Asian and oceanic countries. Rev Environ Contam Toxicol 1997;152:1–55.
10. Albert LA. Persisent pesticides in Mexico. Rev Environ Contam Toxicol 1996;147:1–44.
11. Jamall IS, Davis B. Chemicals and environmentally caused diseases in developing countries. Infect Dis Clin North Am 1991;5:365–375.
12. Salinas M, Vega J. The effect of outdoor air pollution on mortality risk: an ecological study from Santiago, Chile. World Health Stat Q 1995;48:118–125.
13. Hijazi Z. Environmental pollution and asthma. Pediatr Pulmonol Suppl 1997;16:205–207.
14. Donegan F. Consumer guide: water treatment basics. Popular Mechanics 1993;May:61–63.
15. Anonymous. Water-treatment devices. Consumer Reports 1993; February:79–82.
16. Useem RH, Downie RD. Third-culture kids. Today's Education, 1976; Sept-Oct:103–105.
17. Shlim DR, Hoge CW, Rajah R, et al. Persistent high risk of diarrhea among foreigners in Nepal during the first two years of residence. Clin Infect Dis 1999;29:613–616.
18. Taylor DN, Echeverria P, Blaser MJ, et al. Polymicrobial aetiology of traveller's diarrhoea. Lancet 1985;1:383–385.
19. Taylor DN, Houston R, Shlim DR, et al. Etiology of diarrhea among travelers and foreign residents in Nepal. JAMA 1988;260:1245–1248.
20. Taylor DN, Sanchez JI, Candler W, et al. Treatment of traveler's diarrhea: ciprofloxacin plus loperamide compared with ciprofloxacin alone. Ann Intern Med 1991;114:731–734.
21. Hoge CW, Shlim DR, Echeverria P, et al. Epidemiology of diarrhea among expatriate residents living in a highly endemic environment. JAMA 1996;275:533–538.
22. Houston R, Schwartz E. Helminthic infections among Peace Corps volunteers in Nepal. JAMA 1990;263:373–374.

23. Lobel HO, Miani M, Eng T, et al. Long–term malaria prophylaxis with weekly mefloquine. Lancet 1993;341:848–851.

24. Nosten F, ter Kuile F, Maelankiri L, et al. Mefloquine prophylaxis prevents malaria during pregnancy: a double-blind, placebo-controlled study. J Infect Dis 1994;169:595–603.

25. Steketee RW, Wirima JJ, Slutsker L, et al. Malaria treatment and prevention in pregnancy: indications for use and adverse events associated with use of chloroquine or mefloquine. Am J Trop Med Hyg 1996;55;50–56.

26. Balocco R, Bonati. Mefloquine prophylaxis against malaria for female travelers of childbearing age. Lancet 1992; 340:309–310.

27. Smoak BL, Writer JV, Keep LW, et al. The effects of inadvertent exposure of mefloquine chemoprophylaxis on pregnancy outcomes and infants of US Army servicewomen. J Infect Dis 1997;176:831–833.

28. Vanhauwere B, Maradit H, Kerr L. Post-marketing surveillance of prophylactic Lariam® use in pregnancy. Am J Trop Med Hyg 1997;58:17–21.

29. Carroll ID, Carroll JE. Malaria prophylaxis in pregnant, expatriate missionaries. Program and Abstracts of the 47th Annual Meeting of the American Society of Tropical Medicine and Hygiene 1998;59:314–315.

30. Bogel K, Motschwiller E. Incidence of rabies and post-exposure treatment in developing countries. Bull World Health Organ 1986;64:883–887.

31. Baer GM, Lentz TL. Rabies pathogenesis to the central nervous system. In: Baer GM, ed. The natural history of rabies. 2nd Ed. Boca Raton, FL: CRC Press, 1991:116–118.

32. Bernard KW, Fishbein DB. Pre-exposure rabies prophylaxis for travelers: are the benefits worth the costs? Vaccine 1991; 9:833–836.

33. Shlim DR, Schwartz E, Houston R. Rabies immunoprophylaxis strategy in travelers. J Wilderness Med 1991;2:15–21.

34. Centers for Disease Control. Imported human rabies—Australia, 1987. MMWR Morb Mortal Wkly Rep 1988;37:351–353.

35. Valk TH. Repatriation of expatriate employees and families: pitfalls and solutions. Shoreland's Travel Medicine Monthly 1998;2:12.

36. Gomez-Meija L, Balkin DB. The determinants of managerial satisfaction with the expatriation and repatriation process. J Manag Dev 1987;6:7–17.

Chapter 34

EXPEDITION PARTICIPANTS

STEVEN C. ZELL

INTRODUCTION

There is no consensus definition of adventure travel. However, it may be best envisioned as outdoor travel occurring in underdeveloped or remote areas distant from medical care, posing unique dangers related to extremes of environment augmented by high-risk recreational activites. Adventure travel continues to grow, attracting expedition participants of all ages, genders, and abilities. Individuals can choose from among a seemingly endless array of commercial travel companies. Advertisement sources abound in magazines and newspapers and throughout the Internet. Attractively pictured, adventure travel generally depicts outdoor experiences in remote areas enhanced by the excitement of unique recreational activities. Albeit most travelers return safely in good health with a sense of fulfillment, serious medical problems continue to occur during expedition travel. Personal wealth, youth, or athletic ability cannot substitute for proper judgment. Awareness regarding the risks of injury and illness involved with a recreational activity is critical. Even so, underestimating the forces of nature by extending one's self beyond personal limits of skill or endurance may have tragic consequences.

Granted that adventure travel experiences may be as diverse as their innumerable outdoor locations, expeditions generally share the common attribute of being remote from medical care facilities. With medical evacuation being problematic, expeditions mandate that travelers be self-sufficient and innovative. No substitute exists for thorough pretrip planning. Participants need to be aware of endemic diseases unique to their geographic area of travel and take precautions to receive recommended pretrip vaccines and chemoprophylaxis against infectious disease. Traumatic injury and illness are inherent risks related to all outdoor travel, but unique injuries may arise in association with a chosen recreational activity, requiring a heightened sense of appreciation for their prevention and occurrence. Despite the best planning efforts, problems can still arise due to the uncontrollable forces of nature transforming tranquil travel locales into hostile, threatening environments.

Preparing oneself for expedition travel requires adequate preparation time matching one's skill and support mechanisms against the challenges that lay ahead. An in-depth knowledge of a trip's itinerary with attention paid to any specific recreational activities or extremes of environmental exposure is foremost. Knowledge of the latter defines the setting, influencing the epidemiology of injury and illness likely to be experienced during expedition travel. Awareness of such potential risks should lead to a pretrip analysis of support services to permit a participant's informal assessment of the expedition's preparedness for accidental trauma or medical illness. If deficits exist prior to travel, participants must make a conscious effort to personally fill such gaps or withhold travel plans until safety is reasonably ensured. This may require that individuals purchase specialized equipment beyond a standard first-aid kit, carry their own prescription medicines, or seek medical clearance from a physician prior to trip departure.

In summary, steps can be taken prior to expedition travel to maximize success. Itinerary review identifies travel hazards and environmental concerns that influence the patterns of expected injury and illness. Such knowledge then defines essential support services in the form of both equipment and medical supplies commensurate to the task at hand. Assessment of an expedition's preparedness serves to match on-site support services to potential needs while screening for any preexisting medical conditions of participants likely to be exacerbated during adventure travel.

PRETRIP PLANNING: GENERAL PRINCIPLES

Adventure travel encompasses the difficulty of reaching remote locations with the inherent challenges of travel often in a developing nation. Travelers often take for granted getting to their destination safely, yet their greatest threat abroad is death or injury from trauma related to motor vehicle accidents and attacks of personal crime. Pretrip planning needs to address three key issues: travel safety to one's destination, personal protection abroad, and expected support in the event of an unexpected emergency. Expedition participants need to be aware of local emergency medical services available to foreign travelers and make contacts prior to departure. Political stability and personal protection are enhanced by providing a trip itinerary and registering with one's national embassy. After arriving, take appropriate steps to avoid jet lag on long trips to optimize physical performance and endurance. Table 34–1 summarizes general issues of concern for expedition participants to be addressed prior to departure.

An itinerary evaluation then follows to identify specific hazards related to the unique recreational activities

Table 34–1.   GENERAL PLANNING FOR ADVENTURE TRAVEL

ISSUES OF CONCERN	FACTORS TO CONSIDER
Travel safety to and from destination	Established history of commercial service: air, rail, or vehicle
	Age of transportation used/presence of periodic maintenance
	Presence of basic safety features
	Sanctioned per local government or respected travel agency
Inherent socioeconomic problems	Political stability and acceptance of foreigners
	Endemic and epidemic health problems
	Crime rates: types and locations to avoid
	Currency exchange/protection of valuables
Support in the event of injury or illness	Medical expertise of group leader
	Adequacy of equipment and supplies for risks involved
	Distance and duration from organized rescue operations
	Topographic accessibility to rescue: foot, boat, or air

Reprinted with permission from Zell SC. Environmental and recreational hazards associated with adventure travel. J Travel Med 1997;4:94–99.

Table 34–2.   RECREATIONAL HAZARDS ASSOCIATED WITH ADVENTURE TRAVEL

ACTIVITY	PROBLEMS ENCOUNTERED ABOVE AND BEYOND TRAUMA
Summer backpacking	Water-borne diarrheal illness
	Tick-borne and other zoonotic infections
	Acute mountain sickness
	Solar injuries related to sunburn
	Hypothermia from wind and rain exposure
	Injuries related to bites from mammals/reptiles
Mountain climbing	Hypothermia and frostbite of toes and fingers
	High-altitude cerebral edema
	High-altitude pulmonary edema
	Snowblindness
Backcountry winter camping/skiing	Hypothermia and frostbite
	Sunburn and snowblindness
	Suffocation/traumatic injury from avalanche
Freshwater rafting and kayaking	Drowning and cold water immersion/hypothermia
	Water-borne diarrheal illness
Aquatic activities scuba diving/snorkeling	Marine envenomations from invertebrates (jellyfish)
	Punctures and envenomations from vertebrates (stingray)
	Bacterial infections from abrasions/lacerations (coral)
	Decompression and motion sickness

Reprinted with permission from Zell SC. Environmental and recreational hazards associated with adventure travel. J Travel Med 1997;4:94–99.

being undertaken. Expedition travel implies being in a rugged outdoor environment in which soft-tissue injuries, sprains, strains, and contusions are commonplace; however, certain recreational activities pose unique life-threatening problems beyond trauma. Table 34–2 lists outdoor activities participants commonly engage in and additional problems encountered beyond accidental injury.

Finally, attention to the environmental extremes of an expedition's locale is paramount to successful planning. One must know the precise geographic location and have an in-depth appreciation for the travel terrain, altitude, expected temperature ranges and humidity, precipitation patterns, and issues related to air and water quality. A simplified way to conceptualize evaluating an environment locale is to recognize that outdoor travel is influenced by four key factors: the land itself, the local atmosphere, quality of air/water, and expected extremes of temperature. Table 34–3 identifies the latter four, highlighting key factors to consider in order to maximize safe outdoor travel.

EPIDEMIOLOGIC CONSIDERATIONS IN WILDERNESS TRAVEL

It is difficult to make precise statements on the occurrence risk of injuries and illness associated with outdoor travel. There are no structured systems in place that routinely review and require the reporting of medical problems occurring during outdoor travel. Prospective follow-up of special interest groups and retrospective analysis of emergency medical services from national parks have helped to better describe the incidence and types of injuries seen with outdoor travel. Gradually, wilderness epidemiology is evolving to characterize injuries and illness patterns; however, precise incidence rates cannot be given as they likely vary according to a participant's experience level and performance capabilities.

Despite such limitations, the expected proportion of accidental injuries to illness occurring during travel is remarkably constant. Most studies demonstrate that traumatic injury, generally of a minor nature, exceeds medical illness experienced by outdoor participants by roughly threefold. When reviewing injury patterns, most are minor, consisting predominantly of soft-tissue damage (abrasions/contusions/lacerations), sprains, or strains, with serious dislocations or bony fractures accounting for <5% of all trauma. The lower extremities are by far the most likely to be involved in minor orthopedic injury,

Table 34–3.   ENVIRONMENTAL HAZARDS ASSOCIATED WITH ADVENTURE TRAVEL

ISSUES OF CONCERN	FACTORS TO CONSIDER
Terrain characteristics	Ability to traverse safely/maintain orientation
	Exposure to air, wind, and solar radiation
	Suitability for camping/ability to find shelter
	Native animal and insect habitat/risk for injury or infection
The air about you	Outdoor pollutant standard index for large cities
	Poor indoor quality from fossil fuels/inadequate ventilation
	Existing pulmonary disease and airway hyperactivity
	Elevation, rate of ascent, and risk of mountain sickness
The water about you	Contamination and risk of water-borne infectious disease
	Industrial waste dumping and exposure to chemical toxins
	Freshwater infection risk of schistosomiasis/leptospirosis
	Injuries, infections, and toxic envenomation from aquatic life
Extremes of temperature and weather	Risk for hypothermia or frostbite
	Potential for development of heatstroke
	Prevention of dehydration or cramps with extreme activity
	Solar radiation exposure/acute and long-term skin injury

Reprinted with permission from Zell SC. Environmental and recreational hazards associated with adventure travel. J Travel Med 1997;4:94–99.

with the most common mechanism of occurrence attributed to tripping or short falls while trekking. The implication for expedition participants is obvious: select footwear appropriate to the task at hand providing the best stability and protection from lower extremity injury and carry on-person first-aid material to treat minor abrasions and orthopedic problems from strains and sprains.

Granted that persons embarking on adventure travel fear the acquisition of unusual infectious disease, such occurrence is actually rare if one receives appropriate pretravel advice and recommended vaccines. In reality, most infections reported in wilderness travelers are attributable to nonspecific syndromes such as gastroenteritis or upper respiratory illness. Both likely result from crowded conditions, precluding the practice of adequate hygienic measures. Other commonly reported medical problems include headache (exacerbated by high altitude), dyspepsia due to local food intolerance, dermatitis and sunburn, dehydration/heatstroke from inadequate fluid intake, and worrisome allergic reactions related to insect stings. Thus, expeditioners should supplement their first-aid kits with

appropriate analgesics for pain, antacids and antimotility agents for dyspepsia, and anithistamines for allergic reactions while taking appropriate skin care with sunscreens and lotions to prevent drying and cracking.

In reviewing the outdoor travel literature, one finds that the most deaths are attributable to sudden cardiac arrest, which is likely because of the number of older travelers venturing outside. After excluding deaths from cardiac causes, drowning remains the number one cause of accidental death in outdoor participants. In fact, white-water paddling has been noted to have the highest specific-activity injury rate, suggesting that participants engaging in this recreational activity be uniquely prepared for resuscitation of drowning victims in the setting of significant exposure hypothermia. Ice or rock climbing is another activity having its unique array of injuries with concern related to rare traumatic death from severe head trauma. Participants' awareness of such events is critical to make certain that appropriate first-aid equipment, not routinely found in most kits, is on site to deal with such emergencies. Recommendations for such unique supplies are covered in the section on specific equipment purchases.

COMMERCIAL ADVENTURE TRAVEL: PARTICIPANT'S EXPECTATIONS

After performing a thorough itinerary review to elicit potential recreational hazards and characterize expected injury and illness, one should perform an informal inventory to asses the expedition's preparedness to deal with potential emergencies. What can a traveler expect from commercial adventure travel companies? Support services vary from one company to another. In an effort to profile commercial outfitters, the author identified 25 companies offering travel to the highly popular areas of central Africa and Nepal. Companies were contacted by mail and specifically asked to address the following: level of medical expertise and training of group leader and provision of a community first-aid kit and supplies, along with any requirements for pretravel certification. Twenty-three companies responded to the latter queries, providing a better picture of the support available to expedition participants and hence the gaps that individuals must fill for ensuring safe travel.

Only five companies (22%) stated that their group leader was trained in first aid and no commercial company provided either an on-site physician or nurse. Six outfitters (24%) clearly stated that first-aid supplies were the responsibility of the participant, the vast majority providing some type of community medical kit to deal with minor accidental trauma. Carrying a personal emergency kit (Table 34–4) is still advisable primarily for one's support in the event of search and rescue. However, expecting the dispensing of prescription medicines, such as antibiotics, antidiarrheals, or narcotic analgesics, is not realistic; hence, a traveler might wish to obtain prescriptions for the latter from one's personal physician. Also, consideration should be given a medical examination and

Table 34–4. CONTENTS OF A PERSONAL KIT FOR EMERGENCY SURVIVAL

FIRST-AID SUPPLIES	BASIC SURVIVAL EQUIPMENT
Adhesive tape	Swiss Army knife
Band-Aids	Nylon cord
Sterile 4 × 4 dressing pad	Whistle, small reflective mirror
Elastic bandage wrap	Waterproof matches
Triangular bandage	Poncho
Alcohol pads	Reflective thermal blanket
Scissors	High-energy sports snackbar
Extra-strength Tylenol	Canteen with potable water

clearance especially for the elderly or in special patient populations (see final section). Only four adventure travel companies (17%) provided a health screening questionnaire as part of their general application process, making it clearly the responsibility of participants to review their medical fitness for outdoor travel.

UNIQUE HAZARDS ASSOCIATED WITH ADVENTURE TRAVEL

Various recreational activities deserve special attention as they modify the general risk of accidental injury during outdoor travel and necessitate special equipment or medicines beyond those found in a general first-aid kit. For persons traveling to extremes of altitude, a lightweight nylon hyperbaric chamber that can be pressurized by a portable foot pump may be critical to treat expeditioners suffering from pulmonary or cerebral edema. Sustained-release nifedipine tablets and diamox may be useful during high-altitude trekking to manage pulmonary edema, whereas decadron primarily mitigates cerebral edema. Portable oxygen (low-flow 2 L/min) is of value at altitudes above 15,000 feet during sleep when periodic breathing results in alveolar hypoventilation.

For serious cold weather expeditions, consideration should be given to a hypothermic stabilizer bag consisting of a high-pile synthetic fabric with a chest window carved out to allow cardiopulmonary resuscitation. A low reading thermometer (to at least 82°F) helps detect severe exposure hypothermia. Participants may wish to carry warming pads for their hands and feet, commercially available, that on air exposure produce an exothermic reaction generating heat for frostbite prevention.

Whitewater rating and kayaking place one at risk for water-borne infections, making a high-quality and portable filtration system a prerequisite. In light of potential for accidental drowning, an oral airway may be of value to assist in resuscitation efforts.

Mountain and rock climbing activities place one at risk for dislocations, broken bones, and traumatic head injury. Specific equipment purchases such as an air splint, triangular bandage, and soft cervical collar to manage fractures, shoulder dislocations, and head trauma, respectively, are essential during high-risk climbing.

Finally, tropical travel may require the purchase of mosquito nets for sleeping and permethin spray to treat outdoor clothing and netting. In light of expected high heat and humidity, dehydration can occur, quickly necessitating some type of packaged oral rehydration solution having salt and potassium linked to glucose for active transport into the intravascular compartment. Table 34–5 lists specialized equipment purchases to carry as a function of recreational activities chosen.

CONSIDERATIONS FOR SPECIAL POPULATIONS

PULMONARY DISEASE

Persons with asthma and chronic obstructive pulmonary disease (COPD) may experience exacerbations as a result of hypoxia from high altitude or secondary to reactive airway disease from noxious environmental stimuli. Asthmatics may experience wheezing during travel triggered by exercise in the setting of cold, dry air or as a result of poor air quality. Outdoor pollutants such as byproducts of fossil fuel can be irritable to asthmatics provoking attacks. Winds can "stir up" larger particulate matter such as dust or sand. Indoor air quality may be troublesome due to inadequate ventilation and from exposure to second-hand smoke. Besides carrying a beta-agonist metered dose inhaler, asthmatics should carry a 2-week course of an oral steroid (prednisone) along with a wide-spectrum oral antibiotic. Finally, carrying a surgical face mask to pro-

Table 34–5. SPECIALIZED EQUIPMENT FOR RECREATIONAL AND ENVIRONMENTAL ACTIVITIES

High Altitude	*Bicycling*
Gamow Bag™ and accessories	All-terrain Cyclist Kit™
Gamow Tent™	Hydrogel occlusive dressing
The Breathing Bladder™	
Portable air compressor	*Mountain Climbing/Hiking*
EPAP mask with headstrap	SAM® splint
Portable pulse oximeter	Air-Stirrup ankle brace
	Adjustable, cervical collar
Cold Exposure	
External thermal stabilizer bag	*Tropical/Third-World Travel*
Grabber® warmers	Permethin repellent
Hotronic foot warmers	Oral rehydration salts packet
Space® thermal reflective survival bag	TropicScreen mosquito net
	Sawyer Extractor™
Low reading thermometer	
Watersports	
CPR Microshield™	
Disposable airway protector	
Katadyn or PUR Explorer™ filter	

Reprinted with permission from Zell SC, Goodman PH. Wilderness equipment and medical supplies. In: Auerbach PS, ed. Wilderness medicine: Management of wilderness and environmental emergencies. 3rd rev. Ed. St. Louis: Mosby-Year Book, 1995:413–445.

tect against particulates during periods of outdoor travel and strong winds is advisable.

For those with COPD, the real concern for outdoor travel rests with alveolar hypoxia that ensues at high altitudes. Near 8,000 feet, ventilation must increase to prevent arterial oxygen desaturation. Studies of aircraft pressurized to the latter altitude reveal that travelers with COPD having a forced expiratory volume (FEV) 1 of <50% predicted will experience dyspnea and usually demonstrate hypoxemia on room air at sea level (PaO_2 <55 mm Hg). This level of respiratory dysfunction serves as a general guideline regarding what altitude such persons can safely travel to (maximum 8,000 ft). Absolute contraindications to high-altitude travel include persons with pulmonary hypertension and cor pulmonale, recent pulmonary embolism, sickle cell disease, and sleep apnea. In those persons with mild to moderate COPD judged to have adequate pulmonary reserve, it is still advised not to exceed sleeping above the 10,000-foot level due to nocturnal desaturation and to avoid the use of sedative hypnotics that may further depress respirations and increase hypoxia.

CARDIOVASCULAR DISEASE

Outdoor adventure travel places burdens on those with underlying heart disease that adversely limit exercise endurance and can provoke angina. Physiologic responses include a release of catecholamines producing increased pulse and systolic blood pressures. An increased afterload compromises forward blood flow in persons with heart disease unable to effectively augment their cardiac output. There is great debate concerning the evaluation and advice a physician should provide to persons with cardiovascular disease. No controlled studies exist to justify that outdoor travel, especially at high altitude, confers additional risk to such individuals. Cardiac patients with predictable angina of mild to moderate level may travel if able to exercise by Bruce protocol for at least 9 minutes. In such persons, careful attention must be paid to pace themselves proportionately to expected declines in available oxygen since its consumption limits work capacity at a higher altitude. As a guideline, activity levels should be scaled down to a target heart rate that is roughly 75% of one's ischemic threshold. Absolute contraindications to vigorous adventure travel include those with unstable angina and persons with heart disease limiting daily activities at rest or those with congestive failure or valvular disease such as aortic stenosis. Finally, persons with cardiac disease must remember to carry a copy of their most recent electrocardiogram and complete medicine list during foreign travel.

NEUROLOGIC DISORDERS

There are no data to suggest that altitude reduces seizure threshold; thus, epileptics controlled on medicines may travel safely. Persons with a prior history of stroke or transient ischemic attack can participate in outdoor travel if attention is paid to adequate hydration and aspirin is taken to combat decreases in blood viscosity. Persons with recurrent headaches need to be reminded that high-altitude travel may produce headache and, as a result, should travel with appropriate prescription analgesics.

GASTROINTESINAL DISORDERS

Protection against enteric infections is mediated by stomach acid, so persons receiving potent proton pump inhibitors for management of acid reflux are at an increased risk of water-borne enteric infections. Persons with inflammatory bowel disease may suffer blood-borne dissemination of bacterial pathogens more easily when infected. As a result, for the latter two, meticulous attention to water quality is key. Any dubious water sources should be both filtered and then boiled prior to consumption. Consideration should be given to carrying a fluoroquinolone to treat bouts of diarrhea.

MISCELLANEOUS

Antihypertensive medicines taken during travel may exacerbate dehydration and hypokalemia due to fluid loss from exertion or diarrhea. Such persons should carry a packaged electrolyte replacement (oral rehydration solution) and a source of potassium (dried orange slices/bananas). HIV infection should not preclude outdoor travel as long as such persons pay meticulous attention to water disinfection and receive special immunizations to include pneumococcal, influenza, and hepatitis A vaccines. The latter should also be given to the elderly because of their greater morbidity with such infections plus tetanus immunization, since antibodies are often inadequate in this age group. Finally, diabetics deserve special attention (see Chapter 38) as the challenges to outdoor travel include disruption of normal meal schedules, maintenance of adequate supplies, and ability to self-monitor and initiate treatment for extremes of blood glucose.

RECOMMENDED REFERENCES

General Planning

Zell SC. Common questions: environmental and recreational hazards associated with adventure travel. J Travel Med 1997;4:94–99.

Zell SC, Goodman PH. Wilderness equipment and medical supplies. In: Auerbach P, ed. Wilderness medicine: management of wilderness and environmental emergencies. St. Louis: Mosby-Year Book, 1995:413–445.

Epidemiology of Outdoor Injury and Illness

Basnyat B, Litch JA. Medical problems of porters and trekkers in the Nepal Himalaya. Wilderness Environ Med 1997;8:78–81.

Bowie WS, Hunt TK, Allen HA. Rock-climbing injuries in Yosemite National Park. West J Med 1988;149:172–177.

Crouse BJ, Josephs D. Health care needs of Appalachian trail hikers. J Fam Pract 1993;36:521–525.

Gentile DA, Morris JA, Schimelpfenig T, et al. Wilderness injuries and illnesses. Ann Emerg Med 1992;21:853–861.

Johnson J, Maertins M, Shalit M, et al. Wilderness emergency medical services: the experiences at Sequoia and Kings Canyon National Parks. Am J Emerg Med 1991;9:211–216.

Montalvo R, Wingard DL, Bracker M, Davidson TM. Morbidity and mortality in the wilderness. West J Med 1998;168:248–254.

Welch TP. Data-based selection of medical supplies for wilderness travel. Wilderness Environ Med 1997;8:148–151.

Considerations for Special Populations

Backer H. Medical limitations to wilderness travel. Emerg Med Clin North Am 1997;15(1):17–41.

Bartsch P, Maggiorini M, Ritter M, et al. Prevention of high-altitude pulmonary edema by nifedipine. N Engl J Med 1991;325: 1284–1289.

Bia FJ, Barry M. Special health considerations for travelers. Med Clin North Am 1992;76:1295–1312.

Bezruchka S. High altitude medicine. Med Clin North Am 1992;76:1481–1497.

Kidson W. The problems of travel in diabetes. Med J Aust 1979; 1:125–126.

McIntosh IB. Health hazards and the elderly traveler. J Travel Med 1998;5:27–29.

Oelz O, Ritter M, Jenni R, et al. Nifedipine for high altitude pulmonary oedema. Lancet 1989;2:1241–1244.

Van Gompel A, Kozarsky P, Colebunders R. Adult travelers with HIV infection. J Travel Med 1997;4:136–143.

Chapter 35

THE MIGRANT AS A TRAVELER

LOUIS LOUTAN AND HASSAN GHAZNAWI

In the present globalized world, migrants are part of the increasing mobility of individuals and populations shaping a new epidemiologic environment. Travelers and migrants are key elements in the worldwide circulation of germs and pathogens, resistant strains, contributing to the import and export of common or exotic diseases.[1] Mobility not only means crossing geobiologic boundaries, it also implies crossing sociocultural areas and thus has an impact on health services, with health professionals facing problems of different kinds, such as different health beliefs, different cultural interpretations of diseases, communication difficulties, and health consequences of organized violence. In a globally mobile world, it is of key importance to understand the impact of mobility on the health of those moving and of the population who receive them.[2] What are the specificities and commonalities of each group? What specific risks are for what group? How can each be approached to modify risk perception and behavior?

Are travelers migrants or are migrants travelers? In general, *travelers* cross international borders on a two-way ticket, traveling between rich countries or from rich to poor countries for a limited period of time. Their contacts with the local population will be sporadic, living mostly in comfortable hotels. They may be exposed to poor hygiene and foreign germs and bring some home with them. Most travel for leisure, some for business or other professional purposes. As a whole, the traveler is rather well off, moves voluntarily for a short period of time, and returns home as planned. *Migrants*, in essence, are also travelers, but they travel on a one-way ticket, leaving their country of origin, often poor with specific disease burden, for good or for a long period of time, seeking socioeconomic opportunities in richer countries. Their contact with the local population will be long-lasting, primarily with their kin, at kindergartens, schools, and worksites. They face new sociocultural norms, language, and restrictions, with often reduced access to health care and prevention. Migrants represent an inhomogeneous group of culturally and ethnically diverse individuals and communities. In general, the term migrant refers to individuals with modest socioeconomic status. Various categories are referred to such as immigrants, refugees, asylum seekers, migrant workers, and illegal migrants.

International migration is a worldwide phenomenon, not restricted to industrialized nations. According to the United Nations Population Division, there are 120 million international migrants in the world in 1990, rising from 75 million in 1965, with an annual growth rate of 1.9%.[3] In

1990, international migrants accounted for 2.3% of the world's population. They made up 18% of the total population in Australia and New Zealand, nearly 11% in Western Asia, less than 9% in North America, over 6% in Western Europe, and less than 2.5% in Asia, Africa, and Latin America. Net international migration contributed to 45% of the population growth in the developed world for 1990–1995. In Europe, it contributed to almost 88% of the population growth during this period. The number of refugees has increased markedly, reaching a maximum in 1993 of 18.2 million. Since then, the number of refugees has been decreasing to 13.2 million in 1996, a decline due to major repatriations. By January 1997, the total number of persons of concern to the United Nations High Commissioner for Refugees (UNHCR) (including internally displaced persons) was 22.7 million.[4] The number of persons seeking asylum also increased drastically until 1992, then stabilized due to more restrictive policies of the receiving countries. Between 1985 and 1995, over 5 million asylum applications have been registered in industrialized states. Finally, irregular (illegal) migration is on the rise. There is an estimated 5 million irregular migrants in the U.S.A. and 3 million in Western Europe.[5] Trafficking in migrants has become a very lucrative illegal market, with worldwide ramifications. Having no legal status and living with the constant fear of being deported, illegal migrants represent a very vulnerable population with very little access to health care. Table 35–1 gives comparative statistics on international migration.

MIGRATION AND HEALTH

The health of migrants will vary enormously according to specific living conditions, previous exposure to communicable diseases, deprivation or violence, professional risks, degree of integration into the new society, access to health care, ability to communicate, and presence or absence of a community or family safety net. One cannot compare health problems of refugees in camps of a war-torn region to those of well-integrated immigrants in Canada or Europe.

Most of the data on migration and health come from specific surveys on specific groups of migrants or services or through medical screening programs at the time of entry into the host country. Routinely gathered data on the health of ethnic minorities or of foreign-born residents are often lacking in this area. Thus, one should be cautious in not generalizing the conclusions of specific studies to all

Table 35–1. WORLDWIDE MAGNITUDE OF MIGRATION: SOME INDICATIVE FIGURES

International migrants (1990)[3]	120 million
Victims of forced displacement (1997)[4]	50 million
Refugees	13 million
Other persons of concern to United Nations High Commissioner for Refugees	9 million
Internally displaced persons	20 million
Asylum seekers to industrialized countries[4]	5 million
Irregular/illegal immigrants (U.S.A. and Western Europe)[5]	8 million

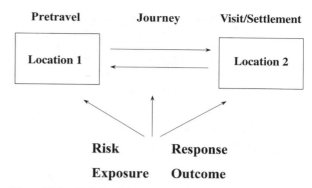

Figure 35–1. Relation between risk and stages of travel.

migrants and, in doing so, contributing to the negative perception of migrants and to some indirect form of discrimination.

A recent review of health issues and problems of migrants in the European Union illustrates that, compared to the host population, migrants have less access to health services and often have a higher rate of certain diseases such as tuberculosis, HIV, hepatitis B, accidental injuries, psychosomatic problems, and depression.[6] Does migration in itself constitute an unhealthy process and put people on the move at higher risk of diseases? Do we have a biased view on the health of migrants through studies uncontrolled for socioeconomic disadvantages or unequal access to health services?[7] No doubt, migration is a very selective process, and those arriving in industrialized nations as immigrants, refugees, or asylum seekers may not be representative of the population they come from. It takes remarkable courage and energy to decide to leave your family and country for good to start a new life abroad in a foreign and unknown environment. Financial resources are also needed to reach the final destination through expensive illegal connections. Thus, those heading for this "adventure" are probably stronger in their mind and body than those staying at home.

TRAVELING AS A MIGRANT

Comparing the process of traveling for travelers or migrants (i.e., leaving one location for another) may encompass very different conditions in terms of duration, environment, exposure, and risks. For travelers, risks and exposure are minimal and travel conditions are comfortable (Figure 35–1).

For migrants, traveling has different implications and content. They often originate from poor countries with lower hygiene standards and with higher prevalence of endemic diseases they may have been exposed to and carry with them (tuberculosis, intestinal parasites). The journey itself may be long, with much hardship and deprivation encountered. Migrants may be exposed to insecurity and abuse; deportation is also feared. Low socioeconomic status in the host country, poor lodging, overcrowding, communication difficulties, and limited access to health care all contribute to an increased risk of poor health outcome.

As immigration and asylum regulations become more restrictive, a growing number of migrants are denied asylum or immigrant status. They then face possible deportation or have to live illegally in the host country. Forced return to their home country may put refugees at high risk not only of infectious diseases but of retaliation by local authorities for having left to go abroad.

There are no studies on the direct impact of the travel process on the health of refugees until they have arrived in the host country. Much information on health comes from medical sceening programs, which are mandatory at the time of entry into the host country. Data show that, according to the region of origin, a significant proportion of refugees and asylum seekers arriving in Europe or in North America have been exposed to tuberculosis and hepatitis B and have a high carriage rate of intestinal parasites[8] (Table 35–2). Screening for exposure to trauma and violence shows an over 60% prevalence rate.[9]

In this chapter, we are not looking at the impact on health of the initial journey of migrants, leaving their home country for a new destination, nor on the asylum

Table 35–2. RESULTS OF MEDICAL SCREENING OF ASYLUM SEEKERS IN SWITZERLAND

	PREVALENCE (%)
Tuberculosis	290/100,000
Hepatitis B	
HBsAg positive	827/13,673 (6)
Anti-ABs positive	3,923/11,137 (35.2)
HBeAg positive	115/756 (15.2)
Syphilis	
VDRL/TPHA positive	78/13,148 (0.6)
Intestinal parasites	
positive	2,539/9,371 (27.1)
Intestinal bacteria	
Salmonella spp	19/8,465 (<0.5)
Shigella spp	29/8,465 (<0.5)

*From HBsAg-positive subjects only.
Adapted from Raeber et al.[8]

seekers being forced to travel back home. We shall concentrate on the migrants being granted residency in the host country, who have an opportunity to visit their home country as travelers. In countries with large ethnic minorities such as England, Canada, and the U.S.A., resident migrants traveling constitute a substantial population.

TRAVEL-ASSOCIATED DISEASES IN MIGRANTS

There are no epidemiologic studies looking prospectively at the risks of migrant travelers of acquiring diseases while returning to their country of origin to visit relatives or conduct business. Data from studies on specific diseases such as malaria or tuberculosis show that residents of foreign origin represent a growing proportion of cases of malaria or tuberculosis, suggesting a higher risk of exposure or insufficient protection taken.[10]

MALARIA

With changing migration and population movements and an increasing influx to Europe of refugees and immigrants from countries where malaria is endemic, an increased proportion of cases of malaria has been recorded in migrants. In Italy, it rose from 14% in 1986 to 40.4% in 1991.[11] In Marseilles (France), Comorians living in this city represented a substantial proportion of imported cases.[12] In an academic medical center in Amsterdam, during the 1991–1994 period a growing proportion of cases of malaria seen is non-Dutch, representing 58% for falciparum malaria compared to only 15% in 1979–1988. Of particular concern were the nonimmune non-Dutch and their children raised in the Netherlands.[13] In England between 1987 and 1992, 49% of 8,355 cases of malaria occurred in ethnic minority travelers visiting friends and relatives. Visitors and immigrants made 19% and 11%, respectively.[10] In a study comparing ethnic minority travelers to U.K. tourists with imported malaria, 51% versus 20%, respectively, were not taking any prophylaxis. It may well be that risk perception in these two groups may be very different. They may believe that they have retained some immunity, having lived at their destination, and thus do not seek pretravel health advice and do not take prophylaxis. The attack rate of those visiting West Africa was three times higher compared to business travelers or tourists. This may be related to a higher rate of transmission in the places visited, rural versus urban, unprotected houses versus-air-conditioned hotels, with less protection. The author reports also on the frequent development of malaria in semi-immune adults who live in malarious endemic countries soon after arrival in the U.K. The development could be stress related (80% of 300 patients studied developed symptoms within 2 weeks of arrival).

Similar observations have been made in hospital-based studies. One prospective study of fever in children in the U.K. who had recently spent time in the tropics showed that most of the cases were among children of former immigrants who had visited their family's country of origin.[14]

TUBERCULOSIS

In North America and Europe, there has been a steady decrease in tuberculosis, whereas it has been increasing worldwide since the late 1980s. In the U.S.A., in 1996, the number of reported cases had still decreased, although there had been an increase in the proportion of cases diagnosed in the foreign born.[15] Similar trends are reported in Europe.[16] In Germany and France, migrants are three to six times, respectively, more likely to be diagnosed with tuberculosis than nonimmigrants.[6] In Denmark, the proportion of foreign-born cases has risen from 18% in 1986 to 60% in 1996.[6] An earlier study in Denmark on childhood tuberculosis had shown a much higher annual incidence rate in the foreign born (68 to 200/100,000) compared to Danish children (5/100,000). Intrafamilial origin of transmission was most frequent, and 10% had visited the country of birth a few months prior to the diagnosis.[17] The incidence rates of tuberculosis in ethnic minority children were lower than those recorded in their country of origin. In England, travelers visiting friends and relatives in Asia accounted for 20% of all notifications, with 80% reported within 3 years of return to the U.K.[18] These data suggest that there is some risk of transmission, particularly in children, when migrants visit family and friends in their country of origin. Recent studies using DNA fingerprinting show a higher level of transmission within subpopulations, particularly immigrants, but a lower level to the receiving population.[19]

HEPATITIS

Hepatitis A is highly prevalent in the developing world with an estimated risk of infection in travelers of 1 case per 300 nonimmune travelers per month. In endemic countries, almost 100% of children by the age of 10 have anti-hepatitis A virus antibodies. Thus, adult migrants who have lived during their childhood in their country of origin can be considered immune and at no risk of acquiring hepatitis A. This is not the case for their children, who are at risk of acquiring it while visiting tropical countries. In the Netherlands, the imported cases of hepatitis A in children (0 to 15 years) are practically all in children from ethnic minority groups after a visit to their country of origin, causing small outbreaks in schools and daycare centers.[20]

In Asia and Africa, hepatitis B (HB) prevalence in the general population is high, with over 5% carriers of the HBs antigen. Migrants and asylum seekers screened at time of arrival have higher carriage rates of the HBs antigen than the host country population. In asylum seekers screened for HB at the time of entry into Switzerland, 34% had a marker for HB, with 6% being carriers of the HBsAg with marked variation in prevalence rates according to origin and age.[8] In countries where HB vaccination in early childhood is not implemented yet, HB vaccination should systematically be proposed to children of ethnic minority origin to prevent maternal and intrafamilial transmission, and also in the case of traveling to their country of origin.

HIV/AIDS AND SEXUALLY TRANSMITTED DISEASES

The HIV/AIDS epidemic hits the hardest developing countries. Migrants coming from these parts of the world are at higher risk of having been or being exposed to the virus. One should be cautious in not generalizing such statements to all migrant groups. Migrants coming from rural areas may be at lower risk than those from urban origin. Furthermore, there are still many areas, particularly in the Middle East and Asia, where the prevalence is much lower than in industrialized countries, putting migrants at higher risk of contamination after arrival in the host country. Nevertheless, the prevalence of the disease in certain migrant communities is higher than in the host population.[21] Traveling back to their country of origin may put migrants at a higher risk of contamination. A survey in six major sexually transmitted disease outpatient clinics in Switzerland showed that 78% and over of patients of foreign origin had acquired a sexually transmitted disease after a recent visit in their region of origin.[22]

Mandatory screening for HIV/AIDS is required by a large number of countries either for long-term residency applicants (students, expatriates) or for those asking for refugee or immigrant status. These requirements are often considered unethical and discriminatory, being implemented more for political or economical reasons than based on sound public health grounds.

MENINGOCOCCAL MENINGITIS

The risk of aquiring meningococcal disease for the standard traveler remains low, estimated at 0.4 per million per month.[23] Although the disease has a worldwide distribution, large-scale epidemics occur in sub-Saharan Africa along the meningitis belt, from Senegal to Sudan, but also in East Africa. Epidemics occurred also in India, Nepal, Mongolia, and Saudi Arabia. Large gatherings of people, particularly refugees, may trigger epidemics of meningococcal disease. This has also occurred during the 1987 pilgrimage to Mecca. During this outbreak, 40 pilgrims among 21,250 who came from England, France, Israel, and the U.S.A. became ill. The overall attack rate was at least 2,000 per million. It was 640 per 100,000 over a 1-month period among American pilgrims. The carriage rate of *Neisseria meningitidis* was 11% of 318 pilgrims who had visited Mecca or Medina.[24] Since this outbreak, vaccination against meningococcal meningitis is required for all pilgrims to Mecca. Migrants visiting their home country, with close contacts with family and friends, particularly in those known for the occurrence of epidemics, should be informed of the risk of aquiring meningococcal meningitis and should be immunized with one dose of polysaccharide vaccine. This applies to West African countries but also East Africa, Nepal, and Mongolia.

ENTERIC DISEASES

Diarrhea and other enteric diseases remain the most frequent health problems encountered by travelers. Coming from countries of endemicity, medical screening programs at the time of arrival have shown that migrants have a high prevalence of intestinal parasites, over 40% depending on the origin.[8] Severe infestation may impair normal growth in children or cause anemia or gastrointestinal symptoms. According to origin, schistosomiasis or liver flukes should be looked for. In areas with large ethnic communities such as California, where Hispanics visit their country of origin, amebiasis is seen frequently. Of 67 amebic liver abscesses treated in a hospital in San Diego, 80% were in patients of Hispanic origin.[25] Typhoid has also become an imported disease in most industrialized countries. A high proportion of cases are imported from the Indian subcontinent. Ethnic minorities from this part of the world are at higher risk of acquiring it. In Scotland, a high proportion of cases are contracted by them (E. Walker, personal communication). In France, up to 69% of imported cases are seen in foreigners, who acquired the diseases mainly in North Africa.[26]

OTHER COMMUNICABLE DISEASES

Visiting family and friends in their country of origin puts migrants at risks of many other parasitic, viral, and bacterial diseases. Loiasis and other types of filariasis should be looked at. Regular visits back home in central African countries, particularly when rural, put migrants at high risk. The majority of cases of loiasis seen in Geneva are imported from Cameroon in foreign African residents visiting their home village. Other parasitic diseases, such as schistosomiasis, echinococcosis, and ectoparasites, can be contracted while returning home, particularly in a rural setting. Schistosomiasis may be a more real risk for children, who have a higher chance than adults of swimming and playing in water. This is particularly the case in Africa but also in certain places in Latin America. In cases of epilepsy, cysticercosis should be looked for. Vector-borne diseases other than malaria should be mentioned. Migrants visiting home, particularly rural areas, should be aware of the potential risk of acquiring them. Japanese encephalitis is one for which an effective vaccine is available. Dengue fever is another, with the increased risk of hemorrhagic complications in case of successive infections, particularly for children. Visceral or cutaneous leishmaniasis is prevalent in many parts of the world. African and American trypanosomiasis are also prevalent. Appropriate vector control personal measures should be taken, such as use of repellants and impregnated bednets at night.

RABIES

Rabies is present in most tropical countries. A review of cases of rabies in Europe shows that 70% of cases were imported.[27] In France, since 1994, five cases have been reported in foreign-born residents returning to visit friends and relatives in their country of origin (Mali, Algeria) and in French travelers.[28] Migrants visiting home with children should be aware of the existing risk of rabies, both in rural and urban settings. Appropriate behavior with dogs and other domestic animals should be respected and pre-exposure rabies vaccination recommended, particularly for children.

ACCIDENTS AND INJURIES

Accidents and injuries remain the main cause of death in travelers. For Peace Corps volunteers living in simple conditions and using local means of transportation, traffic accidents accounted for 48% of all causes of death.[29] Rapid urbanization and an increasing number of vehicles of all sorts in many developing countries have led to a sharp increase in traffic accidents. Visiting home may imply using local public tranportation. The migrant traveler should be aware of these risks and instructed to use a seatbelt when available and a helmet on motorbikes (even better, completely avoid using motorbikes!), check the status of tires and car before renting or using it, and avoid traveling at night or when visibility is reduced.

ARE MIGRANT TRAVELERS AT HIGHER RISKS?

Until good epidemiologic data exist, we should be very cautious in claiming this evidence, as very often we may have preconceived ideas and stereotypes on specific groups' behavior and knowledge. Nonetheless, the increased number of imported cases of malaria, hepatitis A, typhoid, and tuberculosis in migrants visiting friends and relatives or conducting business in their country of origin suggests that they are at high risk of acquiring diseases. It is not clear if they are more exposed or underestimate risks of acquiring communicable diseases and thus do not take adequate preventive measures. This could be due to the fact that they are "returning home," a place they know, which is felt to be safe and familiar. They may underestimate the risks of returning to rural areas with a high level of transmission of vector-borne diseases and enteropathogens due to lower levels of hygiene and clean water. Futhermore, being previously immune or semi-immune to diseases such as malaria or certain enteric germs, they may not be aware of having lost their immunity after a prolonged time living in nonendemic areas such as European and North American countries. Thus, they may not know or feel the necessity of taking prophylactic measures. Also, bringing their children born in Europe with them, who are not immune to malaria or hepatitis A, puts them at risk if not properly protected. Visiting home, particularly in rural areas, may include the risks listed on Table 35–3.

There may also be factors lowering the risks of acquiring diseases. Knowing the places visited, the areas at risk of transmission or insecurity, and having close contacts with people locally for help if needed may reduce risks of exposure.

As for other types of travelers, some groups of migrant travelers are more vulnerable. These are the very young, those with chronic diseases, and the elderly.

CHILDREN

Children visiting relatives in their country of origin, particularly in hot climates, may be at special risk.

Table 35–3.   POTENTIAL RISK FACTORS FOR MIGRANT TRAVELERS VISITING THEIR HOME COUNTRY

Exposure to hot and dry or humid climate with no or little access to air conditioning

Simple conditions of living with little protection from vector-borne diseases

Little control over the safety of food and water while visiting friends and relatives

Eating locally prepared meals

Prolonged periods of exposure in areas of high level of transmission of malaria or other endemic communicable diseases (loiasis, meningitis, leishmaniasis, Japanese encephalitis)

Vacation and visiting time corresponding to the rainy season and time of high transmission of vector-borne diseases

Use of local means of transportation of poor quality with higher risks of traffic accident and injury

Living in areas with little access to medical services

Communicable Diseases   Parents may underestimate the risk of exposure to certain communicable diseases such as malaria and hepatitis A and B, for which they may have full or a certain degree of immunity but which may not be the case of their children. Appropriate chemoprophylaxis or vaccination is needed. Swimming and playing in water may expose children to schistozomiasis. They may be tempted to play with dogs and other domestic animals and be exposed to rabies. Pre-exposure vaccination should be recommended. Parents should be instructed on how to manage cases of diarrhea to avoid dehydration in their children (oral rehydration solution, adequate diet, antibiotics). Possible transmission from close relatives or from other children of hepatitis B, tuberculosis, and meningitis should be discussed and immunization recommended.

Environment   A hot climate, high degree of humidity, and dust may all be causative of various health problems to children: dehydration, skin reaction to sweat and heat, sunstroke and heat exhaustion, skin irritation, infection to dust, etc. Adequate all-cotton and ample clothing, sun protection, and sufficient fluid intake are among the necessary prevention measures that should be provided to children.

Injuries and Trauma   Traffic accidents, riding a bicycle without a helmet, playing in an unprotected environment, contact with garbage, etc. increases the risk of accidents and wounds. Parents should assess potential hazards to their children in their new surroundings.

Access to Care   Access to health professionals and to medicine may be limited. Parents should anticipate and see to what extent some basic medications should be taken with them. Children may be seen by traditional healers and given locally made medicine. There are some risks linked to traditional remedies that parents should be aware of.

MIGRANT TRAVELERS WITH CHRONIC DISEASES

Visiting family and friends living in a tropical environment, with important climatic changes, increased risk of infection, different food and diet, relative isolation, and little access to health services and medicine, may cause difficulties for the migrant traveler with a chronic disease such as hypertension, diabetes, asthma, or bowel inflammatory disease. Compliance to diet and medication at the time of family visits may be difficult because of high expectations and frequent solicitations from relatives and friends, less control on meals offered, culturally determined constraints, etc. Patients should be instructed on how to anticipate and adjust to these constraints and changes in order to avoid decompensation of their underlying condition. Sufficient supply of medicine should be taken, hand carried and in separate luggage in case of delay or loss.

PILGRIMS

Pilgrimages represent a special type of travel in which migrants often participate, many of them being of old age. In various parts of the world, important pilgrimages take place every year, drawing visitors from numerous countries and diverse cultural backgrounds. The Hajj, the annual pilgrimage to Mecca, is one of the most important. Over 10 to 20 days, close to 2 million Muslims from over 80 countries gather in this small area at one time. The sheer number of people, speaking different languages and coming from different cultural and economic backgrounds, makes this a unique event with high risks of health-related problems and an awesome responsibility to the local Saudi health authority. Because the Holy City of Mecca has an average population of only about 500,000, the simultaneous presence of such a huge number of people inevitably results in extreme overcrowding, with all of the attendant health hazards.

Over the centuries, epidemics such as cholera and meningitis have traveled through the Hajj pilgrimage. There is evidence that it was a pilgrim returning from Mecca to Guinea who triggered the cholera epidemic that spread all over Africa in 1971. In August 1987, an outbreak of group A meningococcal meningitis occurred during the pilgrimage. Tracing the specific strain of the causative bacteria by ribosomal DNA typing showed that it was identical to that causing the Nepal epidemic in 1984 and in New Delhi in 1985, and then spreading to West and East Africa.[30] The magnitude of the influx of people causes formidable logistical problems in transportation, accommodation, catering, and provision of health services. Much effort is currently being put into preventing epidemic diseases by implementing preventive measures, early case detection, and treatment by local health authorities.

A study conducted during the 1986 Hajj showed that the most common cause of hospital admissions of visiting pilgrims was by far gastroenteritis (76.6%), with an incidence rate of 4.4/10,000, followed by pneumonia (8.2%) and upper respiratory tract infection.[31] Forty-one percent of patients with gastroenteritis were over 60 years of age. Over this 1-month period, 318 pilgrims died, giving a crude death rate of 3.7/10,000 pilgrims over the 30-day Hajj period. The leading causes of death identified were heatstroke (28.3%) and coronary disease (15.7%). Asphyxia or crushing from overcrowding resulted in 14 deaths (4.4%). Pneumonia had a high case-fatality rate (43.8%) in the 50+ age group. Overall, the majority of deaths (59.2%) occurred in the older age group, 60+ years old.

Much effort has been put into organizing prevention programs. Vaccination against meningitis and yellow fever for pilgrims coming from endemic areas is mandatory. As cholera vaccination is not valid anymore, vigilant and strict care is given to any reported cases of diarrhea, especially rice water, so that an immediate epidemiologic survey is carried out and prophylaxis treatment is given. Health education of visiting pilgrims to prevent heat exhaustion is also offered. Heatstroke centers are available throughout the Hajj sites, and a body cooling unit with special cooling beds has been created in Mecca for severe cases. Currently, there are more than 3,500 hospital beds in the Mecca and Hajj areas with 155 primary health care centers. Of special concern is the significant proportion of older pilgrims, who have a higher risk of health problems and mortality. Specific information on measures to avoid heat exhaustion, overexertion, and dehydration and prevention of diarrheal diseases should be given to all pilgrims, the elderly in particular.

CONCLUSION

As we recognize that a larger than expected proportion of cases of malaria and other diseases such as typhoid fever and rabies are seen in foreign-born residents and that growing evidence of specific risks exists for migrant travelers, travel medicine doctors and public health authorities should respond to their specific needs. Are migrant travelers returning to visit friends and relatives exposed to higher risks of communicable diseases? Is their perception of risks different from that of general travelers? A better understanding of the factors influencing the health of various migrant travelers is necessary in order to adapt prevention messages and their format, stressing specific areas according to needs. Specific risks mentioned above should be addressed and new channels of communication to convey these messages identified. Potential ways to reach migrant travelers could be:

- Leaflets on preventive measures written in the migrants' languages and designed in a culturally sensitive way, taking into account the community's common knowledge and way of expressing messages
- Television and radio programs and Internet information aimed at specific communities, which concentrate on health risks and prevention measures for the most frequent destinations.
- Identifying new ways of reaching specific communities, such as embassies and consulates, local associations and clubs, and local travel agents, which could play a key role in facilitating access to prevention messages.

As societies become more multicultural, with increasing movement of travelers, including migrants, travel medicine doctors and other health professionals need to acquire the appropriate skills to respond to this new demand. The diseases and illnesses that are associated with travel create challenges both for travel medicine providers and those involved in migration medicine. Closer collaboration between professionals involved in these complementary domains will benefit the health of both the traditional traveler and migrants. "In a relative novel manner, migrants may be considered as a cohort of global travelers and their health characteristics, which reflect their geographic origin, can represent a pattern of experience and knowledge for other travelers who may journey in the reverse direction. This wider approach to the health of travelers can expand the scope and increase the coverage and practice of travel and migration health within a shared framework of health risk determination and management."[2] Medical providers today face the challenge of caring for patients from many cultures who have different languages, socioeconomic status, and unique ways of understanding illness and health care. Travel medicine doctors are no exception. They need to acquire more cultural competence to respond to the needs of various types of travelers as individuals coming to see them. This will apply to providing adequate prevention measures and also care when they return. Raising awareness of potential risks of diseases while abroad and promoting access to information through effective channels of communication to reach the various communities of concern are also new fields of travel medicine that need to be developed.

REFERENCES

1. Wilson ME. Population movements and emerging diseases. J Travel Med 1997;4:183–186.
2. Gushulak B. The migrant as traveler. Migration and health newsletter. Geneva: International Organization for Migration, 1998;1:1–3.
3. World Health Organization. The world health report 1998. Geneva: WHO, 1998.
4. United Nations High Commissioner for Refugees. The state of the world's refugees, 1997–1998. A humanitarian agenda. Oxford: UNHCR, Oxford University Press, 1997.
5. Ghosh B. Huddled masses and uncertain shores. Insight into irregular migration. The Hague: International Organization for Migration, Martinus Nijhoff, 1998.
6. Carballo M, Divino JJ, Zeric D. Migration and health in the European Union. Trop Med Int Health 1998;3:936–944.
7. Junghans T. How unhealthy is migrating? Trop Med Int Health 1998;3:933–934.
8. Raeber PA, Billo NE, Rieder HL, Somaini B. Die grenzsanitarische Untersuchung von Asylbewerbern. Ther Umsch 1990; 47:844–851.
9. Loutan L, Bollini P, Pampallona S, et al. Impact of trauma and torture on asylum-seekers. Eur J Public Health 1999;9:93–96.
10. Behrens RH. Travel morbidity in ethnic minority travellers. In: Cook GC, ed. Travel-associated disease. London: Royal College of Physicians of London, 1995:93–100.
11. Di Perri G, Solbiati M, Vento S, et al. West African immigrants and new patterns of malaria imported to North Eastern Italy. J Travel Med 1994;1:147–151.
12. Ruiz JM, Nguyen N, Faugere B, et al. Epidemiological particularities of imported malaria affecting Comorians in Marseille [abstract 143]. In: Fifth International Conference on Travel Medicine. Geneva: International Society of Travel Medicine, 1997.
13. Wetsteyn JCFM, Kager PA, van Gool T. The changing pattern of imported malaria in the academic medical center, Amsterdam. J Travel Med 1997;4:171–175.
14. Klein JL, Millman GC. Prospective, hospital based study of fever in children in the United Kingdom who had recently spent time in the tropics. BMJ 1998;316:1425–1426.
15. Zuber PLF, McKenna MT, Binkin NJ, et al. Long-term risk of tuberculosis among foreign-born persons in the United Sates. JAMA 1997;278:304–307.
16. Rieder HL, Zellweger JP, Raviglione MC, et al. Tuberculosis control in Europe and international migration. Eur Respir J 1994;7:1545–1553.
17. Mortensen J, Lange P, Storm HK, Viskum K. Childhood tuberculosis in a developed country. Eur Respir J 1989;2:985–987.
18. McCarthy OR. Asian immigrant tuberculosis—the effect of visiting Asia. Br J Dis Chest 1984; 78:248–253.
19. Borgdorff MW, Nagelkerke N, van Soolingen D, et al. Analysis of tuberculosis transmission between nationalities in the Netherland in the period 1993–1995 using DNA fingerprinting. Am J Epidemiol 1998;147:187–195.
20. Van Gorkom J, Leentvaar-kuijpers A, Kool JL, Coutinho RA. Jaarlijkse epidemie van hepatitis A in verband gebracht met reisegedrag van kinderen van immigranten in de vier grote steden. Ned Tijdschr Geneeskd 1998;142:1919–1922.
21. De Cock KM, Low N. HIV and AIDS, other sexually transmitted diseases, and tuberculosis in ethnic minorities in United Kingdom: is surveillance serving its purpose? BMJ 1997;314:1747–1751.
22. Swiss Federal Office for Public Health (OFSP). Maladies sexuellement transmissibles contractées lors de voyages à l'étranger. Bull OFSP 1994;(20):314–319.
23. Koch S, Steffen R. Meningococcal disease in travelers: vaccination recommendations. J Travel Med 1994;1:4–7.
24. Moore PS, Harrison LH, Telzak EE, et al. Group A meningococcal carriage in travelers returning from Saudi Arabia. JAMA 1988;260:2686–2689.
25. Katzenstein D, Rickerson V, Braude A. New concepts of amebic liver abscess derived from hepatic imaging, erodiagnosis, and hepatic enzymes in 67 consecutive cases in San Diego. Medicine 1982;61:237–246.
26. Institut de Veille Sanitaire. Bulletin epidémiologique annuel. Saint-Maurice, France: Institut de Veille Sanitaire, 1999.
27. Müller W. Review of reported rabies cases to the WHO collaborating center Tübingen from 1977 to 1992. Rabies Bull Europe 1992;14:14–18.
28. Rotivel Y, Bourhy H, Wirth S, et al. Imported human rabies cases in France. Rabies Bull Europe 1997;21:14.
29. Hargarten SW, Baker SP. Fatalities in Peace Corps. A retrospective study: 1962 through 1983. JAMA 1985;254:1326–1329.
30. Moore PS, Schwartz B, Reeves MW, et al. Intercontinental spread of an epidemic group A *Neisseria meningitidis* strain. Lancet 1989;ii:260–263.
31. Ghaznawi HI, Khalil MH. Health hazards and risk factors in the 1406 H (186) Hajj season. Saudi Med J 1988;9:274–282.

Chapter 36

TRAVELING WITH CHILDREN

KARL NEUMANN AND RON H. BEHRENS

Preparing children for foreign travel requires familiarity with the pediatric aspects of a number of travel-related issues: infectious diseases, immunization protocols, strategies for avoiding and treating diarrhea, insect bite avoidance, preventing sun-related problems, and safety and accident prevention, to mention just a few.[1]

IMMUNIZATIONS

Issues that need to be considered when vaccinating children for travel include modifying routine immunization schedules, administering travel-related vaccines, simultaneous administration of many vaccines, and assessing suitability for immunization.[2]

MODIFYING ROUTINE IMMUNIZATION

Children should be kept up to date for their routine childhood vaccines, especially when traveling to developing countries (Table 36–1). In such regions, infectious diseases are prevalent and close contact with local children and caretakers will put them at significant exposure risk. The fact that a country reports no cases of an infectious disease does not preclude the disease from suddenly reappearing there. Brazil, for example, reported virtually no cases of measles in recent years, the result of intensive vaccination campaigns in the early 1990s. However, an outbreak occurred in 1997 involving tens of thousands of cases, including some deaths. The outbreak was the result of a let-up in the vaccination program and poor vaccination strategy.[3,4] Many children received only one dose of measles vaccine instead of the recommended two, and the vaccine was often given at age 9 months. One dose yields only a 90% to 95% seroconversion rate, whereas two doses give a 98% seroconversion rate. Some 9 month olds have remaining antibodies from their mothers that interfere with the development of immunity from the vaccine. This outbreak demonstrates the risk of epidemics in spite of control programs.

Children in the United States, Canada, and some other industrialized countries generally receive vaccines at the age at which they respond with optimal, long-term protection, not necessarily at the age when susceptibility first occurs.[5] In these countries, most vaccine-preventable diseases are rare or no longer exist. However, many industrialized countries do not have universal vaccination programs against *Haemophilus influenzae* (type B), rubella,

mumps, and hepatitis B, for example. Many developing countries have yet to institute immunization programs to protect all children against diphtheria, tetanus, pertussis, and polio. Many developing countries have also altered their immunization programs to tackle local issues, in particular, hepatitis B, yellow fever, and Japanese B encephalitis.

It therefore follows that infants and young children, when traveling, may require vaccinations earlier than the age selected for an optimal response to ensure protection because of their higher risk. Intervals between doses may have to be shortened, or one or two doses of a three-part vaccine may need to be completed to optimize protection. Although such modifications may decrease the immune response and require an additional dose of the vaccine later, they significantly reduce the risk of infection. Generally, a dose given at an earlier than recommended age should not be counted toward long-term immunity.[2]

For example, in most developed countries, children receive measles vaccine between 12 and 15 months of age (and again at 4 years), usually combined with rubella and mumps (MMR) vaccines. Children traveling to developing countries may need to receive an earlier dose of measles vaccine at 6 months. Mumps and rubella need not be given at this age; these are generally benign diseases in very young children.[5] Parents should check their own immune status for MMR; traveling with children may increase the parents' exposure to local children. These viral infections tend to cause much more serious pathology in adults.[5]

Most children in industrialized countries receive diphtheria, pertussis, and tetanus (DPT) between 2 and 6 months of age. DPT is often given at the same time as *Haemophilus influenzae* b (Hib) vaccine.[6] For travel to developing countries, infants can receive the first dose of DPT at birth (although waiting at least until the infant is 1 month of age is preferable), and the intervals between doses can be reduced to 1 month.[2] Diphtheria and pertussis are prevalent in many developing countries and Eastern Europe, and many cases of pertussis occur each year in industrialized countries.[7,8] In the United States, children receive a fourth dose of pertussis in the second year of life.[9] Tetanus is not a communicable disease and poses no threat to properly immunized individuals at any age. However, worldwide, tens of thousands of children, mostly newborns, die annually of tetanus, nearly all in developing countries.

Close contact with children in developing countries may slightly increase the chance of acquiring Hib infec-

Table 36–1. CHANGES IN SCHEDULE FOR ROUTINE IMMUNIZATION GIVEN FOR TRAVEL

VACCINE	AGE ROUTINELY GIVEN	REVISED SCHEDULE FOR TRAVEL
DTP	2, 4, 6 mo* 2, 3, 4 mo[†]	Birth, 1, and 2 mo[‡]
Polio	2, 4, 6 mo* 2, 3, 4 mo[†]	Birth, 1, and 2 mo[‡]
Hib	2, 4, 6 mo* 2, 3, 4 mo[†]	6 wk, 10 wk, 12 wk[‡]
MMR	12–15 mo*[‡] (12–18 mo)[†]	6 mo* (this dose of measles vaccine should be followed by the routine MMR schedule)[‡]
Hepatitis B	Between birth and 2 mo, 2–4 mo, 6–18 mo* Not routinely given in U.K.	Birth, 1 mo, 2 mo, 12 mo
Varicella	12–15 mo* Not routinely given in U.K.	No change

*Denotes recommendation from the United States of America.
[†]Denotes recommendation from the United Kingdom.
[‡]When vaccinations are given at younger than recommended ages and when the intervals between doses are shortened, vaccinations should be repeated at a later date.

tions.[10] However, the Hib vaccine is poorly immunogenic before 2 months of age.[10]

In the United States and in some other industrialized countries, children receive hepatitis B (HB) at birth, 1 month, and between 6 and 12 months.[5] For travel, the second and third doses can be given at 2 and 3 months, but a further dose should then be given 6 to 12 months later.[2] HB is acquired through exposure to contaminated blood and other human secretions, and possibly from long-term, close contact with HB-infected individuals who have open skin lesions.[11,12] Such lesions, skin ulcers, insect bites, and scratches are especially common in children living in the tropics.

The number of cases of polio worldwide is decreasing.[13] The World Health Organization hopes to eliminate the disease early in the new millennium and would then consider discontinuing polio vaccination programs about 10 years following the last cases. The Western Hemisphere, Western Europe, and other large areas of the world are now polio free. But cases still occur in countries of Southeast Asia, the Indian subcontinent, Central Africa, the countries of the former Soviet Union, and in several countries in the Middle East.[13]

Two types of polio vaccines are available: the oral Sabin (OPV) and an inactivated Salk (IPV) vaccine. Both provide excellent immunity. OPV generates mucosal immunity. This prevents wild polio virus from replicating in the gastrointestinal tract but rarely (1 per 10^6 doses) can result in vaccine-associated paralytic polio (VAPP). IPV generates a systemic immunity. This could allow wild virus to replicate in the gastrointestinal tract and be passed to other susceptible individuals but does not cause vaccine paralytic disease. Infants in diapers are known to spread vaccine polio virus. The new protocol in the U.S. calls for giving IPV only, at 2 and 4 months and at 15 months and 4 years.[14] IPV gives sufficient humoral immunity to prevent VAPP

from subsequent OPV. No data exist for giving IPV to children less than 6 weeks of age.

Tuberculosis (TB) remains a serious problem in most developing countries. The bacille Calmette-Guérin (BCG) is usually offered to infants shortly after birth in such countries. U.S. experts do not believe that there is a useful role for it and it is almost never given. Instead, children are tuberculin tested every few years and before and after extended trips to developing countries. A meta-analysis on the protective efficacy of BCG in preventing TB strongly suggests that BCG does reduce both the incidence of TB infection and extrapulmonary spread.[15] In the United Kingdom and some other European countries, schoolchildren between the ages of 10 and 13 years are offered this vaccine routinely.[16] Where an infant is deemed to be at greater risk of exposure to TB, vaccination will be offered in the neonatal period. The United Kingdom recommends that children intending to live or travel through countries where a greater risk exists (notably Asia, Africa, and Central and South America) for 3 months or longer should be offered the vaccine. A tuberculin skin test should be carried out prior to vaccinating children over 3 months of age.

IMMUNIZATIONS FOR TRAVEL

Administering travel-related vaccines to children requires an understanding of several factors: the risk of infection, which is strongly influenced by the destination; the reason for the trip (visiting family or a stay at a five-star hotel, for example); the duration of stay; and the significance of the lower age limits of the various vaccines.[17]

Cholera vaccine is rarely recommended for travelers and should not be used in infants under the age of 6 months.[18] Presently, no country requires cholera vaccine as a condition of entry.[19] An oral cholera vaccine based on

CVD 103-HgR strain of *Vibrio* is licensed in many European countries and in Canada. (In 1997, the vaccine application for approval in the U.S. was denied by U.S. regulatory authorities.) This vaccine may give better protection with fewer side effects than the parenteral killed whole-cell cholera vaccine.[18] However, protection from the live enteric vaccine is short lived and currently is not recommended for children under the age of 2 years.

Hepatitis A (HA) is highly prevalent in most developing countries. In most of these countries, 90% of indigenous children have anti-HA antibodies by the time they reach the age of 6 years.[20,21] Generally, for children, HA is a subclinical disease that provides lifelong immunity after infection. However, asymptomatic HA-infected children shed virus in their stool and are, therefore, a threat to nonimmune adults in the community.[5] Vaccine against HA is effective and appears to have few and mild side effects. It appears to be immunogenic in children 1 year of age and older. The lower age recommendation for the vaccine varies in different countries and by vaccine manufacturers: in the U.K., the risk of disease (not infection) in infants and children (other than those traveling to the Indian subcontinent is very low, and many experts recommend immunization in travelers who are 10 years and older.[16] In other European countries, infants and children are immunized from the age of 1 year upward, and in the U.S.A., 2 years is the lower limit for immunization. The pediatric preparation contains a smaller dose of antigen than adult formulations of vaccine (Table 36–2).

Japanese encephalitis (JE) is present in a number of rural regions in Southeast Asia and the Indian subcontinent. The disease is rare in travelers.[22] The age-specific incidence is highest in young children in endemic areas. In travelers, susceptibility is probably similar for all ages, although older travelers are more likely to expose themselves to infection. China, Japan, and several other countries in the region protect their children against JE by immunizing them.[22] Children living in rural endemic areas for periods longer than 4 weeks during the rainy season are at most risk and should be considered for immunization. Reactions to the vaccine, which include aches, pains, and fever, are common in children and more serious allergic reactions including anaphylaxis have been reported.[22]

Meningococcal meningitis (MM) is very rare among travelers. Children are at higher risk than adults.[11] MM vaccine is required as an entry requirement for pilgrims to Mecca, Saudi Arabia, for the annual Hajj.[11] The vaccine is recommended for the "MM belt" in sub-Saharan Africa and during periodic outbreaks that occur in India, Nepal, and southern Africa. The vaccine contains antigens against specific serotypes of MM, mostly a combination of the A/C/Y/W135 strains. It is a polysaccharide vaccine and is not immunogenic against serogroup A in children less than 3 months of age or serogroup C in children less than 2 years of age.[23,24] Duration of immunity is variable, and the recommendation is for boosting every 3 years. In many countries, the predominant serotype is B, against which the vaccine provides no protection.

Parents should be encouraged to have their children immunized with pre-exposure rabies vaccine for prolonged stays in countries where rabid animals are common.[27,28] Vaccination may be more important in children than in adults. In many areas, 40% of all human rabies occur in children less than 14 years of age. Children are attracted to animals, which makes them more likely to be bitten. Also, children may not report minor bites or scratches. Pre-exposure rabies vaccine does not negate the need for proper wound care and postexposure vaccination following an animal bite.

Typhoid vaccine manufactured from killed whole cells has been available for many decades. But the vaccine is a crude extract of bacteria and causes frequent and unpleasant side effects such as fever and flu-like symptoms.[27] Two more recent vaccines are now licensed: an oral, live, attenuated strain Ty21a and a parenteral, Vi capsular polysaccharide antigen vaccine, Typhim Vi.[28,29] Ty21a is licensed for use in children 6 years or older. A liquid form of the vaccine is available in some European countries but not in the U.S. or the U.K. Children receive the same dose of Ty21a as adults: four capsules (three capsules in Europe), one capsule every other day. Capsules must be swallowed immediately and are not to be chewed. This may be difficult for children. The duration of immunity is unclear, in part depending on the dose. Following a four-dose primary course, an estimated 5 years of protection are suggested, whereas a three-dose schedule requires annual boosting. As a live bacterium, Ty21a uptake may be compromised by antibiotic use and simultaneous use of mefloquine. Typhim Vi requires a single dose for 3 years protection. This vaccine has not been well studied in children under 5 years but appears to be immunogenic in children 3 years of age and older. The efficacy of these vaccines, especially in younger children, is very variable. A recent meta-analysis of typhoid vaccines in adults suggests that they provide only 53% protective efficacy when used in travelers.[30]

Yellow fever (YF) is endemic in equatorial Africa and tropical South America. Some countries require vaccination as a condition of entry.[11] YF vaccination in infants under the age of 9 months has been associated with encephalitis. Of the 17 reported cases of YF postvaccination encephalitis, 14 occurred in infants under the age of 4 months.[31] Infants between 6 and 9 months of age should be immunized only if they travel to areas of ongoing epidemic YF and a high level of protection against mosquito bites is not possible. Immunization of children 4 to 6 months of age should be considered only under unusual circumstances. An exemption certificate is an official document that can be provided by a physician if there is a concern about side effects.

HUMAN NORMAL IMMUNOGLOBULIN

HA vaccine has reduced the use of human normal immune globulin (HNIG). HNIG at a dose of 0.02 mL per kg is about 90% effective for up to 3 months and 0.06 mL for up to 5 months.[5] Theoretically, HNIG can interfere with the replication of live viruses in vaccines. However, interference has only been confirmed when used concomitantly with MMR vaccine (and is likely with varicella vaccine).[32] Polio and YF vaccines can be used concurrently with HNIG. Therefore, MMR and (varicella) vac-

Table 36–2.   TRAVEL-RELATED VACCINES FOR CHILDREN

IMMUNIZATION	AGE	PRIMARY COURSE	SCHEDULE	BOOSTER	COMMENT
BCG	From birth	Single dose of 0.1 mL ID (<3 mo of age: 0.05 mL ID or use percutaneous dose)			Skin test before vaccination (except neonates)
Hepatitis A vaccine					
Havrix	2–18 yr	Single dose 1 dose (children's formulation)		6–12 mo	Long-term immunity. Limited use in children < 1 yr in U.K.
HavrixMonodose[†]	1–15 yr	Single dose 0.5 mL		6–12 mo	Long-term immunity
HavrixMonodose[†]	>16 yr	Single dose 1 mL		6–12 mo	Long-term immunity
Vaqta	2–17 yr	Single dose 0.5 mL 1 dose (children's formulation)		6-18 mo	Long-term immunity
Hepatitis A immunoglobulin		0.02–0.04 mL/kg 0.06–0.12 mL/kg	Single dose Single dose		Protection up to 3 mo Protection up to 6 mo
Hepatitis A immunoglobulin[†]	<10 yr	125 mg	Single dose		Protection up to 2 mo
Hepatitis A immunoglobulin[†]	<10 yr	250 mg	Single dose		Protection up to 5 mo
Hepatitis A immunoglobulin[†]	>10 yr	250 mg	Single dose		Protection up to 2 mo
Hepatitis A immunoglobulin[†]	>10 yr	500 mg	Single dose		Protection up to 5 mo
Japanese encephalitis vaccine	1–3 yr	3 doses of 0.5 mL SC or 2 doses of 0.5 mL SC[†]	0, 7, 28 days 0, 28 days	2–4 yr 3 mo	Full duration of protection is unknown. Vaccine is unlicensed in U.K. Two-dose regimen (0, 7–28 days) provides immunity for 3 mo in 80% of recipients.
	>3 yr	3 doses of 1.0 mL SC or 2 doses 1.0 mL SC[†]	0, 7, 28 days 0, 28 days	2–4 yr 3 mo	
Meningococcal vaccine* (A, C, Y, W-135 vaccine)	>2 mo	One dose 0.5 mL SC or IM		3 yr	Vaccine is less effective under 18 mo (see text). Duration of immunity is unknown under 4 yr of age. A & C vaccine only available in U.K.
(A & C vaccine)	>2 mo	One dose 0.5 mL SC or IM		3 yr	
Rabies vaccine (pre-exposure) Human diploid cell vaccine (HDCV) Purified chick embryo cell vaccine (PCEC) Rabies vaccine adsorbed (RVA)	All ages	3 doses 1.0 mL IM (or 2 doses 1.0 mL IM)[†]	0, 7, 21 to 28 days (days 0 and 28 days for 2-dose course)[†]	2 yr (6 mo then 2–3 yr)[†]	Inject IM dose into deltoid muscle HDCV may be given by the ID route (0.1 mL) ID route is unlicensed in U.K.[†] Most individuals seroconvert after 2 doses[†]
Tick-borne encephalitis vaccine	No lower age limit Usually >1 yr	3 doses of 0.5 mL SC/IM or 2 doses of 0.5 mL SC/IM	0, 4–12 wks then 9–12 mo (0 and 14 days[‡] for 2-dose course)	3 yr (after 3-dose course)	Not licensed in U.S.A. and U.K. Available in U.K. on named patient basis only. Two-dose regimen gives immunity for 1 yr.
Typhoid vaccine whole cell[‡]	6 mo–10 yr*	2 doses of 0.25 mL SC or IM	> 4 wk (4 to 6 wk)[†]	(3 yr)[†]	All but the 1st dose can be given as 0.1 mL ID (in the U.S.A. the ID route can be used after the primary series of two doses)[†]
Typhim Vi	>2 yr >18 mo[†]	Single dose 0.5 mL SC or IM	2 yr 3 yr		
Oral (Ty21a)	>6 yr	4 capsules* 3 capsule[†]	1 capsule taken every other day	5 yr (full 3-dose course annually)[†]	Vaccine must be stored in refrigerator. Each capsule must be swallowed whole with cool liquid.
Yellow fever vaccine	>9 mo	Single dose of 0.5 mL SC		10 yr	Given at designated centers only.

*Denotes recommendations from the United States of America.
[†]Denotes recommendation from the United Kingdom.
[‡]Indicates the timing of the initial dose; subsequent numbers indicate time period after the initial dose. No longer available in the U.K.

cine should not be given in the period from 2 weeks before until 6 weeks to 5 months after HNIG use. The time interval after HNIG depends on the dose of HNIG administered. There is little interaction between HNIG and inactivated vaccines. Inactivated vaccines can be given at any time before, with, or after HNIG.[5] HNIG is painful to administer, and this makes it less acceptable for pediatric use. In the U.K., the theoretical transmission of prion protein in pooled human blood products has further limited the use of HNIG.

ADMINISTERING VACCINES SIMULTANEOUSLY

Generally, the simultaneous administration of vaccines, live and inactivated, and routine and travel related, does not result in impaired immune response or increased rate of adverse reaction. However, there may be some reciprocal decreased antibody response when YF and cholera vaccines are administered on the same day or less than 3 weeks apart.[11]

Theoretically, if parenteral live vaccines are not administered on the same day, they should be given at least 30 days apart. However, recent thinking suggests that this is not necessary for modern vaccines to be so delayed.[5] Oral typhoid and oral polio vaccines should not be given at the same time on the theoretical grounds of interference in gut mucosal immune response.[33] If a tuberculin skin test is necessary prior to the BCG vaccine, live virus vaccines should be delayed until after this has been read as they may affect the result.[5]

CONTRAINDICATIONS TO VACCINATIONS

Minor illness and fevers do not necessitate deferring vaccination. However, vaccinations are generally deferred with moderate or severe febrile illness (although limited studies indicate that there is no reason to do so).[5] Antibiotic therapy, asthma, and family history of reactions to vaccinations are not contraindications to immunization. Egg allergy from a parent must be fully detailed before deciding whether a YF or MMR should be given. Nearly all 1,209 (99.7%) children with a history of egg hypersensitivity were shown on egg challenge to have no adverse reaction to egg protein.[34]

TRAVELERS' DIARRHEA

A study of travelers' diarrhea (TD) among tourists to developing countries, which unusually included children, showed that the highest incidence, severest disease, and longest duration of TD were in subjects under the age of 3 years. Furthermore, infants may excrete pathogenic organisms for a longer period of time than older children and adults.[35] The stools of an infant in diapers may be an important source of infection to parents and caretakers.[35]

The incidence of TD in children can be reduced by encouraging them to wash their hands frequently and teaching them to avoid placing their hands and other objects in their mouth, swallowing water while swimming or bathing, or eating sand.

TREATMENT

At the first sign of diarrhea, feed children commercial oral rehydration solution (ORS) and continue normal feeding.[36,37] ORS is available in convenient packets and should be mixed with treated water. Such fluids are effectively and rapidly absorbed through the intestinal mucosa via the Na$^+$ linked carbohydrate transport mechanism found in the enterocytes. This mechanism, along with Na$^+$ amino acid coupled transport, requires that both glucose and Na$^+$ be present to enable active transport of the solute, which then drags along water across into the circulation.[36]

Many fluids used to treat children with diarrhea may worsen symptoms.[37] Fizzy or soft drinks that contain 50 to 150 g per L of glucose (recommended is about 25 g/L) and very little sodium will cause loss of water from the body because of the osmotic load exerted by the unabsorbed glucose. On the other hand, chicken broth contains almost three times the needed sodium requirement, but no glucose. Excess sodium can lead to hypernatremia in a dehydrated child. Artificially sweetened soft drinks and tea contain neither sodium nor sugar. Continuing feedings during diarrhea helps prevent dehydration, reduces stool frequency and volume, and shortens the duration of symptoms. ORS should be continued even in the presence of vomiting. Infants should have formula or breastfeeding maintained throughout the illness, supplemented with ORS. For older children, offer cooked rice, maize, wheat, and potatoes, for example, and encourage them to drink ORS. A source of potassium can be obtained through bananas. If ORS is not available, children can be given plain treated water plus salted crackers, mashed potatoes, or banana flakes.

MEDICATIONS

Medications are rarely necessary to treat diarrhea in children.[38] Most substances used by adults are inappropriate for use in small children for the following reasons:

- Kaolin and pectin products are not very effective.[39]
- Bismuth subsalicylate (Pepto-Bismol) contains too much salicylate (although it has been used without ill effects).[40]
- Loperamide (Imodium) and diphenoxylate (Lomotil) are not recommended for children under 2 years of age.[41] In older children, both may lead to toxic megacolon and may cause extrapyramidal problems and hyperactivity.
- Doxycycline stains teeth.
- Quinolones, in animal studies, cause destructive lesions in cartilage of weight-bearing joints and are not licensed for use in children. However, in many recent studies in children, quinolones have been used without any apparent ill effects.[42] If antibiotics are necessary, furazolidone and trimethoprim/sulfamethoxazole (TMP/SMX) are effective against most causes of unknown severe diarrhea.[43] (However, increasingly, there are reports of pathogen resistance to TMP/SMX.)[41] TMP/SMX is

available as a liquid and does not require refrigeration. In the United Kingdom, TMP/SMX has been withdrawn from use because of the high incidence of sulphonamide-related toxicity. Prompt, competent medical attention is essential when children are lethargic, refuse liquids, or have continuous severe vomiting, bloody diarrhea, or a high fever.

MALARIA AND CHILDREN

Infants and children who travel to malarial areas are as susceptible to infection as are adults, but some prophylactic medications used by adults may be inappropriate. Malaria risks can be substantially reduced by:

- Spraying nettings with permethrin-containing insecticide[44];
- Using a pyrethroid-containing flying-insect spray in living and sleeping areas during evening and nighttime hours;
- Placing netting over baby carriages and cribs;
- Dressing children in long-sleeved clothing that fits over neck, wrists, and ankles;
- Covering exposed skin with an insect repellent containing <30% N,N-diethylmetatoluomide (DEET)[45];
- Sleeping in quarters that are air conditioned, when possible;
- Eliminating standing surface water around living quarters; and
- Staying indoors at dusk and after dark.

The use of insect repellents containing <30% DEET is recommended. Toxicity from DEET is very rare.[46,47] The most common problem is skin rash and, very rarely, neurologic symptoms. In the United States, widespread use of DEET has resulted in little evidence of toxicity, which may have been overestimated. Skin reactions to DEET can be minimized by applying it only to exposed skin, never using repellents on irritated skin, and washing off the repellent when protection is no longer necessary. Permethrin and pyrethroid may cause minor skin rashes, but there are no known serious side effects.

CHEMOPROPHYLAXIS

In Table 36–3, the doses and schedule for prophylactic antimalarials for children are given. Preventive medication depends on the region of the world visited and the risk of acquiring malaria, especially chloroquine-resistant falciparum malaria (CRFM).[19,48] Chloroquine is the drug of choice for chloroquine-sensitive malaria. In the United States, chloroquine is available in bitter-tasting tablets. The dosage is optimally calculated by body weight.[11] In Europe and most other countries, chloroquine is also available as a syrup, 50-mg base/5 mL.[49] Check the concentration carefully. It may vary in different countries.

Chloroquine is generally well tolerated by children. Side effects are infrequent and tend to be mild: stomach upsets, headaches, dizziness, blurred vision, and pruritis. Reactions can be reduced by taking chloroquine with meals or in divided, twice-weekly doses.[50] Store chloroquine in a child-proof container out of the reach of children. The ingestion of several tablets can be fatal to a small child.[11]

Mefloquine is effective against most CRFM; however, mefloquine-resistant malaria is widespread, especially in Southeast Asia and Africa.[49] Doses of mefloquine for children are as fractions of one-fourth, one half, or three-fourths of a tablet, depending on the weight of the child. No liquid preparation is available. Tablets are single scored. Accurate dosing of one-fourth or three-fourths doses can be achieved by crushing tablets first and then dividing the powder. The powder can be given with applesauce or a similar substance.[51] Restrictions against using mefloquine in infants and children weighing less than 15 kg have been discontinued.[19] Small children may vomit soon after ingesting mefloquine. Children with a history of seizure or using anticonvulsant should not be prescribed mefloquine or chloroquine. The neuropsychiatric side effects commonly reported to occur in adults taking mefloquine seem to be rare in children.

The combination of daily doses of proguanil with weekly doses of chloroquine is an alternative to mefloquine in areas with CRFM, especially in Africa.[11] Proguanil is not available in the United States but is available in most other countries. Side effects to proguanil include diarrhea, mouth ulcers, and, less frequently, hair loss, which is temporary. Doxycycline is an alternative to mefloquine for CRFM in parts of Southeast Asia. Doxycycline is contraindicated in children less than 9 years of age (12 years in the U.K.), as it inhibits bone growth and stains teeth. It can also cause photosensitivity, manifesting as an exaggerated sunburn reaction. This can be minimized by avoiding prolonged sun exposure and using effective sunscreens.

A new and very promising drug for both treatment and prophylaxis of falciparum malaria is Malarone, a fixed combination of atavaquone and proguanil. The medication is taken once a day starting 2 days before possible exposure and for 7 days after exposure ceases, and is available in both adult and pediatric tablets. In numerous controlled clinical trials, many of them in regions where resistance to other antimalarial drugs has developed, the efficacy of Malarone in preventing malaria is 98.7 percent. Malarone is well tolerated and has few safety concerns. The pediatric tablet contains 62.5 mg atovaquone and 25 mg proguanil.

Lactating mothers taking antimalarials secrete only small amounts of the drug in their breast milk. The amount is insufficient to harm infants or protect infants from malaria.[51] Malaria is the first diagnosis to be excluded in children with unexplained fevers returning from areas where malaria is endemic. Emergency treatment with pyrimethamine/sulfadoxine or quinine can be administered where medical help is unavailable and clear instructions on use have been provided. Emergency treatment may mask other pathology or infections, and parents should be strongly encouraged to obtain a medical opinion before instituting any therapy.[52]

Table 36–3.   DOSAGE AND SCHEDULE FOR PROPHYLACTIC ANTIMALARIALS IN CHILDREN

MEDICATION	ADULT DOSE	U.S.A. RECOMMENDATIONS —PEDIATRIC DOSE	U.K. RECOMMENDATIONS —PEDIATRIC DOSE (FRACTION OF ADULT DOSE)	REMARKS
Chloroquine phosphate (Aralen)* (Avloclor)[†] Chloroquine sulphate (Nivaquine)[‡]	300-mg base weekly* (two tablets weekly)[†]	5-mg/kg base orally once/week up to a maximum of adult dose of 300-mg base	0–5 wk = ⅛ 6 wk – <1 yr = ¼ 1–5 yr (10–19 kg) = ½ 6–11 yr (20–39 kg) = ¾ >12 yr (>40 kg) = adult dose	Bitter-tasting formulation—pulverize tablets and mix with food
Hydroxychloroquine sulphate (Plaquenil)	310-mg base orally once/week	5-mg/kg base orally once/week up to a maximum of adult dose	Not used as a prophylactic antimalarial in the U.K.	May be better tolerated than chloroquine phosphate
Proguanil (Paludrine)	200 mg daily (two tablets)	<2 yr = 50 mg/day 2–6 yr = 100 mg/day 7–10 yr = 150 mg/day >10 yr = 200 mg/day	0–5 wk = ⅛ 6 wk – <1 yr = ¼ 1–5 yr (10–19 kg) = ½ 6–11 yr (20–39 kg) = ¾ >12 yr (>40 kg) = adult dose	Not available in the U.S. Available in Canada, Europe, and Africa. Usually used with chloroquine.
Mefloquine	228-mg base* (250-mg base)[†] One tablet weekly	<15 kg = ⅛ tab wk <5 kg = not used[†] 5–19 kg = ¼ adult dose[†] 15–19 kg = ¼ tab/wk 20–30 kg = ½ tab/wk 31–45 kg = ¾ tab/wk >45 kg = 1 tab/wk	<5 kg = not used 5–19 kg = ¼ adult dose 20–30 kg = ½ tab/wk 31–45 kg = ¾ tab/wk >45 kg = 1 tab/wk	
Doxycycline	100 mg orally	>8 yr = 2 mg/kg orally/day up to adult dose	Not recommended for children under the age of 12 yr	Doxycycline is not yet licensed in the U.K. for malaria prophylaxis
Maloprim (pyrimethamine dapsone)[†]	One tablet weekly (pyrimethamine 12.5 mg and dapsone 100 mg)		1–5 yr (10–19 kg) = ¼ 6–11 yr (20–39 kg) = ½ >12 yr (>40 kg) = adult dose	The adult dose of 1 tablet weekly must not be exceeded because of the risk of agranulocytosis
Malarone (Atovaquone/ Proguanil)	One tablet daily (250 mg atovaquone/ 100 mg proguanil)	62.5 mg atovaquone/ 25 mg proguanil tablets. 11–20 kg = 1 pediatric tablet >20–30 kg = 2 pediatric tablets >30–40 kg = 3 pediatric tablets >40 kg = 1 full-strength (adult) tablet	Same in U.S. and U.K.	Start 2 days before and continue until 7 days after exposure

*Denotes recommendations from the United States of America.
[†]Denotes recommendations from the United Kingdom.
[‡]Nivaquine is available as a syrup in the U.K. (chloroquine base 50 mg/5 mL).

ALTITUDE SICKNESS

The incidence of acute mountain sickness (AMS) in infants and young children is about the same as in adults and, as in adults, the higher the altitude, the faster the ascent, the greater the incidence of AMS. In one study, when 14 children aged 3 to 36 months ascended from 1,609 meters to 3,488 meters, about 20% experienced AMS.[50] AMS-related pulmonary edema seems to develop more often in children who have had recent upper respiratory infections. Identifying AMS in young children can be problematic.[53] Children, whether they climb or not, frequently become ill with vague viral illnesses that give symptoms similar to AMS—headaches (irritability), loss of appetite, inability to sleep, and fatigue, for example—and they cannot verbalize what is bothering them. Parents are advised to avoid high-altitude destinations and, if they do go to such destinations and the children become ill, to assume that it is altitude sickness and descend immediately.

One recent study suggests that the amount of oxygen in the cabin air at the cruising altitude of commercial jets and at higher altitudes in mountains may influence the paO_2 in normal infants.[54,55] The study was undertaken in a laboratory on 40 healthy infants. The infants were subjected to the same oxygen concentrations as those found in an aircraft cabin at normal flying altitudes, which equates to 1,800 meters above sea level. Four of the infants developed irregular breathing patterns and were noted to have rapidly decreasing paO_2. The infants had to be withdrawn from the study. Millions of infants have traveled safely by air without apparent adverse consequences.

CHILDREN AND AIR TRAVEL

Air travel appears to be safe for children with upper respiratory infection (URIs), nasal allergies, and ear infections.[56] Although children occasionally experience pain during flight, permanent damage from barotrauma (abnormal pressure build-up in the middle ear) appears to be extremely rare in children. The use of decongestants and nasal sprays for URIs and nasal allergies may decrease the chances of discomfort, although some studies suggest that these medications have limited effectiveness in children and some decongestants are known to produce drowsiness. Ideally, medications should be started several days before flying. Additional doses of spray should be given on starting descent and then 5 minutes later. Older children should blow their noses before using sprays.

Middle ear infections appear to protect children from pain during flight. Such infections generally produce fluid in the middle ear. The fluid obliterates the middle ear space; therefore, differentials in pressure cannot occur. For children who have aerating tubes through their tympanic membranes, flying appears not to pose an added risk of problems. The tubes equalize the pressure between the middle ear and the outside.

Conventional wisdom recommends nursing infants or giving them bottles during ascent and descent and when crying during a flight. The rationale is that infants cry when experiencing barotrauma (especially during descent) or because of dehydration from the low humidity aboard aircraft. There are no data to show that infants cry more frequently on aircraft than at other times, that they experience barotrauma, or that they become dehydrated. Frequent feeds may worsen crying, as at the cruising altitude, air in the intestine has already expanded by 20% from that at ground level. Sucking and eating increases intestinal gases, causing discomfort and crying. Increased frequency of feeding infants may cause rather than solve problems.

REFERENCES

1. Kennedy BC, Gentile DA. Children in the wilderness. In: Auerbach PS, ed. Auerbach management of wilderness and environmental emergencies. St. Louis: Mosby, 1995.
2. Barnett ED, Chen R. Children and international travel: immunization. Pediatr Infect Dis J 1995;14:982–992.
3. Pan American Health Organization. EPI Newsletter. 1997; 19:1–3.
4. Measles eradication. MMWR Morb Mortal Wkly Rep 1997; 46(RR11):1–19.
5. Report of the Committee on Infectious Diseases. Elk Grove Village, IL: American Academy of Pediatrics, 2000.
6. Centers for Disease Control. Recommendations for use of *Haemophilus* b conjugate vaccines and a combined diphtheria, tetanus, pertussis, and *Haemophilus* b vaccine. Recommendations of the Advisory Commitee on Immunization Practices (ACIP). MMWR Morb Mortal Wkly Rep 1993;42(RR13):1–17.
7. Centers for Disease Control. Diphtheria epidemic—New Independent States of the former Soviet Union, 1990–1994. MMWR Morb Mortal Wkly Rep 1995;44:177–181.
8. Sheldon T. Dutch whooping cough epidemic puzzles scientists. BMJ 1198;316:92.
9. Centers for Disease Control. Recommendations of the Advisory Committee on Immunization Practices (ACIP). MMWR 1993;42:1–15.
10. Global Programme for Vaccines and Immunization (GPV). The WHO position paper on *Haemophilus influenza* type b conjugate vaccines. Wkly Epidemiol Rec 1998;73(10):64–68.
11. Centers for Disease Control. Health information for international travel, 1996–1997. Atlanta: Department of Health and Human Services, 1997.
12. Shapiro CN, McCaig LF, Gensheimer KF, et al. Hepatitis B virus transmission between children in day care. Pediatr Infect Dis 1989;8:870.
13. Centers for Disease Control. One thousand days until the target date for global poliomyelitis eradication. MMWR Morb Mortal Wkly Rep 1998;47:234.
14. Centers for Disease Control. Polio prevention in the U.S. Introduction of a Sequential Vaccination Schedule of inactivated poliovirus vaccine followed by oral poliovirus vaccine. MMWR Morb Mortal Wkly Rep 1997;46(RR3):1–25.
15. Colditz GA, Berkey CS, et al. The efficacy of bacillus Calmette-Guérin vaccination of newborns and infants in the prevention of tuberculosis: meta-analyses of the published literature. Pediatrics 1995;96:29–35.
16. Department of Health, Welsh Office, Scottish Office Home and Health Department, DHSS (Northern Ireland). Immunization against infectious disease. London: The Stationery Office, 1992.
17. Tucker AW, Haddix AC, Bresee JS, et al. Cost-effectiveness analysis of a rotavirus immunization program for the United States. JAMA 1998;279:1371–1376.
18. Behrens RH, Collins M, Botto B, Heptonshall J. Risk for British travellers of acquiring hepatitis A. BMJ 1995;311:193.
19. World Health Organization. International travel and health. Vaccination requirements and health advice. Geneva: WHO, 1995.
20. Steffen R, Kane MA, Shapiro CN, et al. Epidemiology and prevention of hepatitis A in travelers. JAMA 1994;272:885–889.
21. Centers for Disease Control. Prevention of hepatitis A through active or passive immunization. MMWR Morb Mortal Wkly Rep 1996;45(RR15):1–30.
22. World Health Organization. Japanese encephalitis. Wkly Epidemiol Rec 1994;69:113–120.
23. Centers for Disease Control. Control and prevention of meningococcal disease. MMWR Morb Mortal Wkly Rep 1997; 46(RR5):1–21.
24. Petola H. Clinical efficacy of meningococcal group A capsular polysaccharide vaccine in children three months to five years old. N Engl J Med 1977;297:686–691.
25. Fischbein DB, Robinson LE. Rabies. N Engl J Med 1993;329: 1632–1638.
26. Centers for Disease Control. Rabies prevention United States, 1991. Recommendations of the immunization practices advisory committee (ACIP). MMWR Morb Mortal Wkly Rep 1991;40:1.
27. Centers for Disease Control. Typhoid immunizations, recommendations of the Advisory Committee on Immunization Practices (ACIP). MMWR Morb Mortal Wkly Rep 1994;43(RR14): 1–7.
28. Levine MM, Noriega F. Vaccines to prevent enteric infections in children. Pediatr Ann 1993;22:719–725.
29. Engels EA, Falagas ME, Lau J, Bennish ML. Typhoid fever vaccines: a meta-analysis of studies on efficacy and toxicity. BMJ 1998;316:110–116.
30. Health hints for the tropics, 1998. Northbrook, IL: American Society of Tropical Medicine and Hygiene.
31. Centers for Disease Control. Yellow fever vaccine. Recommendations of the Immunization Practices Advisory Committee (ACIP). MMWR Morb Mortal Wkly Rep 1990;39(RP6):1–6.

32. American Academy of Pediatrics. Recommended timing of routine measles immunizations for children who have recently received immunoglobulin preparations. Pediatrics 1994;93: 682–685.

33. Health information for overseas travel. Department of Health Welsh Office, Scottish Home and Health Department, DHSS (Northern Ireland) with the Public Health Laboratory Service Communicable Disease Surveillance Centre. London: The Stationery Office, 1995.

34. Salisbury D, Begg N, eds. Immunization against infectious disease. London: Department of Health, HMSO, 1996:141–142.

35. Pitzinger B. Incidence and clinical features of travelers' diarrhea in infants and children. Pediatr Infect Dis J 1991;10:719.

36. Lanata CF, Black RE, Creed-Kanashiro H, et al. Feeding during acute diarrhea as a risk factor for persistent diarrhea. Acta Pediatr Suppl 1992;381:98–193.

37. Roper WL. The management of acute diarrhea in children; oral rehydration, maintenance, and nutritional therapy. MMWR Morb Mortal Wkly Rep 1992;42(RR-16):1–20.

38. Johnson PC, DuPont HL, et al. Chemoprophylaxis and chemotherapy of travelers' diarrhea in children. Pediatr Infect Dis J 1985;4:620.

39. Ludan AC. Current management of acute diarrheas. Use and abuse of drug therapy. Drugs 1998;36(Suppl 4):18–25.

40. Figuera-Quintanilla D, Salazar-Lindo E, et al. A controlled trial of bismuth subsalicylate in infants with acute watery diarrheal disease. N Engl J Med 1993;329:1653–1658.

41. Bhutta ZA, Molla AM. Safety of loperamide in infants with diarrhea. J Pediatr 1991;119:842–843.

42. Hampel B, et al. Ciprofloxacin in pediatrics: worldwide clinical experience based on compassionate use—safety report. Pediatr Infect Dis J 1997;16:127–129.

43. Ericson CD, et al. Treatment of travelers' diarrhea with sulfamethoxazole and trimethropin and loperamide. JAMA 1990; 263:257.

44. d'Alessandro. Mortality and morbidity from malaria in Gambian children after the introduction of an impregnated bednet programme. Lancet 1995;345:479–484.

45. Fradin MS. Mosquitoes and mosquito repellents: a clinician's guide. Ann Intern Med 1998;128:931–940.

46. Veltri JC, Osimitz TG, Bradford DC, Page BC. Retrospective analysis of calls to poison control centers resulting from exposure to the insect repellent N,N-diethyl-m-toluamide (DEET) from 1985–1989. J Toxicol Clin Toxicol 1994;32:1–16.

47. Goodyer L, Behrens RH. The safety and toxicity of insect repellents. Am J Trop Med Hyg 1998;59:323–324.

48. Lobel HO, Kozarsky PE. Update on prevention of malaria for travelers. JAMA 1997;278:1767–1771.

49. Bradley DJ, Warhurst DC. Malaria prophylaxis: guidelines for travellers from Britain. BMJ 1995;310:709–714.

50. Barry M. Medical considerations for international travel with infants and older children. Infect Dis Clin North Am 1992;6: 389–404.

51. Nahlen BL, et al. International travel and the child younger than two years: 11. Recommendations for prevention of traveler's diarrhea and malaria chemoprophylaxis. Pediatr Infect Dis J 1989;8:735.

52. Miller KD, Lobel HO, et al. Severe cutaneous reactions among American travelers using pyrimethamine/sulfadoxine for malaria prophylaxis. Am J Trop Med Hyg 1986;35:451.

53. Yaron M, Niermeyer S, Nicholas R, Honigman B. The diagnosis of acute mountain sickness in preverbal children. Arch Pediatr Adolesc Med 1998;152:683–687.

54. Pollard AJ, Murdoch DR, Bartch P. Children in the mountains. BMJ 1998;316:874–875.

55. Parkins KJ, Poets CF, et al. Effect of exposure to 15% oxygen on breathing patterns and oxygen saturation in infants: interventional study. BMJ 1998;316:873–874, 887–894.

56. Weiss MH, Frost E. May children with otitis media with effusion safely fly? Clin Pediatr 1987;26:567.

Chapter 37

PREGNANCY, NURSING, CONTRACEPTION, AND TRAVEL

PHYLLIS E. KOZARSKY AND ALFONS VAN GOMPEL

The recent logarithmic increase in international travel has included growing numbers of travelers among special risk groups, including pregnant women. Fortunately, physicians and researchers have gained a better understanding of the physiology of pregnancy, recognizing it as a normal state rather than a disabled condition. This has allowed the development of practical, scientifically based recommendations. An increased awareness of their potential problems and possible solutions are now providing pregnant women with a greater sense of security and enjoyment in their travels. Despite this, however, prior to making decisions about travel, health advisors should consider each pregnant traveler individually and base recommendations on medical history, personal characteristics, itinerary, final destination, and degree of flexibility.[1]

FACTORS AFFECTING THE DECISION TO TRAVEL

Much of what dictates whether a pregnant woman should travel is common sense. If a woman has not traveled previously to the developing world, pregnancy is not the ideal time to undertake such a journey. And, certainly, long-term trips need extra consideration. If the trip is optional, it can be scheduled for a more convenient time or at a site with better facilities. A complete itinerary should be evaluated, with attention specifically to the quality of medical care available at the destination and during transit.

Another consideration prior to international travel during pregnancy is the degree of emotional maturity and flexibility of the woman. Tolerance and a sense of humor are mandatory because of the large number of variables that are not under the traveler's control, particularly in developing world destinations. Whereas a camping out environment with extremes of climate or topography and few or no amenities may at times be desirable and exhilarating, it may not be so while pregnant in a foreign country.

A last general item for consideration prior to decision making is the cultural aspect of traveling while pregnant or nursing. In some countries, business may not be as fruitful if the chief negotiator is a woman who is 7 months pregnant. Similarly, having a nursing infant at the breast may not be conducive to playing power politics. Local customs regarding pregnancy and nursing must also be followed.

According to the American College of Obstetrics and Gynecology, the safest time for a pregnant woman to travel is during the second trimester (between 18 and 24 weeks), when she usually feels best and is least in danger of experiencing a spontaneous abortion or premature labor. Many obstetricians ask women who are over 28 weeks gestation to stay within a few hundred miles (or 500 kilometers) of home because of concerns regarding access to their physicians in case of problems such as hypertension, phlebitis, or false or premature labor. There are, however, relative contraindications to international travel, which are listed in Table 37–1.[2] Even during the second trimester for certain pregnant women, the final decision to travel will require the judgment of health advisors in addition to the women themselves.

GENERAL RECOMMENDATIONS FOR TRAVEL

Once a pregnant woman has decided to travel, there are a number of issues that need investigation and/or clarification prior to departure. Table 37–2 serves as a partial checklist of those items.

It is advisable for pregnant women to travel with a companion. Even the most adventuresome women candidly admit to having the desired assistance and support from a familiar face while traveling during their pregnancies. Furthermore, pregnant women or those with infants should readily avail themselves of services such as boarding aircraft first or using porters to help carry luggage. They may also want air-conditioned hotel rooms, even if this is not their usual mode of travel. Attention not only to the necessities of safe travel but also to more comfortable travel will make trips far more enjoyable.

Motor vehicle accidents are a major cause of morbidity and mortality. When available, seat belts should be fastened at the pelvic area. Lap and shoulder restraints are best; in most accidents, the fetus recovers quickly from the seat belt pressure, but even after seemingly blunt, mild trauma, a physician should be consulted. Infant car seats should be brought from home so that they can be used in aircraft and in cars.

Table 37–1. RELATIVE CONTRAINDICATIONS TO INTERNATIONAL TRAVEL DURING PREGNANCY

PATIENTS WITH OBSTETRIC RISK FACTORS

History of miscarriage
Incompetent cervix
History of ectopic pregnancy (ectopic with present pregnancy should be ruled out prior to travel)
History of premature labor or premature rupture of membranes
History of or present placental abnormalities
Threatened abortion or vaginal bleeding during present pregnancy
Multiple gestation in present pregnancy
History of toxemia, hypertension, or diabetes with any pregnancy
History of infertility or difficulty becoming pregnant
Primigravida greater than age 35 or less than age 15

PATIENTS WITH GENERAL MEDICAL RISK FACTORS

Valvular heart disease or congestive heart failure
History of thromboembolic disease
Severe anemia
Chronic organ system dysfunction requiring frequent medical interventions

PATIENTS CONTEMPLATING TRAVEL TO DESTINATIONS THAT MAY BE HAZARDOUS

High altitudes or extreme travel, particularly where there is difficult access to an adequate medical facility
Areas endemic for or where epidemics of life-threatening food or insect-borne infections are occurring
Areas where chloroquine-resistant *Plasmodium falciparum* is endemic
Areas where live virus vaccines are required and recommended

Adapted from Lee.[2]

Typical problems of pregnant travelers are the same as those experienced at home: fatigue, heartburn, indigestion, constipation, vaginal discharge, leg cramps, increased urination, and hemorrhoids. Signs and symptoms that should take them immediately to a physician are bleeding, passing tissue or clots, abdominal pain or cramps, contractions, ruptured membranes, excessive leg swelling, headaches, or visual problems. The decision to travel internationally while nursing brings another set of challenges. Bearing this in mind, however, breastfeeding has nutritional and anti-infective advantages that serve an infant well while traveling. Cultural factors also play a role. In some societies, nursing in public is not acceptable, whereas in others, breastfeeding is the norm. Supplements are usually not needed by breastfed infants, and breastfeeding should be carried on as long as possible. In case milk output is inadequate, powdered formula that requires reconstitution with boiled water should be carried. Planning to wean after a trip is ideal.

Nursing women need to realize that their eating and sleeping patterns, as well as stress, will inevitably affect their milk output. They need to increase their fluid intake and avoid excess alcohol, caffeine, and, as much as possible, exposure to smoke.

Table 37–2. CHECKLIST FOR THE PREGNANT TRAVELER

1. Make sure health insurance is valid while abroad and during pregnancy. Check to see if the policy covers a newborn should delivery take place. Obtain a supplemental travel insurance policy (compare those available) and a prepaid medical evacuation insurance policy that ensures rapid transportation to adequate medical care and then home.

2. Check destination medical facilities. If in last trimester, medical facilities should be able to handle complications of pregnancy, toxemia, and cesarean sections. The facility should also be able to provide neonatal expertise.

3. Determine ahead of time whether prenatal care will be required abroad and, if so, who will provide it. Make sure prenatal visits that require specific timing are not missed (e.g., amniocentesis, chorion biopsy, blood tests for genetic diseases).

4. Check ahead of time whether blood is screened for HIV and hepatitis B at the destination. Make sure the pregnant traveler knows her blood type. Traveling companions should also know their blood types.

5. Check destination facilities regarding availability of consumable food and beverages, including bottled water and pasteurized milk.

6. Plan on nursing a newborn as this is safest for the infant in a developing world environment.

SPECIFIC RECOMMENDATIONS FOR TRAVEL

IMMUNIZATIONS: WORLDWIDE IMPORTANCE

Because of the theoretical risks to the fetus from maternal vaccination, the risks and benefits of each immunization should be carefully reviewed prior to its administration. Ideally, all women who are pregnant should be up to date on their routine immunizations.[3] Polysaccharide vaccines have been used in pregnancy without adverse events and should be used when benefit outweighs risk.[4] In general, pregnant women should avoid live vaccines or avoid becoming pregnant within 3 months of having received one; however, fetal damage has not been reported from the accidental administration of these vaccines during pregnancy. Nursing women may be immunized for maximum protection depending on the travel itinerary, but consideration needs to be given to the neonate who cannot be immunized at birth and who would not gain protection against many of these infections (e.g., yellow fever, measles, meningococcal meningitis) through breastfeeding.

Diphtheria/Tetanus The combination diphtheria/tetanus immunization should be given if the traveler has not been immunized within 10 years, although preference would be for its administration during the second or third trimesters.

Measles/Mumps/Rubella and Varicella Immunity to measles is essential for all travelers. Many young adults require immunization (and, in some cases, reimmunization) for protection. Specific recommendations for different age groups vary depending on the traveler's country of origin and the epidemiology of measles in that country. The measles vaccine and the measles, mumps, and rubella combination (MMR) are live vaccines and are contraindicated in pregnancy. Because of the increased incidence of measles in children in developing countries, its communicability, and its potential for causing serious consequences in adults, some health advisors recommend delaying travel for nonimmunes until after delivery when immunization can be safely given. However, in cases where the rubella vaccine was accidentally administered, there were no complications reported. If a documented exposure to measles occurs, immune globulin should be given within a 6-day period to a pregnant woman to prevent illness. Varicella vaccine has become available recently and is underused in children and in the adult nonimmune population; varicella can cause significant problems in pregnancy, including congenital defects in the newborn. The epidemiology of this illness is unusual in the tropics, with most children not being exposed. Thus, travelers to the tropics who have not had illness previously add to the pool of susceptibles. Varicella zoster immune globulin should be administered to nonimmune pregnant women who have had contact with varicella.

Polio   It is important for the pregnant traveler to be protected against polio. Paralytic disease may occur with greater frequency when infection develops during pregnancy. Anoxic fetal damage has also been reported, with up to 50% mortality in neonatal infection. If not previously immunized, a pregnant woman should have at least two doses of vaccine prior to traveling (day 0 and at 1 month). Despite being a live vaccine, the oral preparation (OPV) had previously been recommended when immediate protection was needed. (The recommendation for the nonimmune pregnant traveler is one dose of OPV prior to travel followed by completion of the regimen after delivery.) During a nationwide immunization campaign in Finland when several thousand pregnant women received the OPV, there was no increase in the occurrence of congenital malformations.[5] However, for routine boosting or for when immediate protection is not required, the enhanced inactivated vaccine (eIPV) is preferred. OPV may become less available as it is being used less frequently in many countries for routine childhood immunization. Thus, eIPV is most frequently recommended for adult immunization and for immunization of pregant women.

Hepatitis B   Although there are no specific contraindications to its use in the first trimester, as with all vaccines, one would prefer to administer it during the second or third trimester.

The hepatitis B vaccine may be administered during pregnancy but preferably after the first trimester. For short-term tourists or business travelers, it is usually not routinely recommended unless a woman is working in a health care setting, is sexually active with new partners, is planning delivery overseas, or will be a long-term traveler staying over 1 month.[3] It is desirable, however, for everyone to be protected against hepatitis B.

Pneumococcal/Influenza   The pneumococcal and influenza vaccines should be given to all who would otherwise qualify for special protection against these diseases: pregnant woman with chronic diseases or pulmonary problems. Pregnant women have greater morbidity associated with influenza infection. In general, women with serious underlying illnesses should not travel to developing countries when pregnant.

IMMUNIZATIONS: SPECIAL IMPORTANCE

Yellow Fever   The yellow fever vaccine should not be given to a pregnant woman unless travel to an endemic or epidemic area is unavoidable. In these instances, the vaccine can be administered. The first systematic epidemiologic study of yellow fever vaccination in pregnancy found no evidence of congenital infection in 40 exposed infants in Nigeria.[6] Antibody responses of pregnant women and mothers who were vaccinated mainly during the last trimester were much lower than those of yellow fever-vaccinated nonpregnant women in a comparable control group. A 1993 study of women immunized inadvertently during pregnancy found one apparently well neonate with yellow fever viral-specific immunoglobulin M antibody, indicating a vaccine-related congenital exposure.[7] No congenital abnormalities have been reported after administration of this vaccine to pregnant women.

If traveling to or transiting regions within a country where the disease is not a current threat but where policy requires a yellow fever certificate, a physician waiver should be carried along with documentation on the immunization record. In general, travel to areas where yellow fever is a risk should be postponed until after delivery, when the vaccine can be administered without concern of fetal toxicity. A nursing mother should also delay travel, as the neonate cannot be immunized due to risk of vaccine-associated encephalitis. Breastfeeding is not a contraindication to the vaccine for the mother.

Hepatitis A   Pregnant women without immunity to hepatitis A need protection prior to traveling to developing countries, as the risk for nonimmune travelers is between 3 and 6 per 1,000 per month.[8] Rates as high as 20 per 1,000 are seen in overland travelers living and eating under poor hygienic conditions. Hepatitis A is usually no more severe during pregnancy than at other times and does not affect the outcome of pregnancy. There have been reports, however, of acute fulminant disease in pregnant women during the third trimester when there is also an increased risk of premature labor and fetal death.[9] These events did occur in women from developing countries and may have been related to underlying malnutrition. The hepatitis A virus is rarely transmitted to the fetus, but this can occur during viremia or from fecal contamination at delivery. Immune globulin is a safe and effective means of preventing hepatitis A, but immunization with one of the hepatitis A vaccines gives a more complete and prolonged protection. The effect of these killed virus vaccines on fetal development is unknown, but the production methods for the vaccines are similar to that for the eIPV, which is considered safe during pregnancy. Although immune globulin preparations have been used for years in pregnant women, a 1996 report showed an increase in fingertip dermatoglyphic changes in infants whose mothers received >5 mL.[10]

Typhoid   In countries where it is still available, the older injectable typhoid vaccine (heat/phenol inactivated) is not recommended during pregnancy because of febrile reactions that can result in spontaneous abortions, although it can be administered intradermally with less risk of systemic symptoms. The safety of the oral typhoid vaccine in pregnancy is not known. Nonetheless, neither of these is absolutely contraindicated during pregnancy, according to the American Committee on Immunization Practices. The newer Vi capsular polysaccharide preparation may be the vaccine of choice, where available, as it is inactivated and requires only one injection. With any of these, the vaccine efficacy (about 70%) needs weighing against risk of disease. At highest risk appear to be those visiting friends and relatives in the Indian subcontinent or in Central/South America.

Meningococcal Meningitis   The polyvalent meningococcal meningitis vaccine (quadravalent A, C, Y, W135, or A & C) may be administered during pregnancy if the woman is entering an area where the disease is epidemic or during an outbreak. The safety of these vaccines during pregnancy has not been conclusively demonstrated, although a small study published by McCormick et al. in 1980 showed no birth defects in infants whose mothers were vaccinated during an epidemic in Brazil. Results from this study also showed that these children were not immunotolerant to groups A and C vaccines when administered at 6 months of age.[11]

Cholera   Despite an increase in maternal morbidity associated with cholera during pregnancy and an increase in fetal deaths in the third trimester, the older parenteral vaccine should be avoided due to adverse reactions, mainly abortion, and poor efficacy. There are several new cholera vaccines. A newer killed injectable and oral vaccines are available outside the U.S., although their safety during pregnancy has not been established.[12-14] The live oral preparation CVD 103-HgR is available in a number of countries, including Canada. Although it is well tolerated and may be given as a single dose, there are no data regarding its safety in pregnancy. It should thus be avoided on theoretical grounds because it is a live preparation.

Rabies   The cell culture rabies vaccines may be given during pregnancy for either pre- or postexposure prophylaxis.[15] A 1991 review of the literature cited 24 cases of pregnant women exposed to rabid animal bites.[16] Exposures occurred during all trimesters. The women received equine rabies immune globulin and/or vero cell vaccine or duck embryo vaccine. There was one fatality due to inappropriate postexposure prophylaxis. Among the infants, two were born prematurely, and there was one spontaneous abortion. There were no physical or mental abnormalities except in the case described where the child did well after repair of transposition of the great vessels. In this child, the bite occurred weeks after the heart formed embryologically.

Japanese B Encephalitis and Miscellaneous   There is no information available on the safety of the Japanese encephalitis vaccine in pregnancy. It should not be routinely administered during pregnancy, except when a woman must stay within a high-risk area, as infection with Japanese encephalitis virus within the first or second trimester may result in increased fetal mortality. If not mandatory, travel should be delayed. The inactivated tick-borne encephalitis virus vaccine may be administered if indicated. There are no data available on the plague vaccine. The bacille Calmette-Guérin vaccine for the prevention of tuberculosis can theoretically cause disseminated disease and thus affects the fetus[17]; skin testing for tuberculosis exposure before and after travel is preferable when the risk is high.

Malaria   Malaria in pregnancy carries significant morbidity and mortality both for the mother and the fetus.[18-20] The World Health Organization (WHO) advises pregnant women to avoid traveling to areas where transmission of chloroquine-resistant *Plasmodium falciparum* (CRPF) occurs.[21] Because no antimalarial agent is 100% effective, it is imperative that pregnant women use personal protective measures when traveling through a malaria-endemic area. Pregnant women should remain indoors between dusk and dawn, but if outdoors at night, light-colored clothing, long sleeves, long pants, and shoes and socks should be worn. They should sleep in air-conditioned quarters or use screens and permethrin-impregnated bednets.[21] Pyrethrum-containing house sprays or coils should also be used indoors if insects are a problem. Insect repellents containing a low percentage of diethyltoluamide (DEET) (recommendations vary from <10%–35%) can be used on the skin. Nursing mothers should be careful to wash repellents off hands and breast skin prior to handling infants.

Any medication taken during pregnancy carries some risk. A list of antimalarials available and their uses and contraindications during pregnancy can be found in Table 37-3. Because of these potential problems, some travel health advisors recommend that pregnant women avoid travel to regions where CRPF malaria occurs. Nursing mothers should take the usual adult dose of antimalarial appropriate for the country to be visited. The amount of medication in the breast milk will not be helpful or harmful to the infant. Therefore, the breastfeeding child needs his or her own prophylaxis.

Chloroquine has been used by pregnant women for malaria chemoprophylaxis for decades without any documented increase in birth defects.[22] For this reason, travel to areas where chloroquine can be used for prophylaxis is considered relatively safe (Table 37–4). Unfortunately, terminal prophylaxis (or radical treatment) of *P. vivax* or *P. ovale* using primaquine phosphate is not feasible dur-

Table 37–3.   ANTIMALARIAL AGENTS AND THEIR USE DURING PREGNANCY

DRUG	RECOMMENDED USE DURING PREGNANCY	POTENTIAL TOXICITY TO MOTHER AND/OR FETUS
Quinine	For life-threatening infections	Maternal hyperinsulinemia and hypoglycemia Oxytocic effect in very high doses Optic nerve hypoplasia and congenital deafness reported Neonatal thrombocytopenia and hemolytic anemia in G6PD-deficient newborn
Primaquine	Not recommended	Fetal red blood cells relatively deficient in G6PD and glutathione; therefore, fetus at ↑ risk for intravascular hemolysis and methemoglobinemia
Chloroquine	For prophylaxis and treatment of chloroquine-sensitive strains of malaria	When used in prophylactic doses, no ↑ in birth defects reported Chorioretinitis and cochleovestibular damage reported in newborns of mothers given large daily doses
Proguanil	Has been used without problems in pregnancy in combination with chloroquine for prophylaxis Data not available on 200-mg/day dose in pregnancy	Not teratogenic in animals Pregnant women should take folic acid supplement daily (1–5 mg suggested)
Doxycycline	Not recommended	Inhibition of bone growth, teeth discoloration, and dysplasia
Pyrimethamine	Not as a single agent	High doses are teratogenic in laboratory animals Theoretical risk during first trimester but used extensively without fetal abnormalities (including for treatment of toxoplasmosis in pregnancy)
Pyrimethamine/dapsone	Not recommended	Little known about safety of combination, although dapsone used safely in pregnant women with leprosy
Pyrimethamine/sulfadoxine	For emergency standby treatment For treatment of CRPF following quinine Not to be used at term or during first trimester	Sulfonamides associated with kernicterus when used late in pregnancy
Halofantrine	Not recommended	Few data available Embryotoxic in laboratory animals Animal data suggest it is secreted in breast milk and may result in reduced weight gain in offspring; therefore, contraindicated in nursing mothers
Artemisinin derivatives	Not recommended	Few data available Embryotoxicity with low doses demonstrated in animal studies
Mefloquine	For 2nd and 3rd trimesters, prophylaxis against CRPF Some recommend for 1st trimester when travel cannot be postponed	No significant increase in spontaneous abortion or malformations when used for prophylaxis; higher doses used for treatment are of greater concern

ing pregnancy due to the risk of hemolytic anemia in the glucose-6-phosphate dehydrogenase (G6PD)-deficient fetus. A woman who is either at very high risk for a relapse of one of these infections or who is currently being treated for active infection requires weekly chloroquine until delivery. Only thereafter, and with confirmation of a normal G6PD level, can she receive primaquine.

In 1994, the WHO and various national expert groups expanded their indications for mefloquine prophylaxis in areas of CRPF to include pregnant women in their second and third trimesters[23,24] (see Table 37–3). Data showed that mefloquine prophylaxis was well tolerated in Karen women who were >20 weeks gestation, and no significant adverse events were noted in the women or in their offspring.[25] In another study in Malawi where nearly 1,000 pregnant women received mefloquine prophylaxis and 14 received it for treatment during the first trimester, there was also no evidence of abnormalities attributable to the drug.[18] Mefloquine remains controversial for prophylaxis during the first trimester, but in numerous spontaneously reported cases of inadvertent use at the beginning of pregnancy, there was no increase in congenital malformations.[26,27] In fact, mefloquine use in any stage of pregnancy is never an indication for an abortion. Despite these data and despite loosening of restrictions, there continue to be concerns in this regard. A solid understanding of the controversies surrounding mefloquine use is recommended prior to administering antimalarial chemoprophylaxis to a pregnant woman or to someone planning pregnancy who will be traveling to an area endemic for CRPF.[28–31] The pharmacokinetics of mefloquine is not altered by oral contraception. A problem that remains is prophylaxis of pregnant women traveling to confirmed areas of mefloquine resistance, such as the Thai-Myanmar border. Travel should be strongly discouraged, but, if mandatory, the combination of sulfisoxazole and proguanil can be considered for prophylaxis during the second and early part of the third trimester.[32]

Studies done in Africa have shown that semi-immune pregnant women are more likely to develop malaria due to CRPF than are controls, to experience higher levels of parasitemia, and to respond less well to chloroquine.[33] Highest levels of parasitemia and failure to clear parasitemia after chloroquine are seen with greater frequency in primigravidae. Clinical disease with severe complications including cerebral malaria, massive hemolysis, and acute renal failure is also more common in pregnancy. These problems may be seen in conjunction with fetal sequelae such as spontaneous abortions, stillbirths, preterm deliveries, low birthweight infants, and congenital infections.[34] Malaria must be considered in the differential diagnosis of the toxoplasmosis, rubella, cytomegalovirus, herpes, syphilis (TORCHS) syndrome in susceptible infants with fever, anemia, and hepatosplenomegaly.[17]

Any pregnant traveler returning with malaria from an area where CRPF is endemic should be treated as a medical emergency and as if she had illness due to chloroquine-resistant organisms. Because of the serious nature of malaria, quinine or intravenous quinidine should be used and should be followed by Fansidar, or even doxycycline,

Table 37–4.   MALARIA CHEMOPROPHYLAXIS IN PREGNANCY

GEOGRAPHIC REGION	CHEMOPROPHYLAXIS
Chloroquine-sensitive areas (Mexico, Central America, Haiti, North Africa, Middle East)	*Chloroquine
Areas endemic for chloroquine-resistant *Plasmodium falciparum*	†Mefloquine ‡Chloroquine plus proguanil Defer travel in 1st trimester
Mefloquine-resistant areas	#Defer travel

*After travel to high-risk areas for *Plasmodium vivax* or *Plasmodium ovale*, terminal prophylaxis with primaquine must be delayed until after delivery.
†If the risk of malaria is very high, mefloquine is recommended in the first trimester since the risk of adverse events may be smaller than the risk of infection.
‡This regimen has far less efficacy than mefloquine but remains first choice for many authorities because of its safety record. Standby Fansidar (Roche) (25 mg pyrimethamine and 500 mg sulfadoxine) can be given for emergencies.
#Doxycycline is contraindicated in pregnancy and in children <8 years. If travel imperative, consider combination of sulfonamide and proguanil with the understanding that neither has a confirmed saftey record in pregnancy.

despite concerns regarding potential fetal problems. A study from Thailand published in 1985 revealed no oxytocic effect in 12 pregnant women treated with high-dose quinine for severe malaria in their third trimester. Uterine activity was monitored and did not change.[35] Frequent glucose levels and careful fluid monitoring often require intensive care supervision. Mefloquine is an alternative treatment but the high doses required have engendered greater concerns as a recent study reported a significant number of fetal deaths in mefloquine-treated women. There are few data involving treatment of malaria in pregnancy with halofantrine or the artemisinin derivatives; limited experience treating pregnant women with the latter has shown no untoward effects.[36]

TRAVELERS' DIARRHEA

Dietary vigilance should be adhered to while traveling during pregnancy because dehydration due to travelers' diarrhea (TD) can lead to inadequate placental blood flow. Potentially contaminated water should ideally be boiled. Iodine-containing purification systems should not be used long term. Iodine tablets can probably be used for short-term travel up to several weeks, but congenital goiters have been reported in association with administration of iodine-containing drugs during pregnancy.[1] Eating only well-cooked meats and pasteurized dairy products, as well as avoiding preprepared salads, should help avoid diarrheal disease as well as infections such as toxoplasmosis and listeria, which can have serious sequelae in pregnancy. It is not recommended that pregnant women use prophylactic antibiotics for the prevention of TD.[37]

Oral rehydration is the mainstay of TD therapy. Bismuth subsalicylate compounds are contraindicated due to the theoretical risks of fetal bleeding from salicylates and teratogenicity from the bismuth. The combination of kaolin-pectin may be used, but loperamide should be used only when necessary. The antibiotic treatment of TD during pregnancy can be complicated. Ampicillin or ampicillin/clavulanic acid may be used, but many strains of *Escherichia coli* and other TD-causing organisms are resistant to these. Erythromycin is safe but is not effective against many enteric bacteria except *Campylobacter* sp. Azithromycin is an alternative, but data on safety are lacking. Trimethoprim is teratogenic in the first trimester in small mammals and sulfonamides cannot be used early or late in pregnancy; both are highly excreted in breast milk and are contraindicated in lactating women as well. The quinolone compounds are contraindicated due to inhibition of bone growth in the fetus and in children, although these may be safe for very short-term use. Thus, cefixime or other oral third-generation cephalosporins may be the best option for treatment of TD in pregnant women.

In general, mildly symptomatic infections with intestinal parasites during pregnancy can be treated after delivery. Furazolidone may be used for treatment of giardia, although it has been reported to cause fetal hemolytic anemia and thus is not recommended by many physicians. Paromomycin has been shown to be effective in about 50% of cases of giardia. Intestinal ameba may also be treated with paromomycin; however, some may be reluctant to use it because it has not been approved by some regulatory agencies (e.g., the Food and Drug Administration). Metronidazole has been used successfully later in pregnancy for both of these infections, and previous fears about using this drug during pregnancy have been dispelled.[38,39]

Breastfeeding is desirable during travel and should be continued as long as possible due to its safety and its lower incidence of infant diarrhea. A nursing mother with TD should not stop breastfeeding but should increase fluid intake.

HEPATITIS E

Hepatitis E is an illness of growing concern for travelers, particularly for pregnant women whose mortality rate may reach 25% with this infection. Hepatitis E is transmitted by fecal-oral route, similar to hepatitis A, but also may be transmitted from person to person. It has been reported from a number of countries and areas of the world, including India, China, Nepal, Myanmar, Pakistan, African nations, Eastern Europe, Mexico, Central America, and Southeast Asia. Unfortunately, immune globulin is not protective.

AIR TRAVEL

Commercial air travel poses no special risks to a healthy pregnant woman or her fetus. The lowered cabin pressures (kept at the equivalent of 5,000–8,000 feet or 1,524–2,438 meters) affect fetal oxygenation minimally because of the fetal hemoglobin dissociation curve. Severe anemia (Hgb <8.5g/dL), sickle-cell disease or trait, a history of thrombophlebitis, or placental problems are relative contraindications to flying; however, supplemental oxygen may be ordered ahead of time in the former situations.[40] Each airline has policies regarding pregnancy and flying, and these change frequently. Short-haul travel is usually permitted until 36 weeks gestation, whereas long-range travel is curtailed anywhere between weeks 32 and 35. It is always safest to check with the airline when booking reservations, as some will require special medical forms to be completed. Pregnant women should always carry documentation stating their expected date of confinement.

An aisle seat at the bulkhead and in the no-smoking section will provide the most space and comfort, but a seat over the wing in the mid-plane region will give the smoothest ride. A pregnant woman should walk every half hour during a nonturbulent flight and flex and extend the ankles frequently to prevent phlebitis. While the woman is seated, the seat belt should always be fastened at the pelvic level. Fluids should be taken liberally due to the dehydrating effect of the low humidity in aircraft cabins.

Concern has recently been voiced about the possibility of exposure to excess radiation at altitudes of >35,000 feet (>10,000 meters) where radiation levels may be 100 times greater than at sea level. This may be a problem for pregnant crew members on repeated flights, especially during their first trimesters, but should pose no problem to the usual traveler.[41]

Women traveling with infants should keep in mind that those less than 2 weeks old should not fly because their alveoli are not completely functional. Infants are particularly susceptible to pain with eustachian tube collapse during pressure changes, and breastfeeding during ascent and descent relieves this discomfort.

Altitude   There are no risks known for pregnant women who travel to high altitudes for a few days. Some data have shown a progressive decrease in birth weights of infants born at altitudes >7000 feet (2,130 meters). Also, premature babies born at high altitudes have greater mortality rates. It is difficult, however, to separate risks due to high altitude alone and risks due to the combination of altitude with other factors that often coincide such as low temperatures, harsh conditions, and increased enteric infections experienced in travelers in these situations. Furthermore, there are no data on the safety of pregnancy at altitudes greater than 15,000 feet (4,571 meters). Of greater concern, however, than altitude alone is access to good medical care in many of these remote areas.

EXERCISE

There are no contraindications to exercise or to vigorous exercise during pregnancy (heart rates <150 beats/minute).[17] Women need to be careful in their choice of sports, however, and should not begin new activities or increase their intensity of activity during pregnancy. Aerobic exercise is beneficial, but the effects of anaerobic training are not known. Trekking in remote areas is contraindicated, as well as certain water sports.[17] Water skiing has been associated with genital lacerations, and there is a risk of miscarriage or peritonitis from water being forced through the cervix. Scuba diving places the fetus at risk for decompression sickness and congenital anomalies, and hyperbaric oxygen for recompression treatment causes fetal wastage in experimental animals. The high concentration of oxygen may also lead to retrolental fibroplasia. Entry into hot tubs and saunas during the first trimester is contraindicated because of the theoretical possibility of core temperature elevation and neural tube defects. Swimming, however, is ideal. Hypoglycemia, hyperthermia, and dehydration should be avoided. Moderate exercise may also be contraindicated for women who have had any of the following problems: a history of spontaneous abortion, premature rupture of membranes, premature labor, multiple gestation, incompetent cervix, bleeding, placenta previa, or cardiac disease.

THE TRAVEL HEALTH KIT

Additions and substitutions to the usual travel health kit need to be made during pregnancy and nursing. Prenatal vitamins, talcum powder, a thermometer, oral rehydration packets, multivitamins, an antifungal agent for vaginal yeast, acetaminophen, insect repellent containing a low percentage of DEET, and sunscreen with a high sun protection factor should be carried. Women in their third trimester may want to carry a blood pressure cuff and urine dipsticks to check for proteinuria and glucosuria, both of which would require attention. Antimalarial and antidiarrheal self-treatment medications should be evaluated individually depending on the traveler, her trimester, the itinerary, and her health history. Most medications should be avoided, if possible. A review of the safety of a number of commonly used medications can be found in Samuel and Barry's chapter in the 1998 travel medicine edition of the *Infectious Disease Clinics of North America*.[20]

Although not usually part of a travel health kit, a supply of safe foods and beverages may be desirable for some women who are traveling for short periods of time. Natural bran will help counteract constipation. Simple food items such as crackers, canned tuna, peanut butter, and juice boxes may ease developing world travel considerably for the pregnant woman with a busy schedule who is concerned about becoming ill. Nursing women should always carry a supply of bottles, nipples, and formula.

THE DECISION NOT TO BECOME PREGNANT: CONTRACEPTION FOR TRAVEL

To prevent acquisition of sexually transmitted diseases, one should avoid casual sex or practice safe sex by using condoms no matter what other means of birth control is being used simultaneously. Unfortunately, women are often hesitant to carry condoms, and even when they do, are hesitant to insist on their use. The newer female condoms offer an alternative, and U.N. AIDS officials are urging more widespread distribution of female condoms.[42] For the woman traveler with a steady partner, however, there are a number of contraceptive alternatives that

should be considered (Table 37–5).[42,43] These options should be discussed by the traveler and her physician to determine which is appropriate depending on the health history and style of life.

Women wishing to try a new means of contraception should ideally begin months prior to travel, especially if planning to be overseas long term or to be living in a remote area. Sexually active woman living overseas should incorporate a pelvic examination into annual leave, field conferences, or vacation plans.[44] Although nursing an infant generally protects against pregnancy, this is not an adequate means of birth control. Similarly, lack of menses due to alterations in schedule or stress from travel does not protect against pregnancy, as the woman may still be ovulating.

An adequate supply of contraceptives should be brought with the traveler or carried by friends who will be visiting; mailing them later is less reliable. When taking birth control pills (BCP), it is often difficult to find exact brand names in other countries. An empty package of BCP should be saved to show the local pharmacist or physician. Also, because the amounts of hormone may vary in the different varieties of BCP, adverse effects may be experienced when trying a new brand. If diarrhea or stomach upset occurs, there will be decreased absorption of BCP. A barrier method should be used for the duration of the illness and for 2 weeks thereafter. If vomiting occurs within 3 hours of taking BCP, the woman should take another. Antibiotics such as tetracyclines or ampicillin, both frequently used by travelers, decrease the absorption of most BCP. Again, during the time on these antibiotics and for 2 weeks thereafter, another method of birth control should be used. If these 2 weeks coincide with the 7 pill-free days, the woman should not take a break but should carry on with a fresh packet of pills, despite no withdrawal bleeding. Some women choose to continue their oral contraceptive regimens without the week break to prevent menses during travel, although breakthrough bleeding may occur. Antimalarial medications, other than tetracyclines, do not interfere with the action of BCP. If taking doxycycline and BCP, there may be a slightly increased pregnancy risk.

A survey done by the United Methodist Mission groups has indicated that pregnancies and deliveries among missionary women have been successful.[44] This survey was done, however, before the explosion of AIDS and the understandable fears of blood transfusion and the use of unsterile equipment. Depending on the field site, women may want to travel to a major medical center either within the country or to a more developed environment several weeks prior to her due date. A woman expatriate should ideally try to avoid pregnancy and delivery within the first year of posting abroad.

Emergency contraception has increased dramatically, and, according to one manufacturer, the demand for medication for this reason is recently up 124%. Emergency contraception compromises ovulation and may also inhibit implantation. Table 37–6 reviews the various methods.

Table 37–5. CONTRACEPTIVE ALTERNATIVES FOR USE DURING TRAVEL

METHOD	ADVANTAGES AND DISADVANTAGES
Condom	85%–98% effective Offers barrier protection against transmission of HIV and other sexually transmitted diseases Brands and materials differ in quality May break down in heat and humidity
Intrauterine device	Very effective Some effective only 3–5 years Can exacerbate sexually transmitted diseases Heavy bleeding and increased cramps Insertion and removal require trained personnel May be expelled
Diaphragm (with spermicide)	Easily carried Requires spermicide, which may not be available Can breakdown in heat and humidity May not have access to clean water to wash diaphragm Needs fitting
Cervical cap (with spermicide)	Protection against some sexually transmitted diseases but not HIV Requires spermicide Not user friendly Cervical irritation (Pap smear abnormalities)
Contraceptive sponge	Not very effective Does not require a prescription
Female condom	More expensive than male condom Awkward, cannot be used without a man's knowledge Prevents HIV and other sexually transmitted diseases
Birth control pills	Useful for short-term avoidance of menses Convenient, effective, and easy to carry Drug interactions can be a problem Gastrointestinal illness interferes with absorption Needs to be taken every 24 hours
Medroxyprogesterone acetate injections	Injection lasts for 3 months Very effective Can cause irregular bleeding, weight gain, headache Not affected by other medications
Levonorgestrel subdermal implants	Very effective Effective for 5 years Headache, weight gain Removal problems

If a traveler becomes pregnant and wishes to consider terminating her pregnancy, it may be best to return home. Sixty of 128 countries listed by International Planned Parenthood Federation (IPPF) prohibit abortion except in extreme circumstances such as rape or life-threatening illness.

If a woman has a problem or questions regarding contraception in the country to which she is traveling, IPPF keeps a worldwide guide to contraceptives and an address list of family planning agencies. The Federation's address is Regent's College, Inner Circle, Regent's Park, London NW1 4NS, England.

CONCLUSIONS

Because women, and therefore pregnant and nursing women, will continue to travel in greater numbers, it is crucial that they be well educated by their travel health advisors regarding their special risks. No matter how meticulous they may be in their pretravel preparations, however, there are no guarantees that they will not experience complications abroad. Hopefully, the combination of common sense and the guidelines in this chapter will help them to better enjoy their travels by staying healthier.

Table 37–6.   METHODS OF EMERGENCY CONTRACEPTION

REGIMEN	TIME AFTER INTERCOURSE	STATUS OF METHOD	REPORTED EFFICACY
Estrogen and progestin (5 mg of ethinyl estradiol daily for 5 days) 0.5 mg of levonorgestrel given twice, with 12 hr between doses	Up to 72 hour	Licensed in some countries since early 1980 (e.g., United Kingdom, the Netherlands) Available unlicensed in the appropriate combination of oral-contraceptive pills	75%–80%
Levonorgestrel (0.75 mg given twice, with 12 hr between doses)	48 hours (possibly up to 72 hours)	Licensed in some countries in Eastern Europe and Asia	Equivalent to estrogen-progestin
High-dose estrogen (e.g., 5 mg of ethinyl estradiol daily for 5 days) suggested	72 hr	Licensed in the Netherlands; little used elsewhere	Equivalent to estrogen-progestin
Mifepristone (a single 600-mg dose)	72 hr	Widely used in China in a variety of lower doses; being licensed by a number of countries (www.safewebmedical.com)	100% effective
Danazol (400–800 mg given twice 12 hr apart or 400 mg given 3 times at intervals of 12 hr)	72 hr	Used only under research conditions	Reports vary from failure rates of <1% to ineffective
Cooper intrauterine device	Up to 5 days after the earliest estimated day of ovulation	Available worldwide but not licensed for emergency contraception	Failure rates <1%

REFERENCES

1. Macleod CL. The pregnant traveler. Med Clin North Am 1992; 76:1313–1327.
2. Lee RV. The pregnant traveler. Travel Med Int 1989;7:51–58.
3. Health information for international travel 1999–2000. Atlanta: U.S. Department of Health and Human Services, Centers for Disease Control and Prevention, Department of Health and Human Services.
4. Shahid NS, Steinhoff MC, Hoque SS, et al. Serum, breast milk and infant antibody after maternal immunization with pneumococcal vaccine. Lancet 1995;346:1252–1257.
5. Harjulehto-Mervaala T, Aro T, Hiilesmaa VK, et al. Oral polio vaccination during pregnancy: no increase in the occurrence of congenital malformations. Am J Epidemiol 1993;138:407–414.
6. Nasidi A, Monath TP, Vandenberg J, et al. Yellow fever vaccination and pregnancy: a four-year prospective study. Trans R Soc Trop Med Hyg 1993;87:337–339.
7. Tsai TF, Paul R, Lynberg MC, Letson GW. Congenital yellow fever infection after immunization in pregnancy. J Infect Dis 1993;168:1520–1523.
8. Steffen R. Hepatitis A and hepatitis B: risks compared with other vaccine preventable diseases and immunizations recommended. Vaccine 1993;11:518–520.
9. Gilbert GL. Miscellaneous viral infections. In: Infectious diseases in pregnancy and the newborn infant. Chur, Switzerland: Harwood Academic, 1991.
10. Ross JL. Dermatoglyphics on offspring of women given gammaglobulin prophylaxis during pregnancy. Teratology 1996; 53:285–291.
11. McCormick JB, Gusmao H, Nakamura S, et al. Antibody response to serogroup A and C meningococcal polysaccharide vaccines in infants born of mothers vaccinated during pregnancy. J Clin Invest 1980;65:1141–1144.
12. Berger SA, Shapiro I. Re-emergence of cholera vaccine. J Travel Med 1997;4:58–60.
13. Clemens JD, Sack DA, Harris JR, et al. Field trial of oral vaccines in Bangledesh: results from three-year follow-up. Lancet 1990;335:270–273.
14. Sanchez JL, Trofa AF, Taylor DN, et al. Safety and immunogenicity of the oral, whole cell/recombinant B subunit cholera vaccine in North America. J Infect Dis 1993;167:1446–1449.
15. Fescharek R, Quast U, Dechert G. Post exposure rabies vaccination during pregnancy. Vaccine 1990;8:409.
16. Chabala S, Williams M, Amenta R, Ognjan AF. Confirmed rabies exposure during pregnancy: treatment with human rabies immune globulin and human diploid cell vaccine. Am J Med 1991;91:423–424.
17. Bia FJ. Medical considerations for the pregnant traveler. Infect Dis Clin North Am 1992;6:371–388.
18. Steketee RW, Wirima JJ, Slutsker L, et al. Malaria prevention in pregnancy: the effects of treatment and chemoprophylaxis on placental malarial infection, low birth weight, and fetal, infant, and child survival. United States Agency for International Development Africa Regional Project (698–0421), U.S. Department of Health and Human Services, 1996.
19. Steketee RW, Wirima JJ, Slutsker L, et al. Malaria treatment and prevention in pregnancy: indications for use and adverse events associated with use of chloroquine or mefloquine. Am J Trop Med Hyg 1996;55:50–56.
20. Samuel BU, Barry M. The pregnant traveler. Infect Dis Clinic North Am 1998;12:325–354.
21. Dolan G, ter Kuile FO, Jacoutot V, et al. Bed nets for the prevention of malaria and anemia in pregnancy. Trans R Soc Top Med Hyg 1993;87:620–626.
22. Wolfe MS, Cordero JF. Safety of chloroquine in chemosuppression of malaria during pregnancy. BMJ 1985;290:1466.

23. Health Information for international travel 1997. Atlanta: U.S. Department of Health and Human Services, Centers for Disease Control and Prevention, Department of Health and Human Services.

24. World Health Organization. International travel and health 2000. Geneva: WHO, 2000.

25. Nosten FF, ter Kuile F, Maelankiri L, et al. Mefloquine prophylaxis prevents malaria during pregnancy: a double-blind, placebo-controlled study. J Infect Dis 1994;169:595–603.

26. Steffen R, Fuchs E, Schildknecht J, et al. Mefloquine compared with other malaria chemoprophylactic regimens in tourists visiting East Africa. Lancet 1993;341:1299–1303.

27. Phillips-Howard PA, Steffen R, Kerr L, et al. Safety of malaria chemoprophylaxis in pregnancy: indications from exposure in travellers. J Travel Med 1998;5:121–126.

28. Balocco R, Bonati M. Mefloquine prophylaxis against malaria for female travelers of childbearing age. Lancet 1992;340:309–310.

29. Bradley D. Prophylaxis against malaria for travellers from the United Kingdom: malaria reference laboratory and the Ross Institute. BMJ 1993;306:1247–1252.

30. Nosten F, ter Kuile F, Maelankiri L, et al. Mefloquine prophylaxis prevents malaria during pregnancy: a double-blind, placebo-controlled study. J Infect Dis 1994;169:595–603.

31. Phillips-Howard PA, Bjorkman AB. Ascertainment of risk of serious adverse reactions associated with chemoprophylactic antimalaria drugs. Bull World Health Organ 1990;68:493–504.

32. Pang LW, Limsomwong N, Singharaj P, Canfield CJ. Malaria prophylaxis with proguanil and sulfisoxazole in children living in a malaria endemic area. Bull World Health Organ 1989;67:51–58.

33. Mvondo JL, James MA, Campbell CC. Malaria and pregnancy in Cameroonian women. Effect of pregnancy on *Plasmodium falciparum* parasitemia and the response to chloroquine. Trop Med Parasitol 1992;43:1–5.

34. McGregor IA. Epidemiology, malaria, and pregnancy. Am J Trop Med Hyg 1984;33:517–525.

35. Louareesuwan S, White NJ, Karbwang J, et al. Quinine and severe falciparum malaria in late pregnancy. Lancet 1985;ii:4–8.

36. Li GQ, Guo XB, Fu LC, et al. Clinical trails of artemisinin and its derivatives in the treatment of malaria in China. Trans R Soc Trop Med Hyg 1004;88(Suppl 1):S5–S6.

37. DuPont HL, Ericsson CD. Prevention and treatment of travelers' diarrhea. N Engl J Med 1993;328:1821–1827.

38. MacLeod CL. Parasitic infections in pregnancy and the newborn. Oxford: Oxford University Press, 1988.

39. Cook GC. Use of antiprotozoan and antihelmintic drugs during pregnancy: side effects and contraindications. J Infect 1992;25:1–9.

40. Huch R, Baumann H, Fallenstein F, et al. Physiologic changes in pregnant women and their fetuses during jet air travel. Am J Obstet Gynecol 1986;154:996–1000.

41. Maccato M, Hammill H. Travel recommendations during pregnancy and breast feeding. Pediatr Infect Dis J 1992;3:18–21.

42. Hatcher RA, Stewart FS, Trussell J, et al. Contraceptive technology. New York: Irvington, 1994.

43. The female condom. Med Lett 1993;35:123–124.

44. Frame JD. Health common sense for Christian workers overseas. New York: National Journal of the Churches of Christ in the U.S.A., 1991.

Chapter 38

THE AGED, INFIRM, OR HANDICAPPED TRAVELER

BRADFORD L. DESSERY AND MARC R. ROBIN

INTRODUCTION

Although the physical limitations of age, disability, or chronic illness may restrict some activities, they do not normally preclude travel. In fact, the benefits of travel are increasingly available to people with physical limitations, due in part to increased awareness and support for their needs. Whereas some existent illnesses tend rather to aggravate during travel to subtropical and tropical destinations, others tend to improve. Two studies, however, show somewhat ambiguous results, although having been generated by the same group (Figure 38–1).[1,2]

These conditions do, therefore, present a challenge to the travel medicine practitioner to anticipate potential problems and provide for the patient's comfort and safety in a new environment. Advice must be tailored to fit the unique circumstances of each person, including the support available from travel companions, the travel characteristics, and the patient's medical history and condition.

ROUTINE PREPARATIONS

There are a number of routine preparations that all travelers, especially those under treatment for any medical condition, can make to enhance the success of their journey:

1. Travelers should carry a supply of all of their medications to last the entire trip, plus up to a week's extra supply. Equivalent medications may not be available in other countries, and dosage and strength are frequently different without readily discernible conversion factors. Medication names may also differ.

2. Medication should be carried on person or in hand luggage aboard aircraft or ground transport vehicles. This will ensure a supply of medication in case checked luggage is misrouted, lost, or stolen, although even hand-carried bags can be stolen or misplaced.

3. If medications are lost or stolen, patients are advised to replace them with identical medication from the same manufacturer if at all possible. There may be a variation in potency among different brands of the same drugs, even when dosage and strength are otherwise the same.

4. Travelers under treatment for preexisting medical conditions should carry their physician's office and emergency phone numbers, as well as a copy of all pertinent medical records. This should include a summary of medical problems, current therapies, drug allergies, and a list of generic medications and dosages. When appropriate, the physician should also provide a copy of the most recent electrocardiogram and any significant test results.

5. Travelers should carry with them written prescriptions for all of their medications. Prescriptions provide a written record of the medication regimen, help deflect legal or customs inquiries, and may allow quick replacement in case of theft or loss.

6. Prescriptions are advisable for patients carrying syringes or medications apt to be questioned by customs officials. An official document on letterhead stationery detailing the medical need for needles and syringes, injectable medications (including insulin), multiple medications, and narcotics or other con-

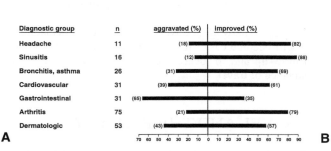

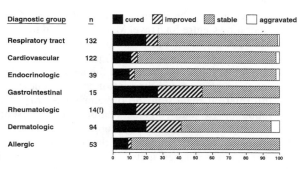

Figure 38–1. Preexisting diseases and travel. *A*, Retrospective analysis of 10,507 tourists returning from developing country. *B*, Follow-up of 664 patients to developing countries.

trolled substances is also advisable. Such a letter might look like the following:

STERILE NEEDLE AND SYRINGE PERMISSION LETTER

Date:
Name:

The above-named traveler is my patient and under my medical care and must carry a supply of medically approved sterile syringes and needles for use in (choose one):

1. a medical emergency,
2. their medical condition (e.g., diabetes), and
3. their medical treatment.

Sincerely,

Dr. _____

7. In tropical countries or when traveling on water, medications have the potential to become moist and break down. They should be kept in a cool, dry place during extended stays abroad. Place them in a sealable plastic container, keep them refrigerated, or add a packet of a drying agent such as silica gel. This is usually available where ammunition is sold. These measures will help prevent breakdown of the medication.

8. Except for very short-term travel (e.g., airline crews), patients traveling across time zones will have to take their medications at different times than at home. Have them gradually adjust their medication times over several days, depending on the length of stay. For insulin adjustments according to time zone changes, see Table 38–2.

9. Travelers with a significant medical condition, especially one that might result in unconsciousness, should consider wearing a Medic Alert necklace or bracelet during travel even if they do not at home. This could save valuable time in an emergency. Cards carried in a wallet or purse are not as accessible during a crisis and are more easily lost or stolen. Information can include medical conditions such as diabetes or seizure disorders, allergies, medication regimens, and other information such as blood type. In North America, contact the Medic Alert Foundation, PO Box 1009, Turlock, CA 95381-1009 or phone 1-800-432-5378. In Europe, the *Health Passport*, created by the Tourist Health Centre, WHO Collaborating Centre for Travel Medicine, based in Italy, has been distributed in 6 million copies. The document consists of three parts: (1) personal identification including blood group and the name of the person to be contacted in the case of an emergency; (2) information regarding the traveler's case history, immunologic status, and medication; and (3) a list of countries visited and health problems that occurred abroad, all to be completed by the traveler. The text is in seven languages, including Arabic and Russian.

10. Travelers should carry spares of any medical items that could be difficult to replace. These include eyeglasses, contact lenses, and batteries for hearing aids or glucose meters. Travelers who wear glasses are advised to carry a copy of their current lens prescriptions.

11. When using contact lenses, travelers should carry solutions for the entire trip. Water purified with iodine should not be used to rinse contacts as some lenses will become stained. A back-up pair of glasses should always be carried in case contacts cannot be worn. On long flights, glasses are preferable to contacts because of dryness from the low humidity.

12. Even more than the usual travelers, the aged, infirm, or handicapped traveler should be encouraged to assemble a first-aid kit, to use protective measures against mosquitoes, to consume only safe food and beverages, to avoid excessive heat exposure, and to drink plenty of nonalcoholic fluids to help prevent dehydration.

13. Encourage patients to be aggressive in self-treating traveler's diarrhea. In addition to the risk of dehydration, diarrhea can reduce absorption of routine medications due to decreased transit time in the gastrointestinal tract. Patients should be advised to seek medical attention for any illness or worsening of pre-existing medical problems.

14. Travelers on a special diet, such as low sodium or diabetic, should be reminded to make requests to airlines 24 to 48 hours in advance.

HEALTH INSURANCE

Elderly travelers and those with chronic medical problems need to be especially attentive to insurance needs. In addition to trip cancellation insurance, additional health insurance including air evacuation is advisable. A call to their current health insurer will ascertain coverage and the availability of optional travel insurance. They can also verify the procedure for filing a claim and obtain the necessary forms.

OVERSEAS MEDICAL ASSISTANCE

If a patient has a particularly complicated medical problem, provide him/her with the name and phone number of a specialist at the destination if at all possible. IAMAT, The International Association for Medical Assistance to Travellers, provides a directory of English-speaking physicians worldwide. Their headquarters address is 40 Regal Road, Guelph, ON N1K 1B5, Canada. Travelers may also contact their local embassy or consulate for physician referrals.

As the network of travel medicine providers matures, it will become easier to arrange medical evaluation and follow-up and to locate specialist medical services in advance of travel.

TRAVEL AND THE ELDERLY

International travel should not be regarded as an experience from which the elderly must be excluded. To avoid risks, the health aspects of the journey should be carefully planned in advance (Table 38–1). The following are the most important aspects to consider.

EXERCISE

With age, there is a decrease in muscle tone and strength, joint flexibility, and cardiovascular performance. Since the level of activity required during travel is frequently greater than at home, it makes sense to begin an exercise program 3 to 4 weeks in advance of travel. Besides this, all travelers may benefit by using luggage with wheels or a collapsible luggage cart.

Another way to cope with the limitations of age and infirmity is to take advantage of organized tours that cater to the elderly. These usually provide a leisurely itinerary, frequent rest stops, help with the luggage, and other services. A cruise is another alternative that allows the traveler to set his or her own pace.

IMMUNIZATIONS

Immunization requirements for the elderly traveler are no different from other adults except for pneumococcal and annual influenza vaccination.

Table 38–1 HEALTH HINTS FOR THE ELDERLY TRAVELER

1. Ask for a medical check-up before starting the journey, particularly if you suffer from a chronic disease. Ask your doctor for personalized advice on preventive measures to be taken.
2. Take with you all health documentation that could be of use to a doctor who may have to be consulted at your destination. If you have been hospitalized, take a recent electrocardiogram and a copy of your case records.
3. Collect information on the health services available in the country that you intend to visit. Give preference to a country that offers better facilities.
4. Take out one or more insurance policies to ensure your right to obtain any health treatment you may require and repatriation by air-ambulance if needed.
5. Avoid physical exertion when preparing for the journey and when moving luggage. Once your destination has been reached, avoid a frenetic pace of life and do not attempt to do things or see places that you have perhaps never done or seen before in the space of only a few days.
6. Take light and easily digestible meals. Avoid or limit the consumption of alcohol. Drink other liquids frequently to avoid imbalances of body fluids.
7. Increase sun exposure gradually and do not subject your body to excessive heat. The elderly are more prone to heatstroke than any other age group.
8. Avoid high mountain areas and rapid ascents to high altitudes.
9. If visiting a spa center, ask for a medical examination complete with electrocardiogram to ensure that no potential complications are involved in the treatments.
10. After returning from an international journey, ask for a medical examination if you have had a high temperature, persistent diarrhea, or other health problems.

There are a few vaccines that may be contraindicated due to certain medical conditions or drug therapies. (See Chapter 22.1 Vaccine-Preventable Diseases: The Commercially Available Vaccines.)

MALARIA PROPHYLAXIS

Malaria mortality rates increase with age. Prophylaxis is also essential for the older traveler facing exposure. Persons over 60 years of age tend to have less adverse events despite the fact that they often use other medication.

MOTION SICKNESS

All medications against kinetosis have similar rates of effectiveness and adverse events[3]; however, transdermal scopolamine patches, frequently used by cruise ship passengers for prevention of motion sickness, should not be routinely prescribed for elderly travelers. The side effects of anticholinergic drugs are more frequent, including confusion, constipation, dry mouth, urinary retention, and narrow angle glaucoma.[4] Scopolamine is contraindicated for persons with narrow angle glaucoma.

AUTOMOBILE ACCIDENTS

Elderly vacationers driving cars can be prone to greater accident risks due to diminished sensorial capacities. As age increases, the sharpness of vision and hearing declines; night vision is impaired, it becomes more difficult to turn the head sideways, and reaction times increase. In addition, the elderly are more likely to use drug therapies that can influence driving capacity (psychoactive drugs, antidepressants, antihistamines, and antihypertensives).

SUN EXPOSURE

Many drugs increase sensitivity to sunlight, including tetracyclines, sulfas, and some oral hypoglycemic, diuretic, and nonsteroid anti-inflammatory medications.

ACCLIMATIZATION

Hot Climates Elderly travelers are less tolerant of hot climates because the ability of peripheral blood vessels to dilate and the skin to perspire is impaired with age. The elderly are less sensitive to thirst. Because of decreased kidney function, they are more susceptible to fluid and electrolyte disturbances from diarrhea.[5] Also, appetite loss, nausea, vomiting, and fever can contribute to dehydration. In turn, dehydration hastens symptoms of heat exposure. If travelers are overweight, have cardiovascular disease or diabetes, or take diuretics or anticholinergics, susceptibility to heat is increased, as is the risk of serious complications.

Medications, particularly diuretics and anticholinergics, beta and calcium channel blocking agents and some antidepressants, antihistamines, and antiparkinsonian drugs, can slow acclimatization to heat.

Adjusting to hot climates may take several days. Rest and avoidance of strenuous activity are desirable initially. Air conditioning, shade, loose-fitting cotton clothing, dark glasses, a wide brim hat, cool baths or showers, and a good fluid intake will ease the transition.

Cold Climates Susceptibility to hypothermia also increases with age. Adequate layers of clothing are essential, including protection for the head, hands, and feet. Cold climates are drying and fluid intake is important, especially with exertion. Skin moisturizers may be required for extended periods outdoors.

Altitude Acute mountain sickness actually is a greater risk for children and young adults than for healthy older travelers. Some antihypertensive medications, such as beta-blockers, may interfere with a compensatory increase in the heart rate at high elevations. This may result in shortness of breath and symptoms that mimic acute mountain sickness. Altitudes above 8,000 feet can also compromise cardiopulmonary function in travelers with preexisting heart or lung disease or severe anemia (see Chapter 13 Medical Problems of High Altitude).

JET LAG

Both jet lag and the adverse side effects of sedatives prescribed to counter jet lag are seen more frequently in the older population.

TRAVELER'S DIARRHEA

Elderly travelers are more likely to suffer fluid and electrolyte imbalances as a result of diarrhea. Prompt therapy is essential, including oral rehydration solutions. Medications and instructions for the prompt treatment of travelers' diarrhea should be included in a first-aid kit. In prescribing treatment for travelers' diarrhea, be aware of potential drug interactions. Trimethoprim/sulfamethoxazole combinations may potentiate oral hypoglycemics. Quinolones prolong the half-life of theophyllines. Ofloxacin, however, reportedly does not have this effect.[6]

CONSTIPATION AND HEMORRHOIDS

Constipation can be exacerbated by the minor ordeals of travel. Constipation may also follow the use of antimotility medications or other constipating drugs, such as codeine or aluminum-based antacids.

VISION

Visual acuity deteriorates with age. As vision declines, there is an increased risk for falling and fractures, especially fractures of the hip. Encourage patients who need glasses to use them during travel.

HEARING

Hearing loss is the most common sensory impairment in the elderly and may predispose to not hearing approaching vehicles, particularly electromobiles. Encourage travelers with hearing loss to use a hearing aid if needed and to take along extra batteries.

DENTURES

Denture adhesive is often difficult to find, and travelers are advised to take along enough for the entire trip. If dentures need to be soaked overnight, use purified water. The best solution for both sterilizing and odor control is a 1 to 10 solution of household bleach and water. Water treated with iodine can also be used, as stains are not likely to occur from the iodine. If a pure water source is not available, beer, soft drinks, or bottled mineral water can be used instead. For short periods of time, up to 3 to 4 weeks, there is usually no harm in leaving dentures in overnight if desired.

Broken dentures can usually be repaired at a dental laboratory, if one is available. If not, clean breaks or cracks are reparable with cyanoacrylate adhesive ("superglue").

DRUG INTERACTIONS

Since many of the elderly use multiple medications, it is important to consider potential drug interactions.

PSYCHOLOGICAL AND PSYCHIATRIC PROBLEMS OF HOSPITALIZATION

Elderly travelers may sometimes be subject to hospitalization. The unknown environment can be associated with disturbances of either the emotive and affective sphere or the cognitive and intellective sphere. The difficulties increase if the elderly patient is unable to contact his or her relatives because they cannot be traced.

TRAVEL WITH CHRONIC ILLNESS

DIABETES

Although diabetes is not a contraindication for travel, newly diagnosed diabetics or diabetics whose blood glucose levels are temporarily uncontrolled should postpone travel until their blood sugars are stable. Diabetics face no travel restrictions, but they should plan for increased blood glucose monitoring and prepare for the potential problems of hypoglycemia and hyperglycemia due to the disruption of daily routine and the stresses of travel.

Diabetics should be encouraged to make the following routine preparations for travel:

1. Pack the following supplies in quantities sufficient to last the entire trip, plus at least an extra week's supply of:
   - insulin;
   - syringes;
   - a supplemental bottle of regular crystalline zinc insulin for emergencies, with instructions for use;
   - blood glucose testing strips and lancets;
   - urine ketone and glucose test strips;

- fast oral sugar source, snacks, and sweet nondiet beverages for treating hypoglycemic episodes;
- food such as crackers and cheese or other snacks in case of meal delays;
- sugar substitutes; and
- extra batteries for glucose meters.

2. Carry a glucagon emergency kit for use in case of hypoglycemia resulting in unconsciousness.[7] Prior to travel, patients should instruct a travel companion both in the signs of hypoglycemia and the use of the kit.

3. Request diabetic diets at least 24 to 48 hours in advance for airline travel.

Ideally, insulin should be refrigerated when in hot climates. However, it will keep for at least 1 month unrefrigerated if protected from freezing or temperatures above 86°F (30°C).[8] If insulin may be exposed to heat above 120°F (approximately 50°C), it can be protected with a wide-mouthed thermos or insulated bottle. Rinse the container with ice water, empty, and place the insulin inside wrapped in paper or a washcloth to avoid breakage. Available commercially is the "Medicool Insulin Protector," 23520 Telo Ave., Torrance, CA 90505, tel: 1-800-433-2469 (in California, 1-800-654-1565) or on the Web at www.medicool.com.

Keep insulin in hand-carried luggage, packed between layers of clothing to protect it from breakage and temperature extremes.[7]

For trips longer than 1 month, diabetics should check in advance the local availability and equivalent brand names of their usual form of insulin. For Humulin (human insulin) or other insulin products from Eli Lily and Co., call customer service at 1-800-545-5979. For products from Novo Nordisk Pharmaceuticals, call 1-800-727-6500.

Medication Adjustment During Flight   Oral hypoglycemics for patients with NIDDM (type 2) can be taken as prescribed according to local time without regard to time zone changes. For IDDM (type 1), dosage adjustment of insulin is made according to the direction of flight and the number of time zones crossed (Table 38–2).

If taking insulin, it is easiest to plan mealtimes by keeping a watch set to the original time zone. Prepare for any delays in transit by having sufficient snacks at hand. When administering insulin in flight, put half as much air in the bottle as normal due to the decreased air pressure at altitude. Check blood glucose frequently after flights across several time zones.

Drink plenty of fluids and avoid alcohol in flight to prevent dehydration in the low cabin humidity. Dehydration may make glucose control more difficult. Diabetes increases susceptibility to heat-related problems. Dehydration also makes glucose more difficult to control. Avoid dehydration and increase blood glucose monitoring. Symptoms of hypoglycemia and hyperglycemia may mimic some of the symptoms of heat exposure, such as weakness, dizziness, headache, and confusion.[9]

Diabetics with autonomic neuropathy, which interferes with sweating, should avoid hot climates or make sure the air-conditioned environments are available.

Illness   If vomiting occurs and Type I diabetics are unable to eat, insulin at a reduced dosage must still be used regularly. During any illness, blood sugar levels should be carefully monitored to accurately determine insulin requirements. During illness, it may be easier to maintain control using regular insulin rather than long-acting formulations.[10]

In treating travelers' diarrhea or other illnesses, Type II diabetics taking oral hypoglycemics should avoid

Table 38–2.   INSULIN ADJUSTMENTS ACCORDING TO TIME-ZONE CHANGES

WESTBOUND, 6 OR MORE TIME ZONES (DAY IS LENGTHENED)*			
DOSAGE SCHEDULE	DAY OF DEPARTURE	18 HOURS AFTER AM DOSE CHECK BLOOD GLUCOSE; IF >240 MG/DL	MORNING OF DESTINATION
Single dose	Usual dose	Take ⅓ of usual dose followed by snack or meal	Usual dose
Two doses	Usual am and pm dose (10–12 hours after am dose)	Take ⅓ of usual am dose followed by a snack or meal	Usual dose

EASTBOUND, 6 OR MORE TIME ZONES (DAY IS SHORTENED)			
DOSE SCHEDULE	DAY OF DEPARTURE	MORNING OF DESTINATION	10 HOURS AFTER AM DOSE CHECK BLOOD GLUCOSE; IF >240 MG/DL	SECOND DAY
Single dose	Usual dose	⅔ of usual dose	Take remaining ⅓ of am dose	Usual dose
Two doses	Usual am and pm dose	⅔ of usual am dose	Take usual pm dose plus remaining ⅓ of am dose	Usual 2 doses

*Adapted from Benson and Metz.[10]

trimethoprim/sulfamethoxazole combinations. They can potentiate hypoglycemic activity, causing a dangerous and unexpected drop in blood glucose levels.[11]

Foot Care Diabetic foot care must be rigorous and common-sense rules obeyed; avoid going barefoot. Never break in a new pair of shoes while traveling. Change socks twice daily if needed to keep feet dry and comfortable.

Inspect feet carefully each day. If a foot infection or nonhealing cut or puncture wound occurs, seek immediate medical attention.

In humid climates, an antifungal powder is a useful addition to the first-aid kit, as is Second Skin™ or moleskin for use on blisters.

Activity Log By keeping a detailed record of activities, blood sugar readings, and insulin requirements and adjustments, travelers will be better able to determine their requirements on subsequent trips.

Other Resources The names and addresses of local diabetes associations can be obtained from the International Diabetes Association (IDF), Rue Washington 40, B-1050 Brussels, Belgium,[12] http://www.idf.org/. Local diabetic associations can provide information on overseas physicians specializing in diabetes, restaurants offering special diets, pharmacies open 24 hours, and other useful information. The international list of local diabetes associations can also be obtained by mail or on the Web from "The Diabetic Traveler" (see reference below) or at www.diabetesnews.com.

The American Diabetes Association (ADA), at 1660 Duke St., Alexandria, VA 22314, provides a wallet-size "Diabetic Alert Card" with emergency information in 13 different languages. They have an extensive Web site with a lot of information for both patients and health professionals. The address is http://www.diabetes.org/, with links to other Internet sites.

Another resource is "The Diabetic Traveler." Subscriptions and reprints can be ordered from PO Box 8223 RWS, Stamford, CT 06905, or on the Web at www.ishops.com/diabetes/.

Free medical alert ID necklaces, diabetes self-management diaries, and educational literature can be obtained from The Diabetes Research and Wellness Foundation, PO Box 3837, Merrifield, VA 22116, tel: 202-298-9211, URL: http://www.charities.org/dirs/health/drwf/index.html. They are publishers of the *Diabetes Wellness Letter*.

Excellent annotated links for diabetic resources on the Web can be found at http://www.mendosa.com/diabetes.htm/.

DIALYSIS AND KIDNEY TRANSPLANT PATIENTS

Dialysis is available in many parts of the world for patients who wish to travel. Appointments must be arranged and confirmed as much as 4 or more weeks in advance. Patients should carry a medical summary and treatment recommendations from their physician, as well as the results of a recent hepatitis B antibody test.[13]

A directory of dialysis facilities worldwide can be obtained from Creative Age Publications, 7628 Densmore Ave., Van Nuys, CA 91406-2088, tel: 818-782-7328. Ask for "The List of Transient Dialysis Centers." This information is also on the Web at http://www.eneph.com/. In Europe, information can be obtained from the International Dialysis Organisation, 153 rue du Port, 69390 Fernaison, France, tel: 33-723-1230. Various tour operators specialize in tours and cruises for dialysis and kidney transplant patients, with access provided to the necessary medical resources.

KIDNEY STONES

There is an increased risk of kidney stones in the tropics due to dehydration. Travelers with a history of stones must pay special attention to hydration requirements.

THE HANDICAPPED TRAVELER

The perfectly legitimate aspiration of handicapped persons is to be able to enjoy the opportunities offered by tourism and travel, both individually and in groups, together with nondisabled persons. However, this aspiration is still confronted with the limits posed by architectural and sometimes even cultural barriers, and with the insufficiencies of tourism and travel at an organizational level.

Accommodation of the special needs of the blind, deaf, or mobility-impaired traveler varies tremendously around the world. The chief factors are acceptance and awareness of these needs and the social commitment and resources available to meet them. In this regard, Scandinavian countries and the Netherlands have been well ahead of the rest of the world.[13]

Many travelers with disabilities will prefer the help of a travel professional to make accessible arrangements. Most travel agencies can handle routine requests for tours, accommodations, and transportation for handicapped individuals in the more progressive areas mentioned above. Some agencies and tour operators have developed expertise in handicapped travel. Tours are available for people with a wide range of special physical or medical requirements. Sporting competitions for the wheelchair bound, adventure travel, and rafting trips have all been extended to those with disabilities.

THE MOBILITY-IMPAIRED TRAVELER

For travel, wheelchair users are usually advised that a lightweight folding chair or "junior" model is most convenient. Tools are helpful for making repairs, as is a "wheelchair tightener" for navigating narrow doorways.

Most newer aircraft were designed for wheelchair access, and some older planes still in service have been retrofitted. Check airline regulations regarding battery transport before making reservations. Gel- or foam-filled batteries in scooters or power chairs are usually accepted by airlines. Acid batteries must be removed and may be damaged in baggage compartments. It is helpful to tape clear disassembly instructions on scooters and power wheelchairs, including battery disconnection instructions.

Many cities throughout the world publish accessibility handbooks. Write to their tourist bureaus well in advance of traveling to obtain access information. In Europe, contact Mobility International, 25 rue due Manchester, B-1070 Brussels, Belgium.

THE SIGHT-IMPAIRED TRAVELER

Transport of guide dogs for the blind across international borders can be a major problem, depending on the destination. Lengthy quarantines may be imposed, especially in island nations such as Australia, New Zealand, Great Britain, and Ireland, as well as Hawaii. Guide dogs may be admitted elsewhere based on a medical certificate of health and proof of rabies vaccination. Check regulations with the embassy or consulate of the destination country prior to travel and obtain all necessary medical and legal documents in advance. Do not forget to inquire about requirements for re-entry into the country of origin.

Resource organizations:
American Foundation for the Blind
11 Penn Plaza, Suite 300
New York, NY 10001
Tel: 212-502-7661
TDD: 212-502-7662
FAX: 212-502-7777
http://www.afb.org/

American Council of the Blind
1155 15th Street, NW, Suite 720
Washington, DC 20005
202-467-5081; 800-424-8666
Fax: 202-467-5085
http://www.acb.org/

THE HEARING-IMPAIRED TRAVELER

Deaf travelers need to inform transportation and hotel staff of their disability or they will miss travel announcements or emergency information and alarms. On airline flights, they should request preloading privileges and notify flight attendants of their hearing problem. Attendants will show the emergency equipment and exit locations and keep them informed of announcements.

Resource organizations:
Alexander Graham Bell Association for the Deaf
3417 Volte Place NW
Washington, DC 20007-2778
Tel: 202-337-5220 voice and TTY
http://www.agbell.org/

National Association for the Deaf
814 Thayer Avenue
Silver Spring, MD 20910
Tel: 301-587-1788 voice

Tel: 301-587-1789 TTY
http://www.nad.org/

National Information Center on Deafness
Gallaudet University
800 Florida Avenue NE
Washington, DC 20002-3695
Tel: 202-651-5051
202-651-5052 TTY
202-651-5054 FAX
http://www.gallaudet.edu/

THE MENTALLY IMPAIRED TRAVELER

No rules restrict travel of the mentally retarded or others with mental disabilities, as long as they are self-sufficient. If the need for assistance is anticipated, requests for help en route at airports or elsewhere should be made well in advance. Tours and excursions exist in many countries for those with special needs.

Some people may become disoriented in a strange town and lose their way. It is helpful if they carry a card with the name, address, and phone number of their hotel or other residence, as well as one showing their destination, so that they can obtain directions or assistance if they become lost.

RESOURCES FOR DISABLED TRAVELERS

Web Resources
For current information on the Web, start at an informative site with links to other Web resources, such as:

1. Access-Able Travel Source, http://www.access-able.com/
2. Global Access, http://www.geocities.com/Paris/1502/
3. MossRehab ResourceNet, http://www.mossresourcenet. org/travel.htm/

Disabled travelers with computer access may benefit from direct networking with one of the following USENET groups:

rec.travel.europe
rec.travel.asia
rec.travel.usa-canada
rec.travel.cruises

Books
Wheelchair Around the World, by Patrick and Anne Simpson, Pentland Press, 5124 Bur Oak Circle, Raleigh, NC 27612, 1997. A personal account with extensive bibliography.
How to Travel: A Guidebook for Persons with Disabilities, by Fred Rosen, Science and Humanities Press, 1023 Styvesant, Manchester, MO 63011-3601, 1998. A how-to guide for wheelchair users, the hearing impaired, or those traveling with oxygen.
Access for Disabled Americans—Guide for the Wheelchair Traveler, by Patricia Smither, Access for Disabled American, PO Box 384, Orinda, CA 94563.

Air Carrier Access—free pamphlet on the Air Carriers Access Act, available from Eastern Paralyzed Veterans Association, 75-20 Astoria Boulevard, Jackson Heights, NY 11370-1177.

India, Wheelchair Journey, by Ed Long, Ed Long Publications, 2503 Lincoln Ave, San Diego, CA 92104, USA. Personal account of a 3-month journey in India.

Smooth Ride Guide to United States Eastern Seaboard and *Smooth Ride Guide to Australia and New Zealand*, by Julie Ramsey, FT Publishing, 4 Talbot Road, Highgate, London N6 4QP, U.K. or Seven Hills Book Distributors, 49 Central Ave., Cincinnati, OH 45202.

Easy Access Australia, by Bruce Cameron, PO Box 218, Kew, Victoria 3101, Australia.

The Wheelie's Handbook to Australia, by Colin James, PO Box 89, Coleraine, Victoria 3315, Australia.

World of Options: A Guide to International Exchange, Community Service and Travel for Persons with Disabilities, 3rd Ed., Mobility International USA, PO Box 10767, Eugene, OR 97440.

Wheelchair Through Europe, by Annie Markin, Graphic Language Press, PO Box 270, Cardiff by the Sea, CA 92007. Personal account plus list of resources, 1994.

Holidays in the British Isles (guide to accommodations in the British Isles), *Long Haul Holidays and Travel* (regional guide), and *European Holidays and Travel Abroad* (information for 32 countries in Europe), three guides published by RADAR (Royal Association for Disabilities and Rehabilitation), 12 City Forum 250 City Road, London EC1V 8AF, U.K.

Holiday Care Guide To Accessible Accommodations & Travel, Holiday Care Service, Imperial Buildings, 2nd Floor, Victoria Road, Horley, Surrey RH6 7PZ, U.K. Lists 1,500 inspected accommodations in the United Kingdom.

Exotic Destinations for Wheelchair Travelers: Hotel Guide to the Orient, Hong Kong, Macau, Singapore, Taiwan, Thailand, by Edmond Hansen and Bruce Gordon, Full Data Limited Publishing, San Francisco, 1994.

Great American Vacations for Travelers with Disabilities Fodors Travel Publications, Inc., 1996, 280 Park Avenue, New York, NY 10017.

Wheel and Waves, Wheels Aweigh Publishing Co., 1993. A directory of ships, ferries, and river and canal barges with detailed information on their accessibility.

Able to Travel: True Stories by and for People with Disabilities, Rough Guides Ltd., 1994. A collection of over 100 accounts by disabled travelers.

Access in London, Access in Paris, Access in Israel (3 books), by Pauline Hephaistos Survey Project, Robert Nicholson Publications, Access Project, 39 Bradley Gardens, West Ealing, London W13 8HE, U.K.

The Wheelchair Traveler, by Douglas Rannand, 123 Ball Hill Road Milford, NH 03055.

Organizations

Mobility International, PO Box 10767, Eugene, OR 97440; Tel. 541-343-1284 V/TDD; Fax: 541-343-6812; E-mail: miusa@igc.apc.org. A nonprofit organization that promotes international educational exchange, leadership and disability rights, and travel for disabled persons. Publishes a quarterly newsletter, *Over The Rainbow*, and maintains information sheets on many areas of the world.

Travelin' Talk, PO Box 3534, Clarksville, TN 37047; Tel: 615-552-6670; Fax: 615-552-1182; E-mail: trvlntlk @aol.com. Membership network providing assistance to travelers with disabilities.

SATH (The Society for the Advancement of Travel for the Handicapped), 347 Fifth Ave. Suite 610, New York, NY 10016. Tel: 212-447-7284, Fax: 212-725-8253; E-mail: sathtravel@aol.com. Publishes an excellent information sheet for members with tips for both the handicapped traveler and for travel agents and other providers of travel services. Also has a computer listing of accessible hotels and publishes a newsletter with current access information, including other sources. Individual memberships cost $25.00.

NICAN (National Information Communication Awareness Network), PO Box 407, Curtain ACT 2605; Tel: 06-285-3713, 06-285-3714; Fax: 06-280-4333 TTY; E-mail: nican@spirit.com.au. A nonprofit organization in Australia providing information for persons with disabilities.

Newsletters

The Accessible Travel Newsletter, published by Emerging Horizons, Candy & Charles Creative Concepts, PO Box 278, Ripon, CA 95366; E-mail: horizons@ candy-charles.com; Web site: http://www.candy-charles.com/horizons.htm.

Access to the Skies, published by the Paralysis Society of America, 801 Eighteenth Street, NW, Washington, DC 20006; Tel: 800-424-8200, 800-795-4327 TDD; E-mail: 74012.1101@compuserve.com. News concerning accessible air travel.

We're Accessible—Travel Service for Wheelchair Users and Slow Walkers, 32-1675 Cypress St.,Vancouver, BC V6J 3L4, Canada; Tel: 604-731-2197; E-mail: lynna@istar.ca. Quarterly newsletter on travel and travel resources.

The Very Special Traveler, PO Box 756, New Windsor, MD 21776. Tel: 410-635-2881; E-mail: tbster@ aol.com.

The Able Informer, 197407 Preston Road, Warrensville Heights, OH 44128; E-mail: 71033.1073@compu serve.com. Web site: http://www.sasquatch.com/ ableinfo/. Quarterly newsletter dealing with disability issues including travel.

Access for Disabled Americans, 436 14th Street, Oakland, CA 94612; Tel: 510-419-0523; Fax: 510-419-0728; E-mail: PSmither@aol.com. Quarterly newsletter with some travel tips and information.

The Handicapped Travel Newsletter is published bimonthly and written "for and by disabled persons." Drawer 269, Athens, TX 75751; Tel: 903-677-1260.

Flying Wheels Travel, a travel agency that specializes in handicapped travel, publishes their own newsletter. 143 West Bridge St., Box 382, Owatonna, MN, 800-535-6790.

Magazines

Access To Travel, PO Box 43, Del Mar, NY 12054; Tel: 518-439-4146; Fax: 518-439-9004.

Open World Magazine, 347 Fifth Ave, Suite 610, New York, NY 10016; Tel: 212-447-7284, 212-725-8253; E-mail: sathtravel@aol.com; Web site: http://www.sath.org/openw.html. A publication of The Society for the Advancement of Travel for the Handicapped.

New Mobility, 23815 Stuart Ranch Road, PO Box 8987, Malibu, CA 90267; Tel: 800-543-4116, 310-317-4522; Fax: 310-317-9644; E-mail: sam@miramir.com; Web page: http://www.newmobility.com/.

Paraplegia News, 2111 E. Highland Ave. Siute 180, Phoenix, AZ 85016; Tel: 602-224-0500; Fax: 602-224-0507; E-mail: pvapub@aol.com; Web page: http://www.pva.org. Published by the Paralyzed Veterans of America.

Disability International, 101-7 Evergreen Place, Winnipeg, MB R3L 2T3, Canada. Tel: 800-749-7773, 204-477-5319; Fax: 204-453-1367; Web page: http://www.dpi.org/di.html. Published quarterly by Disabled Peoples' International.

Accent on Living, PO Box 700, Bloomington, IL 61702; Tel: 309-378-2961; Fax: 309-378-4420; E-mail: acntlvng@aol.com; Web page: http://www.blvd.com/accent/index.html. Published quarterly.

We Magazine, 495 Broadway, PO Box 20553, New York, NY 10012; Tel: 800-WEMAG26, 212-941-9584; Fax: 212-941-6458;

E-mail: editors@wemagazine.com; Web site: http://www.wemagazine.com/. Lifestyles magazine for people with disabilities.

Ability Magazine, 1001 W. 17th Street, Costa Mesa, CA 92627; Tel: 714-854-8700; Fax: 714-548-5966; E-mail: ability@pacbell.net.

Mainstream Magazine, PO Box 370598, San Diego, CA 92137-0598; Tel: 619-234-3138; Fax: 619-234-3155; E-mail: publisher@mainstream-mag.com; Web site: http://www.mainstream-mag.com.

Enable Magazine, 3659 Cortez Road West, Suite 110, Bradenton, FL 34210; Tel: 941-758-4903 or 888-436-2253; Fax: 941-758-4710; E-mail: readenable@aol.com; Web site: http://www.enable-magazine.com/.

Other

Information for Handicapped Travelers; Reference Section, National Library Service for the Blind and Physically Handicapped, Library of Congress, Washington, DC 20540.

REFERENCES

1. Steffen R, van der Linde F. Intercontinental travel and its effect on pre-existing illnesses. Aviat Space Environ Med 1981;52:57–58.
2. Burckhardt M, Steffen R. Voyages lointains: faut-il s'attendre à une aggravation ou à une amélioration des maladies préexistantes? Med Hyg (Geneva) 1995;53:1182–1185.
3. Schmid R, Schick T, Steffen R, et al. Comparison of seven commonly used agents for prophylaxis of seasickness. J Travel Med 1994;1:203–206.
4. Jong EC, McMullen R. General advice for the international traveler. Infect Dis Clin North Am 1992;6:275–289.
5. Patterson JE, Patterson TF. The geriatric traveler. In: Jong EC, Keystone JS, McMullen R, eds. The travel medicine advisor. Atlanta: American Health Consultants, 1991:14.1–14.6.
6. Neumann K, ed. Traveling healthy. 1992;5(July/Aug):1–4.
7. Rosenbaum M, ed. Mastering air travel. The Diabetic Traveler 1991;5:1–6.
8. Neumann K, ed. Mastering air travel. The Diabetic Traveler 1991;5(2):1–6.
9. Rosenbaum M, ed. Adapting to the heat and sun: no sweat! The Diabetic Traveler 1992;6:1–4.
10. Benson E, Metz R. Management of diabetes during intercontinental travel. Bull Mason Clinic 1984–85;38:145–151.
11. Patterson JE. The traveler with chronic illness. Yale J Biol Med 1992;65:317–27.
12. Bia FJ, Barry M. Special health considerations for travelers. Med Clin North Am 1992;76:1295–1312.
13. Weiss L. The handicapped traveler. In: Dawood R, ed. Traveler's health. New York: Random House, 1994:471–477.

Chapter 39

THE IMMUNOCOMPROMISED TRAVELER

CHRISTOPHER P. CONLON

INTRODUCTION

The past two decades have seen an explosion in travel with many millions of people from developed and developing countries voyaging abroad for pleasure and for business. Along with this vast increase in the number of travelers has been a large increase in the number of people who, for one reason or another, have some impairment of the immune system. Increasingly, because of better survival and increased opportunities, these immunocompromised individuals are also traveling more and will seek advice from their physicians. Probably the largest such group are people infected with the human immunodeficiency virus (HIV). There are also other groups with congenital or acquired immunosuppression. In addition, because of advances in medical care, there are increasing numbers of patients who have iatrogenic immunodeficiency—for example, by cancer chemotherapy, organ transplantation, or steroid treatment.

The immunocompromised traveler will need advice and management that may differ from that given to healthy travelers. They should be encouraged to seek advice well in advance of the proposed travel date, not only to allow sufficient time for the necessary immunizations but also because part of the medical advice may be to alter the travel plans in some way. Although the data on travel immunizations in the immunocompromised are limited compared to the information on healthy travelers, there are sufficient data on the responses to various vaccines by patients with different forms of immunosuppression to allow informed extrapolation to the setting of international travel.

Key components of travel medicine are education of the traveler and general advice about the avoidance of risk. Immunocompromised travelers should be knowledgeable about the type of immune defect they have and what types of infections they may be more prone to. They should have a clear understanding of the medicines they are taking and should know what to do if they run into difficulty. It is helpful to supply a letter on the physician's letterhead notepaper outlining the medical problems of the patient and providing contact telephone and fax numbers if medical advice is required abroad. Ideally, patients should be given contact details of physicians at or near their travel destination who have specialist knowledge about the traveler's type of condition. Travelers should also be reminded that some medication they take, such as anti-HIV treatment, may be unavailable at their destina-

tion so they should take care to safeguard their supplies when traveling.

FORMS OF IMPAIRED IMMUNITY

Immunocompromised travelers may be at increased risk of certain infections because of their immune defect. However, this defect may also mean that the response to vaccines used to prevent infections may be impaired. In addition, some immunizations may be potentially hazardous. Protection from infection depends on both cellular and humoral (antibody) immune function along with more nonspecific opsonization and phagocytic functions. Response to vaccines usually requires T lymphocyte function, with or without B lymphocyte function. Although antibody levels are often measured as an index of protection, cellular responses and immunologic "memory" may often be more important but are not so easily measured. In practice, many types of immunosuppression, both natural and iatrogenic, affect several arms of the immune response to some extent.

PREVENTIVE MEASURES— GENERAL PRINCIPLES

IMMUNIZATION

Immunization may be either passive or active. Passive immunization is not commonly used in travel medicine these days but should not be forgotten. It requires no immune response from the recipient and may be the only type of protection that can be offered to some immunocompromised travelers. The main issues to consider are the safety of the product, its efficacy for the traveler, and the durability of protection afforded.

Active immunization, on the other hand, requires the recipient to mount a response against the antigen administered. This varies according to the antigen and according to the degree of immunosuppression. There are some data on the immune responses made by different groups of immunocompromised patients to killed and polysaccharide vaccines. Generally, the responses are less good and less durable than normal. Killed vaccines and polysaccharide and conjugate vaccines appear to be safe in immunocompromised recipients. Live vaccines, however, are generally contraindicated because of concerns that the immunocompromised recipient will not be able to contain the replicating vaccine strain. This carries the risk of illness in the recipient, such as disseminated becille Calmette-Guérin (BCG), or may put contacts of the recipient at risk, particularly if the vaccine strain reverts to wild type (e.g., oral polio vaccine).

MALARIA

There are no data to suggest that the immunocompromised traveler is any more prone to acquire malaria than the immunocompetent one. Although there are suspicions that the disease, if acquired, may be more severe, there are no good data to support these fears. Malaria chemoprophylaxis advice generally does not need to be altered for the immunocompromised, although some groups, such as those with HIV, may be more prone to side effects with some medications.

TRAVELERS' DIARRHEA

Although there is no evidence that the incidence of travelers' diarrhea is increased in the immunocompromised, there is good evidence that the disease may be more severe or prolonged. Thus, advice concerning food and water hygiene is essential for the immunocompromised, and this group may be more likely to benefit from chemoprophylaxis.

THE TRAVELER WITH HIV INFECTION

The HIV pandemic has evolved over the past two decades so that globally, millions of individuals are living with HIV and AIDS. The majority of these people live in developing countries in the tropics and have limited scope for travel; nevertheless, many will journey to other countries and possibly present with problems related to their HIV infection. In this chapter, the emphasis will be on those people with HIV infection in developed countries who seek pretravel advice. There are estimated to be over 1 million people with HIV in North America alone.

Infection with HIV is lifelong and leads, in the absence of specific therapy, to an inexorable decline in immune function. The primary problem in HIV infection is impaired cellular immunity, with declining numbers and function of CD4 positive T lymphocytes, which renders the individual susceptible to opportunist infections, such as *Pneumocystis carinii* pneumonia (PCP) and mycobacterial infections.[1] In addition, gut infections with protozoan parasites are a problem, whereas helminth infections are not. These patients also have B lymphocyte dysfunction and are more susceptible to infection with encapsulated bacteria, such as *Streptococcus pneumoniae* and *Haemophilus influenzae*. The response to new antigens is poor, and, as a consequence, response to immunization is often poor and unpredictable compared to immunocompetent vaccine recipients. Generally, patients with early and asymptomatic HIV infection respond better than those with more advanced disease. The advent of specific anti-HIV treatments has led to a new optimism and prolonged survival of patients with HIV. This highly active antiretroviral therapy (HAART) can lead to dramatic improvements in immune status, even in people with a diagnosis of AIDS.

IMMUNIZATIONS IN HIV

Live Vaccines These are usually contraindicated because of the risk of uninhibited replication of the vaccine strain. For example, nontyphoidal salmonella bacteremia is not uncommon n HIV, and there are concerns that the live typhoid vaccine may disseminate in HIV-positive recipients. Disseminated BCG is another cause for concern. Oral polio vaccine may replicate in the gut and be chronically excreted in HIV-positive recipients. There are theoretical risks of reversion to wild-type polio virus in this setting and transmission to close contacts. However, measles vaccine appears to have been safe in HIV-positive children and is not contraindicated. The need to give this to travelers, however, is questionable. Yellow fever vaccination is controversial. Most physicians would not give yellow fever vaccine to a person with HIV with a CD4 lymphocyte count below 500/mm³, but the World Health Organization does recommend the vaccine for those with asymptomatic HIV infection. The risks of yellow fever vaccine in this setting are probably low but are not known. I usually provide a waiver letter on letterhead paper explaining the need to avoid live vaccines and documenting the patient's knowledge that he/she is not protected against yellow fever. This can be presented to immigration personnel if required.

Other Immunizations Killed vaccines appear to be safe in HIV. Studies of influenza immunization, for example, show no adverse effects. However, the level of antibody and the durability of the response are less good than that obtained in immunocompetent individuals.[2] Recent studies have also shown that responses to the new hepatitis A vaccines are adequate in HIV-positive recipients, but the durability of the antibody response is not known.[3] For patients with advanced HIV disease, the response to hepatitis A vaccination is likely to be poor, and they may be better advised to have passive immunization with gammaglobulin. Patients requiring polio vaccination should receive the killed, parenteral Salk vaccine.

Polysaccharide and conjugate vaccines are also safe but are less immunogenic in this population and poorly immunogenic in advanced HIV disease.[4] Pneumococcal vaccine is often recommended for this group of patients, but there are no efficacy data. Although reasonable responses to the conjugate *H. influenzae* type b (Hib) vaccine can be demonstrated, most infections in patients with HIV are with non-type b *H. influenzae*. The parenteral typhoid vaccine can be shown to produce a response in HIV, but the duration of protective antibody levels is likely to be short. There are no efficacy data.

Various immunizations have been shown to lead to transient increases in HIV viral load in the plasma in patients with HIV. The amplitude and duration of these rises are very small and are considered clinically insignificant.[5] Recent small studies have also demonstrated this phenomenon in patients on HAART receiving hepatitis A or influenza vaccines. Patients should be reassured that there is no evidence of harm from nonlive vaccines but should be warned that they may offer less protection compared to immunocompetent recipients.

MALARIA

There is no evidence to suggest that patients with HIV are more prone to malaria or that they get more severe malaria. Standard malaria advice should be adequate. Although there are some data to suggest that chloroquine is mildly immunosuppressive, this is likely to be clinically unimportant and, if indicated, chloroquine can be used for malaria chemoprophylaxis. Proguanil is also safe, but care should be taken if the patient is taking another folate antagonist, such as co-trimoxazole (for PCP prophylaxis), and it may be prudent to supply folic acid supplements.

Many patients with HIV may have subclinical involvement of the central nervous system, and there is an increased risk of neuropsychiatric disease in this population. Mefloquine, therefore, should be used with caution in HIV, although there are no data available. My own practice is to prescribe the drug for 3 or 4 weeks before the travel date to try and identify any problems before the patient travels abroad. Doxycycline would be a suitable alternative when mefloquine is not tolerated. There are no data to suggest serious interactions between HAART and antimalarial drugs.

Patients with HIV are more prone to a variety of infections, many of which present with fever. In the tropics, these infections may be misdiagnosed as malaria and treated inappropriately. Patients should be warned of this and advised to seek expert help should they become febrile and unwell.

FOOD- AND WATER-BORNE INFECTIONS

Many people with HIV have abnormalities of the gastrointestinal tract, particularly achlorhydria, and may be more prone to gastrointestinal infections. Although there is no increased risk of acquiring salmonella infections, people with HIV may have trouble clearing these infections and have an increased risk of salmonella bacteremia. Probably the largest risk comes from coccidian parasites, such as *Cryptosporidium parvum* and *Isospora belli*. These can cause cholera-like diarrhea, which can be chronic and very debilitating. Cryptosporidiosis may also lead to an ascending cholangitis. Infections with these organisms and others, such as microsporidia and *Cyclospora cayetensis*, are more common in the tropics. People with HIV should be given good advice about avoiding travelers' diarrhea. They may want to use a portable water filter in addition to chemical disinfection of drinking water. Consideration should be given to chemoprophylaxis or empiric therapy for travelers' diarrhea in this patient group. Patients who are already taking co-trimoxazole for PCP prophylaxis may get some protection from this against travelers' diarrhea.

ENDEMIC INFECTIONS AT THE DESTINATION

When individuals with HIV travel abroad, they may encounter new organisms not endemic in their own country.[6] Infections are more likely to be acquired if the HIV infection is advanced but may be acquired early and present later. A variety of fungi are geographically restricted and are known to cause disease in the context of HIV. *Penicillium marneffei* is a particular risk for those traveling to the Far East, whereas *Histoplasma capsulatum* is a problem for those going to the southern United States and northern South America. Equally, travelers from the tropics where PCP is less common may acquire *P. carinii* when they travel to temperate countries in Europe or North America. Even European holidays can be risky. Leishmaniasis is endemic around the Mediterranean coasts of southern Europe and North Africa. Although infection usually results in benign cutaneous disease in immunocompetent people, those with HIV may have disseminated disease and present with visceral leishmaniasis, which can be difficult to treat.

Respiratory infections are more common generally in travelers and may lead to problems in those with HIV. Bacterial infections are more common in HIV, particularly due to *S. pneumoniae*. Those with HIV are also more prone to infection and disease with *Mycobacterium tuberculosis,* which may be a hazard with prolonged stays in countries where tuberculosis is very prevalent. BCG is contraindicated. There is some evidence that isoniazid chemoprophylaxis may be effective for HIV-positive individuals in high-risk areas. This may be appropriate to consider if a person with HIV is going to live or work in a country with a high tuberculosis prevalence for a prolonged period, but this must be weighed against the risks of isoniazid hepatotoxicity, which is significant in those over the age of 35 years. For short trips, isoniazid cannot be recommended, but vigilance is required if the returning traveler develops fevers or lung infiltrates.

SEXUALLY TRANSMITTED DISEASES

There is evidence to show that holiday makers are more likely to engage in risky sexual behavior when abroad compared to when they are at home. There is also good evidence to suggest that sexually transmitted infections act as cofactors for HIV infection and may accelerate disease progression in HIV. There is also the theoretical risk that some strains of HIV may be more virulent than others, so that the acquisition of a new virus strain by someone already HIV positive may be detrimental. In addition, there is the risk of acquiring hepatitis B. The HIV-positive traveler should be warned of the hazards of sexually acquired diseases.

BUREAUCRACY

Although, at the time of writing, no countries require proof of a negative HIV test for entry for tourism, some require HIV tests for people wanting to stay for more than 3 months and for those intending to work or study. It is sensible for anonymous enquiries to be made to the relevant embassy or immigration officials concerning that country's regulations concerning HIV.

THE ASPLENIC PATIENT

The spleen acts as a sort of filter and has an important role in removing circulating particles, such as bacteria or parasitized red cells, that are not opsonized by complement. In addition, the spleen is important in antibody production and produces properdin, associated with complement activation, and another protein, tuftsin, which may have a role in opsonization. Splenectomy removes an important defence against infection; it is estimated that there is a lifetime risk of up to 5% of overwhelming sepsis in the asplenic individual. Most of the risk appears to be with pneumococcal infections, but other encapsulated organisms, such as *H. influenzae* and *Neisseria meningitidis*, may also pose an increased risk.[7]

Spleens are occasionally removed as part of the management of hematologic disease, and splenectomy may add to a preexisting immune impairment. Sometimes spleens are removed following trauma or incidentally during abdominal surgery for other conditions. In this setting, surgeons often leave some splenic cells in the peritoneal cavity in the belief that these will take over the immunologic role of the spleen; there is no evidence that this happens, so such patients should be considered truly asplenic. It should also be remembered that patients with sickle cell disease may become functionally asplenic following repeated splenic infarcts.

IMMUNIZATIONS

The asplenic patient, although at increased risk of bacterial sepsis, responds poorly to polysaccharide vaccines, such as pneumococcal vaccine. Many authorities recommend immunization of the asplenic patient with vaccines against pneumococci, *H. influenzae*, and meningococcus, but the efficacy of the vaccines in this setting is unknown. Most patients will only produce low levels of antibody, and the response may be short-lived. Postimmunization levels tend to be worst in those who have had splenectomy for hematologic diseases such as Hodgkin's disease.[8] If possible, these immunizations should be given at least a month before a scheduled splenectomy. Ideally, the response should be measured, but this may be difficult in practice. Although the response may be poor, immunization in the absence of a spleen is not harmful (except for theoretical risks of live vaccines) and may provide some short-term benefit to the individual traveler. I would generally offer pneumococcal and meningococcal vaccination but would also suggest that travelers take a course of an antibiotic, such as amoxycillin, with them to use empirically if they develop a fever while abroad.

MALARIA

There is no evidence to suggest that the asplenic individual is at an increased risk of acquiring malaria. There are theoretical concerns, because of the filtering role of the spleen, that malaria may be more severe in asplenic travelers. However, there are no data to support these concerns. Circumstantial data from patients with babesiosis are the only reasons for caution. *Babesia* seems difficult to eradicate in the asplenic patient, and there are case reports of overwhelming and fatal babesiosis in patients without spleens, whereas this red cell parasite rarely causes problems in those with intact spleens.[9]

Asplenic patients should be offered standard malaria advice and take standard antimalarial chemoprophylaxis appropriate to the region of travel. It may be prudent to suggest avoiding travel to areas of high transmission rates of falciparum malaria because of the theoretical risks of severe disease. Those people traveling to areas where babesiosis is a risk (e.g., northeastern coast of North American and northern Europe) should avoid tick bites.

SOLID ORGAN TRANSPLANT RECIPIENTS

Solid organ transplant recipients are maintained on immunosuppressive therapy to prevent graft rejection. Most patients receive glucocorticosteroids and cyclosporin or tacrolimus; a few receive azathioprine instead of, or in addition to, cyclosporin or tacrolimus. Steroids have some effects on neutrophil function, but this is probably insignificant unless very high doses are given. Most of the immunosuppressive effects concern inhibition of macrophages and lymphocytes. Cyclosporine and tacrolimus primarily inhibit CD4 positive T lymphocytes ("helper" lymphocytes), whereas azathioprine affects neutrophils slightly in addition to inhibiting lymphocyte function. Such patients are more prone to infections with intracellular pathogens, such as viruses, mycobacteria, and fungi, than they are to bacteria.

IMMUNIZATIONS

These patients will respond less well than normals to immunization. Antibody levels will be lower and will persist less well.[10,11] Nevertheless, many will develop a sufficient response to be useful to cover short trips abroad. There is no evidence to suggest that immunization will adversely affect the graft or increase the risk of rejection. Live vaccines should be avoided because of theoretical concerns about dissemination. At the time of writing, there are no data concerning the response to hepatitis A vaccination in this group of patients. It may, therefore, be prudent to offer gammaglobulin instead of vaccination or to measure the response to vaccination before traveling.

OTHER ISSUES

Organ transplant recipients should be given standard malaria advice. There is no evidence that the immunosuppressive drugs and antimalarial drugs interact in any way. Renal transplant recipients should know about the risks of dehydration in the heat and in the event of diarrhea occurring. All transplant recipients may have an increased risk of bacteremia if they acquire salmonella or campylobacter gastroenteritis. Some may benefit from having a course of ciprofloxacin, or other quinolone, to hand to use as empiric therapy for travelers' diarrhea.

BONE MARROW TRANSPLANTS

Patients receiving bone marrow transplants (BMT) are generally more immunosuppressed than solid organ transplant recipients, even though the maintenance immunosuppression is similar. They often have immunosuppressing diseases for which they are receiving the transplant and are further immunocompromised by the pretransplant conditioning and the antirejection therapy. There are B and T cell defects along with deficits in specific antibodies. Immediately following transplantation, the biggest problem is neutropenia, but this will have resolved before the patient contemplates travel abroad. However, it may take a long time for neutrophil function to fully recover, and it may be a year or longer after transplantation before cell-mediated immunity returns to normal.

IMMUNIZATION

These patients respond poorly to immunization post-transplantation, particularly in the first year.[12] In addition, those who have chronic graft-versus-host disease respond very poorly with low antibody levels. Ideally, patients should receive vaccinations, such as pneumococcal vaccine, before BMT. Live vaccines are contraindicated. Travelers should be given standby antibiotics in case of illness abroad

OTHER ISSUES

Malaria and other tropical diseases are not particularly a problem for BMT patients, so they can receive standard advice. The returning traveler will need careful evaluation should an illness present as opportunist infections are more likely.

PATIENTS WHO HAVE RECEIVED CANCER CHEMOTHERAPY

Some cancers may, in themselves, be immunosuppressive, but problems arise usually because of the effects of chemotherapy. Studies have shown that the response to influenza vaccination is poor compared to normal volunteers. Responses are particularly poor in hematologic malignancies, such as Hodgkin's disease.[13] The responses to typical travel vaccines have not been evaluated, but, by extrapolation, they would be predicted to be less reliable in this patient group.[14] It is likely that patients remain relatively immunosuppressed up to 3 months after completing chemotherapy, so live vaccines are contraindicated during this period.

Patients with myeloma or chronic lymphocytic leukemia are functionally antibody deficient, so immunization is unlikely to protect.[15] Although intravenous immunoglobulin may protect against infection in chronic lymphocytic leukemia,[16] it is probably more cost effective and safer to offer antibiotic prophylaxis or standby empiric antibiotics to these patients when they travel.

Patients who have undergone cancer chemotherapy should be given standard advice about malaria and travelers' diarrhea.

PATIENTS RECEIVING STEROIDS AND OTHER IMMUNOSUPPRESSIVE THERAPY

Improvements in diagnosis and management have led to increased numbers of patients with systemic vasculitis and other diseases, such as systemic lupus erythematosis, surviving and being maintained on immunosuppressive medication. Typical therapies include corticosteroids combined with other agents, such as cyclophosphamide or azathioprine. These patients tend to have defects in cell-mediated immunity and have relatively poor responses to immunization.[17] In terms of their requirements for travel advice and immunization, these patients can be considered to be similar to those with solid organ transplants.

CONGENITAL IMMUNODEFICIENCY

Most children with severe immunodeficiency rarely survive unless they receive a BMT. However, the most common form of congenital immunodeficiency with survival into adulthood is hypogammaglobulinemia. These patients cannot produce antibodies; therefore, immunization is pointless. Episodes of travel should be covered with prophylactic or empiric antibiotics. Consideration should be given to timing their dose of intravenous immunoglobulin to coincide with the immediate pretravel period. Standard malaria advice is adequate.

CHRONIC MEDICAL CONDITIONS

Patients with chronic diseases have better survivals now than ever before, and, as a result, more are likely to choose to travel despite their medical problems. Generally, their main risks will come from exacerbations or complications of their underlying disease rather than from travel-related illness, so they and their physicians should make an objective assessment of these risks before contemplating travel abroad.

CHRONIC RENAL FAILURE

Uremia is moderately immunosuppressing, and patients with chronic renal failure are more prone to bacterial infections. They respond less well than normal to immunization, but most will form adequate antibody responses to standard vaccinations.[18] Antibody levels will be lower and less long-lasting than normal but will still probably provide useful protection. Live vaccines can be used if required.

Malaria chemoprophylaxis can be a problem in renal failure. Chloroquine is metabolized in the liver and is not a problem, but proguanil is largely renally excreted and may accumulate in renal failure and lead to folate deficiency and anemia.[19] This should not be a problem for short trips, but if the patient is staying in a malaria-endemic area for more than a month, the proguanil dose should be halved after the first 4 weeks and folic acid supplements should be taken. Mefloquine is metabolized mainly in the liver, but about 10% is excreted via the kidneys. There are no good data about its use in renal failure. Doxycycline is hepatically cleared and should be safe, but, again, there are no data.

CHRONIC LIVER DISEASE

Patients with chronic liver impairment are more prone to bacterial infections, particularly pneumococcal disease. Pneumococcal vaccine should be offered, although its efficacy in this patient group is not known. Other standard travel vaccines, including yellow fever, may be given. Chloroquine and mefloquine may accumulate in liver disease, and although dose reduction seems reasonable, there is no information to use as a guide.

CHRONIC CARDIAC OR RESPIRATORY DISEASE

Consideration should be given to giving these patients immunization against pneumococci and influenza in addition to the usual travel vaccinations. Respiratory tract infections are more common in travelers and may lead to serious exacerbations of underlying heart or lung disease.

CONCLUSIONS

It should be possible for many immunocompromised patients to travel abroad, providing that they are adequately prepared and understand the risks. In general, live vaccines should be avoided. In most cases, alternative immunizations are available, but consideration needs to be given to yellow fever certification requirements. Other vaccines can be safely given but are unlikely to be as effective as in normal hosts. Nevertheless, most recipients will probably gain short-term benefit. These patients may also benefit from having a course of broad-spectrum antibiotics to have as standby medication should they fall ill abroad and are also good candidates for empiric antibiotic therapy for traveler's diarrhea.

Immunocompromised patients are at increased risk of acquiring infections abroad that are not typical travel-related problems and then subsequently presenting with an illness at home that is not familiar to their physicians. These patients need careful evaluation if they become ill, and infections, such as fungal infections, that are endemic in the country they have visited need to be considered in the differential diagnosis.

REFERENCES

1. Pantaleo G, Graziosi C, Fauci AS. The immunopathogenesis of human immunodeficiency virus infection. N Engl J Med 1993; 328:327–335.
2. Kroon FP, van Dissel JT, de Jong JC, van Furth R. Antibody response to influenza, tetanus and pneumococcal vaccines in HIV seropositive individuals in relation to the number of CD4+ lymphocytes. AIDS 1994;8:469–476.
3. Hess G, Clemens R, Bienzle U, et al. Immunogenicity and safety of an inactivated hepatitis A vaccine in anti-HIV positive and negative homosexual men. J Med Virol 1995;46:40–42.
4. Opravil M, Fierz W, Matter L, et al. Poor antibody response after tetanus and pneumococcal vaccination in immunocompromised, HIV-infected patients. Clin Exp Immunol 1991;84:185–189.
5. Glesby MJ, Hoover DR, Farzadegan H, et al. The effect of influenza vaccination on human immunodeficiency virus type 1 load: a randomized, double-blind, placebo-controlled study. J Infect Dis 1996;174:1332–1336.
6. Wilson ME, von Reyn CF, Fineberg HV. Infections in HIV-infected travelers: risks and prevention. Ann Intern Med 1991; 114:582–592.
7. O'Neal BJ, McDonald JC. The risk of sepsis in the asplenic adult. Ann Surg 1981;194:775–778.
8. Jakacki R, Luery N, McVerry P, Lange B. *Haemophilus influenzae* diphtheria protein conjugate immunization after therapy in splenectomized patients with Hodgkin's disease. Lancet 1980;ii:450–453.
9. Gorenflot A, Moubri K, Precigout E, et al. Human babesiosis. Ann Trop Med Parasitol 1998;92:489–501.
10. Versluis DJ, Beyer WEP, Masurel N, et al. Impairment of the immune response to influenza vaccination in renal transplant recipients by cyclosporine, but not azathioprine. Transplantation 1986;42:376–379.
11. Linnemann Jr CC, First RF, Schiffman G. Revaccination of renal transplant and hemodialysis recipients with pneumococcal vaccine. Arch Intern Med 1986;146:1554–1556.
12. Guinan EC, Morine DC, Antin JH, et al. Polysaccharide conjugate vaccine responses in bone marrow transplant patients. Transplantation 1994;57:677–684.
13. Siber GR, Gorham C, Martin P, et al. Antibody response to pretreatment immunization and post-treatment boosting with bacterial polysaccharide vaccines in patients with Hodgkin's disease. Ann Intern Med 1986;104:467–475.
14. Gross PA, Gould LA, Brown AE. Effect of cancer chemotherapy on the immune response to influenza virus vaccine: review of published studies. Rev Infect Dis 1985;7:613–618.
15. Schmid GP, Smith RP, Baltach AL, et al. Antibody response to pneumococcal vaccine in patients with multiple myeloma. J Infect Dis 1981;143:590–597.
16. Cooperative Group for the Study of Immunoglobulin in Chronic Lymphocytic Leukemia. Intravenous immunoglobulin for the prevention of infection in chronic lymphocytic leukemia: a randomized, controlled clinical trial. N Engl J Med 1988;319:902–907.
17. McDonald E, Jarrett MP, Schiffman G, et al. Persistence of pneumococcal antibodies after immunization in patients with systemic lupus erythematosus. J Rheumatol 1984;11:306–308.
18. Nikoskelainen J, Koskela M Forsstrom J, et al. Persistence of antibodies to pneumococcal vaccine in patients with chronic renal failure. Kidney Int 1985;28:672–677.
19. Tattershall JF, Greenwood RN, Baker LRI, Cattel WR. Proguanil poisoning in a hemodialysis patient. Clin Nephrol 1987;28:104.

Chapter 40

TRAVEL FOR HEALTH

WALTER PASINI

Travel for health is one of the traditional reasons for travel. Travel can be for tourism, business or work, religious pilgrimages, visits to relatives and friends, and many other reasons, but a frequent motive that persuades people to leave their home and travel to some other place is that of conserving or regaining health.

There is a long history of journeys undertaken with the objective of caring for the body and recovering a state of health. In Ancient Greece, journeys were made to places where there were springs attributed with healing powers for many illnesses, and in Roman times, baths were visited not only by local residents but also by outsiders seeking a cure. In the 19th century, doctors would prescribe periods of residence in places with particular conditions of climate as a treatment for tuberculosis and other diseases.

In the late 19th century, hospitals were built in Europe in places with a milder climate, with the intention of providing cures for rickets, various forms of tuberculosis, or other poverty-related diseases. In Italy, these hospitals were called "marine hospices"; one of these was the Ospedale al Mare in Venice.

Italy's "colonie climatiche," or children's health camps, were a similar kind of institution opened for the temporary accommodation of children in summer (Figure 40–1). These colonies were an offshoot of the hygienist positivism that flourished in Italy in medical and social fields during the second half of the 19th century, as a result first of Catholic charity organization and later of public institutions and private philanthropists. During the period when Italy was united under a sovereign, children's health camps were basically hostels and places for the treatment of diseases caused by poverty and urban pollution. Under Fascist rule, these colonies were exploited for propagandistic ends, to "improve" and exalt the Italian "race." The colonies differed not only in their location (by the sea, a river, or a lake or in the mountains) but also by the length of time their young guests stayed. Permanent colonies, open all year, overtly catered for children with chronic diseases like tuberculosis, associated with prolonged periods of hospitalization rather than with brief holidays. Temporary colonies were open for only a few months and generally served as summer camps for prophylaxis and recreation.[1]

Nowadays, travel for health often means visiting other countries for medical treatments not considered to be suitably available in the country of residence. Otherwise, visits can be made to spa resorts or places with a favorable climate for spa or dietary cures, or to wellness centers for exercise programes to regain fitness, or for beauty treatments.

In this chapter, the subject will be divided in two parts: health care travel and spa medicine.

HEALTH CARE TRAVEL

One of the main reasons for health care travel is to seek diagnosis and therapy in foreign hospitals or clinics. The destinations of these "journeys of hope," as they are called by the press, are the United States, France, Switzerland, and the United Kingdom. Patients from the south of Europe, Israel, the United Arab Emirates, and Central and South America set out on journeys that are often long and expensive with the hope of receiving some cure for a disease that in their own country is believed to be incurable.

In Switzerland, every year some 3,000 foreigners visit the country's 2,000 private clinics for check-ups or operations. From the medical point of view, Swiss private clinics cover the entire range of modern medicine at the highest level. Whether patients come for a heart operation or cancer treatment, whether they have orthopedic problems or need an eye specialist, in a Swiss private clinic they can be confident of receiving the best medical care that modern science can offer.

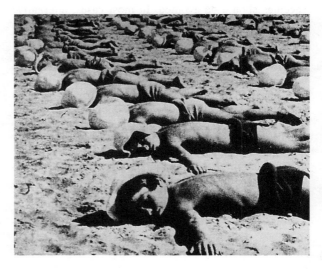

Figure 40–1.   A heliotherapy session.

There are several clinics that specialize in a specific sector, such as oculistics. Some of these have an outpatient program that uses lasers to treat near-sightedness, eliminating the need for glasses or contact lenses. Others use radiosurgical irradiation devices to painlessly remove small brain tumors.

The Clinique de Genolier, located high above Lake Geneva, receives patients from Europe and the Middle East, in particular from the United Arab Emirates. The clinic recently became the European partner of the Memorial Sloan-Kettering Cancer Center in New York, a world leader in cancer prevention, treatment, and research. In Davos, the Alpine Kinderklinik caters exclusively for the health needs of children and adolescents. About half of the young patients, many of whom suffer from asthma, bronchitis, dermatologic problems, and allergies, are from Germany.

Although Italy is one of the world's six most industrialized countries, there is a strong demand for health treatment abroad, and Italian patients suffering cancer are attracted in particular by a number of French hospitals. In 1989, over 2,000 Italians visited the G. Roussy Institute, a center specializing in tumor therapy located at Villejuif on the outskirts of Paris. Italians represent a large proportion of the users of this hospital. In 1988, there were 1,940 Italian patients of an overall total of 12,077 (16%), and with respect to the total number of foreigners (2,673), Italians represented 72.6% of all foreign patients for that year.[2]

Another hospital that is a frequent destination for Italian patients is the Paul Brousse Hospital, a medium-sized center that is also on the outskirts of Paris. A study conducted by researchers at the Genoa Tumour Institute has shown that 67% of the Italians visiting this hospital are from the south of the country or from its islands, with a preponderance of female patients (64%). In this hospital, as in several others in France, the number of Italian patients makes it necessary for the staff to be fluent in Italian as well.

Other oncology centers that attract Italian patients are at Lugano in Switzerland or in the United States at New York (Memorial Sloan-Kettering Institute), Houston (MD Anderson Cancer Center), and Bethesda, Maryland (National Cancer Institute).

Observing the migration of Italian patients toward France, it seems logical to ask if these journeys of hope are justified in medical terms. Does a trip for therapy to Paris, Marseilles, or Lyons correspond to a real need, or is it more the result of a current fad, a psychological necessity, or an economic interest cultivated by private health care centers?

Scientific exchanges, which have been rendered even more intense by information technology and, above all, the Internet, have, for example, resulted in oncology therapy protocols being known by the international scientific community; consequently, there would seem to be no valid justification for seeking treatment abroad.

At times, this phenomenon of journeys of hope damages the reputation of the patient's country of origin, but even more often it damages the health of the patient. The psychophysical stress of the journey, logistical problems, the difficulty of speaking and understanding a foreign language, and the lack of continuity in the relationship between doctor and patient can sometimes lead to results that are not as satisfactory as those that could be obtained at home.

Journeys abroad are often undertaken for diagnostic procedures and surgical treatments that could have been performed just as well in one's own country, if only the patient or doctor responsible for the case had known of the existence of the more advanced centers present on national territory.

There are many reasons for health care migration from one country to another, and the matter is certainly very complex. Here we will attempt to list the main causes of the phenomenon as regards Italy, in the belief that the situation may be very similar in other countries where this problem exists.

DELAYS IN PROVISION OF DIAGNOSTIC AND THERAPEUTIC SERVICES

In a study conducted by the Italian journal *Medico e Paziente*, 37% of the doctors interviewed declared that the reason for health care migration was the better organization and greater efficiency of health services hospitals abroad.[3] The organizational shortcomings of Italy's health care service have even been recognized by the country's legislators. Health Ministry Circular 33 of 12 December 12, 1989 affirmed that "until national hospital services have been reorganized and are able to guarantee promptness with certain specialist procedures and standards of assistance comparable to those of other countries of the European Community, travel abroad in exceptional circumstances for therapy, if this is motivated by objective insufficiencies in the national health service, may not be subject to limitations."

The decree published in the *Official Gazette* on February 5, 1990, entitled "Identification of Classes of Pathology and Services Obtainable at High-Level Specialization Centres," takes for granted the absolute inevitability of long waiting lists, as if this were caused by merely structural problems or some divine malediction instead of by severe organizational malfunctions.

The problem of long waiting lists in Italian hospitals would seem to be the main reason for health care migration. This problem emphasizes the need for a more rational reorganization of work in our hospitals. In many hospitals, it is standard practice to concentrate activities of diagnosis and cure in the morning hours, leaving the rest of the day drastically underexploited. In these conditions, it is easy to understand that the volume of work carried out is insufficient and that long waiting lists are the natural result. The basic problem is that of making full use of available health care facilities and the professional capacities of medical and paramedical personnel.

LACK OF ADEQUATE STRUCTURES

Another reason for these journeys of hope may be the absence or shortage of suitable health facilities. This is particularly true for citizens of developing countries in a medium-high income bracket who can afford to invest considerable sums in a trip abroad to seek treatment. This situation is also true to a certain extent for countries like Italy, which have a more or less marked degree of economic disparity between north and south. It is no mere coincidence that the vast majority of Italians visiting French health care structures (G. Roussy and Paul Brousse hospitals) are from the south of the country or from the islands. This lack of facilities also explains the phenomenon of internal migration from southern to northern Italy for many pathologies, not only tumors and heart complaints but also for orthopedic, pediatric, neurologic, and other problems.

In the case of journeys of hope for children, the cited study reveals that it is doctors themselves who send their young patients north, as the hospitals of southern Italy are considered to offer inadequate medical skills, to lack suitable facilities, or to be without sufficient nursing staff. The most frequent causes for infantile migration include mental retardation, convulsions, neoplasia, renal malformations, asthma, thalassemia, congenital cardiopathy, chronic hepatopathy, and rare neurologic diseases.

LAXNESS OF LEGISLATION

The phenomenon of journeys abroad for health treatments is one that has grown and continues to exist in the context of a legislative system that is perhaps insufficient and incomplete, and certainly erring on the overindulgent as regards both the total sums reimbursed and the extension of these to expenses for travel, board, and lodging for patients and sometimes family members and also the number of pathologies admitted for treatment abroad and the waiting time conceded at Italian health facilities before departure to a foreign treatment center.

MISTRUST OF ITALIAN HEALTH SERVICES

Another possible cause for the preference for treatment abroad may be a basic lack of trust in the Italian health system. An enquiry made in 1988 by the journal *Corriere medico*, cited in "Viaggiare per guarire?" quotes 64% of the Italian population as saying that they would seek help from a foreign doctor were they in a position to do so, while 58% expressed doubts on the professional skills of doctors in Italy, 34.1% maintained that Italian doctors made mistaken diagnoses, and 35% gave a negative assessment of their communicative capacities.[4]

The cases of clamorous hospital errors and incompetence reported with such emphasis by the media are also highly deleterious to the reputation of the Italian health service. By contrast, foreign health care facilities, heard about from friends or in the press, about which little is known and which are far away, can achieve an almost charismatic appeal that attracts the attention of the public.

The lack of trust in Italian health care facilities is not only the result of the mistakes and poor service reported with such prominence by the media. In many cases, it can also derive from negative experiences encountered either directly or by friends and family. It is an indisputable fact, for example, that there are substantial variations in the quality of hospital services between different regions of Italy or between the south, center, and north of the country.

EXCESSIVE IDEALIZATION OF FOREIGN HEALTH CARE FACILITIES

Together with this low appraisal of the Italian health care service, a certain role in health care migration is played by an excessive idealization of foreign structures. Although it is undoubtedly true that some French, Swiss, and American centers are able to work with greater numbers of patients and accumulate a higher number of case studies than Italian facilities, and have a greater amount of modern equipment and medical staff with an extremely high level of professional skill, in many cases, there is also a certain love of all things foreign.

PSYCHOLOGICAL MOTIVES

A journey abroad for treatment may be the result not only of the idealization of the capacities of foreign doctors but also of the attempt to do everything possible before an unfavorable diagnosis must be sadly accepted. In this case, it is more often members of the family than patients themselves who make extensive enquiries of friends and acquaintances to find the best consultant in a particular specialization or the most famous foreign health care center so as to leave no possible option unexplored, thus understandably putting their conscience at ease. In such circumstances, journeys of hope become journeys of hopelessness, distressing odysseys in search of miraculous cures that more often than not are not found.

INADEQUATE KNOWLEDGE OF SPECIALIZED ITALIAN CENTERS

General practitioners often advise patients to seek treatment abroad because they are not adequately aware of available health care centers in their own country that could successfully treat the pathology in question. One of the most probable causes of health care migration might therefore be a lack of national information services that patients could consult to locate the health care facilities they need. In this field, as in many others, the role of the general practitioner is fundamental in assisting patients in their choice.

It is necessary therefore to provide general practitioners with a detailed directory of the health care facilities present in their area, region, and country as a whole so that they acquire the habit of contacting them to discuss the diagnosis and treatment programs of their patients.

A full knowledge of the available options is fundamental for the activity of all general practitioners, especially as regards facilities for cancer therapy, heart surgery, the diagnosis and treatment of rare diseases, and transplants.

CONDUCT OF DOCTORS

Specialists may actively encourage health care migration if they are on the consulting panels of foreign hospitals. Many of these, in France, America, Switzerland, Monte Carlo, or Belgium, have consultants in Italy, who, as a part of their activity, are able to direct a certain number of patients toward the institutes with which they are in contact. Rivalry between doctors may also encourage health care migration.

GROWTH OF THE INTERNATIONAL DIMENSION OF DAILY LIFE

In the past, travel, perhaps for reasons of discovery, trade, colonial conquests, or emigration to a new country, was extraneous to the daily life and common experience of the majority of the population. Local lines of demarcation and more so national ones were rarely crossed, or if they were, it was on a journey with no return. In recent years, however, the international dimension has noticeably entered the sphere of daily life. For many people, the world is something that can be traveled in, a reality that is part of common experience. The processes of international integration in daily life are increasingly present and increasingly complex. Instruments of mass communication (above all television but also films), international tourism, and immigration from underdeveloped countries have brought us all greater experience with the international dimension, bringing distant countries closer to our experience and our lives. However, although mass communication media divulge images and news filtered through the experience of others, and the phenomenon of immigration from countries outside Europe allows us to live the international dimension on our home ground, the growing mobility of persons outside their natural borders, for reasons of tourism, work, pilgrimages, etc., brings ordinary people into direct contact with the international dimension. The increasing availability and speed of means of transport and the growing comfort of hotels allow a greater number of people to directly experience the international dimension. Seen against such a background, a trip abroad for medical reasons no longer seems to be beyond our mental horizon.

LACK OF A CULTURE OF PREVENTION

Given that the diseases (cancer and cardiovascular illnesses) for which treatment is sought abroad are strongly influenced by lifestyles, individual conduct, and environmental conditions (smoking, alcohol, incorrect eating habits, pollution), the development of a culture of prevention both in individuals and in national political authorities would allow the need to resort to medical and hospital treatments to be reduced. As a consequence, the phenomenon of health care migration would also decline.

SPA MEDICINE

Spa medicine is very popular in Europe, particularly in central and southern countries of the continent like Ger-

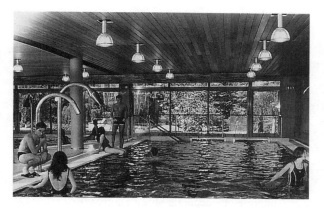

Figure 40–2.   Many European spas were built in the 19th century.

many, Austria, Hungary, the Czech Republic, France, and Italy. Italy alone has around 400 spa centers that attract more than 2 million patients every year. In Europe, spa medicine has ancient traditions and is firmly rooted in popular culture (Figures 40–2, 40–3).[5]

The history of spa medicine is as old as that of civilization itself, and since the dawn of time man has recognized empirically in water, and in particular water with special characteristics, such as temperature, taste, and smell deriving from its mineral contents, a dual capacity both as a defense against illness (prevention) and as a promoter of healing (therapy).[6]

The therapeutic use of water was known to Hippocrates, and thermal springs can still be seen today on the island of Cos. The use made by the Romans of baths is noted, and they were built not only in the capital of their empire, where the ruins of Caracalla give a clear idea of the sheer scale of these constructions, but also in every province and territory that the Romans occupied. Even the legionnaires would use hot springs wherever they found them to recover from the toils of battle and to heal their

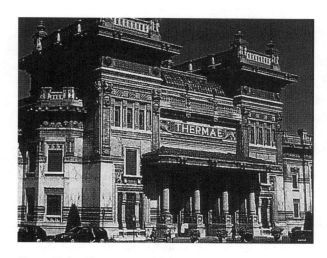

Figure 40–3.   The entrance of Salsomaggiore Terma (Italy).

wounds. This was the start of the immense network of spa centers in Europe that over the centuries has been embellished by architects and town planners.

Over the ages, spa medicine has seen an alternation between periods of splendor and periods of decline and almost total abandonment. The spread of Christianity in Europe marked a halt in the culture of baths, as they were considered to be places for the wanton care of the body in which nakedness was permitted, and therefore put the salvation of the soul at risk. With the rise of the city-states, however, spa medicine recovered a certain importance, but until the 19th century the use of spring water was based solely on empirical concepts, even though these were supported by accurate observation of their effects.

Scientific progress then gradually enabled, on the one hand, the physicochemical characteristics of individual spa waters to be determined, and, on the other, the pathogenesis of the various ailments that were known to benefit from the use of these waters to be identified.

The discovery of a correlation between water characteristics and the effects that could be obtained with each water was a direct consequence of the steps forward made in these two directions. At the same time, the use that had been classically made of spa waters for many centuries, with methods of application that had been established empirically (balneotherapy, crenotherapy, antrotherapy, and water cures), was allied with new and more specific techniques (inhalation, aerosol, irrigation, etc.), made possible by the availability of newly developed instruments.

The use of spa waters to promote human health began to acquire an increasingly rational basis.

Spa waters, with their specific physicochemical properties that vary from spring to spring, are an important instrument for the overall safeguarding of health, as they offer many possible applications:

- treatments for many diseases that have a prevalently chronic course,
- rehabilitation of subjects with potentially invalidating pathologic after-effects from diseases and traumas, and
- prevention of the onset of certain diseases by means of mechanisms capable of prematurely interrupting their pathogenic development before the appearance of significant clinical phenomena (secondary prevention).

To obtain these results, spa waters can be used both internally (by drinking, irrigation, inhalation, aerosol) and externally (baths, mud packs, caves).

Spa medicine does more than provide a range of treatments. It also encourages healthier lifestyles (physical exercise, correct eating, and drinking habits, etc.). Spa centers do not offer a refuge from death or just a treatment during an illness. They represent institutions that promote health in the wider sense indicated by the World Health Organization, which, as is known, considers health to be not merely the absence of disease or infirmity but more a state of complete physical, mental, and social well-being.[7]

Spa cures, often associated with physiotherapy, are of proven efficacy in cases in which there is a definite prognosis, either for the onset of problems of physical health or for subsequent physical limitation resulting in a probable reduction of activity. They also offer the possibility of functional recovery in cases in which limitations are already present. In addition, they offer environments and more leisurely lifestyles that are a beneficial alternative to the stress and pollution to which we are increasingly exposed.

The effectiveness of many spa treatments has by now been clearly demonstrated and derives both from the observation of their effects on the pathology in question and from the plausibility of the existence of direct links between the physicochemical qualities of spa water and the pathogenesis of the disorder.

Spa treatments may have value in the following disorders: arthrosis, aftermath of bone fractures, liver and gallbladder diseases, illnesses related to metabolic disorders, kidney stones, skin diseases, gynecologic disorders, inflammations of the respiratory tract, vascular diseases, and digestive system disorders.

Naturally, the effects that can be obtained for a specific pathology are selectively correlated to the characteristics of individual spa waters. The first consequence of this is that every spa center must be used for the treatment of a specific range of pathologies. The second is that the physicochemical characteristics of water at spa centers must be periodically checked and must remain constant, as it is precisely according to these characteristics that their specific therapeutic effects are classified and also obtained.

In European Union countries, rigorous routine checks are carried out on waters, mud, treatment premises, and equipment, providing adequate safeguards for users.

One of the aspects of spa waters that must be checked is their bacteriologic purity at the sources. Checks must also be made for the possibility of subsequent contamination of waters by opportunistic pathogenic microorganisms, capable of having a harmful action in particular circumstances, or even by nonpathogenic microorganisms that are nevertheless the result of environmental or fecal pollution. The absence of opportunistic microorganisms from spa water is indispensable, as these microorganisms, often present in the environment but not usually pathogenic for humans, may become in contact with particularly receptive subjects, such as the elderly, patients suffering prevalently chronic-degenerative diseases that lower immune defenses, and patients receiving immunosuppressive therapeutic treatments.

As recalled earlier, spa treatments are particularly beneficial in certain chronic-degenerative ailments (arthropathy, turnover disorders, disorders of the digestive or urinary systems) that before manifesting themselves in their definitive form can be predicted by a range of symptoms that clearly indicate their future development. It is in this phase that spa treatments can have the most positive effect, capable of blocking the pathogenic evolution (thus providing secondary prevention) toward more serious clinical situations, often tending to have invalidating outcomes.

Elderly people are often subject to conditions of this kind, and for these subjects, spa treatments can have considerable significance in terms of prevention. As the proportion of elderly persons has progressively increased over the last few decades, with some 20% of our total population now in the over-65 age group, and as elderly people are affected by pathologic events with greater frequency and for a longer duration than the rest of the population, it is clear that the request for health care services is inevitably destined to increase. Basically, a greater number of elderly persons means a greater use of health care services, and this, in turn, means greater expenditure. This situation could be partially alleviated by attempting to reduce the frequency of fully developed pathologies, which not only require particularly expensive treatment but also result in a loss of self-sufficiency.

Spa treatments can be of prime importance in halting the evolution of chronic-degenerative pathologies and thus have a major role to play in reducing the overall number and cost of other medical treatments and hospitalization. This is a field of medicine in which the cost-benefit ratio is particularly favorable.

Given their functions of prevention, therapy, and rehabilitation, spa centers still represent an important heritage that must be defended. In part, this can be achieved with adequate European legislation on aspects such as the protection of spa water catchment areas against contamination, environmental protection in general and more specifically the protection of water, the rational determi-

nation of standards of quality for spa waters, and their classification and indicated applications.

In this way, spa medicine can continue to bring us its benefits well into the new millennium.

REFERENCES

1. Pasini W. Le colonie climatiche: aspetti sanitari, pedagogici ed urbanistici, Proceedings of a National Congress, September 5–6, 1986.
2. Pasini W. Curarsi all'estero perché? Naples: Pagano Editore, 1994.
3. Ma in Italia le strutture ci sono, basta conoscerle. Medico E Paziente, 1995.
4. Morasso G. Viaggiare per guarire? Dati, storia ed interpretazioni delle migrazioni sanitarie in oncologia. Milano: Masson, 1992.
5. Gualtierotti R. Medicina termale. Milano: Lucisano Editore, 1991.
6. Wright L. Clean and decent. London: Routledge & Keagan Paul, 1987.
7. Pasini P. Health promotion through tourism. In: Lobel HO, Steffen R, Kozarsky PEH, eds. Travel medicine. 2: proceedings of the Second Conference on International Travel Medicine. Atlanta: International Society of Travel Medicine, 1992.

Chapter 41

BIOLOGIC AND CHEMICAL TERRORISM

JACK MELLING

INTRODUCTION AND BACKGROUND

Biologic and chemical terrorism is only one of the many potential travel hazards, and although the current risk may be low, the future position is uncertain. Accordingly, for those providing medical advice to travelers, a general understanding of the agents that could be involved and the means of treatment and/or prophylaxis should facilitate appropriate decisions and advice as the level of risk may change. The possibilities of terrorist use of biologic or chemical agents have been the subject of many fictional accounts, especially over the last 25 years. The reality is also of concern, although, fortunately, for reasons that will be discussed below, the number of fatalities or even casualties has been low, especially in comparison with other risks to human health. Nevertheless, the nature of the threat and the possibility that terrorist actions may in future succeed where others have failed has resulted in major expenditure throughout the developed world to put in place contingency plans to counter a disaster.

Chemical and biologic (C/B) terrorism involves the use of poisonous substances or microorganisms to cause harm to humans, livestock, crops, or other resources. It includes using C/B agents to assassinate individuals and to sabotage infrastructures. The effects of such terrorism may be tactical or strategic, short or long term, and may produce physical or mental harm. Except in their motivation, terrorist and ordinary criminal activities are indistinguishable, and when C/B agents are involved, there may also be little difference in the harm that results.

Terrorist use of chemical or biologic agents, as with other weapons such as firearms and explosives, is likely to be based on military research, development, and exploitation. Lone individuals or indigenous groups may, due to resource limitations, adopt particular methods to suit their circumstances. Military use of biologic weapons has a recorded history stretching back more than 2,000 years and includes the low-technology, but no less devastating, use of smallpox against native populations.[1] Chemical weapons were first employed some 75 years ago, almost as soon as their production became feasible.

A Monterey Institute Report[2] identified some 50 politically or ideologically motivated terrorist incidents since 1960 in the U.S.A. that involved chemical or biologic agents. Half of these have occurred in the preceding decade. A striking feature of these incidents is that there has been only one fatality: a person shot with eight cyanide-tipped 0.38 bullets. It may well be that the effect of the cyanide was marginal. The most serious incident (numerically) affected 751 people in 1984 who were poisoned by *Salmonella typhimurium* contamination of food and drink in Oregon restaurants.

Worldwide, there have been numerous reports that politically motivated groups may have attempted to acquire and/or use C/B agents. A few examples are:

- 1970—The Bavarian Interior Ministry referred to rumors of terrorist plans to use nerve agent sprays in aircraft highjackings.[3]
- 1981—A group in the U.K. calling themselves Dark Harvest threatened to distribute soil contaminated with anthrax.[4]
- 1981—Herbicide contamination of food in stores in the U.K.[4]
- 1983—Documents said to have been captured from the Palestinian Liberation Organization indicated Soviet training in the use of chemical agents.[3]
- 1984—Arsenic contamination of Tylenol capsules in the U.S.A.[4]
- 1985—Herbicide contamination of drink dispensers in Japan.[4]
- 1986—Cyanide contamination of Tylenol capsules in the U.S.A.[5]
- 1993—Attempt to smuggle 130 g of ricin into Canada.[6]
- 1995—Extremists in Tajikistan using cyanide killed seven people and injured a number of others.[7]
- 1996—Police in Germany seized computerized directions for producing mustard.[7]

There are many other reports of rumors of threats or intents, but in the absence of details or arrests, these are difficult to substantiate. Overall, it does appear that a combination of effective law enforcement, the technical difficulties involved, and a lack of knowledge by the perpetrators have limited the impact of such attempts.

The most concerted effort at C/B terrorism was probably that perpetrated by the Japanese cult Aum Shiurikyo in the early 1990s, which culminated in the release of sarin in the Tokyo subway in March 1995, killing 12 people and injuring thousands. From the testimony of cult members, it later emerged that the cult had once sprayed botulinum toxin from vehicles. Anthrax was sprayed on several occasions both from the roof of a building and from vehicles. Neither agent had any effect. Aum also tried to acquire Ebola virus in Zaire. In their concealed but fairly sophisticated facilities, the cult also attempted to develop as weapons VX, cyanide, and the microbe that causes Q fever[8,9] and to engineer bacteria.[10]

The Aum cult was probably the best-funded and organized of indigenous groups so far identified. Their failure to inflict major casualties indicates that the technologic requirements for large-scale use of both biologic and chemical agents are not simple and do require types of expertise that are, fortunately, not readily available to such groups.

Expert opinion is divided about the ease with which C/B terrorism could be conducted. A former Commander of the U.S. Army Medical Research Institute indicated in Senate testimony the difficulties with which terrorists are confronted. Somewhat in contrast, a FBI spokesman said "with a little bit of knowledge and a little bit of depravity you have the makings of a horrendous event." This dichotomy between those who focus on the awfulness of a possible event and others who view such an event as being of low probability is at the heart of the debate. Nevertheless, the current reality is that for the average person, biologic or chemical terrorism poses less risk than automobile travel or crossing the street. It cannot, however, be assumed that this state of affairs will continue indefinitely.

POSSIBLE THREAT SCENARIOS

There are many possible forms that terrorist incidents may take. The factors that make up a particular scenario include the agent(s) involved, type of delivery, number and location of people exposed, and state of readiness of the emergency services. The type of agents involved coupled with the level of exposure will determine the magnitude of any incident and the number of people affected. In turn, these factors depend on the capabilities and resources of the terrorists.

There is a wide variety of possible ways to use C/B agents for terrorist purposes, and agents can enter the body by pulmonary, oral, or cutaneous routes. Thus, agricultural sprayers or dusters, explosive dissemination, or introduction of agents into consumables may be delivery mechanisms.

Broadly, terrorists may be state sponsored, an indigenous group, or a lone individual. The state-sponsored group is the most dangerous, since it would be the most likely to have access to major resources for:

- support for research, weaponization, acquisition, and transport of materials;
- training in target reconnaissance, covert entry, self-protection, and escape; and
- funding.

An indigenous group could have a lower but still significant level of capability including:

- collective expertise for agent production/acquisition, attack targeting and planning, and delivery and escape and
- funding.

The lone individual is likely to have:

- limited knowledge concerning agent characteristics, production, and dissemination;
- No support for reconnaissance, targeting, and escape; and
- limited funding.

It is therefore probable that of possible targets, which range from cities, towns, or other large areas through buildings and rooms to individual people, only the better resourced groups could inflict major damage. This pattern is supported from a review of incidents over the last 20 years. Although there is no indication of any state-sponsored activity, groups, as opposed to individuals, have focused on the larger targets.

The type of agents involved coupled with the mode of dissemination would be significant elements in determining the scale of any incident. Table 41–1 summarizes the possible consequences depending on the particular combination of those elements.

For terrorists to inflict major damage, there are, fortunately, significant problems that they must overcome. These include:

- acquisition of samples of agents,
- production and harvesting on a sufficient scale,
- formulation to maintain viability and aid dissemination,
- delivery to obtain appropriate particle size,
- knowledge of the agent's characteristics, and
- knowledge of the target.

The combination of capabilities needed to overcome these problems is unlikely to be found in an individual but becomes more likely in groups and especially state-supported groups. Fortunately, in the case of groups, they are more susceptible to surveillance by both law enforcement and/or military intelligence agencies.

Table 41–1. EFFECT OF CATEGORY OF AGENT AND MODE OF DISSEMINATION ON INCIDENT CONSEQUENCES

AGENT CATEGORY	MODE OF DISSEMINATION		
	LARGE SCALE (AEROSOL)	SMALL SCALE (AEROSOL OR TAMPERING)	INDIVIDUAL ATTACK
Lethal			
Contagious*	Serious consequences on any scale depending on the incubation period, ease of spread, effectiveness of treatment		
Noncontagious†	Casualties probably in the range		
	>10⁵	>10³	>10
Incapacitating†	Serious _____ to _____ Little disruption disruption		

*Only biologic agents; †biologic and/or chemical agents.

POTENTIAL THREATS

Although both chemical and biologic agents may pose a threat, the two categories differ significantly in the scale and nature of that threat. The effect of chemical agents is rapid, and lethality can be high in the absence of readily available antidotes, but only those directly exposed suffer harm. In contrast, biologic agents are generally more insidious in that the effects may take several days to appear and there may be person-to-person transmission during the incubation period, thus amplifying the effect. A further important difference is in the quantities of material required to produce injury or lethality. Table 41–2 illustrates the potency of chemical and biologic agents relative to other weapons.

CHEMICAL AGENTS

There are several categories of chemical agents that can be grouped according to the effects they produce. Tables 41–3 and 41–4 list the various agents and some of their general properties. Although the nerve and blistering agents are liquids at ambient temperatures, their vapor pressures are such that inhalation forms a significant component of the exposure risk, allied to skin penetration.

BIOLOGIC AGENTS

Although some biologic agents have been considered for use against animals or crops, those that affect humans will be considered here.

Biologic agents include viruses, bacteria, rickettsia, fungi, and toxins. Although the natural routes of exposure may differ for the various agents, it is likely that terrorist

Table 41–2. COMPARISON OF CONVENTIONAL, CHEMICAL, BIOLOGIC, AND NUCLEAR WARHEADS*

TYPE OF WARHEAD	NUMBER OF DEAD	NUMBER OF INJURED
Conventional (1 ton of HE)	5	13
Chemical (300 kg of GB)	200–3,000	200–3,000
Biologic (30 kg of anthrax)	20,000–80,000	??
Nuclear (20 kiloton yield	40,000	40,000

?? = no data.
*Missile with 1 tonne warhead against a large city with average population density of 30 unprotected civilians per hectare.[11]

use would involve aerosols or possibly contamination of foodstuffs.

Table 41–5 lists biologic agents that have been considered to have characteristics that make them potential weapons. Of those listed, there is a smaller number that are known or reported to have been weaponized or developed for weaponization in former biologic weapons programs of nation states. Only a few of the agents that formed part of military programs are readily transmissible from person to person.

Indeed, the former Soviet Union program described by Alibek[13] contrasted with the U.S. program (unilaterally abandoned after 1968) in the number of transmissible agents involved. In both of those cases, the range and nature of the agents accorded with a prevailing military doctrine. In the case of terrorist use, accessibility of agents is likely to be the major factor, especially if there is no state support involved.

Table 41–3. CHARACTERISTICS OF SOME CHEMICAL AGENTS

AGENT	BOILING POINT °C	HALF-LIFE IN SOIL (DAYS)	LD$_{50}$ 70 KG HUMAN—CUTANEOUS (G)	BIOLOGIC MODE OF ACTION
Nerve				
GA (Tabun)	230	1.5	1.0	Inhibition of cholinesterase leading to an
GB (Sarin)	158	<1	1.7	excess of acetylcholine and overstimulation
GD (Soman)	198	Persists	0.35	of muscles
VX	298	2–6	0.01	
Blistering				
Mustard	227	Months	7.0	Complex action disrupting cellular functions
Phosgene oxime	128	<0.1		
Lewisite	190	Days		
Cyanide				
Hydrogen cyanide	26	<0.1	7.0	Inhibition of mitochondrial cytochrome
Cyanogen chloride	13	NA		oxidase affecting aerobic metabolism
Pulmonary				
Phosgene	7	NA	??	Damage to cell membranes in the alveoli
Diphosgene		NA		
Riot control				
CS, CN, CR, CA DM, DA, DC	Smokes	NA	NA	Irritant

Table 41–4.   BIOLOGIC EFFECTS OF SOME CHEMICAL AGENTS*

AGENT	ONSET TIME	SYMPTOMS	TREATMENT
Nerve GA (Tabun) GB (Sarin) GD (Soman) VX	Seconds to minutes	Miosis, rhinorrhea, dyspnea, collapse, fasciculations, convulsions	Atropine, pralidoxime, anticonvulsants, ventilation
Blistering Mustard Phosgene oxime Lewisite	Minutes to hours	Erythema, itching, blistering, dyspnea, eye irritation	Decontamination, topical antibiotic, bronchodilators, ventilation
Cyanide Hydrogen cyanide Cyanogen chloride	Minutes	Nausea, weakness, convulsions, apnea	Nitrites and sodium thiosulfate
Pulmonary Phosgene Diphosgene	Minutes to hours	Dyspnea, coughing, suffocation	Oxygen, bronchodilators, ventilation
Riot control CS, CN, CR, CA DM, DA, DC	Seconds to minutes	Severe irritation of eyes, nose, and airways; vomiting	Wash exposed surfaces, bronchodilators, oxygen, ventilation
Opioids Carfentanil Sufentanil	Minutes	Dyspnea, ataxia, catatonia	Naloxone, nalmefane, naltrexone, ventilation

*Data from Institute of Medicine.[12]

PROPHYLAXIS AND THERAPY

The risk of exposure to either chemical or biologic agents is currently considered to be low, particularly for groups other than those in high-risk occupations or areas. Accordingly, prophylaxis for either class of agents is not considered advisable. Further factors militating against prophylaxis are the numbers of agents and their diversity in biologic effect.

CHEMICAL AGENTS

Nerve agent prophylaxis has been achieved using pyridostigmine bromide (PB), which works by (reversibly) occupying sites on the enzyme cholinesterase to which nerve agents would otherwise (irreversibly) bind. Once there is no further risk of nerve agent exposure, ceasing administration of PB allows the functional enzyme once more to be available.

Therapy for nerve agent exposure is aimed at counteracting the resulting blockade of cholinesterase and the effects of increased levels of acetylcholine that causes overstimulation of cholinergic synapses leading to respiratory failure and convulsions.

This is achieved by administration of a combination of atropine, pralidoxime, and diazepam. Atropine, by blocking muscarinic receptors, counteracts the effect of acetylcholine. Pralidoxime reactivates cholinesterase, except in the case of soman, where rapid irreversible binding occurs. Diazepam helps control seizures and prevent brain damage.

There are no proven treatments for blistering or pulmonary agents apart from rapid decontamination for the former.

Cyanide intoxication can be treated by a combination of amyl nitrite inhalation and intravenous administration of sodium nitrite to convert hemoglobin to methemoglobin, which then removes cyanide from cytochrome oxidase. Intravenous administration of sodium thiosulphate detoxifies the cyanide and regenerates normal hemoglobin.

Although most military personnel on active service carry autoinjectors containing atropine, pralidoxime, and diazepam, these are not likely to be readily and rapidly available for civilian use. Similarly, relatively few kits are kept for treatment of cyanide poisoning—usually resulting from occupational exposure. Chemical agent treatments are summarized in Table 41–4.

BIOLOGIC AGENTS

Vaccines have proven to be effective in reducing or even, in some regions, eliminating many common diseases. This success has been achieved because there has been a general public acceptance of the need for vaccination, and the vaccines used have been proven to be safe and effective by means of human trials.

In the case of BW agents, vaccination has limited value for civilian and, indeed, some would argue, even for military populations. The risk of exposure to any one of the potential threats is very low, the costs and risks outweigh the benefits, and a high level of vaccine coverage in the absence of a clear and present danger is unlikely to

Table 41–5.   CHARACTERISTICS OF SOME POTENTIAL BIOLOGIC AGENTS AGAINST HUMANS

AGENT/DISEASE	AEROSOL INFECTIVE DOSE (IF KNOWN)	INCUBATION PERIOD (NATURAL, DAYS)	VACCINE PROTECTION (KNOWN STRAINS)	EFFECTIVENESS OF THERAPY	
				SERO-	CHEMO-
Viruses					
Yellow fever		3–6	+	–	–
TBE		7–14	+	–	–
JE		5–15	+	–	–
Dengue		5–7	–	–	–
VEE*	10–100	2–8	+[†]	–	–
EEE	10–100	7–14	+[†]	–	–
WEE	10–100	7–14	+[†]	–	–
Chikungunya		3–12	+[†]	–	–
O'nyong-nyong		3–12	+[†]	–	–
Rift Valley		3–12	+[†]	–	–
Influenza[‡]		1–3	+	–	+/–
Hanta		14–28	–	–	–
Smallpox*[‡]	10–100	7–17	+	+/–	+/–
Crimean-congo[‡]	1–10	4–21	–	+/–	+/–
Lassa*[†]	1–10	4–21	–	+/–	–
Marburg*[‡]	1–10	4–21	–	+/–	–
Ebola*[‡]	1–10	4–21	–	+/–	–
Bacteria					
Plague*[†]	100–500	5–60	+/–	–	+
Anthrax*	8,000–50,000	1–5	+/–	–	+/–
Tularemia*	10–50	2–10	+[†]	–	+
Brucellosis	10–100	5–60	–	–	+
Glanders	? 1,000	Days–weeks	–	–	+/–
Cholera	(10^6 oral)	2–3	+/–	–	NA
Typhoid		3–90	+	–	+
Rickettsia					
Typhus		7–14	–	–	+
Rocky mountain fever		3–14	–	–	+
Q fever*	1–10	10–40	+[†]	–	+
Fungi					
Coccidioidomycosis		7–28	–	–	+
Toxins					
Botulinum*	LD_{50} 0.05–0.2 mg	1–5	+[†]	+	–
Staphylococcal*	ED_{50} 0.025 m	1–6 hr	+[§]	+[§]	
Enterotoxin	LD_{50} 1–2 mg				
Ricin*	>100 mg	8–24 hr	+[§]	–	–

*Agent was under development and/or weaponized in BW programs; [†]vaccine is experimental—used in humans; [‡]transmissible from person to person; [§]vaccine only tested in animals.
JE = Japanese encephalitis, VEE = Venezuelan equine encephalomyelitis, EEE = eastern equine encephalomyelitis, WEE = western equine encephalomyelitis, LD = lethal dose, ED = effective dose.
+ = suitable good, +/– = moderately effective, – = poorly effective.

be achieved. Use of vaccines is also complicated by a further factor. The natural disease incidence in the case of biologic warfare agents precludes normal epidemiologic trials to determine efficacy, and of the two vaccines licensed in the U.S. (anthrax and plague), there are questions as to how effective they are in protecting humans against aerosol exposure. Development and regulatory approval of other vaccines against BW agents have also been impaired by an inability to conduct human trials and, in many cases, a lack of information on immune correlates of efficacy to allow extrapolation of animal protection data to humans.[14]

If vaccines can be given to laboratory and other at-risk persons as IND products on the basis of informed consent, then, in appropriate cases, immune globulin could be available for emergency civilian use, but again there will be regulatory issues to be addressed.

Another potential drawback to reliance on vaccines is the possibility that vaccine-resistant strains of some agents may have been deliberately created.[13,15]

Treatment and disease control in the aftermath of a biologic attack present significant problems. A study on the civilian medical response to chemical and biologic terrorism[12] categorized response capabilities at local, state, and federal levels as mainly "little or no capability" or "some capability"; only the ability at the federal level for agent detection in clinical samples was rated as "high."

The number of potential agents and the variety of possible therapeutic measures present major logistical problems, especially if large numbers of people have been exposed. Because of the rarity of most of the threats, diagnosis of early casualties is likely to be delayed. If contagious agents, particularly those with long incubation periods, are involved, even if relatively few people were directly exposed, there are likely to be significant problems of patient isolation and contact tracing. For many of the agents, especially viruses (see Table 41–5), there are no clearly proven effective treatments, and intensive supportive care of large numbers of casualties may be impossible. In the case of state-sponsored terrorism, there is also a real possibility that bacterial agents may have been engineered to be multiply antibiotic resistant.

CONCLUSIONS

Where major adverse consequences may result from an incident, even though the probability of such an incident is low, expenditure on contingency planning is a prudent and worthwhile investment. In the case of possible terrorist use of chemical or biologic agents, the ability to cause large-scale damage and the probability of an incident occurring appear low based on past experience. However, in this area, the key to action must be good intelligence assessments.

There is concern among knowledgeable officials in the U.S. about C/B terrorism. The director of the CIA has stated that terrorist groups are increasingly exploring C/B sabotage and expressed the view that this type of terrorism is the most urgent challenge. He also said that it was no longer a question of would a major act of C/B terrorism take place, but when would it happen.[16] In 1997, President Clinton sent to Congress a report describing the system formed to counteract threats of terrorist use of weapons of mass destruction.[17] Concern is not limited to the physical harm that C/B terrorism might cause. A range of adverse psychological responses has also been described, including panic, demoralization, anger, paranoia, social isolation, and loss of faith in social institutions.[18]

In many countries, at national, regional, and city levels, there are contingency plans to deal with terrorist attacks. States of readiness vary in respect to availability of the various medical countermeasures that would be required. At present, maintaining large stocks of many possible treatments does not appear justified both in view of the number and type of agents that could be used, the likelihood of an event, and the limited shelf-life and hence the cost of maintaining large stocks of medicines. For any individual, the risk of death or serious injury from this source remains low, and there are no special precautions that individual citizens or travelers need take.

REFERENCES

1. British Medical Association. Biotechnology, weapons and humanity. Amsterdam: Harwood, 1999.
2. Monterey Institute. Terrorism in the USA involving weapons of mass destruction. Monterey, CA: Center for Nonproliferation Studies, Monterey Institute of International Studies, 1998.
3. Bruck GM, Floweree CC. International handbook on chemical weapons proliferation. New York: Greenwood Press, 1991.
4. Douglas JD, Livingstone NC. America the vulnerable. Lexington, MA: Lexington Books, 1987.
5. Simon JD. Biological terrorism: preparing to meet the threat. JAMA 1997;278:428–430.
6. Kifner J. New York Times 23 December 1995.
7. Oehler GC. The growing chemical and biological weapons threat. Testimony before the Permanent Subcommittee on Investigations of the Senate Committee on Government Affairs, March 20. Accessed at http://www.kimsoft.com/korea/ciachem1.htm, August 18, 1998.
8. Holley D. Japanese sect linked to gene weapons plant. Los Angeles Times, 20 March 1995.
9. Broad WJ. When a cult turns to germ warfare. New York Times 26 May 1998.
10. Marshall E. Bracing for a biological nightmare. Science 1997;275:745–746.
11. Fetter S. Ballistic missiles and weapons of mass destruction: what is the threat? What should be done? Int Security 1991;16:5.
12. Institute of Medicine. Chemical and biological terrorism. Washington, DC: National Academy Press, 1999.
13. Alibek K. Biohazard. New York: Random House, 199.
14. Melling J. Defence-related vaccines: product licencing issues and constraints. In: Price BBS, Price RM, eds. Proceedings of the 2nd CB Medical Treatment Symposium. Portland, ME: Applied Science and Analysis:81–85.
15. Pomerantsev AP, Staritsin NA, Mockov YV, Marinin LI. Expression of cereolysin ab genes in *Bacillus anthracis* vaccine strain ensures protection against experimental hemolytic anthrax infection. Vaccine 1997;15:1848–1850.
16. Washington Times 6 February 1997.
17. Congressional Record. (1997) February 26 H65160.
18. Holloway HC, Norwood AE, Fullerton CS, et al. The threat of biological weapons. JAMA 1997;278:425–427.

Chapter 42

ILLNESS ABROAD AND BACK HOME

42.1 MEDICAL EMERGENCIES ABROAD: INDICATIONS FOR AND LOGISTICS OF AEROMEDICAL EVACUATION

PHILIP ROGENMOSER AND PETER V. SAVAGE

INTRODUCTION

Every traveler experiencing a medical emergency abroad wishes to get competent help and, above all, to return home as quickly as possible.

However, immediate transport back home is often neither possible nor necessary. What happens with the unfortunate traveler in a remote hospital somewhere in the bush? Who is going to help him cope with the problem? What options does he have? Will he require medical evacuation by air-ambulance or is transport on board a commercial airline appropriate? Who will cover the expenses, and when will he finally be back home? The following chapter aims to deal with these questions.

MEDICAL ASSISTANCE SERVICES

Although until relatively recently, a sick or injured traveler abroad was left to his own devices, over the past 10 years or so many insurance companies have set up special assistance services to deal with medical emergencies abroad.

With global tourism on the increase, telemedical assistance from the traveler's home country is becoming more and more important. However, this kind of assistance is not a substitute for competent medical care in the host country but rather complements what is offered locally.

For many decades, Swiss Air-Ambulance (REGA) has been dealing with medical emergencies abroad. Its concept of a differentiated and comprehensive approach to what may be called "In-Travel Emergency Management" (ITEM) has evolved over the past 10 years and reflects the specific needs of injured or sick travelers. The services offered range from telemedical counseling and case monitoring to the organization and execution of aeromedical evacuations and repatriations (Table 42.1–1).

MEDICAL EVACUATION AND REPATRIATION

Although many illnesses and injuries can be efficiently dealt with locally, there are a substantial number of patients who need to be transferred to a medical center where they will receive competent medical care. When talking about patient transport, it is useful to distinguish between medical evacuation and medical repatriation.

Whereas medical evacuation refers to the transportation of a patient to a medical center in the host or a nearby country, medical repatriation means transporting the patient back to his home country. Repatriation is primary when the patient is directly flown home and secondary when this transport takes place after the main medical problem has been resolved abroad.

Taking the example of our unfortunate traveler who is lying in a remote up-country hospital, there are usually three options to consider:

1. Medical evacuation to a competent medical center in the host country (e.g., from any location in Thailand to Bangkok) and secondary repatriation after stabilization.
2. Medical evacuation to a competent medical center in a neighboring country (e.g., from one of the Caribbean islands to Florida, U.S.A.) and secondary repatriation after stabilization.
3. Primary repatriation to the patient's home country (e.g., from Tunisia to Zurich).

Table 42.1–1. ITEM (IN-TRAVEL EMERGENCY MANAGEMENT)

Assistance in locating the nearest appropriate and competent medical care

Assessment of the medical problem through doctor-to-doctor report

Medical counseling

Monitoring progress during treatment

Establishing contacts with family physician or specialist at home/second opinion

Information/reassurance of family members

Organization and execution of aeromedical evacuation or repatriation

Assistance in coping with problems, such as language barriers, insurance coverage, transfer of funds, reticketing, etc.

MEDICAL EVACUATION

The purpose of a medical evacuation is to transport the patient to the nearest competent medical center as quickly and safely as possible. Depending on the geographic region, centers of medical excellence are sometimes a considerable distance away, even outside the host country. It may therefore be worthwhile considering the possibility of a primary/postprimary repatriation instead. Based on our experience with European travelers, we have drawn up a world map showing some of the medical centers with their "drainage areas" (Figure 42.1–1).

Although, theoretically, medevacs can be carried out by air-ambulance or by an airline, the urgency and clinical condition of the patient often make an air-ambulance indispensable. The number of air-ambulance services has increased considerably over the past few years in line with the growth in mass tourism, with the result that now coverage is almost worldwide. Although most of these services cover specific geographic areas, a few companies offer transcontinental and long-haul repatriation flights (Table 42.1–2).

MEDICAL REPATRIATION

Securing immediate medical care for the patient is certainly the primary goal of any doctor dealing with a medical emergency abroad. However, travelers usually ask for more; they want to return home and, in most cases, as soon as possible.

When and by what means a secondary repatriation can be organized depends on many factors: the traveler's medical condition, the geographic region, the operational possibilities, and, above all, the patient's travel insurance or financial means.

TRANSPORT BY AIRLINE

Patients who have been stabilized may be transported on board a commercial carrier. Depending on their clinical condition, they may travel either on their own or with a medical escort. The accompanying medical team usually comprises a doctor and/or nurse. Although most airlines offer special services to sick or disabled passengers, such as early boarding, the use of wheelchairs, and in-flight medical oxygen, they do not provide a medical escort. This is taken care of by the assistance company. Major commercial carriers provide stretcher facilities with curtains for greater privacy. Since the cost of a stretcher transport is quite substantial (e.g., the equivalent of six first-class air tickets), it is reasonable to rule out any other possibility, such as traveling in a sitting position in the business or first-class section of the aircraft.

It is important to know that the airline will require a medical report by the physician treating the patient. The airline's medical consultant will then either give or withhold the medical go-ahead for the flight. Without entering into details of flight physiology, it should be borne in mind that cabin pressure usually corresponds to an altitude of 2,300 m (8,000 feet), which results in a reduced barometric pressure and a decreased partial pressure of oxygen (pO_2). Although this poses no problems for a healthy traveler, it may adversely affect patients with pulmonary, coronary, anemic, or cerebrovascular problems.

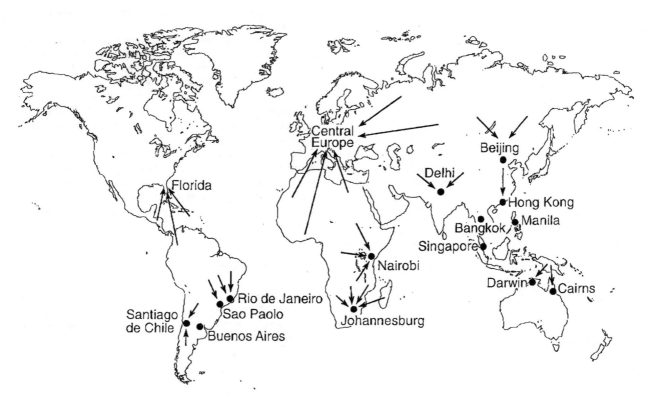

Figure 42.1–1.   Medical centers mostly used by European travelers.

Table 42.1–2.   SELECTED AIR-AMBULANCE ORGANIZATIONS

WORLD REGION	LOCATION	AIR-AMBULANCE
Africa	Nairobi	AMREF Flying Doctor Service
	Nairobi	ICAA Intensive Care Air Ambulance
	Johannesburg	MRI Medical Rescue International
	Johannesburg	National Air-Ambulance
	Johannesburg	MedicAir Edenvale
	Harare	Medical Air Rescue Service
	Douala	Cameroun Assistance Sanitaire
	Dakar	Senegalair
Asia	Singapore, Beijing, Hong Kong, Jakarta, Denpasar, Tokyo, Kazakstan, Kuala Lumpur, Manila, Seoul, Tapei, Bangkok, Ho Chi Minh City, Hanoi	AEA International SOS
	Calcutta	ARMS Asia Rescue & Medical Services
	Delhi	East West Rescue
	Mumbai	India Aeromedical Services
North America/ Caribbean	Fort Lauderdale, FL	Aero Jet International
	Fort Lauderdale, FL	National Air Ambulance
	St. Petersburg, FL	Care Flight
	San Diego	Critical Care Medicine
	Alabama	Medjet International
South America	Sao Paolo	Med Fly Seviços
	Rio de Janeiro	Lider Air-Ambulance
	Buenos Aires	Aeromedicos
	Buenos Aires	Med-Plane
Europe	Helsinki	Euroflite
	Innsbruck	Tyrolean Air-Ambulance
	Stuttgart	DRF German Air Rescue
	Zurich	REGA Swiss Air-Ambulance
Australia/ New Zealand	Sydney	Royal Flying Doctor Service
	Auckland	Pacific Air-Ambulance

If there is any doubt regarding the patient's suitability to fly, the airline company can be contacted for advice.

TRANSPORT BY AIR-AMBULANCE

Given the limited therapeutic possibilities on board a commercial carrier, it is obvious that many patients do not qualify for this kind of transport. There are situations

Table 42.1–3.   INDICATIONS FOR AIR-AMBULANCE SERVICES

Critically ill patients (e.g., on ventilator/catecholamines)

Patients with contagious diseases (TB, hepatitis, varicellosis, measles, meningitis, viral hemorrhagic fever)

Patients requiring transport at sea level (lung cysts, bowel obstruction, undrained pneumothorax, pneumoencephalon)

Patients requiring urgent transport (e.g., acute ischemia in peripheral arterial disease)

Patients requiring special equipment (e.g., incubator for neonates)

Patients with bulky tractions, which are otherwise not manageable

Patients with severe behavioral disturbances (psychoses)

Patients compromising the comfort of fellow passengers (offensively smelling wounds, diarrhea, vomiting)

Operational reasons (overbooking, high season, no stretcher facility)

Short-distance flights with competitive prices

where transport by air-ambulance is the only viable solution. The advantages are clear. As there are no rigid timetables to adhere to, the evacuation can take place at any time, day or night. Moreover, the cabin pressure can be adjusted to the patient's requirements, and, if necessary, flights can even be carried out at sea level. Fully dedicated air-ambulances can guarantee the maintenance of an intensive care environment. The smaller aircraft have access to airports with short airstrips, with the result that they can land closer to the site and to the final destination. Time-consuming and dangerous transfers to and from the airport by road-ambulance can be reduced to a minimum. The main indications for transport by air-ambulance are shown in Table 42.1–3.

Thanks to advanced technology and improved medical expertise, now more or less any patient can be moved to any point on the globe. However, it must be kept in mind that every transport also means destabilization. Therefore, moving critically ill patients over long distances needs careful evaluation. The risk of remaining in a place with limited medical facilities must be weighed against the risk of undergoing a transport. This decision is best left to the professionals—doctors experienced in aviation medicine who are able to judge the quality of the local medical care. Leading insurance companies have realized that they can no longer handle this difficult task themselves. They have wisely decided to "outsource" this service and leave it to specialized assistance companies.

FACTS AND FIGURES

Each country deals with medical emergencies abroad in its own way. Destinations, as well as attitudes, expectations, and financial means, differ from country to country. The following reports from two distinct geographic regions, Switzerland and the U.S.A., illustrate a European and an American approach to the same problem. Whereas the report from Switzerland focuses on what actually happened to travelers during 1998, the U.S. contribution deals with

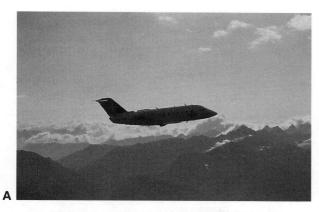

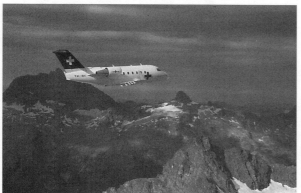

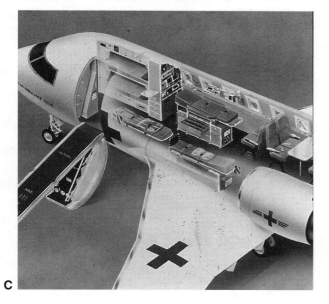

Figure 42.1–2.   A, B, Air-ambulance repatriation flights; *C,* Cutaway showing interior configuration of Challenger CL-601.

pretravel aspects, such as the evaluation of emergency assistance programs and health/travel insurance policies.

SWITZERLAND

The smaller the country, the more people will spend their holidays beyond its borders. This is certainly true for Switzerland. Compared to the country's total population, outgoing tourism in Switzerland is among the highest in the world. It is therefore of little wonder that the idea of repatriation has always been particularly cherished by the Swiss. Already in the early 1950s, REGA dedicated itself to aeromedical rescue. Although initially its activities were limited to Switzerland, these days REGA is active at a global level. Its three fully dedicated ambulance-jets (Figure 42.1–2) operate from Zurich Airport. A team of 12 fully employed doctors and nurses are responsible for the medical counseling and repatriation service.

The following data relating to the in-travel emergency management (ITEM) of Swiss and other European travelers in 1998 give an insight into the way in which REGA operates.

Geographic and General Data   In 1998, 1,525 travelers asked Swiss Air-Ambulance for assistance; 652 (43%) cases could be solved by telemedical assistance (counseling/case monitoring), whereas 873 (57%) patients were repatriated with a medical escort. In presenting thess data, the focus is placed on the group of patients who were repatriated. When interpreting these figures, it must be remembered that REGA serves an international clientele. Disease patterns do not necessarily reflect the actual incidence of medical emergencies among Swiss travelers.

The geographic distribution of travelers repatriated in 1998 is shown in Figure 42.1–3.

Clinical Data   Forty percent of the repatriated travelers had sustained a trauma, whereas 60% were suffering from a disease. The trauma and disease patterns are shown in Figure 42.1–4.

Number of Days of Hospitalization Prior to Repatriation   Patients are keen to know when they will be able to return home. The days spent in hospital prior to repatriation are a good criterion for judging the efficiency and quality of a travel or health insurance (Figure 42.1–5).

Practical Considerations   There is no doubt that travelers who wish to benefit from such services must have good travel and health insurance. The following points are worth considering before departure:

1. Check your health insurance to make sure that you are covered for illness and injury abroad. All too frequently, coverage is inadequate, especially for countries such as the United States, where medical care can be extremely expensive.
2. If you decide to buy travel insurance, make sure that it also covers medical evacuation and repatriation. Read the small print regarding restrictions and limitations and ask who is responsible for carrying out the evacuation in an emergency. Remember that the quality and reliability of insurers, assistance companies, and air-ambulances vary considerably.
3. If, despite all of your precautions, the sometimes unavoidable occurs, contact the alarm center of your

WORLDWIDE

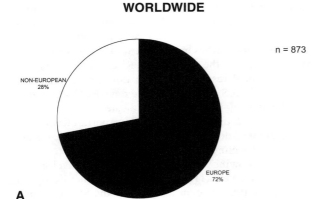

n = 873

A

NON-EUROPEAN REGIONS

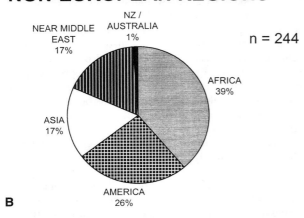

n = 244

B

Figure 42.1–3. Geographic distribution of repatriated travelers in 1998.

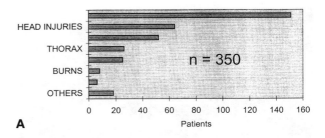

n = 350

A

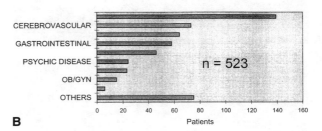

n = 523

B

Figure 42.1–4. Trauma patterns of repatriated travelers in 1998.

ening cases—to travelers who cannot show that they have cash, credit, or emergency assistance coverage of up to $10,000. Counseling on such matters by a travel medicine professional may well prove to be life-saving advice for his or her traveling clients.

It is not the job of travel medicine professionals to know the ins and outs of emergency medical assistance insurance. However, they can enhance their services by being in a position to inform their clients of the benefits of emergency medical assistance. This section is designed to show a travel medicine specialist how to do just that.

What kind of traveler's medical assistance is currently available on the market?

Credit Cards. Many major credit card companies and international travel agents (AMEX, Carlton, AAA) offer some kind of traveler's emergency medical assistance to cardholders and travel customers. This can be procured by means of a telephone call or by ticking a box on a travel tour application form. However, travelers should first find out exactly who is responsible for providing which services.

As regards travel medical services in connection with a traveler's credit card, there is an important difference between (a) using the emergency telephone number indicated by the credit card company (e.g., AMEX or VISA) to get help, when no prior emergency assistance insurance has been procured by the cardholder, and (b) calling the same telephone number when credit card payment has already been made in advance to cover emergency medical assistance provided by the credit card company's supplier.

Under (a), a traveler calling the credit card emergency number will be provided with a service that may be limited by the maximum credit of the card, with the result that a costly air evacuation would probably not be covered. If it is covered, the cost of the evacuation will be subsequently charged to the traveler's credit card. Under (b), the traveler will have been charged (perhaps auto-

insurance company and be prepared to answer the questions shown in Figure 42.1–6.

UNITED STATES

U.S. Guide to Emergency Medical Assistance Often American travelers—unlike European ones—do not consider carrying additional emergency medical insurance when they are on a trip abroad. American insurers and health maintenance organizations frequently do not cover medical problems outside the U.S. Medicare does not cover assistance outside the U.S., and if it is covered, it is on a reimbursement basis, which is effected long after the medical emergency. Failure to procure additional insurance can be ruinously expensive if a traveler requires emergency medical evacuation and has to be flown home from some distant land. Coverage for emergency medical assistance, including air evacuation, is something no traveler should be without, and it is definitely not a topic one wishes to first encounter during a medical crisis in a foreign country and in a foreign language.

In some European countries, a medical facility will refuse to provide medical services—even in life-threat-

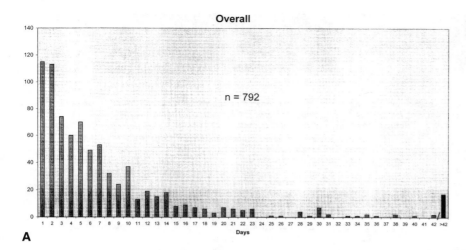

A

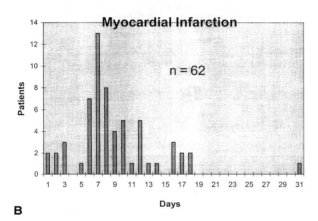

B

Figure 42.1–5. Days in hospital prior to repatriation in 1998.

matically, if the card is used for international travel) for an insurance or assistance fee. This fee will provide wider assistance coverage, usually including air evacuation, by the credit card company's designated emergency assistance supplier.

In the first case, the traveler is activating a service for which he will pay. In the second case, he is activating an insurance policy that covers an emergency service. Some credit card companies offer a "referral service" (outlined below) instead of emergency assistance services.

Direct Medical Assistance Program. The most comprehensive emergency medical assistance coverage is included in an insurance policy or assistance service known as a direct medical assistance program. This program provides around-the-clock telephone access to a reputable assistance company, which, in the case of an emergency, will take the appropriate action, including finding a suitable doctor or clinic, sending funds, or arranging medical evacuation to a competent medical facility.

Referral Service. A direct medical assistance program should be distinguished from a referral service or a travel accident insurance policy. Several credit cards provide referral services whereby, when alerted to a crisis, the company's emergency center will refer the traveler to someone on an approved list. The traveler is then left to

contact that person and decide for himself what action should be taken. Unless otherwise agreed on beforehand, all expenses are payable by the traveler and will be charged to his credit card after the crisis.

Travel Insurance Policy. A travel insurance policy often has no emergency contact provision, and the traveler is reimbursed for any expenses (as stated in the policy) resulting from a medical emergency that occurs during a trip abroad. Medical evacuation with a specified maximum amount may be included, but it is up to the traveler to take the appropriate action, including choosing an evacuation company.

For a travel medicine professional, it is important to stress that travelers should be aware in advance who is going to do what and what is paid for if they are injured or incapacitated while they are abroad. The most comprehensive response is provided by a direct medical assistance program.

What assistance companies and insurers exist in the emergency medical assistance market? The basic elements of emergency medical assistance are straightforward. In the case of a medical emergency, the traveler calls the international number of the assistance company, quotes his card number, and explains the nature of the emergency. The assistance company, in consultation with

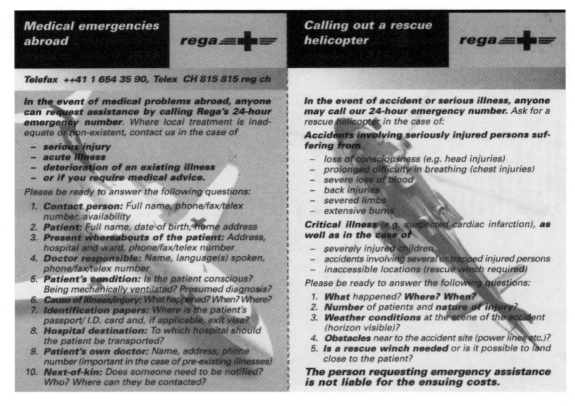

Figure 42.1–6. REGA's Emergency Card: 10 points to remember.

its medical director or medical staff (and, wherever possible, the traveler's own physician), will decide what steps need to be taken on the traveler's behalf. The assistance company may alert a local doctor from its contact list to attend to the traveler and arrange for him to be taken to an appropriate medical facility. If cash is needed, the assistance company will provide it.

If an evacuation is required, the assistance company will determine the location of the nearest suitable medical facility and arrange for either transportation on board a commercial aircraft or the services of an air evacuation company. The assistance company may decide that the traveler should be flown home to the U.S. for treatment and coordinates the repatriation with the traveler's doctor, its own medical staff, and the local physician assigned to the traveler. The cost of the operation will be covered by the insurer up to the limits and terms set out in the insurance policy or agreement.

A travel medicine professional can also help travelers by suggesting a number of questions that they should ask about an assistance company and by advising them where the answers can best be found. First and foremost, is the assistance company experienced in providing emergency medical assistance? Are its staff well trained? Does it have up-to-date records of doctors and reliable medical facilities to contact? Second, do its staff have the discretion and authority to approve assistance services and evacuation, if necessary late on a Sunday evening, when the traveler may not have his card or policy number with

him? The brokers listed below can help to answer questions such as these (Table 42.1–4).

Although there has been a shake-out and consolidation in the emergency assistance company market recently, there are several well-established companies that have been in business for many years (Table 42.1–5). These companies serve major corporations and institutions that send employees abroad. They also have individual policies that cover tourists, students, and pleasure trippers. Coverage for individuals usually runs for a period of a year.

This list is not definitive, and there are other reputable companies, both in the U.S. and abroad, which provide such services. Many other providers or brokers offer a wide range of coverage, but travelers requiring a direct medical assistance program are well advised to purchase their policy through an established emergency response company, such as those listed above.

How can a travel medicine professional determine what a traveler needs and match him to the appropriate assistance company? A travel medicine professional who wants to direct a traveler with individual needs to the most appropriate assistance company and policy may refer him to a health/medical coverage broker. Some assistance company policies, for example, exclude coverage of a traveler's preexisting health conditions. A broker can find a policy that will include such coverage. There are several well-known providers in this field (see Table 42.1–4).

Table 42.1–4.   U.S. BROKERS

COMPANY	ADDRESS	PHONE/FAX	REMARKS
Thomas W. Snyder & Company	552 Pewter Drive, P.O. Box 718, Exton, PA 19341-0718	++1 610-363-6450 phone ++1 888-396-8888 phone ++1 610-363-0247 fax	Uses AIG Assist as an assistance company
Wallach and Company	107 West Federal Street, Suite 13, P.O. Box 480, Middleburg, VA 27118	++1 800-237-6615 phone	Often uses MEDEX for assistance
Travel Guard International	1145 Clark Street, Stevens Point, WI 54481-9970	++1 715-345-0505 phone ++1 800-826-1300	Has its own Mercury Assistance Company
CMI Insurance Specialists	1447 York Road, Lutherville, MD 21093-6032	++1 410-583-2595 ++1 410-583-8244	Contact: E. Gay Persons

This list, too, is not definitive and there are many other brokers who specialize in travel groups, students, long-term overseas residents, and adventure travel.

Armed with these lists of insurance providers, assistance companies, and brokers, a travel medicine professional is in a position to advise a travel customer requiring a direct medical assistance program to reputable providers, as well as to brokers who can analyze and meet individual travel needs.

CONCLUSION

For the international traveler, the starting point is very often total ignorance about emergency medical assistance: what it is, the consequences of failing to buy coverage, and what determines a good service from a bad or incomplete one. A travel medicine clinic is probably the first place a traveler will go where the risk of illness during a trip will be explained. For this reason, the travel medicine professional at a clinic is in a unique position to educate and guide a traveler to an intelligent decision about emergency medical assistance and medical evacuation insurance.

This section is designed to give a travel medicine professional the tools to evaluate the services, companies, and brokers in this business. Passing such information on to your travel clients is a valuable service to them and is likely to add to their esteem of your professionalism and your clinic.

Table 42.1–5.   U.S. EMERGENCY ASSISTANCE COMPANIES

COMPANY	ADDRESS	PHONE / FAX	REMARKS
AIG Assist (formerly AIAS)	Regency Square, 6464 Savoy Road, Houston, TX 77036	++1 800-237-0072 phone ++1 713-267-2540 phone	Corporate and individual policies
AXA Assistance, U.S.A.	200 West Jackson Suite 1100, Chicago, IL 60606	++1 312-935-3500 phone ++1 312 -935-3590 fax	Successor to USAssist, affiliated with American Express Gold Card
International SOS Asistance/ AEA International	Eight Neshaminy Interplex, P.O. Box 115568, Trevose, PA 19053-6956	++1 215-244-1500 phone ++1 800-523-8661 phone ++1 215-244-2227 fax E-mail: corporate@intsos.com	Corporate and individual policies; recently merged (1998)
MEDEX Assistance Corporation (MEDEX)	9515 Deereco Road, 4th Floor, Timonium, MD 21093	++1 410-453-6300 phone ++1 410-453-6301 fax ++1 800-537-2029 phone	
Worldwide Assistance Service, Inc.	1133 Fifteenth Street, NW, Suite 400, Washington, DC 20005-2710	++1 202-331-1609 phone ++1 800-821-2828 phone ++1 202-828-5896 fax E-mail: info@worldwide assistance.com	
Access America	6600 W. Broad St., Richmond, VA 23230	++1 804-673-1159 phone Web site: www.access america.com	Affiliated with VISA credit card
MedPass/Global Emergency Medical Services (GEMS)	2001 Westside Parkway, Suite 120, Alpharetta, GA 30004	++1 770-475-1114 phone ++1 800-860-1111 phone ++1 770-475-0058 fax	Offers direct calls to medical professionals with insurance as an add on

42.2 MEDICAL CARE FOR INTERNATIONAL VISITORS TO THE UNITED STATES AND CANADA

EDWARD R. RENSIMER

OVERVIEW

Travel medicine issues most usually involve problems facing individuals passing through or temporarily residing in developing countries and who are subjected to health care systems operating below Western standards of care. There are several conditions that define travel medicine concerns differently for a foreign traveler or expatriate to the North American continent. As will become evident, although some problems encountered with less developed medical care systems become irrelevant, a number of issues still must be proactively considered and addressed in order for "a stranger in a strange land" to achieve optimal medical management and outcomes.

First, we must consider those issues unique to U.S./Canadian travel. They will define the context for the traveler's planning and subsequent actions.

SOPHISTICATED HEALTH CARE SYSTEM

High-quality health care providers are widely available throughout North America. Strict professional credentialing, licensing, and continuing education processes regulate quality control. Of course, training and experience of physicians and support medical services are most commonly directed toward those medical issues of the resident population. Nevertheless, with deliberate research, one can locate individuals and institutions equipped to deal effectively with virtually any problem from anywhere in the world. This assertion is qualified by the fact that such broad expertise is realistically centered in major urban areas, often within academic or affiliated medical institutions. However, centers of medical excellence are quite widespread and accessible. It may be presumed that, except for repatriation for personal, elective reasons, evacuation is not a medical necessity for anyone who becomes ill while in North America.[1]

The U.S. and Canadian systems are fee-for-service models, the latter tightly regulated by the federal and provincial governments since the Canada Health Act of April 1, 1984.[2] Canada's system is one of universal, broad health services/benefits coverage prepaid by citizen members. Still, it is not a socialized medicine program since physicians are not employed by the government. Nevertheless, fees are highly regulated. For health services non-insured by the government, individuals may pay providers directly or purchase private insurance coverage.

The U.S. system is entirely fee for service and functions under a myriad of prepaid health plan models. These include managed care situations, such as health maintenance organizations, preferred provider organizations, and point of service plans. Otherwise, private indemnity coverage is used. U.S. residents commonly obtain their health coverage policies by way of their employers.

Both U.S. and Canadian systems are structured to provide access to care. Individuals who do not have private insurance in the U.S. and who are not covered by the government-sponsored, prepaid Medicare/Medicaid plans are expected to work within the local county/state-supported and regulated system of public health care hospitals and clinics for the indigent. Such care is provided based on the individual's ability to pay—sometimes pro rata charging, but usually free. Although the diagnostic and treatment capabilities in the public health sector may be sufficient, the burden of uninsured and indigent patients creates a system always operating at extreme limits and minimum efficiency. It is not a preferred option.

SOPHISTICATED INFORMATION INFRASTRUCTURE

Information on medical care options and technical/operational considerations regarding such care is available from a number of sources, as shown in Table 42.2–1.

The U.S. and Canadian federal and local governments provide information on government-sponsored and supported medical institutions both by telephone and on the Internet. Again, except for public health system patients, such programs require citizenship status and sometimes other requirements, such as prior military service and age criteria.

The agent sponsoring an individual's presence in a country, such as a corporation or employer, often can provide very specific, effective recommendations for local medical care since the agent often has had to solve such problems previously.

The embassy/consulate of the country of origin also can be of invaluable assistance, as well as any existing expatriate and/or ethnic communities, in directing travelers to appropriate medical care providers. The International Association for Medical Assistance to Travelers (IAMAT), operating out of Lewiston, NY, U.S.A., or Guelph, Ontario, Canada, maintains a list of physician

Table 42.2–1. MEDICAL CARE RESOURCES

Government
Sponsoring agent
Embassy
Expatriate community
Ethnic community
IAMAT
Travel medicine advisor
Travel insurance carrier
Internet

providers who frequently deal with travelers.[3] These physicians have set their fees for travel medicine services and list languages with which their organizations can work. Another such directory, *Travel Medicine Advisor*,[4] published by American Health Consultants in Atlanta, GA, also provides information on travel health clinics throughout the U.S., Canada, and Israel. Also, the American Society for Tropical Medicine and Hygiene publishes a directory of travel medicine clinics with descriptions of services.[5]

Travel medicine insurance carriers may also direct travelers to those who are both qualified and comfortable with the unique needs of the traveling ill.

Finally, the Internet is a growing source of institutions, medical organizations, and specific physician providers. It is becoming increasingly common for individual physicians in North America to have a specific Web site containing their professional credentials, training, achievements, unique capabilities, and practical medical practice policy information. Specific, detailed information on the Internet as a travel medicine resource is available in other sections of this textbook and other sources.[6]

A relatively brief search of these pathways can produce a variety of specific, useful facts for structuring a personal medical response system while in North America.

NORTH AMERICAN MEDICAL RISKS

Traditionally, the dividing point for travel medicine discussions has been infectious and noninfectious diseases. This is relevant to the origins of travel medicine as a discipline, concerning itself mainly with diseases acquired while in developing countries. Communicable diseases are less of an issue in the North American travel context since public health controls on waste disposal and water purification, along with epidemiologic containment of communicable diseases, have been successful in an unprecedented way. The exception to this for any traveler, anywhere, is sexually transmitted diseases. Certain risk factors (Table 42.2–2) make acquisition of sexually transmitted diseases a much increased possibility, particularly for travelers, since they are more prone to change behavior patterns while on the road.

Notwithstanding this exceptional consideration, the traveler to North America should be more concerned with noninfectious disease problems that threaten health (Table 42.2–3).

The dominant medical occurrences are cardiovascular, trauma/injury-related, and routine major medical/surgical problems, as opposed to "exotic" diseases, and suggest the risk profile specific to travel in North America and thus the priorities in medical planning.

PAYMENT FOR SERVICES

Travelers to North America will likely not be covered for medical services by their prepaid government-sponsored systems. They will be expected to cover their expenses with cash unless their travel sponsors have provided cov-

Table 42.2–2. **TRAVELER SEXUAL ACTIVITY CHARACTERISTICS**

Up to 50% of travelers
Male
Youth
Non-family travel
Alcohol use
Lengthier trips
Infrequent barrier sex: 30% to 50%

erage or the traveler has arranged for private insurance coverage for the trip. Otherwise, nonurgent care of the uninsured is directed to the public health care system, although in a true medical emergency, "Good Samaritan" laws encourage and/or require provision of services to the ill by both individual health care providers and institutions.

It cannot be assumed that the insurance system extant in the traveler's country of origin provides benefits in North America. Such may be the case, as with Australian and Canadian Medicare national insurance, but benefits should be specifically verified for each country.

Finally, travelers with a specific trip sponsor may have medical benefits provided by way of the sponsor. Some U.S. corporations maintain the traveler/expatriate on a payroll plan within the company such that the employee retains the health benefits of the insurance system of his country of origin. Some agents purchase a private medical policy for the traveler to cover the length of stay in North America. It must be emphasized that these issues are extremely important in the care of nonurgent, but necessary, medical care. Medical systems throughout North America will mobilize in a medical crisis irrespective of ability to pay. However, careful planning and comprehensive insurance coverage will ensure an optimally efficient and pleasant encounter with the health care systems.

NORTH AMERICA TRAVEL MEDICAL PLAN

Medical planning for a North America sojourn involves measures on two levels:

1. *Non-System.* Those things a traveler should attend to in order to minimize the need for engagement of the medical care system. Every traveler should do this.

Table 42.2–3. **NON-INFECTIOUS TRAVEL ILLNESS RISKS**

Accidents/trauma
High-risk behavior
Medical/surgical problems
Psychiatric events

2. *System.* This planning covers items that expedite efficient, optimal interaction with the local medical care system. Again, some issues pertain to any traveler, but others are relevant to very specific, complex, or unusual preexisting medical situations (i.e., special patients).

Please note that the principles and approach to pretravel "non-system" preparation are clearly stated in other sections of this textbook.

SYSTEM PLANNING (TABLE 42.2–4)

PROVIDERS

Prior to departure, it would be optimal for the traveler to locate physicians who are medically, culturally, and operationally capable of handling ongoing and unanticipated need for medical care. This is clearly indicated for those who have preexisting illnesses or who are deemed at increased risk for medical catastrophe. Such a search could be conducted through destination-located ethnic groups, travel sponsor, local embassy, travel medical insurance carrier, and destination-itinerary-oriented medical Internet Web sites.

FACILITIES

As with providers, health care facilities at the destination should be assessed for any required special capabilities and for reasonableness of access. Such information may be obtained beforehand.

Although hospital emergency departments may be used both for routine and emergent care, time waiting to be seen can be substantial, and emergency room physicians are basically triage specialists who are not skilled in long-term management aspects of disease. They will start the process of diagnosis and treatment but then refer the patient to another physician to ultimately complete case management. So, this venue tends to be inefficient and cost intensive since it is based in the hospital.

When a nonurgent medical problem requires attention, it is best to start with a primary physician who is in private medical practice or who practices at an academic (university-affiliated) medical center. North American private practice physicians, if selected after diligent screening for both problem-specific medical expertise and orientation to the patient's country of origin and culture, should provide high-quality service. But prospective payment will be mandatory to cover not only professional time but also all expenses related to diagnostic testing and treatment. Although institutionally based medical

practice, such as at teaching hospitals and clinics, may be less business oriented since their staff physicians are often salaried employees, the competitive health care marketplace and declining federal subsidies in recent years have increasingly forced such institutions to tighten their business operations. The acceptability of the trade-off of receiving medical case material for physician trainees in lieu of payment for services provided is no longer a given, particularly in the U.S. So, from the patient's perspective, except in public health (charity) teaching hospitals, expectations of payment will likely be as much a priority in academic institutions as in private practice. It is characteristic of academic facilities that physician trainees are providing most or all patient care services. On the other hand, some academic institutions, because of international patient referrals, have developed cross-cultural services departments that may be advantageous in the total care/management of the foreign traveler in trouble.

INSURANCE

The traveler must clarify whether he/she will be covered by the country of origin national medical plan, by a travel sponsor arranged plan, or by a personally procured policy. It should be noted that there are usually document execution requirements in order to extend country of origin insurance for overseas travel or residence. For instance, travelers originating from member countries of the European Union must fill out International Health Insurance Certification E111 from their home country insurer to continue their benefits while away if their trip will be no longer than 12 months. Other countries have similar requirements or reciprocity agreements for underwriting foreign medical care for their respective citizens. Finally, many credit cards, especially the more exclusive ones, provide travel health coverage for a limited period of usually 48 days.

SPECIAL PATIENTS[7–9]

Obviously, certain travelers will require ongoing medical services or will be at substantial risk for developing problems while away from home. This would apply to anyone with a chronic, active disease such as cancer, heart disease, diabetes mellitus, chronic renal or liver failure, and neurologic disorders. Likewise, extremes of age increase the risk of acute medical deterioration. Reasonable preparations include all of the aforementioned plus contact with appropriate disease-specific local organizations (such as the American Diabetes Association and the American Cancer Society) for special advice and direction about local medical capabilities. More detailed information on the special patient travel medicine considerations are provided elsewhere in this text.

Table 42.2–4.   SYSTEM PLANNING

Providers
Facilities
Insurance
Special patients

SOLUTION: PERSONAL RESPONSE SYSTEM

In the face of medical care systems unreliably prepared to manage medical problems of foreigners optimally, including communication with significant individuals in the country of origin, it is essential that travelers take steps to construct their own personal "medical response system." Of course, an individual traveler can always dial "911" on a telephone in the U.S. or Canada for immediate, unconditional response of the medical care system to a crisis. But in otherwise urgent or nonurgent medical situations, the traveler can substantially improve his/her encounter by proactively defining the location(s) for medical care and under what circumstances that care will be given.

Many physicians in traditional practice situations in North America will be insufficiently equipped to deal with the following:

- *Foreign Language Communication.*
- *Medical Records Transfer.* Real-time exchange of information from overseas may be problematic unless a medical practice is Internet linked.
- *Communication Overseas.* Real-time, ongoing contact with overseas family and medical providers can be impractical, again, unless the practice has direct Internet connectivity.
- *Logistical Barriers.* Working with other medical care providers across time zones and locations may present obstacles such that a traveler with a mobile itinerary may well receive disjointed, suboptimal care unless a physician and his/her support staff are set up and oriented to routinely provide this kind of service.
- *Payment.* Physicians may be reluctant to deal with special payment arrangements with a traveler for fear of nonpayment unless their business staff are accustomed to nontraditional arrangements.

For all of these reasons, it is important to organize a medical response system or mechanism prior to traveling or expatriating.

In addition to all of the previously mentioned information, three areas of inquiry remain:

- Travel health insurance
- Nonurgent care sources
- Travel medicine clinic services checklist

TRAVEL HEALTH INSURANCE

About 1 per 1,000 travelers ultimately submit a medical claim for travel-related problems; 8 per 100,000 die.

In evaluating health insurance policy features, a traveler should consider a number of issues:

- *Assistance*
  - Physician location: finding a doctor for the traveler,
  - Contacting the traveler's family,
  - Translators,
  - Physician referral policies/restrictions,
  - Prescription medication coverage,
  - Hospitalization expenses,
  - Medical case management/monitoring (by insurer),
  - Medical evacuation coverage: not covered by most major medical policies, and
  - Legal aid/posting bond.

- *Health Payments*
  - Direct: on-the-spot reimbursement to care providers by the patient,
  - Reimbursement (to patient after he/she has paid for services), and
  - Accidental death/dismemberment coverage (repatriation).
- *Other*
  - Trip interruption/cancellation coverage and
  - Baggage damage/loss.

Each of the above items should be investigated fully with regard to amount of coverage, restrictions, limitations, defaults, and exclusions, and the insured's responsibilities (financial and otherwise) under the terms of a policy (Table 42.2–5).

NONURGENT CARE SOURCES

There are a number of options for routine medical care in the United States and Canada. Care can be obtained from a local, traditional private practice physician, local hospital emergency department, or a referral medical center (such as an academic institution). Recommendations for where to go for care may come from contacting hotel officials, travel sponsor company officials, embassy staff, local medical society officials, local hospital emergency department staff, and local ethnic community contacts. Each of these traditional entry points to North American health care likely suffers multiple previously noted inefficiencies and incapabilities, particularly for the traveler suddenly in trouble.

Another option for the traveler is to look into the availability of full-service travel medicine clinics in the area. Many travel medicine clinics are basically "shots" clinics, specializing in preparing North American residents for overseas travel to underdeveloped countries with immunizations and medications mainly directed at "exotic," endemic infectious diseases. But some travel medicine clinics are developing expansive capabilities for handling international medicine issues and medical care for both North America-originated travelers and those transiting through North America. A full-service travel medicine operation offers a number of advantages to individuals temporarily in North America:

- Familiarity with foreign medical care systems and records;

Table 42.2–5. POTENTIAL INSURANCE EXCLUSIONS

Against medical advice travel
Preexisting illness
Risky activities (i.e., sports, etc.)
Manual labor tasks
Substance abuse problems
Mental illness
Sexually transmitted diseases
Medical problems from acts of God/insurrection

- Established linkage to necessary institutions and groups
  - embassies,
  - multinational corporations,
  - ethnic communities, and
  - overseas medical support services, such as evacuation providers liaison;
- Proficiency with foreign, exotic diseases and medications;
- Flexibility—staff tend to be open to "global thinking," both medically and operationally; and
- Internet connectivity.

Attention to these areas will create the foundation for the most effective entry into and use of the North American health care systems by travelers in medical distress.

REFERENCES

1. Smith MAH Jr. Medical care for foreign visitors to the United States of America and Canada. In: DuPont HL, Steffen R, eds. Textbook of travel medicine and health. Hamilton, ON: BC Decker, 1997:333–336.
2. Health System and Policy Division. Canada's Health System. www.hc-sc.gc.ca/main/hc/web/datapcb/datahesa/hlthsys/Ehlthsys.htm. Accessed October 1998.
3. IAMAT directory. International Association for Medical Assistance to Travellers. Lewiston, NY, 1995.
4. Travel medicine advisor, the physician's update on international health. Atlanta: American Health Consultants, 1997.
5. The American Society of Tropical Medicine & Hygiene. 1997 ASTMH Clinical Consultants Directory. Lawrence, KS: Allen Press, 1998.
6. Freedman DO. Keeping current: travel medicine resources available on the Internet. Infect Dis Clin North Am 1998;12:543–549.
7. Jong EC, McMullen R. General advice for the international traveler. Infect Dis Clin North Am 1992;6:275–289.
8. Patterson JE. The traveler with chronic illness. Yale J Biol Med 1992;65:317–327.
9. Bia FJ, Barry M. Special health considerations for travelers. Med Clin North Am 1992;76:1295–1312.

42.3 MEDICAL EMERGENCIES FOR INTERNATIONAL VISITORS TO DEVELOPING COUNTRIES

SANTANU CHATTERJEE

Medical emergencies are inevitable during travel. Studies reveal that although there is a 60% to 75% chance of reporting physical symptoms or suffering minor illness per month of travel in Asia, there is only a 5% chance of the need to seek medical help.[1] Many of these medical conditions are self-limiting and resolve with first-aid measures. Defining specific health risks can be difficult, but it is evident that disease frequency varies with the type of travel and region visited.[2] Tourists are ill more often than people traveling on business.[3] Diarrhea and upper respiratory tract infections are common in visitors to most developing regions.[4] Other medical problems range from hepatitis and malaria to accidents.[5,6]

If we consider the chances of mortality abroad, they seem reassuringly small and are mainly attributable to heart attacks and accidental injuries. Infections account for relatively few deaths. Although cardiovascular deaths are the most common cause of death in tourists traveling outside their country,[6] they occur mostly in older travelers with preexisting disease and are often unrelated to travel. Accidental deaths, however, are directly travel related, involve younger travelers, and comprise mainly road accidents and drownings. A study of Peace Corps volunteers confirmed that motor vehicle accidents are the leading cause of death in younger travelers.[7] Accidents and injuries involving tourists are largely preventable.[8,9] Driver error, excessive alcohol intake, fatigue, or unfamiliar road conditions are common reasons for error. Developing countries have higher motor vehicle crash death rates in comparison to developing countries.[10] For example, India accounts for nearly 6% of all road accidents worldwide and has one of the highest accident rates at 34.6 per 10,000 persons.[11] A survey involving 216 travelers seeking medical assistance in Calcutta revealed 34% requesting help for emergencies, of which 7% was attributable to trauma (Figure 42.3–1).

The developing world is experiencing a remarkable growth rate in travel, and with this comes a growing demand for the highest level of medical care. There is also a marked increase in tourists choosing exotic destinations where medical facilities are still limited. Moreover, increasing business opportunities in the developing world necessitate many corporations to relocate their staff. The health and safety of these employees remain an area of utmost concern. Expatriate employees and travelers now expect medical facilities of international standards. In addition, we need to assure them that, in a crisis situation, their health will be managed by competent professionals. Contrary to expectations, urban health systems in Asia are going through radical changes with government prefer-

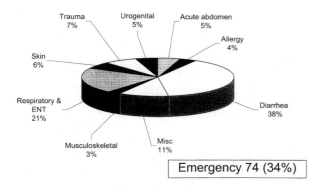

Figure 42.3–1.   Health problems (N = 216).

ences tending toward spending more for primary health care and encouraging the private sector to enter the health business and provide advanced medical care. As a result, private health care is booming, with consumer spending on nongovernment medical treatment growing in many areas at an average of 20% every year.[12] Most cities in these regions can now offer a wide range of medical care from simple diagnostic clinics to sophisticated private hospitals where efficiency and quality care merge with high technology.

HOW TO ACCESS HEALTH CARE IN THE DEVELOPING WORLD

In this region, recommending medical care that is satisfactory in terms of cost, quality, and access is often difficult. Standards of health care are changing and may even differ in the same hospital over a given period. Private health care is usually more expensive, and, given an optimum level of care, costs vary widely between different regional centers. General health care is usually available but options for specialized treatment may often be inadequate. In urban areas, there are many choices, especially in the private sector, but locating quality health care in many smaller towns and remote rural districts can be a problem. In situations needing urgent medical attention, the best chances are definitely with the nearest hospital. Mobile emergency services are rare and ambulance services virtually nonexistent in some regions. It is therefore advisable to use any form of available transport to reach the hospital.

Health care providers in host countries play a pivotal role in providing medical assistance to travelers, especially at primary care levels. They are usually the first to be called in during emergencies. Professional competence, bedside skills, and quality of health advice may differ from what the traveler is accustomed to at home. The essential prerequisites for a health care provider are listed in Table 42.3–1.

Although individual preferences, past experiences, and varying confidence levels in local health care can influence the decision, there are several possible options for medical assistance abroad. These include the following:

- *Diplomatic missions.* The local embassy or consulate provides referral lists of hospitals and English-speaking physicians on request including clinic addresses, fee schedules, and emergency contact numbers. Information can be obtained from the consular office during working hours and from the duty officer at other times. They normally do not recommend any particular doctor, but approaching a sympathetic staff member for suggestions may prove worthwhile in urgent situations.
- *Hotels.* Major tourist hotels in most developing countries have in-house physicians who provide medical assistance to both resident and nonresident guests. Smaller hotels and guesthouses have a doctor on call, as part of the services provided to their guests. Alternatively, hotels can arrange appointments with local physicians and help with directions to the nearest hospital. In case of any need, the receptionist or lobby manager is the contact person, since he or she is usually responsible for coordinating the medical service. The prescribed medications can also be arranged from local chemists. Most physicians have a fixed fee and agree to make "house calls" to the hotel room on a priority basis. For minor illnesses, this is a convenient arrangement, but a visit to the doctors' office is preferable especially when dealing with wounds or accidents.
- *IAMAT.* The International Association for Medical Assistance to Travelers (IAMAT) is a Canada-based nonprofit foundation promoting the coordination of medical care abroad. They identify and recruit qualified physicians in various cities and tourist destinations. IAMAT physicians are usually on 24-hour call, agree on a set fee schedule, and maintain a high professional standard of medical practice. When contacted, they provide comprehensive medical care, which includes an appropriate medical examination, arrange for the medicines, make specialist and hospital referrals if needed, and provide a full medical report. Membership to IAMAT is open to all, and members are provided with an updated worldwide directory, which lists qualified English-speaking physicians, hospitals, and health care centers. (IAMAT office address: USA: 417 Center Street, Lewiston, NY 14092; Tel: 716-754-4883; Canada: 40 Regal Road, Guelph, ON NIK IBS; Tel: 519-836-0102; E-mail: iamat@sentex.net

Table 42.3–1.   **ESSENTIAL PREREQUISITES FOR HEALTH CARE PROVIDERS IN HOST COUNTRIES**

Proper professional training and language skills

Comprehensive knowledge of regional health risks

Competence in attending both routine and emergency cases

Developing resources for prompt hospital referrals

Good communication links and easy availability

Coordinating with insurance and assistance organizations

Organizing and implementing evacuation protocols

- *Tourist offices.* The local tourist office is a good option to seek appropriate medical referrals. Travel-associated health risks, particularly health scares, have substantial commercial implications for the tourism industry in host countries.[13] The plague outbreak in parts of India during 1994 is one example of a health scare having a tremendous economic impact.[14] Realizing this, tourism authorities in most destinations make conscious efforts to be helpful and usually recommend the best options during emergencies.

- *Pharmacies.* Given the boom in private health care, most areas have a pharmacy catering to the needs of the local population. General practitioners frequently have their consulting rooms either within or adjoining these premises. The pharmacist is often a local man who is acquainted with the medical infrastructure of the region and usually provides the basic medical advice, especially in remote areas, where doctors may not be easily available. Backpackers trekking through such places are known to rely on them for suggestions, although the appropriateness of certain remedies may sometimes be questioned.

- *Credit card assistance.* Major credit card companies provide a 24-hour telephone hotline facility for their premium cardholders. This operates as an emergency medical assistance service where each case is dealt with on an individual basis. Apart from providing physician and hospital referrals, they can organize translators in case of language difficulties, notify the office and family on request, and make appropriate travel arrangements.

- *Travel insurance with assistance.* Comprehensive health and travel insurance endeavors to provide on-the-spot medical help together with aeromedical repatriation, if indicated. This is advantageous, especially in cases requiring hospitalization. Although costs and coverage can vary, most insurance plans have round-the-clock telephone access to an emergency center and facilities for immediate physical referral or telephonic medical advice. Others provide additional benefits like monitoring of medical conditions by multilingual staff from the assistance center, which includes physician-assisted advice, liaison with the treating physician, renewal of prescriptions, coverage for air-ambulance repatriation, and on-site emergency medical payment. Nonmedical assistance like emergency cash transfers, travel arrangements, legal assistance, replacement of lost prescriptions, and reporting of lost or stolen credit cards are also provided to clients. Some insurance policies have limits to medical reimbursement that include dental treatment, pregnancy-related problems, or accidents involving adventure sports like skiing and scuba diving. Others may reimburse treatment costs only if prior approval is taken or treatment availed from an approved list of physicians or hospitals. Preexisting illnesses may require additional coverage.

- *Publications.* Regional newspapers often have a section on emergency public services that lists the telephone numbers of local ambulance services and hospitals. Travel guides like Lonely Planet publications or the Rough Guide Series are particularly informative and frequently contain contact addresses of health providers in popular tourist destinations. The Yellow Pages in the local telephone directory are a valuable source of information. They provide listings of regional medical clinics, hospitals, diagnostic centers, and emergency services. The clinics often rent space to attending doctors. Telephoning the office of the local newspaper can also prove helpful in emergencies. In addition, the International Society of Travel Medicine publishes a Travel Clinic Directory that lists clinics run by the members of the Society. This covers 44 countries worldwide and aims to assist people in locating appropriate health care professionals overseas.

- *Hospitals.* Medical colleges and university-affiliated or teaching hospitals in cities have qualified specialists and English-speaking staff members. As a rule, private hospitals are known to offer better service than state-run hospitals, where outpatient clinics are busy and queues for appointments expected. The medicines prescribed may need to be purchased from adjoining pharmacies, unlike private clinics, which have in-house dispensing facilities. In semiurban or rural areas, one can enquire for the local missionary hospital or non-government organization-funded clinic, as they are reasonably well equipped and provide standard medical facilities. Some have only outpatient and diagnostic care, whereas others have indoor facilities. On weekends, emergency admissions and formalities can be tedious and ambulance service unavailable. Moreover, some clinics often require a letter of introduction from the referring physician before admitting a patient. It is thus advisable to check beforehand the facilities and admission procedures, especially for those planning a longer stay.

- *Corporate and professional medical networks.* Most business corporations have provisions for on-site medical services that include a well-equipped first-aid center and ambulance facility as part of their occupational health service. In rural areas where medical services are limited, the industrial medical center serves the needs of the local community, especially for emergencies. However, this may not be the case in urban locations, where corporate health care is more specifically oriented toward catering to the needs of their own employees. Professional organizations like the Rotary or Lions Club in many towns have members from the medical fraternity and could be contacted during emergencies.

- *Personal recommendations.* This is arguably the best method of locating a qualified physician, since the most reliable recommendations are those from satisfied patients. Friends, colleagues, or other expatriates living in the area can provide reliable suggestions. This is particularly applicable in long-term visitors or expatriates with families planning to relocate overseas for extended periods where provisions for health care remain a crucial issue.

- *International clinics.* International clinics have recently been established in many large cities of this region. They are staffed by local and foreign physicians and offer a comprehensive range of services incorporating both corporate health screening and emergency medical care primarily targeted at the expatriate clientele and business traveler. Since this is perceived as a growing market, wherein they function as health care providers in cross-cultural settings, they are extremely customer oriented and service driven in approach. Facilities usually include a well-stocked pharmacy, routine laboratory service, basic radiology, and primary dental care. Emergency beds with life-support systems are available in some centers, where critical cases are stabilized and then assessed for appropriate medical treatment. This includes arranging referrals to specialized regional hospitals and planning for medical evacuations if the situation so demands.

AREAS OF CONCERN

QUALITY OF CARE

Inadequate emergency medical care at the accident site, particularly cardiorespiratory resuscitation measures and delays in hospital transfers, are problem areas in trauma care. In a study looking at road accidents in New Delhi, 85% of the crash victims took more than 15 minutes to reach the hospital and 4% were transported by ambulance.[15] Poor quality of prehospital care in India was responsible for the 2.5 times higher mortality in head injury cases when compared to an intensive care center in the United States.[16] In certain places, the quality of available care may not be up to satisfactory levels, as revealed by an American study where only 50% travelers felt that the treatment received from local sources for diarrheal illness was beneficial.[17]

BLOOD

Professional blood donation is a reality in developing countries. Commercial blood banks are often unlicensed and ill-equipped, have poor quality control, and use cheaper screening tests that are less sensitive. In the subcontinent, post-transfusion hepatitis is well recognized as an entity.[18] Estimates of nationwide blood testing for HIV antibodies vary from 30% to 80%.[19] Voluntary blood banks like those managed by the Red Cross Society or lists of voluntary donors available with the local Rotary or Lions Club are reasonable alternatives. Efforts have been made to develop a "walking expatriate" blood donor panel for emergency needs at some centers.

MEDICAL EVACUATION

The ability to judge and plan the need for evacuation requires considerable knowledge of the region, past experience in handling such situations, and, more importantly, a high degree of professionalism. This makes risk appraisal the key element in the decision-making process. Moreover, organizing this complex procedure requires a well-coordinated team effort. A thorough assessment of the possible treatment options and identifying the location of the nearest health care facility are essential prerequisites. In

remote areas, this poses the biggest challenge logistically. Another problem is with obtaining a quick, reliable, and expert on-site medical evaluation quickly, especially if the case merits immediate medical evacuation. It is therefore imperative that assistance companies have a dependable network of heath care providers to coordinate this procedure. There are limited resources for chartering private aircraft in some areas of this region. In inhospitable mountain terrain like the Himalayas or from inaccessible regions like oil rigs and gas exploration sites, helicopters are ideally suited to evacuate the sick or injured.

DENTAL CARE

Dental hygiene is a low priority in developing countries, and finding appropriate dental care, especially within the public health system, is often a problem. Availability of certain dental hygiene products like dental prosthesis may vary considerably. Sterile disposable equipment may be limited, and there is a possibility of transmitting infection from contaminated instruments. However, most private clinics have reasonable infection control standards, although charges tend to be expensive. Travel insurance provides some coverage for emergency dental expenses overseas, although they normally do not cover for preexisting problems.

NOTIFICATION

Most insurance companies need to be notified within 24 hours in cases of hospital admissions and frequently request an emergency medical report from the treating physician. Failure to get the necessary authorization may lead to nonpayment, especially for those cases where the existing health policies also provide coverage for non-emergency overseas care. It is always advisable to check the coverage available with the insurance company before departure as few countries in this region have reciprocal arrangements with regard to emergency medical treatment. For expatriates and long-term travelers, it is essential that the travel insurance covers emergency evacuation and does not exclude psychiatric emergencies.

PAYMENTS

Many hospitals and physicians prefer that all major payments for medical services be settled in cash since billing the insurance company directly is often a difficult and time-consuming process. Although few private hospitals do accept credit cards, this may not always be possible. Furthermore, in emergency cases requiring hospital admission, a cash deposit is usually required. Travel insurance can help in such situations by providing emergency medical payment either by arranging an on-site medical advance or a standing guarantee for hospital payments.

CONCLUSION

Illness during travel in developing countries needs serious consideration. In such situations, coping with medical emergencies can be quite stressful for the traveler. There are many options to source health care, although medical skills and quality of available care can vary throughout the region. It is evident that emergencies are best managed through a network of health care providers in conjunction with local hospitals, travel clinics, and emergency care services. Physicians, particularly those involved in primary care at tourist destinations, are pivotal to this network. Given the diverse nature of training and core values in the developing world, one cannot expect a uniform professional standard. However, it is essential that efforts are made to develop a system of accreditation and thus ensure benchmarking in the practice of travel health in host countries. Travel medicine practitioners, working together with the travel industry, are ideally placed to initiate this process in their endeavor to promote safe and healthy travel.

REFERENCES

1. Rose SR. International travel health guide. Northampton, MA: Travel Medicine Inc., 1995:1–12.
2. Caumes E. Health and travel. Lyon, France: Pasteur Mérieux, 1994:11–15.
3. Reid D, Dewar RD, Fallon RJ, et al. Infection and travel: the experience of package tourists and other travellers. J Infect 1980;2:365–370.
4. Steffen R, Van der Linde F, Gyr K, Schar M. Epidemiology of diarrhea in travelers. JAMA 1983;249:1176–1180.
5. Steffen R, Rickenbach M, Wilhelm U, et al. Health problems after travel to developing countries. J Infect Dis 1987;156:84–91.
6. Hargarten SW, Baker TD, Guptill KS. Overseas fatalities of United States citizen travelers: an analysis of deaths related to international travel. Ann Emerg Med 1991;20:622–626.
7. Hargarten SW, Baker SP. Fatalities in the Peace Corps. JAMA 1985;254:1326–1329.
8. Hargarten SW. Injury preventon: a crucial aspect of travel medicine. J Travel Med 1994;1:48–50.
9. Steffen R. Travel medicine: prevention based on epidemiological data. Trans R Soc Med Hyg 1991;85:156–162.
10. International Road Federation. World road statistics 1987–1991. 1992.
11. Anonymous. Head injuries: a neglected field in India. Natl Med J India 1991;4:54.
12. Chatterjee S. Emergency care in the subcontinent. In: Program and Abstracts, Second Asia-Pacific Travel Health Congress. Taipei, July 10–13, Chinese Association of Travel Medicine, 1998:57.
13. Berfield S. First-class cure. Asiaweek 15 March 1995:48.
14. Behrens RH, Grabowski P. Travellers' health and the economy of developing nations. Lancet 1995;346:1562.
15. Grabowski P, Chatterjee S. The Indian plague scare of 1994—a case study. In: Clift S, Grabowski P, eds. Tourism and health—risk, research and responses. London: Pinter, 1997:80–96.
16. Maheshwari J, Mohan D. Road traffic injuries: a hospital based study. In: Proceedings of the 11th World Congress of the International Association for Accident and Traffic Medicine. Dubrovnik: International Association for Accident and Traffic Medicine, 1988:307–310.
17. Colohan ART, Alves WM, Gross CR, et al. Head injury mortality in two centres with different emergency medical services and intensive care. J Neurosurg 1989;71:202–207.
18. Hill DR. Illness associated with travel to the developing world. In: Second Conference on International Travel Medicine. Atlanta: International Society of Travel Medicine, 1991:71–73.
19. Desai DC. Post-transfusion hepatitis—how many more? J Assoc Physicians India 1993;43:190–191.
20. Bollinger RC, Tripathy SP, Quinn TC. The human immunodeficiency virus epidemic in India: current magnitude and future projections. Medicine 1995;74:97–106.

42.4 DIAGNOSTIC AND MANAGEMENT APPROACHES IN RETURNING TRAVELERS

MARGARETHA ISAÄCSON AND JOHN A. FREAN

In this chapter, three aspects of travel medicine that relate to the returning traveler will be presented. First, the patient with fever without localizing findings will be the focus of discussion. Second, diagnosis and evaluation of the returning patient with eosinophilia will be considered. Finally, the value and limitations of performing a post-travel examination in the returning traveler will be discussed.

FEVER WITHOUT FOCAL SYMPTOMS

Pyrexial illness during or after travel is very common. It is usually due to infection, caused by a cosmopolitan agent such as influenza virus or by a pathogen of more limited prevalence, such as *Rickettsia tsutsugamushi*, the causative agent of scrub typhus. Immunodeficiencies are becoming more common, largely due to the rising prevalence of infection with the human immunodeficiency virus (HIV). Therefore, opportunistic infections should also be expected to be seen with increasing frequency in travelers.

PAST MEDICAL HISTORY

A general medical history should be obtained. Special attention should be paid to the presence of previous and underlying illnesses (e.g., diabetes, chronic cardiac, renal and/or respiratory disease, malignant conditions, AIDS/HIV infection), surgery (e.g., splenectomy), blood disorders (e.g., thalassemia, sickling), and physiologic conditions such as pregnancy. Splenectomized persons are especially vulnerable to severe malaria, babesiosis, and infections caused by pneumococci, meningococci, and *Haemophilus influenzae*. Persons suffering from AIDS are not only susceptible to common infections with more severe manifestations than immunocompetent individuals but may also develop infections due to microorganisms that are not usually pathogenic.

HISTORY OF THE CURRENT ILLNESS

Fever   Different types of fever patterns may facilitate the diagnosis. A consistently low-grade fever is common in several parasitic and chronic bacterial infections. Sustained fever, often high and with small fluctuations, occurs in acute systemic infections such as typhoid fever, typhus, and plague. A relative bradycardia, although not diagnostic, is characteristic of typhoid. In overwhelming infections, especially of the gram-negative bacterial kind, the temperature may fall to subnormal levels, and other signs of severe endotoxemia such as peripheral vascular collapse, hypotension, and hemorrhagic tendencies occur. Similar fever patterns also occur in some overwhelming viral and protozoan infections.

Associated Signs and Symptoms   Many symptoms, although nonspecific, are more pronounced in some diseases than in others. Headache, common in pyrexial illnesses, is especially intense in malaria, rickettsioses, and psittacosis. Myalgia is particularly marked in some viral hemorrhagic fevers such as Lassa fever and Marburg/Ebola hemorrhagic fevers. Photophobia occurs in arboviral infections, rabies, and leptospirosis.

Skin rashes are valuable diagnostic indicators. They are usually present in infections caused by most rickettsias (usually absent in African tick-bite fever[1]), arboviruses, and filoviruses (Marburg and Ebola viruses), but less frequent in trypanosomiasis, typhoid fever, brucellosis, leptospirosis, relapsing fever, and arenaviral infections (Lassa fever and Argentinian, Bolivian, and Venezuelan hemorrhagic fevers).

Rashes may be transient and sparse like the "rose spots" seen on the upper abdominal skin in typhoid fever, or they may be profuse as in smallpox, now an extinct disease. The distribution of the rash is helpful. The vesicular rash of smallpox is centrifugal but centripetal in chickenpox. Papular and maculopapular rashes are common in the spotted fevers in which, unlike many other rash-associated infections, the palms of the hands and the soles of the feet are usually involved. Sindbis fever is characterized by a fine papular rash with minute vesicles topping individual papules. Petechial and other hemorrhagic rashes occur in septicemias (classically meningococcemia), Rocky Mountain spotted fever, and other spotted fevers (in the latter, usually at the extremes of age), viral hemorrhagic fevers, several arboviral infections such as dengue and chikungunya fever, and in African trypanosomiasis. In Crimean-Congo hemorrhagic fever, bleeding into the skin typically presents as large, confluent ecchymotic areas.

Localized skin lesions are useful in diagnosis. The tender primary chancre of African trypanosomiasis appears at the bite site within days after an infected tsetse fly bite. In American trypanosomiasis (Chagas' disease), a skin lesion (chagoma) results from wound contamination with feces of an infected reduviid bug. The early primary lesion of cutaneous anthrax, usually on the face, hands, or forearms, has a central, black, necrotic area surrounded by a raised rosette of vesicles (malignant pustule). Extensive pressure necrosis due to severe associated edema later effaces these early characteristics.

Some localized skin lesions may be obscure and missed if a thorough physical examination is not performed. A common example is the eschar at the site of an infected tick bite in most spotted fevers when concealed in scalp or body hair. An associated and painful regional lymphadenopathy found in many cases may provide a clue to the location of the eschar.

Localized, painless lymphadenopathy occurs late in West African (Gambian) trypanosomiasis, typically in the posterior triangle of the neck where it is known as Winterbottom's sign. The peripheral lymphadenopathy of bubonic plague, which is very painful and tender, usually is localized to the inguinal, femoral, axillary, or cervical glands.

Several febrile infectious diseases may present with jaundice. Hepatitis A was found to be the most common type of infectious hepatitis in travelers.[2,3] In undiagnosed malaria, hemolytic jaundice has sometimes been mistaken for viral hepatitis, occasionally with a fatal outcome. Hemolytic jaundice also occurs in visceral leishmaniasis, bartonellosis, and other infections. Jaundice due to hepatocellular dysfunction is seen in viral infections (caused by hepatitis viruses, cytomegalovirus, herpes viruses, arboviruses, and Epstein-Barr virus), bacterial infections (typhoid fever, leptospirosis, syphilis, relapsing fever, and Q fever), and parasitic infections (toxoplasmosis).

TRAVEL HISTORY

When Did the Patient Travel?   It is not enough to ask patients about recent travel only, since several travel-related fevers can have an incubation or latent period of several months or even years. Incubation periods of selected febrile diseases in Table 42.4–1 serve as a rough

Table 42.4–1.   USUAL INCUBATION PERIODS OF SELECTED FEBRILE DISEASES THAT MAY AFFECT TRAVELERS

SHORT ≤ 10 DAYS	INTERMEDIATE ± 7–28 DAYS	LONG > 4 WEEKS	VARIABLE WEEKS TO YEARS
Anthrax	Bartonellosis	Brucellosis	AIDS
Boutonneuse fever	Brucellosis	Hepatitis A, B, C, E	Melioidosis
Crimean-Congo HF	Chagas' disease	Leishmaniasis	Rabies
Chikungunya fever	Ehrlichiosis	Loiasis	Schistosomiasis
Colorado tick fever	Hepatitis A, C, E	Lymphatic filariasis	Tuberculosis
Dengue	HF with renal syndrome	Malaria (malariae)	Amebiasis
Histoplasmosis	Lassa fever	Trypanosomiasis gambiense	
Legionellosis	Leptospirosis		
Marburg/Ebola fever	Lyme disease		
Plague	Malaria (falciparum, ovale, vivax)		
Psittacosis			
Rat-bite fever	Q fever		
Relapsing fever	Rocky Mountain spotted fever		
Rocky Mountain spotted fever	Smallpox		
	South American HFs		
Tularemia	Toxoplasmosis		
Yellow fever	Trichinellosis		
Yersiniosis	Trypanosomiasis rhodesiense		
	Typhoid fever		
	Typhus fevers		

HF = hemorrhagic fever.

guide only, as various factors can shorten or lengthen incubation periods beyond the usually accepted norms.

Duration of Travel. Risk of infection is often directly related to the duration of exposure. Also, diagnostic options can be excluded when their minimum incubation period exceeds the interval between arrival at a travel destination and the onset of symptoms. For example, a patient who develops a febrile illness 1 day after arrival in a malaria area is unlikely to have malaria.

Where Did the Patient Travel? Details of the area visited may be helpful as infections often are limited to a small part of a country. Visits to rural as opposed to urban areas are associated with a greater risk of exposure to certain infections, especially those associated with animal and/or arthropod reservoirs. In some regions, contact of intact or broken skin with water may result in schistosomiasis or leptospirosis, respectively.

Type of Travel. Most tourists follow the well-trodden tourist routes, overnighting at reputable, air-conditioned hotels. However, they are usually exposed to mosquito bites for several hours after sunset and eat in a cross-section of restaurants. An increased risk of exposure to infections such as travelers' diarrhea, viral hepatitis, malaria, dengue,[4] and upper respiratory tract infections therefore exists. These risks are higher for the adventurous traveler who is also subject to less common diseases. For example, African trypanosomiasis tends to be more common in big game hunters than in the 3-day package tourist taking

in Nairobi and Mombasa with a half-day game park visit in an air-conditioned bus squeezed in between. Game viewing in open vehicles, on the other hand, encourages attack by tsetse flies. Cross-country hikers and campers are especially at risk of arboviral and rickettsial infections and viral hemorrhagic fevers. "Adventurous eating" poses an additional hazard of acquiring unusual pathogens. Expatriate contract workers such as road builders may similarly be intensely exposed to local disease vectors. Expatriate workers in refugee camps or in other situations involving frequent contact with underprivileged persons are at increased risk of acquiring infections, such as measles, tuberculosis, and louse-borne typhus fever, which are more common in such communities.

Insect Bites Sustained. Most patients recognize mosquito bites as such but are less adept at identifying other insect bites. To identify a possible arthropod-borne illness (Table 42.4–2), a history of pain (marked and immediate with tsetse fly bites), adhesion by arthropods (ticks), and itchy bites (fleas, bed bugs) may be helpful.

Animal Contact. Infections following exposure to animals are listed in Table 42.4–3, which is not intended to be all-inclusive but shows the more common types of animals incriminated in human infections. The risk of exposure to rabies tends to be proportional to the duration of sojourn in endemic areas, particularly if the latter are rural. Arbovirus infections, several systemic mycoses, babesiosis, trypanosomiasis, and ehrlichiosis are excluded

Table 42.4–2. ARTHROPOD-BORNE FEBRILE DISEASES BY VECTOR

VECTOR	DISEASE
Mosquitoes	Malaria
	Filariasis
	Arbovirus infections
	Yellow fever
	Dengue fever
	Chikungunya fever
	Sindbis fever
	Various encephalitides
	Rift Valley fever
Flies	African trypanosomiasis
	Bartonellosis
	Onchocerciasis
	Loiasis
	Tularemia
	Leishmaniasis
	Sandfly fever
Ticks	Spotted fevers
	Rocky Mountain spotted fever
	Boutonneuse fever
	African tick bite fever
	North Asian spotted fever
	Queensland tick typhus
	Oriental spotted fever
	Arboviral infections
	Crimean-Congo hemorrhagic fever
	Kyasanur Forest disease
	Omsk hemorrhagic fever
	Various encephalitides
	Colorado tick fever
	Tularemia
	Ehrlichiosis
	Endemic relapsing fever
	Lyme disease
	Babesiosis
Mites	Scrub typhus
	Rickettsial pox
Fleas	Plague
	Endemic (murine) typhus fever
Lice	Epidemic typhus fever
	Epidemic relapsing fever
Bugs	American trypanosomiasis
	Hepatitis B

from the table as their association with animals is often indirect and unrecognized by patients.

IMMUNIZATION HISTORY

Effective vaccines are available against some febrile illnesses (e.g., yellow fever). Some vaccines, like those against typhoid and cholera, are of limited usefulness in that protection may not be absolute. Pretravel cholera vaccine is often administered in order to avoid difficulties at some border posts. In such cases, the necessary follow-up dose is usually not administered, resulting in a further reduction of efficacy.

Until the advent of specific vaccines, immune globulin afforded the only means of protection against hepatitis A and B. Such passive protection is of short duration and may not cover the full length of time during which travelers will be at risk of exposure. Hepatitis B vaccination is important for travelers to developing countries where hospitalization and blood transfusion, for example, following a road accident, may carry a high risk of exposure to hepatitis B. An accurate history covering details of immunizations should therefore be obtained.

Travelers with AIDS or other immunodeficient states may not have been immunized with live vaccines. If potential exposure was possible, conditions such as yellow fever should be included in the differential diagnosis of their illness. Conversely, immunocompromised and splenectomized persons may, unlike most other travelers, have been immunized against pneumococci, meningococci, and *Haemophilus influenzae.*[5]

DRUG HISTORY

The history should include information on any type of prescribed and over-the-counter medication taken during travel. This should include details on chemoprophylaxis against malaria and travelers' diarrhea. Information on drug and alcohol abuse is also important.

PHYSICAL EXAMINATION

A thorough physical examination of a returned traveler with a febrile illness is essential and does not differ markedly from that of any other patient with a fever. Provided that a good history has been obtained, the examining physician is likely to have a good idea of the underlying cause of illness.

Illness suspected to be highly infectious, such as the viral hemorrhagic fevers, plague, and tularemia, necessitates elementary precautions to protect health care staff likely to have contact with the patient. Wearing gloves, gown, and mask while examining the patient, provision of a private room, and practicing universal precautions with all blood, body fluids, and tissues are usually effective. Diagnostic laboratories should be alerted to the arrival of any potentially biohazardous samples, and the appropriate health authorities must be informed. Prophylactic antibiotics may be considered for health care personnel dealing with air-borne bacterial pathogens such as those causing plague or tularemia.

SPECIAL INVESTIGATIONS

Hematology   A complete blood count (CBC), including a white blood cell count (WBC) and hemoglobin estimation, should be done in all cases. Leukocytosis, usually with a preponderance of polymorphonuclear leukocytes, is common in acute bacterial infections. A

Table 42.4–3.   ANIMAL SOURCES AND ROUTES OF TRANSMISSION OF SELECTED ZOONOSES AND OTHER ANIMAL-ASSOCIATED INFECTIONS

DISEASE	DOGS	CATS	RODENTS	HERBIVORES	RABBITS	PIGS	MONKEYS	BIRDS	BATS	FISH	REPTILES
Anthrax				acm							
Bacillary angiomatosis		c									
Bacillary peliosis		c									
Balantidiasis						i					
Brucellosis	ac			acm		ac					
Campylobacteriosis	i	i	i	i	i			i			i
Cat scratch disease		bsv									
Cowpox		c		c							
C-CHF				cv				c†			
Cryptococcosis								a			
Endocarditis				m*		c#					
Erysipeloid						c				s	
Hantavirus infection			a								
Haverhill fever			i								
Hepatitis B							c				
Histoplasmosis								a	a		
Lassa fever			aci								
Leishmaniasis	v		v								
Leptospirosis	aci		aci	aci		aci					
Listeriosis				m							
Lyme disease			v	v							
Lymphocytic choriomeningitis			ai								
Marburg/Ebola Viral HFS							c				
Monkey pox			c				c				
Ornithosis/psittacosis								a			
Pasteurellosis	bl	bl	b			b					
Plague		bav	v								
Q fever		ac		amv							
Rabies	b	b		b					b		
Rat-bite fever			b								
Relapsing fever			v								
Rift Valley fever				cv							
Salmonellosis	i	i	i	i	i			i			i
Shigellosis	i				i		i				
Simian B virus infection							b				
Rickettsioses	v		v	v							
Toxocariasis	i										
Toxoplasmosis		i		m							
Trichinellosis						m					
Tuberculosis				m			a				
Tularemia			acv		acv						
Yersiniosis	i	i	i	i	i	i					i

a = aerosolized excreta/secretions (inhalation)
b = bite
c = contact (direct or indirect)
i = ingestion of food/water contaminated by
* = caused by *Streptococcus zooepidemicus*
# = caused by *Streptococcus suis*
C-CHF = Crimean-Congo hemorrhagic fever
l = lick
m = ingestion of milk/meat from infected animal

s = scratch
v = via arthropod vector animal excreta
† = single ostrich abattoir-based outbreak (17 cases) in South Africa

notable exception is typhoid fever, which is characterized by a low WBC. This feature, together with the clinical picture, resembles that found in malaria and in systemic viral infections such as the viral hemorrhagic fevers. Eosinophils tend to be conspicuous by their absence in typhoid fever. A preponderance of mononuclear cells is common in many viral infections and may be accompanied by the presence of atypical lymphocytes, as in infectious mononucleosis. Falciparum malaria is usually characterized by a thrombocytopenia, but frank bleeding is unusual.

Anemia is a diagnostic indicator in some infections. Hookworm disease is characterized by a microcytic, hypochromic type of anemia due to intestinal blood loss. In all types of malaria, anemia is principally hemolytic in nature. Hemolytic anemia is also a feature of acute bartonellosis (Oroya fever). A megaloblastic anemia is found in some patients with infestation by the fish tapeworm, which competes with the host for vitamin B_{12}.

Microscopy and Culture   Ideally, antibiotics should not be given for suspected bacterial infections before all of the necessary samples have been taken for bacteriologic analyses. In practice, this is not always feasible, especially if the patient has recently seen another physician for the same illness or has practiced self-therapy. Contamination of samples with members of the normal bacterial flora must be avoided. Special techniques are required for virus isolation and fungal cultures.

Blood.   When the diagnosis is not immediately apparent, blood cultures should be performed. These are especially useful in the diagnosis of septicemia, bacterial endocarditis, enteric fevers (such as typhoid fever), brucellosis, plague, tularemia, melioidosis, listeriosis, anthrax, bacterial pneumonia and meningitis, rat-bite fever, leptospirosis, and bartonellosis.

Blood films must be microscopically examined for the presence of malaria and other blood parasites such as trypanosomes, microfilariae, and borreliae if the patient has returned from an area where such infections are prevalent. A single negative malaria result does not exclude this diagnosis, and the examination must be repeated several times if necessary. Chemoprophylaxis can extend the incubation period, modify the clinical picture, and markedly reduce the level of parasitemia in malaria. A positive malaria result must be expressed quantitatively as a high parasite load is one of the criteria of severity of infection. On the other hand, a low parasite load does not exclude severe malaria. Quantitative results also facilitate monitoring of therapeutic efficacy. If *Plasmodium falciparum* is detected, monitoring of blood glucose should be commenced. This is especially important in pregnant patients. Falciparum malaria infections, quinine or quinidine therapy, and pregnancy all contribute to hypoglycemia, which is an important complication to be recognized as early as possible during the management of malaria. The case fatality rate of falciparum malaria is low even in nonimmune persons, provided that they are diagnosed and treated promptly, but rises sharply to levels of 25% and higher if treatment is delayed. Malaria in non-immune patients, therefore, must always be regarded as a medical emergency.

Direct microscopy of blood films also confirms babesiosis, trypanosomiasis, visceral leishmaniasis, loiasis, lymphatic filariasis, relapsing fever (darkfield), and bartonellosis: anthrax bacilli, *Capnocytophaga canimorsus* (DF-2), and ehrlichiae may occasionally be seen. Coexisting bacterial infections, especially bacteremia,[6] are not uncommon in some of these infections, especially in malaria, and diagnosis of the latter does not necessarily exclude a need for bacterial cultures of blood, urine, sputum, or cerebrospinal fluid (CSF).

Bone Marrow.   In problem cases, bone marrow microscopy and culture may be indicated for the diagnosis of tuberculosis, brucellosis, typhoid fever, leishmaniasis, or histoplasmosis. A bone marrow aspirate may yield *Salmonella typhi* in patients who have received antimicrobial therapy when other biologic fluids are negative for the organism.

Skin.   Microscopy of skin snips is performed for the laboratory confirmation of onchocerciasis. In patients with suspected rickettsial infections such as Rocky Mountain spotted fever, immunofluorescent techniqes are useful to visualize these tiny bacteria in biopsied skin lesions.[1,7]

Cerebrospinal Fluid.   CSF microscopy, cell count, culture, and chemical analyses should be done in all febrile patients with symptoms and signs of meningitis or meningoencephalitis. The central nervous system (CNS) infections seen commonly in general practice may also be acquired during travel. This applies especially to meningococcal meningitis.

Prior partial or inappropriate antimicrobial therapy may modify the CSF cellular and chemical constituents to resemble those seen in tuberculous or viral CNS infections.

Less common bacterial infections of the CNS include anthrax and plague meningitis, the latter often in patients treated with an inappropriate choice or inadequate dosage of antibiotic. Other, less common infections in travelers demonstrable by CSF examination include advanced African trypanosomiasis (sleeping sickness), cerebral toxoplasmosis, eosinophilic meningitis or meningoencephalitis, and primary amebic meningoencephalitis.

CNS involvement in African trypanosomiasis is diagnosed by the finding of trypanosomes and raised IgM levels in the CSF. Confirmation of primary meningoencephalitis is by microscopic observation of motile amebae (*Naegleria fowleri*) in a purulent CSF. Early diagnosis may be life saving, and this infection should be suspected when swimming, usually in heated water, is followed by a fulminating pyogenic meningoencephalitis.[8]

Sputum.   Microscopy of representative sputum samples is of special value in the diagnosis of bacterial pneumonias and tuberculosis. Persons whose travel involved close and prolonged contact with refugees and other disadvantaged communities in developing countries, as well as travelers with AIDS and other cellular immune deficiency states, are at increased risk of contracting tuberculosis. Sputum cultures may be indicated in such cases.

Urine. Microscopy should be included in the investigation of patients with urinary tract infections or suspected of having schistosomiasis (ova), leptospirosis (spirochetes), or trichomoniasis (trophozoites). When appropriate, the urine should also be cultured for isolation and antimicrobial susceptibility of the causative bacteria or chlamydia.

Stool. After the first week of illness, stools will often be positive for *Salmonella* in cases of typhoid and paratyphoid fever. A positive stool culture, without other supportive evidence such as characteristic illness, should be interpreted with some caution since the patient may be a typhoid carrier with a current illness of different etiology.

Serology Blood samples for specific antibody demonstration should be obtained from a febrile patient at the first visit and again about 3 to 5 days later. This will show seroconversion from negative to positive. If both samples are positive, a fourfold increase in antibody titer is diagnostic for most common infections.

Traditional serology (e.g., the Widal test) for antibodies to typhoid fever are often positive in vaccinated persons or those living in typhoid endemic regions and are then of limited diagnostic value unless a significant (fourfold) rise in titer can be demonstrated.

For uncommon or rare infections (e.g., plague or a viral hemorrhagic fever), it may be acceptable to obtain a single positive antibody test for the diagnosis to be considered likely.

Radiography Chest films are indispensible in the diagnosis of lower respiratory tract infections. Some parasitic lesions, such as amebic liver abscesses, also are readily visualized radiologically.

Scanning Techniques Ultrasound, computed tomography, and magnetic resonance imaging occasionally may be required. Isotope scans (gallium, indium, etc.) may be useful in locating foci of inflammation.

MANAGEMENT

Specific therapy and general management of febrile patients are determined by the etiology and severity of illness in each case.

EOSINOPHILIA

Eosinophilia refers to absolute eosinophil counts above the upper limit of normal values that range from 0.04 to 0.44×10^{10} per L (40–440 per μL) of blood.[9] Marked diurnal variation in the circulating eosinophil concentration occurs, with highest counts in early morning and lowest in the afternoon. For an accurate evaluation of quantitative variations, it is therefore important to perform consecutive eosinophil counts at comparable times of day. Reliance on relative eosinophil counts can be misleading, as such values are expressed in terms of total WBC. A "high" eosinophil ratio of 10% may be normal in a patient with a WBC of 4,000 per μL blood, whereas a "normal" eosinophil ratio of 4% may be excessive in association with a WBC of 20,000 per μL of blood. The significance of percent values must be interpreted, therefore, in the context of the total WBC.

DISORDERS ASSOCIATED WITH EOSINOPHILIA

Allergies and helminth infections are not only the most common causes of peripheral blood eosinophilia in travelers, but they are often likely to be a direct consequence of travel.

Many nematode (round worm) and trematode (fluke) infections are characterized by tissue invasion at some stage in their life cycle. This stimulates a circulatory eosinophilia and, in certain cases, a local eosinophilia in affected organs such as the lungs or CNS. There may not be a significant eosinophilia when the parasite is well walled-off in the host, as seen with hydatid cysts, or when it is entirely intraluminal, as happens with adult tapeworm infections. Eosinophilia is not produced by protozoan infections, with the exception of the coccidian parasite *Isospora belli*[10] and the ameboflagellate *Dientamoeba fragilis*.[11] When reported in association with protozoan infections such as malaria or toxoplasmosis, eosinophilia is likely to be due to another, coexisting parasite, which should be identified by appropriate laboratory tests.[12] In this context, it should be remembered that mixed parasitic infections occur frequently. Parasites consistently associated with eosinophilia and their approximate geographic distribution are listed in Table 42.4–4.

Less common disorders associated with eosinophilia include a wide range of conditions (Table 42.4–5) involving one or more organ systems, which may be the sole site or sites of eosinophil infiltration. Table 42.4–6 lists parasitic and nonparasitic causes of eosinophilia by organ systems.

SOME COMMON EOSINOPHILIC SYNDROMES

Tropical eosinophilia (TE) and Löffler's syndrome (LS) are two common syndromes associated with nematodes that have a larval phase involving the lungs of the human host. The essential differences (Table 42.4–7) between these syndromes are to a certain extent determined by the degree of tissue involvement. Hypereosinophilia is a third syndrome, of unknown etiology. When it affects the heart, it is known as Löffler's disease, not to be confused with LS, which would be better designated as transient parasitic pneumonitis (TPP).

Tropical Eosinophilia Tropical eosinophilia occurs mainly in Asia and Africa in association with Malayan and bancroftian filariases.[13] Larvae are produced continuously within the host, resulting in more intense, often chronic or recurrent eosinophilia than in LS, as well as more severe and persistent asthma-like symptoms with marked wheezing, dyspnea, paroxysmal cough, fatigue, fever, anorexia, and weight loss. IgE levels, total WBC, and antifilarial antibody titers are typically high in the absence of a demonstrable microfilaremia. The condition usually responds to treatment with diethylcarbamazine.

Table 42.4–4. SELECTED PARASITOSES ASSOCIATED WITH EOSINOPHILIA AND THEIR DISTRIBUTION

NAME OF DISEASE	APPROXIMATE GEOGRAPHIC DISTRIBUTION
Intestinal nematode infections	
Ascariasis	Cosmopolitan
Hookworm disease	Tropics and subtropics worldwide
Strongyloidiasis	Cosmopolitan
Tissue nematode infections	
Lymphatic filariasis	Tropics worldwide
River blindness (onchocerciasis)	Tropics of South and Central America, Africa, Yemen
African eye worm (loiasis)	West and Central Africa
Mansonellosis	West Indies, Central America, Northern South America, West and Central Africa
Dracunculiasis (Guinea worm)	Tropical Africa north of equator, Pakistan, India
Trichinellosis	Worldwide wherever undercooked pork or game meat consumed
Infections due to nonhuman nematodes	
Cutaneous larva migrans	Tropics and subtropics worldwide
Visceral larva migrans	Cosmopolitan
Eosinophilic meningitis	Southeast Asia and Pacific Islands
Tremadode infections	
Schistosomiasis japonica	China, Taiwan, Philippines, Sulawesi (Indonesia)
Schistosomiasis mansoni	Africa, Madagascar, Arabia, Brazil, Suriname, Venezuela
Schistosomiasis haematobium	Africa, Madagascar, Mauritius, Middle East
Fasciolopsiasis	India, Southeast Asia, China
Fascioliasis hepatica	South America, Caribbean, Europe, Australia, Middle East, Asia
Fascioliasis gigantica	Africa, Western Pacific, Hawaii
Clonorchiasis	Far East, Southeast Asia
Paragonimiasis	Far East, Southwest Asia, Africa, the Americas

Based on data from Benenson.[8]

Löffler's Syndrome (Transient Parasitic Pneumonitis) By contrast, Löffler's syndrome is caused primarily by intestinal nematodes such as *Ascaris lumbricoides* and less commonly hookworms and *Strongyloides stercoralis*, all of which have a short-lived pulmonary larval phase. LS is usually transient, and larval activity tends to be localized to the lungs, causing manifestations that are fewer and less severe than in TE. In light infections, the larval presence in the lungs is often asymptomatic, whereas a transient eosinophilia, when present, may remain undetected or recognized only as a chance laboratory finding. The total WBC is normal and filarial serology negative.

Hypereosinophilia This syndrome is defined by the prolonged duration (≥6 months) of an unexplained eosinophilia exceeding a count of 1,500 per μL in the presence of end-organ involvement affecting the heart in more than 75% of cases.[14] Typically, it is found in males in their fourth decade who are living in a temperate climate. Late-stage eosinophilic endomyocardial disease presents as a restrictive cardiomyopathy and is also known as Löffler's endocarditis parietalis fibroplastica, or Löffler's disease.

APPROACH TO THE INVESTIGATION OF A RETURNED TRAVELER WITH EOSINOPHILIA

Eosinophilia may be found during routine post-travel examination of asymptomatic persons or in patients complaining of one or more symptoms. After determining that a true eosinophilia exists, the following questions need to be answered:

Where Did the Patient Travel? Parasites such as the intestinal nematodes are cosmopolitan, whereas others, such as schistosomiasis and loiasis, are less widely prevalent.

When Did the Patient Travel? Some parasitic causes of eosinophilia, such as loiasis and onchocerciasis, have a latent or incubation period that may be as long as several years. Knowledge of their incubation periods allows early exclusion of some infections.[8] Ectopic schistosomal granulomas (e.g., in the spinal cord) may also take years to manifest clinically. Many patients do not associate the appearance of symptoms with travel to the tropics that may have occurred many months or even years earlier. It is important, therefore, not to confine travel-related questions only to the recent past.

Duration of Travel? Short-term travelers rarely acquire filariasis or hydatid disease. Repeated exposure to the causative agents of these parasitoses are more likely to result in clinical illness.[12]

Is There an Association with Travel-Related Recreational or Occupational Pursuits? A typical example is bathing in natural fresh water in rivers, dams, or pools. This is associated with a high risk of acquiring schistosomiasis in endemic areas. If prompted, the patient may remember having had "swimmer's itch" on areas of the skin that were in contact with the suspected water. Swimmer's itch is, however, more commonly caused by non-human schistosomes.

Going about barefoot in tropical areas may result in invasion by hookworm larvae. Likewise, such a patient

Table 42.4–5. NONPARASITIC EOSINOPHILIA-ASSOCIATED DISORDERS

Allergies	Atopic dermatitis
	Urticaria
	Bronchial asthma
Nonparasitic infective agents	Chronic tuberculosis
	Resolving scarlet fever
	Acute coccidioidomycosis
	Bronchopulmonary aspergillosis
Drugs	Pulmonary infiltrates (nonsteroidal anti-inflamatory drugs, nitro-furantoin, sulphonamides)
	Hepatitis (semisynthetic penicillins, tetracyclines)
	Vasculitis (allopurinol, phenytoin)
	Bronchial asthma (aspirin)
Malignancies	Lymphomas, especially Hodgkin's
	Some adenocarcinomas
	Some myeloid leukemias
	"Eosinophilic leukemia"
	Necrotic secondaries of some tumors
Toxins	Toxic oil syndrome
	Eosinophilia-myalgia syndrome
Idiopathic	Hypereosinophilic syndromes Löffler's disease (fibroplastic parietal endocarditis) "Eosinophilic leukemia"
	Eosinophilic gastroenteritis
	Dermatitus herpetiformis
	Pemphigus
	Polyarteritis
Hereditary	Hereditary eosinophilia

Based on data from Weller.[13]

Table 42.4–6. ETIOLOGY OF EOSINOPHILIA BY ORGAN SYSTEM

ORGAN AFFECTED	DISEASE	
	PARASITIC	NONPARASITIC
Skin	Onchocerciasis	Urticaria
	Masonellosis streptocerca	Bullous pemphigoid
	Strongyloidiasis	Toxic erythema of newborn
	Cutaneous larva migrans	Eosinophilia-myalgia syndrome
	Schistosomal dermatitis	
	Scabies	
Subcutaneous tissue	Onchocerciasis	Eosinophilic cellulitis
	Loiasis	Eosinophilia-myalgia syndrome
	Sparganosis	
	Cysticercosis	
	Gnathostomiasis	
	Dracunculiasis	
Muscle	Trichinellosis	Eosinophilia-myalgia syndrome
	Cysticcercosis	
Blood and lymphatics	Lymphatic filariasis	Various lymphomas and leukemias
	Mansonellosis perstans and ozzardi	
Heart	Loiasis (rare)	Idiopathic hypereosinophilic syndrome
	Trichinellosis	
Pulmonary system	Larval migration (Löffler's syndrome, e.g., in ascariasis, hookworm disease, strongyloidiasis)	Bronchopulmonary aspergillosis
		Coccidioidomycosis
	Tropical pulmonary eosinophilia	Aspirin-sensitive asthma
	Paragonimiasis	Churg-Strauss syndrome (vasculitis)
	Echinococcis	Hypersensitivity pneumonitis
		Drug-induced pneumonitis
		Chronic eosinophilic pneumonia
		Eosinophilia-myalgia syndrome
Gastrointestinal tract	Strongyloidiasis	Eosinphilic gastroenteritis
	Ascariasis	Inflammatory bowel disease
	Human hookworm infection	
	Cat and dog hookworms	
	Trichiuriasis	
	Capillariasis philippinensis	
	Anisakiasis	
	Hymenolepiasis	
	Fasciolopsiasis	
	Schistosomiasis	
Liver	Echinococcosis	Drug-induced hepatitis
	Fascioliasis	
	Clonorchiasis	
	Schistosomiasis	
	Visceral larva migrans	
	Capillariasis hepatica	
Urinary tract	Schistosomiasis	Beta-lactam-induced interstitial nephritis
Central nervous system	Angiostrongyliasis	Coccidioidomycosis
	Baylisascariasis	Ventriculoperitoneal shunts
	Gnathostomiasis	Various malignancies
	Trichinellosis	
	Cysticercosis	
	Coenurosis	
	Ectopic parasitosis e.g., echinococcosis paragonimiasis schistosomiasis myiasis	Hypersensitivity reactions to contrast media, antibiotics Eosinophilia-myalgia syndrome

Adapted from Philpott and Keystone.[12]

may have had a localized itchy papular dermatitis ("ground itch") at the time and at the site of penetration, commonly on the feet. In such cases, there may be a history of a Löffler's-type syndrome, or this may be the reason for the current consultation. In persons with hookworm infestation who have not previously been exposed to hookworm larvae, gastrointestinal symptoms are more common than respiratory complaints.[13]

Was There Exposure to Pet Animals at Home or Abroad? Exposure to dog and cat feces in the immediate environment is a risk factor for cutaneous and visceral larva migrans (CLM and VLM). VLM, affecting any organs, occurs almost exclusively in children and is especially marked by eosinophilia, often of a very high order. On the other hand, invasion of the eye (ocular larva migrans), associated with a normal eosinophil count, may be the only manifestation of infection. The ocular form has often been mistaken for a retinoblastoma. The importance of a good history (pica, exposure to sand boxes) is, therefore, self-evident if inappropriate therapy and/or loss of vision is to be avoided.

Table 42.4–7. DISTINGUISHING FEATURES OF TROPICAL EOSINOPHILIA, LÖFFLER'S SYNDROME, AND HYPEREOSINOPHILIA

FEATURE	TROPICAL EOSINOPHILIA	LÖFFLER'S SYNDROME	HYPEREOSINOPHILIA
Common associated infections	Lymphatic filariasis Dirofilariasis	Pulmonary phase of Ascariasis Hookworm disease Strongyloidiasis	Unknown, if any
Eosinophilia	High (>3,000/µL)	Moderate (1,000–3,000/µL)	Moderate to high (>1,500/µL)
White blood count	Often high	Normal	Often normal
Wheezing	Common	Rare	Absent
Systemic involvement	Common	Rare	Always
Filarial serology	High titers in absence of microfilaremia	Negative	Negative
IgE levels	High (often ≥10,000 ng/mL)	Moderate	Low to moderate
Duration	Recurrent	Transient	≥6 months
Response to diethycarbamazine	Positive	Negative	Negative

Based on Ottesen[14] and Felice et al.[15]

Was There Exposure to Mosquito Bites? If no anti-mosquito measures were taken to prevent malaria in tropical areas, the risk of acquiring other mosquito-borne parasitoses, such as filarial infections, could have been considerable.

Drug History? Many travelers take medication, if only to prevent some of the travel-associated diseases such as travelers' diarrhea and malaria. Commonly used drugs that may induce eosinophilia include penicillin, ampicillin, cephalosporins, streptomycin, nitrofurantoin, sulfonamides, para-aminosalicylic acid, diphenylhydantoin, and phenothiazines.[12]

Did the Patient Indulge in "Adventurous Eating?" Increasingly, travelers sample strange and exotic foods such as crocodile meat, roasted caterpillars and beetles, giant snails, snakes, and other local "delicacies" that, if not thoroughly cooked, may harbor viable and equally exotic parasites. An example is *Angiostrongylus cantonensis*, the agent of eosinophilic meningitis or meningoencephalitis. Its larvae, together with their hosts such as snails, slugs, and certain earth worms, may be ingested in raw or undercooked vegetables, fish, prawns, or land crabs.[16] In areas where some seafood is traditionally served raw, such as in the Far East, this may be a major risk factor. CLM, which more commonly follows penetration of the skin by infective, nonhuman hookworm larvae, and VLM may also be caused by eating raw or undercooked meat of fowl, fish, or frogs infested with larvae of *Gnathostoma spinigerum*.[17]

PHYSICAL EXAMINATION

In addition to confirming some of the above symptoms, important signs to be elicited include anemia, abdominal or muscular tenderness, hepatomegaly, splenomegaly, lymphadenopathy, and neurologic deficits.

LABORATORY AND OTHER SPECIALIZED INVESTIGATIONS

An approach to the laboratory investigation of patients with eosinophilia is presented in Figure 42.1–1.

Hematology Complete and differential blood count and hemoglobin concentration should be estimated in all cases. A need for serum iron estimation (low in hookworm disease) may be indicated by the blood picture. Some authors consider the degree of eosinophilia important in specific parasitic infections, but it varies and is not always a reliable diagnostic indicator. Thus, conditions typically associated with very high eosinophil counts may in some patients present with relatively low counts and vice versa.

Microscopy *Blood.* Thick and thin blood films and membrane-filtered blood should be microscopically examined for malaria parasites and microfilariae, respectively.

Stool. *Ascaris*, hookworm, schistosome and other fluke ova; *Strongyloides* larvae.

Urine. Schistosome ova.

Sputum. Eosinophils; larvae of *Strongyloides*, *Ascaris*, and hookworm; ova of *Paragonimus*.

CSF. Eosinophils; larvae of *Angiostrongylus cantonensis*. In eosinophilic meningitis, eosinophils may comprise up to 100% of CSF cells in the absence of a peripheral blood eosinophilia.

Biopsy Material. Skin (onchocerciasis, mansonellosis streptocerca), muscle (trichinellosis), rectal mucosa, and other suspected ectopic sites (schistosomiasis).

Serology Serologic tests to demonstrate antibodies are useful adjuncts to the diagnosis of many parasitoses. They are not recommended in isolation, as cross-reactions are common and positive results may be obtained after exposure to nonhuman parasites, which may be of little or no consequence. However, current developments in this field are likely to result in more specific diagnostic procedures becoming available in the near future. Currently available serologic tests for *Strongyloides* and *Toxocara* have been shown to be useful.

Serologic and other techniques are also used for the identification of parasite antigens or nucleic acids. These include various enzyme-linked immunoassays, immuno-fluorescent microscopy, polymerase chain reactions, and nucleic acid probes.

Radiology X-rays of the chest are useful in the diagnosis of tropical eosinophilia, Löffler's syndrome, and hydatid disease. X-rays of the skull and soft tissues may reveal calcified cysts in patients with cysticercosis. Calcified schistosomal ova may be demonstrated on x-rays of the bladder and other sites. The use of a contrast medium in the intestinal tract sometimes and fortuitously shows up a filling defect caused by some of the larger helminths such as *Ascaris*.

Scanning Techniques Parasitic cysts and granulomas in brain and spinal cord, liver, lungs, and other sites can be demonstrated by means of ultrasound, computed tomography, or magnetic resonance scanning techniques.

TREATMENT

The treatment of eosinophilia is determined by its etiology. In cases where the etiology cannot be established, presumptive treatment with anthelminthics frequently has been successful and saved the patient the discomfort and expense of more invasive and protracted investigations. In all cases, follow-up eosinophil counts to assess the effect of treatment are mandatory.

ROUTINE POST-TRAVEL MEDICAL EVALUATION

Medical evaluation of the asymptomatic returned traveler is not recommended as a routine measure, except for certain defined categories where either the traveler or his/her community may be at increased risk of developing serious illness.

Infected but asymptomatic travelers who potentially endanger members of their community by virtue of their occupational activities include employees in the food-handling industry, those who work in close contact with infants, such as in daycare centers, and those whose occupation involves close contact with immunocompromised patients. In these categories, post-travel medical evaluation is recommended with the main emphasis on infections that are transmissible by the fecal-oral route.

Travelers who recovered from an illness during their trip, especially if they did not seek medical advice at the time, may also benefit from retrospective evaluation.[18] The geographic history is important in selecting specific infections, for example, malaria, schistosomiasis, or cholera, for consideration.

Persons at risk of sexually transmitted diseases should also undergo medical evaluation. Tests for HIV infection may need to be repeated for a period of up to 1 year after return.[19]

Refugees are a group with special considerations different from those of most other travelers. The need for medical evaluation of refugees is dictated by the high

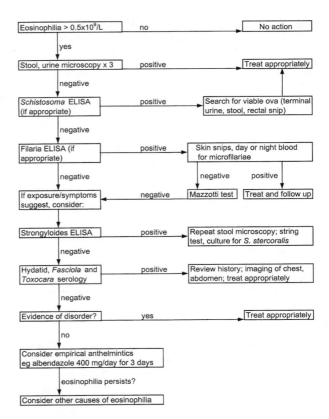

Figure 42.4–1. The investigation of eosinophilia in the returned traveler. Reproduced with minor modifications by courtesy of Churchill et al.[15]

level of physical and psychological stress, lack of sanitation, overcrowding, and insanitary and often inadequate food and water during travel. Additionally, refugees, especially children, are frequently not or incompletely immunized against childhood infections. These factors contribute to enhanced transmission of and susceptibility to infectious agents. To avoid outbreaks of disease among refugees and to protect the health of the host community, medical evaluation should be carried out routinely at the earliest opportunity during travel (i.e., on arrival in the first available refugee reception center with appropriate facilities).

The vast majority of travelers do not belong to these categories and should be advised to see their physician only if and when symptomatic illness manifests itself.

HISTORY AND PHYSICAL EXAMINATION.

A full medical and travel history should be obtained and a physical examination performed. Although this rarely yields signs referable to asymptomatic tropical diseases, abnormalities unrelated to recent travel are commonly found.[18]

LABORATORY INVESTIGATIONS

Laboratory investigations are essential for the diagnosis of most infections, especially those caused by parasites.

Table 42.4–8.   APPROACH TO ROUTINE LABORATORY SCREENING OF THE ASYMPTOMATIC RETURNED TRAVELER

SAMPLE	EXAMINATION	FINDING	INTERPRETATION/ACTION/THERAPY
Blood	FBC	Anemia	Investigate and treat appropriately
		Eosinophilia	Investigate and treat appropriately
	Microscopy	Microfilaremia	Identify and treat accordingly
		Plasmodia	Identify and treat accordingly
	Serology	Not applicable	Freeze and store serum for later use only
Stool	Microscopy	Tapeworm ova	Anthelminthic of choice
		Nematode ova	Anthelminthic of choice
		Nematode larvae	Strongyloidiasis: albendazole or ivermectin
		Schistosome ova	Praziquantel
		Other trematode ova	Praziquantel
		E. histolytica	Metronidazole
		Giardia lamblia	Metronidazole
	Culture	*Salmonella* spp	Antibiotics only indicated for persistent shigella.
		Shigella spp	Do follow-up cultures and counseling re. sanitary
		Vibrio spp	practices.
		Yersinia spp	
Urine	Microscopy	Schistosome ova	Praziquantel if re-exposure unlikely.
		Trichomonas vaginalis	Metronidazole; also for sexual partner(s).

An approach to the laboratory investigation of asymptomatic returned travelers is presented in Table 42.4–8.

A CBC with a differential WBC and microscopy for blood parasites is essential. Although this will often clear up spontaneously, a finding of eosinophilia after travel is an indication for further investigations to identify the etiology. Any anemia should be further investigated as to its type, which may indicate a possible etiology. For example, hemolytic anemia is classically seen with malaria, iron deficiency anemias are characteristic of hookworm disease, and megaloblastic anemia occurs in infections with the fish tapeworm *Diphyllobothrium latum.*

Stool should be cultured for bacterial pathogens and examined microscopically for parasitic ova and larvae of *Strongyloides stercoralis*. It is important to submit an adequate and representative sample. Rectal swabs, although satisfactory for bacterial culture, carry insufficient material for a reliable parasitic examination. If blood and/or mucus are present in the stool (unlikely in otherwise asymptomatic patients), these constituents should also be present in the stool sample submitted to the laboratory. Asymptomatic hookworm infections in otherwise healthy patients need not be treated, but the risk of severe and life-threatening strongyloidiasis hyperinfection in later life demands the complete eradication of this parasite even in asymptomatic infections.

Microscopy and/or dipstick examination of urine is useful, but bacterial culture is unlikely to yield significant results in asymptomatic persons. In travelers who are sexually active with casual and/or multiple partners, an effort to demonstrate asymptomatic infections with gonococci, chlamydia, and treponemes may be justified.

Routine HIV screening, after appropriate counseling, is advised for any traveler who has engaged in sexual intercourse with potentially promiscuous partners or in intravenous drug abuse.

Serologic baselines in the asymptomatic returned traveler may be very valuable for the interpretation of results obtained during subsequent illness. These tests need not be done at the time of screening when storage of a frozen serum sample is a cost-effective precaution in case of future illness. In the latter event, the stored serum will enable the performance of baseline serologic tests relevant to the patient's illness.

REFERENCES

1. Fournier PE, Roux V, Caumes E, et al. Outbreak of *Rickettsia africae* infections in participants of an adventure race in South Africa. Clin Infect Dis 1998;27:316–323.
2. Hall AJ. Hepatitis in travellers: epidemiology and prevention. Br Med Bull 1993;49:382–393.
3. Steffen R. Hepatitis A and hepatitis B: risks compared with other vaccine preventable diseases and immunization recommendations. Vaccine 1993;11:518–520.
4. Wittesjö B, Eitrem R, Niklasson B. Dengue fever among Swedish tourists. Scand J Infect Dis 1993;25:699–704.
5. Conlon CP. The immunocompromised traveller. Br Med Bull 1993;49:412–422.
6. Prada J, Alabi SA, Bienzle U. Bacterial strains isolated from blood cultures of Nigerian children with cerebral malaria. Lancet 1993;342:1114.
7. Dumler JS, Gage WR, Pettis GL, et al. Rapid immunoperoxidase demonstration of *Rickettsia rickettsii* in fixed cutaneous specimens from patients with Rocky Mountain spotted fever. Am J Clin Pathol 1993;93:410–414.
8. Benenson AS, ed. Control of communicable diseases in man. Washington, DC: American Public Health Association, 1995.
9. Hoffbrand AV, Pettit JE. Essential haematology. Oxford: Blackwell Scientific Publications, 1993.
10. Trier JS, Moxey PC, Schimmel EM, Robles E. Chronic intestinal coccidiosis in man: intestinal morphology and response to treatment. Gastroenterology 1974;66:923–935.

11. Moore TA, Nutman TB. Eosinophilia in the returning traveler. Infect Dis Clin North Am 1998;12:503–521.

12. Philpott J, Keystone JS. Eosinophilia: an approach to the problem in the returning traveller. Travel Med Int 1987;5:51–56.

13. Weller PF. Eosinophilia in travelers. Med Clin North Am 1992;76:1413–1432.

14. Ottesen EA. The filariases and tropical eosinophilia. In: Warren KS, Mahmoud AAF, eds. Tropical and geographical medicine. New York: McGraw-Hill, 1990:407–429.

15. Felice PV, Sawicki J, Anto J. Endomyocardial disease and eosinophilia. Angiology 1993;44:869–874.

16. Stark ME, Herrington DA, Hillyer GV, McGill DB. An international traveler with fever, abdominal pain, eosinophilia, and a liver lesion. Gastroenterology 1993;105:1900–1908.

17. Harinasutha KT, Bunnag D. Gnathostomiasis. In: Goldsmith R, Heyneman D, eds. Tropical medicine and parasitology. London: Prentice-Hall, 1989:421–423.

18. Churchill DR, Chiodini PL, McAdam KPWJ. Screening the returned traveller. Br Med Bull 1993;49:465–474.

19. Yung AP, Tilman AR. Travel medicine. 2. Upon return. Med J Aust 1994;160:206–212.

42.5 DERMATOLOGIC PROBLEMS ABROAD AND ON RETURNING

ERIC CAUMES AND LESLIE C. LUCCHINA

EPIDEMIOLOGIC DATA

In travel medicine, the importance of dermatoses is overshadowed by the greater frequency of travelers' diarrhea and the greater severity of malaria. However, dermatoses were the fifth (1.2%) most common cause of health problems related to travel among 7,886 (short-term) Swiss visitors to developing countries.[1] Sunburns and insect stings were reported by 10% and 3%, respectively, of 2,665 Finnish travelers worldwide.[2]

On-site studies of health impairment during travel to Nepal or tropical islands showed that dermatoses are one of the three main reasons for consultation in travelers abroad. In Nepal, dermatoses were the third most frequent presenting illness among tourists, accounting in one study for 12% of 860 health impairments among 838 French tourists[3] and in another report for 10% of 19,616 presentations of patients of all nationalities at a clinic.[4] Moreover, in the Maldives and Fiji, dermatoses were the most frequent presenting illness, with sunburns and superficial injuries documented most often.[5,6] Similar features were observed in U.S. military troops during a 33-day exercise in Thailand where dermatoses were the most frequent reason for consultation, accounting for 19% of 1,299 patient visits to three military clinics.[7]

On-site studies have also more specifically identified the spectrum of travel-associated dermatoses. Bacterial and fungal skin infections as well as scabies infestation were the most significant travel-associated dermatoses in Nepal, accounting for 4.35%, 1.86%, and 2%, respectively, of 860 health impairments in French tourists.[3] In Fiji, injuries (including those due to contact with marine life) and skin rash (frequently attributable to sunburn)

each accounted for 10% of clinic visits by tourists, whereas skin infections accounted for 13%.[5] In the Maldives, superficial injuries (often caused by contact with coral and shells) and "sun allergies" accounted for 14% and 13%, respectively, of health impairments among tourists.[6] Overall, these on-site studies reveal that dermatoses are a common reason for consultation while traveling abroad and that the dermatoses occurring while abroad are cosmopolitan.

In contrast, reports of travelers returning from tropical countries showed that approximately 50% of the dermatoses observed after return were tropical diseases. A prospective study evaluated 269 patients who presented to a tropical disease clinic in Paris with a travel-associated dermatosis.[8] Skin lesions appeared while the patient was still abroad in 61% of cases and in 39% after the patient's return home. Among the latter group of patients, the median time of onset after departure from the tropics was 7 days. A firm diagnosis was made in 260 (97%) of the 269 cases (Table 42.5–1). Of these 260 firm diagnoses, 137 (53%) involved an imported tropical disease.

Travel-related dermatoses are closely related to the geographic location visited and the onset of signs and symptoms relative to the date of return. Sunburns and superficial injuries are prominent in hot seaside areas and are most often seen during the patient's stay abroad than on return. Also, arthropod-related reactions usually occur while abroad. Skin infections, most particularly pyoderma, are ubiquitous and are likely the most common cause of dermatoses after return. It is noteworthy that tropical dermatoses are usually seen after the traveler returns given the prolonged incubation period of these diseases.

Table 42.5–1. TRAVEL-ASSOCIATED DERMATOSES DIAGNOSED IN 269 FRENCH TRAVELERS PRESENTING TO A TROPICAL DISEASE UNIT IN PARIS IN 1991–1993[8]

DIAGNOSIS	NUMBER OF CASES (%)
Cutaneous larva migrans	67 (24.9)
Pyodermas	48 (17.8)
Arthropod-related pruritic dermatitis	26 (9.7)
Myiasis	25 (9.3)
Tungiasis	17 (6.3)
Urticaria	16 (5.9)
Rash with fever	11 (4.1)
Cutaneous leishmaniasis	8 (3.0)
Scabies	6 (2.2)
Injuries*	5 (1.9)
Cutaneous fungal infections	5 (1.9)
Exacerbation of preexisting illness	5 (1.9)
Sexually transmitted disease	4 (1.5)
Cutaneous herpes simplex	3 (1.1)
Septicemia	3 (1.1)
Acute venous thrombosis	2 (0.7)
Pityriasis rosea	2 (0.7)
Mycobacterium marinum infection	2 (0.7)
Acute lymphatic filariasis	1 (0.4)
Traumatic abrasion	1 (0.4)
Miscellaneous†	3 (1.1)
Undetermined	9 (3.3)
Total	269 (100)

*Injuries included local envenomation (one case), superficial injuries caused by contact with marine creatures (two cases), and cellulitis-like reactions presumably caused by arthropods (two cases).
†Miscellaneous diagnoses were lichen planus, erythema nodosum (manifesting infection with *Salmonella enteritidis*), and Reiter's syndrome (of unknown etiology).

The incubation period is usually a few days. Among 67 cases of CLM observed in French travelers and 60 cases in Canadian travelers, the cutaneous lesions appeared after their return in 51% and 55%, respectively,[8,9] with the median time of onset being 8 days (range 0 to 28 days)[8] and 5 days (range 0 to 30 days).[9] The eruption usually lasts between 2 and 8 weeks but has been reported to last up to 2 years.

Apart from pruritus, the most frequent clinical sign of CLM is an erythematous, linear, or serpiginous lesion that is approximately 3 mm wide and may be up to 15 to 20 mm in length (Figure 42.5–1). Lesions may be single or multiple. The larva advances a few millimeters to a few centimeters daily. Given the pruritic nature of CLM, excoriation and impetiginization are common. Edema and vesiculobullous lesions are less frequent, being observed in 6% and 9% of the French patients[8] as opposed to 17% and 10% of the Canadian patients in the above-mentioned report.[9] The lesions are located 3 to 4 cm from the penetration site. The most frequent anatomic locations of CLM lesions are the feet, followed by the buttocks and trunk. Systemic signs and symptoms such as urticaria, dry cough, and wheezing have been reported in extensive infection. Blood eosinophilia varied from 0% to 37% (mean 5%) among 40 German patients with CLM.[10]

The diagnosis is based on the characteristic clinical findings and a history of possible exposure. The differential diagnosis includes the other causes of serpiginous or linear migrating cutaneous lesions such as dracunculiasis, gnathostomiasis, strongyloidiasis (larva currens), loiasis, and myiasis due to *Hypoderma* sp or *Gasterophilus* sp. There is a particular form of hookworm-related cutaneous larva migrans, known as hookworm folliculitis, that usually occurs on the buttocks (Figure 42.5–2). The diagnosis is made clinically where the serpiginous tracks are seen among the lesions of folliculitis or on histopathologic grounds when the hookworm larva is found in the sebaceous follicular canal.

TROPICAL DERMATOSES IN THE TRAVELER

HOOKWORM-RELATED CUTANEOUS LARVA MIGRANS

Cutaneous larva migrans (CLMs), also called creeping eruption, creeping verminous dermatitis, sandworm eruption, plumber's itch, and duck hunter's itch is one of the most frequent travel-associated dermatoses. CLM is widely distributed and most commonly found in tropical and subtropical geographic areas worldwide. CLM is caused most often by the larvae of hookworms of dogs, cats, or other mammals. *Ancylostoma braziliense*, the dog hookworm, is the most common cause of CLM in humans. CLM is acquired by skin contact with infective larvae in the soil. Activities such as walking barefoot on a beach or playing in sand contaminated with animal feces increase the risk of CLM.

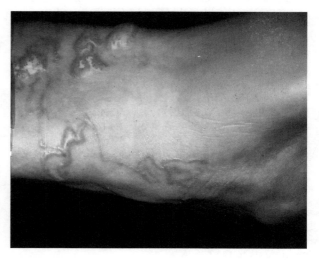

Figure 42.5–1. Cutaneous larva migrans.

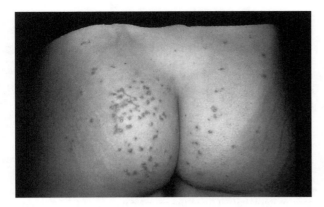

Figure 42.5–2. Hookworm folliculitis.

The treatment of choice for CLM is the topical application of a 15% liquid suspension of thiabendazole applied three times per day for at least 7 days. Topical thiabendazole may be difficult to use in cases of multiple lesions. Oral thiabendazole (50 mg/kg/day) for 2 to 3 consecutive days is effective, although its use is limited by the incidence of moderate to severe adverse events such as dizziness, nausea, vomiting, and headaches. Oral albendazole (400–800 mg/day) for 3 consecutive days is also effective and well tolerated. However, of the anti-helminthic agents available, ivermectin has the advantage of being well tolerated with nearly 100% efficacy when taken in a single dose.[8] A single 12-mg oral dose of ivermectin was significantly more efficacious in a prospective comparative study than a single 400-mg oral dose of albendazole (100% versus 46%; *p* = .017).[11] Prevention against CLM includes avoiding direct contact with fecally contaminated soil.

LOCALIZED CUTANEOUS LEISHMANIASIS

Localized cutaneous leishmaniasis (LCL) occurs in tropical and warm temperate countries and is transmitted by sandflies of the genera *Phlebotomus* (Old World) and *Lutzomyia* (New World). Old World LCL is caused primarily by *L. major* and *L. tropica*. Old World LCL is found in the sub-Saharan and North Africa, the Mediterranean basin, the Middle East, the Indian subcontinent, and China. New World LCL is caused primarily by the species of *L. braziliensis* and *L. mexicana* complexes. However, up to 15 *Leishmania* species are known to cause New World LCL in the Americas from southern Texas to northern Argentina. Workers in the Amazon forest are particularly at risk for LCL. In the U.S.A., 59 cases of cutaneous leishmaniasis were reported to the National Institutes of Health from 1973 to 1991. These included 42 cases of LCL (23 Old World, 19 New World), 4 cases of recurrent cutaneous leishmaniasis (RCL), 2 cases of mucosal leishmaniasis (ML), and 10 cases of diffuse cutaneous leishmaniasis (DCL).[12] LCL was mainly observed in American travelers. RCL, ML, and DCL occurred essentially in immigrants to the U.S.A.

Between January 1, 1985 and April 30, 1990, the Centers for Disease Control provided a pentavalent deriv-ative of antimony for 59 American travelers with New World LCL. Twenty-six (46%) of those treated were expatriates and 23 (39%) were tourists. At least 15 (26%) had stayed in a forest region for a week or less and at least 6 of these patients were at risk for exposure for a maximum of 2 days.[13] The median time interval between return from the tropics and the onset of cutaneous lesions has been estimated to be 15 days (range 7 to 30 days) in one study,[12] whereas the median maximum possible incubation period was 30 days (range 1 day to 5 months) in another report.[13] Typically, the time of exposure to onset of symptoms is 2 weeks to 3 months or longer.

The clinical presentation is variable. Typically, the lesion begins as a papule at the site of the sandfly bite and slowly progresses to a nodule, a plaque, then a painless ulcer, 3 to 12 cm in diameter, with a violaceous and well-circumscribed border and a granular base (Figure 42.5–3). Cutaneous lesions tend to be multiple in Old World LCL, whereas one to few primary lesions are usually seen in New World LCL. Common features of all cases of cutaneous leishmaniasis include the anatomic location on exposed skin (face, arms, legs), chronicity (more than 15 days duration), failure of antibiotics (which are often prescribed, given that it commonly looks like pyoderma), and absence of pain. Late, destructive ML may be seen if the patient is infected with a *Leishmania* species such as *L. braziliensis* complex and past treatment was inadequate. It is therefore important to identify the *Leishmania* species involved in that some species have the potential for late complications that may occur despite spontaneous regression of a LCL lesion. The differential diagnosis includes pyogenic infection, furuncular myiasis, tropical ulcer, spider bite, and tick eschar.

Limited knowledge of leishmaniasis among Western physicians can delay the diagnosis and effective treatment. This is illustrated by a study where the median time interval from when LCL lesions were first noticed to when treatment was instituted was 112 days (range 0 to 1032 days).[13] Diagnosis is made by evaluating a slit skin smear of the cutaneous lesion stained with Giemsa under light microscopy. Skin biopsy from the edge of the ulcer reveals the characteristic finding of amastigotes within macrophages. *Leishmania* species are cultured on Novy-MacNeal-Nicolle (NNN) media. DNA and monoclonal

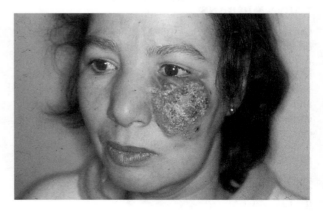

Figure 42.5–3. Cutaneous leishmaniasis.

antibodies are used for *Leishmania* antibody analyses and species identification.

The mainstay of treatment is pentavalent antimonial agents given intramuscularly in New World LCL and intralesionally in Old World LCL.

MYIASIS

Cutaneous myiasis (also called furuncular myiasis) is the infestation of human tissues by *Diptera* fly larvae. Furuncular myiasis is caused primarily by *Cordylobia anthropophaga* (the tumbu fly) and *Dermatobia hominis* (the human botfly). Depending on which fly is involved (the tumbu fly or the botfly), the presentation of myiasis differs by the place of acquisition, duration of maturation, number and anatomic location of cutaneous lesions, and the ability to manually extract the larvae. *C. anthropophaga* is found in sub-Saharan Africa and *D. hominis* is found in Central and South America. *C. anthropophaga* larvae penetrate the skin after hatching from eggs deposited on clothing and bed linens hung to dry outdoors that have not been ironed. The infestation by *D. hominis* larvae develop from fly eggs carried to the human by a biting mosquito. In both cases, the larvae develop by successive moults. The incubation period varies from days to weeks (7 to 10 days for the tumbu fly and 15 to 45 days for the botfly).

The clinical features include a 1- to 2-cm furuncle-like lesion with a central punctum through which serosanguinous or purulent fluid discharges (Figure 42.5–4). Movements of the spiracles of the larvae are seen within the lesion. The patient complains of pruritus and a crawling sensation within the lesion. *C. anthropophaga* lesions are painful, more commonly multiple, and usually located on areas of the body covered by clothing, such as the trunk. *D. hominis* lesions usually number from one to three and are commonly located on exposed areas of the body such as the scalp, face, forearms, and legs. The largest number of lesions ever reported in a patient was 94 This was in a child from Ghana who was infected by *C. anthropophaga*.[14]

The diagnosis of myiasis is made by the identification of the larva from the lesion. The differential diagnosis primarily includes pyogenic infection and tungiasis. Treatment is removal of the larvae. It is important to avoid breaking the larvae in that incomplete removal may result in a hypersensitivity or foreign body reaction to the larvae antigen. In the case of *C. anthropophaga*, manual pressure to the lateral aspects of the lesion may allow the expression of the larva. With *D. hominis*, placing an occlusive agent (e.g., paraffin, petrolatum, fingernail polish, adhesive tape, pork fat, toothpaste cap) onto the lesion may cause the larva to migrate to the skin surface and allow for extraction.[15]

TUNGIASIS

Tungiasis is the infestation by the female sand flea *Tunga penetrans* (also called chigoe flea, jigger flea), which is widely distributed throughout Latin America, the Caribbean, Africa, and Asia up to the west coast of India.[16]

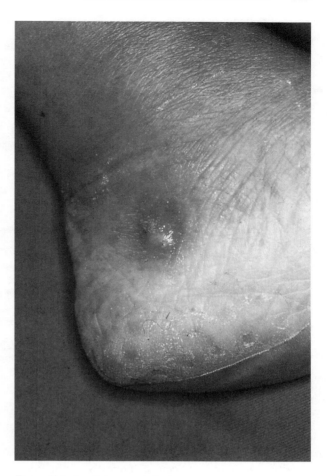

Figure 42.5–4.   Cutaneous myiasis.

The female sand flea penetrates human skin, feeds on blood, and produces eggs within its abdomen. The time of exposure to the onset of cutaneous lesions varies from 7 to 15 days. The flea may survive up to 1 month. The clinical features include a black dot at the site of penetration that develops into a nodule through which the eggs of the flea are expelled (Figure 42.5–5). There is a limited number of nodules (1 to 10) that are usually located on the feet (sub-

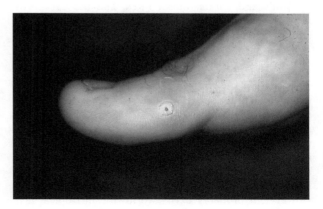

Figure 42.5–5.   Tungiasis.

ungual, sole, toe) and lower extremities. There is pruritus at the time of sand flea penetration.

The diagnosis is made by the characteristic clinical findings and morphology of the flea. The differential diagnosis includes myiasis, pyogenic infection, and foreign body reaction. The treatment is the removal of the flea by excision and curettage.

COSMOPOLITAN DERMATOSES OF INTEREST IN TRAVELERS

CERCARIAL DERMATITIS

Cercarial dermatitis (also called clam digger's dermatitis, schistosome dermatitis, sedge pool itch, swimmer's itch) is caused by the infestation of the skin by cercariae (larvae) of nonhuman schistosomes whose usual hosts are birds and small mammals.[17] Cercarial dermatitis is acquired by skin exposure to fresh and salt water infested with cercariae. The cercariae penetrate intact human skin and die without invading other tissues. Cercarial dermatitis occurs in swimmers and those with occupations that include water exposure. The geographic distribution is worldwide, involving both salt and fresh water that is inhabited by the appropriate molluscum hosts. There are sporadic reports from all continents.

The time of exposure to onset of symptoms varies from a few minutes to hours after exposure. If there is a history of previous contact with the infective cercariae, the clinical findings may begin sooner, with increased severity and a prolonged course. Typically, the eruption peaks in 2 to 3 days and lasts 1 to 2 weeks.

The clinical features include a prickling sensation during or shortly after exposure to the infective cercariae. Approximately 1 hour later, a pruritic macular erythematous eruption occurs that develops into a papular, papulovesicular, and urticarial eruption. The anatomic distribution typically includes skin surfaces that are exposed to water with sparing of the skin surfaces that are covered by clothing.

The diagnosis is made by the characteristic clinical findings and the history of appropriate epidemiologic exposures. The differential diagnosis includes seabather's eruption, contact dermatitis secondary to marine plants, hydroids and corals, insect bites, and the causes of urticaria. Cercarial dermatitis is self-limited. Oral antihistamines and topical steroids may reduce the symptoms.

SEABATHER'S ERUPTION

Seabather's eruption (also called sea lice) is acquired by skin exposure to salt water inhabited by larvae of the adult sea anemone and jellyfish.[18] Seabather's eruption is caused by the larvae discharging toxin from nematocysts into human skin. Seabather's eruption has been reported on the Atlantic coast of the U.S.A., the Caribbean, Central and South America, Singapore, and the Philippines. However, it probably exists worldwide in tropical and subtropical marine environments.

The time from exposure to onset of symptoms is usually minutes to 24 hours. Individuals with a history of previous exposures may develop a prickling or stinging sensation or urticarial lesions while in the water. The clinical features include pruritic erythematous macules, papules, vesicles, and urticarial lesions on an anatomic distribution that typically includes skin surfaces covered by swimwear. The eruption is more pronounced in areas that are more confined (e.g., waistband) and uncovered skin surfaces where there is friction (e.g., axillae, medial thighs, surfer's chest). The eruption can last for 3 to 7 days but may be longer. Children and rarely adults may have chills, malaise, headache, and nausea. The diagnosis is made by the characteristic clinical findings and the appropriate epidemiologic exposure. The differential diagnosis includes cercarial dermatitis, contact dermatitis secondary to marine life inhabitants, and the causes of urticaria. Seabather's eruption is self-limited. Oral antihistamines and topical steroids may reduce the symptoms.

MARINE LIFE DERMATITIS

Marine life dermatitis results from human skin contact with a marine creature. This is a frequent cause of envenomation and infection in travelers to tropical islands.[5,6]

The *Cnidaria,* which are found worldwide in tropical and subtropical waters, have nematocysts on their appendices or tentacles that contain a spiral-coiled thread with a toxin-containing barbed head.[19] Contact with nematocysts of Portugese man of war, fire coral, jellyfish, and sea anemone immediately produce a stinging sensation that varies from a slight burning sensation to excruciating pain. The cutaneous lesions that appear within a few minutes include macules, papules, vesicles, and ulcers and are at the site where the skin was exposed to the envenomation. Contact with a jellyfish may result in systemic symptoms such as hypotension, muscle spasm, and respiratory paralysis and may be fatal.

Sea urchins and other echinoderms are covered with venomous spines and pedicellariae. They may produce similar cutaneous and systemic symptoms as observed with *Cnidaria.*

The other dangers of tropical and subtropical marine environment include shark and moray eel bites, stone- and firefish stings, sea leech burns, and coral cuts and scratches. Some bites or stings may be fatal when occurring at a great distance from the seashore and medical assistance. (See also Chapter 14 Marine Hazards.)

PHOTOSENSITIVITY AND PHOTO-INDUCED DISORDERS

Ultraviolet irradiation may have both acute and chronic effects on the skin. In the traveler, skin changes due to acute sun exposure are common and numerous, including sunburn, phototoxic reactions, both drug and plant induced (phytophotodermatitis), photoallergic reactions, both drug induced and solar urticaria, as well as eruptions such as polymorphic light eruption, actinic prurigo, and hydroa vacciniforme. Sun exposure may also result in an exacerbation of chronic diseases such as acne, atopic der-

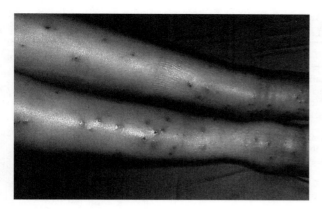

Figure 42.5–6.   Arthropod bites.

matitis, lupus erythematosus, dermatomyositis, pemphigus foliaceus, and several of the porphyrias.

Chronic sun exposure over the years may result in dermatoheliosis, chronic actinic dermatitis, lentigines, actinic keratoses, and skin cancer. (See also Chapter 16 Diseases and Disorders Caused by the Sun.)

ARTHROPOD-RELATED DERMATOSES

Exposure to an arthropod is one of the most common causes of skin lesions in tropical areas.[20] Attempts to identify the implicated arthropod are often difficult in that arthropods of different species give rise to similar dermatologic manifestations. Epidemiologic exposures suggested by history are useful.

The clinical picture varies according to the nature of skin injury (e.g., traumatic injury, local envenomation, hypersensitivity reaction).[21] The predominant feature of the arthropod reaction is an eruption of intensely pruritic erythematous and excoriated papules (Figure 42.5–6). This reaction is considered to be an evolving stage of papular urticaria. It is the dermatologic manifestation of a hypersensitivity reaction to the bites of insects such as fleas, bedbugs, and, less commonly, mosquitoes, chiggers, and rat mites.[21] Arthropod bites may also result in vesiculobullous

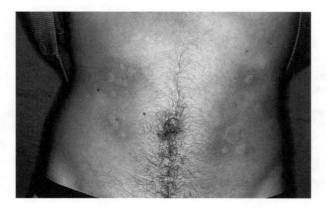

Figure 42.5–7.   Acute urticaria associated with invasive schistosomiasis.

Table 42.5–2.   RELEVANT HISTORICAL DATA IN THE EVALUATION OF SKIN LESIONS IN THE TRAVELER

Travel history
    Duration of travel
    Duration of time since return
    Geographic locations visited
    Recent outbreaks of disease in locations visited
    Means of transportation
    Housing
    Lifestyle
    Dietary habits, including food and water
    Clothing and shoes worn
    Exposures: beach, fresh or salt water, plants, insects, animals, field trips
    Personal and sexual contacts
    Medications: therapeutic and prophylactic
    Use of personal preventive measures: insect repellent, mosquito net
    Previous medical care
    Fellow travelers with similar signs and symptoms

Dermatologic history
    Time of onset relative to potential exposures
    Time of onset relative to return
    Description of initial presentation of lesion(s)
    Anatomic distribution of lesion(s)
    Local and systemic signs and symptoms
    Description of progression of lesion(s)
    Alteration of skin integrity during travel
    Underlying skin diseases

General history
    Age
    Current and past medical history
    Immunizations

lesions. Arthropod bites are self-limited. Oral antihistamines and topical corticosteroids may improve the symptoms. (See also Chapter 30 Envenoming and Poisoning Caused by Animals.)

GENERALIZED PRURITUS

Scabies is one of the most common causes of pruritus in travelers. Scabies is the infestation by the *Sarcoptes scabiei* var *hominis* mite that is acquired by skin-to-skin contact. Clinically, the patient complains of pruritus within 4 weeks of exposure and then a generalized hypersensitivity reaction 1 to 2 weeks later. In the patient with a history of previous scabies exposure, pruritus may occur within 24 hours. Skin findings include lesions at the site of infestation (burrows) and a generalized cutaneous hypersensitivity reaction to the mite. Secondary skin changes such as excoriation, lichenification, and impetiginization are common. The diagnosis is made by the light microscopic identification of the *S. scabiei* var *hominis*

Table 42.5–3.   DERMATOSES ENCOUNTERED BY TRAVELERS ACCORDING TO CLINICAL PRESENTATION AND DURATION OF TRAVEL

CLINICAL PRESENTATION	SHORT-TERM TRAVELER	LONG-TERM TRAVELER AND IMMIGRANT
Papules and nodules	Adverse drug reaction, acne exacerbation, milaria rubra, sea urchin granuloma Arthropod bites, tungiasis, myiasis, tick granuloma, lice Pyodermas, mycobacterial infection Leishmaniasis, scabies, cercarial dermatitis, gnathostomiasis, seabather's eruption Sporotrichosis	Leprosy, tuberculosis, mycetoma, pinta, bartonellosis, glanders, yaws Orf, milker's nodules Onchocerciasis, cysticercosis, schistosomiasis, dirofilariasis, sparganosis, African trypanosomiasis, American trypanosomiasis Paracoccidioidomycosis, paragonimiasis, chromomycosis, West African histoplasmosis, lobomycosis
Erythematous plaque	Bacterial cellulitis, pyoderma, Lyme disease Leishmaniasis	African trypanosomiasis
Vesicles and bullae	Sunburn, blister beetle dermatitis, contact dermatitis, irritant dermatitis, phytophotodermatosis, milaria rubra, fixed drug eruption Arthropod bites Bullous impetigo Herpes simplex infection Cutaneous larva migrans, cercarial dermatitis, seabather's eruption	Varicella infection (in adult) Dracunculiasis
Ulcers	Spider bite Ecthyma, pyodermas, tache noire (tick eschar) Herpes simplex infection Leishmaniasis Sporotrichosis	Cupping Mycetomas, tropical ulcer, anthrax, tuberculosis, mycobacterial infection, cutaneous diphteria, glanders, melioidosis, plague,* yaws,* tularemia* Cutaneous amebiasis, dracunculiasis West African histoplasmosis, North American blastomycosis, paracoccidioidomycosis, chromomycosis
Genital ulcers/lesions	Syphilis, chancroid Herpes simplex infection	Granuloma inguinale, lymphogranuloma venereum
Nodular lymphangitis with or without ulcer	Bacterial lymphangitis, mycobacteriosis, tularemia, cat-scratch disease Leishmaniasis Sporotrichosis	
Linear or serpiginous lesions	Blister beetle dermatitis, phytophotodermatitis Cutaneous larva migrans, myiasis (due to *Gasterophilus* and *Hypoderma* spp), gnathostomiasis	Strongyloidiasis (larva currens) loiasis, dracunculiasis
Migratory lesions	Cutaneous larva migrans, gnathostomiasis, myiasis (*Gasterophilus* and Hypoderma spp)	Strongyloidiasis (larva currens) loiasis, hookworm ("ground itch"), sparganosis, American trypanosomiasis (secondary chagomas)
Facial edema	Bacterial cellulitis Trichinosis	Onchocerciasis, American trypanosomiasis (eyelid)
Limb edema	Bacterial cellulitis Onchocerciasis	Lymphatic filariasis, loiasis
Localized pruritus	Contact dermatitis, irritant dermatitis, phytophotodermatis, arthropod bite, lice, seabather's eruption Cercarial dermatitis, cutaneous larva migrans, enterobiasis (perianal), gnathostomiasis	Loiasis, strongyloidiasis (larva currens)
Generalized pruritus	Adverse drug reactions, ciguatera fish poisoning, atopic dermatitis exacerbation Scabies Schistosomiasis, ascariasis, hookworm, trichinosis, strongyloidiasis	Varicella (in adults) Loiasis, onchocerciasis, African trypanosomiasis

(continued)

Table 42.5–3. Continued

CLINICAL PRESENTATION	SHORT-TERM TRAVELER	LONG-TERM TRAVELER AND IMMIGRANT
Urticaria	Adverse drug reaction Hepatitis A infection Schistosomiasis, ascariasis, hookworm, trichinosis, strongyloidiasis	Fascioliasis
Fever and rash	Adverse drug reaction Acute meningococcemia, typhoid fever, syphilis, rat-bite fever, leptospirosis, rickettsial infections Measles, dengue, viral hemorrhagic fevers	Brucellosis African trypanosomiasis

Any of the diseases listed above that may affect the short-term traveler may also affect the long-term traveler and immigrant and vice versa.
*Primary inoculation site.

mite, eggs, or feces on skin scraping. Treatment includes permethrin cream 5% or lindane lotion 1% (*gamma benzene hexachloride*) or benzyl benzoate lotion (in Europe). Bedding and clothing must be laundered or removed from contact for no less than 3 days. Personal and household contacts must also be treated.

Another significant cause of pruritus is ciguatera fish poisoning, which is acquired by the consumption of certain tropical marine reef fish in tropical and subtropical regions in the world. Marine fish implicated in ciguatera fish poisoning contain a toxin transmitted through the ingestion of smaller marine organisms that contain a toxic substance or its precursor. Within minutes to 30 hours, the patient has gastrointestinal signs and symptoms (diarrhea, vomiting, abdominal pain), fatigue, myalgias (particularly of the lower extremities), pruritus, and neurosensory manifestations (perioral and distal extremity paresthesias and altered temperature sensation). Unique to ciguatera fish poisoning, temperature sensation to cold is reversed; thus, cold beverages and objects are described as feeling hot. There may be cardiovascular impairment. Gastrointestinal symptoms typically resolve in less than 24 hours. However, myalgias, pruritus, and neurosensory symptoms last days and may occur for as long as 6 months after the initial event. Treatment is supportive.

URTICARIA

Acute urticaria is a common reason for dermatologic evaluation. The travel history may provide epidemiologic clues such as exposure to freshwater acute schistosomiasis) (Figure 42.5–7), ingestion of undercooked meats (trichinosis), ingestion of raw vegetables (ascariasis), or walking barefoot (hookworm and strongyloidiasis). Hypersensitivity reaction to drugs, not only daily medications but prophylaxis associated with the patient's travel, must always be considered in the differential diagnosis of urticaria in travelers.

DIAGNOSIS OF A SKIN LESION IN THE TRAVELER

Skin lesions in the traveler, both during and after travel, often present a diagnostic dilemma.[22,23] The evaluation of

the traveler with skin lesions must include an extensive patient history with a focus on possible epidemiologic exposures as well as a complete physical examination.[23] The differential diagnosis is broadened and depends on factors such as geographic location visited, length of stay, and many other entities as listed in Table 42.5–2.[22]

For many infections acquired during travel, skin lesions may be the only clinical finding that provides important diagnostic clues. The appearance of cutaneous lesions is of particular interest because dermatologic diseases are classified according to their morphologic characteristics such as type (e.g., macule, papule, nodule, vesicle, ulcer), color (e.g., skin colored, red, brown, blue, black, hyperpigmented, hypopigmented, depigmented), shape (e.g., round, oval, annular, serpiginous), configuration (e.g., linear, annular, serpiginous, zosteriform, reticulated), and distribution (e.g., localized, generalized, limited to a specific anatomic location). In the evaluation of the traveler with skin lesions, further diagnostic studies such as blood tests and serologies, skin biopsy and cultures, and imaging techniques may be warranted. Diseases with dermatologic manifestations that are encountered by travelers are listed by characteristic clinical morphology and duration of travel in Table 42.5–3.

With the marked increase in international travel to tropical and developing countries over the past decades, physicians must be well informed of the many travel-associated dermatoses in order to allow for prompt diag-

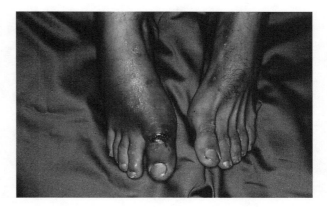

Figure 42.5–8. Necrotizing cellulitis.

nosis and treatment. Travelers should receive the appropriate immunizations and vaccines for the location to be visited. Travelers must be aware of the well-known diseases and ailments affecting visitors to specific geographic areas. Individuals traveling abroad must be instructed to take precautions to prevent common skin diseases during travel. Patient instructions should include specific details in the prevention of and skin care for the following: adverse drug reactions (daily and prophylaxis medications), skin infections (Figure 42.5–8), sunburn, miliaria rubra, frostbite, plant-related dermatoses, arthropod bites, insect larvae and parasite penetration into the skin, and water-related dermatoses.

REFERENCES

1. Steffen R, Rickenbach M, Wilhelm U, Helminger A, Schar M. Health problems after travel to developing countries. J Infect Dis 1987;156:84–91.
2. Peltola H, Kironseppa H, Holsa P. Trips to the south; a health hazard. Morbidity of Finnish travelers. Scand J Infect Dis 1983;15:375–81.
3. Caumes E, Brücker G, Brousse G, et al. Travel associated illness in 838 french tourists in Nepal in 1984. Travel Med Int 1991;9:72–76.
4. Shlim DR. Learning from experience: travel medicine in Kathmandu. In: Lobel HO, Steffen R, Kozarsky PE, eds. Travel medicine 2: Proceedings of the Second Conference on International Travel Medicine. Atlanta: International Society of Travel Medicine, 1992:40–42.
5. Raju R, Smal N, Sorokin M. Incidence of minor and major disorders among visitors to Fiji. In: Lobel HO, Steffen R, Kozarsky PE, eds. Travel medicine 2: proceedings of the Second Conference on International Travel Medicine. Atlanta: International Society of Travel Medicine, 1992:62.
6. Plentz K. Nontropical and noninfectious diseases among travelers in a tropical area during five year period (1986–1990). In: Lobel HO, Steffen R, Kozarsky PE, eds. Travel medicine 2: proceedings of the Second Conference on International Travel Medicine. Atlanta: International Society of Travel Medicine, 1992:77.
7. Sanchez JL, Gelnett J, Petruccelli BP, et al. Diarrheal disease incidence and morbidity among United States military personnel during short-term missions overseas. Am J Trop Med Hyg 1998;58:299–304.
8. Caumes E, Carrière J, Guermonprez G, et al. Dermatoses associated with travel to tropical countries: a prospective study of the diagnosis and management of 269 patients presenting to a tropical disease unit. Clin Infect Dis 1995;20:542–548.
9. Davies HD, Sakuls P, Keystone JS. Creeping eruption. A review of clinical presentation and management of 60 cases presenting to a tropical disease unit. Arch Dermatol 1993;129:588–591.
10. Jelineck T, Maiwald H, Nothdurft HD, Loscher T. Cutaneous larva migrans in travelers: synopsis of histories, symptoms and treatment of 98 patients. Clin Infect Dis 1994;19:1062–1066.
11. Caumes E, Carrière J, Datry A, et al. A randomized trial of ivermectin versus albendazole for the treatment of cutaneous larva migrans. Am J Trop Med Hyg 1993;49:641–644.
12. Melby PC, Kreutzer RD, McMahon-Pratt D, et al. Cutaneous leishmaniasis: review of 59 cases seen at the National Institutes of Health. Clin Infect Dis 1992;15:924–937.
13. Herwaldt BL, Stokes SL, Juranek DD. American cutaneous leishmaniasis in US travelers. Ann Intern Med 1993;118:779–784.
14. Biggar RJ, Morrow H, Morrow RH. Extensive myiasis from tumbu fly larvae in Ghana, West Africa. Clin Pediatr 1980;19:231–232.
15. Brewer TF, Wilson ME, Gonzalez E, Felsenstein D. Bacon therapy and furuncular myiasis. JAMA 1993;270:2087–2088.
16. Sanusi ID, Brown EB, Shepard TG, Grafton WD. Tungiasis: report of one case and review of the 14 reported cases in the United States. J Am Acad Dermatol 1989;20:941–944.
17. Gonzalez E. Schistosomiasis, cercarial dermatitis and marine dermatitis. Dermatol Clin 1989;7:291–300.
18. Freudenthal AR, Joseph PR. Seabather's eruption. N Engl J Med 1993;329:542–544.
19. Auerbach PS. Marine envenomations. N Engl J Med 1991;325:486–495.
20. Wirtz RA. Azad AF. Injurious arthropods. In: Strickland GT, ed. Hunter's tropical medicine. 7th Ed. Philadelphia: WB Saunders, 1991:893–910.
21. Shatin H, Canizares O. Dermatoses caused by arthropods. In: Canizares O, Harman RRM, eds. Clinical tropical dermatology. 2nd Ed. Boston: Blackwell Scientific, 1992:372–403.
22. Lucchina LC, Wilson ME, Drake LA. Dermatology and the recently returned traveler: infectious diseases with dermatologic manifestations. Int J Dermatol 1997;36:167–181.
23. Lockwood DNJ, Keystone JS. Skin problems in returning travelers. Med Clin North Am 1992;76:1393–1411.

Chapter 43

INVESTIGATION AND MANAGEMENT OF INFECTIOUS DISEASES ON INTERNATIONAL CONVEYANCES (AIRPLANES AND CRUISE SHIPS)

SUSAN A. MALONEY AND MARTIN S. CETRON

INTERNATIONAL TRAVEL

Over the past two centuries, the world's population has grown from 1 billion to more than 6 billion persons, and the time to circumnavigate the globe has decreased from 365 days to less than 3 days (Figure 43–1). In recent years, international travel has increased substantially. For the period covering 1990–1997, world tourist arrivals increased by an annual average percentage of 4.3%.[1] In 1997, 612,835,000 tourist arrivals were registered worldwide. The speed and volume of international travel is cited by the Institute of Medicine as one of the principal factors contributing to the global emergence of infectious diseases. Most international travel occurs on airplanes and cruise ships, making travel on these conveyances of substantial public health significance. Travelers on commercial flights can travel between any two cities in the world in less than 36 hours, which is shorter than the incubation period of many infectious diseases and makes detection of disease transmission aboard these conveyances difficult for many communicable diseases. The cruise ship travel industry is also burgeoning, with an increasing volume of passengers traveling to international destinations and an expansion in the range of global destinations for cruise ship itineraries (Figure 43–2). The large numbers of persons traveling on international airplanes and cruise ships annually and expansion of travel to a greater number of international destinations have increased the potential for exposure to infectious disease and its transfer across international boundaries.

CURRENT REGULATIONS GOVERNING INFECTIOUS DISEASE REPORTING AMONG INTERNATIONAL TRAVELERS

Preventing the spread of infectious disease across international borders has long been a topic of public health concern. Countries have struggled to stop the spread of infection through travel since the 14th century, when the

city-state of Venice developed legislation aimed at preventing shipboard rats from introducing plague.[2] It was the plague of the 14th century (the Black Death) that gave rise to one of the first formal systems of quarantine. Italian ports at the time were important hubs in the growing trade routes between Europe and the Orient, and with the arrival of plague, measures were instituted to control the entry and spread of disease inland from coastal cities. As early as 1348, a system for managing infected ships, passengers, and cargo existed in Venice, and in 1485 a requirement that ships arriving from infected ports sit at anchor for 40 days before landing was adopted. The word "quarantine" was used to describe this requirement; it is derived from the Latin word *quaresma,* meaning forty. Numerous international treaties followed, but they were not standardized until 1951, when the World Health Organization (WHO) adopted the International Sanitary Regulations. These regulations were amended and renamed

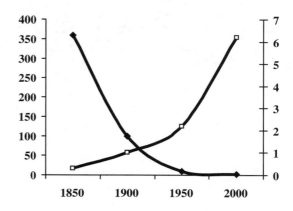

Days to circumnavigate the globe
World population in billions

Figure 43–1. Global travel time and world population growth. Adapted from Murphy FM, Nathanson N. The emergence of new virus disease: an overview. Semin Virol 1994;5:87–103.

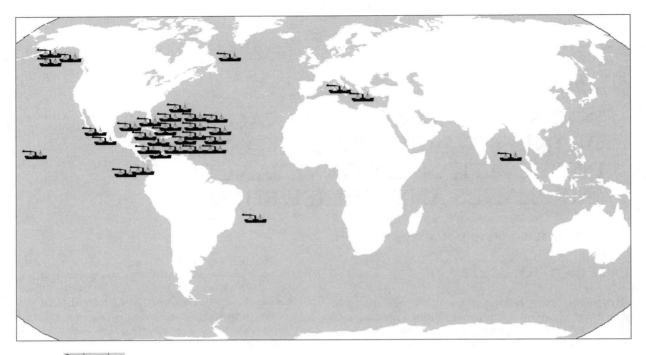

= 500,000 passenger bed-days

O   = New destinations (<500,000 passenger bed-days)

A

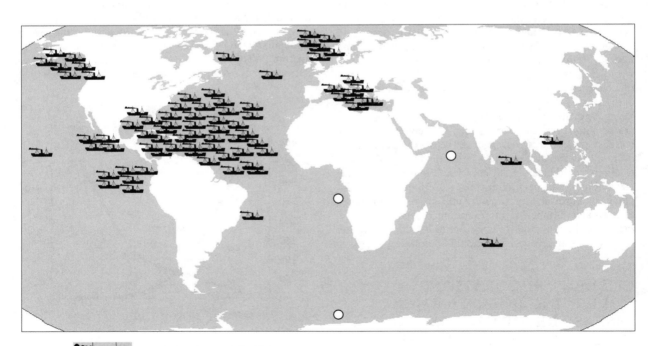

= 500,000 passenger bed-days

O   = New destinations (<500,000 passenger bed-days)

B

Figure 43–2. Cruise ship growth in volume and destinations of port calls: *A*, Cruise destinations, 1987; *B*, Expanding cruise destination, 1997.

the International Health Regulations (IHRs) in 1968.[3] The objective of these regulations is to provide maximum protection against the spread of infectious diseases while endeavoring to create minimum interference with world traffic. These regulations set standards for sanitation at air and seaports to prevent the importation and spread of infectious diseases. Plans to revise the IHRs are under way; the revised version may require reporting of disease by syndromes associated with the major types of infectious diseases that have potential for international spread.[4]

In the United States, legislation gives the U.S. Public Health Service responsibility for preventing the introduction, transmission, and spread of communicable diseases from foreign countries into the United States. Under its delegated authority, the Division of Quarantine of the Centers for Disease Control and Prevention (CDC) implements and administers regulations found in the Code of Federal Regulations (42 CFR Parts 34 and 71).[5] The Division of Quarantine is a part of CDC's National Center for Infectious Diseases, with headquarters in Atlanta, Georgia. Eight quarantine stations are located in New York, Miami, Atlanta, Chicago, Los Angeles, San Francisco, Seattle, and Honolulu. Quarantine stations have responsibility for all ports (air and sea) in an assigned region of the United States and are staffed by quarantine inspectors who respond to incidents of public health importance identified during their inspection of arriving passengers and cargo. The Division of Quarantine is empowered to apprehend, detain, medically examine, or conditionally release individuals (including U.S. citizens) suspected of having a "quarantinable" disease. The list of "quarantinable" diseases, contained in a 1982 Executive Order of the President, includes cholera and suspected cholera, diphtheria, infectious tuberculosis, plague, suspected smallpox, yellow fever, and suspected viral hemorrhagic fevers. Foreign quarantine regulations also require that death or illness in an arriving international passenger or crew member be reported by the captain of an arriving international conveyance (airplane, cruise ship, rail, or vehicle) to the quarantine station having responsibility for the particular port of entry.

Although current regulations provide an important structure for addressing infectious disease transmission among countries, they must be supplemented by strong global partnerships to strengthen international cooperation in infectious disease surveillance, prevention, and control. In practice, modern quarantine measures are only infrequently effective in preventing or controlling disease outbreaks. Therefore, strong national surveillance systems and rational public health practices are essential for addressing the potential threat of spread of infectious diseases on a global basis. Virtually any infectious disease is a candidate for global spread, and transfer from one location to another typically occurs while the infection is still in its incubation period. Public health infrastructure, practices, and response at ports of entry and in local communities can determine whether imported infectious diseases are recognized and controlled, create localized outbreaks, or result in massive epidemics.

EPIDEMIOLOGY OF INFECTIOUS DISEASES ON INTERNATIONAL CONVEYANCES (AIRPLANES AND CRUISE SHIPS)

INFECTIOUS DISEASES ON INTERNATIONAL AIRPLANES

In the past decade, international air travel has grown dramatically; in 1998, 1.4 million persons traveled internationally by air every day, and more than 500 million travelers cross international borders annually by commercial aircraft alone.[6] The speed and availability of air travel increase the potential for rapid dissemination of disease by travelers returning to their home communities. Travelers who have been exposed to infectious diseases may not appear ill when they arrive at their travel destination, and travelers who become ill after their arrival must be identified through surveillance efforts at the national and local levels. Knowledge of the most commonly reported infectious diseases on international aircraft and common modes of transmission can facilitate early identification and response to illness among international airplane travelers.

Modes and Sources of Transmission of Infectious Diseases on Airplanes *Food- and Water-borne Diseases (Common Source Transmission).* Gastroenteritis from contaminated food and water is among the most commonly reported illnesses in international travelers, including international aircraft passengers. Foodborne disease outbreaks on international airplanes have been well documented, including salmonellosis,[7-9] staphylococcal food poisoning,[10] shigellosis,[11] and cholera.[12] Most of these outbreaks have been traced to contaminated food items and food-handling errors, particularly improper temperature for food preparation or for holding food in flight. Subsequent person-to-person spread has been strongly suspected or documented in several outbreaks. Recognition of these outbreaks and tracing of an outbreak source have been facilitated by the high attack rates among passengers and/or crew members, the relatively short incubation periods of implicated pathogens, the severity of illness among affected persons, and the occurrence of an illness, such as cholera or typhoid fever, which is likely to be investigated by public health officials.[11]

These outbreak reports likely underestimate the risk of occurrence of airplane-associated outbreaks; many outbreaks do not come to attention due to (a) lower attack rates among passengers, which makes detection difficult, and (b) diseases with incubation periods longer than flight time, which allow exposed persons to disperse widely, making passengers, crew, and implicated foodstuffs difficult to identify and locate. Transmission of food-borne diseases on airplanes, although infrequent, is of substantial public health importance because a large number of persons may be exposed before the outbreak is recognized, and these outbreaks have the potential for rapid and wide geographic dissemination; these incidents merit swift intervention and may require rapid and coordinated response by numerous agencies and public health authorities in several countries. For example, in a salmonellosis outbreak reported by Burslem et al.,[8] which affected almost 1,000 passengers, aircrew, and ground personnel (and included two deaths), the authors likened the outbreak investigation and response to a major aircraft disaster in the number of national and international agencies and scientific disciplines involved.

These outbreaks emphasize the importance of appropriate methods and protocols for preventing food-borne illness on aircraft and highlight several important preventive measures. Travelers to areas where hygiene and sanitation are inadequate have long been advised to eat only foods that have been thoroughly cooked and are still hot. Such precautions are also advisable for air flights originating from or stopping in such countries. Additionally, commercial airlines should monitor the practices of their catering services. Prepared foods should be obtained from reliable sources and must be maintained either cold or hot; room-temperature storage is not safe. Aviation catering workers involved in food preparation should be trained to follow hygienic measures, including established hand washing and food preparation guidelines. Physicians should obtain a travel history from patients with gastroenteritis and recognize the possibility of food-borne diseases common to airplane outbreaks or endemic to countries of travel.

Direct Contact and Air-borne Transmission. Passenger and crew proximity in a confined space and the closed aircraft ventilation system create the potential for exposure to and transmission of numerous infectious diseases, particularly those spread by direct contact or air-borne transmission. Reported instances of potential or actual transmission of pathogens spread by direct contact or air-borne spread on international aircraft have included measles,[13,14] influenza,[15] and tuberculosis.[16–21] In these outbreaks, transmission of disease was traced to an infected index passenger or crew member, emphasizing the role of passengers and crew members as disease carriers during international travel and the potential for extensive disease transmission in the closed aircraft cabin environment. Disease transmission may be even more dramatic if the ventilation system within the aircraft is turned off or is working improperly. For example, in the reported outbreak of influenza aboard a commercial airliner, over 72% of passengers became ill, with symptoms appearing within 72 hours of exposure to the index case. This high attack rate was believed to be caused by a 3-hour delay in Alaska, during which the ventilation system was inoperative.

Response and management protocols for infectious diseases will differ depending on the suspected pathogen involved. For measles and other vaccine-preventable diseases (VPDs), retrospective passenger notification of potential exposure may be undertaken, particularly for passengers at high risk for complications from infection. The best means to prevent these diseases among travelers is through immunization programs for susceptible persons, travelers, and crew members. In the case of meningococcal exposure, prompt chemoprophylaxis is generally recommended for close or household contacts of a person with meningococcal disease because of an increased risk of contracting the disease.[22] However, scant data are available to determine if fellow passengers on prolonged air flights have a similarly increased risk. In the absence of any other data, CDC recommends that chemoprophylaxis be offered to passengers seated immediately adjacent to the index case if the total flight duration (including delays) is longer than 8 hours. In the case of tuberculosis transmission on airplanes, from 1992 through 1994, CDC, together with state and local health departments, investigated seven instances of potential tuberculosis (TB) transmission, involving one flight attendant and six passengers with active TB. The number of potentially exposed passengers and crew members was approximately 2,600 on a total of 191 air flights. Although the index case in each of the outbreaks was considered to be highly infectious, only two investigations documented transmission of TB aboard the aircraft, and in both cases transmission occurred after more than 8 hours exposure on the aircraft. These investigations have led to formal CDC recommendations for notification and follow-up of potentially TB-exposed passengers, based on infectiousness of the index case and duration of air flight, including ground delays.[19] Guidelines for the prevention and control of tuberculosis during air travel have also recently been published as a joint WHO and CDC effort.[23]

Other Modes of Transmission (Insect- and Vector-borne Transmission). International travel can also facilitate the global spread of insect- and vector-borne diseases, specifically by transporting insect vectors from one global destination and introducing them into another. Clusters of airport malaria are increasingly being recognized and reported,[24] and a real concern of tropical countries where yellow fever is not endemic is the potential introduction of its mosquito vectors by international aircraft. Selective disinsection of aircraft and cargo and vector control in the area surrounding airports have thus far been reasonably effective in preventing the introduction of *A. aegypti* and the outbreak of disease. However, the true impact of disinsection policies remains difficult to assess as the global spread of many vectors occurs via routes other than airplanes. Vector control by surveillance, spraying, and open-water control at international airports are also effective methods to prevent potential introduction of insect vectors.

INFECTIOUS DISEASES ON INTERNATIONAL CRUISE SHIPS

From 1987 to 1997, the number of passengers traveling aboard North American cruise ships more than doubled, growing from approximately 2.5 million passengers in 1987 to more than 5 million passengers in 1997.[25] Over this same period, there has also been an increase in the volume of passengers traveling to international destinations and an expansion in the range of global destinations for cruise ship itineraries (Figure 43–2). The large numbers of persons traveling on cruise ships annually and expansion of travel to a greater number of international destinations have increased the potential for exposure to infectious disease and its transfer across international boundaries. These factors make it important to understand trends in growth of the cruise ship travel industry and to monitor the composition and health status of cruising travelers. Additionally, knowledge of the most frequently reported diseases on international cruise ships and common modes of transmission can facilitate early identification and response to illness among international cruise ship travelers.

Modes and Sources of Transmission of Infectious Diseases on Cruise Ships   *Food- and Water-borne Diseases (Common Source Transmission).*

Cruise ships have long been associated with outbreaks of bacterial and viral gastrointestinal diseases, including typhoid fever,[26] shigellosis,[27-30] cholera,[31] staphylococcus food poisoning,[32] Norwalk virus,[33-35] other small round structured viruses,[36] entertoxigenic and enteroinvasive *Escherichia coli*,[37,38] trichinosis,[39] and Brainerd diarrhea.[40] These outbreaks have typically been transmitted by contaminated food or water, most served aboard ship; however, illnesses have also been associated with onshore exposures during the cruise vacation. Subsequent person-to-person spread has been strongly suspected or documented in several outbreaks. Similar to outbreaks on airplanes, the identification of these outbreaks was facilitated by the high attack rates among passengers and/or crew members (typically greater than 30%), the severity of associated illness, and the occurrence of unusual or reportable diseases. In 1975, in response to reported outbreaks, CDC's Vessel Sanitation Program (VSP) was established to assist the cruise ship industry in raising the standard of sanitation on cruise ships and lowering the risk of outbreaks. The VSP requires captains of cruise ships with international itineraries that call on ports in the United States to report the number of passengers who consulted the ship physician for diarrhea at least 24 hours before arrival. The captain notifies CDC if 3% or more of passengers or crew members have diarrhea during the cruise, which may prompt an investigation. In addition to these surveillance activities, twice a year the VSP staff performs unannounced inspections of all international cruise ships arriving at U.S. ports. Each ship is assigned a sanitation score, and these scores are published biweekly in CDC's Summary of Sanitation Inspections of International Cruise Ships. These reports are also available on the Internet through the CDC Web page (www.cdc.gov/travel).

Outbreaks of gastroenteritis on cruise ships have decreased steadily since the VSP was established,[41,42] and the surveillance system has documented a decreased occurrence of water- and ice-associated outbreaks. In the most recent review of VSP surveillance data describing the epidemiology of cruise-associated diarrheal disease outbreaks from 1986 through 1993, Koo et al.[42] estimated a risk of 2.1 outbreaks per 10 million passenger-days. An etiologic agent was implicated in 21 (68%) of 31 investigated outbreaks. The most common vehicles of transmission were undercooked scallops (enterotoxigenic *E. coli*), eggs (*Salmonella enteritidis* and Norwalk-like virus), and food items provided by caterers during onshore excursion (*Shigella sonnei*). This report determined that observance of two simple precautions, cooking seafood thoroughly and using pasteurized eggs, could have prevented almost one-third of the outbreaks investigated. Preventing food handlers from working while ill and not using onshore caterers might have prevented at least an additional third of these outbreaks. The reported data likely underestimate the risk for cruise-associated outbreaks because many outbreaks do not come to attention due to their small magnitude or the fact that passengers have disembarked and returned home prior to diagnosis of illness. Further reduction in the risk for shipboard outbreaks will require continued surveillance for diarrheal illness and cooperative efforts between the cruise ship industry and CDC, prompt identification and investigation of outbreaks, careful attention to food-handling practices and shipboard sanitation, and an ongoing program of ship inspection. Passengers on cruise ships should be sure that all food items they eat are thoroughly cooked and carefully evaluate the risk of eating food while off the ship, as during any travel overseas.

Environmental Reservoirs. Cruise ships have long been known as sources of diarrheal diseases; more recently, several outbreaks of legionnaires' disease affecting cruise ship passengers have been reported.[43-47] For a number of reasons, cruise ships may be the foci of legionnaires' disease and other forms of pneumonia. Various ports of call may pose risks for this disease, which can occur in association with seasonally used tourist facilities, and tropical regions may pose a greater risk of legionnaires' disease than nontropical regions because of the greater concentration of air-conditioning systems and the potential for bacterial growth in warm potable water.[48-52] Additionally, ships' water systems and recreational whirlpool spas may not be designed and maintained for optimal reduction of *Legionella* species contamination, and passengers may be at higher risk than the general population for legionnaires' disease because of their age and underlying chronic medical conditions. The reported *Legionella* outbreaks have implicated ship potable water supply systems and whirlpool spas as the source of the outbreaks and have been characterized by delayed outbreak recognition resulting in prolonged disease transmission occurring during multiple cruises. Delayed recognition of these common-source outbreaks is multifactorial; the incubation period is so long that passengers often disperse before symptoms develop and physicians may fail to recognize that travel is a risk factor for legionnaires' disease. In addition, there is a relative lack of qualified laboratories available to perform tests (urine antigen) for legionnaires' disease.

Cruise ship-associated legionnaires' disease is ultimately preventable. Knowledge of the environmental ecology of *Legionella pneumophila* has led to the design of water-containing devices that can be used and maintained to reduce colonization by the bacterium.[53-55] Specific guidelines for maintenance of ship water supplies and spas have been published.[56-58] The general principles for reducing the risk of *Legionella* exposure through water systems include proper disinfection, filtration, temperature monitoring, maintenance and storage of source water, and proper cleaning, disinfection, and maintenance of whirlpool spas. Because outbreak detection is so difficult, vigorous attention to reports of *Legionella* pneumonia is important in detecting outbreaks. Ship travel should be included in the travel history, and a high index of suspicion for *Legionella* pneumonia should be maintained. Reporting of travel-related cases of pneumonia to public health authorities is essential, and a centralized system for reporting radiographically confirmed pneumonia in cruise ship passengers may be useful for future prevention efforts.

Direct Contact and Air-borne Transmission.
Cruise ships have been the site of numerous recent outbreaks of VPDs among crew members and passengers.[59–62] Four cruise ship outbreaks (Table 43–1), investigated by CDC, highlight the potential role of international cruise travel in the dissemination and global spread of VPDs. In two rubella outbreaks aboard cruise ships, crew members (most of whom came from countries without routine rubella vaccination programs) were infected with rubella virus over the course of numerous cruises. A rubella serologic survey during the second outbreak indicated that at least 12% of the crew were acutely infected with or susceptible to rubella at the time of the outbreak. Further, although no rubella infections were identified in passengers, surveys during the outbreak indicated that 33% of the passengers were women of child-bearing age, a group at high risk, if infected during pregnancy, for serious adverse health outcomes, such as congenital rubella syndrome. Both outbreaks were terminated after the institution of active surveillance, crew isolation procedures, and mass vaccination of crew members. The varicella outbreak among crew members revealed that almost 13% of crew were infected or susceptible to varicella virus. Most crew members were foreign born, many from tropical climates, and the proportion of varicella-susceptible crew was two to three times higher than expected in a comparable U.S.-born population. Institution of isolation measures and vaccination of crew members were associated with interruption of disease transmission. In an influenza outbreak that occurred aboard a cruise ship sailing from Canada to New England on a U.S.-Canadian "fall colors" cruise, 32 of 493 (6%) crew members and 52 of 1,284 (4%) passengers surveyed had symptoms consistent with influenza-like illness (ILI); among passengers, 994 (77%) were ≥65 years of age (many with chronic underlying medical conditions), the group at highest risk for serious complication and death from influenza infection. This investigation documented substantial morbidity among passengers and crew and determined that influenza A was introduced aboard ship by travelers from the Southern Hemisphere, where influenza was in season. Instituting surveillance and isolation procedures, vaccinating crew members, treating ill persons with antiviral agents, and administering antiviral chemoprophylaxis to all crew and to high-risk passengers were associated with interruption of the outbreak.[61] Another influenza outbreak recently occurred among cruise ship and land travelers to Alaska and the Yukon Territory during the summer of 1998.[63,64] A CDC investigation identified more than 2,500 cases of ILI and 270 cases of pneumonia among Alaskan cruise ship passengers and crew members. Control measures were insufficient to control the outbreak, likely because it was widespread among land and sea travelers; cases of illness abated only after the tourist season ended and travelers and cruise ships left the region.

Outbreaks of all infectious diseases aboard cruise ships are of public health importance. Cruise ships are a semi-enclosed environment conducive to the transmission, amplification, and dissemination of infectious diseases (Figure 43–3). The nature of cruise ship travel (with an average length of cruise of 6.4 days) provides the type of prolonged and repeated contact among passengers and crew needed to amplify transmission of disease aboard the vessel and can allow subsequent dissemination of disease to home communities. In addition, passengers frequently take trips ashore to ports where infection may be acquired and spread aboard ship. The crew may serve as a reservoir for continuing disease transmission beyond a single cruise. Many passengers are at high risk for serious morbidity associated with these infections, and medical facil-

Table 43–1. OUTBREAK INVESTIGATIONS OF VACCINE-PREVENTABLE DISEASES ABOARD INTERNATIONAL CRUISE SHIPS, CENTERS FOR DISEASE CONTROL (CDC), 1997–1998

PATHOGEN	AUTHOR (REF)	YEAR	CRUISE REGION	NO. CREW INFECTED/ NO. CREW (%)	NO. CREW SUSCEPTIBLE/ NO. CREW (%)	NO. PASSENGERS INFECTED/ NO. PASSENGERS (%)	CONTROL MEASURES A	B	C	D
Rubella	CDC59	1997	Caribbean	6/900 (<1%)	Unknown	Unknown	x	x		
Rubella	CDC59	1997	Caribbean	16/366 (4%)	25/366 (8%)	Unknown	x	x		
Varicella	CDC60	1998	New York Harbor	3/398 (<1%)	17/138 (12%)	Unknown	x	x	x	
Influenza A	CDC61,62	1997	Canada-New England	32/493 (6%)	Unknown	*52/1284 (4%)	x	x	x	x

A = crew isolation, B = crew vaccination, C = crew treatment (acyclovir for varicella-infected crew members and rimantidine for influenza-infected crew members and as chemoprophylaxis), D = passenger treatment (rimantidine treatment for influenza-infected passengers and as chemoprophylaxis for passengers at high risk for influenza complications [age ≥65 years or chronic underlying medical condition]).
*Number of passengers voluntarily reporting to the ship's medical infirmary for acute respiratory infection (ARI). When passengers were queried directly for symptoms of ARI via a cabin-based survey, the attack rate of ARI was actually fourfold higher.

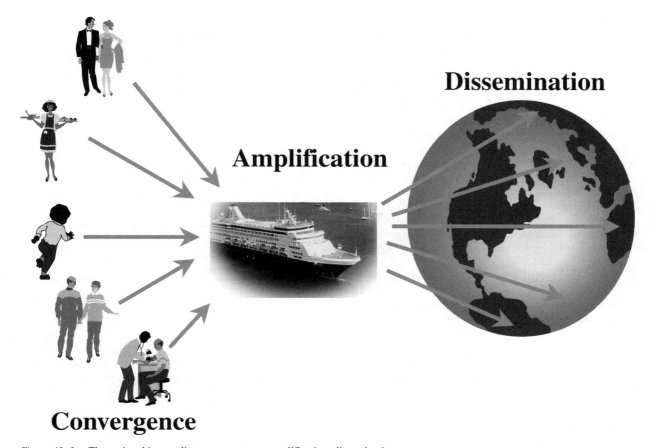

Figure 43–3.   The cruise ship paradigm: convergence, amplification, dissemination.

ities and supplies on the ship may be insufficient to control the outbreak and provide adequate medical treatment to affected individuals. The importance of appropriate and thorough pretravel counseling and the administration of all routine and travel-indicated vaccines to prospective travelers during pretravel visits cannot be overstated. Recent outbreaks also highlight the need for the establishment of routine vaccination policies for cruise ship crew members, formalized surveillance programs to monitor illnesses among passengers and crew members, and a standard response sequence when levels of illness rise above a defined level. CDC, working in collaboration with various cruise ships lines, has recently issued guidance on surveillance for influenza-like illnesses and response and control measures for suspected respiratory illness outbreaks among passengers and crew members on international cruise ships.[65]

Other Modes of Transmission.   Recently, ballast water of cruise ships has been implicated in the introduction of nonindigenous and often harmful species into naive marine ecosystems and in the movement of pathogens from one geographic location to another.[66] Increasing vessel capacity and faster transit times have increased the potential for ballast water to spread pathogens around the globe. The recent cholera outbreak in Peru (which subsequently spread to many countries in Latin America) has been postulated to be due to the dis-

charge of ballast water from Asian tankers delivering goods to Latin America.[67] This hypothesis has been strengthened by molecular evidence linking numerous entry points on the South American Pacific seaboard with Bangladesh.[68] Recommendations and guidance for reducing the risk of disease spread through ballast water by judicious embarkation and exchange of ballast water have recently been developed and issued.[69,70]

INVESTIGATION AND RESPONSE TO SUSPECTED INFECTIOUS DISEASE OUTBREAKS ON INTERNATIONAL CONVEYANCES

RESPONSE TO ARRIVING ILL PASSENGER WITH SUSPECTED INFECTIOUS DISEASE

When an illness or suspected outbreak of illnesses occurs on an international conveyance, it is a public health concern requiring swift intervention; the large numbers of travelers involved and the potential for rapid transport and dissemination of pathogens and vectors across international borders make efforts to control and prevent further illness imperative. U.S. regulations require that death or illness in an arriving international passenger or crew member be reported by the captain of an arriving international conveyance (airplane or cruise ship) to the port authority and quarantine station having responsibility for the particular port of entry. This notification should be sent at the earliest opportunity and should include detailed information regarding the affected passenger's or crew member's symptoms and their severity. Early notification will allow adequate time for planning a response and minimize delays to passengers and conveyances. In addition to such reporting, a systematic response sequence for ill passengers is essential for ensuring appropriate individual case management, as well as effective public health response to the suspected illness. Table 43–2 outlines important steps in response to an arriving ill passenger that can be initiated at the time of identification and often before arrival at the port of entry. Two key aspects of the risk assessment are (1) evaluation of the clinical syndrome and (2) knowledge of the detailed travel itinerary taken in the context of global distribution of endemic diseases and disease outbreaks. This requires a combination of clinical and epidemiologic skills and is dependent on solid global surveillance information.

RESPONSE TO SUSPECTED INFECTIOUS DISEASE OUTBREAKS ON INTERNATIONAL CONVEYANCES

If more than one instance of suspected illness occurs among passengers or crew members of an international conveyance, a more formalized and comprehensive approach to initial investigation is warranted and is outlined in Table 43–3. Responses will vary by type of investigation and type of conveyance. International cooperation by public health authorities in several countries may be required to investigate and control the outbreak.

Steps in An Outbreak Investigation Aboard An International Conveyance (Airplane or Cruise Ship)   The steps outlined below are guidelines that may be followed in investigation and response to a suspected or potential infectious disease outbreak on an international conveyance. In practice, several of these steps are often initiated and performed simultaneously.

Notification of Public Health Authorities.   When an outbreak aboard an international conveyance is suspected, the Division of Quarantine at CDC (and/or other national public health authorities, depending on the jurisdiction) should be notified. Early notification will allow adequate time for public health planning and response and minimize delays in identifying the source of the outbreak and instituting appropriate control measures.

Case Identification and Review.   One of the initial steps in any response to a potential infectious disease outbreak on an international conveyance is to gather information about potential case-patients. Case-finding methods will differ by type of investigation and type of conveyance, but in all investigations, a line-listing of probable case-patients should be developed from personal or telephone interviews with passengers, from questionnaires, or from review of medical log data (for interna-

tional cruise ships). Passengers can be located using the addresses they have written on declaration cards submitted to the U.S. Custom Service upon arrival in the U.S. News media appeals can also be used to ask passengers to contact local health authorities. The investigator should review passenger and crew member information from probable case-patients to define the clinical and epidemiologic characteristics of this patient population and then formulate a case definition. The case definition usually should include clinical, laboratory, and/or other pertinent characteristics. Data collected during interviews and medical record review should include information that allows the investigator to characterize the epidemic in terms of person (patient characteristics), place (geographic distribution), and time (epidemic curve).

Table 43–2.   **RESPONSE TO AN ARRIVING ILL PASSENGER WITH SUSPECTED INFECTIOUS DISEASE**

Assess and manage ill passenger

Collect ill passenger information

   Clinical status

   Age, sex, history of present illness, symptoms, and symptom onset date/time

   Travel itinerary

Notify port authority and quarantine station

Assess the likelihood that a public health intervention is required based on clinical syndrome and detailed travel itinerary

Collect/obtain passenger contact information (i.e., passenger manifest, questionnaires)

Notify passengers as appropriate (e.g., health alert notices, telephone, direct mailing)

Table 43–3.   **STEPS IN AN OUTBREAK INVESTIGATION ON AN INTERNATIONAL CONVEYANCE (AIRPLANE OR CRUISE SHIP)**

Notification of public health authorities

Case identification and review

   Case finding (passenger manifest)

   Case definition: person, place, time (epidemic curve)

Epidemiologic analysis (hypothesis testing)

Specimen collection

Environmental sampling

Laboratory investigation

Control measures

   Active surveillance

   Other appropriate interventions

Notification of passengers

Public health information and messages

Case-Patient Characteristics (Person). Thorough description of the potential case-patient population is important in any epidemic investigation. The case-patient interview and/or medical record review should attempt to define specific host exposures (i.e., travel history including conveyance and passenger itinerary; items of food consumed aboard the conveyance and in transit; if food-borne outbreak is suspected, exposure to other ill passengers, crew members, or other persons; exposure to contaminated water or whirlpool/aerosolized water for *Legionella*) that may be risk factors for disease and specific host characteristics that predispose to infections (e.g., age, underlying illnesses, inadequate vaccination/immune status). Both animate and inanimate exposure factors should be explored, and common exposures to food items, whirlpools, or other ill persons should be reviewed to assess the possibility of person-to-person transmission.

Geographic Distribution (Place). In an investigation of infectious disease on an international conveyance, common exposures prior to embarkation on the conveyance and while on the conveyance (including excursions for cruise ships) should be assessed. Passenger seat/cabin assignment and location should also be collected to determine if there is spatial/geographic clustering of infections.

Epidemic Curve (Time). An important step in an epidemic investigation is the construction of an epidemic curve, a graph depicting the number of infections occurring over time by date of onset of infection symptoms in each case-patient. This visual representation of the magnitude and time course of an outbreak provides valuable epidemiologic information. The characteristics of an epidemic curve can suggest the mode of transmissions of infection and assist in differentiation between common vehicle or source exposures, contact, and person-to-person exposures, or even varying forms of transmission within the same outbreak. In a common vehicle or source outbreak transmitted by exposure to a common contaminated food item or environmental exposure (i.e., aerosolized water for *Legionella*), the epidemic curve usually rises sharply and then gradually declines. In epidemics caused by person-to-person or air-borne transmission, the epidemic curve usually rises gradually, has a flatter peak than does a common-source outbreak, and then decreases (Figure 43–4). In the example presented in Figure 43–4, both epidemiologic and laboratory evidence supported the hypothesis of person-to-person transmission of influenza A from among cruise ship passengers and crew members.

Epidemiologic Analysis. After a thorough review of case-patient information and medical records for host exposure and susceptibility factors, the investigator should develop and test reasonable hypotheses for the cause of the outbreak. In most epidemic investigations, the most effective means for refining and testing hypotheses is a case-control or cohort study. Case-control studies are more frequently used in epidemic investigations because cohort studies are usually more difficult, expensive, and time consuming. In the instance of a specific air flight or cruise, however, the number of passengers may be small enough to reasonably allow for undertaking a cohort study. The purpose of such a cohort study is to compare case-patients (affected/infected patients) to unaffected patients (control or non–case-patients). From the

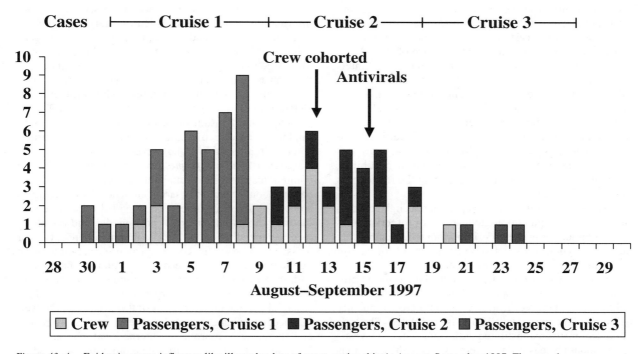

Figure 43–4. Epidemic curve: influenza-like illness by date of onset, cruise ship A, August–September 1997. The open boxes represent cases among crew members, the closed boxes represent cases among passengers on three successive cruises as delineated. Note the spread from passengers to crew and then to successive passengers.

cohort study, the investigator can calculate the frequencies of various host exposure and susceptibility factors among case and control patients, focusing on significant differences between the two groups. These differences often support or suggest hypotheses about the mode of disease transmission and the source of the outbreak. If performing a case-control study, care should be taken to ensure that case and control patients have an equal opportunity for exposure to relevant and suspected risk factors.

The findings of these epidemiologic studies may also suggest sources of exposure that should be investigated further and/or laboratory tested. The results of such epidemiologically initiated environmental or personal laboratory testing often clarify or support hypotheses of disease transmission suggested by the epidemiologic analyses.

Environmental Sampling and Patient Specimen Collection. Because a substantial proportion of outbreaks is associated with contaminated food and water or environmental reservoirs, a systematic review of food procurement and preparation and disinfection and maintenance protocols and procedures for drinking and bathing water should be undertaken when a common exposure is suspected. In addition, frequently during the course of outbreaks, environmental laboratory testing is undertaken to identify a common source or reservoir. It is important that the investigator ensure that critical specimens that might be needed for analysis are preserved until the epidemiologic studies are completed. Patient and/or environmental isolates believed to be implicated in the epidemic should be saved. The investigator should collect samples of any materials likely to be relevant to disease transmission, especially materials that will be discarded or cleaned and disinfected before completion of the epidemiologic studies. In addition, appropriate laboratory specimens should be obtained from all passengers and crew members identified as potential case-patients.

Laboratory Investigation. Laboratory evaluation is used to support epidemiologic evidence of spread of a common organism among passengers and crew. All interviewed passengers or just suspected case-patients can be asked to submit stool or other appropriate samples for culture or serum for antibody titers. Strain clonality can confirm the association between patients and sources of reservoirs of implicated microorganisms. Traditional laboratory methods have used phenotypic characteristics such as biochemical typing, antimicrobial susceptibility, phage typing, or serotyping to determine the relatedness of epidemic strains.

Molecular typing methods are increasingly used to supplement the epidemiologic analysis of infectious disease outbreaks. However, it is important to remember that molecular typing does not supplant the need for careful traditional epidemiologic assessment.

Control Measures. Initial control measures to prevent further disease transmission are often instituted immediately upon recognition of an outbreak, frequently before the epidemic investigation is completed. The type of control measures instituted at the outset of the investigation should be based on the seriousness of the infections and previous experience with similar outbreaks, if available. For example, in outbreaks of respiratory infection with influenza where transmission usually occurs by person-to-person spread, investigators should consider institution of appropriate isolation procedures for ill passengers and crew members. These interventions have been effective in terminating similar outbreaks. For VPDs aboard cruise ships, isolation of crew members and vaccination campaigns have been largely successful in controlling the outbreak. At times, it may even be reasonable to institute these control measures and evaluate their effectiveness before the decision to embark on a full epidemic investigation is made. As the results of the epidemiologic studies are available, additional control measures targeting implicated exposure factors should be instituted. It is important for surveillance to continue throughout and beyond the outbreak investigation in order to document the success of control measures and to confirm the validity of the proposed hypothesis as the cause of the epidemic.

Notification of Passengers. As part of an outbreak (or suspected outbreak) investigation it is frequently necessary to contact passengers of the airline or cruise ship. The purpose of passenger notification is manifold but principally serves two purposes: (1) informational—to provide notice regarding the outbreak occurrence, time frame, etiology, risk factors, and prevention or control recommendations and (2) investigational—to find additional cases or to request additional information from case-patients. Depending on the epidemiologic assessment of ongoing transmission and the incubation period, passenger notification may either be retrospective (disembarked passengers), concurrent (existing passengers), prospective (future passengers), or any of the three. Given the variable points of origin and widespread dispersal of international travelers after disembarkation, the greatest challenge is often obtaining adequate passenger contact information to mount an investigation and complete notification. Assistance and cooperation of a variety of agencies and jurisdictions may be required. Airlines and cruise lines need to recognize their critical role in facilitation of these investigations and should be urged to maintain electronic copies of passenger manifests with sufficient contact information in a readily accessible format. Timely passenger notification often determines the success of implementing effective interventions to control further spread, limit morbidity, and prevent deaths.

Public Health Information. It is often necessary to communicate information about outbreaks aboard international conveyances to a larger audience than passengers alone. The information can be provided on a variety of platforms including Internet, print media, and broadcast media, depending on the desired target audience, type of message, and message content. The information in these public health messages needs to be tailored to the target audience in easily understood language and carefully worded to avoid unnecessary panic or confusion. It is essential that the dissemination of these messages be well planned, coordinated with all partners in the investigation, and shared with appropriate international, national, and local public health authorities who might be impacted by the news. Ideally, a single point of contact through the agency's public affairs office should be established.

REFERENCES

1. World Tourist Organization. Yearbook of tourism statistics, 1998. Vol. 1, 50th Ed. Madrid, 1998.

2. Fidler DP, Heymann DL, Ostroff SM, O Brien TP. Emerging and reemerging infectious diseases: challenges for international, national, and state law. Int Lawyer 1997;31:773–800.

3. World Health Organization. International health regulations (1969). 3rd annotated Ed. Geneva: World Health Organization, 1983.

4. World Health Organization. Revisions of the international health regulations. Wkly Epidemiol Rec 1996;71:233–235, 1997:72:9–11, 72:213–215 and 1998;73:17–19.

5. U.S. Government Printing Office. Code of federal regulations, October 1, 1996. Title 42, Vol. 1, Parts 1–399:501–510.

6. Cetron M, Keystone J, Schlim D, Steffen R. Travelers' health. Emerg Infect Dis 1998;4:405–407.

7. Tauxe RV, Torney MP, Mascola L, et al. Salmonellosis outbreaks on transatlantic flights: foodborne illness on aircraft 1947–1984. Am J Epidemiol 1987;125:150–157.

8. Burslem CD, Kelly MJ, Preston FS. Food poisoning—a major threat to airline operations. J Soc Occup Med 1990;40:97–100.

9. Back E, Romanus V, Sjoberg L, et al. An epidemic of *Salmonella typhimurium* infection among aircraft passengers. Scand J Infect Dis 1977;9:175–179.

10. Eisenberg MS, Gaarslev K, Brown W, et al. Staphylococcal food poisoning aboard a commercial aircraft. Lancet 1975;2:595–599.

11. Hedburg CW, Levine WC, White KE, et al. An international food borne outbreak of shigellosis associated with a commercial airline. JAMA 1992;268:3208–3212.

12. Eberhart-Phillips J, Besser RE, Torney MP, et al. An outbreak of cholera from food served on an international aircraft. Epidemiol Infect 1996;116:9–13.

13. Amler RW, Bloch AB, Orenstein WA, et al. Imported measles in the United States. JAMA 1982;248:2219–2233.

14. Centers for Disease Control. Epidemiological notes and reports. Interstate importation of measles following transmission in an airport—California, Washington 1982. MMWR Morb Mortal Wkly Rep 1983;32:210–216.

15. Moser MR, Bender TR, Margolis HS, et al. An outbreak of influenza aboard a commercial airliner. Am J Epidemiol 1979;110:1–6.

16. Caspari D, Wittes RC. Public health approach to infectious disease imported by plane. Can Med Assoc J 1989;140:893–894.

17. Driver CR, Valway SE, Morgan WM, et al. Transmission of *M. tuberculosis* associated with air travel. JAMA 1994;272:1031–1035.

18. McFarland JW, Hickman C, Osterholm MT, MacDonald KL. Exposure to *Mycobacterium tuberculosis* during air travel. Lancet 1993;342:112–113.

19. Centers for Disease Control. Exposure of passengers and flight crew to *Mycobacterium tuberculosis* on commercial aircraft, 1992–1995. MMWR Morb Mortal Wkly Rep 1995;44:137–140.

20. Miller MA, Valway SE, Onorato IM. Tuberculosis risk after exposure on airplanes. Tubercle Lung Dis 1996;77:414–419.

21. Kenyon TA, Valway SE, Ihle WW, et al. Transmission of multi-drug resistant *Mycobacterium tuberculosis* during a long airplane flight. N Engl J Med 1996;67:1097–1100.

22. Hansman D. Meningococcal diseases in the 1980's: epidemiology, prevention and control. Med J Aust 1988;149:349–350.

23. World Health Organization. Tuberculosis and air travel: guidelines for prevention and control. Geneva: World Health Organization, 1998.

24. Van den Ende J, Lynen L, Elsen P, et al. A cluster of airport malaria in Belgium in 1995. Acta Clin Belg 1998;53–4:259–263.

25. Cruise Lines International Association. The cruise industry: an overview. CLIA marketing edition, New York, July 1997.

26. Davies JW, Cox KG, Simon WR, et al. Typhoid at sea: epidemic aboard an oceanliner. Can Med Assoc J 1972;106:877–883.

27. Merson MH, Tenney JH, Meyers JD, et al. Shigellosis at sea: an outbreak aboard a passenger cruise ship. Am J Epidemiol 1975;101:165–175.

28. Finch M, Rodney G, Lawrence D, Blake P. Epidemic Reiter's syndrome following an outbreak of shigellosis. Eur J Epidemiol 1986;2:26–30.

29. Lew JL, Swerdlow DL, Dance ME, et al. An outbreak of shigellosis aboard a cruise ship caused by a multi-antibiotic-resistant strain of *Shigella flexneri*. Am J Epidemiol 1991;134:413–420.

30. Centers for Disease Control. Outbreak of *Shigella flexneri* 2a infections on a cruise ship. MMWR Morb Mortal Wkly Rep 1994;42:657.

31. Boyce TG, Mintz ED, Green KD, et al. *Vibrio cholerae* Bengal infections among tourists to Southeast: an international foodborne outbreak. J Infect Dis 1995;172:140–144.

32. Waterman SH, DeMArcus TS, Wells JG, Blake PA. Staphylococcal food poisoning on a cruise ship. Epidemiol Infect 1987;99:349–353.

33. Gunn RA, Terranova WA, Greenberg HB, et al. Norwalk virus gastroenteritis aboard a cruise ship: an outbreak on five consecutive cruises. Am J Epidemiol 1980;112:820–827.

34. Khan AS, Moe CL, Glass RI, et al. Norwalk virus-associated gastroenteritis traced to ice consumption aboard a cruise ship in Hawaii: comparison and application of molecular method-based assays. J Clin Microbiol 1994;32:318–322.

35. Herwaldt BL, Lew JL, Moe CL, et al. Characterization of a variant strain of norwalk virus from a food-borne outbreak of gastroenteritis on a cruise ship in Hawaii. J Clin Microbiol 1994;32:861–866.

36. McEvoy M, Blake W, Brown D, et al. An outbreak of viral gastroenteritis on a cruise ship. Commun Dis Rep CDR Rev 1996;13:R188–R192.

37. O'Mahony MC, Noah ND, Evans B, Harper D. An outbreak of gastroenteritis on a passenger cruise ship. J Hyg 1986;97:229–236.

38. Snyder JD, Wells JG, Yashuk J, et al. Outbreak of invasive escherichia coli gastroenteritis on a cruise ship. Am J Trop Med Hyg 1984;33:281–284.

39. Singal M, Schantz P, Werner S. Trichinosis acquired at sea—a report of an outbreak. Am J Trop Med Hyg 1976;25:675–681.

40. Mintz ED, Weber JT, Guris D, et al. An outbreak of Brainerd diarrhea among travelers to the Galapagos Islands. J Infect Dis 1998;177:1041–1045.

41. Addiss DG, Yashuk JC, Clapp DE, Blake PA. Outbreaks of diarrhoeal illness on passenger cruise ships, 1975–85. Epidemiol Inf 1989;103:63–72.

42. Koo D, Maloney K, Tauxe R. Epidemiology of diarrheal disease outbreaks on cruise ships, 1986–1993. JAMA 1996;275:545–547.

43. Jernigan DB, Hoffman J, Cetron MS, et al. Outbreak of legionnaires' disease among cruise ship passengers exposed to a contaminated whirlpool spa. Lancet 1996;347:494–499.

44. Guerrero IC, Filippone C. A cluster of legionnaires' disease in a community hospital—a clue to a larger epidemic. Infect Control Hosp Epidemiol 1996;17:177–178.

45. Joseph C, European Working Group on Legionella Infections. Outbreak of legionnaires' disease among British tourists associated with Rhine cruise. Available at: http//www.phls.co.uk EUROSURV 1997 971030.html#rhine.

46. Christie P, Joseph C, European Working Group on Legionella Infections. Legionella on board a cruise ship. Available at: http//www.phls.co.uk EUROSURV 1998 989702.html#leg.

47. Castellani-Pastoris M, Monaco RL, Goldoni P, et al. Legionnaires' disease on a cruise ship linked to the water supply system: clinical and public health implications. Clin Infect Dis 1999;28:33–38.

48. Rosmini F, Castellani-Pastoris M, Mazzoti MF, et al. Febrile illness in successive cohorts of tourists at a hotel on the italian Adriatic Coast: evidence for a persistent foci of *Legionella* infection. Am J Epidemiol 1984;119:124–134.

49. Bhopal RS, Fallon RJ. Seasonal variation of legionnaires' disease in Scotland. J Infect 1991;22:153–160.

50. Anonymous. Cluster of cases of legionnaires' disease associated with travel to Turkey. Commun Dis Rep CDR Wkly 1995; 5:175.

51. Joseph CA, Hutchinson EJ, Dedman D, et al. Legionnaires' disease surveillance: England and Wales 1994. Commun Dis Rep CDC Rev 1995;5:R180–R183.

52. Ostroff SM, Kozarsky P. Emerging infectious disease and travel medicine. Infect Dis Clin North Am 1998;12:231–241.

53. Brundett GW. Legionella and building services. 1st Ed. Oxford, UK: Butterworth-Heinemann, 1992.

54. Chartered Institution of Building Services Engineers. Minimising the risk of Legionnaires' disease [technical memorandum]. London: Chartered Institution of Building Services Engineers, 1991:1–24.

55. Health and Safety Executive. The control of legionellosis including legionnaires' disease. London: Health and Safety Executive, 1991.

56. Department of Transport. Recommendations to prevent contamination of ships' freshwater storage and distribution systems. Notice to shipowners, masters, fishing vessel skippers, shipbuilders and repairers. Notice M.1214. Merchant Shipping Notice. Edinburgh: Her Majesty's Stationary Office, 1986.

57. Department of Transport. Contamination of ships air conditioning systems by *Legionella* bacteria. Notice to shipowners, masters, fishing vessel skippers, shipbuilders and repairers. Notice M.1215. Merchant Shipping Notice. Edinburgh: Her Majesty's Stationary Office, 1986.

58. National Center for Environmental Health, National Center for Infectious Diseases. Final recommendations to minimize transmission of legionnaires' disease from whirlpool spas on cruise ships. Atlanta: Centers for Disease Control and Prevention, 1995.

59. Centers for Disease Control. Rubella among crew members of commercial cruise ships—Florida, 1997. MMWR Morb Mortal Wkly Rep 1998;46:1247–1250.

60. Ostrowski SR, Zane SB, Seward J, et al. Varicella zoster virus seroprevalence among multinational cruise ship crew, 1998. Centers for Disease Control unpublished report.

61. Miller, Tam T, Maloney SA, et al. Cruise ships: a travel destination for high-risk passengers and new influenza viruses. Clin Infect Dis 2000 (in press).

62. Centers for Disease Control. Update: influenza activity—United States, 1997–98 season. MMWR Morb Mortal Wkly Rep 1997;46:1094–1098.

63. Centers for Disease Control. Update: outbreak of influenza A infection—Alaska and the Yukon Territory, July–August 1998. MMWR Morb Mortal Wkly Rep 1998;47:685–688.

64. Zane S, Uyeki T, Bodnar U, et al. Influenza in travelers, tourism workers, and residents in Alaska and the Yukon Territory, summer 1998 [poster]. Presented at the 6th Conference of the International Society for Travel Medicine, Montreal, Canada, June 6–10, 1999.

65. Bodnar U, Maloney SA, Fielding K, et al. Preliminary guidelines for the prevention and control of influenza-like illness among passengers and crew members on cruise ships. Atlanta: Division of Quarantine, National Center for Infectious Diseases, Centers for Disease Control and Prevention, August 1999.

66. Murrison AW. Marine hitch hikers—the transport of pathogens in ballast water. J R Navy Med Serv 1996;82:40–43.

67. Anderson C. Cholera epidemic traced to risk calculation. Nature 1991;354:255.

68. Faruque SM, Albert J. Genetic relation between *Vibrio cholerae* 01 strains in Ecuador and Bangladesh. Lancet 1992; 339:740–741.

69. International Maritime Organization. Marine Environment Protection Committee resolution 50 (31), 1991.

70. Department of Transport. Merchant shipping notice M.1533. Edinburgh: Her Majesty's Stationary Office, 1993.

43.1 EPIDEMIOLOGIC ALERT AT INTERNATIONAL AIRPORTS

ERIC L. WEISS

INTRODUCTION

Those in the field of travel medicine are quite aware of the recent increases in international travel. More and more people are traveling, and destinations are becoming increasingly exotic. Over the last 20 years, the world's population has been estimated to grow at approximately 2% per annum; however, the traveling population has grown at three times that rate, or 6% per annum. Clearly, this number is even greater if one looks at more recent history.

With this increase in both the frequency and scope of international travel, it has become clear that "tourists" are not the only globetrotters. Infectious agents and their vectors are quite capable of traveling the globe. Recent mortalities from "imported" infections such as yellow fever in California and Lassa fever in Germany have attracted significant attention. Also, high-profile epidemics (Ebola) or possible epidemics (plague) have focused public policy on this issue: just how can we limit the spread of potentially devastating infectious diseases by modern-day conveyances or their passengers?

HISTORY

The first official effort at regulating passage, with an intent to preserve public health, was in 1377. The City of Venice passed quarantine legislation directed at the devastating "black death" or epidemic bubonic plague of the 14th century. Navigators were detained for a period of 40 days, from which derives the word "quarantine" (*quaranti giorni*). The first International Sanitary Conference followed much later in 1851, which introduced the philosophy of "maximum protection with minimum restriction" of the traveler. Although uniform quarantine measures were adopted, it took the passage of 100 additional years and the formation of the World Health Organization (WHO) to bring more productive organization to this international challenge. In 1951, the International Health Regulations (IHR) were adopted, which stressed (1) strong epidemiologic principles, (2) improved sanitation around ports and airports, and (3) prevention of vector dissemination. Note that despite an emphasis on epidemiologic principles, the principle tool of the IHR was physical quarantine.

AIRPORT MEDICINE

Although the history of the IHR is based on travel by ground or sea, it is clear that in today's world, the challenges lie in regulating and protecting a population that travels largely by air. The numbers speak largely for themselves. It is estimated that over 50 million North Americans will travel across borders this year, with more than 10 million of them traveling to tropical destinations with significant infectious disease risk. Ten percent of Japanese citizens travel abroad each year.

The challenges of such regulations become apparent upon examination. Article 15 of the IHR prescribes "in as many of the ports and airports in a territory as practicable an organized medical and health service with adequate staff, equipment and premises, and in particular facilities for the prompt isolation and care of infected persons, for disinfection, disinsecting and deratting, for bacteriological investigation, for the collection and examination of rodents for plague infection, for collection of water and food samples and their dispatch to a laboratory for examination." Clearly, how this is both interpreted and, more importantly, implemented is going to vary from country to country and culture to culture.

In the United States, such responsibilities fall to the U.S. Public Health Service, which, in turn, delegates implementation of such a program to the Centers for Disease Control and Prevention (CDC), National Center for Infectious Diseases, Division of Quarantine. Quarantine stations are located at major international airports in seven U.S. cities (Los Angeles, San Francisco, Miami, Honolulu, Chicago, New York, and Seattle). These seven stations are responsible for all ports in the United States. At airports that do not have a formal Division of Quarantine presence, officials of the Immigration and Naturalization Service (INS) and/or Division of Quarantine contract physicians serve as quarantine officers.

Division of Quarantine staff are not physically able to screen all arriving passengers. Critical to the implementation of this program is the participation of the airline industry. There are federal regulations that require flight crews to notify officials of passengers who appear ill. Specifically, arriving passengers are to be observed for "signs and symptoms of illness, such as rash, unusually flushed or pale complexion, jaundice, shivering, profuse sweating, diarrhea, and inability to walk without assistance." Airport officials are then instructed to "hold ill passengers and crew, and ask for details about symptoms and itinerary. At a port of entry where a quarantine station is staffed, that station should be notified and a quarantine inspector will investigate. If there is no quarantine inspector at your port, the appropriate quarantine station should be notified. The quarantine station will release or conditionally release the ill person, or if the circumstances warrant, call a physician to conduct an examination and recommend appropriate action."

PUT TO THE TEST

In September 1994, India reported cases of plague for the first time in 28 years. By the end of the month, more than 300 unconfirmed cases of pneumonic plague and 36 deaths had been reported from Surat, a city of 2 million residents. As a result of these reports, hundreds of thousands of Surat residents fled, many to the major cities of Bombay, Calcutta, and New Delhi. The potential for national and international spread of disease was obvious, and several countries closed their borders to Indian travelers and cargo and stopped their domestic airlines from flying to or from India. Those countries wishing to take less drastic measures but eager to prevent the introduction of a potentially deadly disease turned to the IHR for direction. Note that such reasoned measures were subsequently shown to be appropriate as, in retrospect, the entire plague "epidemic" in India has come under considerable question of having occurred at all.

MODEL RESPONSE?

Governments around the world responded quickly and efficiently, building on systems put in place by national policy, often based on IHR guidelines. As reported by Fritz et al., the better responses were built on the dual approach of education and information, as well as intensified active and passive surveillance.

Alarmed by the recent news, the U.S. public and medical community turned to the CDC for information. The CDC produced five separate information pieces: (1) a general plague outbreak notice, (2) a plague alert notice for international travelers from India, (3) a plague advisory for travelers bound for India, (4) plague treatment and prophylaxis guidelines for physicians, and (5) guidelines for diagnosis and biosafety for persons handling samples from patients with suspected plague. Information was also made available on the CDC's Voice and Fax Information Service. Last, all passengers arriving at U.S. airports from India were given a plague alert notice that described plague symptoms and directed them to seek medical attention (and notify CDC authorities) if they developed any febrile illness within the next 7 days.

An active surveillance program was also initiated based on the existing U.S. Division of Quarantine program outlined earlier. All crews of aircraft originating from or passing through India were reminded to be especially vigilant for passengers with fever, cough, or chills. Existing regulations require aircraft crew to notify the quarantine officer at the destination airport of such passengers. Upon notification, the quarantine officer, with a physician, would greet the arriving plane, and before passengers were allowed to disembark, would examine the suspect passenger(s). The medical officer on call at the CDC Division of Vector-Borne Infections Diseases was available by telephone consultation if needed.

If the passenger was deemed not likely to have plague, then he or she would be released but placed under surveillance of the local health department and instructed to consult a physician and to monitor his or her temperature for the next 7 days. All other passengers would be permitted to deplane and were given a copy of the CDC plague alert notice for their information.

If plague could not be sufficiently ruled out, then the unfortunate passenger would be placed in isolation at the airport until they could be safely transported to a designated hospital. Once hospitalized, the patient would be placed in respiratory isolation and the diagnosis would be facilitated by the CDC plague laboratory. In this situation, the other passengers would be informed that they were under surveillance under federal quarantine regulations. Locating information would be obtained from all passengers, and they too would be asked to consult a physician and monitor their temperature for the next 7 days. Additionally, passengers seated within 2 meters of the patient would be advised to begin prophylactic antibiotics because of their presumed risk of infection. If the patient actually had plague, then all proximal passengers would be contacted to confirm completion of course of prophylactic antibiotics, and all remaining passengers would be contacted to ensure none developed symptoms consistent with disease (Figure 43.1–1).

In addition to the above "active surveillance" program, a system of "passive surveillance" was also used.

In this system, private physicians, hospitals, and public health officials were relied upon to identify travelers from India who fell ill within a few hours to 7 days after their arrival. Local physicians, in consultation with medical officers from the CDC, would then determine the appropriate course of action (Figure 43.1–2).

During the 30 days in late 1994 in which this heightened level of surveillance was in effect, 13 airline travelers from India were identified and evaluated for having plague. Six were evaluated in their arriving airport and the remaining seven during the next few days by private physicians. None were found to have plague.

LESSONS LEARNED

It is clear from the experience in 1994 that any national surveillance system is a substantial undertaking requiring an enormous amount of coordination. It makes sense to use an already existing system and network, one that has a preexisting structure yet can be flexible to adapt to the situation at hand. Having such a system be centrally coordinated by an agency like the CDC makes sense, but even here many others played key roles in the success of this program. Federal, state, and local officials, as well as airline staff, medical practitioners, the INS, and the U.S. Customs Service, played critical roles. Note that the first line of defense in such a system relies on personnel with no or very minimal medical training (airline staff including flight attendants, INS, and customs officials). Thus, the system has some weaknesses, and the sensitivity would be less if there had been no opportunity to bring the situation to people's attention and provide additional or refresher training.

Additionally, this situation brought attention to the WHO's IHR, which had not been revised since 1981 when smallpox was removed from the list of quarantinable dis-

Figure 43.1–1. Adapted from Fritz CL, Dennis DT, et al. Surveillance for pneumonic plague in the United States during an international emergency: a model for control of imported emerging diseases. Emerg Infect Dis 1996;2(1):30–36.

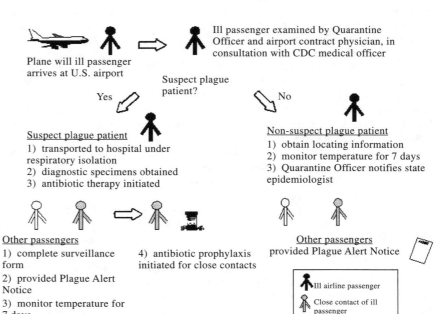

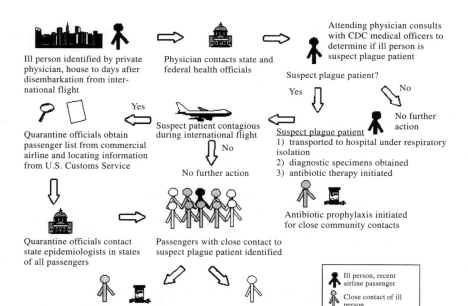

Figure 43.1–2. Adapted from Fritz CL, Dennis DT, et al. Surveillance for pneumonic plague in the United States during an international emergency: a model for control of imported emerging diseases. Emerg Infect Dis 1996;2(1):30–36.

eases (leaving only plague, cholera, and yellow fever). It was clear that the IHR needed to be updated.

In 1995, the Director General of the WHO summoned an international group of experts to re-examine the program's IHR. It became clear that certain assumptions should be changed. The basic principle of "ensuring maximum security against the international spread of disease, involving minimum interference with world traffic and trade" should remain. However, the focus on specific disease states and reportable infections will be replaced with a philosophy of "immediate reporting of defined *syndromes* of urgent international importance." Such syndromes may include:

- Acute neurologic syndromes (e.g., rabies),
- Acute respiratory syndromes (e.g., pneumonic plague, hantavirus),
- Acute diarrheal illness,
- Hemorrhagic fevers,
- Diseases targeted for eradication (e.g., polio), and
- Diseases associated with drug resistance (e.g., malaria, tuberculosis).

Additionally, other triggers may include (1) the occurrence of an unusual number of cases of a known syndrome, (2) a more severe course for a known syndrome, or (3) an unusual and unknown syndrome.

Program information including epidemiologic updates will be included on a regular basis in the WHO's *Weekly Epidemiological Record*, and information on the entire IHR program will be distributed in an easily available handbook. Also of importance, information will be included on inappropriate or unnecessary interventions with clear indications as to why these actions would not be required. Finally, the emphasis on quarantine will be replaced with an emphasis on sensible public health measures including the appropriate use of technology and improved surveillance and intervention strategies.

SUMMARY

The world has seen an explosion in international travel, trade, and tourism. A traveler can now easily return home from most anywhere on the planet within 24 hours. Unwanted souvenirs may include infectious agents with significant public health impact or threat. By using a multidisciplinary, but centrally coordinated, approach to "airport epidemiology," such potential disasters may be averted. The appropriate resources, training, and support must be committed by our respective governments for such programs to be effective. The World Health Organization is learning from recent experience and is currently refining its IHR for the new millennium.

BIBLIOGRAPHY

Fritz CL, Dennis DT, et al. Surveillance for pneumonic plague in the United States during an international emergency: a model for control of imported emerging diseases. Emerg Infect Dis 1996;2(1):30–36.

Ohtaka M. Epidemiological approach to the prevention of imported infectious diseases in the age of globalization. Kansenshogaku Zasshi 1997;71(1):18–25.

Royal L, McCoubrey I. International spread of disease by air travel. Am Fam Physician 1989;40:129–136.

U.S. Department of Health and Human Services. Public health screening at U.S. ports of entry. U.S. Government Printing Office. Revised October 1995.

World Health Organization. International Health Regulations. 3rd Ed. Geneva: WHO, 1983.

World Health Organization. Revision of the International Health Regulations, progress report. Wkly Epidemiol Rec 2000;January(4):35–36.

Chapter 44
TRAVEL MEDICINE 2010

ROBERT STEFFEN AND HERBERT L. DUPONT

TRAVEL MEDICINE HERE AND THERE

Travel medicine—the term was essentially created in preparation of the first international conference held in Zurich in 1988—will be "mature" by the year 2010. Although rapid evolution of travel medicine will continue, there will also be signs of consolidation. Hopefully, the field will be included in the medical curricula in all countries in which a substantial proportion of the population travels to destinations where infrastructure and hygiene are suboptimal. Obviously, to be successful, more scholars must become professors of travel health or travel medicine.

In many countries, this will lead to questions as to the department in which this new field should be integrated: infectious diseases or general internal medicine, tropical medicine, or preventive medicine or public health? Each of these associations is possible but also unsatisfactory, as the interdisciplinary field of travel medicine goes far beyond any of these academic or clinical areas. Different solutions will be taken as the field will remain mainly preventive (travel health) in some places and preventive and therapeutic (travel medicine) in others.

In the new decade, many countries will progress toward consistent quality in travel health services by introducing examinations for those practicing in the field. In view of the fact that most national opinion leaders belong to an international network based on a common scientific approach and common goals to keep travelers healthy, there is hope that these examinations as far as legally possible will be standardized and made relevant to a majority of industrialized countries. To achieve that, further steps toward uniform recommendations are needed not only within countries but globally. To achieve this, it would be beneficial if the World Health Organization (WHO) would take a stronger lead, for instance, by issuing more precise recommendations for pretravel measures in its annual publication *International Travel and Health.*

For the future, negative developments are also possible. Probably, new International Health Regulations will be adopted by the World Health Assembly in the next decade. These are likely to allow practicing physicians of all countries to perform yellow fever vaccinations. This is certainly justified, as yellow fever vaccine handling is no more difficult than handling of other live vaccines, but so far the obligation to visit specialized centers has had the advantage that these centers at the same time were able to give competent advice in other travel health-related fields. If restrictions for yellow fever vaccination are lifted, other mechanisms—such as examinations or requirements for continued medical education—should guarantee that quality of travel health practice is maintained.

GENERAL TRENDS IN THE PRACTICE OF TRAVEL MEDICINE

Increasingly, those working in the field of travel medicine will be able to profit from electronic media. The media will inform travel clinics of new risks, such as epidemics or increasing drug resistance. They also will inform travel health professionals on preventive measures recommended by national or international expert groups, thus allowing for standardized travel health advice and setting an end to the difficult situation where different healthy family members who for the same trip consulted the same travel clinic on different days and obtained different advice, different immunization, or different medication. Such equipment will also allow large clinics to survey the health of their customers after they have returned from their journey. It will also be possible to provide printouts with the most relevant medical information on travelers' health. Obviously, this does not replace eye-to-eye advisory sessions.

Since—after some hesitation—the pharmaceutical industry has detected travel health as a profitable market, many new products are to be expected (see below). This results in quite a challenge for travel health professionals. The goal of travel medicine is not to sell as many of the available vaccines, drugs, and other products as possible to future travelers, sometimes resulting in a ridiculous ratio of travel health costs versus total travel costs, anecdotally in some "victims" exceeding 20%(!). More is not always better, and besides an increase in costs because of the practice, an increase in rates of adverse reactions may occur. Experienced travel health specialists with extensive knowledge, not just from books but also from personal travel on various continents, will realize that recommendations issued nationally or internationally are sound, and less experienced professionals should resist the fear of missing something and should also stick to those recommendations.

Unless somebody has an elegant solution, one serious problem will remain. Travel medicine, although affordable to visitors of multistar hotels and expensive trips, is sadly often too expensive for those at highest risk, such as backpackers.

In developing countries, a few physicians caring for foreigners are taking advantage of their affluent customers. Unnecessary hospitalizations for trivial infections occur; deliberate misdiagnosis of malaria is often observed to be able to bill higher charges.

TRAVEL RISKS IN THE YEAR 2010

No dramatic changes in the means of travel are to be expected in the next 10 years. Although aircraft manufacturers are now designing both super-jumbos, with a capacity of over 800, and possibly new supersonic passenger planes, the physiologic implications for travelers will remain the same as in the past. At most, a few tourists will need advice for outer space. Faster trains will be introduced in various countries. Ships, buses, and cars will continue to become more comfortable, and this should have a positive impact on travelers' health especially with regard to increased safety. Despite sophisticated safety tools, however, risks may persist or even increase if maintenance and handling are inadequate in countries with a weak economy, as illustrated recently by crashes of aircraft, some of them brand new, in India, China, and the former Soviet Union.

Travelers have already now conquered almost the entire world. New destinations will be developed, however, for some of these new destinations, serious ecologic damage may occur as a result of travel patterns. Ultimately, this can create health risks to tourists, as recently illustrated during and after heavy rainfalls on the Kenya coast where rapid expansion of resorts was not accompanied by the necessary improvements in sewage and other infrastructure, resulting not just in floods but in contamination of freshwater sources, which caused epidemics of gastrointestinal disease. High-class resorts will decline to middle and lower class status after some time unless stringent environment controls are observed. Such degeneration occurred in the Italian Adriatic where the European aristocracy once vacationed at the turn of the century. This area is now urbanized, polluted, and deserted for most of the year where remaining visitor groups are primarily low-budget bus tours from Eastern Europe.

We cannot exclude the emergence of new or re-emerging infections anywhere. On the other hand, the efforts of WHO and national Expanded Programs of Immunization may lead to the eradication or drastic reduction of the incidence of certain infections, such as poliomyelitis or hepatitis B.

Traveler characteristics will strongly influence risk patterns, and populations newly discovering exotic travel may be at extremely high risk. Eastern Europeans of all age groups now are beginning to tour Africa and Asia on a budget that is much lower than the one used by Western European or North American travelers. This forces them to live under substandard, slum-like conditions; thus, these travelers may acquire infections rarely seen so far, such as cholera. Travelers from postcommunist countries are unlikely to be protected by the full complement of vaccinations and other preventive measures, which constitute a further risk factor. Other groups whose travel

horizons will continue to broaden include populations in the Far East. For the most part, this population will not be put at high risk, since their principal destinations are usually in industrialized countries. One continuing risk is that Japanese travelers might ask for raw fish (e.g., sushi) dishes even in the less developed world, just as persons from the U.S. love hamburgers everywhere and even in places without quality control such as is customary in international chains. Both practices may result in high rates of gastrointestinal infections, and in the case of raw fish consumption, cholera may result.

Increasingly, customers will opt for international experiences during holidays rather than local beach vacations. As long as this is limited to golfing, tennis, etc., no more than an increased rate of sports accidents will result. Although many opt for a safe life at home, many tend paradoxically to take risks abroad, mountaineering, trekking, participating in motorbike expeditions, racing cars or mopeds, or playing roulette in unprotected casual sexual contacts.

In various Islamic countries, travelers may rarely be political targets for fundamentalists who try to destabilize the political system by destroying the tourism industry. Such terrorist activities are likely to increase and to lead to higher rates of assault victims in those who do not remain in well-protected tourist areas. Unless the economic situation improves and criminality associated with drug abuse is better controlled, visitors in North America and Western Europe may also become a more frequent target of assaults.

Resistance of various pathogenic microbial agents to available medication will also lead to major concern in travel medicine within the next decade.

TOOLS TO PROTECT TRAVELERS' HEALTH IN 2010

VACCINES

Within the next 10 years, various new mixtures of currently used vaccines will be marketed. There also will be new options to improve travelers' health:

- Vaccines against gastrointestinal infections: enterotoxigenic *Escherichia coli* vaccine, *Campylobacter* vaccine, *Shigella* vaccine, and hepatitis E vaccine, probably combined with hepatitis A vaccine.
- Vaccines against systemic viral infections: dengue vaccine and HIV vaccine (it is doubtful whether one will be available).
- Vaccine against Lyme borreliosis in Europe.
- Vaccines against malaria; however, it is unlikely that a vaccine offering better protection than chemosuppression will be available before the year 2010.

Also, we will probably have to wait longer to use revolutionary new vaccines, such as naked DNA vaccines or such with new vectors, time-releasing formulations with polymers, or vaccines hidden in bananas or other food items produced by bioengineering. It is unlikely that by

2010 oral preparations of the traditional vaccines will have completely replaced injections.

DRUGS

Against malaria, there are drugs on the horizon, such as tafenoquine (formerly etaquine or WR238605). Malarone™ may become attractive for chemoprophylaxis. *Plasmodium falciparum* may become increasingly resistant to all currently used agents. If drug resistance continues to increase, we may be forced to rely on more drug combinations for prevention or treatment. The choice of agents available for self-treatment of malaria falls short of ideal at present, and as this strategy is difficult to explain or understand, it may become obsolete if simple and well-tolerated prophylactic options become available.

There will be various new agents available for the self-therapy of travelers' diarrhea. Although the currently available treatment options effectively shorten most episodes of diarrhea among travelers, increasing resistance among bacterial enteropathogens will encourage the development of new antibacterial drugs with unique value in enteric disease. Nonabsorbable or poorly absorbed drugs have safety advantages and should be effective. In addition

to possible improvements in antimicrobial therapy, novel antisecretory drugs could be available in the near future that reduce diarrhea without antimotility effects. These drugs should improve symptoms of illness and have a low potential for worsening invasive diarrheal disease and producing post-treatment constipation.

CONCLUSION

Travelers' diseases are moving targets since with time and place epidemiology and etiology, the travelers' destinations, infrastructure, and behavior vary. Epidemiologic data on travelers' diseases are now at least 20 years old and need to be reassessed. For the main infective threats, such as travelers' diarrhea and malaria, continuous monitoring of etiology and antimicrobial resistance is of value. There is a complete lack of data on influenza and on respiratory tract infections. Additionally, there is still a need for the study of host factor-related medical problems, including long-term residents, elderly and handicapped, and travelers using continuous medication, such as drugs reducing gastric acidity or diuretics.

AUTHOR INDEX

SUBJECT INDEX